Oxford Textbook of

Spirituality in Healthcare

Oxford Textbook of Spirituality in Healthcare

Edited by

Mark Cobb

Sr. Chaplain and Clinical Director at Sheffield Teaching Hospitals NHS Foundation Trust; Honorary Research Fellow, Academic Palliative and Supportive Care Studies Group, University of Liverpool; Honorary Lecturer, University of Sheffield (UK)

Christina M. Puchalski

Professor of Medicine and Health Sciences at The George Washington University School of Medicine and Director of the George Washington Institute for Spirituality and Health, Washington, DC (USA)

and

Bruce Rumbold

Director, Palliative Care Unit, School of Public Health and Human Biosciences, La Trobe University (AUS)

OXFORD
UNIVERSITY PRESS

OXFORD
UNIVERSITY PRESS

Great Clarendon Street, Oxford OX2 6DP

Oxford University Press is a department of the University of Oxford.

It furthers the University's objective of excellence in research, scholarship, and education by publishing worldwide in

Oxford New York

Auckland Cape Town Dar es Salaam Hong Kong Karachi
Kuala Lumpur Madrid Melbourne Mexico City Nairobi
New Delhi Shanghai Taipei Toronto

With offices in

Argentina Austria Brazil Chile Czech Republic France Greece
Guatemala Hungary Italy Japan Poland Portugal Singapore
South Korea Switzerland Thailand Turkey Ukraine Vietnam

Published in the United States
by Oxford University Press Inc., New York

First published 2012

British Library Cataloguing-in-Publication-Data
Data available

Library of Congress Cataloging-in-Publication-Data
Data available

Typeset by Cenveo, Bangalore, India
Printed in China on acid-free paper through C&C Offset Printing Co., Ltd

ISBN 978–0–19–957139–0

10 9 8 7 6 5 4 3 2 1

Foreword

Edmund D. Pellegrino

Experienced clinicians have long known that true healing extends beyond the artful use of medical knowledge. They grasped intuitively that serious or fatal illness was an ontological assault, an existential assault on the whole of the patient's lived world. To heal, the physician must recognize the starkness of the patient's encounter with his own finitude, i.e. with his mortality and inherent limitations. Healing of the psychosocial-biological is of itself insufficient to repair the existential disarray of the patient's life without recognition of the spiritual origins of that disarray.

In centuries past, little genuinely scientific therapy was available. The causes and treatment of disease were often sought in frankly spiritual forces. For many centuries spiritual and 'scientific' medicine were practiced side-by-side. In the West, clinicians practiced their art with varying degrees of cooperation between Hippocratic and religiously oriented views of health and disease. Similar confluences of religious and secular treatments existed in the Eastern world as well.

As the era of scientifically effective medical practice expanded, the humane and spiritual dimension of illness and healing were more clearly separated. A certain degree of hubris on both sides led many to deprecate the connection between 'scientific' and religious or spiritual notions of healing. Today, even as scientific medicine expands in therapeutic potency, there is a renewed awareness of what the experienced clinicians never neglected. The modern emphasis on 'wholistic' medicine recognized the disarraying effect of illness on the whole life of the patient. Once again whatever term is used to define the phenomenon, the significance of illness as a disarray of the patient's life is now becoming more precisely recognized.

This comprehensive, authoritative, multicultural volume edited by Mark Cobb, Christina Puchalski, and Bruce Rumbold provides an indispensable guide to clinical practice, research and education in the realms of healing beyond the capabilities of modern scientific medicine alone.

The three editors have assembled an impressive representation of clinicians, investigators, and teachers engaged in the practice and research in the place of spirituality in medicine. Taken together they illustrate the significance, and breadth of definitions of 'spirituality' across a wide spectrum of cultures, medical theories, and historical precedents. The significance for patients of all kinds is extensively explored—in acute and chronic illness, palliative, terminal, and geriatric care.

In each contribution the authors have provided a wide range of discussions crossing cultural, historical, theoretical boundaries. The practical dimensions of diagnosis, modes of therapy and cooperation at the bedside are well documented. The differences in definitions of spirituality, and clinical usage of relevant terms and modes of therapy are well delineated.

The editors have had long experience bringing considerations of spirituality in medical care to the attention of the medical profession, as well as all other health professionals. This volume is encyclopedic, culturally, and historically. It should prove to be an authoritative source for years to come. It provides the kind of serious combination of practice and theory essential to our understanding of what 'healing' really means to patients and the health professionals who sincerely want to use scientific medicine along with a true wholistic approach to the care of those they commit themselves to as authentic healers.

Preface

This is a book about the dimension of life that we refer to as spiritual and its place in healthcare. The conjunction of the two is historical, intellectual, and practical, because both intersect around the human concern and critical interest we have in health. Bringing together a volume dedicated to spirituality and healthcare is therefore never far removed from a dialogue on the meaning and character of health, on the human capacity for sustaining health, and on the ingenuity and creativity we have to respond to those things that disrupt our health and cause us to renegotiate what it means to be human. Spirituality is for many people a way of engaging with the purpose and meaning of human existence and provides a reliable perspective on their lived experience and an orientation to the world. As spirituality engages healthcare it becomes inextricably linked with human suffering and therefore integral to the lives of patients, their families and their caregivers. Inevitably, if healthcare has any regard for the humanity of those it serves it is faced with spirituality in its experienced and expressed forms. How is healthcare to engage and respond, how does it understand and interpret spirituality, what resources does it make available and how are these organised, and how does spirituality shape and inform the purpose and practice of healthcare? These questions are the basis for this book and outline a coherent field of enquiry, discussion and debate that is interdisciplinary, international and vibrant. We have aimed to capture this through a collection of writings involving authoritative and leading-edge writers to provide a unique resource and a stimulating discourse.

Anyone who reads healthcare journals, attends healthcare conferences, or receives course brochures cannot fail to have noticed that spirituality is on the agenda. Similarly, an awareness of current affairs is a reminder that religion is back in the public square, if it were ever absent. Religions bring people into relationship with the spiritual dimension and with others seeking the same; they provide social structures and identity, and maintain living traditions of practice and wisdom. The innate human capacity for spirituality means that many of these religious traditions are ancient relative to healthcare and have therefore contributed to current globalized understandings of health, healthcare, and spirituality. The opening section of the book therefore considers key traditions and explores particular strands of thought, many religious, and their contribution to these contemporary perspectives. Some chapters outline ways in which living traditions underlie and continue to support values important to contemporary views of health and healthcare. Others look at ways in which these values have been received, adapted, challenged, or reinterpreted by modern social thought or post-modern revivals of neglected traditions. Notable alongside chapters on religious traditions are those on the humanist tradition, secularism and philosophy, all of which expand and challenge conventional notions and are topics of contemporary relevance.

An exploration of spirituality and healthcare is premised upon concepts and constructs that often go unexamined. Terms are used that may not be commonly understood and the language of spirituality and healthcare is replete with vocabulary that is underpinned by assumptions. We therefore devote a section of the book to significant concepts in this field with the aim of developing clarity in the discourse. By unpacking and critically reflecting on terminology we discover new insights, helpful differentiations and possible inter-relationships that can further the discursive knowledge of this developing field. However, spirituality and healthcare have practice as their primary mode and it is inevitable that the largest section of the book addresses ways in which the spiritual is addressed in the practice of healthcare. No one discipline has an exclusive claim because many are involved in caring relations, although some have a greater historic perspective, social validation, training, and formation. Practice has also developed around the specialist subdivisions of healthcare and this has resulted in particular approaches described in some of the chapters. Significantly, spirituality has been a challenge to healthcare practice particularly in terms of its attentiveness to the person, its responsibility and responsiveness to the ways we make sense of life, and its capacity to cultivate the co-creation of health in situations of vulnerability. We are therefore faced with questions about whether and how spirituality should be incorporated into developed disciplinary practices, whether it should it be a specialist adjunct, and how spirituality may relate to the vocational and humanistic intentions of healthcare practitioners.

Healthcare is a seedbed of research, substantially in the physical sciences related to the immediacy of problematic human bodies, and to a much lesser extent in the social and behavioural sciences related to the lived experience and social environment of being human. Research inquiries are driven by questions about what disrupts health and how it can be restored and therefore the relationship between spirituality and health has become an obvious subject of study, although not one as current as people assume. Francis Galton's prayer study was originally published in 1872 and he asserts that,

'The efficacy of prayer seems to me a simple, as it is a perfectly appropriate and legitimate, subject of scientific inquiry. Whether prayer is efficacious or not, in any given sense, is a matter of fact ...'(1). Contemporary research has an array of techniques and instruments available to it by which it can scrutinize spirituality in relation to health, but many results are far from conclusive or uncontested. Research provides intelligible, rigorous and systematic methods to investigate and describe claims about the world that spirituality cannot avoid for ethical reasons alone. However, research in this field is relatively immature, and whatever the use of explanatory empirical inquiries there is also a need to develop and be confident in methods of inquiry that help us to better describe and understand the experience and expressions of particular spiritualties and the actual practices of spiritual care.

If spirituality in healthcare is to move beyond the *ad hoc* arrangements and particular interests of individuals that it commonly relies upon then it must become better integrated within health systems. This purposeful approach requires explicit policy directed at improving spiritual care through the allocation and organisation of resources, the attainment of standards related to the structures, processes, and outcomes of healthcare, and the development of consensus and shared understanding. We have examples of this approach within the book, but this agenda needs development, and lessons need to be learnt from health systems that have adopted and implemented policy in this field. Alongside policy development healthcare practitioners need opportunities to learn about spirituality and develop their skills and capacities to attend to the spirituality of patients as well as that of their own. This means not only developing ways of attending to suffering with deep compassion and altruism, but also doing so in careful and competent ways. Training is therefore critical and requires intentional programming, appropriate educational methods, such as inter-professional education and collaborative learning, and its incorporation into professional formation. Without this healthcare practitioners are likely to be uncertain of their response, anxious of failure, ineffective in practice and unaware of ethical consequences.

Spirituality and healthcare share another common characteristic: both have deep historic roots, but remain highly dynamic and adaptive. In the last section of the book we therefore explore some of the challenges within this field and consider how some of the dynamic interactions might play out. No discussion can take place without considering the future of religion, which presents a range of scenarios, and the need to understand the shifting place of religion in society. Similarly, discussions must include secular, humanistic, and cultural perspectives. These social contexts are the place of healthcare and therefore they become an important backdrop and influence on how spirituality is conceived, located and practiced in healthcare organizations. What is evident is that the spiritual within healthcare is far from homogenous and includes conventional religious forms, secular spirituality and therapeutic forms of spirituality each with their own possibilities and contentions. What seems undeniable therefore is that spirituality has opened up a dialectic space in healthcare, often dominated by reductionism, that allows people to make some sense of the transcendent aspects of health and humanity. The engagement of spirituality with healthcare can thus be seen as a core strategy for humanizing healthcare through its focus on inner meaning, approaches to suffering, and compassionate practice. It can also be seen as a core strategy for grounding spirituality in the encounter with human finitude.

Finally, in presenting a subject with the depth and breadth evident in this book has required working with a large group of expert individuals across the world and this has presented its own rewards and challenges. We are indebted to all our contributors for their commitment to this book, to our colleagues world-wide whose perspectives have challenged our thinking and broadened our views, and to our patients and those for whom we care, who are the reason for our passion and commitment to create more compassionate and holistic systems of care. We also thank Amber Morley Rieke for her administrative assistance and the team at Oxford University Press for their perseverance and guidance in making this book a reality.

Mark Cobb, Christina Puchalski and
Bruce Rumbold, August 2012

References

1 Galton, F. (1876) Statistical inquiries into the efficacy of prayer. *The Fortnightly Review Rev* **xii** (lxviii): 125–135. Available at: http://galton.org/ (accessed 24 November 2011).

Contents

List of contributors

Hisham Abu-Raiya
Bob Shapell School of Social Work, Tel Aviv University (ISR)

Lodovico Balducci
Medical Director of Affiliates and Referring Physician Relations and Program leader of Senior Adult Oncology at Moffitt Cancer Center and Professor of Oncologic Sciences at the University of South Florida College of Medicine (USA)

Rodger K. Bufford
Professor of Psychology, George Fox University, Oregon (USA)

Stephen Bullivant
Lecturer in Theology and Ethics, School of Theology, Philosophy, and History, St Mary's University College, Twickenham (UK)

Laurie A. Burke
Department of Psychology, University of Memphis (USA)

Arndt Büssing
Professor of Quality of Life, Spirituality and Coping, Center for Integrative Medicine, University of Witten/Herdecke (DEU)

Lindsay B. Carey
Lecturer and Research Fellow in Public Health, Bioethics and Pastoral Care, Palliative Care Unit, La Trobe University; RAAF Chaplain, Royal Australian Air Force, RAAF Base Williams, Victoria; Director of Australian and New Zealand Chaplaincy Utility Research, Melbourne (AUS)

Nathan Carlin
Assistant Professor in the McGovern Center for Humanities and Ethics at The University of Texas Health Science Center at Houston (USA)

Harvey M. Chochinov
Professor of Psychiatry, Community Health Sciences, and Family Medicine (Division of Palliative Care), University of Manitoba, and Director of the Manitoba Palliative Care Research Unit, CancerCare Manitoba (CAN)

Mark Cobb
Sr. Chaplain and Clinical Director at Sheffield Teaching Hospitals NHS Foundation Trust; Honorary Research Fellow, Academic Palliative and Supportive Care Studies Group, University of Liverpool; Honorary Lecturer, University of Sheffield (UK)

Jeffrey Cohen
Visiting Senior Research Fellow in the School of Public Health and Community Medicine at the University of New South Wales (AUS)

Dan Cohn-Sherbok
Professor Emeritus of Judaism at the University of Wales; Visiting Professor at St Mary's University College, London, and Honorary Professor at the University of Aberystwyth (UK)

Thomas Cole
McGovern Chair in Medical Humanities and founding Director of the McGovern Center for Humanities and Ethics at The University of Texas Medical School at Houston (USA)

Grace Davie
Professor of Sociology emeritus, University of Exeter (UK)

Douglas J. Davies
Professor in the Study of Religion and Director of the Centre for Death and Life Studies, Durham University (UK)

Catherine del Ferraro
Sr. Research Specialist, Nursing Research and Education at City of Hope Medical Center in Los Angeles (USA)

Prakash N. Desai
Professor of Clinical Psychiatry at the University of Illinois at Chicago (USA)

Jaklin Eliott
Social Scientist, Cancer Council Australia, and Affiliate Lecturer, Discipline of Public Health, School of Population Health and Clinical Practice, The University of Adelaide (AUS)

Jacqueline Ellis
Research Associate, Academic Palliative and Supportive Care Studies Group, University of Liverpool (UK)

Gary B. Ferngren
Professor, Department of History, Oregon State University (USA)

Betty Ferrell
Professor, Nursing Research and Education at City of Hope Medical Center in Los Angeles (USA)

George Fitchett
Associate Professor and Director of Research, Department of Religion, Health and Human Values at Rush University (USA)

Patricia Fosarelli
Associate Dean, The Ecumenical Institute of Theology, St. Mary's Seminary & University, Baltimore (USA)

Gregory Fricchione
Director Division of Psychiatry and Medicine and the Benson-Henry Institute for Mind Body Medicine at Massachusetts General Hospital; Professor of Psychiatry, Harvard Medical School (USA)

Fiona Gardner
Senior Lecturer, Social Work and Social Policy, School of Rural Health, La Trobe University (AUS)

Catherine F. Garlid
Director of Spiritual Care and Clinical Pastoral Education, Maine Medical Center (USA)

Kathleen Gregory
Lecturer and Course Convenor, Department of Counselling and Psychological Health, School of Public Health and Human Biosciences, La Trobe University (AUS)

James L. Griffith
Professor of Psychiatry and Behavioral Sciences; Interim Chair and Director, Psychiatry Residency Training, Department of Psychiatry and Behavioral Science, The George Washington University Medical Centre (USA)

George Handzo
Senior Consultant for Chaplaincy Care Leadership & Practice, HealthCare Chaplaincy, New York (USA)

Nigel Hartley
Director of Supportive Care, St Christopher's Hospice, London (UK)

Graham Harvey
Reader in Religious Studies, Open University (UK)

Paul Heelas
Senior Research Professor in Sociology of Contemporary Spirituality, Department of Sociology, Erasmus University Rotterdam (NLD)

Margaret Holloway
Professor of Social Work, University of Hull; Social Care Lead, National End of Life Care Programme (UK)

Brandon Horn
Deputy Director of the Children's Hospital of Los Angeles Acupuncture Program; Professor at Yosan University; Faculty at UCLA School of Medicine (USA)

Rosalie Hudson
Honorary Senior Fellow, School of Nursing and Social Work, University of Melbourne (AUS)

David J. Hufford
Senior Fellow in Brain, Mind and Healing, the Samueli Institute; University Professor Emeritus, Penn State College of Medicine; Adjunct Professor, Religious Studies Department, University of Pennsylvania (USA)

Marek Jantos
Director, Behavioural Medicine Institute of Australia (AUS)

Michael Kearney
Medical Director of Palliative Care Service at Santa Barbara Cottage Hospital and Associate Medical Director at Visiting Nurse & Hospice Care (USA)

Ewan Kelly
Senior Lecturer, School of Divinity, The University of Edinburgh and Programme Director for Healthcare Chaplaincy and Spiritual Care, NHS Education for Scotland (UK)

Russell Kirkland
Professor of Religion, Department of Religion, University of Georgia (USA)

Emmanuel Y. Lartey
Professor of Pastoral Theology, Care and Counseling, Candler School of Theology, Emory University (USA)

Mari Lloyd-Williams
Consultant in Palliative Medicine and Professor and Director of the Academic Palliative and Supportive Care Studies Group at the University of Liverpool (UK)

Elizabeth MacKinlay
Director, Centre for Ageing & Pastoral Studies, St Mark's National Theological Centre, Professor School of Theology Charles Sturt University, Canberra (AUS)

Alister E. McGrath
Professor of Theology, Ministry and Education, and Head of the Centre for Theology, Religion and Culture at King's College, London (UK)

Wilfred McSherry
Professor in Dignity of Care for Older People Staffordshire University and Shrewsbury and Telford Hospital NHS Trust (UK)

Robert A. Neimeyer
Professor of Psychology, Department of Psychology, University of Memphis (USA)

Shamim Nejad
Department of Psychiatry, Massachusetts General Hospital (USA)

Holly Nelson-Becker
Associate Professor, School of Social Work, Loyola University Chicago (USA)

Eleanor Nesbitt
Professor Emerita, Institute of Education, University of Warwick (UK)

Graham Oppy
Professor, Philosophy Department, Monash University (AUS)

Raymond F. Paloutzian
Professor Emeritus of Psychology, Westmont College, Santa Barbara (USA)

Kenneth I. Pargament
Professor of Clinical Psychology, Bowling Green State University (USA)

Edmund Pellegrino
John Carroll Professor Emeritus of Medicine and Medical Ethics, Senior Research Scholar, Kennedy Institute of Ethics and Interim Director, Center for Clinical Bioethics, Georgetown University (USA)

Neil Pembroke
Senior Lecturer, The School of History, Philosophy, Religion & Classics, The University of Queensland (AUS)

Martyn Percy
Principal of Ripon College Cuddesdon and the Oxford Ministry Course, Professor of Theological Education at King's College London, and Professorial Research Fellow at Heythrop College London (UK)

Christina M. Puchalski
Professor of Medicine and Health Sciences at The George Washington University School of Medicine and Director of the George Washington Institute for Spirituality and Health, Washington, DC (USA)

Linda Ross
Senior Lecturer, Faculty of Health, Sport and Science, University of Glamorgan (UK)

Susan A. Ross
Professor of Theology and a Faculty Scholar at Loyola University Chicago (USA)

Bruce Rumbold
Director, Palliative Care Unit, School of Public Health and Human Biosciences, La Trobe University (AUS)

Abdulaziz Sachedina
Frances Myers Ball Professor of Religious Studies, University of Virginia (USA)

Kevin S. Seybold
Professor of Psychology, Grove City College, Pennsylvania (USA)

Shane Sinclair
Postdoctoral Fellow, Canadian Institutes of Health Research, Manitoba Palliative Care Research Unit, University of Manitoba; Spiritual Care Coordinator, Tom Baker Cancer Centre, Alberta Health Services; Adjunct Lecturer, Faculty of Medicine, Department of Oncology, University of Calgary (CAN)

Peter Speck
Researcher, Cicely Saunders Institute of Palliative Care, King's College London (UK)

Trevor Stammers
Program Director, Bioethics and Medical Law, St Mary's University College, Twickenham (UK)

Henry W. Strobel
Professor of Biochemistry and Molecular Biology, The University of Texas Medical School at Houston (USA)

Margaret L. Stuber
Vice Chair for Education in Psychiatry and Daniel X. Freedman Professor at the David Geffen School of Medicine and the Semel Institute for Neuroscience and Human Behavior at University of California, Los Angeles (USA)

Mary Pat Sullivan
Senior Lecturer, School of Health Sciences and Social Care, Brunel University (UK)

Daniel P. Sulmasy
Kilbride-Clinton Professor of Medicine and Ethics in the Department of Medicine and Divinity School; Associate Director of the MacLean Center for Clinical Medical Ethics at the University of Chicago (USA)

Chris Swift
Head of Chaplaincy and Chaplaincy Research, Education and Development Office at The Leeds Teaching Hospitals NHS Trust and Lecturer at Leeds Metropolitan University (UK)

John Swinton
Chair in Divinity and Religious Studies and Professor in Practical Theology and Pastoral Care, School of Divinity, History and Philosophy, King's College, University of Aberdeen (UK)

David Tacey
Associate Professor, Department of Arts, Communication and Critical Enquiry, Faculty of Humanities and Social Sciences, La Trobe University (AUS)

Carol Taylor
Professor of Medicine and Nursing, Senior Research Scholar, Center for Clinical Bioethics, Georgetown University (USA)

Peter van der Veer
Director of the Max Planck Institute for the Study of Religious and Ethnic Diversity at Göttingen (DEU)

Stan van Hooft
Professor of Philosophy, School of International and Political Studies, Deakin University (AUS)

Antonia van Loon
Senior Research Fellow RDNS, Adjunct Faculty, School of Nursing and Midwifery, Flinders University, Adelaide (AUS)

Bella Vivat
Research Lecturer, School of Health Sciences and Social Care, Brunel University (UK)

Susan Walker
Administrative Director, Diabetes Institute, Walter Reed Health Care System and adjunct faculty at George Mason University School of Health and Human Services, Washington, DC (USA)

Radhule Weininger
Clinical Psychologist, Santa Barbara (USA)

William West
Reader in Counselling Studies, University of Manchester (UK)

Ashley J. Wildman
Department of Counselor Education and Counseling Psychology, Western Michigan University (USA)

Angelika A. Zollfrank
Director of Clinical Pastoral Education, Massachusetts General Hospital (USA)

SECTION I

Traditions

CHAPTER 1

Medicine and religion: a historical perspective

Gary B. Ferngren

Introduction

To many who live in a modern secular society a connection between medicine and religion is not readily apparent. To associate religion with healing seems to be an anachronism that is incompatible with scientific medicine. In fact, the two have had a close association since the earliest human attempts to heal the human body. In the ancient world, when little was known about medicine or the structure of the human body, healers realized that they could do little to restore health to those who were ill. The causes of disease were mysterious and often ascribed to magic or divine beings. Of common diseases only the symptoms could ordinarily be treated; for more serious conditions, healers hoped that by appealing to supernatural forces they might gain help. Those who attempted healing did not need to be priests or physicians to understand that where they could do so little, the best (and perhaps the only) hope of physical restoration came from the gods. Religion today still intersects with medicine in surprisingly diverse ways, some of them assuming roles not very different from the forms they took in the ancient world: helping the sick to live with pain and suffering, providing compassionate care for those who are ill, and offering spiritual consolation to the sick and dying.

Concepts of health

Concepts of health reflect the culture in which they develop. Health is a concept that is imprecise. Words that denote health are semantically related in many languages to concepts of physical wholeness, and are synonymous with health and wellbeing. They may refer to the body, the mind, or the soul. Health and physical wholeness were thought by the Mesopotamians and Egyptians to be present so long as life remained in harmony with the forces of nature. Illness reflected disharmony between the individual and the total environment. *Shalom,* which is often translated as *peace,* was a Hebrew concept that denoted a broad and inclusive concept of health that included spiritual well-being. This may be seen in the Hebrew Bible, where health is consistently described in spiritual, rather than in medical terms.[1] In contrast, the Greek medical view of health (*hugieia*) was that it represented an equilibrium or harmony of various elements of the body, such as bodily fluids or matter taken into the body. The Greeks viewed disease as a disturbance of that equilibrium. Their best-known theory of physiology was based on the supposed existence of four humours or bodily fluids (blood, phlegm, yellow bile, and black bile), borrowed by physicians from the pre-Socratic philosopher Empedocles (fl. 444–441 BCE). When the balance of humours was disturbed or upset, medical treatment consisted of restoring them to their correct proportions, in harmony with nature, rather than contrary to it.[2]

The Greek view of health furnished an analogy for the soul, in which moral virtue (*arête*) was considered a balance of the elements of the soul. Philosophers sometimes referred to the soul as sick or diseased. A healthy individual guarded against diseases of the soul by practicing moderation and self-control (*sophrosune*). Hence, medicine and philosophy complemented each other and enabled one to lead a balanced life whose end was happiness[3] (*mens sana in corpore sano*, 'A sound mind in a sound body').[4] The body–soul analogy was used by writers of nearly all Greek philosophical schools. The Christian belief that pain and suffering had a redemptive or sanctifying purpose was unknown in the classical world, in which health was so basic to the enjoyment of life that a life without it was not thought to be worth living. Health was never regarded by early Christians as a virtue, as it had been for the Greeks, but a blessing that was given by God. The World Health Organization defines health as a 'state of complete physical, mental, and social well-being, and not merely the absence of disease or infirmity'.[5]. This is a broad conception that appears to make health nearly indistinguishable from happiness, and is not far removed from those ancient views of health which emphasized a wholeness that encompassed physical, mental, and spiritual health. It is also reflected in definitions of health that one finds in New-Age and 'holistic' healing movements associated with complementary and alternative medicine, in which well-being is achieved by creating a balanced personality in which mind, body, and spirit are in harmony.

Disease: its causes and cure

The ancient world was animistic or polytheistic with a few exceptions, notably Israel, which was monotheistic, and Persia, whose religion, Zoroastrianism, was dualistic. Each locale (village, city) had its own cults and deities, but the syncretistic nature of polytheism resulted in local deities being merged with others over time to form national pantheons. Their view of the world was predominantly an organicist or vitalist one; they viewed it as animated by vague numinous or spiritual presences, which could be manipulated through a complex variety of magico-religious mechanisms that could be employed to maintain or restore health. The earliest historical (that is, literate) civilizations of the Near East arose in Egypt and Mesopotamia at the beginning of the third millennium BCE. Egyptians and Mesopotamians viewed any but the most common diseases aetiologically, rather than symptomatically. Disease could be inflicted by both pernicious supernatural powers and humans who had access to the use of malicious magic. Disturbances to one's health could be understood only by discerning the identity and motives of the responsible agent. Medical craftsmen (the *asu* in Mesopotamia, the *swnw* in Egypt), who mingled empirical methods in treating acute symptoms with prayers and incantations, were consulted. Magical healing employed amulets, incantations, or occult objects like herbs and gems, which manipulated hidden preternatural forces that were within nature, but outside its normal course. While folk medicine, a component that is found in every culture, including our own, and empirical treatments were used, treatment reflected a magico-religious classification of disease in which the aims of medicine were subordinated to those of religion. Since everything that was not readily explicable was believed to have happened for a purpose, sickness had meaning that could be ascertained by its interpreters. Breaking a taboo could occasion divine anger and bring about disease, but the gods sometimes struck capriciously. The Babylonians attributed some disease to demons, as did the Egyptians and their neighbours. Common physical ills that aroused no awe were viewed symptomatically, and treated with herbs or other natural substances.[6]

In the fifth century BCE Greek medicine began to take on the form of a science as well as a craft. A science requires the existence of a body of theoretical knowledge, which until the late fifth century did not exist in medicine. Many empirical techniques had been collected and transmitted by empirics or folk healers, but they could not be called a body of knowledge. There had been no previous attempt to understand disease in general terms or to frame broad theories that could be applied to particular cases. It was the addition of theory to medicine and concepts of disease that made it possible to explain disease in terms of natural causation, which became a feature of Greek medicine in the fifth century. Physicians who sought a theoretical understanding of disease turned to philosophy, which alone could provide universal formulations. We term these physicians (*iatroi*) *Hippocratic* physicians after the celebrated father of medicine, Hippocrates.

Although Hippocrates was the subject of much legend, we know almost nothing about him. Only two contemporary references to him exist, both in the dialogues of Plato. He probably became the subject of widespread interest during Hellenistic times, when a number of anonymous medical works came to be attributed to him. They are known as the Hippocratic Corpus and they number about 60 treatises. None of them can be attributed to Hippocrates with any certainty. They are a disparate group of medical writings, most of them probably having been composed in the fifth and fourth centuries BCE, but some as late as the second century BCE. They reflect a variety of points of view. Many Hippocratic treatises reveal an approach to medicine that is both rational and empirical: rational in its freedom from magic and demons, and in its belief in the natural causes of disease; and empirical in the collection of case histories with careful descriptions of symptoms.[7]

Side by side with the development of a naturalistic tradition of medicine in classical Greece, there existed a parallel tradition of religious medicine in which the sick sought healing directly from a god, rather than a physician. Those who desired divine help for healing could appeal to a wide variety of gods, demigods, and heroes. Originally, there were no special gods of healing. Any deity could be invoked by the sick. But one hero, Asclepius, came to be the chief healing god of the classical world. By the fourth century BCE the northern Peloponnesian city of Epidaurus became the centre of a healing sanctuary of Asclepius and from there his cult spread throughout the Greek and Roman world. The sick came to his temples seeking supernatural healing, often for diseases that physicians could not cure. Pilgrims first underwent a rite of purification and offered a small sacrifice. The actual healing process involved incubation, the practice of having pilgrims spend the night in the *abaton*, where they were to lie on a couch and wait for a dream or a vision of the god, in which Asclepius would appear to heal or advise them. The god often appeared holding a staff with a snake coiled around it (the caduceus), which became associated with him. Sometimes he merely touched patients, sometimes he operated on them or administered drugs, and sometimes a sacred serpent or dog would lick the wounds. When patients awoke the next morning they might find themselves cured. Those who were healed left votive offerings, which have been found in abundance and testify to actual cures. They include terracotta models of eyes, ears, limbs, and other organs that had been healed.

However, Asclepius also healed through physicians by natural means just as he did by miraculous means through incubation. He became the patron of physicians who practiced secular medicine, as well as of their patients. Physicians swore oaths by Asclepius and other healing gods. They had no objections to religious healing; rather they viewed it as complementing their own work. When Greek physicians believed they could not help a patient they refused to provide treatment. The patient might then seek the direct help of Asclepius. The two traditions existed side by side, often with little contact, but with no apparent tension. During the Hellenistic period (323–30 BCE) that followed the death of Alexander the Great a number of foreign deities entered Greece from Egypt, Syria, and Asia Minor. While several of them (such as Serapis) inspired healing cults, none seriously challenged the primacy of Asclepius.[8,9]

Medical ethics

The best known of the Hippocratic collection is the so-called Hippocratic Oath. It is uncertain when it was written, although the earliest mention of it was in the first century CE. There is no evidence that it was used in the pre-Christian era. Those who took the Oath swore by Apollo, Asclepius, and other gods and goddesses of healing to guard their life and art 'in purity and holiness.' Some of its injunctions (e.g. prohibition of abortion, euthanasia, and perhaps surgery), together with its religious tenor, suggest that it originated among a limited group of physicians. The oath was regarded by some pagan medical writers during the Roman imperial period as setting forth an ideal standard of professional behaviour, but at no time was it used in the classical world to regulate the practice of more than a minority of physicians.[9]

The deontological treatises of the Hippocratic Corpus (e.g. *Precepts, Decorum, Law*) provide the earliest writings that deal with medical etiquette. They define a distinct identity for the physician and establish guidelines for professional conduct. They are rooted in the culture of the medical craftsman, rather than in any religious or moral values. In defining the obligations of the physician, they both created a tradition of medical ethics and formulated an ideal of competent practice, which were subsequently adopted in late Roman antiquity, and in the Middle Ages by Christian, Jewish, and Muslim physicians. They have influenced the Western medical tradition up to the present day and remain one of the greatest legacies of Hippocratic medicine.[10]

In the medical-ethical literature of the early Middle Ages, the religious and philanthropic ideas of monastic medicine were merged with the earlier secular tradition of Hippocratic medical ethics. Both came to form important strands in Western medical ethics. With the introduction of the Christian emphasis on compassion as an essential motive of the physician, one can speak of something new in medical ethics—an element that cannot be said to have been represented as an ideal in pre-Christian medicine.[11]

Beginning in the Middle Ages moral theologians in the Western (later Roman Catholic) church created and modified over time a highly intricate system of ethics based on canon law. In the area of medical ethics it historically focused on issues at the beginning and end of life, such as contraception, abortion, and euthanasia. Since the Council of Trent (1545–1563) there has been a strong emphasis placed on the natural-law tradition, which views God's purposes as evident in the nature of every human act. The concept of natural law, which owes much to Aristotle, has been basic to Roman Catholic medical ethics. It is capable of great subtlety and has produced much ingenuity in defining its application to medical ethics. For example, the Catholic position historically stressed an intrinsic connection between the unitive and procreative purposes of sexual expression in marriage. Because it regarded the natural intent of sexual intercourse to be to conceive children, the prevention of conception by artificial contraception was believed to be unnatural and therefore sinful.[12]

Protestantism differed from both the Roman Catholic and Orthodox churches in resting the church's authority on Scripture alone (*sola scriptura*). The Bible has been the touchstone by which all matters of theology, morals, and ecclesiastical practice were to be tested. Protestantism has tended to reject the formulation of a detailed system of ethics and to roll ethics back into systematic theology. Protestant medical ethics arose more directly from religious considerations of health and disease, as well as from biblical themes like providence, justification, law and grace, covenant, and the place of suffering in the Christian experience. Hence, Protestantism never produced a tradition of casuistry similar to that of Roman Catholic canonists. Instead, Protestants stressed 'commandment and conscience' (or 'norm and context') as the twin pillars on which ethics should be based: the application of general biblical principles to particular situations. The individual alone before God was a basic Protestant theme. The cultivation of the private conscience, which sought to apply the text of Scripture to concrete ethical situations, became its characteristic emphasis. On a number of questions in medical ethics that did not admit of easy solution because the biblical evidence was not clear, Protestants took divergent approaches. Thus, against the traditional Roman Catholic position that suicide was a violation of the sixth commandment and a sin that precluded repentance, some Protestants (like John Donne in his famous essay *Biothanatos* [1607–1608]) argued that God might forgive suicides and that one could not judge the state of the mind or heart that led them to take their own lives. In the last third of the twentieth century liberal and conservative Protestants became deeply divided in their attitudes to a variety of issues in medical ethics, particularly abortion and euthanasia. The divide reflected their disagreement over whether biblical prohibitions were merely culturally conditioned, or absolute and binding on modern societies. On ethical issues raised by new medical technologies, such as cloning and stem-cell research, consensus among Protestants has been lacking, given the insistence within the tradition on the exercise of private conscience. One issue that both have agreed upon is opposition to genetic engineering.[13]

Theodicy

In every culture societies have attempted to account for suffering in general and sickness in particular. We term these attempts *theodicies*. In the ancient world the most common explanation for suffering was that misfortune was retributive. When the gods were angry they sent plague, drought, famine, flood, defeat in battle, or some other calamity, which could only be removed by sacrifice or purificatory rites that would propitiate the gods or spirits (*numina*) by appeasing their anger. Homer's *Iliad* (Bk 1, lines 43 ff.) provides a well-known example. The epic begins by describing a plague that has afflicted the Greek forces besieging Troy. The Greeks attribute the calamity to Apollo, who has for been aiming pestilence-carrying arrows at his victims for 9 days, with the result that piles of corpses were being burnt. On the 10th day a seer is consulted to determine why the god is angry. Once he discovers the cause, Apollo is propitiated and the plague ends. Throughout antiquity devastating natural disasters, such as plague, stimulated not only popular religious fervour, but also the tendency to look for scapegoats. Thus natural disasters evoked persecution of early Christians on the ground that toleration of these 'atheists' had provoked the wrath of the gods.

The tendency to moralize sickness by rendering its victims as sinners in need of repentance was a late development in Egyptian and Mesopotamian religion, but it came to be widely held in antiquity that the sick were suffering deservedly because their disease was retributive. A sick person was not viewed compassionately, but as the recipient of deserved punishment. One finds this attitude everywhere in the Ancient Near East, including the Hebrew Bible. One does not pity the sick, but encourages the person to repent. This is the attitude of Bildad the Shuhite, one of Job's comforters, who warns Job that Yahweh acts justly. Job and his sons have sinned against him, but if he repents and remains upright in his behaviour, Yahweh will prosper him (Job 8:1–10). Bildad's attitude transcends cultural boundaries and one finds it everywhere in the ancient world.[14] So deeply rooted was this cultural prejudice that it hindered the establishment of any charitable concern for the sick.

Early Christians formulated a view of the human condition in which suffering assumed a positive role that it had previously lacked. They believed that, rather than bringing shame and disapproval, disease and sickness gave to the sufferer a favoured status that invited sympathy and compassionate care.[15] In the classical world neither philosophy nor religion encouraged a compassionate response to human suffering. During times of plague, the sick and dying were abandoned, and corpses often left unburied in order to prevent the spread of contagion. This may be seen in a contemporary account by Dionysius, Patriarch of Alexandria, of the Plague of Cyprian in the mid-third century.

> The heathen behaved in the very opposite way. At the first onset of the disease, they pushed the sufferers away and fled from their dearest, throwing them into the roads before they were dead, and treating unburied corpses as dirt, hoping thereby to avert the spread and contagion of the fatal disease; but do what they might, they found it difficult to escape.[16]

This description can be paralleled by several passages that describe popular reaction to plague in the classical world. Christians viewed suffering as an opportunity to provide care of the sick and dying, while at the same time they saw in it an opportunity for personal self-examination that could bring spiritual illumination. While Christians believed that suffering might be God's chastisement for sin, they did not posit a simple correlation between sin and suffering. Rather they viewed it as a means of grace for the spiritual benefit of the sufferer. So universal, however, has been the connection between moral failing and sickness that it has remained a dominant theodicy in many societies, including our own.[17]

Beneficence

Classical society saw in philanthropy (*philanthropia*, 'love of humanity') a potential motive for the practice of medicine, but it was never believed to be an essential virtue. The Greek physician Galen (CE 129–ca. 210 or later), in discussing the several motives that might cause individuals to engage in the medical art, listed a variety of possible incentives. They included philanthropy, as well as a desire for money, honour, and immunities from taxation. However, he thought that only competence was essential. Greek and Roman philanthropy excluded pity as a motive for medical treatment and thereby differed markedly from Christian concepts of medical charity in both motive and practice. The larger cultural values of Graeco-Roman society also militated against medical philanthropy. They included the Stoic conception of *apatheia* (insensibility to suffering) and a spirit of quietism that thought it impossible to improve the world. We can assume that many pagan physicians, in fact, demonstrated compassion towards those whom they treated. Nevertheless, in the classical world there existed no virtue or ideal of compassion that was urged upon physicians. One finds a few, such as Scribonius Largus, a first-century medical writer, who believed that it is essential, but in general the virtuous physician was not expected to display philanthropy in his medical practice. Christianity introduced a very different set of values from those that dominated the classical world, which over time came to underpin the ethics of medical practice.[18]

Basic to Christianity was a philanthropic imperative that sought to meet physical needs. Whereas Graeco-Roman values included no religious impulse for charity that involved personal concern for those who required help, Christianity based its charity on *agape*, which reflected the incarnational and redemptive love that God had displayed in Jesus Christ, who by his death on the cross provided a model for the sacrificial love of one's fellow human beings. Of Jesus' teachings none was more influential in this regard than the parable of the Good Samaritan (Lk. 10:25–37), which served as an encouragement to care for the sick. The imperative of the parable became a motivating ideal of the Christian physician: 'Go and do likewise' (v. 37). Compassion, hitherto unknown in Greek medical ethics, became an inspiration for the care of the sick.[19] While ordinary Christians were enjoined to visit the sick and aid the poor, the early church established congregational forms of organized assistance. Each congregation (*ecclesia*) maintained a clergy of presbyters (priests) and deacons, who cooperated in the direction of the church's ministry of mercy. The relief of physical want and suffering was assigned to deacons, who regularly visited those who were sick, while presbyters had charge of the administration of funds to aid them. Once each week alms were collected and distributed among the sick and the poor. Widows formed a special group to visit women and the office of deaconess grew out of the practice. Early Christian medical charity was developed while the churches were small, scattered, and experiencing persecution by the Roman government. Yet it was both effectively organized and extensively practiced. In the first two centuries of its existence, the Christian church created the only organization in the Roman world that systematically cared for its sick.[20]

There were no pre-Christian institutions in the ancient world that served the purpose that hospitals were created to serve, namely, the offering of charitable aid, particularly health care, to those in need. Roman infirmaries, called *valetudinaria*, were maintained by Roman legions and large slaveholders, but they provided medical care to a restricted population (soldiers and slaves), and were not charitable foundations. The earliest hospitals (*nosokomeia*, *xenodochia*) grew out of the long tradition of the care of the sick in Christian churches. The best known, and the earliest, was the Basileias, begun about 369 and completed by about 372 by Basil the Great, who became bishop of Caesarea in Cappadocia (Turkey). His hospital employed regular live-in medical staff who provided not only aid to the sick, but also medical care in the tradition of secular medicine. It included a separate section for each of six groups: the poor, the homeless and strangers, orphans and foundlings, lepers, the aged and infirm, and the sick. Hospitals spread rapidly in the Eastern Roman Empire in the fourth and fifth centuries, with bishops taking the initiative in founding them. They appeared in the Western Empire a generation after they were established in the East, but their growth was much slower in the West owing to economic difficulties. Hospitals and other charitable medical institutions were recognized as peculiarly Christian institutions. Only a minority of them had the resources to employ physicians, and they existed in the Byzantine East. In Western Europe there were few physicians in hospitals until the end of the Middle Ages. Early hospitals and related institutions grew out of the monastic movement, and the widespread existence of monastic orders provided much of the personnel to staff them. Hospitals were founded specifically to provide care for the poor (Basil called his hospital a *ptōchotropheion* or poorhouse). The pattern persisted until the mid-nineteenth century, and hospitals remained for centuries what they had been intended to be from the beginning, institutions for the indigent. Those who could afford a physician's care received it in their homes.[21] The large number of faith-based hospitals that were founded in North America indicates how seriously religious traditions took their call to medical philanthropy.

In the sixth and seventh centuries lay charitable orders came to be attached to large churches in the major cities of the Byzantine Empire. The best known were the *philoponoi* ('lovers of labour') and *spoudaioi* ('the serious ones'). They were largely drawn from the lowest class and had no medical training, but they sought out the homeless who could be found everywhere in the large cities of the eastern Mediterranean, bathed and anointed them, and provided them with palliative care.[22] Many similar movements have existed in the history of Christian philanthropy. Roman Catholics have excelled in organizing and institutionalizing their medical charities, including hospitals, most of them maintained by religious orders of women. The Sisters of Charity, founded by St Vincent de Paul (1580–1660), became a major force in caring for the sick.[23] A Lutheran order, the deaconess movement, was founded in the nineteenth century by two German pastors, Theodore Fliedner and Wilhelm Loehe, who were influenced by a Mennonite deaconess movement in Holland, and by the English Quaker Elizabeth Fry. It began at Kaiserswerth and soon spread throughout Europe. Florence Nightingale took her training at Kaiserswerth before opening a school of nursing in England.[24] Medical missions constituted another branch of Christian medical philanthropy. Missionaries to European colonial possessions often established medical facilities and much of their work was invested in the founding of hospitals, leprosaria, and other health-related institutions.[25] Medical philanthropy has spread to many other faith traditions, most particularly, Jewish and Muslim.

Religious healing

The New Testament Epistles indicate that early Christians experienced ordinary illnesses, of which they were sometimes healed and sometimes not. Biblical writers do not condemn secular medicine; in fact, although the evidence is slight, it appears that early Christians routinely employed it, as did most other religious and non-religious populations within the Mediterranean world.[26] Belief in religious healing has, however, always existed in Christianity, less frequently in the mainstream and more often on the sectarian fringe. Origin (ca. 185–ca. 254) maintained that Christians who wished to live in an ordinary way should use medical means, while those who wished to live in a superior (i.e. more spiritual) way should seek prayer for healing (*contra Celsum* 8.60). While there is little evidence that religious healing was prominent in the first three centuries, by the fifth century it had emerged as an element in Christian practice. Claims of miraculous healing were ubiquitous in the Middle Ages, especially focused on the tombs and relics of saints, which were believed to possess miraculous healing properties. Miracles became part of ordinary life, most of them claimed for the healing of a physical affliction. Pilgrimages to these shrines became enormously popular.[27] The Roman Catholic and Orthodox churches have continued to claim that miraculous healing occurs in the modern world as a demonstration of God's working in his church. Protestants by contrast have historically held that miracles ceased after apostolic or early Christian times. While they believed that God healed in answer to prayer, they considered miraculous healing (i.e. healing apart from medical means) to be rare. In the mid-nineteenth century, however, faith healing gained credence in some circles of American Protestantism, largely through Methodist influences, although most mainstream Protestant traditions rejected it.[28]

At the turn of the twentieth century a new movement, Pentecostalism, claimed that supernatural gifts of the Holy Spirit, such as glossolalia (i.e. speaking in unknown languages) and supernatural healing, were normative for the church in every age. The movement began in 1901 with Charles Fox Parham, a faith healer. His teachings were carried to Los Angeles, where they led to the Azusa Street revival, widely regarded as the beginning of Pentecostalism in America. Pentecostalism grew rapidly in the first two decades of the twentieth century. It taught that Jesus' death on the cross atoned not only for sin, but for disease as well. Hence, Christians could claim supernatural healing as a result of the 'prayer of faith.' Pentecostalism produced many itinerant healers who claimed to possess the gift of miraculous healing, with some practicing exorcism, regarding demons as a cause of illness. A minority of Pentecostals recognized medicine as an alternative to supernatural healing, albeit an inferior one. Many rejected medicine as unfaithful to God's unconditional promise to heal. In the latter half of the twentieth century some Pentecostals modified their categorical rejection of medicine. Since the 1950s, Pentecostal influences, often without their sectarian trappings, influenced mainstream Protestant and even Roman Catholic churches. The 'charismatic renewal,' as it came to be called, gained widespread influence as it introduced healing, sometimes in a sacramental fashion, to churches that had not traditionally practiced it, particularly in liturgical traditions, such as Anglican and Lutheran.[29]

Much popular Roman Catholic piety remained outside the control of the institutional structure of the Church. While educated Catholics might consider some manifestations of Catholic piety, especially those that syncretized pagan survivals, as superstitious, they reflected an important aspect of Catholic piety. There existed within the Church a tendency, which was not limited to post-tridentine Catholicism, to blur the distinction between ecclesiastically-sanctioned (usually sacramental) rites and folk practices. The approved observance of venerating relics and blessing animals, for example, has seemed to some Catholics not very different from popular cults that attributed healing to statues of the Virgin Mary. Hence, there remained a place for religious healing within the larger confines of the Church, such as that which existed within Pentecostalism. Chief among them was the miraculous healing offered at pilgrimage sites. Beginning in the nineteenth century, Lourdes in France, Fatima in Portugal, and Guadalupe in Mexico drew huge numbers of pilgrims year after year, in spite of the revolutionary advances of medicine that were taking place.[30]

Secularization and alternative healing

In the late nineteenth and early twentieth centuries Western societies underwent rapid secularization in nearly every public sphere. The professionalization of medicine eliminated from medical practice those without formal training in medicine, including clergymen who had practiced medicine, particularly in areas that were without physicians. A new emphasis on training in the sciences resulted in raising standards considerably for students entering medical schools. As medicine became a secular profession, it moved away from a religious emphasis on vocational calling and compassionate care. The new model of science became a naturalistic evolutionary one in which spiritual values were diminished as traditional religion found itself pushed to the margins of society in the academy and the professions. By the mid-twentieth century medicine no longer had formal ties to religious values. No appeal was made to spiritual values in medical treatment except in cases where health-care providers themselves felt a vocational calling. Hospitals and charitable medical facilities became secularized as well, with the decline of religious medical orders and the transition of faith-based hospitals to community-based or for-profit corporations. Mainstream medical ethicists in the last three decades of the twentieth century adopted utilitarian or consequentialist perspectives in place of implicitly religious ones.[31]

Concurrent with the growth of secularism has been the widespread following accorded New Age spirituality that developed in the latter half of the twentieth century.[32] The movement drew on Eastern pantheistic religions and metaphysical traditions, as well as naturopathy, spiritism, anthroposophy, and theosophy, which appealed to the newly-fashionable motifs of religious inclusivism and pluralism. It claimed to merge science (which often appeared to outsiders to be pseudoscience) with an alternative spirituality and sought to create an approach to healing that was both holistic and vitalistic (the view that the body is animated by a life force).[33] New-Age spirituality became popular in the 1970s and continues to attract widespread support, even if in a diffused and attenuated fashion. Indeed, it might be considered a component of the spirit of the age. Because it rejects defined theology and creedal formulations in favour of more pantheistic views, it has coalesced easily with modern secularism, and has influenced education and the professions, including medicine. Complementary and alternative medicine (CAM) is very much a component of New-Age belief, which rejects 'biomedical ethnocentrism' and allopathic medicine in favour of self-healing and self-realization (the two are often intertwined) that are intended to create a harmony of body, mind, and spirit. They include elements of traditional Chinese medicine (TCM), such as T'ai Chi, acupuncture, and herbal remedies, as well naturopathy and various forms of psychic healing. While some of these practices remain marginal, others (such as yoga and acupuncture) have been incorporated into routine medical practice. There is a strong spiritual component in much of CAM, sometimes derived from Hindu or Tibetan roots, sometimes from Native American or European pagan backgrounds. However, it more commonly appears as an amorphous patchwork of folk-healing practices drawn from a wide variety of 'spiritual' sources, rather than traditional religious communities, and is little noticed because it operates outside conventional medicine. In this sense, it resembles nineteenth-century American religions that had an alternative medical component, such as Seventh Day Adventism and Christian Science.

Consolation

In the intersection of religion and medicine, religion has played no greater role than that of providing consolation in sickness and death. It is an ancient tradition. When Job had been afflicted with the destruction of his family and possessions, and was covered with boils, three of his friends came to console him. For 7 days they sat with him in silence in a traditional attitude of mourning before they spoke (Job 2:11–13). Consolation enjoyed a role, as well in Greek philosophy. Consolatory essays in the form of letters to bereaved friends were a genre that dated back to the fifth century BC. Two of the best known were written by the Stoic philosopher Seneca (4 BCE–CE 65) on the death of family members (*De consolatione ad Polybium, ad Marciam*). The tone of these philosophical essays is (in the Stoic manner) emotionally detached, however, and they display little sympathy for the personal loss of the recipients. More focused on spiritual comfort was the consolatory literature of a long Christian tradition, which tried to bring solace to bereaved family members by urging that they seek their help in Christ and employ spiritual remedies to assuage their loss. A strong traditional belief in providence gave many religious believers a confidence that God controls every aspect of life and death, and that nothing happens by chance. The decline in a belief in providence in the twentieth century has weakened this certainty, which consoled generations of religious believers.

For Christians, suffering had a positive role that it lacked in classical paganism. For the Greek philosopher, physical suffering had no redeeming qualities. In Stoicism, sickness was one of those indifferent matters (*adiaphora*) that must be endured. Stoics urged impassibility in the face of the death of even the closest family members. By contrast, in the Hebrew Bible, Jews who suffered sought consolation from Yahweh, a theme that one sees often in the Psalms (Psalms 27, 46, 121,138; cf. Is. 61:1–3). Christianity went further, focusing on suffering as an element that God used in the process of sanctification. When suffering was accepted as sent from God, it possessed great spiritual value. Sickness invited self-reflection and, if it was the result of sin, the possibility of confession, repentance, and restoration of fellowship with God. Painful and chronic disease brought not self-pity, but the opportunity for drawing closer to God. Job could say at the end of his trials, 'I had heard of you by the hearing of the ear, but now my eye sees you' (Job 42:5).

'I was sick and you visited me' (Mt. 25:36). Jesus' words were a summons to a ministry of pastoral care of the sick. Consoling those who suffer has been one of the most important duties of pastors and priests who were charged with the cure of souls. A concern for pastoral care caused some mediaeval monks and secular priests to study medicine in order to combine medical care with spiritual solace. Similarly, when many towns had no physicians, some Protestant pastors, as educated men who could understand medical books, acquired knowledge of medicine in order to treat the sick in their communities. Cotton Mather (1663–1728) of Boston was one such minister. He became the focus of controversy when, during an epidemic of smallpox in 1721, he supported the physician Zabdiel Boylston in advocating inoculation. Conservative physicians and the local press opposed the practice, but several members of the local clergy supported Mather. Mather called the care of the soul *and* the body the 'angelical conjunction.' In his *Magnalia Christi Americana* (1702) he devoted a major section to biographies of New England's founders, many of which detail their suffering as contributing to their Christian character.[34]

'In the midst of life we are in death.'[35] The care of the dying was an extension of the ministry of consoling the sick. In the fifteenth century a genre of literature grew up that was intended to prepare one for a Christian death. Treatises on the 'art of dying' (*ars moriendi*) became popular in Europe during the Black Death. A later example of this genre, and the best known in English, is Jeremy Taylor's classic devotional work, *The Rules and Exercises of Holy Dying* (1651). Taylor's treatment of his subject differs from the mediaeval approach by his making the whole of life a preparation for dying. John Wesley, who admired the work, made it a practice in his itinerant preaching of visiting jails to offer spiritual counsel to men facing the gallows. It was not only compassion for their lot that pastors offered, but concern for the souls of those about to die. Were they ready to meet their Maker? If they were, the pain of this world and the death that awaited them had its sting removed by anticipation of heaven, which would bring release from their suffering, the hope of meeting their loved ones, and the certainty of seeing their Maker face to face. Of the benefits that religious certainty offered the dying, none was greater than the hope it gave of the life to come.

Bibliography

On the relationship of medicine and religion

Sullivan, L.E. (ed.) (1989). *Healing and Restoring: Health and Medicine in the World's Religious Traditions*. New York: Macmillan.

Ferngren, G.B. (2013). *Medicine and Religion: A Historical Introduction*. Baltimore, Johns Hopkins.

On the relations of Christianity to medicine and healing

Numbers, R.L., Amundsen, D.W. (eds), (1986). *Caring and Curing: Health and Medicine in the Western Religious Traditions*, reprinted Baltimore, 1997.

Sheils, W.J. (ed.) (1982). *The Church and Healing*. Studies in Church History 19. Oxford 1982.

On Asclepius

Edelstein, E., Edelstein, L. (1945). *Asclepius: A Collection and Interpretation of the Testimonies*. 2 vols in 1. Reprint, Baltimore, Johns Hopkins, 1998.

On medicine and healing in the early and medieval church

Amundsen, D.W. (1996). *Medicine, Society, and Faith in the Ancient and Medieval Worlds*. Baltimore: Johns Hopkins.

Biller, P., Ziegler, J. (2001). *Religion and Medicine in the Middle Ages*. Woodbridge, Suffolk and Rochester, NY: York Medieval Press.

Ferngren, G.B. (2009). *Medicine and Health Care in Early Christianity*. Baltimore: Johns Hopkins.

Siraisi, N.G. (1990). *Medieval & Early Renaissance Medicine: An Introduction to Knowledge and Practice*. Chicago and London: University of Chicago Press.

Temkin, O. (1991). *Hippocrates in a World of Pagans and Christians*. Baltimore: Johns Hopkins.

On medical missions

Hardiman, D. (ed.) (2006). *Healing Bodies, Saving Souls: Medical Missions in Asia and Africa*. Amsterdam and New York: Rodopi.

On clergy-physicians in colonial New England

Watson, P.A. (1991) *The Angelical Conjunction: The Preacher-Physicians of Colonial New England*. Knoxville, University of Tennessee, 1991.

On the religious implications of epidemic disease

Duffy, J. (1953). *Epidemics in Colonial America*. Baton Rouge: University of Louisiana.

Rosenberg, C.E. (1962). *The Cholera Years: The United States in 1832, 1849, and 1866*. Chicago: University of Chicago, 1962.

On the Pentecostal movement

Harrell, D.E., Jr (1975). *All Things Are Possible: The Healing and Charismatic Revivals in Modern America*. Bloomington: University of Indiana.

On the history of the hospital

Horden, P. (2008). *Hospitals and Healing from Antiquity to the Later Middle Ages*. Aldershit, England: Ashgate.

Miller, T. (1997). *The Birth of the Hospital in the Byzantine Empire*, second edition. Baltimore and London: Johns Hopkins University Press.

Risse, G.B. (1999). *Mending Bodies, Saving Souls: A History of Hospitals*. New York: Oxford.

For a comprehensive treatment of medical ethics in the world's leading faith traditions

Baker, R.B., McCullough, L.B. (eds) (2009). *The Cambridge World History of Medical Ethics*. New York: Cambridge University Press.

Jonsen, A.R.(2000). *A Short History of Medical Ethics*. New York: Oxford University Press.

On New Age and alternative healing

Sutcliffe, S.J. (2003). *Children of the New Age: A History of Spiritual Practices*. London: Routledge.

On pastoral care

Holifield, E.B. (1983). *A History of Pastoral Care in America: From Salvation to Self-Realization*. Nashville: Abingdon.

McNeill, J.T. (1951). *A History of the Cure of Souls*. New York: Harper and Row.

References

1 Amundsen, D.W., Ferngren GB (2000). Medicine. In: G. Ferngren (ed.) *The History of Science and Religion in the Western Tradition: An Encyclopedia*, pp. 485–87. New York: Garland.

2 Ferngren, G.B. (2009). *Medicine and Health Care in Early Christianity*, pp.18–19. Baltimore: John Hopkins University.

3 Ferngren, G.B., Amundsen, D.W. (1985). Virtue and medicine in pre-Christian antiquity. In: E.E Shelp (ed.) *Virtue and Medicine: Explorations in the Character of Medicine*, pp. 9–12. Dordrecht: Reidel.

4 Juvenal, *Satire* 10, line 356.

5 Preamble to the Constitution of the World Health Organization as adopted by the International Health Conference, New York, 19–22 June, 1946 (Official Records of the World Health Organization, no. 2, p. 100). Geneva: WHO.

6 [1] p. 486.

7 Nutton, V. (2004). *Ancient Medicine*, pp. 53–71. London: Routledge.

8 [7], pp. 103–14; Edelstein, E.J., Edelstein, L. *Asclepius: A Collection and Interpretation of the Testimonies*, especially vol II, pp. 139–213.

9 von Staden, H. (1996). In a Pure and Holy Way: Personal and Professional Conduct in the Hippocratic Oath. *J Hist Med* **51:** 404–37.

10 [7], pp. 155–6.

11 [1], pp. 109–12. On the continuing tradition of Hippocratic medical ethics in the Middle Ages see Galvão-Sobrinho, C.R. (1996). Hippocratic ideals, medical ethics, and the practice of medicine in the early Middle Ages: the legacy of the Hippocratic Oath. *J Hist Med* **51:** 438–55.

12 For the Catholic tradition in medical ethics see Amundsen, D.W. (2008). The discourses of Roman Catholic medical ethics. In: R.B. Baker, L.B. McCullough (eds) *The Cambridge World History of Medical Ethics*, pp.218–84. Cambridge: Cambridge University Press.

13 For the Protestant tradition see Ferngren, G.B. (2008). The discourses of Protestant medical ethics. In: Baker and McCullough [12], pp. 255–63.

14 (a) Garland, R.(1995). The eye of the beholder: deformity and disability in the Graeco-Roman World, pp. 59–61. Ithaca: Cornell University Press. (b) Sigerist, H.E. (1977). The special position of the sick. In: D. Landy (ed.) *Culture, Disease, and Healing*, p. 391. New York: Macmillan.

15 Sigerist, H. (1943). Civilization and Disease, pp. 69–70. Chicago: University of Chicago. Cf. idem [14b], 391–2.

16 Eusebius, *Eccles Hist* **7:** 22 (Williamson translation).

17 Cf. the late historian Tony Judt regarding the diagnosis of his fatal ALS: 'To fall prey to a motor neuron disease is surely to have offended the Gods at some point, and there is nothing more to be said.' Quoted in *The Nation*, **292** (7): Feb 14, 2011, p. 30.

18 Galen, *On the Doctrines of Hippocrates and Plato (De placitis)* IX 5.4. [2] 87–95.

19 [2] 108–12.

20 [2] 113–14.

21 [2] 124–30.

22 [2] 130–6.

23 O'Connell, M.R. (1986). The Roman Catholic Tradition Since 1545. In: R.L. Numbers, D.W. Amundsen (eds) *Caring and Curing*, pp. 135–7.

24 Lindberg, C. (1986). The Lutheran tradition. In: *Caring and Curing* [23], pp. 190–2.

25 Numbers, R.L., Sawyer, R.C. (1982). Medicine and Christianity in the Modern World. In: M.E. Marty, K.L. Vaux (eds) *Health/Medicine and the Faith Traditions: An Enquiry into Religion and Medicine*, pp. 149–51. Minneapolis: Fortress Press.

26 [2] 45–8, 59–61.

27 Amundsen, D.W. (1986). The Medieval Catholic Tradition. In: *Caring and Curing* [23], pp. 79–82.

28 (a) Ferngren, G.B. (1986). The Evangelical-Fundamentalist tradition. In: *Caring and Curing* [23], pp. 491–5; (b) Wacker, G. (1986). The Pentecostal tradition, in *Caring and Curing* [23], pp. 516–18.

29 [28b], pp. 520–32.

30 [23], pp. 135–7.

31 The secularization of medicine is a theme in [25]. For a survey of trends in bioethics since the mid-twentieth century see Jonson, A.R. *A Short History of Medical Ethics*, pp. 99–114. New York: Oxford University Press.

32 Sutcliffe, S.J. (2003). *Children of the New Age*, pp. 174–94. London: Routledge.

33 The term *holism* was coined by the South African statesman and philosopher, Jan Smuts (1870–1950), in his book *Holism and Evolution* (1926).

34 Smylie, J.H. (1986). The Reformed Tradition. In: *Caring and Curing* [23], pp. 212–13.

35 From a Latin antiphon attributed to Notker, a monk of St. Gall, in 911.

CHAPTER 2

Buddhism: perspectives for the contemporary world

Kathleen Gregory

Introduction

Buddhism approaches the human being from the perspective of impermanence and, as a consequence, the inevitability of illness, ageing, and death is stressed. In this way, rather than defining health in terms of the physical domain, Buddhism emphasizes mental health in terms of the kinds of attitudes we have to the most immediate and direct experience of impermanence—the decline and death of the human life process. To live within these conditions from which none of us can escape, Buddhism suggests, is not to be pessimistic, but to have a 'healthy attitude' of mind. As a result, the central role that mind plays in terms of our wellbeing is at the heart of Buddhism. Appreciating who the Buddha was and how the philosophies and practices he taught arose from his own experience becomes the basis in this chapter for understanding health from a Buddhist perspective. Further, within the contemporary context, Buddhism will be shown to be not only the religious domain of many Asian communities living in Western countries, but also the site of both religious and spiritual meaning for many Westerners to varying degrees of commitment, which itself brings challenges to healthcare workers and systems. Moreover, the evident interface of Buddhism with the fields of palliative care, psychotherapy, and general wellbeing further demonstrates the significant role Buddhism is already playing in relation to healthcare within the contemporary Western context.

Exemplifying this, recently, a friend was diagnosed with cancer and her prognosis was not good. She had learnt meditation in a secular context many years ago and asked for any Buddhist meditations that might be helpful. As a long-time Buddhist practitioner I gave her some instruction at this time. She had found a picture of a Buddhist shrine from somewhere and this was in her hospital room when she died. She had been raised in an atheist household and had little exposure to Buddhism, yet it came to mean something to her in the last few months of her life. It is well recognized that approaching death can bring a 'spiritual crises'. With the focus on mental health this chapter explores what in particular Buddhism can offer, both for living and dying in the contemporary Western context.

The aim of this chapter is to assist Western health practitioners to appreciate that the central concern of Buddhism is how to live well within the conditions that circumscribe our lives as human beings. Health is a concept in Buddhism that can be understood first, in relationship to the unavoidable sufferings and inevitability of sickness, ageing, and death; and secondly, in terms of developing a healthy attitude of mind characterized by understanding, mental stability, and compassion. To this end, the Four Noble Truths will be elucidated in relation to these factors. Furthermore, the fear of death is understood as natural and, in Buddhism, the importance of the living in dying is stressed in relation to developing a peaceful and calm state of mind.

Terminology

The notion of the *West* is defined not only in relation to geography but perhaps more importantly, by ideology. In the contemporary context the West is characterized by secularization and universality as dominant ideological forces.[1] This ideological context has played an important role in the rise of the concept of spirituality in the West, and in both the appeal and popularization of Buddhism within that.

Religion and *spirituality* are terms that, to a certain degree, have become oppositional. For example, formal versus informal, collective versus individual, public versus private, tradition versus modern, closed versus open.[2] However, it also remains that people continue to think very differently about what these terms mean. In relation to Buddhism, the question is often asked, 'Is it a religion or spirituality;' as if, as Traleg Kyabgon says, there is a distinction to be made. To consider Buddhism in relation to these terms, he suggests the religious refers to the external aspects, such as prayer, ritual, chanting, a belief system, and where the spiritual is the 'internal aspect of the whole religious phenomenon'.[3] From this perspective, the religious aspect is the method to attain spiritual realization. It is beyond the scope of this chapter to explore this distinction; however, it does provide an example of the enduring difficulty of translation and the application of Western terminology to another tradition like Buddhism.

Buddhism is a system that can be distinguished in relation to geography, historical time, and/or doctrine. Identified within Buddhism are the traditions or schools of Theravada, Mahayana, Vajrayana, and Zen, and within these further distinctions can be made. However, this concept of Buddhism in terms of schools can result in an over-determination of differences at the expense of the essential or basic teachings that are the 'unifying link between the various Buddhist traditions'.[4] In this chapter, Buddhism is presented from the essential perspective; inclining towards 'a universal approach', which characterizes the practice of Buddhism irrespective of time, place, or school. This perspective places emphasis on the mind in terms of wellbeing.

Buddhism and Buddhists in the contemporary Western spiritual context

Buddhism is now without doubt, on 'Western ground'.[5] In the last 40 years or so an explosion of interest in Buddhism has been well-evidenced in Europe and America; Brazil, Canada, South Africa, New Zealand, and Australia have all earned chapters in a relatively recent publication concerned with the spread of Buddhism 'beyond Asia'.[6] From the increase of Buddhist Centres in the West to the proliferation of books about Buddhism or with a Buddhist theme, from popular cultural images to the iconic status of His Holiness the Dalai Lama, to the fact that some of its concepts have entered everyday parlance (for example, *karma*); Buddhism itself has become a signifier that encompasses multiple images and meanings within the contemporary Western context.

Two factors can be identified which have been crucial in shaping Buddhism on Western ground in the late twentieth-century. First, Buddhism is but one tradition that has become incorporated in the rising trend of consumerist spirituality as outlined by Heelas (Chapter 11), resulting in individualistic and 'hybrid' spiritual orientations and identities. Secondly, the increased diaspora of Eastern Buddhists from first East Asia, and then South and Southeast Asia, have seen Buddhist migrants and their descendents settling in most Western countries. This has resulted not only in the establishment of Buddhist temples, which often act as important ethnic centres for their communities, but has also created a unique context for Western contact with all forms of Buddhism on home ground. Asian Buddhists living in the West have been distinguished as 'cradle' Buddhists as opposed that is, to 'converts,' although for many Asian Buddhists the meaning or significance of Buddhism, in fact, may be subsumed under their ethnic identity.[7] Moreover, the term cradle Buddhist needs now to include second generation Western (particularly American) Buddhists who are the children of first generation Western converts to Buddhism from the 1970s.

The notion of a convert suggests a self-conscious religious conversion to the extent that a previous religious identity is eradicated (if there was one), and a commitment to the new tradition undertaken. To be a Buddhist or more rightly to *practise* Buddhism, from a traditional view entails three aspects:

- a way of viewing the world
- a matrix of meditations, or ways of cultivating the mind
- a way of life.[8]

There is a small but ever-increasing number of Westerners who more rightly fit this definition, especially within the Tibetan and Japanese traditions, where the formal structure of a teacher–student relationship is the basis of this commitment. The convert population of Westerners can, in the main, be described as householders; having taken lay precepts they undertake a commitment to certain practices and are actively involved members of a Buddhist Centre, whilst still maintaining their everyday life. There is also a significant number of Westerners who have 'taken up robes', many of whom continue to work, especially in professions such as palliative care or psychology, where their Buddhist orientation can be a self-conscious part of their working life.

However, aside from the population of Western converts to Buddhism whose identity can be said to meet the traditional criteria, there exist numerous forms of engagement with Buddhism within which people themselves may or may not identify with 'being a Buddhist'. For example, there are those who participate occasionally in Buddhist meditation retreats, initiations, or group activities, many of whom may still retain another religious identity.[9] In trying to capture the diverse forms of Western engagement with Buddhism, Tweed makes the distinction between 'night-stand Buddhists', who may or may not identify themselves as Buddhists in some way and whose engagement is limited more to reading Buddhist literature; and 'Buddhist sympathizers', who may have had little actual engagement with Buddhism, but are sympathetic to its philosophies and may even see themselves incorporating some Buddhist ideas in their own lives.[10] These identities are, of course, fluid and in terms of the hybridity of spiritual identity as suggested above, in which Buddhism may be just one component, the necessity of understanding the meaning an individual attributes to and thus gains from the tradition(s) within which they are engaging is stressed.

In general, 'to our Western eyes Buddhism has come to be seen as beneficent or at least inoffensive'; and for the many that are drawn to it, Buddhism is predominately seen in relation to 'gentleness, to its compassion towards all forms of life, to its tolerance, to its non-violence'. It may in fact have come to be seen as a remedy or a 'kind or therapy'.[11] Within the context, that is, of an identified lack of tradition in the West; many Westerners have come to romanticize the East, Eastern people, and Eastern religions, to the extent that there is a projection of Western 'yearnings' associated with the 'values of tradition, community, wisdom, religion, and modesty'.[12] At the same time, some Westerners have come to regard Buddhism as an ethnic 'other' tradition, which is neither reflective of nor responsive to modern Western experience. The ensuing Westernization of Buddhism has seen the religious aspects (for example, rituals, the status of monastics) rejected and even central beliefs such as *karma*, *rebirth*, and *nirvana* have become either de-emphasized or abandoned. Authors such as Stephen Batchelor[13] and Joseph Goldstein[14] are examples of this modernizing of Buddhism, who have placed emphasis on the practice, for example, of mindfulness decontextualized from its broader doctrinal context and then re-contextualized it as primarily a means of psychological healing and spiritual awakening within a kind of 'secular spirituality'.[15]

Thus, in all kinds of ways Buddhism is assuredly on Western ground. Whether it is in a traditional religious form engaging both ethnic and Western populations; whether it has become Westernized as a kind of secular spirituality; or in the myriad ways Buddhism is part of individuals' spirituality or philosophy of life or, indeed, co-exists with another religious identity (for example, being a Christian and attending Buddhist meditation retreats); Buddhism is both *in* and *of* the contemporary Western context.

Buddhism's interface with health in the contemporary West

It is evident that many people attracted to Buddhism have suffered a life crisis of some kind, often of a health nature. Indeed, many work within the health professions. This increasing interest in Buddhism and, in particular, the practice of mindfulness, is testament to the practical application it is seen to have not only in relation to general wellbeing, but for helping people live with and manage all kinds of physiological and psychological clinical presentations, popularized, for example, in the work of Kabat-Zin.[16]

In the work of psychotherapy, the practice of mindfulness has increasingly become accepted and often incorporated with another therapeutic modality, for example, cognitive therapy.[17] The application of Buddhist ideas and practices to psychotherapy reflects the different Western engagements with Buddhism as outlined above; as a result many can be described as incorporating more casual to hybrid understandings. At the same time from within the tradition of Tibetan Buddhism there have developed a number of institutes that have sought to bring traditional Buddhist 'psychology' together with Western psychotherapy. For example, in Denmark and now established in a number of other European countries the Tarab Institute founded by the late Tarab Tulku Rinpoche has developed a comprehensive 'Unity in Duality' psychotherapy training programme; and in the USA the Naropa University founded by the late Chogyam Trungpa Rinpoche has an extensive graduate contemplative psychotherapy programme. Both institutions have a long history reflecting the fact that, in first coming to the West, traditional Tibetan Buddhist teachers saw Western psychology as an appropriate 'tool for communicating' Buddhism, since it is essentially a method for 'investigating the nature of one's own mind'.[18]

In addition, mindfulness has been identified as helpful to health practitioners themselves and, more recently, the benefits of mindfulness in relation to the therapist and the therapeutic process has been explored, suggesting that the therapist's 'ability to be mindful positively impacts his or her ability to relate to patients'.[19] Teaching mindfulness meditation has been shown to enhance qualities such as empathy, openness, acceptance, and compassion that are core therapist qualities.

However, as we now turn to consider the Buddhist approach to health and explore the fundamental emphasis on mental health in terms of healthy attitudes to the experiences of ageing, sickness, and dying; it becomes evident that Buddhism offers unique, relevant, and helpful perspectives for healthcare workers. In the last section this will be demonstrated in relation to working with dying and death. The context in which to understand the development of this view lies in the origin of Buddhism within the experience of the Buddha, which we will now consider.

The tradition of Buddhism

As is well known, Siddhartha Gautama/Siddhattha Gotama (Sanskrit/Pali), who is known as the *Buddha*, lived approximately 2500 years ago. He began his life as a prince living in privileged circumstances protected from the hardship of the world. When he ventured past the palace walls as an adult and saw for the first time the all-pervasive suffering human beings endured, he began a quest to discover how human beings found meaning and solace in the face of the difficulties that circumscribed their lives. He engaged with the religious traditions around him and experimented with many ascetic practices in his search for spiritual realization. After exhausting the myriad of spiritual practices available to him, he concluded two things: first, no spiritual or religious practice could safeguard a person against the inevitability of sickness, old age, death, and the ever-changing nature of human circumstance. Secondly, although it was self-evident that these were all unavoidable sufferings, human beings compounded their suffering through all kinds of misperceptions about their condition. From this the Buddha identified that it was, in fact, the human mind that creates 'avoidable' sufferings, when in truth all human beings desire happiness. At this point he abandoned engaging in ascetic practices and simply sat in meditation to work with his mind. It was through his efforts in this way that the Buddha is then said to have overcome erroneous beliefs and, as a result, insight was born in him. Insight can be described as 'seeing things as they are', which relates to the realities of our lives as human beings.[20] The word *buddha* actually means 'awakened', so in this sense the Buddha moved from a state of ignorance or not-knowing, to a state of being awakened; thus, it is said that the 'Buddha saw the world as it is and that was his enlightenment'.[21]

A number of points can be highlighted here that clarify Buddhism in relation to its content and purpose. Foremost, the Buddha is neither the incarnation of a higher being nor an intermediary or messenger of any kind; he demonstrated through his example that anyone who spent the time and made the effort could gain the insights he had realized.[22] That is, since the insights he gained arose from his own human experience without reliance on the 'supernatural powers of any being or creator', the teachings of the Buddha are 'related to the actual lives of all people' and, consequently, reflect 'natural principles'.[23] In this way, Buddhism can be understood as a tradition sourced in human experience and as a consequence, its primary orientation is to offer practical help to human beings.[24]

The story of the Buddha as presented above in fact outlines the development of the Four Noble Truths, which form the basic orientation of Buddhism.[25] The First Noble Truth the Buddha realized was the truth of the nature of suffering—our human life is circumscribed by impermanence, which reflects the nature of all things and results in kinds of unavoidable and, indeed, intractable sufferings (decline, the inevitability of change). However, the suffering we inevitability face as human beings become compounded by our misperceptions of the reality of impermanence. That is, the cause of avoidable sufferings is related to our attitudes and beliefs that he identified in the Second Noble Truth: the 'main suffering that afflicts us is created by our own mind and attitude'.[26] From his own experience as outlined, the Buddha discovered that it was possible for the mind to attain peace and contentment, even in the face of unavoidable sufferings, encapsulated in the Third Noble Truth—that is, the truth of the cessation of suffering. Finally, the Fourth Noble Truth outlines the Path to this cessation. The Eightfold Noble Path describes the practices that develop the three aspects considered exemplary of an ideal person:

- having wisdom as to the nature of the human condition
- being moral in action and thought
- demonstrating mental fortitude in the face of unavoidable sufferings.

From a Buddhist view, these three aspects in fact exemplify a healthy mind, which will be demonstrated in the examples that follow.

Sickness, old age and death: developing healthy attitudes

As suggested in the First Noble Truth the truth of suffering is to be understood in relation to the fact of impermanence. Just by having been born a human being we suffer the inevitable disease of 'decline, degeneration, and breakdown of the life process.'[27] Deterioration and death are merely the natural processes of the life cycles of all sentient creatures and living matter; as, too, is the deterioration of 'non-living' phenomena. In traditional teachings, the example of mountains that appear so solid, stable, and enduring are given as subject to change; how much more so our own bodies it can be asked. Our physical bodies, that is, are 'completely vulnerable and exposed to the elements, to external forces and to internal disease and breakdown of the organism.'[28] Even in the moment-to-moment pattern of our lives, our cells are dying and being replaced in never-ending cycles of birth and death; thoughts and emotions are arising, abiding for a time, and then dissipating. Once something comes into being, its passing is said to be certain.

Everything is said to be marked in this way; in the sense that 'impermanence is a universal reality.'[29] As a result, impermanence is to be understood as 'neutral, neither good nor bad', since it is the 'common nature of all things'. However, as identified in the Second Noble Truth, the Buddha identified ignorance of the 'nature of things' as the basis of avoidable suffering. That is, to not know 'things according to their nature is to lack fundamental knowledge and understanding of important questions: "What is life?", "What is old age and decay?", "How should we act in the face of old age?" When people lack knowledge and a correct way of thinking, then when they think about or come face to face with old age, various foolish, cowardly, and depressing feelings, and symptoms arise.'[30] Without a doubt, it is understood from the Buddhist point of view, it is a person's mental attitude that makes sickness, ageing, and dying 'unbearable.'[31] Simply from the Buddhist view, when it comes to attitude it is said: 'Whatever is destructive to you is unhealthy. Whatever integrates your life is healthy.'[32] Two common unhealthy attitudes to ageing, sickness, and death; and their alternative healthy attitudes represented in Buddhism can illustrate this.

First, it is evident that, without understanding the universal reality of impermanence and its manifestation in human beings as sickness, ageing, and death, people take these personally. They feel that in some way they are 'being singled out' and, as a result of this, their anxiety and suffering increases.[33] Buddhism identifies the fact that when things are felt personally then a person 'increases their attachment to the pain and suffering they are experiencing. The more a person focuses on the pain and discomfort, the deeper the suffering.'[34] A well-known story within the Buddhist Canon is of the woman overwhelmed by grief at the death of her baby through illness; she asked the Buddha to bring him back to life. In response, the Buddha said before he would talk further with the woman she was to bring him an ordinary mustard seed from any household she visited, which when she enquired, had not suffered the loss of someone through accident, sickness, or old age. Of course, the woman returned empty-handed and, in the process, awakened to the reality of death within the human condition; this is what helped her overcome attachment to her own grief.

This story demonstrates the 'all pervasiveness of death ... If you think only of the person you have lost and concentrate on your own grief about them, your focus becomes very narrow and your loss may seem overwhelming. But if you think of all the mothers in the world who have also lost their children and experienced the same grief as yourself, then the experience is more encompassing, it is no longer such a personal problem.'[35] From a Buddhist view, it is in the universality of our individual experiences that we can take comfort. In fact, because of the universality of our human experience in relation to sickness, ageing, and death, there is nothing 'particularly special or terrible' within it. From the perspective of Buddhism this attitude does not undermine the relative suffering of an individual human being or, indeed, the actual suffering experienced in sickness, ageing, and death; but rather serves to support genuine openness to our experience and circumstance. In this way, a healthy mind can be said to be associated with 'some kind of psychological openness' to experience.[36] A healthy attitude is one that understands the universality of impermanence and this understanding is what will increases the ability to relate to situations in a much more positive manner. 'Recognizing and acknowledging where one is and working with whatever situation life presents—accepting it just as it—is an important step towards mental and spiritual maturity.'[37] Understanding the universality and non-personal nature of impermanence in the most immediate and direct way—in relation to the demise of ourselves and others—is the basis for a more open and positive attitude to both life and death. As a result, the mind also becomes more stable; in the sense that one is 'ready to move forward in life, to face up to and deal with everything in the world with determination and joy.'[38] From a Buddhist view, it is this attitude that reflects a healthy mind. Otherwise, as the story of the woman and the mustard seed exemplifies the attachment and aversion that arises from our desire for things to be a certain way or other than they are, compounds the suffering we experience in the face of ageing, sickness, and death.[39]

Secondly, it is evident that rather than appreciating sickness, ageing, and death as natural consequences of the life process, increasingly in our modern Western context, these have come to be seen as 'something extra' or even an enemy to human beings.[40] As a result metaphors such as fighting, killing, cheating, or taming sickness, old age, and death are commonly employed. These examples suggest sickness, ageing, and death are in some way 'external events imposing themselves upon us' to which, in turn, we have mistakenly come to view 'our desire to get rid of disease as a desire to live'.[41] It is evident that worrying about sickness, old age, and death is neither going to improve one's health or 'make dying any less eventual'. At the same time, 'applying fixation' cannot 'cure change;' nor should we spend our time 'feeling sorry for ourselves' in the face of the inevitable deterioration and death of our life cycle.[42] Rather, the focus in Buddhism is on cultivating an attitude that helps us relate to the circumstances within which we find ourselves without going to these kind of 'extremes'.

The Buddha's teachings are summarized as the Middle Way; and serve as a practical instruction for living without extreme. From the Buddhist view, this is the most fundamental healthy attitude we can adopt since extremes create attachment and aversion (for example, wanting things to be a certain way or not wanting things to be a certain way), and result in fixation (for example, 'if I only had *x*, then everything would be perfect'), thus leading to further suffering. The Middle Way is thus a practical instruction to relate to the circumstances and conditions that circumscribe our lives as human beings. For most of us living in the contemporary West, we have what Buddhism would call the good fortune to be born in a time and place where there are unprecedented advances in medical technology and treatment. Having a healthy attitude to sickness, ageing, and death in this context does not presuppose at the one extreme denying oneself access to medical intervention and adopting some kind of fatalistic attitude. One can adopt an appreciative attitude, which expresses an acknowledgment of the good circumstance one has to be able to access treatment for illnesses, which at one time in history (and still in some parts of the world) were untreatable. At the other extreme it does not mean clinging to treatment (and thus to life) at all costs and denying the realities that our medical condition may present. Death and sickness are not enemies to be fought; nor is physical health a sovereign right. A healthy Middle Way attitude rests between these extremes to relate both appreciatively with what treatment is available and realistically, with the inevitability of unavoidable suffering. Furthermore, maintaining a positive frame of mind and sustaining realistic hope in relation to one's condition is important; whereas 'cutting off all hope' may, in fact, be counterproductive to feeling empowered to deal with our situation [43]. 'Trying to live with sickness is a much healthier attitude than doing something that is not conductive to our own wellbeing, such as denying the reality of the illness or having misguided confidence in our powers of recovery' [44]. From a Buddhist view, adopting a Middle Way attitude serves the foundation for increased mental fortitude in the face of whatever circumstance encountered in our human condition.

These two examples of 'healthy attitudes' demonstrate the teaching of the Buddha when he said that we must train ourselves to think: 'Even though my body is plagued with illness, my mind will remain healthy.'[45] As these examples illustrate, Buddhism is orientated to fostering a 'healthy mind' in practical terms, in relation to what to both refrain from and cultivate in terms of attitudes. Buddhism can be described as providing methods to cleanse the 'mind of all mental illnesses, eliminating all knots and impediments to its smooth functioning'; resulting in a 'general sense of healthiness, or intrinsic goodness in your state of mind.'[46] A healthy mind in Buddhism is one that reflects understanding in relation to the impermanent nature of our condition as human being and, as a result, mental fortitude can develop to help us face the circumstances in our living and dying as they arise.

The analogy between mental and physical health can be applied here to further elaborate the perspective of mental health from the Buddhist view. A 'state of perfect mental health can be compared to a body in perfect health, when in the absence of any disturbing illness; all of its organs function smoothly, to full capacity with complete efficiency.'[47] In this way, like the body, if the mind is not properly trained it becomes lethargic and lazy: 'a lazy mind is an irritable mind. Everything becomes irritating, there is no resilience, and so everything becomes a source of discomfort.'[48] Thus, as the body requires care in the form of discipline, nourishment, and 'exercise designed to sharpen its abilities and maintain healthy tone', the mind too needs the discipline of restraint to protect it from harmful attitudes that destabilize and compound suffering; nourishment in the form of healthy attitudes, which bring a sense of peace and contentment to the mind; and exercise in the form of meditation and contemplation.[49] As has been demonstrated in the examples above, this notion of restraint and cultivation can be applied. That is, one needs to learn to refrain from the mental habits of taking things personally and falling into 'extreme thinking' and, at the same time, cultivate understanding of the universal reality of impermanence and adopting a Middle Way view.

Buddhism, in fact, emphasizes preparing ourselves for the inevitable suffering of sickness, ageing, and death; understanding impermanence is, in fact, the best preparation for the time of death. From a Buddhist perspective we need to 'familiarize ourselves with our sense of mortality and impermanence.'[50] Buddhism recognizes that, in particular, the situation of death may indeed be painful and frightening; as a result it is preferable to come to it with some preparation through cultivating 'the kind of attitudes that we and others need when faced with death.'[51] We now turn to consider the Buddhist approach to death.

Working with the dying: the role of compassion

This chapter began with the assertion Buddhism is a religious/spiritual tradition on 'Western ground' in a variety of forms representing diverse meanings. Within the healthcare context a survey of the literature reveals that the primary emphasis has been on the spiritual needs of Ethnic Buddhists.[52] More recently, there has been recognition that the first generation of Western Buddhist converts is the ageing 'baby boomer' generation and as a consequence, their health and dying needs will reflect their religious and spiritual preferences.[53] However, some general points can be made that reflect Buddhism's main focus in relation to death: 'Dying at peace is dying skilfully'. This can be related to three aspects:

- letting go of the things that attach one to this life
- letting go of past wrongs and mistakes
- being emotionally undisturbed.[54]

In these ways, it can be said that, in Buddhism, the process of dying is more about life than 'death' as such. As Sogyal Rinpoche says: 'The most important thing is not so much the kind of preparation that you have had [to die], but the life that the dying person has left to live. If that life is well spent, if it is meaningful, shared, celebrated, that leads to a meaningful death.'[55]

Thus, as it is in living, so too it is in dying: 'it is a person's attitude and the whole orientation of their being that has the biggest effect when they come to die.'[56] It is acknowledged in Buddhism that death raises particular difficulties for human beings, given as Chogyam Trungpa suggests the 'vanguard of death is uncertainty and complete bewilderment'; even our attempts to 'hold onto life' are described as having the 'sense of death rather than life.'[57] At the same time within the contemporary Western context, death has become sanitized to the point of seeming unnatural. Even the dying in movies which is 'acted out by people who then get up and star in another movie' creates a 'kind of illusion' around death suggests Tai Situpa.[58] However, it can be simply said that a 'fear of death arises precisely because of the fact that we die.'[59] As a result of this fear, 'at the moment of death we need so much help'.[60] Within this context it is then the attitude towards death of those who are caring for the dying person, whether a family member, friend, or health professional, that is critical. The most important attitude we can adopt when being with someone who is dying is to help make them 'feel real, rather than some kind of species apart.'[61] As Sogyal Rinpoche reiterates, 'some kind of physical show of love and acceptance is very important, because one fear that many dying people have is that they will become an outcast or no longer loveable.'[62] In Buddhism, the development of compassion is crucial to working with others in sickness and death.

Compassion in Buddhism engenders the positive desire for the pain and suffering of others to cease, in the Eight-Fold Noble Path (the Fourth Noble Truth) compassion is associated with the development of morality, since it concerns how we relate through our thoughts and actions to others. Within Buddhism, the emphasis is on learning to 'extend compassion to others not because we are attached to them or afraid of their pain but because we know that all beings want happiness, just like ourselves. Just like us, they do not want pain.'[63] In Buddhism, compassion is understood to arise from the understanding of our impermanent nature. As a result, compassion is in fact the genuine understanding 'that one has to become one with the situation.'[64] To do so entails overcoming our own barriers to certain experiences like pain and death; it is a process of 'learning how to soften and open' to what 'is there' in our human condition.[65] In this way, it can be seen that understanding the impermanent nature of our existence and the inevitability of ageing, sickness, and death, can become the basis for an 'open heart.' In Buddhism, the knowledge that arises from this understanding assists us to be compassionate: with more clarity we can look for 'ways in which we can actually be of help ... We need to apply compassion intelligently.'[66] This is particularly relevant when working with sick and dying persons, 'intelligent compassion' expressed, for example, in kindness and concern can inspire confidence and trust in patients.[67]

Conclusion

The Buddha's insight was into the nature of the human condition, giving primacy to the human mind in discriminating what can bring a sense of either suffering or real happiness; concluding that 'everything has to do with attitude.' It is then right to say that 'Buddhism promises nothing. It teaches us to be what we are, where we are, constantly, and it teaches us to relate to our living situations accordingly.'[68] From this, the notion of spirituality can be further elucidated: the Buddhist view of spirituality is one that is 'based on a realistic approach to oneself and to the world.'[69] Since this approach corresponds to mental dispositions and attitudes, the notion of health in Buddhism is then relative to a healthy mind, which can be characterized as one that prepares 'us for suffering and death.'[70] From the perspective of Buddhism, when we understand and relate realistically and with an open heart to our human condition, in essence, we ennoble both our own life and death, and that of others.

References

1 Latouche, S. (1989/1996). *The Westernization of the World: the Significance, Scope and Limits of the Drive Towards Global Uniformity*. R. Morris, (transl). Malden: Polity Press.

2 Heelas, P. (1996). Introduction: detraditionalization and its rivals. In: P. Heelas, S. Lash, P. Morris (eds) *Detraditionalization: Critical Reflections on Authority and Identity*, pp. 1–20. Oxford: Blackwell.

3 Kyabgon, Traleg (2010). Buddhism: religion or spirituality (transcript of talk). In: *The wheel of time*, pp. 1–8. Kagyu E-Vam Buddhist Institute Newsletter (winter). Melbourne, Australia.

4 Tiradhammo, Thera Ven Ajahn (1989). Forward. In: K. Jones (ed.) *The Social Face of Buddhism: An Approach to Political and Social Activism*, pp. 11–17. Wisdom Publications, London.

5 Aronson, H. (2004). *Buddhist Practice on Western Ground*. Boston: Shambhala.

6 Prebish, C., Baumann, M. (eds) (2002). *Westward Dharma: Buddhism Beyond Asia*. Berkeley: University of California Press.

7 Tweed, T. (2002). Who is a Buddhist? Night-stand Buddhists and other creatures. In: C. Prebish, M. Baumann (eds) [6], pp. 17–33.

8 Wallace, B. (2002). The spectrum of Buddhist practice in the West. In: C. Prebish, M. Baumann (eds) [6], pp. 34–50.

9 [8].

10 [7].

11 Droit, R-P. (1997/2003). *The Cult of Nothingness: The Philosophers and the Buddha*. D. Streight, P. Vohnson, P (transl.) 1. Chapel Hill: University of North Carolina Press.

12 Kyabgon, Rinpoche Dagyab (2001). Buddhism in the West and the image of Tibet: In: T. Dodin, H. Rather (eds) *Imagining Tibet: Perceptions, Projections, and Fantasies*, pp. 385–6. Boston: Wisdom Publications.

13 Batchelor, S. (1997). *Buddhism Without Beliefs: A Contemporary Guide to Awakening*. New York: Riverhead Books.

14 Goldstein, J. (2002). *One Dharma: The Emerging Western Buddhism*. New York: Harper Collins.

15 [8], p. 37.

16 Kabat-Zin, J. (1990). *Full Catastrophe Living: Using the Wisdom of Your Body and Mind to Face Stress, Pain, and Illness*. New York: Delacorte.

17 Segal, Z., Williams, M., Teasdale, J. (2002). *Mindfulness-Based Cognitive Therapy for Depression: A New Approach to Preventing Relapse*. New York: Guilford Press.

18 Trungpa, C. (2005). Editor's introduction. In: C. Gimian (ed.) *The Sanity We are Both With: A Buddhist Approach to Psychology*, pp. xvii–xxxi. Boston: Shambhala Publications.

19 Bruce, N., Manber, R., Shapiro, S., Constantino, M. (2010). Psychotherapist mindfulness and the psychotherapy process. *J Psychother Theory Res Practice Training* **47**(1): 83–97.

20 Kyabgon, Traleg (2001). *The Essence of Buddhism*. Boston: Shambhala, 2.

21 Trungpa, C. (1976). *The Myth of Freedom and the Way of Meditation*. Boston: Shambhala.

22 [20].

23 Payutto, Prayudh (1995). *Buddhadhamma: Natural Laws and Values for Life*. G. Olson (transl). Albany: State University of New York.

24 Rinpoche, Samdhong (2006). In: D. Roebert (ed.) *Uncompromising truth for a compromised world: Tibetan Buddhism and today's world*, Bloomington: World Wisdom.

25 Gethin, R. (1998). *The foundations of Buddhism*. Oxford: Oxford University Press.

26 [20], p. 5.

27 [23], p. 105.

28 Kyabgon, Traleg (2003). *The Benevolent Mind: A Manual in Mind Training*. New Zealand: Zhyisil Chokyi Ghatsal Publications.

29 Rinpoche, Kalu (1993/1997). *Luminous Mind: The Way of the Buddha. An Anthology of Teachings Complied under the Direction of Lama Denis Tondrup*. M. Montenegro (transl). Boston: Wisdom Publications.

30 [23], p. 67.

31 Rinpoche, Chokyi Nyima (2004). *Medicine and Compassion: A Tibetan Lama's Guidance for Caregivers*. Boston: Wisdom Publications.

32 Kyabgon, Traleg (1993). *The Abhidharmasamuccaya* (transcript of talk). Melbourne: Kagyu E-Vam Buddhist Institute.

33 Mipham, Sakyong (2005). *Ruling Your World: Ancient Strategies for Modern Life*. New York: Doubleday.

34 [31], p. 139.

35 Kyabgon, Traleg (1998). Death, dying and reincarnation (transcript of talk) in Ordinary Mind. *E-Vam Inst Q* 4–6.

36 Trungpa, C. (2005). In: C. Gimian (ed.) *The Sanity We are Born With: A Buddhist Approach to Psychology*, p.154. Boston: Shambhala.

37 Situpa, Tai (1992). *Relative World Ultimate Mind*. Boston: Shambhala.

38 [23], p. 268.

39 [33], p. 125.

40 [37], p. 21.

41 [36], pp. 155–6.

42 [33], p. 126.

43 [31], p. 148.

44 [20], p. 33.

45 [23], p. 270, n.160.

46 [36], p. 161.

47 [23], p. 269.

48 Kyabgon, Traleg (2009). The Triple Gem (transcript of talk). In: *The Wheel of Time*. Melbourne: Kagyu E-Vam Buddhist Institute Newsletter, pp. 1–10.

49 [37], p. 61.

50 [48], p. 5.

51 Hookham, Lama Shenpen (2006). *There's More to Dying than Death: A Buddhist Perspective*. Birmingham: Windhorse Publications.

52 Nakasone, R. (2008). A brief review of literature of Buddhist writings on spirituality and aging. *J Relig Spiritual Aging* **20**(3): 220–6.

53 Ai, A., McCormick, T. (2010). Increasing diversity of American's faiths alongside baby boomers' aging: implications for Chaplain intervention in health settings. *J Health Care Chaplaincy*, **16**(1–2): 24–41.

54 [31], pp. 146–50.

55 Rinpoche, Sogyal (1998). Death and dying (transcript of talk). In: *Ordinary Mind*. Melbourne: E-Vam Institute Quarterly, pp.16–23.

56 [51], p. 136.

57 [36], p. 31.

58 [37], p. 59.

59 [35], p. 5.

60 [55], p. 18.

61 [51], p. 132.

62 [55], p. 19.

63 [33], p. 110.

64 Trungpa, C. (2009). In: C. Gimian (ed.) *Smile at Fear: Awakening the True Heart of Bravery*. Boston: Shambhala, p. 49.

65 Chodron, Pema (1991). *The Wisdom of No Escape and the Path of Loving-Kindness*. Boston: Shambhala.

66 Rinpoche, Khenchen Thrangu (2002). *Essential Practice*. J. Levinson (transl). Ithaca: Snow Lion Publications.

67 [31].

68 [21], p. 93.

69 [36], p. 21.

70 [51], p. 5.

CHAPTER 3

Chinese religion: Taoism

Russell Kirkland

Introduction

Taoism (sometimes written Daoism) is a Chinese religious tradition that coalesced during the fifth century CE, integrating numerous strands of earlier Chinese culture. Over time, Taoism incorporated an array of distinct concepts about the nature of human life, and a wide variety of interrelated moral values and religious practices. It is neither a founded tradition, like Christianity or Buddhism, nor a generic rubric for the disparate beliefs and practices throughout a diverse society, like Hinduism. Rather, Taoism is a fluid religious organization conceived by learned members of the Chinese aristocracy who had witnessed the successes of Buddhism (which had been imported across Inner Asia from India in the first centuries CE) and felt compelled to preserve and fortify China's indigenous spiritual traditions in response.

More broadly, the term 'Taoism' can be regarded as a rubric for a holistic worldview and ethos, which originated among unknown minds in 'classical' times, around the 4th century BCE. In classical Taoist texts, to live a proper life is to live in such a way that one restores the world's holistic unity. The ideals expressed in those ancient texts were meant more to inspire than to instruct, so it was only in mediaeval times that they were developed into a sociocultural framework allowing sensitive, dedicated men and women eager to put those ideals into *practice* within their lives. That mediaeval framework, denominated *Tao-chiao* (*Daojiao*, 'the Teachings of Tao'), was founded and led by socially prominent members of the literate class—just like its more humanistic counterpart, Confucianism—and has endured to the 21st century.

The Taoist understanding of personal identity and human values has long been contrasted with that of Confucianism. Confucians have generally insisted that fulfilling one's role in society is necessarily grounded in moral self-cultivation, and that one's proper goal should be to develop oneself in order to strengthen and enhance society and the political order. Confucians tacitly assume humans to be innately distinct from, and superior to, other lifeforms, because of humans' social inclinations and moral consciousness. (Confucius himself was clearly a theist, but later Confucians minimized his religious thrust of his teachings, particularly when explaining them to modern Westerners.) Taoism, by contrast, locates humanity's value not in what separates humans from the rest of the natural world, but rather in what they share with it.

However, Taoism was never truly the opposite of Confucianism: each tradition presented distinct models for pursuing ideals that were, in general, common to both. Indeed, until the changes that swept Chinese society after the Mongol conquest (13th century), Confucians and Taoists characteristically agreed that their traditions shared key perspectives on life's most basic issues:

- the need for living a moral life
- the need for personal self-cultivation
- the need for society and government to be transformed by the effects of people who fulfill the tradition's ideals of moral/spiritual self-cultivation.

What distinguishes the two traditions is that Confucians have typically located life's most crucial values squarely within humanity itself. In contrast, the Taoist approach to life sprang from a holistic worldview, so its ethos concentrates upon holistic transformation of self, society, and the natural cosmos through a variety of interrelated moral activities and religious practices.

Taoism in proper perspective: correcting 20th century misunderstandings

Though Europeans had occasional contact with China throughout history, virtually all of what modern Westerners think about China's religions, including Taoism, dates from the late 19th century: throughout the 20th century, Westerners still understood 'Taoism' simply as a set of ideas that 19th century missionary scholars had taught them to associate with two texts of late-classical China: the *Lao-tzu* (*Laozi*) or *Tao te ching* (*Daode jing*), and the *Chuang-tzu* (*Zhuangzi*). For instance, the first English translations of 'Taoist classics' date from the 1870s. The man who chose which Chinese texts should be imagined to represent 'the Taoist classics' was not a Taoist, nor someone who interacted meaningfully with Taoists or studied the hundreds of writings that Taoists had honoured and preserved. Rather, the man who effectively 'founded' Taoism as a construct in the Western mind was a Scottish missionary, James Legge (1815–1897). Single-handedly, Legge caused all later Westerners to imagine that China's religions should be understood in the terms that Victorian Englishmen understood their own religion—that Taoism (and Buddhism), like Christianity, originated in the wisdom of one 'enlightened mind' of long ago, then 'degenerated' into centuries of superstitious nonsense, just as the 'purity' of the Christian Gospel had supposedly degenerated into what the Victorian Protestant mind regarded as the 'superstitious nonsense' called Catholicism.

In addition, the 19th century creators of the Western mind's 'Taoism' were steered by Confucian informants, who fed gullible Westerners like Legge slanderous deceptions about how 'enlightened' we Confucians have always been, and how dangerously superstitious those Taoists have always been. For instance, 20th century minds imagined that in traditional China, all concern with ethical ideals or service to society was an exclusive province of Confucians, and that Taoists never even entertained an idea of developing any social ethic, much less involvement with health or medicine. As the 21st century opened, scholars have been able to demonstrate the truth about Taoism—that within the rich heritage of imperial China, there were in fact not just one or two ancient philosophical texts, but a wide variety of profound Taoist writings designed to guide how we live our lives within society, as well as within our bio-physical environment.

Some Taoist texts were reputedly revealed by spiritual beings that are conscious and active in our world—quite like comparable Jewish, Christian, and Muslim writings. For instance, since the 2nd century, Chinese emperors venerated 'the Old Lord' (Laojun), an eternal being who periodically descends into the mortal world to aid us. The emperors understood the Old Lord as the revealer of the text known in the West as the *Tao te ching*. However, in late antiquity, the Old Lord saw that mortals had fallen into improper behaviours, so he also revealed ethical instructions known as 'The 180 Precepts'. The behaviours enjoined in those Precepts include proper restraint in eating and drinking; proper respect for women; and proper engagement with the natural world: one should not improperly fell trees, drain rivers or marshes, abuse animals, or even frighten birds or beasts, much less cage them. Of course, the Old Lord forbade taking any human life, including that of the unborn (Precept 13). In other words, people should restrain all impulses to act in a thoughtless or self-indulgent manner, thereby ensuring that we do no harm to others or to the world in which we live. But 20th century minds never knew that centuries of Chinese emperors recognized divine beings who guide us in understanding how to manage our lives. For Taoism to be palatable to modern minds, it was necessary for it to be portrayed as simply an ideal of 'being one with Nature' (or some comparable tenet of modernist faith), which never offered any teachings about the social dimensions of life, the moral dimensions of life, the realities of the human body, including our need for healthcare.

In reality, Taoists over the centuries not only presented the social and moral dimensions of life as integral to the spiritual life: Taoists even provided the conceptual framework in which *all* traditional Chinese *medical* practitioners have done their healing work. We now know of thousands of Taoist writings by the centuries of learned men—and women—that articulate a wide array of nuanced models for understanding reality and the nature of human life. Within those models, the conscientious practitioner learns the true nature of our own reality, and with that knowledge, is empowered not only to preserve one's own health and wellbeing, but also to revive and enhance the health and wellbeing of others.

The Taoist worldview

Throughout history, members of the Taoist tradition have shared certain common assumptions, foremost of which is that human life is grounded in deeper realities: we are components of a *cosmos*, a harmonious universe in which all things are subtly, but actively interrelated. Taoists teach that the lives of all embodied beings extend into spiritual realities that far transcend the life of any species, yet which form the basis on which individuals should consider their decisions and actions pertaining to life, including questions regarding healthcare.

Another common Taoist assumption is that most people live fundamentally unaware of the true nature of the reality within which our lives take place. Hence, they live their lives on terms that are not in accord with the true nature of their own reality. Such lives are inherently flawed, so ultimately fruitless. However, while members of other religious traditions, including Buddhism, share those assumptions, Taoists historically believed that misguided life decisions rob one's life not only of meaning and depth, but of health as well. In Taoism—more clearly than in any other non-Western tradition—the body is important, and it is fundamental not only to one's spiritual practice, but to all our interaction with others.

It is here, in what might be called the affirmation of the body's spiritual reality, that we see something shared by Taoists and not by most of the world's other religious traditions, including Confucianism. For Taoists, it is not only an individual's own 'real-life' bodily realities that have profound relevance for one's transformational practices: so indeed does our natural environment, which, properly understood, is *not* 'dead matter'—just like the human body, our entire cosmos is a world in which the spiritual and the material are not only subtly intertwined, but profoundly interactive. Understanding these facts is essential for traditional Chinese healthcare.

Since classical times, Taoists have insisted that we must focus our concern upon (re)integration with the deeper realities of the cosmos through a process of personal refinement (*lian*). In classical texts, that process was expressed in 'bio-spiritual' terms; in imperial times, it was often couched in terms of the ideal of 'fostering life' (*yang-sheng*). But, despite 20th century misconceptions, fostering life never implied simply trying to prolong a patient's physical life. In fact, Taoists of all periods would be puzzled by the dogged conviction of many modern minds that the prevention of biological death, in and of itself, morally trumps all other concerns: to Taoists—as indeed, for members of most other religious traditions—the reality of anyone's life extends far beyond the mere biological activity of one's body, so extending the latter *for its own sake* hardly seems even desirable. The Taoist goal is always healthy integration with the deeper dimensions of life, and on those terms a medical model that defines 'life' in purely material terms appears quite perverted.

Moreover, the Taoist ideal has never simply involved pursuit of individual wellbeing: the life that a Taoist is taught to foster is not just his or her own, but the wellbeing of other persons, other living beings, and indeed the whole cosmos.[1]

Taoist spiritual practice

The Taoist religious tradition that emerged among China's mediaeval aristocracy presents an array of teachings and practices designed to facilitate a meaningful personal transformation. The nature of those practices, and the nature of that transformation, are rooted in the act of learning to experience, and work with, the true structures and energies that subtly link an individual's personal experience to the rest of our living world. Among Taoists, those practices are perceived to lie directly within the subtle informing structure of one's own being, within what might be called the individual's own bodily energies. The fundamental activity in which one should ideally engage is a 'cultivation of reality' (*xiu Zhen*) that occurs as a practitioner forges a newly-experiential engagement with the subtle forces, structures, and energies inherent to our reality. In that process, one learns that all such structures and energies actually stretch throughout all that is real, both within one's own personal form and throughout what unperceptive minds regard as the external universe.

The earliest known model of what we now call Taoist cultivational practices is presented vaguely in a classical text called the *Neiye* (4th century BCE), and more fully particularized in the *Huainanzi* (2nd century BCE).[2–4] The *Neiye* and related texts influenced fundamental concepts of traditional Chinese medicine—which is still widely practiced today, not only in China, but around the world—as well as many elements of later Taoist imagery and practice.[5] Within such theory—if the word theory may even be applied to such a vague set of ideas—the term *dao* was simply a nebulous marker for 'the realities that one ought to cultivate.' In that context, the term *tao* was also used synonymously with the word *ch'i/qi*—the salubrious life-forces inside and around all living beings—and with the term *shen*, which corresponds almost perfectly with the English word 'spirit.' I have termed these practices 'bio-spiritual cultivation'.

In later centuries, the dedicated men and women who developed the tradition they called *Daojiao* articulated a wide range of additional conceptual frameworks and practices. Those new frameworks never fully displaced the early traditions of bio-spiritual cultivation. The core of Taoist practice—from classical times to the twenty-first century—has involved practices of self-cultivation within a cosmos full of subtly linked forces.

Yet, we must beware misinterpreting such ideas in terms of modern individualism: Taoist theory never assumed any dichotomization of 'self' and 'other.' That is, Taoists did not assume that anyone's 'self' could be fulfilled without reference to the fulfillment of other persons, other living beings, and the broader realities in which all beings (embodied and unembodied) are naturally and properly embedded. Taoist self-cultivation does not assume that each human being has some enclosed, individualized self that is more worthy of value and attention than what is outside that enclosure. On the contrary, every embodied being—human and non-human—lives within a matrix of unseen forces that Taoists usually came to term *Zhen*, a term connoting 'the reality of which non-practitioners remain unaware.'

Modern medicine tends to assume that human life takes place entirely within a materialistic framework. Though some practitioners are devout Jews or Christians, the theoretical framework of modern medicine—including the very concept of what the body is—does not, for instance, acknowledge spiritual energies suffusing a patient's being, or seek to treat illness by correcting/removing blockages of those energies through holistic means, as in traditional Chinese medicine.

Yet, regardless of any medical practitioner's personal religious beliefs, even the most materialistic scientists today must, for instance, acknowledge that our bodies:

- exist within the flow of the earth's *invisible* magnetic sphere
- are constantly affected by *invisible* radiation from the sun
- are also permeated, every second, by *invisible* man-made radiations, including messages being sent and received—right *through* each person's physical body—within radio waves of all kinds.

Yet very few people have any *awareness* that such *invisible forces* are actively present, permeating not only our individual bodies, but also the continuum of time/space/matter/energy in which all such persons exist.

Traditional Chinese medicine developed in tandem with Taoist expositions of the vital significance of *natural* invisible forces for the health and wellbeing of all persons. However, for any person to become aware of any such invisible forces—much less to gain proper benefit from them—it is necessary for one to have a correctly tuned receiver. That receiver must be properly designed and manufactured, and its user must see that it is correctly powered and tuned. In Taoism, each person's personal life matrix may be understood as just such a receiver. The practices articulated in each sub-tradition of Taoism are designed to effect the proper tuning of the practitioner's bio-spiritual receiver.

Yet, we must remember that tuning one's own receiver is not somehow a turning inward upon oneself, a rejection of one's interconnectedness with others: to lose sight of our interconnectedness inevitably reduces one's awareness of true reality and diminishes one's health. Yet, the only person who can learn to do the tuning necessary for one to gain the benefit of the unseen natural forces that flow around and through us all is, logically, each individual. Hence, the spiritual practices envisaged by Taoists are, logically, practices that only the individual can undertake. Yet, in so doing, he/she is intrinsically working to engage him/herself more fully with a set of invisible realities that connect the individual with all of reality.

For these reasons, the Taoist tradition has held a special place for men—and indeed women—who have mastered such processes, and can tune their own beings in such a way as to extend the resulting benefits to others around them—benefitting all beings universally. Taoist temples have traditionally been staffed by such persons—men and women who accept the responsibility of working to bridge the gaps between the skilled spiritual practitioners who have mastered life's invisible forces and those who have not. For Taoist priests and priestesses, the basis on which their other activities are founded has always been a life of self-cultivation: that life requires them to labour productively—through moral discipline, meditation, and appropriate ritual action—to participate fully in the reality of life's subtle, unseen forces, the forces called *Zhen*.

The Taoist foundations of Chinese concepts of health

A fundamental Taoist assumption is that disorder is a result of imbalance, whether physical or spiritual, individual or social. In traditional Chinese medicine, physical illness is understood as a symptom of some kind of bio-spiritual imbalance. In most presentations of Chinese medicine, disease is ultimately explained as a result of a misalignment of *ch'i/qi*, the natural life force that permeates our natural bio-physical world, as well as one's individual body.

In a broad theoretical context, the imbalances that result in disease might be attributed to a natural entropy: ancient Chinese thought assumed that the present state of the world represents a degeneration from an earlier state of universal harmony, called *taiping*. The goal of life for Taoists is to restore that universal harmony and certain Taoists took profound interest in the problem of restoring the harmony of individuals through treating physical maladies. However, disease and healing have never been understood in purely materialistic terms, and the goal of medicine was never simply the alleviation of physical suffering. Like healers in other traditional cultures (such as Native Americans like the Navajo), Taoists generally assume that all physical symptoms remit when one restores the biospiritual integrity of the individual and re-establishes a state of balance and harmony with the deeper realities of life. Consequently, some Taoists worked to restore patients' health through therapeutic ritual activity, while others studied the pharmacological effects of various substances that co-exist with humans within earth's interactive matrix.

Classical texts, like the *Neiye* and the *Daode jing*, teach that personal self-cultivation, done correctly, results in a beneficent transformation of other living things, a transformation that reaches ultimately to the furthest extent of the world. In other words, by pursuing the proper ideals, one participates in a holistic project that actually benefits 'self' and 'others' alike, on a universal basis. The process of personal cultivation is thus not to be regarded as something that takes place solely within—or solely for the benefit of—one's own individual life. Rather, because of the holistic nature of the world in which we live, that process results in a transformative effect that allows others—human and non-human alike—to be benefitted. By engaging in that transformative process, rather than in interventional acts, one effects a therapeutic metamorphosis throughout the world, while avoiding the harmful effects that, as the *Daode jing* insists, are intrinsic to interventional action, however well-intentioned.

A seldom-noticed teaching of the *Daode jing* is that *self-restraint* is its prime behavioural ideal. The *Daode jing* argues that it is morally necessary for humans to restrain their impulse to 'go out and make the world as it should be' because in reality, the world in which we live is produced from *an unseen matrix* that is not only *beneficent*, but also worthy of our *trust*, like a loving Mother who gives life and nurtures all things without ever engaging in any kind of controlling behavior.[6] The *Daode jing* urges its reader to be benevolent, loving, and caring—without presuming that our personal thoughts, emotions, or actions should be imposed on others' lives. Instead of endorsing a behavioural ideal that 'dares to take action,' the *Daode jing* urges us to *dare to restrain ourselves*, and learn to recognize the world's unseen realities that, like water, give life freely to all, without thoughts, emotions, or actions—an ideal that the *Daode jing* calls *shan* or 'goodness.' The *Daode jing* teaches that an 'enlightened' person is one who is wise enough and caring enough to participate in producing meaningful change in the world by boldly foregoing self-righteousness, refraining from interventional activity, and allowing the inherent beneficent forces of the world to hold sway.

From the Taoist holistic perspective, that ethic of benefitting others by allowing the natural world to operate as it is designed to operate is the only *true* goodness possible, *if* one respects the true nature of reality. That is because there are actually subtle, imperceptible beneficent forces ceaselessly at work in the world at all times; and those forces are constantly benefitting all things selflessly, the way that water does, without 'doing' anything. Rather than needing human ingenuity or heroic action to 'make the world (or any being, including a medical patient) as it should be,' life is *already* being guided by the greatest and most beneficent force in the world, the invisible, but inexhaustible force called Tao.

The *Daode jing*'s editors gave it a socio-political relevance by expanding its teachings to provide guidelines for leaders in the fields that were essential to the intended audience ca. 300 BCE: rulers and military leaders. Since medicine was not essential to that audience, the *Daode jing* was not framed to explain its pertinence for practical issues of healthcare. However, that fact should not lead one to imagine that Taoists, or the people of pre-modern China in general, were opposed to science or medicine in the modern sense. In fact, until quite recent times, the development of the life sciences in China—as indeed, the physical sciences—was frequently far in advance of what existed in Europe during comparable periods.[7] The history of Chinese science and medicine (as well as the outlook on such matters within the very *un*-traditional society of China today—i.e. under a political system rooted in Marx and Lenin) have been explored by leading Western scholars, such as Nathan Sivin.[8] Here we are concerned with the theoretical assumptions that undergird both Taoist religious practice *and* traditional Chinese medicine, both of which are based squarely on the teachings found in the *Neiye*—the earliest extant text that explains self-cultivation through daily, practiced regulation of the forces of life.

For instance, the *Neiye* teaches that good health begins with dietary self-restraint, as well as restraint from excessive passion and excessive cogitation. Such self-restraint—which is simultaneously moral, emotional, psychological and physiological—allows life's beneficent unseen forces—'life-energy' (*ch'i/qi*) and 'spirit' (*shen*)—to fill one's being. In the *Neiye*, 'life-energy'—the universal force that gives life to all things—is equated with 'Vital essence' (*ching/jing*), which traditional Chinese medicine often explains as the individual's innate reservoir of life-energy. But within this theory of life, every individual tends to lose his/her 'essence'—and consequently, to develop health problems of *every* kind—because of careless mismanagement, not only of our physical form, but more importantly of our 'heart/mind' (*hsin/xin*).

Within all Chinese thought, the heart/mind is the ruling agency in the individual's biospiritual nexus, i.e. in the entire personal complex of body, mind, heart, and spirit. Each individual's heart/mind is held to have been originally pure, but it becomes agitated by excessive activity, which leads to dissipation of one's vital essence, and hence to confusion, sickness, and death. To preserve one's vitality, one must maintain a tranquil heart/mind, thereby becoming an efficient receptor of life's salubrious energies; without tranquility, those healthy energies leave and one's health, and very life, will become threatened. Quieting the heart/mind is an ideal of personal moral and spiritual perfection that remained constant in later Taoism, as well as in Confucianism, though the idea that doing so is essential for health became lost in Confucian thought.

Healing in the history of Taoism

Over the very long course of Chinese history, different segments of the Taoist tradition addressed issues of health and healing, from varying distinct perspectives.

During the Han dynasty (206 BCE–221 CE), imperial advisers produced a scripture called the *Taiping jing*, 'Scripture of Great Peace', which—like nearly all Taoist texts—remained unknown in the West until the past few years.[9] The *Taiping jing* teaches that the (mythical) rulers of highest antiquity maintained an 'ambience of Great Peace' or 'Grand Tranquility' (*taiping*) by practicing self-restraint and trusting to the world's natural order.[10] When rulers began meddling with the world, Grand Tranquility was disrupted. Until a wise ruler returns us to that halcyon condition, each of us should endeavour to return to that natural state of harmony by practicing self-restraint and following the *Taiping jing*'s teachings, which include recommendations for enhancing health through breath control, medicine, acupuncture, and even music therapy.

The *Taiping jing* inspired certain social movements, such as the 'Heavenly Master' (*Tianshi*) organization (ca. 2nd–7th century CE). *Tianshi* thought assumed that a healthy society depends upon the moral, physical, and spiritual health of all its members, so the organization's male and female officiants healed the sick by performing expiatory rituals. The ideal of therapeutic ritual was shared not only by many later Taoists, but by many rulers and most East Asian Buddhists, as well as by the Navajo and other traditional cultures. In addition, in imperial China some Taoists were active in both the theoretical and the practical dimensions of the physical and biological sciences. Chinese pharmacology and medicine evolved largely through efforts of mediaeval Taoists intent upon 'nourishing life.' Mediaeval Taoist texts on the physiological aspects of nourishing life are still used today in the training of Chinese physicians, although they have never been translated into English, and are known today only to a handful of scholars and Taoist practitioners in China. One example is the *Fuqi jingyi lun* ['On the Essential Meaning of the Absorption of Life-Energy'] by the 8th century Taoist leader Sima Chengzhen. Like several other texts by mediaeval Taoist theorists (such as the physician Sun Simo), Sima's work methodically explains the nature of biospiritual reality, providing guidelines for the practitioner to sublimate personal deficiencies and establish a healthy, *qi*-filled personal existence.

Through later centuries, Taoists retained that focus on personal cultivation, though some little-known traditions emerged to turn the skills of the fully developed spiritual leader into therapeutic techniques. The earliest of those, called Qingwei ('Clarified Tenuity'), was reportedly founded a young woman ca. 900 CE. Qingwei 'thunder rites' (*leifa*) were designed to empower a priest/priestess to internalize the spiritual power inherent in thunder; then, using that power, the priest/priestess could aid others by performing healings. A contemporary tradition of ritual healing, called Tianxin ('Heart of Heaven') Taoism, was established by a retired official. Tianxin scriptures teach priests how to heal illness by drawing down the spiritual power that inheres in the stars.

However, those movements that featured ritual therapeutics eventually blended into the traditions that emphasized the personal attainment of 'spiritual transcendence' (*shenxian*): by offering models of self-cultivation that men or women of higher social/cultural classes can practice either in seclusion or in a monastic setting, these traditions tended to attract followers from all levels of society. Eventually, all those groups merged into one, which became the form of Taoism that has predominated throughout modern times: Quanzhen, 'Complete Perfection' Taoism. The 12th century founder of Quanzhen, a scholar from a well-to-do family, taught that 'spiritual immortality' can be attained within one's present life, by cultivating one's internal spiritual realities (*xing*), and harmonizing them with the realities of one's external life (*ming*). One of his leading disciples was a woman, and women have remained prominent in Quanzhen life to the present day.

Despite tribulations during the Cultural Revolution (1966–76), Quanzhen Taoism flourished throughout modern times. In the late 20th century, China's current government not only began sanctioning the revival of such religious institutions: it has also sponsored the expansion of traditional Taoist temples, and even established a Taoist College. Throughout China, Quanzhen leaders have preserved not only the Taoist institutions of imperial times, but also the age-old self-cultivation practices, e.g. explaining 'the Way of Immortality' in the ancient terms of cultivating spirit (*shen*) and vital-energy.

Healing in modern Taoism

Quanzhen Taoism not only embodies the full range of traditional Taoist ideals and practices, but reveals their intimate connection with the principles of Chinese traditional medicine. In Quanzhen Taoism, 'The full freedom and power of the immortal Spirit cannot be recovered without the proper care and training of the body.'[11,12] As in earlier Taoist traditions, Quanzhen self-cultivation constitutes a holistic integration of what Western minds have traditionally regarded as incommensurable—the body, the personal consciousness, the spiritual energies that suffuse the natural world, and the spiritual realities that transcend *all* material existence. The goal of Taoist practice is therefore neither simply to prolong bodily life indefinitely, nor to separate oneself spiritually from the body. Rather, the Taoist goal is to perfect oneself fully within the body, thereby both maintaining good health throughout one's natural life and, hopefully, attaining a transcendent spiritual condition, such that one's perfected self will endure as long as the universe itself does, despite the inevitable demise of all corporeal forms.

In Taoist thought and practice, attaining stillness or tranquility within the heart/mind involves not some stylized meditational regimen, in which a practitioner takes time out of everyday life to *separate* consciousness from activities like eating, drinking, and sexual activity. Rather, the Taoist process of stilling the heart/mind takes place within everyday life, although self-perfection cannot occur until a person has learned to refrain from all *self-indulgent* activity, physical and psychological alike. The Quanzhen founder reportedly said: 'you must first uphold the [ethical] precepts. Be pure and still ... and practice goodness.'[13] The term 'goodness' sounds vapid to modern ears, but simply translates the ancient word *shan*, which the *Daode jing* employs as a technical term for selfless nonintervention, by which one enhances others' lives as one enhances one's own. To Quanzhen Taoists, 'the pursuit of health and longevity requires morality and mental discipline.'[14]

The reason that all these ideals are so deeply intertwined is that in the Chinese worldview—among Neo-Confucians, as well as Taoists—the vital energy called *qi* is explained as the fundamental reality underlying all existence. A principle assumption of both Taoism and traditional Chinese medicine is that 'the leakage of the body's vital *qi* (is) the prime cause of disease and death. This leakage, in turn, was blamed on ignorance and lack of discipline.'[15] That is to say, one's susceptibility to disease and injury is attributed, in the first instance, to a person's failure:

- to understand the world in terms of its holistic unity
- to commit oneself to a life of moral and religious self-discipline;

through which one both preserves one's health and attains spiritual perfection.

Of course, Taoists have always been quite aware that disease and injury can also 'occur as a result of outside influences or circumstances beyond one's control.'[16] In fact, some Taoist texts suggest that a person's health deficiencies, or susceptibility to specific maladies, can even begin *in utero*, when the mother can be affected by unwholesome factors. Hence, prenatal care for both mother and unborn child is urged, to ensure that the child will be born healthy enough that, when grown, he/she will be able to repel health challenges from external influences, by means of both a healthy lifestyle and biospiritual cultivation—both considered components of 'nourishing life.' Through biospiritual cultivation, the skilled practitioner 'refines and transforms the body's vital substances. This purified *qi* is circulated through the body's various psychic channels, ... and one's innate connection with, and personal manifestation of the Dao is awakened.'[17]

Nonetheless, the goal of Taoist practices is never simply to benefit oneself, but also to benefit others:

> The Quanzhen masters possessed and transmitted a great deal of knowledge on how to prevent, cure and anticipate diseases. With this knowledge, they expected to be ... at least capable of curing their own diseases ... without the aid of a physician or medicines. However, [they] also saw it as their responsibility to heal the diseases of others.[18]

However, as seen earlier, many Taoist sub-traditions over the centuries featured therapeutic practices intended to assist individuals afflicted by health problems that they had difficulty managing themselves. More concretely, mediaeval Taoists, like Chinese Buddhists, even turned their religious establishments to social services, including medicine and public health:

> In fact, ... hospitals, orphan care, and community quarantine procedures [in imperial China] were linked to the activities of the Taoist and Buddhist monasteries ... The root of this concern for community health care ... could be interpreted as an aspect of the selfless kindness and concern for human health extended to all persons in the practice of *wu-wei* [non-intervention].[19]

Conclusion: healing in the context of the holistic Taoist worldview

China's Taoists, down to the present, are—by tradition and temperament alike—men and women who acknowledge the true value of all aspects of human life. Models that focus on the individual are complemented by acknowledgment of the importance not only of human society, but even of non-human creatures, and models that focus on cultivation of personal awareness or the transformation of consciousness are complemented by teachings explaining the true meaning of our bodily existence. In that sense, the term 'Tao' refers to the spiritual realities that underlie every aspect of such transformational practices, whether focused upon:

- the configurations of an individual's mind/body
- the community within which any person's life takes place or
- the broader world of seen and unseen forces within which all processes take place.

In summary, the Taoist life requires dedication to an ongoing process of selfless personal refinement, which constitutes one's contribution to the health and well-being of nature as well as society. To live the Taoist life is thus to accept personal responsibility for taking part in a universal healing, doing one's full part to restore the health and wholeness of all individuals, as well as society and the natural cosmos.

References

1 Kirkland, R. (1986). The roots of altruism in the Taoist tradition. *J Am Acad Religion* **54**: 59–77.

2 Kirkland, R. (1997). Varieties in Taoism in ancient China: a preliminary comparison of themes in the Nei Yeh and other 'Taoist Classics'. *Taoist Resources* **7**(2): 73–86.

3 Kirkland, R. (2008) Nei Yeh. In: F. Pregadio (ed.) *Encyclopedia of Taoism*, vol. 2, pp. 771–3. Abingdon: Routledge.

4 Major, J.S., Queen, S.A., Meyer, A.S., Roth, H.D. (transl/eds) (2010). *The Huainanzi: A Guide to the Theory and Practice of Government in Early Han China, by Liu An, King of Huainan*. New York: Columbia University Press.

5 Wallner, F. (ed.) (2010). *The Way of Thinking in Chinese Medicine: Theory, Methodology, and Structure of Chinese Medicine*. Frankfurt: Peter Long.

6 Kirkland, R. (2002). Self-fulfilment through selflessness: the moral teachings of the Daode jing. In: M. Barnhart (ed.) *Varieties of Ethical Reflection*, pp. 21–48. New York: Lexington Books.

7 Needham, J. (ed.) (started in 1954). *Science and Civilisation in China*, 7 vols. Cambridge: Cambridge University Press.

8 A starting point for the study of Chinese science and Chinese medicine is the website of Nathan Sivin, Professor of Chinese Culture and of the History of Science, Emeritus, University of Pennsylvania http://ccat.sas.upenn.edu/~nsivin/pers.html. Among the invaluable 'selected writings' are: 'Science and medicine in Chinese History'; 'Taoism and Science'; 'Text and experience in classical Chinese medicine'; and 'Reflections on the situation of medicine in the People's Republic of China, 1987.'

9 Hendrischke, B. (2006). *The Scripture on Great Peace*. Berkeley: University of California Press.

10 Kirkland, R. (2010). Taoist political thought. In: M. Bevir (ed.) *Encyclopedia of Political Theory*. Thousand Oaks: SAGE Publications.

11 Eskildsen, S. (2004). *The Teachings and Practices of the Early Quanzhen Taoist Masters*. Albany: State University of New York Press.

12 Kirkland, R. (2005). The teachings and practices of the early Quanzhen Taoist masters (review). *China Rev Int* **12**(1): 88–97.

13 Eskildsen, S. (2004). *The Teachings and Practices of the Early Quanzhen Taoist Masters*. Albany: State University of New York Press, p. 94.

14 [13], p. 62.

15 [13], p. 74.

16 [13], p. 74

17 Komjathy, L. (2007). *Cultivating Perfection: Mysticism and Self-transformation in Early Quanzhen Daoism*. Leiden: Brill.

18 Eskildsen S (2004). *The Teachings and Practices of the Early Quanzhen Taoist Masters*. Albany: State University of New York Press, p. 88.

19 Girardot, N. (1979). Taoism. In: W.T. Reich (ed.) *Encyclopedia of Bioethics*. New York: Macmillan; p. 1636.

CHAPTER 4

Christianity

Alister E. McGrath

Introduction

Christianity is the world's largest religion, with a highly developed understanding of the impact of religious belief and commitment on personal and social wellbeing. Although the basic elements of such understandings of the relation of spirituality and wellbeing are found in the New Testament, the foundational document of the Christian faith, the full development of these ideas dates from later periods, most notably the Middle Ages in western Europe. [1,2] This period witnessed substantial growth in reflection on the relationship between Christian spirituality and healthcare, physically demonstrated in the establishment of hospitals within monastic communities,[3] and intellectually manifested in a significant number of treatises dealing on the relation of faith with what is now recognizable as issues in mental health and emotional wellbeing.

This connection between Christian commitment and healing continues to the present day. The category of the 'medical missionary' remains an important witness to the Christian belief that spiritual, mental, and physical wellbeing are interconnected.[4,5] Particularly during the nineteenth and early twentieth centuries, substantial numbers of Christian missionaries melded both spiritual and medical skills in their 'care of souls.' The inner dynamics of the Christian faith posit a natural connection between salvation and healing,[6] traditionally traced back to the healing ministry of Jesus of Nazareth, continued and extended in the early church.

According to Christian tradition, Luke—the author of both the gospel bearing his name and the Acts of the Apostles—was a physician, often leading to his being spoken of as a 'physician of the soul' in Christian spiritual and devotional writings. Although routine assertions to the effect that the churches opposed medical advancement—such as the use of chloroform to relieve pain in childbirth—are still encountered in more popular discussions of pain relief or medical history,[7] these have long since been discredited in the scholarly informed literature.[8]

This article sets out to assemble the various ways in which the rich Christian spiritual tradition relates to issues of healthcare. This takes a number of forms, including the inculcation of values and attitudes that are conducive to wellbeing and care for the ill. Readers who are not familiar with the Christian tradition need to appreciate that it is complex and multifaceted, and hence difficult to summarize adequately. What follows is, however, a representative account of some important themes, values, and practices that are of direct relevance to the themes of this volume.

The personal ministry of the founder of Christianity

There are a number of components to the gospel accounts of the ministry of Jesus of Nazareth. Two of the most important are teaching and healing. According to the gospel accounts, Jesus of Nazareth both taught the values of the 'kingdom of God' and undertook a healing ministry, seeing these as two sides of the same coin. This dual emphasis was, in turn, passed on to 'the Twelve'—the group of disciples closest to Jesus of Nazareth, who would play a decisive role in shaping the ethos and beliefs of the early church. Luke records that Jesus gave authority to these disciples to teach and to heal, and 'sent them out to proclaim the kingdom of God and to heal' (Luke 9:1–2).

Jesus of Nazareth played a critical role in establishing and consolidating the ethical and pastoral values of the Christian faith.[9] The nature of this influence must be understood as operating at several levels. First, the early Christian community regarded the memory of Jesus, including his teachings and actions, as determining its identity. Yet this essentially historical understanding of the formation of attitudes and values must be supplemented at a more rigorously theological level. The doctrine of the incarnation—that is, that God chose to enter into human history in the person of Jesus of Nazareth—led to certain decisive aspects of his teaching and ministry being understood to be divinely mandated and authorized, including the importance of promoting healing and personal wellbeing. A commitment to the importance of healing did not, of course, directly lead to an interest in the scientific discipline of medicine; rather, this development is better seen as preparing the ground for such a development, by emphasizing the spiritual importance of the pursuit of personal health as an aspect of authentic Christian existence.[10]

The importance of the example of Christ for the church's commitment to a ministry of healing can be illustrated from countless documents throughout its history. A good example lies to hand in the statements concerning healthcare of the United States Conference of Catholic Bishops, which ground this commitment explicitly in the ministry of Christ, and the benefits this is understood to convey:[11]

> The Church has always sought to embody our Savior's concern for the sick. The gospel accounts of Jesus' ministry draw special attention to his acts of healing ... Jesus' healing mission went further than caring only for physical affliction. He touched people at the deepest level of their existence; he sought their physical, mental, and spiritual healing (John 6: 35, 11: 25–27). He 'came so that they might have life and have it more abundantly' (John 10: 10).

The interconnection of salvation and healing

The understanding of salvation set out in the New Testament is complex, involving the intertwining of notions, such as reconciliation with God, the forgiveness of sins, the achievement of true human potential, the restoration of humanity to its proper condition, and the transformation of its understanding of its own situation and its future destiny.[12] The Greek term *sōtēria*, normally translated as 'salvation', bears a rich range of meanings, including 'healing', 'restoration,' and 'rescue'.

The Christian tradition has developed these ideas extensively, at both the theological and pastoral levels. Theologically, the transformative impact of the Christian gospel upon individuals is often articulated using medical models. Augustine of Hippo (358–430), widely regarded as the western church's greatest theologian, made extensive use of medical images in exploring the many aspects of the Christian gospel. God's grace healed spiritual blindness and restored people to spiritual health. Augustine thus argued that the Christian church was to be conceived as a hospital—a place in which wounded and broken people might receive care and healing.[13] While Augustine insisted that the ultimate healer of humanity was God, he considered human beings to be involved in this process of healing and restoration.

Augustine's approach was consolidated during the theological renaissance of the early Middle Ages, and played an important role in laying an intellectual foundation for the development of hospitals as an integral aspect of the ministry of monasteries and churches. While not reducing the full Christian understanding of the nature of salvation to the promotion of wellbeing and the achievement of healing, Augustine ensured that these elements would be fully integrated within an overall understanding of the preaching and ministry of the church.

An issue of particular importance concerns how the crucifixion and resurrection of Jesus of Nazareth are implicated in this vision of salvation. Traditional Christian theology takes its cues from the New Testament, which sees the suffering and death of Christ as possessing a transformative significance for humanity: 'by his wounds you have been healed' (1 Peter 2: 24). Christians traditionally understand Christ as God incarnate, thus establishing a connection between the sufferings of Christ and the Godhead.

This theme was expressed visually in what many regard as one of the finest pieces of art of the early sixteenth century—the Isenheim altarpiece by Matthias Grünewald (ca. 1475–1528). Around the year 1515, Grünewald was commissioned to produce an altarpiece for the hospital chapel of Saint Anthony's Monastery at Isenheim, about 20 miles south of Colmar, in Alsace. The hospital specialized in the treatment of skin diseases, such as leprosy, which often caused terrible disfigurement to those affected by them. The central panel depicts the crucifixion in a dramatic manner, portraying Christ as emaciated, pock-marked, and discoloured. Christ is thus portrayed as 'a man of suffering and acquainted with infirmity [who] has borne our infirmities and carried our diseases' (Isaiah 53: 3–4). The theological message is unambiguous: this is the one who bears human afflictions, and is the ultimate hope of human renewal.

The Christian conception of salvation is also future-orientated, shaped by the resurrection of Christ. An integral aspect of Christian hopes of salvation focuses on the idea of the final renewal of all things in the 'New Jerusalem.' The New Testament holds that faith ensures that believers will share in the resurrection of Christ. This has important consequences for attitudes to illness, suffering and death. Many early Christian writers considered the resurrection of the body as being like the recasting of a metal statue, which had lost its original beauty, and was now damaged and tarnished beyond any hope of human repair. Methodius of Olympus (died ca. 311) asked his readers to imagine that the same craftsman who had made the original statue in all its beauty and glory, melted it down, and recast it, with all its blemishes and defects removed, and all the damage repaired. This process of recasting affirmed both the continuity between the old and the new, while insisting upon the transformation brought about by the resurrection. The hope of the resurrection is thus linked with that of renewal: 'See I am making all things new' (Revelation 21: 5). The human physical body may become ravaged and disfigured by age, sin, and illness. Yet it is possible to live with this debilitation in the hope of future renewal and transformation.

The interconnected themes of 'resurrection' and 'eternal life' play an important role in shaping Christian attitudes towards suffering and death,[14] and their relevance to healthcare should be noted. Christianity holds that believers will share in the resurrection of Christ. This idea is often conceptualized in terms of being 'citizens of heaven', with a right to return to the homeland. Although located in this world, the hope of being in a better place illuminates and transforms the way in which the present is understood and perceived. Christianity thus casts the present life as a prelude to something greater, with the hope of the latter enabling believers to deal with the ambiguities and tribulations of the former.[15] As Karl Marx noted with some reluctance in the 1850s, such beliefs enabled people to cope with physical suffering and social deprivation. For Marx, this was an irritation, in that it discouraged radical social action against the political and economic system that caused many of these problems in the first place.[16]

Yet Marx's judgement is misplaced. The New Testament refers to Christ's resurrection as the 'first fruits of the new creation' because it demonstrated that the realities of new creation could be realized, however imperfectly, in the old, giving a role to human agency in bringing these about, however imperfectly. This framework of belief thus gives a powerful intellectual and spiritual motivation for political action on the one hand, and commitment to healing and pastoral ministries on the other.[17] Both are seen as an attempt to actualize the values of the 'New Jerusalem' on earth, providing a motivation and inspiration for action. Far from disempowering political engagement or commitment to a ministry of healing, belief in the resurrection—when rightly understood—enables and encourages both.

At a more popular level, Christian ideas about salvation find their expression in sermons, homilies, hymns, and spiritual songs. These affirm the leading themes of a Christian approach to salvation in accessible terminology and imagery, often accentuating the hope that religious belief and commitment brings to those experiencing illness or mental despair. One of the most familiar of these is the Afro-American spiritual 'There is a balm in Gilead', whose origins are thought to date to the 1850s. This simple spiritual uses the biblical image of a medicinal 'balm' (Jeremiah 8:22) to emphasize the hope and transformation brought to the human situation by God:

> There is balm in Gilead,
> To make the wounded whole;
> There's power enough in heaven,
> To cure a sin-sick soul.

Pastorally, considerations such as these have led Christian community to embrace with particular concern those who are seen to be wounded, damaged, and marginalized. Theologically, this is often expressed in terms of a 'theology of the wounded', which speaks of a wounded saviour bringing salvation and renewal to a wounded people.[18] Pastoral commitment to such groups of people is thus informed and directed by a theological belief that something can and should be done to help them.

Christianity and post-traumatic growth

In recent years, there has been growing interest in the way in which the specific features of the Christian faith relate to traumatic experience, and establish a framework for post-traumatic growth.[19] Psychological accounts of trauma generally place an emphasis upon the psychological and existential threats that trauma poses to human wellbeing. Not only does the experience of trauma pose a threat to human wellbeing and survival; it also calls into question core positive beliefs about the world or the individual through the shattering of personal assumptions that relate to the meaning of life and the value of self. Developing means of engaging and transforming such shattered assumptions is thus of therapeutic significance.[20, 21] The central Christian narrative of the crucifixion and resurrection of Christ provides what is, in effect, an exemplary metanarrative of post-traumatic growth, with the potential to illuminate and transform the human situation.

While Christianity shares a belief in a single God with Judaism and Islam, it offers a distinctive understanding of the nature of that God that sets it apart from the other Abrahamic religions. Knowledge of God is held to be linked to (and shaped by) the crucifixion of Christ. The gospel narratives depict this act of violence and brutality against Christ as leading to distress, incomprehension, and hopelessness on the part of the disciples, accompanied by radical questioning of existing ways of thinking that are now held to be inadequate in the wake of events.

The New Testament shows how this traumatic development shattered certain existing ways of thinking, particularly concerning the way in which God acts in history and in personal experience. Yet this questioning of existing modes of understanding leads to reconstruction and renewal, enabling people to make more sense of things, and cope with the paradoxes of experience. The resurrection of Christ is depicted as initially engendering fear, partly on account of its unexpectedness, but partly also on account of the challenge that this event poses to existing mental maps of reality (or 'schemas'). Both the gospels and some of the epistles of the New Testament speak of the radical changes in thinking that are required in response to this event, and the challenges to 'wisdom' that it brings.

The distinctive Christian capacity to cope with suffering and trauma is ultimately grounded in the historical origins of the church in a traumatic paradigmatic context. In the aftermath of the shattering of certain unrealistic expectations arose a new way of thinking, which enabled Christians to face the paradoxes of suffering in a new light and with a new confidence. This point has not been overlooked by those working in the field of post-traumatic growth. One leading authority in the field begins their discussion of the phenomenon by highlighting a section in a New Testament letter, which illustrates this response:[22] 'but we also boast in our sufferings, knowing that suffering produces endurance, and endurance produces character, and character produces hope, and hope does not disappoint us' (Romans 5: 3–5). Although Tedeschi and Calhoun omit Paul's reference to the ultimate grounding of this radical revision of ideas in what J. R. R. Tolkien terms the *eucatastrophe* of Christ's resurrection, they correctly identify the radical alteration that ensues from it. Within a Christian context, this revision of ideas is grounded in the narrative of crucifixion and resurrection, which both acts as its foundation, and shapes its values.

Given the importance of trauma in contemporary western culture and its implications for healthcare professionals, on the one hand, and the fabric of society at large, it is clear that such a spirituality has potential to encourage post-traumatic growth. Although grounded in (and ultimately dependent upon) a specifically Christian metanarrative, this approach clearly has wider potential. If it is true that 'growth occurs when the trauma assumes a central place in the life story,'[23] then the Christian community's constant recollection and celebration of the trauma of the crucifixion in its regular rehearsal of the narrative of Christ's death in the liturgy of the eucharist must be considered to generate a potentially therapeutic community for those now affected by such trauma.

Coping with suffering

The centrality of the image of the crucified Christ within Christianity is reflected in its willingness to engage with suffering as both an existential and intellectual issue. Dealing with suffering is of significance at two distinct levels in relation to human wellbeing. First, a feeling that suffering is devoid of meaning or purpose—especially if it is held that its presence points to a meaningless universe—is often destabilizing, leading to depression or disengagement. If suffering can be understood within a greater context, this can lead to more positive mental attitudes conducive to good health.[24,25] We have touched on this issue already in relation to the question of trauma. Secondly, suffering is not simply something to be understood or rationalized. It is something that has to be endured, raising the issue of how people can cope successfully with such situations.[26,27] The question thus arises as to whether the Christian tradition offers resources that enable people to cope with suffering—for example, long-term illness, or the illness and death of a close relative, friend, or colleague. In this section, we shall consider both these issues.

The philosopher Iris Murdoch (1919–99) is one of many writers to emphasize the 'calming' and 'healing' effect of ways of looking at the world that suggest it is rational and meaningful.[28] Christian theologians have, since the earliest times, argued that the presence of suffering in the world does not constitute a challenge to its rationality, nor to the notions of meaning and purpose that are embedded within the Christian faith. Augustine of Hippo (358–430), for example, set out an approach to the presence of evil within the world that affirmed the original integrity, goodness, and rationality of the world. Evil and suffering arose from a misuse of freedom, the effects of which are being remedied and transformed through redemption.[29] Augustine argues that the believer is enabled to make sense of the enigmas of suffering and evil in the world by recalling its original goodness, and looking forward to its final renewal and restoration in heaven.

Other Christian writers have developed different explanations to account for the origins of evil and suffering, and their persistence within the world (for a summary, see [30]). Such approaches are essentially concerned with resolving the mental enigmas and intellectual puzzles arising from suffering. Yet many regard such approaches as inadequate to deal with the real problem caused by suffering and evil, which is better understood as *existential*, rather than *rational*. An example will make this point clearer.

In his 1940 work, *Problem of Pain*, the noted Christian apologist C. S. Lewis (1898–1963) argued that belief in God was consistent with the existence of pain in the world. Pain, he famously argued, was God's 'megaphone to rouse a deaf world.' Yet Lewis's reconciliation of faith and experience was rational, not existential.[31] It was at the level of abstract ideas, not the harsh, brutal realities of suffering and death. To its critics, Lewis's approach in *Problem of Pain* amounted to an evasion of the reality of evil and suffering as experienced realities; instead, they are reduced to abstract ideas, which require to be fitted into the jigsaw puzzle of faith.

Two decades later, Lewis published (initially under a pseudonym) *A Grief Observed*. This moving work consisted of the painful and brutally honest reflections of a man whose wife has died, slowly, and in pain, from cancer.[32] One of the most moving and memorable features of this work is Lewis's description of his dawning realization that his rational, cerebral faith has taken something of a battering from the emotional crisis that has overwhelmed him. The slow death of Lewis's wife did not lead him to reject his belief; it did, however, reveal the precarious nature of a faith based only on ideas, and disconnected from the harsh realities of life.[33] Lewis recovered both his faith and sense of determination to get on with life. However, he realized that his earlier approach to suffering had been rationally adequate, but existentially unsatisfactory.

The point here is that rational frameworks of reality often collapse under severe emotional and existential pressure. As we noted earlier when considering the importance of post-traumatic growth, this implosion of mental schemas often results in their reassembling in more optimal and viable forms. This process, often described in terms of growth in 'maturity' or 'wisdom', can be seen as the outcome of provisional schemas being challenged by experience, and subsequently being rebuilt in more accommodated and robust forms.

Perhaps on account of such issues, more recent approaches to such questions within the Christian tradition have dealt with the question of how faith enables believers to cope with suffering, illness, and trauma. Approaches of this kind dominated Christian spirituality during the Middle Ages, when there was a widespread acceptance that suffering was simply a fact of life that did not require explanation; it did, however, need to be engaged. Many writers of the age explore the question of how someone can grow in wisdom and maturity through suffering, often using images of the crucified Christ as an imaginative gateway to reflection.[34] Where academic theologians wrote about the cognitive tensions arising from suffering, most writers focused on how people could deal with such pain and perplexity, using them as stepping-stones to wisdom and maturity.

These more pragmatic approaches have re-emerged in western Christianity, with an increased emphasis upon the importance of enabling people to survive suffering and pain, and find these as pathways to personal growth. Perhaps the most discussed of these is Jürgen Moltmann's *Crucified God* (1974), which argues that reflection on the crucified Christ allows the believer to be reassured of God's solidarity with people in their pain, and God's presence with them as they struggle to make sense of it and cope with it.[35] Earlier, Dietrich Bonhoeffer had developed a similar approach, finding that such a form of meditation enabled him to cope with life in a 'godless world' as he awaited execution in a Nazi concentration camp.

Ultimately, the issue raised by the existence of evil, suffering, and pain focuses on the question of *meaning*. Is the world merely a random, meaningless, accumulation of accidental events? Or may a deeper picture be discerned, which enables the issues of human existence to be brought into sharper focus. We shall therefore consider this issue in more detail in the following section.

Finding purpose and meaning in illness and trauma

One of the more significant questions concerning life relates to the attribution of purpose, meaning or value to actions and individuals.[36,37] A distinction is drawn between 'surface' or 'empirical' readings of situations and more significant interpretations that are held to lie beneath their surface. Resilience in the face of illness, suffering or trauma is widely agreed to be enhanced if this is seen as purposeful, intentional, or productive. A religious belief system, such as Christianity or Judaism, provides a framework of meaning and interpretation, which allows such an interpretation to be placed on these events, thus facilitating individual believers to cope with their distress and anxiety.[38,39]

This point was emphasized by Erich Fromm (1900–80), who was shocked by the insanity and destructiveness of the First World War. Fromm began to reflect deeply on what people really needed if they were to remain sane. The answer, he argued, lay in developing what he called a 'framework of orientation and devotion,' a way of thinking about the world that endows existence with purpose and significance.[40] The specific framework that Fromm himself developed is secondary to his recognition that we need such frameworks if we are to live and act in the world without going insane. Living purposefully and meaningfully requires a frame of reference, which offers us a secure foundation and focus for our lives.

These insights were further developed by Viktor Frankl (1905–97), whose experiences in Nazi concentration camps during the Second World War led him to realize the importance of discerning meaning in coping with traumatic situations.[26] Survival depended on the will to live, which in turn depended on the discernment of meaning and purpose in even the most demoralizing situations, which were directly experienced as threats to survival and self-preservation. Those who coped best were those who had frameworks of meaning that enabled them to accommodate their experiences within their mental maps. Without the capacity to make sense of events and situations, and to attribute meaning to them, people are unable to cope with reality.

The importance of such points in considering the relevance of religious faith in general, and Christianity in particular, to issues of healthcare and wellbeing will be clear.[41] A sense of coherency in life appears to engender emotional stability and promote wellbeing.[42] Christianity provides a series of possible mental maps that position illness and suffering in such a manner as to allow them to be seen as coherent, meaningful, and potentially positive, allowing them to foster personal growth and development. Some of these maps—such as those offered by Augustine of Hippo, Ignatius Loyola (1491–1556), and Edith Stein (1891–1942)—portray illness as something that is not part of God's intentions for humanity, but can nevertheless be used as means of growth; others, such as that offered by Martin Luther (1483–1546), tend to see suffering as something intended by God, with the objective of stripping away illusions of immortality and confronting human beings with the harsh reality of their frailty and transiency.

This provision of a framework of meaning engenders a positive expectation that something may be learned and gained through illness and suffering. It discloses the true human situation; it makes available new ways of thinking about life; and it catalyses the emergence of more mature judgements and attitudes. Although this consideration has clear implications for attitudes to illness and their outcomes, it is increasingly being recognized as being of significance in coping with ageing, including its associated medical conditions.[43,44)

There are evidential grounds for suggesting that wellbeing and successful recovery from illness and trauma are both influenced by positive mental attitudes on the part of patients.[45] While it is potentially simplistic to propose a direct correlation between religious belief and such positive outlooks, the issues discussed in this section nevertheless point to the importance of such mental maps in fostering recovery from illness and injury.[46]

Values and practices for living

Finally, it is important to consider the personal and social values and practices that arise from religious commitment, which are often prosocial.[47] Once more, it is important not to overstate this factor, as individual believers tend to adopt core values of their faith somewhat selectively, whether this is informed by theoretical judgements or personal inclinations. Nevertheless, it remains clear that the personal and social moral visions associated with the Christian faith from the outset have important consequences for issues of wellbeing and healthcare.

From the outset, the Christian churches saw a resilient link between their faith and the care of the sick, weak, and socially marginalized—such as the 'widows and orphans'. The practice of care for the ill was envisioned as an integral part of the ministry of the church, to be supplemented—not contradicted—by the development of medicine. The close semantic and theological links between salvation and healing were reflected from the outset in a concern for the development of healing ministries as part of the mission of the churches.[10]

Value systems that emphasize moderation or disengagement from substances or practices which could be physiologically damaging—such as the excessive consumption of alcohol—have clear implications for health. Other values, however, may be argued to have more questionable outcomes for healthcare, such as the traditional Catholic refusal to condone artificial contraception, even in situations where population growth leads to health issues. Traditional Christian emphases upon monogamy arguably lessen the risk of sexually-transmitted diseases within populations.

The role of prayer in healing remains empirically unclear,[48] yet is seen as an integral part of the practice of faith. Pentecostal communities, for example, often regard physical health and personal prosperity as the natural outcome of faith and prayer as the means of securing them both. Others adopt more nuanced approaches, tending to regard prayer as an expression of a relationship of dependency and intimacy with God.

Yet, perhaps most significantly, the values and beliefs of the Christian tradition affirm the importance of healthcare as a calling, and the positive role of the church in encouraging such a profession—an attitude admirably summarized in the traditional Collect (appointed prayer) for the feast of St Luke:

> Almighty God,
> you called Luke the physician,
> whose praise is in the gospel,
> to be an evangelist and physician of the soul:
> by the grace of the Spirit,
> and through the wholesome medicine of the gospel,
> give your Church the same love and power to heal;
> through Jesus Christ your Son our Lord,
> who is alive and reigns with you,
> in the unity of the Holy Spirit,
> one God, now and for ever.

References

1 Amundsen, D.W. (1996). *Medicine, Society, and Faith in the Ancient and Medieval Worlds*. Baltimore: Johns Hopkins University Press.

2 De Souza, M. (ed.) (2009). *International Handbook of Education for Spirituality, Care, and Wellbeing*, 2 vols. New York: Springer.

3 Kliewer, S., Saultz, J.W. (2006). *Healthcare and Spirituality*. New York: Radcliffe.

4 McGrath, A.E. (2004). *Christian Spirituality: An Introduction*. Oxford: Blackwell.

5 Numbers, R.L., Amundsen, D.W. (1998). *Caring and Curing: Health and Medicine in the Western Religious Traditions*. Baltimore: Johns Hopkins University Press.

6 Simmons, P.D. (2008). *Faith and Health: Religion, Science, and Public Policy*. Macon: Mercer University Press.

7 McGinn, B., Meyendorff, J. (eds) (1985). *Christian Spirituality: Origins to the Twelfth Century*. New York: Crossroad.

8 Raitt, J. (ed.) (1987). *Christian Spirituality: High Middle Ages and Reformation*. New York: Crossroad.

9 Risse, G.B. (1999). *Mending Bodies, Saving Souls: A History of Hospitals*. Oxford: Oxford University Press.

10 Fitzgerald, R. (2001). 'Clinical Christianity': the emergence of medical work as a missionary strategy in colonial India, 1800–1914. In: P. Biswamoy, M. Harrison (eds) *Health, Medicine and Empire: Perspectives on Colonial India*, pp. 88–136. London: Sangam Books.

11 Hardiman, D. (ed.) (2006). *Healing Bodies, Saving Souls: Medical Missions in Asia and Africa*. New York: Rodopi.

12 Wells, L. (1998). *The Greek Language of Healing from Homer to New Testament Times*. New York: de Gruyter, pp. 120–209.

13 Dormandy, T. (2006). *The Worst of Evils: The Fight Against Pain*. New York: Yale University Press.

14 Numbers, R.L. (ed.) (2009). *Galileo Goes to Jail: And Other Myths About Science and Religion*. Cambridge: Harvard University Press, pp. 123–30.

15 Burridge, R.A. (2007). *Imitating Jesus: An Inclusive Approach to New Testament Ethics*. Grand Rapids: Eerdmans.
16 Ferngren, G.B. (2009). *Medicine and Health Care in Early Christianity*. Baltimore: Johns Hopkins University Press.
17 United States Conference of Catholic Bishops (2009). Ethical and Religious Directives for Catholic Health Care Services, 5th Conference of Catholic Bishops, Washington, DC.
18 McGrath, A.E. (2011). *Christian Theology: An Introduction*, 5th edn. Oxford: Wiley-Blackwell, pp. 315–47.
19 Alexander, D.C. (2008). *Augustine's Early Theology of the Church: Emergence and Implications*, 386–91. New York: Peter Lang, pp. 274–94.
20 Bauckham, R., Hart, T.A. (eds) (1999). *Hope Against Hope: Christian Eschatology at the Turn of the Millennium*. Grand Rapids: Eerdmans.
21 Lincoln, A.T. (1981). *Paradise Now and Not Yet: Studies in the Role of the Heavenly Dimension in Paul's Thought with Special Reference to His Eschatology*. Cambridge: Cambridge University Press.
22 Lash, N. (1982). All shall be well: Christian and Marxist hope. *New Blackfriars* **63**: 404–15.
23 Wright, N.T. (2008). *Surprised by Hope: Rethinking Heaven, the Resurrection, and the Mission of the Church*. San Francisco: HarperOne.
24 Park, A.S. (2004). *From Hurt to Healing: A Theology of the Wounded*. Nashville: Abingdon Press.
25 Collicutt, J. (2006). Post-traumatic growth and the origins of early Christianity. *Ment Hlth Religion Cult* **9**: 291–306.
26 Calhoun, L.G., Tedeschi, R.G. (1999). *Facilitating Posttraumatic Growth: A Clinician's Guide*. Mahwah: Lawrence Erlbaum Associates Publishers.
27 Calhoun, L.G., Tedeschi, R.G. (2006). *Handbook of Posttraumatic Growth: Research and Practice*. Mahwah: Lawrence Erlbaum Associates.
28 Tedeschi, R., Calhoun, L. (1995). *Trauma and Transformation: Growing in the Aftermath of Suffering*. Thousand Oaks: Sage Publications.
29 [28], p. 85.
30 Joseph, S., Linley, P.A. (eds) (2008). *Trauma, Recovery and Growth: Positive Psychological Perspectives on Posttraumatic Stress*. Hoboken: Wiley.
31 Snyder, C.R., Lopez, S.J. (2009). *Oxford Handbook of Positive Psychology*. New York: Oxford University Press.
32 Frankl, V. (1963). *Man's Search for Meaning*, Boston: Beacon Press.
33 Pargament, K.I. (1997). *The Psychology of Religion and Coping: Theory, Practice and Research*, New York: Guilford Press.
34 Murdoch, I. (1992). *Metaphysics as a Guide to Morals*. London: Penguin.
35 Evans, G.R. (1990). *Augustine on Evil*. Cambridge: Cambridge University Press.
36 Kreeft, P.J. (1987). *Making Sense out of Suffering*. London: Hodder and Stoughton.
37 Lewis, C.S. (1940). *The Problem of Pain*. London: Bles.
38 Lewis, C.S. (1961). *A Grief Observed*. London: Faber & Faber.
39 Loades, A. (1989). C. S. Lewis: grief observed, rationality abandoned, faith regained. *Lit Theol* **3**: 107–21.
40 Ross, E.M. (1997). *The Grief of God: Images of the Suffering Jesus in Late Medieval England*. New York: Oxford University Press.
41 Moltmann, J. (1974). *The Crucified God: The Cross of Christ as the Foundation and Criticism of Christian Theology*. London: SCM Press.
42 Baumeister, R. (1991). *Meanings of Life*. New York: Guilford Press.
43 Warren, R. (2003). *The Purpose Driven Life: What on Earth Am I Here For?* Philadelphia: Running Press.
44 Kushner, H.S. (1981). *When Bad Things Happen to Good People*. New York: Avon Books.
45 Harrington, D. (2000). *Why Do We Suffer? A Scriptural Approach to the Human Condition*. Dublin: Sheed & Ward.
46 Funk, R. (2003). *Erich Fromm: His Life and Ideas*. New York: Continuum International Publishing Group.
47 McGrath, A.E. (2006). Spirituality and well-being: some recent discussions, brain. *J Neurol* **129**: 278–82.
48 Eriksson, M., Lindström, B. (2005). Validity of Antonovsky's 'Sense of Coherence' Scale: a systematic review. *J Epidemiol Comm Hlth* **59**: 460–6.
49 MacKinlay, E. (2006). *Ageing, Spirituality and Palliative Care*. London: Haworth Press.
50 Atchley, R.C. (2009). *Spirituality and Aging*. Baltimore: John Hopkins University Press.
51 Ai, A.L., Park, C.L. (2005). Possibilities of the positive following violence and trauma: informing the coming decade of research. *J Interpers Violence* **20**: 242–50.
52 Koenig, H.G., Cohen, H.J. (2002). *The Link between Religion and Health: Psychoneuroimmunology and the Faith Factor*. Oxford: Oxford University Press.
53 Wells, S., Quash, B. (2010). *Introducing Christian Ethics*. Malden: Wiley-Blackwell, pp. 209–335.
54 Francis, L., Robbins, M., Lewis, C.A., Barnes, L.P. (2008). Prayer and psychological health: a study among sixth-form pupils attending Catholic and Protestant schools in Northern Ireland. *Ment Hlth Religion Cult* **11**: 85–92.

CHAPTER 5

Feminist spirituality

Susan A. Ross

Introduction

The women's movement, which emerged in the 1960s and 1970s, has had an enormous impact on society. From the earliest days of 'women's lib,' with demands for equality in pay, to the present day, where the presence of women on police forces, construction crews, and in political office is no longer even worth comment, feminism has changed the ways that we understand ourselves and our gendered roles in society. In the academic world, feminist theory has challenged such issues as the literary canon, the autonomous self of the Enlightenment, the distinction between 'craft' and 'art,' and what constitutes a historical event. The fact that half of medical students today are women testifies to the increasing 'feminization' of the healthcare field.

Religious thought is no exception to these changes. In what was perhaps the earliest feminist theological essay, published in 1960, a young woman theological student asked whether women's experiences make a difference in the ways that such issues as sin and grace are understood.[1] When religious leaders criticize human beings as sinful and filled with pride, and encourage humility as the correct response to God, she asked, does this have the same significance for women as it does for men? One of her conclusions was that because women have long been socialized to put others first, they probably need to be encouraged to be less humble, not more, so that their gifts are not 'hidden under a bushel.' What feminist theology and spirituality challenge, then, is the idea that men's experiences are the standard by which to judge all human behaviour. While pride may be the 'sin of man,' it is questionable whether women's characteristic failing is the same.

This chapter will focus on feminist spirituality and its significance in a healthcare context. That is to say, women's lived experiences and reflections on their spiritual lives will affect the ways that they take care of themselves and others. Feminist spirituality holds that women's neglected experiences and ideas need to be brought to the center not only of women's religious lives but also to their personal and social lives. Healthcare is no exception. In this chapter I will focus primarily on the feminist dimensions of the Jewish and Christian traditions; there is a growing literature on feminist spirituality in Islam, Hinduism, and Buddhism, as well as newer religious movements, but space precludes my doing justice to all the world religions. I will venture to say, however, that much of what characterizes feminist spirituality in Judaism and Christianity is in some way applicable to other religious traditions.

The chapter will proceed along the following lines: first, I will provide a description of the major themes of feminist spirituality, particularly as they challenge, reject, or reform traditional religious ideas, and with an eye to those themes that have particular relevance to healthcare. I will give examples of the ways that these themes have been developed in spiritual and religious feminist thinkers. Secondly, I will relate these ideas to healthcare, with particular attention to how healthcare and healthcare providers can be more attentive to feminist spiritual concerns.

Major themes in feminist spirituality: relation, embodiment, and nature

In a 1985 essay, Margaret Farley, a Sister of Mercy who spent her academic career at Yale University, and who specializes in bioethical issues, identified three key characteristics of feminist theology as relevant for bioethics: patterns of relation, human embodiment, and the world of 'nature.'[2] Farley's essay is very helpful in sorting out the issues that concern feminist theologians and ethicists and it is worth the time here to spell out these key themes.

First, by 'patterns of relation,' Farley means that all forms of feminism 'oppose discrimination on the basis of sex.'[2] She notes the long history of patriarchal structures and traditions in religion, and includes a number of examples: the domination of women by men, the association of women with evil (e.g. blaming Eve for the 'Fall' into original sin), the identification of the divine as male, and the relationship of submission to God on the part of humanity. All of these examples reveal 'oppressive patterns of relationships and ideologies which foster them,' patterns that are not only based on sex, but permeate many other dimensions of human life.[2] In response to this critical analysis of religion, feminists, as I noted above, either reject the tradition or attempt to reform it.

Both the 'rejecters' and the 'reformers' of religion agree that these destructive patterns of relationship of domination and subjugation need to be overturned in favour of relationships of equality and reciprocity.[2] Within these relationships, women's agency is also emphasized. That is, women must claim the power to name themselves and their experiences.

The second point that Farley emphasizes is the significance of embodiment. Feminists are critical of the ways that the human body has been devalued in religious traditions, particularly those in the West. Women are often identified as being 'more bodily' than men in traditions that see the spiritual as superior to the bodily. Farley notes: 'Central to the association of women with bodiliness has been the interpretation of their sexuality as more "carnal" than men's, again "closer to nature," more animal-like, less subject to rational control.'[2] In contrast to this position, feminist thinkers emphasize the goodness of the body and its creation by God, as well as the ways that embodiment is not just something that human beings *have*, but rather what they *are*. For Christian theology, the Incarnation—God becoming human in the person of Jesus—is one way of showing how the body is central to human spiritual and religious life, although the fact that God became incarnate in a male is also held to be definitive.[3] For the Jewish tradition, the many laws and rituals that concern the body are, similarly, an expression of the value that the body has and its participation in the divine economy.[4] For spiritual feminists, the body has a holiness all of its own and, in particular, the woman's body is revered as the source of life.

Womanist theologians, among others, take up the point that the body cannot be considered outside of its social context.[5] While it is a good thing to value the body as intrinsically good, one cannot assume that the body's location or its history always contributes to women's wellbeing. The bodies of women of colour have been deemed less worthwhile than the bodies of women of privilege; the fact that African-American women die of breast cancer at much higher rates than white women is an issue that deserves much more research.[6] Recognizing the significance of embodiment means recognizing the worth of all people, particularly those who are most vulnerable: women, children, the poor.

The third theme that Farley develops is 'the world of nature.'[2] The western tradition has tended to view the world of nature, especially over the last 300 years, as a place for human beings to subdue and dominate; moreover, 'nature' has often been described in feminine terms, which 'mirror similar identifications of the essence of woman.'[7] That is, nature is irrational, needs to be controlled, and is understood largely in utilitarian terms. Here, again, a critique of hierarchical structures that pit 'nature' against 'human' is characteristic of feminist thought, which holds an alternative view of nature as valuable in its own right. Feminist thinkers seek a more holistic relationship with nature; a number of feminist thinkers draw on nature for inspiration and rituals. As we will see below, feminist spiritual and religious writers argue that human beings need to see themselves as a part of nature, enmeshed in nature, and not in opposition to it.

Women's experiences, ritual, and the divine

I noted above that one of the first feminist writers on religion raised the issue of women's experiences. Women's experiences play a central role in feminist spirituality, but what is meant by the term 'women's experience?' The question is actually more complex than it may initially appear. In the early years of feminism—a movement largely dominated by white middle-class women—certain assumptions were made about 'women's experience.' For example, in her book *The Feminine Mystique*, Betty Friedan wrote about 'the problem that has no name,' that is, the boredom and depression of the (white) middle-class housewife.[8] In 1980, Carol Gilligan, a psychologist trained at Harvard, wrote a book about women's experiences of moral decision-making, arguing that women's tendency to define themselves relationally, rather than individualistically, gave women a 'different' mode of being moral, one that deserved greater recognition and was not inferior to a rights-based understanding of morality.[9] By the mid-1980s the category of 'women's experience' became problematized, as both activists and scholars asked whether the experiences of women of colour or of a lower class, were adequately represented in feminist theory. Thus, generalizing about 'women's experience' is a very risky endeavour.

Women of colour often have different experiences than white women, both in their lives, and in their encounters with the healthcare system. The middle-class women who spoke of 'boredom' assumed a situation of economic stability, a situation that many poor women and women of colour could not assume. 'Women's experience' tended to be somewhat psychological and personalized, in that the social and economic conditions of women's lives were not critically analysed. Womanist theologians have taken up the issue of women's health and have argued for a critical focus on the whole context of healthcare.[10] I will return to these issues below.

Looking to feminist spiritual practices is another way of exploring feminist spirituality, although these practices encompass different dimensions of women's experiences. Religious and spiritual feminists find a way of expressing their deepest convictions in ritual practices. In her book *Ritualizing Women: Patterns of Spirituality*, Lesley Northup identifies some 'emerging patterns' in women's ritualizing.[11] In terms of ritual themes and images, Northup names the circle, which is symbolic of the womb and of a non-hierarchical arrangement of space; use of nature, the body, and women's experiences, such as childbearing and mothering; valuing the 'ordinary,' women's work in crafts (often not identified as 'art'), the community, and the naming of women influential to participants. Women's ritual actions tend to be spontaneous and informal, with no clear ritual leader, and seldom rely on traditional 'sacred texts.'[11] In many cases, feminists rely on religious practices and traditions that are often considered marginal by dominant religious groups. What is important to note in these practices is their rejection of hierarchical structures and their concern for inclusivity. Hierarchy is identified with male power structures of which feminists are highly critical; practices of exclusion (i.e. those who do not profess 'right belief' or who belong to marginalized groups) are also rejected.

Perhaps the strongest expression of feminist spirituality is its critique and often rejection of male ideas of the divine. One who chose to reject the tradition is the feminist philosopher Mary Daly (1929–2010). While she began her academic career as a Catholic theologian, and wrote her first book about how the church should change to be more inclusive of women, she soon came to realize that the Catholic church and, in fact, all religions were, as she saw it, hopelessly patriarchal.[12] In her ground-breaking book *Gyn/Ecology*, Daly identified the ways that religions systematically oppress and even destroy women. She described Christianity in particular as a religion based 'on a dead man hanging on a dead tree.'[13] In an often-quoted remark from another book, *Beyond God the* Father, Daly writes, 'If God is male, then the male is God.'[14] Daly's sharp observation that the language and imagery used of God have profound effects on how people perceive the divine is key for feminist thought. However, Daly still held to the importance of the spiritual, and in her later writings focused on ways that women could find spiritual significance outside of institutional religion.[15]

Other thinkers who have rejected institutional religion and male ideas of the divine include Charlene Spretnak, Carol Christ, and Margot Adler.[16–18] Their efforts are often focused on ways of retrieving the divine feminine. Many 'goddess feminists' argue that the original form of religion was matriarchal and that human beings saw in women's power to give life a divine quality. However, the original feminine dimension of the divine was eventually overturned by patriarchal religious ideas, which saw the divine as a transcendent and disembodied male figure, and which also supported the domination of women by men.[19] While the historicity of this thesis is questionable, goddess feminists point out that, for the most part, women in male-dominated religions are often seen as temptresses, leading the more spiritual men into sin, or as spotlessly perfect women, known as the 'virgin/whore' dichotomy.

In an essay entitled 'Why Women Need the Goddess,' feminist thealogian (note the change in vowel) Carol Christ argues that there are not only religious, but also psychological and political dimensions to naming the divine in female terms.[20] Such an identification of the divine allows women to see themselves as powerful ('like God') and provides a symbolic foundation for women's ability to take on leadership roles. It is not by accident that most religious leadership roles have traditionally been held by men; those traditions that do not allow women in these roles, such as the Roman Catholic Church, appeal to divine authority to substantiate such claims.[3]

The lack of female imagery of the divine in western religious traditions tells women that men are closer to the divine than they are and thus has a powerful effect on women's capacity to image the divine. And even in eastern traditions, such as Hinduism, the fact that there are many goddesses and devotional practices related to goddesses is no guarantee that women have a more privileged place in these traditions than in traditions that have a male divine figure.[21]

Christian theologian Elizabeth Johnson has offered a way of approaching God that retrieves dimensions of theology that have been suppressed by the traditions. In her influential book *She Who Is*, Johnson argues that Christians need to 'take long draughts' of female language for God and to leave behind images of God as impassible (incapable of feeling and passion), distant, and disconnected from humanity.[22] Sallie McFague, in her book *Models of God*, proposes that Christians conceive of God as Mother, Lover, and Friend.[23] Both McFague and Johnson make a strong case for the necessarily metaphorical dimension of all God language, and note that this dimension is hidden when language for God is primarily in male terms. It becomes more visible when female terms are used: the very naming of God as 'She' suggests, by its unusual nature, that language for God cannot be taken literally.

A final dimension of feminist spirituality that cannot be ignored is an emphasis on women's agency or subjectivity. In most religious traditions, women have been the objects, not the subjects, of religious ideas. Consider how the tenth commandment prohibits coveting one's 'neighbor's wife,' among the other goods of the neighbour. Women's behaviour has been dictated by male leadership, male leaders have told women how to dress (e.g. by requiring hats in church), women's education has not been a priority, and in its worst forms, women have been described as those responsible for the evils of the world Thus, the capacity for action, particularly moral action, on the part of women is a significant feminist concern. While feminist spirituality values mutual and equitable relationships, feminists are critical of hierarchical and authoritarian relationships.

Feminist spirituality and healthcare

The context of women's healthcare

Healthcare, by definition, is how societies treat those who are physically or mentally ill, dependent, and in need. The very term *care*, as I noted above, has emerged as central in feminist thought about relationships with others. Some feminist ethicists have turned to care as a basic concept in human relationships, particularly in the way that we treat those among us who are vulnerable.[24] Other feminist theorists are concerned that care not be seen as simply a 'woman's issue,' since all human beings require care at some point in their lives.[25] How can feminist spirituality best inform ideas and practices of healthcare?

One of the first issues to take into consideration is the issue of access to healthcare. Feminist spirituality asks how conceptions of human life and wellbeing affect women and their children. If women do not have access to basic healthcare, not only their own health suffers, but also that of their families. In the USA, for example, healthcare has not been considered a basic right, but rather as a service to be purchased by the individual consumer; therefore, the market dominates healthcare in the USA. While it is beyond the scope of this chapter to analyse and critique the healthcare systems of various countries, healthcare professionals need to consider the broader context of their patients' lives.

In her book *Women, Ethics, and Inequality in U.S. Healthcare*, theologian Aana Marie Vigen writes of Black and Latino women with breast cancer who encounter the healthcare system in New York City.[26] She uncovered racial bias, intransigent systems, and multiple personal indignities that these women encountered through her interviews and the analysis of their situations. As a feminist theologian, she is concerned about the dignity of these women, how they are respected or not as embodied and spiritual persons, and how both religious traditions and healthcare providers need to be more attentive to the wellbeing of all, not just the privileged. Paying attention to the most vulnerable is a way of testing the adequacy of healthcare: if those among us who have the least power are also those with the poorest care, the system fails. This kind of feminist analysis is attentive not only to women's concerns as women, but also to the broader contexts of women's lives. Thus, 'spiritual' wellbeing cannot be detached from one's situation in life, but is rather attentive to all the relationships and contexts that affect their wellbeing.

A second example of context, feminist spirituality, and healthcare comes from eastern Africa. In sub-Saharan Africa, the spread of HIV/AIDS is a monumental social issue. Because of patterns of employment and traditional cultural practices, women are particularly vulnerable to infection. Indeed, as a young scholar who writes about risk factors for HIV/AIDS, marriage is the main risk factor for women.[27] Many men are employed in areas far from their homes and only see their wives every few months, if that often. Whilst away, they have sex with other women, while their wives are expected to be faithful to their husbands. This double standard means that many men think it is their right to have as many sexual partners as they want. Thus, single women find it easier to demand that a man use a condom, whereas a married woman who asks her husband to use a condom is suspected of being unfaithful—when, in fact, it is the husband who is the unfaithful one and who spreads infection. When religious traditions urge fidelity and condemn the use of condoms, as is the practice of the Roman Catholic Church, women are the ones who suffer.[27]

Thus, two of the main concerns of feminist spirituality—to value mutuality and equality in relationships, and to value everyone's embodied personhood—cannot be practiced in a context that works against these values. To be sure, the healthcare system of the USA and the cultural practices of eastern Africa are different and complex situations, but they show how feminist spiritual values go far beyond what could be seen as 'only women's concerns.' Women's concerns are human concerns, as has often been said, and when these concerns go unaddressed, all of human life suffers.

Feminist spirituality and sexuality

The fact that women are the ones who conceive and bear children accounts for many of their encounters with healthcare. Feminist spirituality values embodiment and the natural world, and sees sexuality and reproduction as good and natural. It also sees religious traditions' views of these issues to be greatly in need of critique. That is to say, religious traditions, dominated by male leadership, have defined the meaning of sexuality, regulated its use in relationships, and either valorized or condemned ways of being sexual in ways that have often been harmful to women. A prominent feminist ethicist writing on the issue of abortion comments: 'We have a long way to go before the sanctity of human life will include genuine regard and concern for every female already born, and no social policy discussion that obscures this fact deserves to be called moral.'[28]

The focus of this section will be on the significance of women's agency in relation to their sexual and reproductive lives. First, let us recall that feminist spirituality emphasizes mutually and equality in relationships. This mutuality works out in relationships in different ways. In terms of women's sexuality, the importance of women's agency is foremost. Girls and women are socialized in most cultures to please others, especially men. It is important for women to be able to act sexually in ways that are safe and mutual, and also in ways that respect women's subjectivity and desires.

The incidence of sexual violence against women remains a worldwide problem. While there has been increased recognition of the problems of sexual violence against women in the global north, violence against women still remains epidemic in many parts of the world.[29] Healthcare providers can play a significant role in the prevention of sexual violence. First, they have a duty to treat everyone with dignity and respect. They can also communicate the importance of this dignity and respect to their women clients. In the USA, healthcare providers are obliged to ask their clients whether or not they feel safe in their environment.[30] Such attentiveness is not merely personal, but is intended to convey to the patient that she or he is entitled to safety and that there are resources available if this is a concern.

Secondly, healthcare providers can play a role in the education of their girl and women patients regarding their bodily integrity. In many parts of the world, sex education is taboo; it is not discussed in families or in educational settings, and misinformation results in unplanned pregnancies and the spread of sexually-transmitted diseases. Healthcare providers' attentiveness to the importance of communicating accurate information in sensitive ways can help to increase women's wellbeing. Feminist spirituality emphasizes the goodness of the body and the delight that a positive sexual life can bring to one's life; healthcare providers can help to communicate this understanding to their women and girl patients.

In her book *Body, Sex, and Pleasure*, Christian ethicist Christine Gudorf makes the point that religious traditions need to shift their emphasis from sex as being primarily significant for the generation of life to one that stresses the 'sustaining of life.'[31] While her primary examples come from the Christian, and specifically Roman Catholic, tradition, which teaches that sex—which can only be licitly experienced within marriage—must always be open to the transmission of life,[32] her point is applicable to other religious traditions as well. Her point is that sex is a way of creating and maintaining bonds between people and ultimately contributes not only to the individual, but also to the social, good. In addition, she makes the point that sexual pleasure for women needs to be valued as a social good.[31,33]

The practice of female genital cutting, sometimes referred to as female genital mutilation (FGM), Gudorf notes, is deliberately intended to ensure that women do not experience clitoral sexual pleasure; in addition, it 'removes from women any incentive to infidelity, makes them undemanding sexual partners, and also supposedly increases the pleasure of men by making the vaginal entrance permanently "tight."'[31] FGM is a complex cultural practice, and there has been a great deal of literature on the importance of having women who come from cultural traditions that practice FGM be the ones to raise awareness of its devastating physical and emotional effects.[34–35] Nevertheless, healthcare providers can work within these cultural traditions to educate communities about the consequences of this practice. In some cases, healthcare providers are asked to perform the cutting in hospital settings. In such cases, healthcare providers are in a position to raise questions about the practice, and its psychological and physical effects.

Even in countries where FGM is not practiced, the possibility of women's sexual pleasure has rarely been seen as a necessary good. Most religious traditions have little if anything to say about it. Feminist spirituality emphasizes the goodness of the body; the subject of women's sexual pleasure offers healthcare professionals a way of raising the topic of women's sexual health and wellbeing. Healthcare providers need to consider a woman's wellbeing as inclusive of her sexual health and her potential for a satisfying sexual life—that is, satisfying not only her partner, but also herself.

Feminist spirituality and reproduction

Women's experiences of pregnancy and childbirth have been deeply invested with religious significance. Consider the many portrayals of the Virgin Mary with the baby Jesus. Motherhood is often seen by religion as the most significant vocation for a woman; indeed, Jewish and Christian biblical narratives of the barren woman suggest that childlessness is the worst possible fate for a woman [see the examples of Sarah (Genesis 16) and Rachel (Genesis 30)]. In some parts of the world, this is still the case.

Pregnancy and especially childbirth are two experiences where feminist spirituality has had a great deal to say. There are countless books available on the spiritual dimensions of pregnancy, with most of them emphasizing the joyful participation of the pregnant woman in the sacred dimension of life.[36] However, this is also one of the places where feminist spirituality and traditional practices of healthcare, particularly in the West, may come into conflict. Feminist spirituality emphasizes the goodness of natural processes and their spiritual dimensions, where traditional western medical practices are concerned with the physical health of the mother and child, but also with the potential dangers that may occur in childbirth—and fears of malpractice lawsuits. In her classic book *Of Woman Born: Motherhood as Experience and Institution*, Adrienne Rich sharply criticizes the way that childbirth has been 'medicalized' in the West, particularly in the USA.[37] In tracing the history of childbirth, showing how the male-dominated field of obstetrics demonized midwives and brought childbirth into hospitals—where initially, maternal death rates surged before antiseptic practices were understood—Rich argues that, in the present, women need to take a more active role in childbirth. While she is aware of the vast improvements in maternal and infant mortality that has been made possible by improvements in the care given to women in childbirth, Rich nevertheless points out that the 'medicalization' of childbirth has made women passive recipients of the obstetrician's method and timing, rather than active participants in the process.

It is certainly the case that with the growth in the numbers of women in the medical profession, as well as the encouragement of fathers in the delivery room, the process of childbirth is no longer practiced the way it was done in the 1960s when Rich gave birth to her two sons. However, it is worth consideration for healthcare professionals to think about how childbirth is medically 'managed.' Recent reports of the inability of midwives to practice or to have a connection with a hospital are examples of the continued medicalization of childbirth.[38] Movements for 'spiritual' childbirth are critical of medical interventions (e.g. inducing labour, foetal monitoring) and emphasize the importance of women connecting with their own spirituality in the birthing process.[39,40] Healthcare professionals should be in conversation with pregnant women about their hopes and desires for childbirth, and ask whether all of the medical interventions practiced in the context of a hospital birth are always necessary.

Abortion is also an issue that feminist spirituality addresses. As noted above, many feminists are critical of the way that religions have taken on abortion as being the central moral issue of the present day.[41,42] Feminist spiritual writers are concerned that the wider context of abortion is given little attention: that is, the circumstances in which women find themselves unhappily pregnant, and the demonization of women for their choices in a way that men are not, for example, the taking of life in war.[43] For some feminist spiritual writers, abortion is a sad choice that is understood within a larger cycle of birth and death. There are a number of rituals that feminists have developed to recognize the sadness and loss in both miscarriage and abortion.[44] Other feminist writers take issue with the primary focus on women's choice and argue that the feminist concern for life and relationship should take priority even in the case of an unwanted pregnancy.[42] Healthcare providers should be sensitive to women's spiritual concerns at the time of an unplanned pregnancy and help the woman in question to sort through her own hopes and values.

Finally, the increased use of artificial reproductive technologies (ART) raises critical questions for feminist spirituality. As Margaret Farley notes, there is no unanimity of opinion on this topic. An early feminist writer, Shulamith Firestone, found in ART a solution to what she saw as the enslavement of women to the 'tyranny of their reproductive biology' and that these developments would result in greater gender equality with women freed from their tie to biology.[45] Other feminist writers would disagree; Farley notes that '[f]or many feminists, the sundering of the power and process of reproduction from the bodies of women would constitute a loss of major proportions.'[2] However feminist thinkers value ART, the significance of their agency and decision-making power remains primary.[2]

Caring and feminist spirituality

Feminist religious and spiritual writers have also taken up the issue of 'care', as at least an alternative, if not a more adequate way of conceiving of human ethical relationships.[24] Traditionally, women have been the primary caregivers of dependent others—children, the ill, the frail elderly—and have often been seen as more 'naturally' disposed to care for others than men. While feminist spirituality values nurturing, feminists also ask why women and those on the margins of society have been the ones to take on the often poorly-paid and undervalued work of caregiving.[46] Caring for others raises questions about the relationship between the one being cared for and the care-giver: Is the autonomy of the one cared for being adequately recognized? Does an ethic of caring challenge more traditional conceptions of an ethic of justice? One helpful observation on the relationship between care and justice suggests that 'An ethic of justice, in which persons are treated as autonomous individuals, presupposes an ethic of care, in which dependent persons are nurtured to autonomy.'[47]

Healthcare providers are in the position of both nurturing autonomy and providing care for those who depend on their expertise. Feminist spirituality values not only the professional training that is brought to caring for those in need, but also the recognition of the relationship between the caring one and the one cared-for. Ultimately, the goal is holistic healing, in which the person in need of care is able to move forward, knowing that both body and spirit have been recognized and respected by the caregiver, even when physical healing is not possible. In any situation in which women are the recipients of care, including both the illnesses and dependencies women share with men, and those that affect women in unique ways, such as reproduction and female cancers, feminist spiritual writers emphasize the importance of caring for the *whole person* and respecting the unique gifts that women contribute both as carers and the cared-for.

Conclusion

Feminist spirituality offers a perspective on healthcare that brings to the fore the fact that women historically have lacked power and agency in both religious traditions and in healthcare systems. It recognizes as well the historical connections between religious and healing powers. Feminist spiritual writers seek to empower women to be more active in their own healthcare, to value themselves as both physical and spiritual beings, to be attentive to the kinds of relationships that they encounter in their healthcare, and to be sensitive to the broader context of their own and others' need for healthcare.

Ultimately, what religious and spiritual feminists and healthcare providers seek is the same thing: care for the whole person.

Understanding and valuing feminist spirituality can enable healthcare providers to be aware of and sensitive to issues unique to women, and also to the contributions that feminist spirituality can make to a healthcare system that values human life in all its diversity.

Acknowledgment

I would like to thank my graduate assistant, Daniel Dion, for his help in preparing this essay and my sisters, Mary Ross Osborn, RN, BSN, MSN, Kathleen Ross Larkin, RN, BSN, MSN, and Sarah Ross Davis, RN, BSN, as well as James M. Larkin, MD, for their comments.

References

1 Saiving, V. (1960). Human experience: a feminine view. *J Religion* Jan: 40. Reprinted in Christ, C.P., Plaskow, J. (eds) (1979). *Womanspirit Rising: A Feminist Reader*, pp. 25–42, New York: Harper.

2 Farley, M. (1994). Feminist theology and bioethics. In: L. Daly (ed.) *Feminist Theological Ethics: A Reader*. Louisville: Westminster/J. Knox.

3 The Sacred Congregation for the Doctrine of Faith. *Inter Insigniores* **Oct 15:** 1976. Available at: http://www.papalencyclicals.net/Paul06/p6interi.htm (accessed 6 November 2010).

4 Greenberg, B. (1981). *On Women and Judaism: A View from Tradition*. Philadelphia: Jewish Publication Society of America. Plaskow, J. (1990). *Standing Again at Sinai*. San Francisco: Harper & Row.

5 Walker, A. (1983). *In Search of our Mothers' Gardens: Womanist Prose*. San Diego: Harcourt Brace Jovanovich.

6 Wilson, B. (2009). For Black Women, Breast Cancer Strikes Younger, *NPR* Dec 7. Available at: http://www.npr.org/templates/story/story.php?storyId=120985060 (accessed 18 November, 2010)

7 White, L. (1967). The historical roots of our ecological crisis. *Science*, **155**: 1203–7.

8 Friedan, B. (1983). *The Feminine Mystique*. New York: Dell Publishing Co.

9 Gilligan, C. (1982). *In a Different Voice: Psychological Theory and Women's Development*. Cambridge: Harvard University Press.

10 Townes, E.M. (1998). *Breaking the Fine Rain of Death: African American Health Issues and a Womanist Ethic of Care*. New York: Continuum.

11 Northup, L.A. (1997). *Ritualizing Women: Patterns of Spirituality*. Cleveland: Pilgrim Press.

12 Daly, M. (1985). *The Church and the Second Sex*. Boston: Beacon Press.

13 Daly, M. (1990). *Gyn/Ecology: The Metaethics of Radical Feminism*. Boston: Beacon Press.

14 Daly, M. (1975). *Beyond God the Father: Toward a Philosophy of Women's Liberation*. Boston: Beacon Press.

15 Daly, M. (1992). *Outercourse: The Be-dazzling Voyage*. San Francisco: HarperSanFrancisco.

16 Spretnak, C. (2004). *Missing Mary: The Queen of Heaven and Her Re-emergence in the Modern Church*. New York: Palgrave Macmillan.

17 Christ, C.P. (2003). *She Who Changes: Re-imagining the Divine in the World*. New York: Palgrave Macmillan.

18 Adler, M. (1979). *Drawing Down the Moon: Witches, Druids, Goddess-worshippers, and Other Pagans in America*. New York: Penguin Books.

19 Starhawk (1979). *The Spiral Dance: A Rebirth of the Ancient Religion of the Great Goddess*. San Francisco: Harper and Row.

20 Christ, C.P. (1982). *Why Women Need the Goddess: Phenomenological, Psychological, and Political Reflections*. In: C. Spretnak (ed.) *The Politics of Women's Spirituality*, Garden City, NY: Anchor Books.

21 Pintchman, T. (1994). *Rise of the Goddess in the Hindu Tradition*. Albany: State University of New York Press.

22 Johnson, E.A. (2002). *She Who Is: The Mystery of God in Feminist Theological Discourse*. New York: Crossroad.

23 McFague, S. (1987). *Models of God: Theology for an Ecological, Nuclear Age*. Philadelphia: Fortress Press.

24 Gilligan, C. (2006). In a different voice. In: V. Held (ed.) *Ethics of Care: Personal, Political, Global*. New York: Oxford University Press.

25 Tronto, J. (1993). *Moral Boundaries: A Political Argument for an Ethic of Care*. New York: Routledge.

26 Vigen, A.M. (2006). *Women, Ethics, and Inequality in U.S. Healthcare, To Count Among the Living*. New York: Palgrave Macmillan.

27 Browning, M. (in press). *Patriarchy, Christianity and the Aids Pandemic*. Dissertation, Loyola University, Chicago.

28 Harrison, B.W. (1994). Theology and morality of procreative choice. In: L. K. Daly (ed.) *Feminist Theological Ethics: A Reader*, pp. 213–32. Louisville: Westminster John Knox Press.

29 United Nations Department of Economic and Social Affairs (2010). *The World's Women 2010: Trends and Statistics*, United Nations Publication, 2010 Oct 20. Available at: http://unstats.un.org/unsd/demographic/products/Worldswomen/WW_full%20report_color.pdf. (accessed 6 November 2010).

30 American College of Emergency Physicians (nd). *Violence Free Society*. Available at: http://www.acep.org/Content.aspx?id=29848 (accessed 18 November, 2010)

31 Gudorf, C. (1994). *Body, Sex, and Pleasure: Reconstructing Christian Sexual Ethics*. Cleveland: Pilgrim Press.

32 Catechism of the Catholic Church, 2nd edn (1997). *United States Catholic Conference*. Washington: Libreria Editrice Vaticana.

33 Jung, P.B., Hunt, M.E., Balakrishnan, R. (2001). *Good Sex: Feminist Perspectives from the World's Religions*. New Brunswick: Rutgers University Press.

34 UNICEF (2005). Changing a harmful social convention: female genital mutilation/cutting. In: A. Lewnes (ed.) *Innocenti Digest*. Geneva: United Nations Children's Fund. Available at: http://www.unicef-irc.org/publications/396 (accessed 6 November, 2010).

35 OHCHR, UNAIDS, UNDP, UNECA, UNESCO, UNFPA, UNHCR, UNICEF, UNIFEM, WHO (2008). *Eliminating Female Genital Mutilation*, an Interagency Statement. Geneva: World Health Organization. Available at: http://www.unicef.org/media/media_38229.html. (accessed 6 November, 2010).

36 Frymer-Kensky, T.S. (1995). *Motherprayer: The Pregnant Woman's Spiritual Companion*. New York: G.P. Putnam Sons.

37 Rich, A. (1976). *Of Woman Born: Motherhood as Experience and Institution*. New York: Norton.

38 Goodman, S. (2007). Piercing the veil: the marginalization of midwives in the United States. *Soc Sci Med* **65**: 610–21.

39 Gaskin, I.M. (2002). *Spiritual Midwifery*, Summertown: Book Publishing Company.

40 Hopkins, J. (1999). *Welcoming the Soul of a Child*. New York: Kensington Books.

41 Harrison, B.W. (1983). *Our Right to Choose: Toward a New Ethic of Abortion*. Boston: Beacon Press.

42 Callahan, S. (1986). Abortion and the sexual agenda: a case for prolife feminism, *Commonweal* **Apr 25**: 232–8.

43 Gudorf, C. (1996). To make a seamless garment, use a single piece of cloth. *Conscience*, **17**(3): 10–21.

44 Ruether, R.R. (1985). *Women-church: Theology and Practice of Feminist Liturgical Communities*. San Francisco: Harper & Row.

45 Firestone, S. (1970). *The Dialectic of Sex: The Case for Feminist Revolution*. New York: Morrow.

46 Noddings, N. (1984). *Caring: A Feminine Approach to Ethics & Moral Education*. Berkeley: University of California Press.

47 Clement, G. (1996). *Care, Autonomy, and Justice: Feminism and the Ethic of Care*. Boulder: Westview Press.

CHAPTER 6

Indian religion and the Ayurvedic tradition

Prakash N. Desai

Introduction

For Hindus, history is a lived-in reality. The survival of major treatises for centuries, written down perhaps only after the development of the Brahmi script (considered to have been finished in about 300 BCE), attests to the emphasis placed on memory—remembering the past and interpreting it to serve the present.[1] This gives to the Hindu culture both a paleocentric and mythopoetic character.

Hindus revere the past, but not only in a religious sense; the past inspires and guides social and personal conduct. The ancient Vedic literature, the later epics, and the medieval tales of the past *(puranas)* illustrate through myth-making the essential relationship between people and institutions. In both private and public contexts ancient heroes and their deeds are recalled, and the present compared with the past. The outcome is flexible rules of ethical and moral conduct. Although Hindus recall their early past to guide them in actions, the narrative of the conduct of their ancestors is not fixed. As new myths are generated, the heroes of the legends are given new forms, and stories are adapted to the needs of the present. Different versions of ancient texts exist, and different texts always tell slightly altered accounts of particular events. This constant accommodation gives the Hindus their amazing diversity yet keeps them in the fold.

One difficulty in speaking about Hindu 'faith' as a distinct object of study is that Hinduism is more a tradition than a faith. In the daily practices of Hindus, traditions are faithfully observed. What might be considered an aspect of secular life in the west, Hindus would assert to be a part of their religion—what they eat, for example, or with whom they eat or who cooks for them. One also finds religious life pervaded with matters considered profane elsewhere—for example, couples in sexual congress depicted on the outer walls of a temple. It is difficult to draw lines between that which is tradition, handed down from generation to generation, and that which is derived from religious doctrines. Obligations and duties that direct behaviour can probably be traced to some idea about human relationship with God, but more often than not the actor attributes the behaviour to the force of *pranalika* (originally meaning a channel or a course flowing down a reservoir) or tradition. No actions can be viewed outside the moral or religious sphere, and a Hindu scholar can always trace the origin of a ritual or a custom to some spiritual imperative, or to some Hindu scripture. However, for a layperson, no conscious knowledge of such a command is required nor does it often exist.

A distinctly identifiable Hindu medical tradition, the Ayurvedic, exists both in theory and in practice, stretching back two millennia over all of India. The theory is inseparably intertwined with the theological and liturgical discourses of the time. The medical texts articulate religious beliefs, and the religious texts incorporate diagnoses and therapies. Hindu medicine never became divorced from the rest of life's pursuits, especially not from religious practice, as did medicine in the West.

Apart from the dominant Ayurvedic tradition, a second medical tradition, *siddha*, has a following in the south of India. The theoretical principles are largely derived from the Ayurvedic tradition, but siddha's use of oxides of metals in therapies was influenced by Greek apothecary.

Astrology also has an influence. The houses of the horoscope represent sectors of life, designated variously as the seats of health, illness, marriage, progeny, and so on. The heavenly bodies have specific domains, including those of health and well-being. Astrologers are called on to make predictions, which may lead to specific ritual performances or the wearing of certain stones to ward off or alleviate illnesses. An Ayurvedic physician may draw on the horoscope in calculating the treatment of a particular disorder.

One difficulty in demarcating the medical and health concerns of Hindus is the introduction of medical systems from the West. It is clear that the Greek Hippocratic medical tradition interacted with the later Ayurvedic tradition, as did the Arabic medical tradition (the Unani), especially in the north of India. The Unani tradition (from the word Ionian), was developed by the Islamic tradition and has a following both among the Muslims and Hindus. More recently, allopathy (the Western modern medical tradition)[2] has come to India and taken its place alongside competing ideologies and health ideals.

All these influences allow for a complex interplay between pragmatic health concerns and help-seeking behaviours. It is again a measure of the assimilative strength of the Hindu tradition that these contradictory systems coexist, often borrowing from each other at the periphery. The receiver of care is hardly concerned with these traditions. Just as an Indian uses history for his or her immediate ends, the patient chooses his or her healer to match pressing concerns.[3]

Sources of Hindu tradition

A vast collection of Hindu literature has been compiled over centuries. The Vedas, from the word *vid*, 'to know,' are the repository of ancient knowledge about the Hindus and their experiences. The *Rig Veda*, the earliest of Hindu texts, is usually regarded as having been composed around 1500 BCE. It is a compendium of about 1080 hymns—invocations of the gods who preside over the earthly realms and songs in praise of their power. More imaginative than contemplative, they show poetically the Aryan's awe before nature.

Later Vedas contained liturgical treatises, meditations, and philosophical commentaries, as well as hymns. The liturgical treatises (*brahmanas*) present narrations of rituals, detailing principally the sacrificial work of the priests. In a world where temples had not yet been built and gods had not assumed iconic forms, the performance of the sacrifice involved the propitiation of the Vedic gods and an invitation to them to reside in the ritual fire. The *aranyakas* are the meditations of forest dwellers and are a starting point for the philosophical commentaries known as the Upanishads.

The Upanishads are writings about the inner meaning of life and death, as given by a father or teacher to his most advanced students. The major Upanishads were composed before 500 BCE and were not taught widely or published, but rather passed on orally in secret. They discuss meditation, the true nature of person and world, states of consciousness, and human fulfillment. They were considered as *shruti*, that which was heard and thus revealed, rather than *smriti*, that which is remembered. This latter category is considered derivative of the Vedas, and includes the epics *Mahabharata* and *Ramayana*, and the *dharmashastras*, or law texts. A principal law text is the *Laws of Manu*.

The *Laws of Manu* is a systemization of the Hindu view of society, containing such categories as the four goals of mankind, the four stages of life, and the four castes (*varnas*). It seeks to unify the two opposing religious goals of Hindus: social obligation (*dharma*) and personal liberation (*moksha*). These are located at different stages of life in *Manu*, and can thus coexist, as division of labour coexists in the caste systems.

Another major system of works is that of *darshana*, or philosophy. The three systems most relevant to the issues of health and medicine are those of yoga, Nyaya-Vaisheshika (two traditions, often paired together) and *samkhya* philosophies. The origins of these philosophies are traced to early Indian thought and practices. Classical yoga is based on the *Yoga Sutra* of Patanjali (second Century BCE), which describes methods to bring the yogin's body and mind under the control of his spirit. The goal is control of the modulations of the yogin's mind-the suppression of states of consciousness. This is done by stages—positive and negative moral rules, postures and breath control, disengagement of the senses from worldly things, concentration and meditation, and perfectly balanced consciousness. The goal of Patanjala yoga is isolation (*kaivalya*), in which the person becomes a pure observer, without attachment.

Nyaya-Vaisheshika puts forward a substantialist and materialist view of the universe. Its realist ontology, with discourses upon substances, qualities, and inherence among others, lays the foundations of Indian Sciences, both physical and psychosocial.

Yoga is based on the `*samkhya* system of philosophy, which emphasizes the dissociation of spirit from matter. Its most important text is the *Samkhya Karika* of Isvarakrishna (200 CE). According to samkhya, the world is real, but it is based on ignorance of the spirit. The spirit is enslaved by its participation in nature, which is eternally changing and disintegrating. Liberation (*moksha*) means an escape from suffering and attachment, knowledge of one's true situation, and a renunciation of matter in favour of spirit.

Another significant text is the *Bhagavad Gita*, which occurs within the epic *Mahabharata* (400 BCE–400 CE). This epic is the story of the great war in which relatives within the family of the Bharatas fight over succession to the throne. Its most famous segment is the *Gita*, the 'Song of God,' in which warrior prince Arjuna doubts the value of this warfare, and his charioteer (the god Krishna in human form) discusses why Arjuna can and must fight. Within this discussion arise the topics of duty, action, love spiritual growth, and religious vision. The *Gita* shows the ideal relationship between god and devotee, mentor and pupil.

The Ayurvedic literature also begins in the pre-Christian era and consists of several texts on health and medicine, the three major ones being the Carakaksamhita (100 CE), the Sushrutasamhita (200 CE), and the Ashtangahridaya samhita (700 CE). Pain and suffering, illness and its cure, and the conduct of the caregiver are the subjects of these treatises.

Much in Hindu literature deals with the goals of *kama*, love and desire, and *artha*, wealth and power. The most famous *kama* text is probably the *Kamasutra* of Vatsayana, from the third century CE. It includes such topics as sexuality, courtship and marriage, prostitution, the 64 arts, and the lifestyle of the man-about-town. Other *kama* texts discuss spells, potions, and further variations of sexual relationships. The most famous text on *artha* is probably the *Arthashastra*, which discusses diplomacy, warfare, and politics.

All these works and others are part of the great Sanskritic, or classical, tradition of India. They interact on the local level with folk and village beliefs in ancestor worship, spirit possession and exorcism, and worship of local deities. These local traditions are called the 'little traditions,' and they have affected the interpretations of the texts of the 'great tradition.'

The history and development of Hindu thought is as long as it is varied. It is not possible to tease out the antecedents of current practices to locate their origins, nor to establish authorship and dates. Without a central defining authority of a prophet, book or priestly order, the evolution of Hindu civilization took a variable course. This course was further complicated by geographic diffusion and the entry of hitherto unassimilated groups of people. New religions arrived; new sects were formed as new ethics and practices emerged. A continuous process of interpenetration of the great tradition with little traditions gave way to local specialization and a way of life that could call upon convenient sources of justification. Yet underneath all these complexities and elasticities lies a fountain-source of conceptions about the self, the body, and the life course. These often unspoken assumptions lend coherence to Indian life and are responsible for its continuity.

Traditions, customs, rituals, beliefs, and laws enunciated in the law books are as alive today as they were when the texts were composed. In contrast to earlier Vedic formulations, which have been incorporated and subsumed into traditional Hindu life and lore, the ideas and practices of the *dharmashastras* are an explicit and integral part of Hindu traditions in their near-original forms. Many scholars suggest that the *dharmashastras* capture the spirit of proper Hinduism and that the older Vedic literature may be regarded as a philosophical backdrop to them.[4] Others bemoan the corruption of the ancient Vedic religion in later Hindu practices.[5] The principles of Order (Rita, the origin of the concept of dharma), connectivity and relationship (interconnectedness of all things), and permeability and boundaries (much like a cell membrane, with pollution as a danger), are the psychological categories of the evolved system.

The four aims of life

Virtue (*dharma*), purpose or wealth (*artha*), and pleasure (*kama*) motivate human actions. For an ordinary human being, the pursuit of self-realization rests in the acceptance of these three ends. Although disagreement prevailed regarding their hierarchical ordering, the *Laws of Manu* concluded that all three were to be equally pursued.[6] The fourth and supreme end of life is *moksha*, release, or liberation from the cycle of rebirth.

Dharma, artha, kama, and *moksha* are principles of human action throughout the course of life. To each person the goals of virtue, wealth, and pleasure are assigned according to his or her situation, especially in relation to caste, status, age, and gender. These aims of life not only guide personal action vis-à-vis God, but more stringently ordain relationships with other persons. Husband–wife, parent–child, and teacher–pupil relations, kinship networks, and inter-caste relations—all require specific transactions. From early childhood one prepares for these mutual obligations in the family network as well as outside it. Mutuality does not presuppose symmetry: an order of hierarchies in relationships is established. Nurturing this sense of place in a child is a mark of good parenting.

Artha is interpreted as both intention and object. It means the pursuit of livelihood not as an end in itself, but as necessary for the sustenance of life. Wealth and material wellbeing do not violate religious obligations, and a life of poverty is neither comfortable nor enhances self-esteem. *Kama* reflects acceptance to the realities of human nature, and refers broadly to the affectional aspect of persons through which they bind themselves to each other. From another vantage point, it is also an effort to integrate and regulate passions. The twin dangers of wild expressions of desire and indiscriminate suppression of impulses are acknowledged. *Artha* and *Kama* are thus subsumed under *dharma*, but their separate status attests to the here-and-now attitude in Hindu transactions. These are not just another set of duties, they are entitlements within the scope of a moral life. The legitimation of material goals and the fulfillment of desires permit inclusion of such activities within the ethical domain.

Moksha is different. It is otherworldly, an end in itself, a release from the bondage of works and the cycles of birth and rebirth. It aims to go beyond the body, beyond the physical nature, and it connects the search for immortality with the quest for cohesion. *Moksha* stands for freedom from the experience of pain, old age, and death, but also for merger with the original principle of creation. It is the culmination of appropriately conducted *dharma*.[7]

These four ends of Hindu life are incorporated into the Ayurvedic medical literature. As the *Carakasamhita*, the source book of Ayurveda, declares wellbeing ('a disease-free state') is to be pursued for the attainment of 'virtue, wealth and gratification'.[8] The authors of the medical texts show rare practical wisdom in their ability to sidestep confrontation with the priestly order. They did this without divorcing the body from intentions and behaviours, or wellbeing from considerations of habits, personality, and relationships.

A long list of good conduct and virtuous behaviours is offered in the *Carakasamhita* without distinctions among physical, psychological, social, and spiritual considerations. Duties include worshipping gods and Brahmins, keeping the sacred fire and offering oblations, respecting the teacher, performing the rites for dead ancestors, not telling a lie or desiring the women or property of others, not being critical of others, and not swimming in strong currents.[9]

Desire for long life, desire for wealth, and desire for the other world are the principal motivations of Ayurvedic prescriptions. The desire to live is first, 'because on departure of life, everything departs.' Next to life, wealth is sought because 'there is nothing more sinful than to have a long life without means (of sustenance).'[10] The Ayurvedic text then goes on to present arguments for and against the notion of rebirth. It decides in favour of a theory of rebirth on the basis of authority, recognizing the limitations of perception, inference, and reasoning.

The four classes

The division of people into four classes or castes is one of the oldest aspects of the Hindu tradition, originating in the creation myth of the *Rig Veda*. The four classes were created from different parts of the body of the cosmic giant Purusha and were also differentiated on the basis of skin colour. The Vedic myth has continued to shape Indian society to the present day. The original four classes were the Brahmins (priests, scholars and teachers, the kshatriyas (rulers and warriors), the vaishyas (traders, bankers and agriculturalists), and the shudras (the toilers and menial workers). The untouchables, a later designation, were outside the system and performed the most menial jobs. The modern division of Indian society is into jatis, or subcastes, a proliferation of the original divisions, and also incorporating new immigrants. The increasing and changing stratification of castes attests that neither have these categories been fixed nor has social organization been static.

Debate continues on whether the four classes were hereditary or determined by the qualities and occupations of people. There is hardly any doubt that further subdivisions of the castes were necessitated by mixed marriages. The *Laws of Manu* gives an elaborate list of the categories resulting from such mixtures, which are seen as posing danger to society and threatening the loss of status and occupation.[11] Rules for the exchange of cooked food were also well-established, including prohibitions against receiving cooked food from physicians and surgeons, people in low occupations and without virtue, and those with undesirable physical or psychological qualities.[12]

The concept of equality is not Indian: social reform movements in India have borrowed moral values from the outside. The Sikh religion borrowed from Islam the idea of brotherhood and the abolition of *sati* and, more recently, the Gandhian movement to eradicate untouchability showed Western influence. To many scholars, the Indian constitution and the changes promoted by secularism presented ideas alien to Indian culture.[13]

Secularism in the West means that in political and economic life, and before the law, individuals of different faiths will not be treated differently. However, the Indian problem is that even those who believe in the same God are essentially different and unequal. These inequalities flow from the religious tradition itself.

Health and medicine

Hindu ideas about health and illness spring from the construction of the Hindu universe. Unlike Western notions of religion, Hinduism is not primarily about the relationship of human beings with a divinity. The religion accounts for the relationships among all that is contained in the universe and the universe itself. Hinduism has survived as a continuous tradition because of its understanding of relationships. This Ayurvedic worldview continues both to inform and limit the health expectations of patients, and the healing practices of physicians.

In the evolution and spread of medical knowledge and practice, Buddhist and later Jain scholars made vital contributions. Antibrahminical spirit permitted the Buddhist medical men to investigate, experiment, and break caste barriers freely (one interpretation holds that *carak* 'the legendary author of *Carak Samhita*' or 'itinerant' applied most aptly to Buddhist monks). At the early stages, Buddhist thought was in many important respects a continuation of Hindu beliefs and practices, and in turn influenced later Hindu thought and medicine.

The Ayurvedic texts place the medical tradition squarely within the larger province of traditional religious pursuits and philosophy. The survival of accounts of the transmission of medical knowledge attests that medical theory and practice both affected, and were affected by, the Hindu tradition. Thus, a body free from disease is essential to the realization of life's tasks, including the spiritual. Ayurveda for the early physician was eternal knowledge created before the creation of the world. The potential for the protection of health and removal of disorders was built into the act of creation. Health-seeking was a religious obligation, and traditional prescriptions were medicinal ones.

In Ayurvedic medicine illness is viewed simply as a state of imbalance. The physical, psychological, social, and spiritual realms are parts of the all-encompassing realm of Ayurveda. Illness and wellness are not mutually exclusive; circumstances and intentions determine the proportions of illness and wellness.[14] The pathophysiology is based on a theory of humors: the functional aspect of the body is governed by three biological humors, Tridosha. Wind and Ether (Vata), Fire and Water (Pitta), and Water and Earth (Kapha) pervade the body in distinct channels, their concentrations determining both normal and abnormal functions. This theory is similar to the Greek system, but of separate origin. The pharmacopeia is essentially botanical, with some animal products and metal oxides also used, and is dispensed with consideration of gender, age, place.

The Hindu world can be seen as a series of ever-widening circles extending into infinity. At the centre is the private self. Each circle exerts an influence on the centre in direct proportion to the size of the influencing object and in inverse proportion to its distance from the centre. The kind and degree of illness may be visualized as a product of disturbance in any circle or in a combination of them. In contrast, a state of health is a balance of bodily substances, a humoral balance that gives comfort and pleasure to body, mind, and senses. The balance of physical, sensory and mental dispositions also is vital.

In a system that changes with every kind of input and tends toward imbalance, remaining in a state of equilibrium is a daunting task. Disequilibrium of the humors are seen by authors of the Ayurvedic texts as implicated in anger, jealousy, excessive desire, laziness, and so forth. In the same way, outside influences, like dietetic input, may alter psychological states.

Food or diet on which 'the *prana* rests,' is a central concern. Rarely would an Indian patient not ask his or her physician for a diet, matched to the disease, to go along with the medical preparations. Almost every pill has to be accompanied by a compatible fluid (like water, milk, or honey) used to swallow the pill. The compounding of mixtures, a lost art elsewhere, is an essential skill of a general practitioner in India because medicine in fluid form is more acceptable to most Indian patients.

The health and illness language of Hindu patients is remarkably Ayurvedic. Hot and cold, light and heavy, dry and wet are the idioms of diets, disease, drugs, and temperamental dispositions. The Ayurvedic physician is bound by the same medical paradigm from which patients' idioms have emerged. Occasionally, however, a few step out of the fold. A sign in one Ayurvedic dispensary advises his patients that in cases of children's fever (often from infections), it is permissible to mix injections (meaning antibiotics) with his treatments. Much to the chagrin of purists, many Ayurvedic doctors (*valdyas*) resort to allopathic medications, even administering injectable antibiotics. Some Ayurvedic medical colleges teach both Ayurvedic and allopathic medicine.

In much of modern medical practice (for example, in the West), scientific and technological imperatives have caused a dissociation of medical practice from the faith traditions of patients and doctors. In India a variety of medical traditions exist, and only a few patients patronize a particular tradition exclusively. Patients go from a practitioner of one tradition to a practitioner of another, sometimes in the treatment of the same disorder. This 'picking and choosing' is not only consistent with the Hindu orientation to life; it also protects against too obvious a fracture between a patient's tradition-informed help-seeking behaviour and the health practitioner's ministrations. Of greater concern than a fracture between faith and medicine in India may actually be the degree to which medicine has been captive to the paradigms of the Hindu philosophical and religious ethos. The successful introduction and widespread acceptance of allopathic medicine point to some unmet medical needs and significant gaps in the effectiveness of traditional medicine against a variety of diseases.

Hindu medicine repeatedly stresses the common origin of humanity and the universe. The human relationship with the environment is intrinsic. The elements that compose the universe also constitute the human body and, hence, the laws that govern the elements govern the human world. The five elements, or *bhutas*, having been created and therefore subject to dissolution, are also a source of misery. In health and illness, the qualities of these constituents are the same inside and outside the body, and the interaction between the two may explain disease, as well as cure.

The principles of transformation of the body's material constituents and the continuity of the cosmic elements into the human body were firmly established in Hindu thought at the time of the composition of the first medical compendia. *Space* gives rise to the faculty of hearing, carries the spoken word, is the connectivity of all parts. *Wind* becomes the tactile sensory organ; it is responsible for all movements of the body and lightness is its property. *Fire* is associated with the sense of sight, the eyes, and the form. It gives rise to emotion and luster, alacrity and bravery, and is the principle of digesting (or cooking) food. *Water* is associated with taste; it is heavy and cool. It is the source of fluids in the body, including semen, and has the property of being viscous. *Earth*, the fifth element of the body, is linked to smell and has the property of hardness and heaviness. The elements also acquire physiological and psychological properties.

Later Hindu thought, belief, and practice were profoundly influenced by Ayurvedic formulations. So deep and lasting has been the impact of medical theory that not only are contemporary health-related ideas and behaviours continuous with Ayurvedic constructions, but so is the social and psychological life of the modern Hindu.

Maintaining a balance of substances in the body and the environment becomes the major task of those who desire a healthy state for themselves and also for the physician, Pundit Shiv Sharma, an Ayurvedic physician and historian, suggests that Ayurveda contains the principles of both allopathy and homeopathy, for it propounds the principle of treatment with both contrary *(allo)* and similar *(homeo)* substances.[15] For Hindus every contact, human or non-human, has the potential to alter the balance positively or negatively, with simultaneous and inseparable implications for moral and physical wellbeing. Persons, drugs, diets, and so on can be further modified by the forces of time and geography, and an extremely contextual relativistic universe emerges. Any contact between any two items in the cosmos therefore has to be appropriate.

The business of wellbeing is a full-time occupation. Physical health can easily be disturbed by the wrong kind of food, a change in habits, or disturbed sleep, although strict adherence to the order of input and output can usually maintain a state of balance. The social world is also in a state of constant flux. The universe of family and caste is so finely knit and rules are so clearly defined for almost every situation that only in the private world can a person be totally free. The task of seeking spiritual wellbeing in India is therefore a very private affair. As McKim Marriott observed after his time in a village in North India, "Extreme stability of caste and kinship leaves individuals fairly free to think and to believe as they please. Thus, within one family there may be devotees of as many different gods as there are members; one member of the family may know nothing and care nothing about the god worshipped by another member".[14]

Within the stream of Hindu life lie the subjective realities of Hindu persons. Where Ayurveda and *dharma*, along with other constructions of the cosmos, govern the aims of Hindu life, a fluid interpersonal world emerges. Human activities and relationships are a grid of intricate hierarchies and boundaries, not always fixed. Such a grid may be visualized as a template for wellbeing.

The body is viewed as a vertical axis in which the head and foot are the two poles. Head is high, foot is low, higher is purer and more subtle, lower is impure and gross. Who the head of a family is, to whom the headship passes, what one may or may not touch with the feet, to whom and when one bows the head, and at whose feet one sits—all these are connected with the maintenance of wellbeing.

Instead of the ego-boundaries of an individual, Hindus erect social and geographic boundaries. Prescriptions for the egress of impulses seek to regulate otherwise volatile substances. Limitations are placed on sexual and social intercourse in order to create conditions of social and physical wellbeing. Crossing the boundaries brings ill-health and pollution. Limits, order, and control are essential for human welfare, and trust is founded on the understanding of these boundaries.

Hindus allow many ways of being religious, yet there is an orthodoxy in the context of a group like a family, sect, or caste. Religion does not enforce absolute laws, either in worship or relationship. Hindu gods do not demand an absolute adherence to particular modes of being. It is the social consideration of belonging to a group that tends to codify behaviour. Medical beliefs and native cures constitute the forces that provide continuity between the past and the present. They cut across geographic, as well as group boundaries, for they grow out of a common and enduring heritage of notions about context and relationships. Hindus would readily agree that their medical concerns are rooted in their common religious beliefs.

The future of the tradition

In the transitional society of modern India, the old norms of relationships no longer work well. The nature of work has changed and a democratic polity rests on egalitarian not hierarchical values. Industrial and urban growth has curtailed group cohesion and discouraged traditional behaviours, aspirations, and expectations. A new ethic has not yet emerged, but in the family, where health is a shared phenomenon and connectedness a prime virtue, there is hope for new norms to grow.

A more difficult problem is the lack of legitimization of secular life and institutions. There is a massive mistrust of public institutions. When only religious institutions have power and justification, these institutions involved with daily life may be trivialized or even ignored. Little emphasis is placed on the justice and dignity of all. People of lower castes and outcasts continue to be treated badly, shunned, sometimes beaten, barred from the wells and houses of towns, in spite of constitutional guarantees. With few ways to negotiate and resolve conflicts among competing interests, violence is never far from the surface.

Next only to the untouchables, women bear the brunt of problematic beliefs and attitudes shaped by the forces of history. Women are seen as having powerful, uncontrollable urges and lacking self-regulation. Thus, the society has constructed roles for them in which they are externally governed, especially in the area of sexuality. They seem to have little control over their bodies and little to say in the choice of marital partner in traditional India. Only when they contribute to generational continuity by giving birth to a male child do they rise in power and status. The problems of women and untouchables continue to be two of India's greatest problems today.

In Hindu psychology, the forces of the Self, the body-self, and the body give shape to spiritual and secular quests. The fear of being alone, without another to respond, generates hunger for contact. Two separate dramas get played out, one a need for intense intimacy, and another a nagging disbelief in the affective profusion of the moment. The environment never fully satisfies one's need for admiration and idealization. Detachment *(vairagya)* always looms on the horizon as an ideal. Suspicion about the genuineness of responses and the persistent demand for affirmation can display an alienation from the body and from others, which results from the Hindu construction of the self, the mind, and the body. Any physician must take these forces into account when dealing with Indian patients.

The Hindu tradition and the west

Hindu tradition continues to engage western societies in a variety of ways. In India itself western allopathic medicine increasingly shapes health policy and health service delivery, particularly in cities, but is, in its turn, shaped by Indian assumptions about good care that derive from Ayurveda. Thus, a consultation with an allopathic practitioner may reflect an Ayurvedic understanding of the interaction between doctor and patient.[17] Ayurvedic medicine continues to be an important health resource in rural areas of India, although even here acute illness will be more likely taken to allopathic practitioners. This pattern of coexistence of allopathic and traditional medicine is common in most Asian countries.[18] Ayurveda, a traditional practice within India, has expanded on a global level as a complementary therapy in recent years.[19,20]

Sizeable communities of expatriate Indians now live in most major western cities. In particular, Indian physicians form a significant part of the medical workforce in most western countries. These expatriate communities comprise, for the most part, educated professional people, well assimilated into their new countries. Nevertheless, their foundation in Hindu tradition continues to shape personal beliefs and practices concerning health and illness, including interactions with the health system.[21] For example, people's initial strategies in coping with illness are usually dietary, even if not strictly along Ayurvedic lines. Family and community remain an important resource, and when experiencing illness it is common for people to consult a member of their extended family before consulting their own physician. Medical decisions too will involve family consultation where possible, perhaps using a trusted family physician as an intermediary.[22]

The traditions that in India were part of everyday community life can, in expatriate communities, take on a more formal or ceremonial status. Festivals become times at which community members can gather, celebrate their heritage, and reinforce their cultural identity. Thus the western context constructs Hinduism more as a religion than a way of life. Yet the Hindu notion of being religious encompasses at once every aspect of existence and the hereafter. It is possible to be an atheist, to cease to believe in anything divine or sacred, but it is difficult to cease to be a Hindu. It would not be an exaggeration to state that to be a Hindu is to have a particular psychic organization. More than anything else, it is the continuity between doctrines, ideas, and beliefs revealed in their richness and variation in Indian medicine and religion.

Conclusion

The Hindu tradition is a constantly changing, adapting and, innovative tradition. In India itself with geographic dispersal and the passage of time, interpenetration of the great Sanskritic tradition, and the little local indigenous traditions, as well as new influences from the outside of the tradition has made a variety of local adaptations, variations, and amalgamations. However there are enduring principles and threads that give continuity and cohesion to the Hindu tradition. Some of the principles are the primacy of order and hierarchy, of connectivity and relationships, inputs and outputs for example of diet, thought, and action, and fluidity and boundaries in interpersonal relationships.

With its own distinct medical tradition, India had an evolved system of diagnoses and therapeutics but has conveniently added and combined with both Unani as well as the modern Western (allopathic tradition). However medical ethics has largely remained intact from the original as well as the tradition informed help seeking behaviours, practices, and doctor-patient relationships.

Indian immigrants to the West and elsewhere have been able, on the strength of the tradition to preserve and adapt, and successfully meet new challenges.

Acknowledgement

Adapted from Prakash Desai, *Health and Medicine in the Hindu Tradition*. New York: Crossroad.

References

1 Chatterji, S.K. (1938 (70)). Linguistic survey of India: languages and script. In: Chatterji, S.K., Dutta, N., Pusalkar, A.D., and Bose, N.K. (eds) *The Cultural History of India* (1), pp. 53–75. Calcutta: Ramakrishna Mission.

2 Dunn, F. (1976). Traditional Asian medicine and cosmopolitan medicine as adaptive systems, In: C. Leslie (ed.) *Asian Medical Systems*, pp. 137–58. Berkeley: University of California Press.

3 Daniels, S. (1983). The tool-box approach of the Tamil to the issues of moral responsibility and human destiny. In: C. Keyes, E.V. Daniel (eds) *Karma: an Anthropological Enquiry*, pp. 27–62. Berkeley: University of California Press.

4 Gonda, J. (1987). Indian religions: an overview. In: M. Eliade (ed.) *Encyclopaedia of Religion*, (7). New York: Macmillan.

5 Chaudhari, N. (1979) *Hinduism*. New York: Oxford University Press.

6 Buhler, G. (1969). The Laws of Manu trans. New York: Dover. (Hereafter Manu) Chapter 2 verse 224.

7 Radhakrishnan, S. (1940). *Eastern Religion and Western Thought*. London: Oxford University Press.

8 Carak Samhita trans. *Priyavrat Sharma* 2 vols. Varanasi, India: Chaukhamba Orientalia. Chapter 1 section 1 verse 15 (Hereafter Car).

9 Car, 1.8.17–29.

10 Car, 1.11.3.4–5.

11 Manu, 10.1–73.

12 Kane, P.V. (1968–77). *History of Dharmasastra*, (5). Poona: Bhandankar Oriental Research Institute.

13 Nandy, A. (1985). An anti-secularist manifesto. *Seminar* **314:** 14–24.

14 Wujastyk, D. (2001). *The Roots of Ayurveda: Selections from Sanskrit Medical Writings*. New Delhi: Penguin.

15 Sharma Pundit, S. (ed) (1979). *Realms of Ayurveda*. New Delhi: Arnold-Heinemann.

16 Marriott, M. (1955). Western medicine in northern India. In: B.D. Paul (ed.) *Health, Culture and Community*, pp. 239–68. New York: Russell Sage, p. 248

17 Khare, R.S. (1996). Dava, daktar, and dua: anthropology of practiced medicine in India. *Soc Sci Med* **43**(5): 837–48.

18 Bodeker, G., Burford, G. (eds) (2007). *Traditional, Complementary and Alternative Medicine: Policy and Public Health Perspectives*. London: Imperial College Press.

19 Reddy, S. (2002). Asian medicine in America: the Ayurvedic case. *Ann Am Acad* **583**: 97–121.

20 Wujastyk, D., Smith, F.M. (eds) (2008). *Modern and Global Ayurveda: Pluralism and Paradigms*. Albany: State University of New York.

21 Desai, P. (2006). Health, faith tradition, and South Asian Indians in North America. In: L.L. Barnes, S.S. Sered (eds) *Religion and Healing in America*. New York: Oxford University Press.

22 Mysorekar, U. (2006). Eye on religion: clinicians and Hinduism. *Sthn Med J* **99**(4): 441.

CHAPTER 7

The western humanist tradition

Stan van Hooft

Introduction

Western humanism is not a single strand of thought. Indeed, so various is the use of the term 'Humanism', that it is almost impossible to give a single and unequivocal definition of it. It first came to prominence in the Renaissance of the fourteenth to seventeenth centuries when it was discovered that ancient philosophers and writers could be as inspirational and informative as to the values by which to live as could the sacred texts of established religion. The study of the 'humanities' inaugurated at that time still undergirds the traditional idea of the university as a seat of higher learning. Today, however, the term is often associated with a militant form of secularism that utterly rejects religion, mysticism, and the sacred.[1,2] Secular humanists of this stripe can be found arguing against religious instruction in schools, and defending science against creationists and other religious dogmatists. However, not all forms of modern humanism are polemical in this way. There are also forms of psychology and psychotherapy that describe themselves as 'humanistic'. Describing itself as a 'third force' in psychology alongside behaviourism and psychoanalysis, humanistic psychology fully acknowledges individual autonomy and the pursuit of self-actualization in the lives of all individuals.[3] Such an acknowledgement also marks the discourses of the 'medical humanities', which are sensitive to the existential and personal attributes of clinical patients. Nor was humanistic psychology unaware of the significance of spirituality. Some of its practitioners, such as Abraham Maslow (1908–1970), were instrumental in developing the field of 'transpersonal psychology', which 'is concerned with the study of humanity's highest potential, and with the recognition, understanding, and realization of unitive, spiritual, and transcendent states of consciousness.'[4]

My aim in this chapter is not to describe any of these humanistic movements in detail. Nor is it to provide a detailed narrative in the history of ideas which would explain their emergence. Rather, it is to explore certain themes in the Western philosophical tradition upon which humanism in its many forms has drawn. This, in turn, will reveal that some of these themes offer considerable potential for a humanistic spirituality.

Plato

The Athenian philosopher, Plato (427–347 BCE), saw the world as unstable and dangerous. It was full of variation and unreliability and he longed for a realm of eternal changelessness. The metaphor that he used to express the nature of our world was that of mud: a substance that weighs one down and prevents free movement; that obscures, endangers, and pollutes the realm of existence. If the world seemed inhospitable to us in this way, then a new realm of reality would have to be posited to be the object of our longing. Accordingly, behind the deceptive and hazardous appearances of worldly things there lay a realm of eternal 'Forms', which were posited as the timeless and flawless archetypes of the things of this world. Each individual thing was what it was by virtue of its drawing its reality from an archetypal essence that existed in the realm of Forms. However, it could never be a perfect example of that essence. It could only be a pale copy. Being immersed in the material substance of this realm of beings, it could only aspire to the quality of perfect Being, which the realm of Forms represented.

Plato's conception of knowledge drew upon these metaphysical theories. The problem that he faced in this domain was that of uncertainty and irreconcilable disagreement. His mentor and friend, Socrates, has been put to death by the citizens of Athens because those citizens had not been able to understand the intellectual work that Socrates had been doing amongst them. They were immersed in a socially-constructed sphere of opinion, while Socrates had sought to open them to a rationally constructed sphere of wisdom. The citizens of Athens had rejected '*Philo-Sophia*', the love of wisdom, and preferred their mythical beliefs in the gods of tradition. No agreement could be reached, it seemed, by debate alone. People were too readily swayed by rhetoric and by their desire for comforting beliefs. How could true and certain knowledge be established then? By turning away from this world and discovering non-worldly objects of knowledge, the clarity, beauty, and primordiality of which would convince even the most sceptical. Such objects of knowledge included the Forms, especially the Forms of Goodness, Beauty, and Truth. Wisdom and certainty could not be found in this world because it was full of distractions and obscurity. Even our senses can be deceived by so simple a phenomenon as a straight stick that looked bent in water. How much more could our ideas be swayed by the force of public opinion and the skills of wily orators? Better to concentrate on the eternal and certain Forms.

However, with what could we exercise such concentration? If our physical bodies were the seat of appetites and desires, and if these appetites and desires, in turn, were the source of the distractions that draw us away from the Forms, then what hope have we of attaining wisdom? Plato's answer was that we were possessed of a soul that was not only the source of our rational powers, but also of a unique desire and enthusiasm: namely, the longing for wisdom. This inner fire, unique to human beings, burned with a love of Truth, Beauty and Goodness. It yearned for union with those other-worldly Forms—a union that, if achieved, would ensure the attainment of true knowledge, spiritual beauty, and moral goodness. The existential task of life, then, was to seek to extricate the soul from its bodily and worldly entrapments, and set it free to fly to that metaphysical space beyond this world where it could enjoy its fulfilment in spiritual rapport with the Forms.

Plato created images and metaphors to express these theories that have resonated throughout the Western tradition. Most notable was *The Republic's* story of the cave in which we are asked to imagine human beings imprisoned and held in such a way that they could only see the shadows of objects cast upon the wall of the cave by a fire within it. One day a prisoner breaks free of his chains and sees the real objects, the shadows of which he had thought constituted reality. However, even this revelation is not enough for him. He ventures out of the cave and sees reality as it is illuminated by the sun and he realizes that only in this bright light can the world be known for what it is. The most important reality to come to know is the other-worldly light in the light of which this-worldly things can be known. This man's soul has achieved a kind of freedom, enlightenment, and wisdom that the other prisoners in the cave could not even dream of.

Then there is the story of Diotima, the prophetess who, through the mouth of Socrates, provides the final speech on love in the *Symposium*. Diotima's teaching is that love between human beings in this world is but a preliminary lesson in the ascent to wisdom, which our souls long to pursue. While worldly physical love give us a taste for beauty, and a passionate and partial experience of it, we should grasp this mere glimpse and use it to acknowledge our need of a fuller, purer rapport with Beauty as such. In this way, worldly love can be a first step on a spiritual ascent in which the soul sets itself free from mortal and physical involvements in order to secure a vision of the Form of Beauty. The love that would blossom when that vision is achieved would be more glorious than any flawed and worldly love between bodily beings. It would be a love of the Forms.

However, the most striking figure in Plato's oeuvre is Socrates himself. Socrates has guided his life by the nostrum that the unexamined life is not worth living. Self-knowledge and rational critique are of crucial value to him. See him now in his prison cell condemned to drink the poisonous hemlock for having tried to dissuade the youth of Athens from their mythical beliefs in the gods of Olympus. He comforts his friends and assures them that, despite his condemnation, the life of a lover of wisdom is a worthy one. He convinces them that his soul is immortal and speculates that the souls of good men go on to places of bliss and contemplation. If one has spent one's life in the pursuit of Goodness, Beauty, and Truth, then one will enjoy communion in the afterlife with others who have also attained such wisdom. One's soul will then, at last, be free from the distractions and temptations of worldly existence, and will enjoy a peace and fulfilment that it is difficult for human beings enthralled by this world to even imagine.

Plato's philosophy was assimilated by the fathers of the early Christian church in order to provide the conceptual framework for the Christian religion. Indeed, it could be said to echo in its structure and basic concepts the metaphysical beliefs of almost all of the great world religions. These religions all teach that we have a soul the destiny of which is more important than that of our bodies and whose nature is akin to, and destined for, a realm of reality more perfect and more glorious than this material world. Most religions are Platonic in form.

However, this is not the theme I wish to explore here. My point is that, despite Platonism's affinity to religious thinking, it can also support certain strands of humanism. This strand of humanism sees human existence as containing, or aspiring to, a 'transcendental' dimension. Such humanists argue that human beings have dignity and value because their existence opens them to a transcendental realm, which takes them out of the everyday realities of quotidian existence. This dimension need not take the form of religious faith, but it nevertheless constitutes a love which gives truth to the claim that 'man does not live by bread alone'. On this conception, human beings are seen as beings whose spiritual nature places them midway between the animality of beasts and the divinity of gods.

A further crucial point is that the capacity of human beings to be open to a transcendental dimension is inherent in those human beings themselves. Whereas Christianity asserts that human beings can seek to attain the ultimate transcendence: God, only with the assistance of God's grace, and whereas Judaism envisages God as reaching down towards humanity in order to enter into a covenant with the people He had chosen, humanists believe that our longing for transcendence and our openness to it are features of the human condition that are not dependent upon any supernatural or metaphysical agencies or initiatives. It is humanity itself that is open to the transcendental dimension. At no point does Plato appeal to anything like divine revelation or grace. Whereas more ancient Greek thinkers and those of many other traditions sought to discern the truths whereby we should live in mythological texts and narratives, and whereas the 'religions of the book'—Judaism, Christianity and Islam—depended upon what was believed to be the written revelation of God to his people, Plato inaugurated the tradition of using human reason unaided by myth or dogma to discover wisdom and ascend to the transcendent. He distrusted written texts and presented his philosophy in the form of dialogues in which anyone of normal intelligence could engage in discussion with a view to achieving insight. There was need for neither divine inspiration nor the unique access to wisdom claimed by gurus or the spiritually enlightened.

I would submit, however, that what the Platonic tradition has in common with religion, and where it is not consistent with the spirit of humanism, is that it is driven by fear of the threats that a changeable world contains, by distrust of desire and of the appetites of the body, by a need for certainty in knowledge, by a longing for moral assurance, by a desire for immortality, and by a tendency to turn spiritual intuition into metaphysical doctrine. For a more fully humanistic account of spirituality we will have to turn to that other great philosopher of ancient Greece—Aristotle.

Aristotle

Aristotle (384–322 BCE) was a scientist, as well as a philosopher. He spent years of his life in minute and painstaking studies of living organisms and plants. He described the intricacies of the many sea creatures that he found in the rock pools of Lesbos. He made studies of the anatomies of human beings and other animals. (He never doubted that human beings were indeed animals.) He postulated explanatory hypotheses about the motions of planets and stars, as well as of earthly bodies. He was fascinated by rock formations and by the patterns of the weather. He was not persuaded by a bent-looking straight stick to distrust his senses, but sought to explain such phenomena. A lifetime of such studies could not have been engaged in by a thinker who thought that the world was nothing more than a dangerous and doleful staging point for a more perfect form of life in a realm of transcendence.

Aristotle was also interested in the arts and gave an account, still recognizable by modern psychology, of the effect that drama had on its audience. His theory of politics recognized the interdependence of human beings, and his ethics urged us to fulfil the better parts of our human natures so as to achieve worldly happiness. When he turned to metaphysics and to the ultimate explanations of reality, he did posit a 'Prime Mover' in order to account for motion, but at no point did he give this entity the characteristics of personality or divinity. Aristotle's world was *this* world: a quotidian world of natural processes, understandable change, human interactions, and achievable hopes. Most importantly this was a world in which human beings could, if they used their rational capacities, improve their lot, ameliorate their condition, and achieve happiness. It was a world that was deeply meaningful without having to be consecrated by metaphysical or religious entities in order to be a home for human beings.

Nevertheless, Aristotle did acknowledge, and indeed, celebrate, the transcendental dimension of human existence. His analysis of human subjectivity makes this clear. His conception of the human soul was not that of some pilgrim presence in the body whose destiny was to continue in a blissful, eternal, disembodied existence in an afterlife, but of an energizing principle that moved the body towards the fulfilment of four teleological functions—to live, feel, think, and contemplate. Living involved biological processes and instinctive appetites. Feeling involved desires, emotions, and motivations—both those of which we were aware and those of which we were not. Thinking involved practical understanding of the world and those rational, means-end calculations that enable us to attain what we desire and to make a success of our worldly enterprises. Contemplation involved reflection upon those realities that we could not change by our own means: realities like the rules of logic and the laws of nature, the values inherent in ethics and politics, the beauty of art, and the nature of the gods. These were matters the contemplation of which would take us out of our everyday existence and into a spiritual realm in which we would fulfil the potentialities of our human natures. If happiness is achieved by fulfilling our human potentials and if the capacity for contemplation is one of those potentials, then no human life would be complete without some engagement with transcendence.

A happy human being, for Aristotle, is one who lives a life free of bodily deprivations, in harmony with others, with responsibility towards her environment and community, with equanimity, and with sensitivity to the ultimate realities and values that give meaning to such a life. Human beings have within themselves and amongst themselves the spiritual resources to live such a life without recourse to any other-worldly, metaphysical, or divine sources of insight.

Prometheus

Another strand in the traditions of humanism is represented by a mythical figure of ancient Greece—Prometheus. As described by the ancient poet, Hesiod (active between 750 and 650 BCE), Prometheus is a semi-divine Titan who stole fire from the gods in order to give it to humankind. For giving to human beings this supposedly divine power, Prometheus was condemned to be chained to a rock where an eagle's talons would eternally claw at his ever-renewing body. Many writers and artists have celebrated the deeds and suffering of Prometheus in gratitude for the capacities that he is said to have bestowed upon humanity. Given these capacities, human beings could now control their own destinies. Rather than living at the behest of the gods or at the whims of fate, human beings could develop the knowledge and technologies that would allow them to bend the forces of nature to their wills and harness the resources that the world offered them.

The most striking implication of this myth was the vision of humanity that it fostered. Human beings were seen as having stolen power from the gods, and as having acquired the ability to control and improve their own lives. This vision of human strength and self-affirmation, of defiance of the gods, and of power over nature has been bequeathed to us in the spirit of modern science and technology.

Humanism and modernism

We have now seen the development of at least three traditions of humanism: the Platonic, the Aristotelian, and the Promethean. These traditions have developed and intermingled so as to produce the complex and multifaceted face of humanism today.

The first, Platonic tradition involves a turning away from the world in order to find wisdom and spirituality in a metaphysical realm. Even in the cases where this realm did not comprise religious entities and events, it postulated such abstract and idealized human capacities as free will, pure reason, and the moral law, and hoped for the realization of such perfectionist ideals as complete release from suffering, absolute purity of heart, a bond of love with the infinite, an irrefutable scientific theory of everything, world-wide unanimity in beliefs and values, perpetual peace, and the total elimination of injustice everywhere in the world. These concepts and ideals are Platonic in that they devalue anything that is imperfect, changeable, or uncertain. The Aristotelian tradition is more complex. It stresses the need to be at home in the world and happy in life even as we contemplate their unchangeable realities. It speaks of the perfectibility of human beings in muted tones and shows a reverence for the changeable world, as well as for the fragile, vulnerable, fallible, and mortal condition of being human. [6] However, it is the Promethean tradition, with its celebration of science, progress, and technology, that has had the greatest effect upon modern civilization and spirituality.

The history of how these three traditions interacted and influenced each other, and of how Prometheanism emerged triumphant, is fascinating. Despite the work of such philosophers as Epicurus (341–270 BCE) and Seneca (ca. 1 BCE–65 CE), the celebration of human, worldly existence that Aristotle inaugurated was all but driven underground in the West by that religious graft onto Platonism called Christianity. However, with the rediscovery of the ancient Greek and Roman legacies in the Renaissance, new explorations into the human condition and into the workings of nature without the strictures of biblical authority were begun by Petrarch (1304–1374) in the humanities and Galileo (1564–1642) in the natural sciences. Erasmus of Rotterdam (1466–1536) rejected the authority of tradition and studied the bible as a human historical document. The culmination of these various streams of thought was the Enlightenment: a movement that its greatest philosopher, Immanuel Kant (1724–1804), interpreted as giving humanity permission, for the first time, to think for itself.

Once the Enlightenment had taken hold there was no stopping its development into the Promethean modernism with which we are familiar today. It was soon taken for granted that human beings had both the capacity, and the right to take hold of nature and of history in order to make a better world in accordance with human standards of happiness and progress. In politics the divine rights of kings and hereditary rulers were replaced by liberal ideas of the rights of man, the sovereignty of the people, and uncoerced, democratic participation in politics. The idea that the moral standing of all human beings was equal despite race, class, ethnicity, gender, religion, or language was the fulfilment of an Enlightenment dream for all humanity. The sciences flourished and gave rise to technological wonders that have lightened the burden of daily living for millions around the world, and created an effluorescence of comforts and gadgets to delight consumers everywhere. Modernism is, above all, a belief in progress and in the human ability to harness that progress for the betterment of humankind.

However, this unquestioning faith in technological, political, and social progress is waning today. The exploitation of the environment and of third world peoples that has come in the wake of technological developments constitutes a dark undercurrent of this so-called progress. As the costs of modernism and the problems of technological development mount, new solutions will have to be found. The key point, however, is that it is human beings that will have to find these solutions. The modern Promethean belief is that time and human ingenuity will eventually solve these problems. No one today seriously believes, as Martin Heidegger had put it, that 'only a god can save us.'[7]

One reason for this is that Promethean modernism has 'disenchanted' the world, to use Max Weber's phrase. A modern scientific explanation is typically 'reductionist' in the sense that it seeks to reduce natural phenomena to push-pull causal mechanisms, and 'materialist' in the sense that it accepts as cogs in those mechanisms only entities or forces that can be described in physical and measurable terms. There is neither mystery nor meaning in such mechanistic conceptions, even as they deliver to human beings the power to harness their new knowledge to the purposes of technology. While modern science has freed us from belief in magic, miracles, or the healing power of shamans, it has robbed nature of any inherent depth or beauty. Infinity has been reduced to very large numbers and mystery to a problem yet to be solved.

Even the social sciences have sought to explain human and social events in causal and quantifiable terms. The positivist sociology of Auguste Comte (1798–1857) and the behaviourist psychology of B.F. Skinner (1904–1990) sought to reduce human reality to the play of blind forces on the model of the physical sciences. In the hands of many analytic philosophers this led to a conception of human reality in which anything that could not be explained by science was seen as the mere expression of emotion. Moral norms, aesthetic values and political ideals were reduced to the desires and preferences of individual human beings. And these desires and preferences, in turn, were nothing more than manipulable dispositions towards self-serving behaviour. In this way Promethean thought unknowingly delivered mechanisms of social control into the hands of political power and the advertising industry.

Today, we tend to approach the world and one another as resources. We have come to understand nature and people in largely instrumental terms. We have lost the Aristotelian capacity to contemplate them in their essence. We have silenced the Platonic love of the transcendent. As a result, the only joys we are left with are the fleeting seductions of consumerism and the infantile distractions of popular entertainment.[8] We have a human world—a world whose conceptual construction is based on human knowledge systems[9] and whose functional efficiency is based on human ingenuity[10]—but it is a world that lacks a spiritual dimension.

Towards a humanist theory of spirituality

What resources for spirituality can humanism give us then? Can the Platonic and Aristotelian traditions be revived to enrich and spiritualize the Promethean ethos that dominates our lives? What would a humanist theory of spirituality look like?

Three answers to that last question can be gleaned from Plato. First, it would be a theory that was rationally understandable and discursively accessible to anyone of average intelligence, rather than one handed down by mystery-mongering manipulators or new-age gurus. Secondly, it would understand human subjectivity in ways that showed it to be open to transcendence. Thirdly, it would point to forms and sources of transcendence that answer to our love and yearning for goodness, truth and beauty. From Aristotle we would learn that human subjectivity has the capacity to contemplate such forms of transcendence, but that they are to be found in this world, rather than in the realm of metaphysics. They are not to take the form of supernatural entities or powers with which we would stand in a relationship of subservience or worship. We must not reject the lessons of the scientific legacy that Aristotle inaugurated and seek a theory that would allude to magic, miracles, or any agencies not amenable, in principle, to human understanding. Our humanism must ground a theory that allows us to engage thoroughly with the material world, rather than escape into a spiritual ivory tower.

In order to understand such a humanist theory of spirituality we need to explore the word 'transcendence'. We might begin by saying that it refers to what we cannot know. What we can know is the world we live in. Knowledge is the way we structure that lived world through our empirical experiences, conceptual classifications, and scientific explanations. Knowledge is a form of possession of the world. Of course, the world may contain cognitive and scientific puzzles to which we have no ready solutions, but we know why they are puzzles and we know, more or less, how to go about solving them. The Promethean outlook that modernism has bequeathed to us assures us that human knowledge and human progress are without limit so long as we focus on what is objective, real, and given us in worldly experience. Our known and lived world is a world of objects understood, social formations adhered to, and rules followed. It is a world in which things have a use, others have a role, and I have obligations. It is a world of productivity, efficient service delivery, and economic growth.

However, we are dimly aware of something more. We are aware that beyond the Promethean structures of knowledge that we use to apprehend, classify, and possess this world, there are things that cannot be known. I use the word 'things' because grammar requires a noun to be placed in this sentence, but what I am referring to are not things. If they were they would be included in the inventory of worldly items and would be assimilated into my practical-Promethean way of thinking as objects to be known or problems to be solved. No, these 'things' are beyond the world, ungraspable, and unassimilable. They are, from the point of view of worldly knowledge, mysteries. They are transcendent.

The first of these transcendent mysteries is my own subjectivity. Why do I love those whom I love? Why am I committed to certain moral values? Why do I love the music I love? Why do I find the world so awe-inspiring? Who is the 'I' in these formulations? These questions have no satisfactory answers. The selves that are the object of such reflections are psychological constructs at least one step removed from our existential inwardness. Our subjectivity is not structured by our concepts and understandings, and cannot be rationally grasped or explained. It cannot even be intuited through reflection or seen through introspection. It is manifested by how we experience the world rather than by how we understand ourselves. It is the hidden depth of who we are. We can have no cognitive grasp of ourselves because we are not objects to ourselves. Subjectivity cannot be an object of experience.[11] Even if I were to reflect on myself, the subject of that reflection would not be the object of that reflection, and so I would always escape myself. Accordingly, there can be no direct awareness of subjectivity. We cannot be aware of awareness as such. We can only know the quality and forms of our subjectivity by reading them off the objects that appear to us in experience. It is because I experience visual objects that I know that I can see. It is because I am delighted to see my beloved that I know I love her. It is because of what I do that I know what my commitments are.

However, I can infer what the existential quality of my subjectivity is. Let us return to Plato's cave, but this time imagine that there is no light in it at all. It is so dark that I cannot see anything. There are no visual objects that I can see. Darkness is, after all, not a thing that I see, but the absence of any seen things. While there may be objects that I am experiencing non-visually—sounds, movements of air, or the touch of my clothes on my body—my visual field is empty. I can be aware that my eyes are open, but this awareness makes my eyes—not my seeing—into an object of my proprioception. What then is happening here? It is not only that, objectively, my eyes are open and functioning. It is also that I am open to my empty visual surroundings. I am looking. As soon as the lights come on, that looking will be rewarded by alighting upon objects that I can then see. However, without the light, my sight is in a pure state of emptiness, lack, and seeking. Accordingly, looking in total darkness is an accurate analogy for pure subjectivity. My subjectivity is a reaching out to the world and is already in a relationship to it of longing. However, this relation is transcendent in that it is not itself an object of knowledge. My subjectivity is a transcendent reality.

Plato envisaged subjectivity as imprisoned in a dark cave and seeking the light by which it could attain knowledge. However, then he turned that seeking subjectivity into a metaphysical entity called the soul and suggested that it had an eternal destiny in a life hereafter. In this way, he turned a transcendent mystery into an object of knowledge. He gave the status of a knowable, metaphysical entity to the inner core of our being. Moreover, this metaphysics gives us a life-long responsibility for the destiny of our immortal souls. Accordingly, it also gives us a self-centred mission in life—a mission that involves our souls controlling the inclinations of our bodily existence, directing our attention to the realm of Forms, and thereby deflecting us from responding to the transcendent and spiritual dimensions of the world we live in. If only Plato had retained Diotima's conception of the soul as a lack and emptiness which we seek to fill with such objects of love as Beauty, Truth, and Goodness.

A second transcendence to which the lives of all of us are attuned is 'the Other'. This phrase, with its capital 'O', comes from the writings of Emmanuel Lévinas (1906–1995).[12] He describes human encounters as a meeting between our hidden subjectivity and the face of another person. When we are conversing with someone—especially someone we know well—we look into their face and experience a remarkable epiphany. We think we know this person—and in everyday terms we do—but we also feel that their face discloses an unknowable mystery. We experience a depth and an infinity, as Lévinas calls it, which tells us that we are in encounter with a reality that cannot be known. That Promethean form of cognitive possession is not possible in response to a disclosure of the infinite mystery of the Other. The irony is that the better we know someone in an everyday psychological sense, the less we know them in this deep sense. The person from whom we buy our railway ticket might as well be a machine—and nowadays often is—but the person we love is a transcendence to us. Our relation to the Other is not one of cognitive possession, but one of longing and openness. Indeed, Lévinas argues that the Other draws us out of our own egoistic self-preoccupation so that we become a being-for-the-Other. Our very subjectivity—that transcendent mystery to ourselves—becomes a real self and a social being insofar as it is drawn towards the Other.

For Lévinas the implications of this are ethical. He concludes that what turns our empty subjectivity into an active participant in the world is our responsibility for others—a responsibility that has been evoked in us by the epiphany in our lives of the Other. Rather than our existential selfhood being constituted by a Promethean act of self-affirmation, it is constituted by our responsibility for the Other—a responsibility born of responsiveness to that Other. The term 'Other' becomes here a name for that transcendence our love of which constitutes both myself as an ethical person and the other person as the object of my ethical responsibility. As Lévinas puts it, the Other evokes in me my goodness. Note the echo here of the Platonic thought that Goodness is one of the transcendent objects of our longing. However, while Plato locates that object in the realm of metaphysics, Lévinas locates it in the human world. Rather than taking Diotima's path away from love of others to a metaphysical realm, Lévinas urges us to find goodness and beauty here in the world through authentic encounters with others.

Notice also how the themes of Beauty and Goodness have come together here and have become further names for transcendence. To include Truth in this synthesis we will need to return to Aristotle. What we need is a non-Promethean, non-possessive conception of knowledge of the world. Such a conception can arise from Aristotle's notion of contemplation. Aristotle realized that of all the things we think about there are some that are beyond our capacity to possess or to manipulate for our own purposes. Our Promethean reach does not extend to the laws of nature themselves or to the immensities of the universe. We cannot change the laws of logic and mathematics, the human goal of happiness, the demands of sociality, and the nature of beauty or goodness. If we have a capacity to think about such things at all it must be in a mode of thinking that is marked by awe and reverence. Such contemplation would allow us to love the world without seeking to possess it: to understand the world without turning it into an object of technological manipulation.

Aristotle included the gods amongst the objects of this capacity for contemplation, and theologians have elaborated on this by describing a pantheon of supernatural beings for us to worship. Humanism would reject such objects, but not the capacity for contemplation that is posited with them. This capacity provides us with a mode of knowing, the objects of which are transcendent. If the objects of worldly knowledge are defined as truths, then we may call the transcendence which is an object of non-Promethean, contemplative knowledge, 'Truth'. This does not explain very much, but then we are talking about a mystery. It is a mystery, however, to which we respond with yearning. It is this yearning that pushes us to ever greater efforts at discovery and understanding. It is what leads us to reject creationist explanations for the existence of reality, for example, as lacking, not only intellectual warrant, but also any respect for the mystery of existence. Such putative metaphysical explanations close off our yearning for Truth and give us a pseudo-certainty.

Conclusion

Spirituality is reverence, love, and humility in the presence of transcendence. While religions give the names of their gods to this transcendence, humanism gives it other names: Subjectivity, the Other, Beauty, Goodness, and Truth. Humanism's deepest intuition may well be that these names signify but one reality.

References

1 Dawkins, R. (2006). *The God Delusion*. London: Transworld Publishers.

2 Hitchens, C. (2007). *God is not Great: How Religion Poisons Everything*. New York: Hachette Books.

3 Association for Humanistic Psychology. (2001). *Humanistic Psychology Overview*. Available at: http://www.ahpweb.org/aboutahp/whatis.html (accessed 4 April, 2011).

4 Lajoie, D.H., Shapiro, S.I. (1992). Definitions of transpersonal psychology: the first twenty-three years. *J Transpers Psychol* **24**(1): 79–98.

5 Nussbaum, M. (2001). *The Fragility of Goodness: Luck and Ethics in Greek Tragedy and Philosophy*, rev edn. Cambridge: Cambridge University Press.

6 Ricoeur, P. (1986). *Fallible Man*, Charles A. Kelbley (transl). New York: Fordham University Press.

7 Heidegger, M. (1981). 'Nur noch ein Gott kann uns retten' *Der Spiegel* 30 Mai, 1976, pp. 193–219, W. Richardson (transl) as 'Only a God Can Save Us'. In: T. Sheehan (ed.) *Heidegger: The Man and the Thinker*, pp. 45–67. Chicago: Precedent Publishing.

8 Carroll, J. (2004). *The Wreck of Western Culture: Humanism Revisited*. Melbourne: Scribe.

9 Cooper, D.E. (2002). *The Measure of Things: Humanism, Humility and Mystery*. Oxford: Clarendon Press.

10 Ellul, J. (1978). *The Betrayal of the West*, Matthew J. O'Connell (transl). New York: Seabury Press.

11 Larmore, C. (2010). *The Practices of the Self*, Sharon Bowman (transl). Chicago: University of Chicago Press.

12 Lévinas, E. (1979). *Totality and Infinity: an Essay on Exteriority*, Alphonso Lingis (transl). The Hague: M. Nijhoff Publishers.

CHAPTER 8

Indigenous spiritualities

Graham Harvey

Introduction

Indigenous spiritualities are as various as the cultures and/or lifeways of which they are integral elements. However, while it would be a serious error to imagine a single form of indigeneity, there are some common themes shared among diverse indigenous knowledges and experiences worldwide. Some of these are a result of similar experiences of colonial assaults and the consequent marginalization and dispossession suffered by most indigenous peoples. More positively, however, some are a result of matters that are implicit, at least, in the term indigenous. As a near synonym of aboriginal, indigenous immediately suggests a long-lasting and celebrated (not merely accidental) link to place, land, or country, and to previous generations (sometimes called 'ancestors'). It almost automatically conjures up ideas about community, rather than individuality. Indeed, one challenge for those concerned with indigenous health knowledges and issues, even those committed to holistic therapies, is to fully engage with the widespread understanding among indigenous peoples that 'community' not only involves ancestors, the present generation, and those yet to be born, but may also embrace other-than-human species dwelling locally.

This chapter introduces some key facets of indigenous knowledge (usually best seen in practice or performance) that are necessary features of an understanding of what health and healthcare might mean in relation to indigenous peoples. In particular, it engages with what can (with some care) be called animist worldviews, a reference to the pervasive relational ontologies and epistemologies of many indigenous peoples. It considers some definitions of health as 'good living', which call on people to live with respect for others. The activities and practices of traditional diviners, healers, shamans, and medicine people are introduced. Understanding relationships also leads to understanding the widespread notion that ill-health has relational causes, sometimes caused by breaches of tabu, sometimes by the machinations that might be called 'witchery'. Even when dispossessed from land and communal belonging, indigenous people's health needs are often still tied in to more relational than individualist notions of what it means to be a person. This may be true either because such people maintain 'traditional' habits of living and knowledge or because they are stereotypically treated as 'different' by the dominant society. In short, this chapter tries to consider a range of ways in which health and indigenous spiritualities might intersect and require further consideration.

Defining indigeneity

Perhaps it is necessary to say that the definitional priority of land or place is clear to indigenous people who use terms like 'indigenous'. In contrast, emphasis on time, antiquity, or originality seems most obvious in more dominant discourses. However, the underlying contention in both indigenous and modernist discourses about aboriginality is about land ownership, rather than merely historical priority. European peoples' geographic expansionism has inevitably and obviously ruptured or shattered indigenous belonging and ownership. Claims to have discovered, explored, and settled in places where others were already 'at home' or indigenous, are clearly not objective value-free statements, but assertions about ownership and belonging. Their impact on indigenous health continues to be immensely damaging.

Simultaneously, by their determined avowal of full participation in the contemporary era, indigenous peoples reject their ghettoization as fossils of some fictional pre-contact or 'primal' culture, or as strange beings that cannot move or migrate. Forced exile, dislocation, and alienation from place, land, or country (often understood as community) are common facts of recent and continuing indigenous experience. However, so too are the ability to travel, migrate, and connect with other communities (indigenous or otherwise) globally. In various ways and in various forums, indigenous people commonly reject the notion that movement negates indigenous identity, heritage, culture, or needs.

The terms indigenous and indigeneity are currently the subject of fierce academic debate. Trigger and Dalley[1] helpfully elaborate on the contrast between those who see indigenous as a relational term, necessarily contrasted with various 'others' (e.g. colonialists, settlers, modernists, nation states) and those who seek 'criterial' qualities that can be identified only among those appropriately labelled indigenous. My approach, drawing from elements of both relational and criterial approaches, may suggest an unresolved fuzziness, but it deliberately engages with both indigenous and academic rhetorics in which ebb and flow between relational and criterial, theoretical and activist, critical and polemical, and other uses of these terms are evident. I assert that this fluidity of usage is necessary because indigeneity in lived reality is itself more fuzzy than neatly theoretical. In particular, indigeneity labels diverse realities that are more appropriately labelled and engaged with under specific locally appropriate names that refer to nations, peoples, clans, families, and other social collectives. While indigenous peoples share many common experiences, not all of their responses, protocols, needs, and wishes are applicable or evident elsewhere, let alone everywhere. Just as it would be wrong to assume that all indigenous people have a single experience of colonialism, it would be equally misleading to categorize groups according to a single social, cosmological, epistemological, or religious model. Not all indigenous societies are small scale (especially if the Yoruba nation and its diaspora are considered 'indigenous,' which is a topic of debate in several political arenas) and not all of them face the same degree of cultural-genocide or linguistic-extinction as, undoubtedly, others do.

All of this is to say that indigenous spiritualities need to be approached carefully with a view to understanding how particular, local and inherited notions of belonging (to place, ancestry and community)—ones that do not fix people in alien structures, but do recognize the impact of larger social and political collectives—might enhance people's wellbeing or, when damaged, contribute to their ill-health. In this necessarily brief overview, I focus on some commonalities, but encourage a more robustly localizing engagement in dialogue with indigenous knowledge holders. Vicki Grieves'[2] discussion paper, *Aboriginal Spirituality: Aboriginal Philosophy, The Basis of Aboriginal Social and Emotional Wellbeing*, is an excellent example (in its methods and its results) of the kind of work that is absolutely necessary for a fuller understanding both of local and global indigenous knowledge in this context.

Indigenous knowledges

There is now a large and growing interest in 'indigenous knowledge' related to local, regional, and global concerns and movements. In particular, environmental and botanical knowledge are receiving intense international attention. Attempts to deal with global climate change include carbon-sink trading and hydroelectric projects, for example, that immediately threaten indigenous sovereignty over land-use and even the existence of land itself. It is important, however, to note that the current growth in interest in indigenous knowledges coincides with the rising confidence of indigenous peoples that their cultures do indeed contain important knowledge that is worthy of careful research and testing, and that these can and do provide secure foundations for confronting pollution, poverty, disease, and other global problems.

It is noteworthy that 'indigenous knowledge' can act as a synonym for 'tradition,' but does not carry the baggage of the latter term's suggested reference to the past. Among many indigenous peoples, tradition is that which has been passed to the current generation by ancestors (remote or recent) for further elaboration and investigation. Its robustness in changing circumstances requires that 'tradition' be understood not as inflexible rules handed down by unchallengeable ancestors, but as paradigms and protocols that have served previous generations well and might, when tested, be applicable in the future. Evidence of the flexibility of tradition is provided in the ways in which many indigenous health care systems creatively adopt or adapt ideas, practices, and solutions drawn from other cultures. For these reasons, the term tradition will be used here in ways that resonate with indigenous ways of speaking, rather than with Eurocentric rhetorics.

Importantly, too, 'indigenous knowledge' avoids the errors generated by talking about 'belief' or 'believing.' This is not only to indicate that belief is usually an alien category to most traditional indigenous people, or at least to acknowledge that someone else's innermost ideas and thoughts are usually treated as their own business—at least until they act on them in ways that affect other people. Perhaps more provocatively, it is also to resist the implication that 'we know, they only believe'. Derived from a peculiarly European historical contrast between religion and science, this use of 'believe' allows the speaker to find a place in their own preferred knowledge system for the ideas and practices of 'others,' but this is necessarily a subservient, rather than challenging place. Believers are people who have not yet grasped the knowledge 'we' offer. Beliefs are, allegedly, untested or authoritarian ideas or dogmas that contrast with the experimentation that is claimed as 'scientific method'. However, if 'we' were to recognize 'them' as having knowledge, rather than mere belief we might have to take such knowledge seriously, test its value, and perhaps (at an extreme) we would find that it is preferable to what we previously thought we knew.[3,4] Thus, speaking of 'knowledge', rather than alleging 'belief' seems most appropriate in any attempt to understand indigenous perspectives, experiences, and contributions to debate.

That this is relevant, indeed vital, to understanding indigenous spirituality is revealed by a consideration of the late Maori academic Te Pakaka Tawhai's[5,6] discussions of 'ancient explanations'. Tawhai demonstrates that ancestral knowledge are not about the past nor are they endlessly repeated, verbatim, purely to preserve particular words. Far from it. Users of inherited narratives use their flexibility and rich potential to engage fully with the issues of the present moment. They are spoken freshly and with improvizations each time so that new possibilities, new life can emerge. Precisely by taking narratives about creative beings and processes, and using them as illustrations for his discussion of contemporary Maori spirituality (i.e. doing something with them that is not typical of their previous usage), Tawhai demonstrates his point. Traditional indigenous knowledges address the present in ways that might have surprised the ancestors who passed them down. They may seem to be about the past, but they exist only to be spoken/performed into new contexts where they will make a difference. They are not primitivist or romanticizing 'just so' stories, disguising or purveying ignorance of the world. Rather, they are complex multi-layered encouragements to explore, test, consider, and, ultimately, enrich others by enhancing the potential emerging in the present moment, especially in the areas of health, sustenance, and happiness. Tawhai is far from alone in applying 'traditional' themes, ideas, practices, and protocols to the late modern era—or what several indigenous people have described to me, only partly jokingly, as 'most-modernity'. Practiced application is the intended purpose of indigenous knowledges and the protocols for knowing (coming to know/perform) that are embedded in such systems.

Relating in the larger than human world

Among the most common leitmotivs of shared discourse among indigenous peoples is the theme of relationship. While the societies of European origin have increasingly privileged individuality, indigenous nations and groups have tended to act on the assumption that people are defined by relationships. In contrast with Descartes' slogan 'I think therefore I am', it is possible to sum up much that is important to indigeneity in the phrase 'we relate, therefore we are'. While the imperative call to relate well (appropriately and to mutual and wider benefit) with others is at least implicit in this, something absolutely foundational is involved. In recent studies of cultures as diverse as the Indian Nayaka,[7] the Amazonian Araweté,[8,9] the Siberian Yukaghir,[10] and the First Nation Canadian Mi'kmaq,[11] a radical definition of 'person' has been debated and elaborated. Drawing on what Irving Hallowell learnt among the Ojibwa of the Berens River, Canada, in the 1940s, scholars have proffered a 'new animism'[12] to replace the exhausted and misleading theory of Edward Tylor (first professor of anthropology at Oxford University) that religion is, by definition, an error based on a belief in the existence of non-empirical beings. This false 'belief in spirits' was called 'animism' by Tylor.[13] It is not what the 'new animism' is about and deserves no further consideration here. Rather, 'animism' is now more helpfully used to label varied ways of treating the world as a community of persons, most of whom are not human, but all of whom deserve respect (even the unlikable ones). ('Animism' in its new usage has not yet received a universal welcome among indigenous peoples, and those who wish to avoid sounding colonialist and primitivist will find it best used with care.)

Indigenous knowledge does not typically put humanity at the centre of the cosmos or of local ecosystems. Rather, they conceive of humans as one species among many. We are not merely or accidentally co-inhabitants of environments, but co-citizens of multi-species communities. Indigenous traditions often speak of humans as engaged in important relationships with members of other species, maintained by appropriate etiquette, respectful ritual, constrained consumption, and narratives that iterate the needs and desires of this wider community. Many of the processes by which respect for others is inculcated among traditional indigenous people involve encouragement to pay attention to the interests of other-than-human persons. As a foundation for living, the idea that 'non-humans' or even objects might have such needs, desires, and interests can appear quite radical. That humans should not only notice these, but also take care to make their fulfilment possible (where this is in their control) is an outright challenge to the typically Western/modernist assumption that human needs always take priority. The contrast is encoded in indigenous uses of words like land or country, rather than ill-fitting words like environment (suggesting, as this often does, a mere backdrop to the important business of human lives). Similarly, the structuring of academia around a contrast between 'natural' and 'social' sciences encodes a separation between humanity and the world that probably does not work for anyone,[14] but certainly contradicts indigenous intimations of the social nature of the world.

A common theme implicit in many Native American and other indigenous narratives and ritual protocols is that humans are weak, and in need of considerable help from animals, birds, plants, and others. Only because others are considered to be willing to give up their lives can humans survive (whether in hunting or agricultural communities). Due to an inherent emphasis on human relationships with putative deities in the dominant Western religion, Christianity, many outsiders assume that indigenous people also privilege human relationships with 'spiritual beings' (e.g. deities, ancestors, spirits). However, some of the most significant inter-species relationships, according to indigenous knowledge systems, are between humans and other entirely mundane and ordinary co-inhabitants of particular (earthly, this-worldly) locations. Debbie Rose, for instance, encapsulates much that is important when she writes (in relation to some Aboriginal Australian ecological knowledge), 'there is a clear recognition that the lives of these beings are enmeshed in perduring relationships which bind people and certain animal or plant species together and thus differentiate them from others.'[15] The originally Ojibwe (Native American) word 'totem' is often translated as 'clan' and understood to indicate that an animal or plant symbolizes a human kinship group somewhere between a family and a tribe. However, a totemic clan is, in indigenous reality, a cross-species group in which some humans have a closer relationship with some animals or plants than they do with other humans. Their 'perduring relationships' commit them to mutual aid and to policing activities that might over-burden the ability of a place/community to sustain the well-being of its community. In short, it is not so much that 'animals are good to think' (as Claude Lévi-Strauss [16] summed it up), but that they are good relations. Their knowledge of the world and their many gifts to us (not only of meat, fur, and bone, but also of wisdom and wonder) deserve gratitude.

Wellbeing is, therefore, best understood in the context of the continuous negotiation of the needs and desires of persons (human and other-than-human) bound together by mutual dwelling, belonging to and/or emerging from a location. This being so, land rights are not an optional addition to indigenous culture, a mere desire to claim ownership over resources or boundaries. They are an integral element of identity in a far more profound sense than any 'settler' community has yet achieved. Similarly, ritual performances are not merely colourful expressions of cultural life, dramatic representations of deeply-held beliefs, or peculiar diversions from the everyday necessities of making a living. Rather, they are the currency that maintains and enhances the relationships of all persons (human and other-than-human) whose gift-giving to one another is definitive of life.[17] The banning of indigenous ceremonies by colonial powers in many nations served as one more assault on the communities constructed by the regular enactment of respect and gratitude towards those beings who made life possible. The revitalization of ceremonial life as one strand in the ongoing reassertion of the value of indigeneity and 'tradition' is not about romanticism, heritage, or attracting 'tourist dollars,' but about seeking to live properly in a world that should not be so thoroughly under human domination or so obsessively economic or consumerist. Since indigenous peoples and the larger-than-human multi-species community are usually the first victims of ecological devastation (including the current anthropogenic climate change and mass-extinction disasters), rituals re-asserting human participation in (rather than domination over, or distinction from) what the English language names 'nature' are a major part of the business of contemporary indigeneity as activism. (An important article about Aboriginal Australian 'labour' by Elizabeth Povinelli [18] provides another vital resource for thinking again about what it is that indigenous people do when they do ritual.)

Another Ojibwe term, *minobimaatisiiwin*, can be translated as 'live well', combining the thoughts 'have good health,' 'lead a good life' and 'prosper.'[19] Health and success, in the perspective of speakers of this and many other indigenous languages, are entangled with acting respectfully towards others. They are immediately and necessarily relational. It is not possible to be healthy or 'good' as a solitary individual. Indeed, many indigenous narratives ('myths' perhaps) present extremes of individualism not only as arrogant, but as threats to the world: they are antisocial not only in the sense normative in the West (impolite behaviours disturbing the peace of the polite majority), but undermining the foundations of sociality. Cannibals and other monsters seek their own way regardless of the needs of others.[20] Good people, in contrast, give and receive gifts, and share sustenance with those around them, those to whom they mutually committed by virtue of joint membership of an emplaced community. This complex of resonant associations with words for a 'good life' is a core reason for the prevalence of the word 'respect' in indigenous discourses about how people should act.

It is easy to mistake talk about relationship and respect as moral encouragements to relate. However, far more is at stake. The core point is that relating is definitive of personhood. Animism and, more broadly, indigenous knowledge, involves a statement about ontology: persons are relational. Thus, in one classic intercultural encounter, Irving Hallowell asked an unnamed old Ojibwe man 'are all the rocks we see around us here alive'?[21] In Ojibwe grammar, Hallowell had learnt, the word for rocks is marked as grammatically animate in much the same way that tables are marked as grammatical feminine in French. Do these peculiarities of speech arise from some deeper ontology or result in behaviours in which people might be observed acting towards rocks as persons or tables as females? Hallowell's teacher answered the question somewhat enigmatically, 'no, but some are'. He and other Ojibwe told Hallowell various ways in which they and their compatriots engaged in relationships with some rocks. Resolving the enigma, they showed that, as is often the case, the researcher was asking the wrong question. For the Ojibwe the issue is not whether or not rocks might be alive, animated, conscious, or active. It is not even how one might know or observe animation (in the sense of aliveness). Personhood is not a quality that is inherent in an individual's interiority. Rather, it is relational. Humans and rocks (and any other potential 'person') are only persons as and when they act relationally towards others. Gift-giving (or exchange), and rituals of greeting and respect are among the prime expressions of relational personhood towards others. A solitary individual is not properly a person. Perhaps an experiment in which we speak of 'personing' would provoke a reassessment of what it might mean to have such a thoroughly relational ontology.

Relational ill-health and healing

Among many indigenous peoples, it does not make sense to talk about accidents. This would not be an explanation, but a failure to explain. Things do not just happen. People do not get ill randomly, they do not die without cause. Illness is relational. This must be so because the world and cosmos are so thoroughly relational. Things happen because someone wills them to happen or acts in ways that cause them to happen.

Across sub-Saharan Africa it is commonly understood that the only 'natural' deaths are those of venerable old people who have led successful lives and produced heirs who will honour them. All other deaths are caused either by some fault of the person concerned or by some ill-wishing by another. Getting ill is also a result either of a fault or of another's bad intentions. A person might, for instance, have failed to show proper respect to a deserving being, or they might have breached a taboo or trespassed (inadvertently perhaps) into a separated-off domain. Sickness may result from attempting to refuse to follow one's destiny (perhaps without even knowing it). If illness or injury is the result of another's malevolent actions, the victim might have incurred the wrath of a witch or insulted someone who has asked a witch or a deity to direct punishing illnesses. Certainly contemporary traditional healers have adopted and adapted the Western originated knowledge of bacteria as causes of disease. However, perhaps it would be more accurate to speak of bacteria as the causative agent of disease: persons who act against others in ways that are detrimental to their well being. Mechanisms for regaining health include seeking understanding from a trained diviner (someone who manipulates diagnostic tools), offering sacrifices or other gifts that initiate the restoration of harmonious relations, and taking prescribed curative remedies.[22] More combative acts may be deemed necessary against witchcraft.

In many indigenous cultures, ritual experts are required to deal with the relational causes of illness (and of hunger and other threats to well-being). The term 'shaman' is perhaps now so widely used that it loses some of its power as a critical term. Nonetheless, it is too late to insist that only Tungus-speaking Siberians (among whom the term originated) can properly be said to employ shamans (and then only when they are truly 'traditional', rather than having been influenced by Western neoshamans). Some generalities about shamans are helpful as long as they are received with the increasingly necessary refrain that specific, local practices and ideas are of crucial importance. Thus, shamans are ritualists who are called upon to mediate between their communities and other-than-human persons (e.g. animals, deities, witches, spirits). Sometimes humans come under assault because they have offended someone or because they have been noticed by a predatory being. Perhaps a hunter has treated an animal with a degree of disrespect. Perhaps someone has offended an animal by cooking it with an inappropriate utensil. Perhaps a disease-causing other-than-human person ('spirit' maybe, but 'bacteria' might be as good a term as any) has determined to attack someone. In these and other cases, a shaman can be required to determine the cause(s) of problems (ill-health, failure in hunting). Often utilizing altered states of consciousness, but most frequently employing the adjusted styles of communication that rituals entail, shamans seek to understand the causes of aggression and find a means of dealing with the cause.

If they are unable to resolve a situation or to find a way to restore harmonious relationships, shamans may engage in spiritual combat themselves. In many places the difference between powerful healer and powerful causer of illness is thin. As with 'terrorists'/'freedom fighters,' so 'our shaman' may be 'someone else's sorcerer.' The chief job of a shaman may be to cure, but sometimes that is deemed possible only by attacking the person (human or other-than-human) who causes the problem. This may seem like a contradiction to the oft-repeated claim that 'respect' sums up the ethic of indigeneity. However, just as 'to respect' is not necessarily the equivalent of 'to like,' so it is not necessarily contradicted by 'to attack.' There are usually rules of engagement here, too; combat with those who cause a patient's illness is intended to restore the way the world should work. If someone (human or other-than-human) has transgressed too many boundaries and done too much damage to others, the appropriate demonstration of respect for life may be to prevent them from doing so again.

There are healers in most traditional indigenous communities. Their practices vary considerably because their role in treating individual problems is an aspect of the maintenance and furtherance of the cosmos as understood in their culture. Disruptions and imbalances are threats to communities and to the world and generally require the kind of interventions the Western world labels 'holistic,' rather than 'atomistic.' It is, perhaps, important to note here that the practices of shamans, medicine-people and other indigenous healers have too often been psychologized in Western academic and popular understandings. The problems that people employ such experts to deal with can include, but are not limited to those originating in or manifesting as psychological difficulties. Physical ailments, injuries, hunger, and ignorance are among the concerns of healers (including diviners and other medicine people). Treating the whole person when 'persons' are definitively relational requires different methods and solutions to treating beings understood (as they are in radically Cartesian systems) as primarily interiorized individuals.

Purity

A significant element in both causing and curing illness may be labelled 'purification'. Perhaps due to the legacy of the European Christian Reformations (Protestant and Catholic), rites of purification—and indeed the very notion of 'ritual purity'—can be misunderstood. They seem archetypical of the supposedly 'empty' or 'vain' repetitions that are so often vilified in polemics against (other) religions—or religion itself. (Anti-ritualism is a core aspect of the regular denigration of Judaism by Christians and of religion by secularizing atheists.) However, just as handshakes remain important, ritualized greetings even among the most rationalist European, so purification rituals can be of immense significance among many peoples, not only indigenous ones. Their centrality in at least some healing rituals is important; they are key to the effort to place humans (patients or otherwise) in right relationships with others (human, other-than-human, earthly, cosmic, mundane, and divine). Such rituals may include preliminary acts of larger ritual complexes (such as smudging or censing with the smoke of herbs or sprinkling with sacred water) or may form the entirety of a ritual (e.g. the sweat-lodges in which some Native Americans commit themselves to sacrificial efforts to pray for others' well-being, while suffering extreme heat in an enclosed space). In some contexts, as in some Amazonian rituals, the emetic aid of particular plants is a vital stage in bringing people into the correct state for engaging more fully with the world revealed to them ceremonially and in more discursive teaching methods. By vomiting out illnesses and other negativities, people are freed to perceive the world and themselves more clearly. Often these emetics are also inspirers of visions (for which the term 'hallucination' is unhelpful if it is supposed to interpret indigenous understandings) and are treated as persons in their own right. It is not as active ingredients or chemicals that they play roles in the pharmacology and therapy, let alone the spirituality, of indigenous groups, but as agents of change, and givers of insight and wisdom. Once again, the all-too-easy focus on interiority of the West is probably the reason why most literature about such matters of dramatic plant–human encounters predominantly attend to the mind- or consciousness-altering effects. Emetic results are, however, often as important in their indigenous contexts because purification precedes inspiration. To put it another way, people have to be prepared for life-changing experiences and encounters. Changes of costume, demeanour, posture, and speech may be expected, alongside ritual vomiting of impurities, as a foundation for visions of how the world really works.

Conclusions

This chapter has surveyed some of the key themes in contemporary indigenous spiritualities that aid an understanding of the broader complexes of indigenous knowledges. It has drawn on themes and practices from indigenous cultures in most continents, but it has insisted that indigenous knowledge prioritizes the specific and local over the general and global. This is not to say that indigenous people are trapped by small scale myopia and have nothing to say of international or global import. On the contrary, it is to insist that rootedness and belonging, specificity and emplacement, are key features of the urgent messages offered by many indigenous communities to their neighbours. These might be encapsulated in a phrase such as: find yourself where you are, among your neighbours (human and otherwise) and you and the larger-than-human community may live better, more fulfilled lives.

One of the consistent errors of people of European descent (anthropologists included) is their mistaken assumption that indigenous people live in a different world or an earlier time.[23] Indigenous knowledges are not survivals from previous or ancient eras. They are as contemporary as the people who continue to develop, inculcate, and live by them. Indigenous spiritualities, then, are not romantic hangovers of a putatively better time. They were never fixed and uncontested monoliths in unchanging, pristine communities discrete from all other possible ways of being human. They always required teaching, testing, and application. Now they are contemporary provocations of good living in a world that, practitioners insist, is not as it seems from the perspective of settlers. Rather, the world we all live in is relational and we only survive—and thrive to the extent that we do thrive—because of the efforts of others. All this is implicit in the Aboriginal Australian preference for the term 'law' over any other (more mystifying?) reference to the foundational principles of the cosmos and the teachings about living that arise from them in specific places or countries. Indigenous spiritualities invite responsible and relevant engagement with communal and inherited norms and values. In many places, indigenous people are finding increased meaning in traditional understandings and practices as they seek ways to live more fulfilled lives in the contemporary world.

The flexibility of indigenous law, knowledge, and spirituality has proved valuable in relation to the markedly different circumstances in which many indigenous people find themselves. A still emerging diversity of liberationist movements that challenge the construction of a consumerist, individualist, anthropocentric, Eurocentric world, includes vibrant expressions of indigeneity—or indigenization. These seem to offer distinctive ways of seeking wellbeing in dwelling in lands, countries, bioregional communities of mutual respect and responsibility. They encourage a fusion of localization that builds on the most positive senses of 'indigenous' with a celebration of global links with other people engaged in similar struggles and energized by similar values and hopes. This, at least, is a part of what 'indigenous spirituality' means in the varied local, regional, national, international, and global forums in which indigenous people are currently engaged.

The key themes focused upon here have been the relational nature of personhood and the world (as community), the centrality of dwelling or emplacement, the necessity of respect among citizens of the larger-than-human community of which human persons are members, and the generative power of gifts and gifting, rituals, and etiquette. Greater understanding of indigenous spirituality requires some odd uses of seemingly familiar terms (such as person as a reference to animals, plants and rocks) and some learning of indigenous terms (including terms like *totem* from Ojibwemowin, and 'law' from Aboriginal English). Attention to indigenous protocols, including the centrality of ritual and oratory ('myth-telling' perhaps) may immediately challenge the norms of dominant Euro-global 'most-modern' culture, but promise to enrich the lives of those who make the effort as well as serving the needs of indigenous people in their many and varied circumstances. Much of importance in all these domains is far better represented in the many excellent indigenous novels, plays, films, and cultural performances than in academic, political or legal documents. These convey more fully both the negative (anger and horror) and the positive (humour and passion) of indigenous experiences that inform and erupt into contemporary indigenous spiritualities.

References

1 Trigger, D.S., Dalley, C. (2010). Negotiating indigeneity: Culture, Identity and Politics. *Rev Anthropol* **39**(1): 46–65.

2 Grieves, V. (2009). Aboriginal spirituality: *Aboriginal Philosophy, The Basis of Aboriginal Social and Emotional Wellbeing,* Discussion Paper No. 9. Darwin: Cooperative Research Centre for Aboriginal Health.

3 Ruel, M. (1997). *Belief, Ritual and the Securing of Life*, pp. 36–59. Leiden: Brill.

4 Latour, B. (2002). *War of the Worlds: What about Peace*? Chicago: Prickly Paradigm Press.

5 Tawhai, T.P. (1988). Maori religion. In: S. Sutherland, P. Clarke (eds) *The Study of Religion, Traditional and New Religion*, pp. 96–105. London: Routledge. Reprinted in Harvey, G. (ed.) (2002). *Readings in Indigenous Religions*, Continuum, pp. 237–49. London.

6 Tawhai, T.P. (1996). Aotearoa's spiritual heritage. In: P. Donovan (ed.) *Religions of New Zealanders*, 2nd edn, pp. 11–19. Palmerston North: Dunmore Press.

7 Bird-David, N. (1999). 'Animism' revisited: personhood, environment, and relational epistemology. *Curr Anthropol* **40:** 67–91.

8 Viveiros de Castro, E. (1992). *From the Enemy's Point of View: Humanity and Divinity in an Amazonian Society*. Chicago: University of Chicago Press.

9 Viveiros de Castro, E. (1998). Cosmological deixis and Amerindian perspectivism. *J Roy Anthropolog Inst* (NS), **4**: 469–88.

10 Willerslev, R. (2007). *Soul Hunters*: Hunting, Animism, and Personhood Among the Siberian Yukaghirs. Berkeley: University of California Press.

11 Hornborg, A.C. (2009). *Mi'kmaq Landscapes:* From Animism to Sacred Ecology. Aldershot: Ashgate.

12 Harvey, G. (2005). *Animism:* Respecting the Living World. London: C. Hurst.

13 Tylor, E. (1871). *Primitive Culture*. London: John Murray.

14 Latour, B. (1993). *We Have Never Been Modern*. New York: Harvester Wheatsheaf.

15 Rose, D. (1998). *Totemism, Regions, and Co-management in Aboriginal Australia*. Draft paper for the Conference of the International Association for the Study of Common Property. Available at: http://dlc.dlib.indiana.edu/dlc/bitstream/handle/10535/1187/rose.pdf (accessed 28 December, 2010), p. 8

16 Lévi-Strauss, C. (1969). *Totemism*. Harmondsworth: Penguin, p. 89.

17 Grimes, R. (2006). Performance is currency in the deep world's gift economy: an incantatory riff for a Global Medicine Show. *Interdisciplin Stud Lit Environ* **9**(1): 149–64.

18 Povinelli, E.A. (1995). Do rocks listen? The cultural politics of apprehending Australian Aboriginal labor. *Am Anthropol* **97**(3): 505–18.

19 Nichols, J.D., Nyholm, E. (1995). *A Concise Dictionary of Minnesota Ojibwe*. Minneapolis: University of Minnesota Press.

20 Morrison, K. (2002). *The Solidarity of Kin:* Ethnohistory, *Religious Studies, and the Algonkian-French Religious Encounter*, pp. 68–70. New York: SUNY.

21 Hallowell, A.I. (1960). Ojibwa ontology, behavior, and world view. In: S. Diamond (ed.) *Culture in History:* Essays in Honor of Paul Radin, pp. 19–52. New York: Columbia University Press.

22 Jegede, O. (2010). *Incantations and Herbal Cures in Ifa Divination*. Ibadan: African Association for the Study of Religion.

23 Fabian, J. (1983). *Time and the Other: How Anthropology Makes its Object*. New York: Columbia University Press.

CHAPTER 9

Islam

Abdulaziz Sachedina

Introduction

The word *islām,* which designates the last of the Abrahamic religions, literally means 'submission to God's will.' Muḥammad (born 570 CE), the Prophet of Islam and the founder of Islamic public order, proclaimed Islam in the seventh century CE in Arabia. The beginning of Islam in 610 CE was marked by a struggle to establish a monotheistic faith and create an ethical public order embodying divine justice and mercy. Muḥammad as a statesman instituted a series of reforms to create his community, *umma*, on the basis of religious affiliation.

Within a century of Muḥammad's death in 632 CE, Muslim armies had conquered the region from the Nile in North Africa to the Oxus in Central Asia up to India. This phenomenal growth into a vast empire required an Islamic legal system for the administration of the highly developed political systems of the conquered Persian and Byzantine regions. Muslim jurists formulated various methodological and conceptual devices to set up a comprehensive legal code. They extracted and utilized the ethical and legal principles set forth in the Qur'an, the collected revelations of Muḥ ammad; the precedents set by the Prophet and the early community, the Sunna; and the local customs of the conquered regions.

Differences of opinion on critical issues emerged as soon as Muḥammad died in 632 CE. The question of succession to Muḥammad was one of the major issues that divided the community into the Sunnī and Shī'a. One candidate for the position of caliph (political 'successor') was Abū Bakr (d. 634), an elderly associate of the Prophet who gained the support of the majority of the community, who gradually came to be known as the Sunnis (followers of communal 'tradition'); those who acclaimed 'Alī (d. 660), Muḥammad's cousin and son-in-law, as the 'Imām' (religious and political leader) designated by the Prophet formed the minority group, known as the Shī'a ('partisans' or 'supporters' of 'Alī).

The dispute had profound implications beyond politics. The Qur'an's persistent injunctions of obedience to the prophet endowed him with enormous personal power in shaping the present public order and, hence, the future course of Muslim life. In the post-prophetic period the dispute left the community endlessly searching for a paradigmatic authority: the Sunnis located it in the 'tradition' and the 'community,' whereas the Shī'ites found it in the charismatic person of an Imam. The full title used by the Sunni Muslims to designate themselves as the bearer of the only true and real Islam is *ahl al-sunna wa al-jamā'a*, meaning the 'people of tradition and community.' The Shī'ites use *sh`īat 'Alī* as their proper designation, meaning 'supporters' of 'Alī. Hence, their claim to validity is connected with the acknowledgement of a rightful Imam from among the descendants of the Prophet. The last in the line of these Imams is believed to be living an invisible existence since his disappearance in 940 CE.

Fundamental teachings

The two authoritative sources of Islamic teachings are the Qur'an, regarded by Muslims as the 'Book of God,' and the Sunna (the Tradition), the exemplary conduct of the Prophet. The Qur'an consists of the revelations Muḥammad received intermittently from the time of his call as the prophet in 610 CE until his death in 632 CE. Muslims believe that the Qur'an was directly communicated by God through the archangel Gabriel; accordingly, it remains an infallible text for Muslims. The Qur'an is not a book of systematic theology or ethics; nevertheless, it has been the key source of Islam's theological and ethical doctrines, and its principles of public organization. The Sunna (meaning 'well trodden path') has functioned as the elaboration of the Qur'anic revelation, providing interpretive counsel about every precept and deed, with ostensible precedents in the Prophet's own practice. The narratives that carried such information were designated as *ḥadīth* ('report, narrative'). In the ninth century Muslim scholars developed an elaborate system for the theological and legal classification, and verification of these *ḥadīth* reports, deducing from them various prescriptions for belief and practice.

The 'Five Pillars'

The tradition describes the Muslim creed and practice as 'The Five Pillars of Islam.' These include fundamental doctrines and religious practices that all Muslims endeavour to perform as part of their commitment to the faith community.

The *First* Pillar is the *shahāda* ('bearing witness'), the profession of faith. The *shahāda* consists of two statements: 'There is no deity, but God, and Muḥammad is the messenger of God.' These two avowals are repeated by anyone who wishes to join the community of the faithful. Belief in God is the foundation of the individual's private and social existence. The Qur'an speaks about God as the being whose presence suffuses all worldly things and events. Faith in God engenders security and peace of mind.

Life is the gift of God, and the body is the divine trust given to humankind to enable it to serve God fully. The Qur'an describes a humble origin for humans, who were created from 'dry clay of black mud formed into shape' (Q. 15: 26). Through the well-proportioned creation of human beings in God's image (*'alā Ṣūratihi*) [1] and the perpetual guidance to strive for moral and spiritual perfection, human beings have been given the trusteeship of their bodies. On the Day of Resurrection, all parts of the human body will have to account for the actions of the person whose bodily organs they formed (Q. 36: 65). God has set limits on what human beings may do with their own bodies. Suicide, homicide, and torturing one's body in any form are deemed acts of transgression against God.

Muslims believe in resurrection of the dead on the Day of Judgment, when they will account for their deeds, and reap the rewards or punishments warranted by their life on earth. The Day of Resurrection or Reckoning is a central doctrine in the Qur'an, reminding human beings of their ultimate return to God. The belief in bodily resurrection has determined many a religious-ethical decision regarding cadavers. Dead bodies should be buried reverently as soon as possible. The Qur'an affirms reverence for human life in a commandment similar to those that govern other monotheists: 'We decreed for the Children of Israel that whosoever kills a human being for other than manslaughter or corruption in the earth, it shall be as if he had killed all humankind, and whoso saves the life of one, it shall be as if he saved the life of all humankind' (Q. 5: 32).

Belief in God's guidance entails the responsibility to further God's purposes on earth. Human beings are endowed with the innate disposition (*fiṭra*) or ability to know right from wrong and the will to accept the responsibility for perfecting their existence by understanding and working with the laws of nature. The Qur'an emphasizes God's benevolence, all-forgivingness, and mercy. However, it also highlights God's justice and stresses that humanity should develop moral and spiritual awareness (*taqwā*) in fulfilling everyday requirements of life.

Human existence is not free of tension and inner stresses; they result from the rejection of truth (*kufr*) and impairment of moral consciousness. To help humanity, God sends prophets 'to remind' humanity of its covenant with God (Q. 7: 172). There have been 124,000 prophets from the beginning of history, among whom five (Noah, Abraham, Moses, Jesus, and Muḥammad) are regarded as 'messengers' sent to organize their people on the basis of divine revelation.

The *Second* Pillar is daily worship (*Ṣalāt*, lit. 'to pray, to invoke'). The Islamic concept of 'worship' or 'serving' (*'ibāda*) God is much broader. Any good deed or thought is regarded as 'service' to God. However, *Ṣalāt* is a prescribed ritual that is performed as a 'service' to God with an explicit intention of 'drawing close to God.' All Muslims who have attained the prescribed age of maturity (fifteen for a boy and nine for a girl) are required to offer their prayers five times a day: at dawn, midday, afternoon, evening, and night. These prayers are very short, and require bowing and prostration. A Muslim may worship anywhere, preferably in congregation, facing Mecca. Muslims are required to worship as a community on Fridays at midday and on two major religious holidays. The congregational prayer gives expression to the believer's religious commitment within the community. Women are exempt from this obligation of congregational participation, and the tradition recommends that they worship in the privacy of their homes. Although segregated from men, they have always worshipped at designated areas in the mosque.

The Qur'an prescribes a state of physical purity for the worshipper prior to prayer, requiring the performance of ablutions and a full washing after sexual intercourse or a long illness. Women are required to perform a full washing after the menstrual cycle and childbirth because blood is regarded as ritually unclean. Islamic law prescribes regular cleansing and physical hygiene as expressions of one's faith.

In Islam prayer is therapeutic. In addition to seeking medical treatment, Muslims are encouraged to seek healing, especially for psychological problems, by invoking God's mercy through supplication. Many illnesses, according to the teachings of the Prophet, are caused by psychological conditions like anxiety, sorrow, fear, loneliness, and so on. Hence, prayer restores the serenity and tranquility of the soul.

The *Third* Pillar is the mandatory 'alms-levy' (*zakāt*, literally 'purification,' but more broadly 'sharing of one's wealth by practicing charity'). The Muslim definition of the virtuous life includes charitable support of widows, wayfarers, orphans, and the needy. Islamic law includes technical regulations about how much *zakāt* is due and upon what property it is to be levied. These legal rulings, which originated in early Islam, before the disintegration of the Islamic public order, do not necessarily prevail in contemporary Muslim nations. Although *zakāt* has for the most part been left to the conscience of Muslims, the obligation to be charitable remains an important ethical imperative of Islam.

The *Fourth* Pillar is the fast of Ramaḍān, the ninth month of the Islamic lunar calendar, in which Muḥammad received the Qur'an. During the fast, which lasts from dawn to dusk for each day of the month, Muslims are forbidden to eat, smoke, and drink; they must also refrain from sexual intercourse and acts leading to sensual behaviour. The fasting alters the pattern of life for a month generating a spiritual state that leads to mental and bodily health. The end of the month is marked by a festival, *'Id al-fiṭr*, after which life returns to normal. The discipline engendered by Ramadan varies from individual to individual. It certainly helps individuals to cultivate spiritual and moral self-control. The communal aspect of Ramadan provides a community experience in which families and friends share both fasting and evening meals in a spirit of thanksgiving. Like prayer, fasting also has a therapeutic effect. Prophetic guidance prescribes fasting for treating various ailments, including psychological problems, such as fear, anxiety, and overactive sexual drive.

The *Fifth* Pillar is the annual pilgrimage, the *ḥajj*, to Mecca, which all able-bodied Muslims are required to undertake at least once in their lives, if they can afford to do so. The pilgrimage takes place at a fixed time during the twelfth month of the lunar calendar. This collective ritual performed by thousands of Muslims in Mecca lasts for three days, culminating in the Festival of Sacrifice, which marks the end of *ḥajj*. The three-day rituals that commemorate Abraham's sacrifice of his son Ishmael have the essential spiritual objective of inculcating a form of asceticism by teaching the pilgrims to learn self-control in pursuing worldly desires. The rituals and the special prayers during the *ḥajj* are a source of spiritual healing and inner peace. The experience brings together Muslims of diverse cultures and nationalities to achieve a purity of existence and a communion with God that exalts the pilgrim for the rest of his/her life.

Healing through spiritual morality

Because suffering can result from either natural or moral evil, we are obliged to examine the concept of good health in Islam, especially insofar as this is regarded as part of a person's obligation to avoid undue pain and suffering. The Arabic word *Ṣiḥḥa* ('sound' or 'health') is rich in connotations. Like the word *salāma* (also 'sound' or 'health'), it conveys the wholeness and integrity of a being that generates a sense of security. Furthermore, it connotes a life of balance and moderation that avoids behavioural extremes. Disturbing this balance of *Ṣiḥḥa* causes physical ailment. The Qur'an lays down the golden rule about moderation: 'O children of Adam,... eat and drink the good things you desire, but do not become wasteful' (Q. 7: 31). Imbalance or overindulgence in the enjoyment of God's bounty will lead to both physical and moral suffering. In the moral sense, human volition may result in the overconsumption of certain foods because of sensual indulgence rather than attention to good health. The Prophet is reported to have advised his disciples to avoid overeating and recommended that one stop eating before feeling full.[2] Another tradition traces all sickness to a lack of moderation in eating. On this view, it is physical or psychological conditions beyond one's own control that dictate lifestyle adjustments in the interests of physical wellbeing.

The Qur'an prescribes the pursuit of self-knowledge as a part of maintaining good health. Physical and psychological health cannot be taken-for-granted—they are a divine benefaction that depends on human moderation in food and drink, and regular physical activities, including swimming and horse riding, as the Prophet instructed his followers. Yet there are people who suffer from illnesses that are genetically inherited, in which they have exercised no choice whatsoever. It is this kind of suffering that raises questions about God's will and the existence of evil in the world.

Islamic spirituality

The belief in God's omnipotence is the most important idea in Muslim theology. God is the creator of all things, including human destiny on earth, and rewards and punishments in the hereafter. Such a deterministic concept of human action gives rise to the problem of reconciling divine predetermination of human action with divine justice, which entails God's punishment of the wicked and his rewarding of the righteous. This aspect of the problem of theodicy arose out of statements from the Qur'an and the Tradition. In the context of health care, the idea of God's omnipotence has enormous implications, breeding a quietism that discourages the ill from prying into God's unfathomable ways and encourages resignation to suffering.[3] With modern medicine's enormous strides in healing the sick and alleviating suffering, the inexorability of God's decrees provides little comfort to those who want to see an end to agonies of incurable diseases.

Yet, despite the phenomenal advancement in medical treatment today humans need to come to grips with what I constantly hear in my duties as a hospital chaplain: undeserved suffering. The need to understand the divine decree and cultivate necessary faith in God's goodness brings me face to face with the role of Islamic spirituality.

In Islam the realm of spirituality is located within human experience of transcendence. It does not matter whether one is anchored in an organized religious tradition or not. The experience of transcendence is positioned in the depth of the human heart, which needs to be explored by each individual through the natural endowment that all humans have been created with. This endowment—the innate capacity (*fiṭra*) to incline towards transcendence—is the source of human spiritual and moral awareness (*taqwā*), which is created the moment humans are fashioned as humans (Q. 97: 7–10). At various points in their journey toward spiritual and moral perfection humans receive portents that are present both in their own selves (*anfus*) and in the environment (*āfāq*) for them to realize the stages of their journey towards becoming perfected (Q. 16: 78). In this sense, their personal perfection is tied to the perfection of environment that requires the undivided attention of humanity since its preservation and its beautification is existentially connected with humanity's own survival and internal beauty. The more one understands this indispensable connection between internal and external sources of human spiritual and moral development the more one commits oneself to achieve the equilibrium that this understanding generates in actual life situations. This is the universal dimension of one's nature and spiritual and moral journey.

In this sense, spirituality and morality are intertwined because the former is the internal dimension of the being's identity, and hence, individual and subjective; whereas the latter is the external aspect and grounds for a person's overall performance in corporate existence, and hence, collective and objective. Claims of being spiritual can coexist with the calamity of self-righteous attitudes in faith communities, and are ultimately inaccessible to outsiders for scrutiny. It is for this reason that, in Islam, morality (doing what is right and avoiding what is wrong) must accompany spirituality as its consequence, and take objective and accessible forms for others to establish the validity of the claim to be moral. If spirituality generates peace and confidence, then morality becomes its objective manifestation when one deals with other humans as equals, endowed with the same dignity regardless of one's faith connection. In this estimation, then, spirituality is not only a precondition to one's inner peace and healthy state of mind; it is functionally indispensable to developing moral sensibilities, which enable a person to deal with others in fairness and justice.

However, this morality-orientated spirituality is overshadowed by exclusionary Muslim theology, which finds its major application in the Islamic religious law. The juridical tradition is founded upon this theology, which, paradoxically, also advances the idea of a common human family that can be traced back to the first human couple on earth, Adam and Eve. Human beings need one another to enable them to live in peace and harmony—the very foundation of human wellbeing. Hence, the critical need for spirituality is underscored by the mystical tradition in Islam, namely, Sufism, which neutralizes the exclusionary theology in its emphasis upon the Prophetic teaching that the Children of Adam are like one body, because they share the same essence in their creation. One of the striking features of religiously-based spirituality is its emphasis on human relationships and the ethics that governs these. By its very emphasis on the ethics of relationship, this spirituality is dialogical. It is not only to dialogue with other humans that it inevitably leads;

it also leads to dialogue with the entirety of nature. It requires humans to engage not only in beautifying nature in a reciprocal mode (if I am beautiful, so is my environment); it also mandates its preservation, in the same way as it treats one's own preservation as a moral and religious duty. Dialogue allows the relationship of equality to emerge, which is potentially able to confront the sources of conflict generated by the culturally advanced dichotomy of superiority/inferiority, saved/damned theology. To defeat the negative forces of this cultural theology, human endeavours need to be equipped with the spirituality that orientates a person to ethical action. The Prophet of Islam was asked about the meaning of religion and he is reported to have replied: 'It is obedience to God and kindness to creation (*makhluq*).' The 'creation' is used here in its generic sense to include the entirety of created beings, not just humans. It is for this reason that when human relationships are fractured they need to be mended through healing that comes by way of reaching out to fellow humans qua humans.

The correlation between spirituality and morality provides a unique way of estimating the relationship between faith and law. Law is certainly connected with the human experience of living with one another and in community. In Islam, God's will is expressed in God's commandments delivered through the supernatural medium of revelation. God's law guarantees salvation to those who obey God's commandment. In some unique sense, fulfillment of the legal-ethical rulings restores total human wellbeing leading to a blissful hereafter. In order to fully appreciate this interdependent relation between spiritual and moral wellbeing, we need to turn our attention to the normative legal system in Islam, which functions as a divinely ordained scale of what it means to be a spiritually and morally healthy community.

Islamic law

Islamic law covers all the actions humans perform, whether toward one another or toward God. The Sharī'a is the norm of the Muslim community. It grew out of Muslim endeavours to ensure that Islam pervaded the whole of life. Two essential areas of human life define its scope: acts of worship, both public and private, connected with the pillars of faith; and acts of public order that ensure individual and collective justice. The first category of actions, undertaken with the intention of seeking God's pleasure, is collectively known as 'ritual duties' toward God (*'ibādāt*, literally 'acts of worship'). These include all religious acts, such as daily prayers, fasting, alms-giving, and so on; the second category of actions, undertaken to maintain a social order, is known as 'social transactions' (*mu'āmalāt*, literally 'social intercourse'). The religious calibration of these two categories depended upon the meticulous division of jurisdiction based on the ability of human institutions to enforce the Sharī'a and provide sanctions for disregarding its injunctions. In Islamic law all actions should be performed to secure divine approval, but human agency and institutions have jurisdiction only over the social transactions that regulate interpersonal relations.

In order to create such an all-comprehensive legal system founded upon revealed texts, Muslim scholars went beyond the Qur'an to the person of the founder and the early community. The Qur'an required obedience to the Prophet and those invested with authority, which included the idealized community made up of the elders among first and second generations. In this way, the Qur'an opened the way for extending the normative practice beyond the prophet's earthly life. Such an understanding of the normative tradition was theoretically essential for deriving the legal system that saw its validity only in terms of its being extracted from the Prophet's own paradigmatic status. Hence, the Prophet's life as understood and reported by the early community became an ethical touchstone for what the Muslims call the Sunna, the Tradition. The intellectual activity surrounding the interpretation of God's will expressed in the Qur'an and the evaluation of the *ḥadīth* reports that were ascribed to the Prophet and the early community became the major religious–academic activity among Muslims, laying the foundation for subsequent juridical deliberations—what became known as *fiqh* ('understanding'), or jurisprudence.

By the 9–10th centuries, Muslim community was affiliated with one or the other leading scholars in the field of juristic investigation. The legal school that followed the Iraqi tradition was called 'Ḥanafī,' after Abū Ḥanīfa (d. 767), the 'imām' (teacher) in Iraq. Those who adhered to the rulings of Mālik bin Anas (d. 795), in Arabia and elsewhere, were known as 'Mālikis.' Al-Shāfi'ī, who is also credited as being one of the profound legal thinkers, is the founder of a legal school in Egypt whose influence spread widely to other regions of the Muslim world. Another school was associated with Aḥmad bin Ḥanbal (d. 855), who compiled a work on *ḥadīth* reports that became the source for juridical decisions of those who followed him. Shī'ites developed their own legal school, the Ja'fari school, whose leading authority was Imam Ja'far al-Ṣādiq (d. 748). Normally, Muslims accepted the legal school prevalent in their region. Today most of the Sunni Muslims follow Ḥanafī or Shāfi'ī rite; whereas the Shī'a Muslims follow the Ja'farī school. In the absence of an organized 'church' and ordained 'clergy' in Islam, Islamic legal rite is inherently pluralistic. The determination of valid religious practice is left to the qualified scholars of religious law, collectively known as ulema.

Muslim legal theorists were thoroughly aware of moral underpinnings of the religious duties that all Muslims were required to fulfil as members of the faith community. In fact, the validity of their research in the foundational sources of Islam (the Qur'an and the Tradition) for solutions to practical matters depended upon their substantial consideration of different moral facets of a case that could be discovered by considering conflicting claims, interests, and responsibilities in the precedents preserved in these authoritative sources. What ensured the validity of their judicial decision regarding a specific instance was their ability to deduce the universal moral principles like 'there shall be no harm inflicted or reciprocated' (*lā ḍarar wa lā ḍirār*)[4] that flowed downward from their initial premise to support their particular conclusion without any dependence on the circumstances that would have rendered the conclusion circumstantial at the most. However, the power of these conclusions depended on the ethical considerations that were operative in the original precedents and the agreement of the scholars that sought to relate the new case to the original rationale as well as rules.

Customarily, when faced with a moral dilemma juridical-ethical deliberations are geared toward a satisfactory resolution in which justifications are based on practical consequences, regardless of applicable principles. For instance, in deciding whether to allow dissection of the cadaver to retrieve a valuable object swallowed by the deceased, Muslim jurists have ruled in favour by simply looking at the consequence of forbidding such a procedure. The major moral consideration that outweighs the respect for the dignity of the dead is the ownership through inheritance of the swallowed object for the surviving orphan. Dissection of the cadaver is forbidden in Islam; and, yet, the case demands immediate solution that is based on consequential ethics. Or, in the case of a female patient who, as prescribed in the Sharī'a must be treated by a female physician, in an emergency situation the practical demand is to override the prohibition because the rule of necessity (*ḍarūra*) extracted from the revealed texts outweighs the rule about the sexual segregation extracted from rational consideration. There are numerous instances that clearly show the cultural preferences in providing solutions to the pressing problems of health care in Muslim societies in which communitarian ethics considers the consequence of any medical decision on the family, and community resources and interests.

Health-related beliefs and values

People with different backgrounds approach suffering through illness and death with a wide range of diverse attitudes about its causes and consequences, attitudes that often have been cultivated and transmitted by their respective cultures and religions. Sometimes these attitudes undermine the efficacy of those treatments which require the patient to have the necessary will to fight the disease. A holistic medical approach, which treats both psychosomatic and physical conditions, necessitates that clinicians be aware of the patient's emotional condition and cultural background in order to formulate an accurate diagnosis and successful treatment plan. [5] What should the health care worker know about her Muslim patient's religious and moral presuppositions about the nature of suffering?

Generally, a situation that is negatively described as suffering refers to an objective state of affairs ('It is unbearable!') and the subjective response ('It is harmful for the patient!') of a judging individual. In other words, when one assesses suffering as a form of evil—either objectively or subjectively, one needs to take into account the agent, the act of suffering, and the resultant harm that is objective enough for a positive or a privative understanding of evil. When both subjective and objective elements are present, suffering in the context of illness is described as the experience that is undesirable and maleficent. Both physically and morally, the description immediately captures an objective standard that most people would judge as tragically harmful to the agent, without reference to any ontology or complex metaphysical or theological explanation. We are in a realistic way able to assert that a person is suffering unrequited pain and destruction. Evil then reveals the undesirable and maleficent aspects of human suffering. Understood in this way, we can now probe into theodicy and begin to unfold the divine mystery regarding the infliction of destruction upon innocent life through natural evil.

The quest to unfold the divine mystery about human suffering paves the way for a meaningful conversation between the religious beliefs and medical aspects of illness where metaphysical and physical dimensions of medical care struggle to come to terms with the human condition and the limitations of human undertakings to alleviate that suffering. The difference between religious and medical assessment of the situation is stark. Whereas faith in the divine will nurture humility and reveal human limitations in comprehending the ways of the powerful God who gives and takes life, medicine, taking the responsibility for removing the evil of pain and suffering, continues its search to find the cure and prolongs dying. The stark difference is further underscored by the way religion inculcates personal piety in dealing with illness, which is to inculcate faith in God's goodness and accept suffering as part of the overall divine plan for humanity's spiritual and moral development. Although medicine enters the field of human suffering with enormous confidence and determination to treat ailments by undertaking necessary training and research, religion emphasizes the finitude of human life. It reminds humanity not to arrogate God's functions of taking life at a fixed point in history, whose knowledge rests with God alone.

'How fortunate you are that you died while you were not afflicted with illness.' Thus said the Prophet addressing the person whose funeral rites he was performing. Such an assessment of death without illness coming from the founder of Islam indicates the value attached to a healthy life in Muslim culture. To be sure, good health is God's blessing for which a Muslim, whenever asked: 'How are you?' (lit. 'How is your health?') responds: 'All praise is due to God!' This positive appraisal of good health might, however, seem to suggest that illness is an evil that must be eliminated at any cost. No doubt, illness is regarded as an affliction that needs to be cured by every possible legitimate means. In fact, the search for a cure is founded upon unusual confidence generated by the divine promise that God has not created a disease without creating its cure.[6] Hence, the purpose of medicine is to search for that cure and provide the necessary care to those afflicted with diseases. The primary obligation of a Muslim physician is to provide care and alleviate suffering of a patient. Decisions about ending the life of a terminally ill patient at her/his request are beyond his moral or legal obligations. The Qur'an states its position on the matter in no uncertain terms that 'it is not given to any soul to die, save by the leave of God, at an appointed time.' (Q. 3: 145) Moreover, 'God gives life, and He makes to die' (Q. 3: 156). Hence, 'A person dies when it is written' (Q. 3: 185, 29: 57, 39: 42).

Death, then, comes at the appointed time, by God's permission. In the meantime, humans are faced with the suffering caused by illness. How is suffering viewed in Islam? Is it part of the divine plan to cause suffering? With what end? These general questions about the meaning and value of suffering should lead us to appraise the suffering caused by prolonged illness in an individual's personal and family life. The need to take the decision to end one's life arises precisely at that critical point when the sick person is undergoing severe discomfort and desperation, and when all forms of advanced medical treatments have failed to restore hope in getting better.

Closely related to such a consideration on the part of the sick person is whether the unbearable circumstances caused by one's interminable illness makes existence worthwhile at all. Does such an existence that is almost equivalent to non-existence because of an intense sense of helplessness in managing one's life, possess any value for its continuation? Beneath these concerns remains a deeper question about the quality of life that individuals and society regard as worth preserving.

The discussion about quality of life points to the cultural and religious attitudes regarding human existence and the control over life and death decisions when an individual is overcome by suffering. Furthermore, it underscores the view that a human being has the stewardship, not the ownership, of his body to enable him to assert his right to handle it the way he pleases. He is merely the caretaker, the real owner being God, the Creator. As a caretaker, it is his duty to take all the necessary steps to preserve it in a manner that would assist him in seeking the good of both this world and the next. In light of such a stipulation about human duty toward his earthly existence in Muslim theology, the problem of human suffering through illness assumes immediate relevance. The Qur'an provides essential philosophy behind human suffering by pointing out that suffering is a form of a test or trial to confirm a believer's spiritual station:

> O all you who believe, seek your help in patience and prayer; surely God is with the patient ... surely. We will try you with something of fear and hunger, and diminution of goods and lives and fruits; yet give thou good tidings unto the patient who, when they are visited by an affliction, say, 'Surely we belong to God, and to Him we return'; upon those rest blessings and mercy from their Lord, and those—they are the truly guided. (Q. 2: 153–7.)

Suffering in this situation is caused by the divinely ordained trial. More pertinently, it functions as an instrument in revealing God's purpose for humanity and in reminding it that ultimately it is to God that it belongs and to God it will return. Accordingly, suffering from this perspective cannot be regarded as evil at all. In a well-known tradition, the Prophet is reported to have said: 'No fatigue, nor disease, nor sorrow, nor sadness, nor hurt, nor distress befalls a Muslim, even if it were the prick he received from a thorn, but that God expiates some of his sins for that.'[7]

Hence, understanding suffering is central to Islamic understanding of health and illness. As pointed out earlier, in Muslim theology human suffering in any form raises the question about God's power and knowledge over what befalls human beings. The belief in God's overwhelming power is the most important doctrine in Muslim theology. God is not only the Creator of all things, including human destiny (*qadar*), God also determines the ultimate outcome of human decisions. Such a deterministic theology primarily gives rise to the problem of reconciling God's justice with existing evil. It has tendencies toward resignation and almost passivity in dealing with illness and other forms of afflictions. Our everyday experience with death and disease provides us with plenty of grounds to complain about the sad fact that, in view of what modern medicine promises to do for the sick, faith in the inscrutable ways of God's decree provides little comfort to those who want to see an end to the agonies of incurable diseases.

Muslim theologians have striven to comprehend the rationale for the suffering, for instance, of children or even animals. Explaining the causes of suffering of bad people, even if unconvincing, has been easier because of the causal link drawn between sins and suffering by the majority of Muslim theologians. But what sins can account for the suffering of innocent children? The suffering of children in reproductive technologies and genetics, and the unprecedented devaluation of defective foetuses in contemporary biomedical advancement await full accounting of the ethics of fertility clinics and prenatal genetic screening.

Islamic bioethics[8]

Secular bioethics in the Muslim world today has severed its partnership with faith communities in providing solutions to the moral problems that have arisen in clinical situations as well as public health around the world. International bodies like WHO and UNESCO, which support local efforts in developing culturally sensitive bioethical curriculum, still appear to be unaware of the essentially religious nature of bioethical discourse in the Muslim world and the need to engage religious ethics in the Muslim context to better serve the populations whose cultures take religion more seriously. Examining the emerging literature on Muslim bioethics, mostly authored by interested Muslim physicians, it is obvious that those who represent Muslim bioethics do not take local cultures, and their religious ingredients seriously enough to speak with necessary acumen and sensitivity about Muslim culture-friendly bioethics. Secular bioethics, with its emphasis on liberal Western values does not fully resonate with local and regional Muslim values.

Fundamental principle of public good in Islamic bioethics

The principle of public good consists of each and every benefit that has been made known by the purposes stated in the divine revelation. Because some jurists have essentially regarded public good as safeguarding the Lawgiver's purposes, they have discussed the principle in terms of both the types and the purposes they serve. The entire Sharīʿa is instituted in the interests of Muslims, whether these interests pertain to this life or to life in the hereafter. In order to safeguard these interests and achieve God's purposes for humanity the Sharīʿa seeks to promote three universal goals. The three goals are discussed under the following universal principles whose authority is based on a number of probable instances and supporting documentation in the revelation:

1. *The essentials or the primary needs* (al-ḍarūriyāt): these are indispensable things that are promulgated for the good of this and the next world, such as providing health care to the poor and downtrodden. Such actions are necessary for maintaining public health and the good of people in this life and for earning reward in the next. Moreover, without them, life would be threatened, resulting in further suffering for people who cannot afford even the basic necessities of life. According to Muslim thinkers, the necessity to protect the essentials is felt across traditions among the followers of other religions, too. The good of the people is such a fundamental issue among all peoples that there is a consensus among them that when one member of a society suffers, others must work to relieve the afflicted[9–12]

2. *The general needs* (al-ḥājiyāt): these are things that enable human beings to improve their lives, removeing those conditions that lead to chaos in one's familial and societal life in order to achieve high standards of living, even though these necessities do not reach the level of essentials. These benefits are such that, if not attained, it leads to hardship and disorder, but not to corruption. This kind of common good is materialized in matters pertaining to the performance of religious duties, managing of everyday life situations, maintaining interpersonal relationships, and upholding a penal system that prevents people from causing harm to others[13]

3. *The secondary needs* (al-Taḥsīnāt): these are the things that are commonly regarded as praiseworthy in society, which also lead to the avoidance of those things that are regarded as blameworthy. They are also known as 'noble virtues' (*makārim al-akhlāq*).[14] In other words, although these things do not qualify as 'primary' or 'general' needs, they improve quality of life. The goal is to make them easily accessible to average members of a society,

and even embellish them in order to render these noble virtues more desirable.[15]

One of the issues in the Muslim world that is assessed in terms of the principle of public good is sex selection, particularly in assisted reproduction. Sex selection is any practice, technique, or intervention intended to increase the likelihood of the conception, gestation, and birth of a child of one sex than the other. In the Muslim world, some parents prefer one sex above the other for cultural or financial reasons. Some jurists have argued in favour of sex selection, as long as no one, including the resulting child, is harmed. However, others have disputed the claim that it is possible for no harm to be done in sex selection. They point to violations of divine law, natural justice, and inherent dignity of human beings.[16,17]

The principle of public good has also been examined in terms of collective or individual goodness. When the juristic rule of *istiḥsān* (i.e. choosing between two possible solutions of a case within the context of recognized sources of Islamic law) is evoked to justify a legal–ethical solution, the actual rationale is considerations of common welfare that is unrestricted and that reaches the largest number. However, it is sometimes likely that an individual benefit could become the source for a ruling that could clash with another ruling that entails morally superior consequences. To put it differently, the only criterion for legislation on the basis of public good is that the ruling must lead to the common good even when it is prompted by a specific individual good. The underpinning of primary ordinances (e.g. saving human life or maintaining just order) in the revelation is this kind of good. However, the consideration of individual welfare is provided by the context of change for a ruling from primary to secondary (e.g. prolongation of life without any hope for cure), so that it can benefit that particular individual in that particular situation. To be sure, elimination of the primary ordinance that requires saving life, and its change to a secondary ruling which allows discontinuing extraordinary care, takes place in the context of a particular situation. In this sense, common interests function as criteria for legislation, whereas individual interests function as the context for secondary rulings. This change from common to individual good causes disagreement among Muslim jurists in determining the benefits and harms of the situation under consideration.[18]

Autonomy and piety

There has been a growing interest in the international community Islamic perspectives on bioethics. It is important to keep in mind that it was in the West that autonomy as an overriding right of a patient found institutional and legal–ethical support. Western notions of universal human rights rest on a secular view of the individual and of the relations between such individuals in a secularized public sphere. The idea of individuals as bearers of something called rights presupposes a very particular understanding and reading of the self essentially as a self-regulating agent. The modern idea of the autonomous self envisions social actors as self-contained matrices of desires who direct their own interests. In Islamic communitarian ethics autonomy is far from being recognized as one of the major bioethical principles. The Islamic universal discourse conceives of a spiritually and morally autonomous individual capable of attaining salvation outside the nexus of community-orientated Sharīʿa, with its emphasis on integrated systems of law and morality. The Sharīʿa did not make a distinction between external acts and internal states because it did not regard the public and the private to be unrelated in the totality of individual salvation. Islamic communal discourse sought to define itself by legitimizing individual autonomy within its religiously-based collective order by leaving individuals free to negotiate their spiritual destiny, while requiring them to abide by communal order that involved the play of reciprocity and autonomy upon which a regime of rights and responsibilities are based in the Sharīʿa. Practical piety and reliable character are emphasized in connection with all professions. Although a physician does not have to be a pious individual in order to be a competent physician, because a physician's work is essentially to take care of his/her patient; nevertheless, piety and good character aid in the general acceptance of the physician's advice. Bad character would detract from its value. A physician should be a cultured person, aware of the sensibilities of the people among whom he/she works. In Muslim culture, a physician has to work hard to gain the trust of the patient and cultivate professional confidence.

Islam lays great emphasis on virtues and obligations in connection with medical profession because medicine deals with the most valued aspect of existence, namely, preservation of human life. Bad character in a physician is seen as a mortal poison and a sure path to perdition. The sicknesses of heart and the diseases of soul are regarded as a great threat to the normal professional role assumed by a physician. Moreover, the society and the institutions that provide medical care have certain expectations of a person to whom they entrust their physical wellbeing. Muslim ethicists lay down canons by which virtues become ingrained in the practice of a skillful physician. Techniques of meditation and prayers are suggested for medical professionals to focus their attention on the wholeness of human care, and not simply their physical condition. In this way a medical professional in a Muslim community is expected to learn not only the origins and causes of sicknesses, which cause loss of corporeal life, but also pay attention to the diseases of heart and soul. In this latter diagnosis, the Muslim physician goes beyond role-related technical skills, and equips him/herself with a character built on a virtuous life to understand the religious/psychological dimensions of the profession. The two most important virtues emphasized in Islamic professional ethics are: spiritual and moral consciousness (*taqwā*), and patience (*Ṣabr*). The physician must cultivate these two virtues by leading a balanced and moderate life, and not waste time and energy indulging in pleasure and amusements.

The question of professional ethics is directly connected to a religious problem of the relationship between action and its impact upon human conscience. To state it briefly, human acts have a direct impact upon the development of conscience that, in Islamic tradition, is regarded as the source for determining the rightness or wrongness of human undertakings. The conscience must constantly guard against becoming corrupted. When conscience becomes corrupted as a result of neglecting ethical matters related to the production of daily sustenance, then there is no moral safeguard left to prevent these professionals from engaging in more serious acts that could lead to the destruction of the very fabric of social relations founded upon a divinely ingrained sense of justice and fairness. Both intention and reflection must precede all human acts that infringe upon the spiritual and physical wellbeing of others.

Here, it is important to keep in mind that both patient and physician are required by Islam to observe ethical discipline.

Patients should strictly follow their physicians' orders and respect their physicians. Patients are exhorted to regard their physicians better than their best friends. Patients should have direct contact with their doctors and should confide fully in them concerning their sickness. In fact, it is better for people to stay in touch with a physician who can advise them about their health before they actually need treatment.

Spiritual care of Islamic patients

Spiritual care begins in providing settings that permit, and preferably encourage, religious observance and observe the rules of interpersonal behaviour in providing care and carrying out interventions. Spiritual care, however, also involves supporting appropriate decision-making. Healthcare practitioners need the capacity to provide patients and families with information that is appropriate to religious, communitarian ethical decision-making, and to respect the process such decision-making must take. As part of this process it may be necessary for the patient and family to consult a trusted physician and/or imam, and communication protocols may need to be adapted to include these key people. The negotiable and local character of Islamic communitarian ethics should be a reminder to healthcare practitioners that a 'fact file' approach to care is at best inadequate.

References

1 Muḥammad b. Ismā'īl al-Bukhārī, *Sahiḥ* (Beirut: 'Ālam al-Kutub, n.d.), **8**: 91, Ḥadīth 1.

2 Ibn Māja, *Sunan* (Beirut: al-Maktaba al-'Ilmīya, n.d.), **2**: 1111.

3 George, F., Hourani, 'Ibn Sina's. (1966). 'Essay on the Secret of Destiny," *Bulletin of the School of Oriental and African Studies*, University of London, **29**: pp. 25–48.

4 Lane, E.W. (1968). *An Arabic-English Lexicon*, off-print edn. Beirut: Librairie du Liban.

5 Antes, P. (1989). Medicine and the living tradition of Islam. In: L. E. Sullivan (ed.)*Healing and Restoring: Health and Medicine in the World's Religious Traditions*. New York: Macmillan), pp. 173–208.

6 *Saḥīḥ al-Bukhārī, Kitāb al-Marḍā* (1979). Chicago: Ḥadīth No. 582.

7 *Saḥīḥ al-Bukhārī, Kitāb al-Marḍā* Hādīth No. 545

8 Abdulaziz, Sachedina, (2009). *Islamic Biomedical Ethics: Principles and Application*. New York: Oxford University Press.

9 Abū Ḥāmid al-Ghazālī, *Kitāb al-Mustaṣfā min 'ilm al-uṣūl*. Cairo: Bulaq, 1904–7, pp. 174ff.

10 Ibrāhīm b. Mūsā al-Shāṭibī, *al-Muwāfiqāt fi uṣūl al-sharī'a* (Beirut: Dār al-Jīl, n.d.), Vol. 2: 8ff.

11 Ibn Badrān al-Dimashqī, *al-Madkhal ilā imām Aḥmad b. Ḥanbal* (Beirut: Mu'assassa al-Risāla, 1401/1981), p. 295.

12 'Abd Allāh b. Aḥmad Ibn Qudāma, *Rawḍat al-nāẓir wa jannat al-manāẓir* (Riyād: Jāmi' al-Imām, 1399/1978), **3**:170.

13 Muḥammad b. 'Umar al-Rāzī, *al-Maḥsūl fī 'ilm al-uṣūl al-fiqh* (Riyāḍ: Jāmi' al-Imām, 1400/1979), **6**: p. 220.

14 Shāṭibī, *al-Muwāfiqāt*, **2**: p. 9.

15 Ghazālī, *al-Mustaṣfā*, p. 175.

16 Shāṭibī, *al-Muwāfiqāt*, **2**: pp. 9–10.

17 Muḥammad Sa'Id Ramaḍān al-Buṭī, *ḍawābiṭ al-maṣlaḥa fī sharī'at al-islāmīya* (Beirut: Mu'assassa al-Risāla, 1401/1981), p. 219.

18 *al-Muwāfiqāt*, **2**: pp. 23–5.

CHAPTER 10

Judaism

Dan Cohn-Sherbok

Introduction

From ancient times to the present, Judaism has stressed the importance of healing the sick. Such responsibility is viewed as divinely sanctioned. For this reason, Jewish physicians have had an important role in the Jewish community. In numerous ways, the tradition sanctions healthcare and provides a framework for tending the sick and curing the ill. In addition, both biblical and rabbinic sources stress the importance of visiting the sick, curing the ill, and tending those who are dying. Despite the variety of modern movements with their different and conflicting interpretations of the Jewish faith, there is widespread agreement about the general principles underlying such concern.

Theological foundations

According to the tradition, the beginnings of the Jewish nation stemmed from God's revelation to Abraham at the beginning of the second millennium BCE. Known as Abraham, he came from Ur of the Chaldeans, a Sumerian city of Mesopotamia. The Book of Genesis recounts that God called him to go to the land of Canaan: 'Go from your country and your kindred and your father's house to the land I will show you. And I will make of you a great nation' (Genesis 12: 1–2). The Hebrew Bible traces the history of this tribe from patriarchal times to the Exodus from Egypt several centuries later, and eventually the conquest of the land of Canaan by Joshua in about 1200 BCE. In later books of the Bible, the period of the judges, the rise of the monarchy, the emergence of the prophets, and the eventual destruction of the Northern and Southern Kingdoms are described in detail. With the growth of rabbinic Judaism in the Hellenistic period, the Jewish faith underwent a fundamental change that profoundly transformed Jewish life until the present. This long history of the Jewish people—stretching back over nearly forty centuries—provides the historical framework for the central beliefs of the Jewish faith.

Divine Unity and Creation

Of primary importance is the belief in God's unity. Throughout the history the Jewish people, the belief in one God has served as a cardinal principle of the faith. From biblical times to the present, Jews daily recite the Shema prayer: 'Hear O Israel, the Lord our God, the Lord is One.' According to Scripture, God alone is to be worshipped. Continuing this tradition, the sages of the early rabbinic period stressed that any form of polytheistic belief is abhorrent. For thousands of years, Jews have proclaimed their belief and trust in the one God who created the universe and rules over creation. According to Genesis 1, God created the Heaven and the Earth. This belief is a central feature of the synagogue service. In the synagogue hymn before the reading from the Psalms, God is described as the creator of all:

> Blessed be He who spoke, and the world existed:
>
> Blessed be He;
>
> Blessed be He who was the master of the world in the beginning.

Divine transcendence

For Jews, God is conceived as transcendent. Throughout Scripture the notion of divine transcendence is repeatedly affirmed. In the rabbinic period, Jewish scholars formulated the doctrine of the Shekinah to denote the divine presence. Later in the Middle Ages the doctrine of the Shekinah (God's presence) was further elaborated. According to the ninth-century scholar Saadiah Gaon, the Shekinah is identical with the glory of God, which serves as an intermediary between God and human beings during the prophetic encounter.

Divine providence

Judaism stresses, however, that God is not remote from creation. Rather he controls and guides the universe. According to Scripture, there are two kinds of providence: (1) general providence—God's provision for the world in general; and (2) special providence—God's care for each individual. God's general providence was manifest in his freeing the ancient Israelites from Egyptian bondage and guiding them to the Promised Land. The belief in the unfolding of his plan for salvation is a further illustration of such providential care of his creatures. Linked to this concern for all is God's concern for every person. In the Talmud we read: 'No man suffers so much as the injury of a finger when it has been decreed in heaven.'

The chosen people and revelation

Central to this belief in divine providence is the conviction that God chose the Jews as his special people. Through its election, Israel has been given an historic mission to bear divine truth to humanity.

In this regard, the belief in revelation is critical. According to tradition, the entire Torah (the Five Books of Moses—Genesis, Exodus, Leviticus, Numbers, and Deuteronomy) was communicated by God to Moses on Mt Sinai. As the twelfth century Jewish philosopher Moses Maimonides explained in his Commentary to the Mishnah (Sanhedrin, X: 1).

The Torah was revealed from Heaven. This implies our belief that the whole of the Torah found in our hands this day is the Torah that was handed down by Moses, and that it is all of divine origin. By this I mean that the whole of the Torah came unto him from before God in a manner that is metaphorically called 'speaking', but the real nature of that communication is unknown to everybody except to Moses to whom it came.

Divine commandments

According to tradition, God revealed 613 commandments (*mitzvot*) to Moses on Mt Sinai, which are recorded in the Torah. These prescriptions, which are to be observed as part of God's covenant with Israel are classified in two major categories: (1) statutes concerned with ritual performances characterizes as obligations between human beings and God; and (2) judgements consisting of laws that would have been adopted by society even if they had not been decreed by God (such as laws regarding murder and theft). Traditional Judaism also maintains that Moses received the Oral Torah in addition to the Written Law. This was passed down from generation to generation and has been the subject of ongoing rabbinic debate.

The Oral Law

The first authoritative compilation of the Oral Law is the Mishnah composed by Judah Ha-Nasi in the second century CE. In subsequent centuries, sages continued to discuss the content of Jewish Law—their deliberations are recorded in the Palestinian and Babylonian Talmuds. Subsequently, rabbinic authorities continued the development of Jewish Law by issuing answers to specific questions. In time, various scholars felt the need to produce codes of Jewish Law so that all members of the community would have access to the legal tradition. In the eleventh century, Isaac Alfasi produced a work that became the standard code for Sephardic Jewry. Two centuries later, Asher ben Jehiel wrote a code that became the code for Ashkenazi Jews. Moses Maimonides in the twelfth century also wrote an important code that had a wide influence, as did the code of Jacob ben Asher in the fourteenth century.

The Code of Jewish Law

In the sixteenth century Joseph Caro published the Shulkhan Arukh that, together with glosses by Moses Isserles, has served as the standard Code of Jewish law for Orthodox Jewry until the present day. The Shulkahn Arukh is divided into four divisions: (1) Orah Hayyim dealing with everyday conduct, prayer, and festivals; (2) Yoreh Deah concerning the dietary and ritual laws; (3) Even Ha-Ezer, which deals with matters of personal status; and (4) Hoshen Mishpat dealing with courts, civil law, and torts. For the strictly Orthodox, the Code of Jewish Law is binding and serves as the guide to all matters of daily life.

Principles of healthcare

Within Judaism religion and healthcare have been in alliance since ancient times. From the biblical period to the present, the Jewish tradition has focused on the responsibilities of physicians and others to help those in distress. The attitude of Jewish Law is to encourage and facilitate the struggle against and escape from illness, which is regarded as a significant misfortune. Despite the belief in divine providence, there has been a general acceptance that sickness and disease should be combated and cured if possible. Human efforts to mitigate suffering are extolled and procedures for cure are described in detail. According to tradition, it is the prerogative and duty of human beings to use intellectual and physical resources to conquer disease. According to the Code of Jewish Law, 'the Torah gave permission to the physician to heal; moreover this is a religious precept, and it is included in the category of saving life.[1]

Healing

Judaism affirms that it is a moral duty to heal those in need. As the 15th century commentator and philosopher Isaac Arama noted, human effort is critical. Basing his view on the Pentateuchal narrative describing the patriarchs' efforts to save themselves when in danger, and legislation regarding the duty to construct parapets around roofs for the preventing of accidents, he argues that human beings must not rely on miracles or providence only, but must do whatever they can to maintain life and health.[2] In traditional Jewish sources, there is no rejection of medicine as legitimate. The typical attitude toward the legitimacy of healing was expressed by Chayim J. D. Azulay (a younger contemporary of the Baal Shem Tov, the founder of Hasidism): 'Nowadays one must not rely on miracles, and the sick man is duty bound to conduct himself in accordance with the natural order by calling on a physician to heal him. In fact, to depart from the general practice by claiming greater merit than the many saints [in previous] generations, who were cured by physicians, is almost sinful on account of both the implied arrogance and the reliance on miracles when there is danger to life ... Hence, one should adopt the ways of all men and be healed by physicians.'[3]

Healing by faith and prayer

Alongside the Jewish insistence on physical healing, the tradition has stressed the need for prayer. Typical among Jewish teachers was the medieval poet-physician Judah Halevy's supplication for divine help:

> My medicines are of Thee, whether good or evil,
> whether strong or weak,
> It is Thou who shalt choose, not I,
> Of Thy knowledge is the evil and the fair.
> Not upon my power of healing I rely;
> Only for Thine healing do I watch.[4]

Again, the 17th century rabbi-physician Jacob Zahalon wrote a prayer in which he proclaimed his reliance on God:

> I am minded to busy myself with the practice of medicine in Thy Holy Name and through Thy assistance ... I do not rely upon my wisdom, nor do I place my trust in the drugs and herbs and medicaments which Thou hast created, for they are, but the means to fulfil Thy will and to proclaim Thy greatness and Thy providence.[5]

Such utterances illustrate the physician's perception of his role as a divine agent in the alleviation of human suffering. Ultimately, God is viewed as the ultimate healer of disease.

Amulets and incantations

In general rabbinic sources retained the biblical hostility to superstition, as found in Deuteronomy 18:10–11, which forbids sorcery, witchcraft, divination, soothsaying, consulting auguries, magic spells, and necromancy. Nonetheless, it was a frequent practice in the Middle Ages to use incantations and amulets to ward off evil. In Jewish codes frequent mention is made of the use of incantations and amulets. The medical effectiveness of incantations was widely accepted. Incantations to heal a scorpion's bite, for example, were permitted even on the Sabbath. Similarly, it was allowed to charm snakes or scorpions to prevent injury by them, and such acts were not viewed as violations of Sabbath law. Amulets were normally pendants containing a written text. These were generally worn by the user at all times to cure or prevent certain ailments. In this regard, the Code of Jewish Law states:

> It is permitted to make medical use of amulets, even if they contain [divine] names; similarly, it is allowed to wear amulets containing scriptural verses, provided they serve to protect the wearer from falling ill and not to heal him when afflicted with a wound or a disease. However, it is forbidden to write scriptural verses on amulets.[6]

Demons and evil spirits

In contrast with amulets and incantations, the exorcism of demons is only rarely mentioned in Jewish Law. Following the Talmud, the codes affirm the belief in the existence of demons. In the sixteenth century, the belief in the power of such beings was so great that a leading rabbi discussed whether a woman who was alleged to have had intercourse with a demon should be separated from her husband as an adulteress. More reference, however, is made to evil spirits who pursue or possess human beings, and cause mental illness. The matrimonial regulations in the Code of Jewish Law refer to a husband who wishes to divorce his wife who is seized by the evil spirit and turned insane.[7] It was widely believed that a person in whom the evil spirit had breathed could be cured by milk squirted on him by a nursing mother. Jewish Law refers to two remedies against the harmful effects of the evil eye. A special charm could be worn by persons even on the Sabbath; horses could be protected against the evil eye by a fox-tail suspended between their eyes.

Preservation of human life

The Jewish tradition repeatedly affirms the need to preserve life, even if this involves profaning the Sabbath. Hence, the Talmud and subsequent rabbinic works stress that it is lawful to ignore the Sabbath, as well as other religious precepts in order to save life. It makes no difference whether the life of the person saved on the Sabbath is likely to be extended by many years of merely seconds. The principle is that each human life is infinite so that a hundred years and a single second are equally precious. The principle here is that the duty to promote life and health, and any acts performed to that end, are of paramount importance. Thus, it is not merely permitted, but imperative to disregard laws in conflict with life or health. As the Code of Jewish Law explains: 'It is a religious precept to desecrate the Sabbath for any person afflicted with an illness that may prove dangerous; he who is zealous is praiseworthy, whilst he who asks [questions] sheds blood.[8] In this regard, vital decisions must be made quickly when the interests of life conflict with the demands of religious law. A delay could result in fatal consequences. Here, the Code of Jewish Law provides guidance: on the principle that where a doubt exists involving danger to life, the more lenient view should prevail.[9]

Forestalling danger to life

The principle of preserving life extends to any danger to life itself. Hence, the Code of Jewish Law specifies that flames should be extinguished on the Sabbath before they threaten to engulf properties in which human lives could be threatened.[10] Food may be rescued from a conflagration if required for sick, old, or ravenous people.[11] It is permitted to capture snakes, scorpions, or other dangerous creatures to prevent being bitten by them.[12] Animals whose bite is lethal may be killed on the Sabbath, but if the injury they might cause is not usually fatal, their destruction is lawful only if one is actually pursued by them.[13]

Concern for animals

In addition to concern for human welfare, the Jewish tradition stresses the importance of care for animals. Relaxation of Sabbath laws to protect the health of animals includes permission to anoint their wounds provided they are fresh and painful,[14] to place them in water to cool them following an attack of congestion,[15] to ask a non-Jew to bleed them if venesection can save their life,[16] to raise them from water into which they have fallen,[17] and to ask a non-Jew to relieve them of milk causing them distress.[18]

Illness and death

Judaism's concern with health issues, focuses as well on questions dealing with sickness and death. Throughout the religious sources, the rabbis stress that both physical and mental pain should be relieved whenever possible. Such religious consideration permits Jewish Law to be set aside if necessary. This is so with regard to the Sabbath in particular, but also applies in other contexts. Within rabbinic sources, a wide variety of issues, ranging from caring for the sick to the treatment of the dying, are elaborated in detail. Throughout there is a constant concern for correct conduct and moral concern.

Relief of pain

According to tradition, pain in general justifies infractions of the law. Here pain is understood to involve both physical and mental suffering. Rabbinic sources abound with examples: one need not have the Friday evening meal in the glow of the Sabbath candles as normally required, if the light is the cause of undue discomfort.[19] It is permitted to weep on the Sabbath if this may bring relief from mental stress.[20] The nursing mother especially enjoys sympathy within Jewish Law: to relieve herself of excess milk hurting her, she may suckle a non-viable child or squeeze the milk by hand, even in circumstances in which that is not normally allowed. Jewish Law specifies that when circumcision takes place, time should elapse before a person's immersion in a ritual bath so that he will be able to recover from the operation. Even a criminal walking to his execution is to be saved from unnecessary anguish in compliance with the principle: 'Thou shalt love thy neighbour as thyself'—thus the Talmud insists that an individual should be drugged into insensibility during the final ordeal so as to minimize his suffering.[21]

Visiting the sick

The Jewish tradition stresses the importance of visiting the sick. Such visits are viewed as among the most meritorious acts.

Hence, in a talmudic passage that is recited daily by Jews, this duty is listed as one of the ten most important ethical responsibilities.[22] According to the Talmud, a refusal to visit the sick is like shedding blood, since visits to the sick help them to become well. This obligation is a responsibility of everyone in the community.[23] The manner of performing this religious duty is prescribed in precise terms. There is no limit on the frequency with which the sick should be visited on a single day. The more often the better, as long as it does not trouble the patient. Even a personal enemy should go to see his sick neighbour as long as this does not cause anguish to the person who is ill. Close relatives and friends may visit the patient immediately; those more distant should not come until three days have elapsed, unless the illness has come about suddenly. Visits during the first and last three hours of the day should be avoided. Sick visits are permitted even on the Sabbath.[24]

Treatment of the opposite sex

Judaism makes no restriction on a male physician treating female patients. Nonetheless, it is emphasized that medical practitioners should adopt the highest ethical standards. In this regard the Talmud cites the example of the fourth century sage Abba who was noted for his piety, and had separate consulting rooms for men and women. He also gave his patients a special dress for venesection so that no part of the body would be exposed except what was needed for the operation.[25] In this connection the first Hebrew medical writer, Asaf Judaeus, in the seventh century admonished his pupils not to let the beauty of a female patient arouse the passion of adultery.[26] Echoing such a view, the seventeenth century scholar and medical writer Jacob Zahalon warned: 'When the physician visits women, he should be modest and should not follow the evil thoughts of his heart.'[27] In his prayer for physicians to be recited weekly, he declared: 'Cleanse my mind and purify my thoughts that I think no evil about any woman, whether virgin or wife, when I visit her, that I do not go after my own heart and my own eyes.'[28]

Treatment of the insane

The regulations regarding respect to parents is not diminished if they are mentally deranged. Ideally, children should take responsibility for their parents care. However, according to the 12th century philosopher and codifier, Moses Maimonides, if they become excessively insane, it is permissible to employ others to look after them. In his view, an insane person must not be left without due care. If children are unable to exercise this responsibility, they must find and provide others to do so.[29]

Preparation for death

According to the tradition, every caution must take place with the last preparations before death so that the dying person's condition is not affected adversely. Such matters include the ordering of an individual's affairs, as well as his reconciliation with the Creator. The Talmud specifies that he is first to be told to set his mind on his affairs, for example, if he had left a loan or a deposit with others or held a loan or a deposit from them. Later when he feels death is imminent, he should be encouraged to confess his sins. The Code of Jewish Law specifies that he should be told that 'many have confessed, but did not die, while many who did not confess died; and as a reward for your confession you will live, for whoever confesses has a portion in the world to come.'[30] The prayer of confession seeks to reassure a patient: 'I acknowledge before Thee, O Lord, my God, and the God of my fathers, that my recovery and my death are in Thine hand. May it be Thy will to heal me with a perfect healing; but if I die, may my death be an atonement for all my sins ... which I have committed before Thee.'[31] Yet as the end draws near, mention should not be made of death so that the patient should not know the seriousness of his condition and thereby become weaker.[32]

Treatment of the dying

When death appears near, the patient is still to be related to as a living person. It is forbidden to tie his jaws, anoint him, wash him, plug his open organs, remove the pillow from under him, or place him on sand, clay, or the ground. It is also not permitted to lay a vessel or salt on his belly or close his eyes.[33] Such actions are not allowed because they might hasten his death. For this reason the Talmud states: 'The matter can be compared with a flickering flame; as soon as one touches it, the light is extinguished.'[34]

Euthanasia

According to traditional Judaism, any form of active euthanasia is strictly forbidden. In legal terms the tradition decrees that anyone who kills a dying patient is liable to the death penalty.[35] Yet Jewish Law permits the withdrawal of any factors that may artificially delay a person's death. However, it is permitted to expedite the death of an incurable patient in acute agony by withholding such medicines that sustain his life by unnatural means. It should be noted that this traditional ruling is not universally accepted within the Jewish community. In recent times, some non-Orthodox Jewish thinkers have advocated voluntary euthanasia under certain conditions.

Determining death

The rabbis of the Talmud decreed that death occurs when respiration has stopped. However, with the development of modern medical technology, this definition has been subject to alteration. It is now possible to resuscitate those who previously would have been regarded as dead. Thus, the modern rabbinic scholar Mosheh Sofer in his responsum declares that death is considered to have occurred when there has been respiratory and cardiac arrest. Another legal scholar, Mosheh Feinstein, however, has ruled that a person is considered to have died with the death of his brain stem. Despite such disagreements, it is generally accepted that a critically ill person who hovers between life and death is alive. Jewish Law accepts that no effort should be spared to save a dying patient. In this regard, the Talmud lays down that a change of name may avert the evil decree and, hence, the custom developed of altering the formal name of an individual who is seriously ill. Yet despite such a practice, traditional Judaism fosters an acceptance of death when it is inevitable.

Dealing with a dead person

According to tradition, once death has been determined, the eyes and mouth are closed, and if necessary the mouth is tied shut. The body is then put on the floor, covered with a sheet, and a lighted candle is placed close to the head. Mirrors are covered in the home of the deceased and any standing water is poured out. A dead body is not to be left unattended, and it is considered a *mitzvah* (good deed) to sit with the person who has died and recite psalms. It should be noted, however, that these practices are carried out only within Orthodox Judaism; the non-Orthodox branches of the faith have established their own procedures, which largely dispense with these practices.

Burial

The burial of the body should take place as soon as possible. According to tradition, no burial is allowed to take place on the Sabbath or the Day of Atonement. In contemporary practice it is considered unacceptable for it to take place on the first and last days of the pilgrim festivals (Passover, Succot, and Shavuot). After the members of the burial society have taken care of the body, they prepare it for burial. It is washed and dressed in a white linen shroud. The corpse is then placed in a coffin or on a bier before the funeral service. Traditional Jews only permit the use of a plain wooden coffin, with no metal handles or ornaments. The deceased is then borne to the grave face upwards. Adult males are buried wearing their prayer shawl. Again, it should be noted that, amongst non-Orthodox Jews, many of these practices have been altered or omitted. Among Reform Jews, for example, burial practice differs markedly from that of the Orthodox. Embalming and cremation are usually permitted, and Reform rabbis commonly officiate at crematoria. Burial may be delayed for several days, and the person who has died is usually buried in normal clothing without a prayer shawl.

Conclusion: unity and diversity in Jewish healthcare

In the modern world, the Jewish community has fragmented into a wide range of different groupings, each with their own interpretation of the tradition. Nonetheless, all Jews—whether Orthodox or belonging to the various non-Orthodox branches of the faith—embrace the Jewish emphasis on caring for the sick and those who suffer. Even though the central theological tenets of the tradition are no longer universally accepted within the Jewish world, Jews—whatever their religious orientation–endorse the Jewish emphasis on healthcare. Visiting the sick is regarded as a cardinal virtue, and physicians and healthcare workers are viewed with respect and admiration. Amongst the Orthodox, the traditional healthcare practices continue to govern Jewish life. Yet, it must be emphasized that there is a difference of opinion within the Jewish world about a wide range of contentious medical issues. For example, although many Orthodox Jews regard artificial insemination where insemination is by the husband, there are serious reservations about such a practice where there is an outside anonymous donor. Here, Orthodox authorities have argued that this would pose grave moral problems. Such operations, they maintain, disrupt the family relationship. Moreover, a child conceived in this way would be denied its birthright to have a father and other relations who can be identified. Despite this ruling, however, there are many Jews today who favour artificial insemination regardless of the donor. In their view, there should be no moral reservations about artificial insemination by donor (AID): it is a procedure to be welcomed and encouraged for those unable to have a child by normal means.

Abortion, too, is a topic where there is considerable disagreement. According to Orthodoxy, abortion is sanctioned, but only in cases involving a grave anticipated hazard to the mother whether physical or psychological. A former Chief Rabbi of Israel, for example, adopted an even more strict view, expressly proscribing the destruction of any foetus, at whatever age of gestation, even if serious deformities were suspected. However, opposing this view, the head of the Rabbinical Court of Jerusalem, adopted a more lenient approach, and made a distinction between earlier and later periods of the pregnancy. In his view, an abortion on a Jewish mother, even in the absence of any actual danger to her life, is permitted provided there is a serious medical indication, as well as in cases of rape or incest, or of a definite risk that the child may be born physically or mentally handicapped. Within the non-Orthodox world, however, there is a much more flexible approach to abortion. For many Jews, abortion should be viewed a choice for the mother to make without fulfilling such pre-conditions.

Health care workers must thus be aware of the fact that the Jewish community is no longer unified by belief and practice. When dealing with strictly Orthodox patients, Jewish Law should be followed rigorously. However, in the vast majority of cases Jewish patients will not feel bound by prescriptions found in rabbinic sources. In such instances it is important to ascertain the degree to which Jewish Law will need to be followed or could be set aside. Yet despite such differences of approach to the tradition, there is universal agreement in the Jewish community that healthcare is of primary importance and that those who are engaged in this field are to be respected and admired. Judaism and medicine have been allied with each other throughout thousands of years of history, and this continues to be so in the modern world.

Bibliography

Avinoam Bezalel, S. (1971). *Medicine and Judaism*, Tel-Aviv: Forum for Jewish Thought.

Berger, N. (1988). *Jews and Medicine*, Philadelphia: Jewish Publication Society.

Berman, R.E., Kurzweil, A., Mintz, D.L. (2006). *The Hadassah Jewish Family Guide to Health and Wellness*. New York: Arthur Kurzweil Books, Jossey-Bass.

Bleich, J.D. (2002). *Judaism and Healing*. Jersey City: Ktav Publ. Inc., Halakhic Perspectives.

Bulka, R.P. (1998). *Judaism on Illness and Suffering*. Lanham: Jason Aronson.

Cutter, W. (Ed.) (2007). *Healing and the Jewish Imagination:* Spiritual and Practical Perspectives on Judaism and Health. Woodstock: Jewish Lights.

Cutter, W. (2010). *Midrash and Medicine:* Healing Body and Soul in the Jewish Interpretive Tradition. Woodstock: Jewish Lights.

Feldman, D.M. (1986). *Health and Medicine in the Jewish Tradition:* Pursuit of Wholeness. New York: Crossroad.

Freeman, D.L., Abrams, J.Z. (Eds) (1999). *Illness and Health in the Jewish Tradition*. Philadelphia: Jewish Publication Society.

Friedenwald, H. (1944). *The Jews and Medicine*, 2 VOLS, Baltimore: Johns Hopkins University.

Hart, M.B. (2007). *Healthy Jew:* The Symbiosis of Judaism and Modern Medicine. Cambridge: Cambridge University Press.

Heynick, F. (2002). *Jews and Medicine: an Epic Saga*. Jersey City: Ktav Publ. Inc.

Isaacs, R.H. (1998). *Judaism, Medicine and Healing*. Lanham: Jason Aronson.

Jakobovits, I. (1975). *Jewish Medical Ethics*. New York: Bloch Publishing Company*

Koenig, H.G. (2007). *Spirituality in Patient Care: Why, How, When and What*. West Conshohocken: Templeton Foundation Press.

Meier, L. (1991). *Jewish Values in Health and Medicine*. Lanham: University Press of America.

Orchard, H. (2001). *Spirituality in Health Care Contexts*. London: Jessica Kingsley.

Preuss, J. (1995). *Biblical and Talmudic Medicine*. Lanham: Jason Aronson.

Rosner, F. (2000). *Encyclopedia of Medicine in the Bible and Talmud*. Lanham: Jason Aronson.

Rosner, F. (1972). *Modern Medicine and Jewish Law*. New York: Department of Special Publications, Yeshiva University.

Sinclair, D.B. (2003). *Jewish Biomedical Law: Legal and Extra-Legal Dimensions*. Oxford: Oxford University Press.

Spitzer, J. (2002). *A Guide to the Orthodox Jewish Way of Life for Healthcare Professionals*. London: Dr J. Spitzer.

Spitzer, J. (2003). *Caring for Jewish Patients*. Oxford: Radcliffe Publishing Ltd.

Zohar, N.J. (Ed.) (2006) *Quality of Life in Jewish Bioethics*. Lanham: Lexington Books.

Zoloth, L. (1999). *Health Care and the Ethics of Encounter: A Jewish Discussion of Social Justice*. Chapel Hill: University of North Carolina Press.

*I would like to acknowledge my indebtedness to this important work which has provided information and numerous references throughout this chapter.

References

1 Code of Jewish Law, Yoreh Deah, cccxxxvi.1.
2 Arama, 'Akedath Yitzhak, Sha'ar xxvi (ed.) Frankfurt a/Oder, 1785, p. 57a.
3 Azulay, Birkei Yoseph, Code of Jewish Law, Yoreh Deah, cccxxxvi.2.
4 Friedenwald, H. (1944). *The Jews and Medicine*. Baltimore: John Hopkins Press.
5 [4], p. 273ff.
6 Code of Jewish Law, Yoreh Deah, clxxix.12.
7 Code of Jewish Law, Even-Haezer, cxxi.1.
8 Code of Jewish Law, Orah Hayyim, cccxxviii.2.
9 Code of Jewish Law, Orah Hayyim, cccxxviii.10.
10 Code of Jewish Law, Orah Hayyim, cccxxix.1.
11 Code of Jewish Law, Orah Hayyim, cccxxxiv.5.
12 Code of Jewish Law, Orah Hayyim, cccxvi.7.
13 Jakobovits, I. (1959). *Jewish Medical Ethics*. New York: Bloch, p. 70–1.
14 Code of Jewish Law, Orah Hayyim, cccxxxii.2.
15 Code of Jewish Law, Orah Hayyim, cccxxxii.4.
16 Code of Jewish Law, Orah Hayyim, cccxxxii.4.
17 Code of Jewish Law, Orah Hayyim, cccv. 19.
18 Code of Jewish Law, Orah Hayyim, cccv. 20.
19 Code of Jewish Law, Orah Hayyim, cclxxiii.7.
20 Code of Jewish Law, Orah Hayyim, cclxxxviii.2.
21 Sanhedrin 43a.
22 Shabbat, 127a.
23 Nedarim 40a.
24 [13], p. 109.
25 Ta'anith 21b.
26 [4], p. 22.
27 [4], p. 273.
28 [4], p. 277.
29 [13], op. cit. pp. 117–18.
30 Code of Jewish Law, Yoreh Deah, cccxxxviii.1.
31 Code of Jewish Law, Yoreh Deah, cccxxxviii.2.
32 Jakobovits, p. 120.
33 Ibid., pp. 121–122.
34 Shabbat 151b.
35 Sanhedrin 78a.

CHAPTER 11

'New Age' spirituality

Paul Heelas

Introduction

Incontestably, what might be thought of as 'New Age tradition' underpins great swathes of spirituality in the contemporary world. In countries ranging from Sweden to Pakistan, resources are to be found, resources that are neither secular nor sacred in the form of the God-on-High so typical of religious tradition. Elucidation of the characteristics of this 'New Age tradition' is called for—what health and healthcare mean in this context; the nature of the dynamics linking spirituality with the shift from ill-being, to normal ('I'm feeling okay') wellbeing, to even better-being ('feeling on top of the world'), ultimately, for some, to the experience of perfect health.

'New Age' and 'spiritualities of life'

Although the term 'New Age' has now entered common parlance in many countries, and although it has retained a measure of academic credibility, the term has become sullied by negative associations. Previously used to refer to the ideals of the 'Age of Aquarius' of the counter-cultural 'sixties', when the term highlighted the expectation that the world was moving away from the dystopic towards something akin to a humanistic heaven on earth, the expression is now frequently used to refer to what are considered to be the trivial, superficial, ridiculous hangovers of the days of the hippy.

To be as neutral as possible, the expression 'spiritualities of life' is a far better way of capturing what the 'New Age' of the sixties—and much else besides—is about. As well as being non-judgemental, a huge advantage of this expression is that it can be used cross-culturally. It can be used to refer to cultural settings where the 'New Age' is anything but new—the 'old age' of South Asia or China, for instance.

Thinking of South Asia, spiritualities of life are exemplified by numerous passages, which can be drawn from the works of the great spiritual virtuosi—Ghandi, Tagore, the Dalai Lama, Sufis, Bauls, a great many others of Hindu or Buddhist persuasion. The basic teaching of this path to ultimacy is straightforward. Fundamentally, humans are spiritual beings by virtue of their very nature. Life, at the pre-social time of birth, is sacred, that is, perfect. Inevitably, though, what humans are at birth becomes overlain by what they acquire by way of socialization; by what they acquire from sources other than their birth right. Taken to be the realm of the imperfect, the secular (as it has increasingly come to be called worldwide) contaminates the person. Socialization generates division. On the one hand, there is the perfect of the sacred self, while on the other hand, the imperfections, the unhealthy condition, of the socialized self (in modern day parlance, the 'ego' or 'lower self').

For spiritual virtuosi, the great majority of people have been socialized to the extent of losing all contact with what lies at the core of their being. Accordingly, teachers aim to help people liberate themselves from attachments to the secular realm of the imperfect. Those who experience their inner being, it is maintained, come to 'know'—'sense', 'feel', 'intuit', 'hear'—the 'true' unsullied nature of the values, sentiments, dispositions, passions, sense of the worthwhile, those purposes of life that *really* count, which really enable the participant to believe *in* what life has to offer. Those who come into contact with their inner being, it is maintained, encounter the intensity of agency, power, energy, the dynamism of perfect health. These are the forces that are unleashed to flow as currents into the realms of the imperfect—the damaged body, the inconsequential or interrupting mind, the negative emotion—to transform. Just as the *virtuous* reality of the sacred is expressed, that is, put to work, so is the *energetic* reality of what lies within. Frequently, the virtuous and the 'kinetic' are experienced as inseparable. Gandhi spoke of 'the force of love', for example, a great deal of the complementary and alternative medicine (CAM) of the contemporary west is profoundly ethical with causal agency. Overall, life, itself, is brought to life. 'I felt the sentiment of Being spread', as Wordsworth wrote in the *Prelude*.[1]

Healthcare

For believers, 'true' healthcare means making contact with the sacred within. For them, healthcare has to be spiritual, in the sacred sense of the word, to be 'truly' effective. Healthcare—in the general sense of looking after one's health, the health of others, the health of the social, the cultural and the natural—thus takes its 'true' course by the way of all those activities, for example, yoga, which are held to facilitate contact with the inner life. The three foci of healthcare, namely the preventive, the process of healing disease and the process of perfecting health as much as possible, are then informed by what lies within: not by the actions of the flawed 'ego'.

Directed by the wisdom of those who have already made contact with the sacred, the process of going within itself involves healthcare, largely with a preventative focus. Teachers point out that liberatory progress cannot be made by those who indulge in ego-desires, like gluttony or unjustified anger, to abuse themselves or others. Minimally, the ego has to be prevented from running riot. At least in measure, it is also held that ego-sickness is diminished by taking the preventative step of addressing the ill-being of those established socio-cultural activities which harm the ego. Gandhi's inner-informed, judged assaults on the caste system can be seen in this light. So can modern day attempts to transform the workplace, including preventative steps in connection with that 'parcelling-out of the soul' of which Max Weber wrote.[2]

As for healing and optimization of health foci, believers hold that the key lies with letting the sacred do its work. Already present in the entire person, including her or his body, from birth, but disrupted and repressed by contaminating socialization, the aim is to enable sacred currents to move again. Ameliorating the dominance of the 'ego' permits the dissolution of those 'blockages' generated by the clogging effect of socialization. Once dissolved, it is maintained, and once sacred currents have flowed to purify, transform, or eradicate ego-emotions, desires, values, and the like, the person experiences 'balance', 'harmony', 'integration'; something closely akin to Aristotle's 'golden mean'; something very much to do with 'wholeness'. 'Only connect' is the cry.

In short, due care is paid to the health, the enhancement of health, in all its aspects. Holistic spirituality of an inner-informed variety serves as a particular exemplification of what the World Health Organization's Constitution states, namely that 'Health is a dynamic state of complete physical, mental, spiritual and social well-being' ('spiritual' was added in 1999).[3]

However, this is not all. A great deal of distress is often generated, especially when people are gravely ill or (say) dying too young, by the 'why me?' question. More generally, people often seek some sort of account of why their lives 'don't feel right'. Those with faith in holistic spirituality quite naturally desire to know why the sacred, as the guide to perfect healthcare and with perfect (or absolute) power, does not prevent grave illness or other forms of imperfect health. A theodicy is called for. By attributing less than perfect health to the powerful influence of the malfunctions of the socio-cultural order, spiritualities of life go at least some way to address such matters. What is more, the theodicy provides believers with things to do. They can address the malfunctions; they can tackle the 'why me?' issue by way of the realization that disease has a purpose. As so many of the Romantics so emphasized, often drawing on the Book of Genesis in the process, the purpose of suffering is to serve as a 'practice' on the path to the sacred. Suffering can provide an opportunity for reflecting on what is 'really' important and unimportant in life, thereby putting ego distractions in their place; the approach of death can provide an opportunity to cultivate perspectives, like reflecting on what is harmonious in one's life, perhaps what could be in tune with the sacred.

'Traditions' of spiritualities of life

To flesh out what spiritualities of life have to do with health, healing, and healthcare, concrete illustrations are now provided from the historical record.

South Asian

To provide some exemplifications of the themes under consideration, it is clearly best to begin with those who are widely acknowledged as having mastered the arts of spiritual humanism. Perforce, this means turning east. Historically and geographically, spiritualities of life are more intimately connected with, most fully-developed, and most popular, in South Asia than virtually anywhere else. (Traditional China is the major exception, contemporary Japan being a more arguable one.) Albeit frequently tinged with references to an over-and-above-the-human-and-anything-that-the-human-can-be-or-become Godhead, the thrust of major figures (like Gandhi and Tagore) and mystics who are much less-well known in western circles (like the Sufi Bulleh Shah and the Baul singer-poets) very much revolve around the themes of spiritualities of life.

Essentially, spiritualities of life are about 'true' experience arrived at by way of practice, what is experienced being expressed accordingly. With human language being calibrated, organized, in terms of the realm of the secular, where *the* perfect cannot exist, it is not surprising that the sacred is ultimately taken to be ineffable. Accordingly, believers are hostile to intellectualization; to vigorous, logically coherent conceptual analysis; to propositional beliefs. With the basis of their teachings taken to be the immediacy of first-hand experience, inaccessible to the non-believer, what now follows has to call upon the equally first hand expressions—however elusive they might be—of participants.

Born in 1680, the most famous of all Punjabi Sufi poets of humanist persuasion, Bulleh Shah, tended cattle during his earlier days, to move to near Lahore to practice the Sufi path. In common with so many of the South Asian giants, there is a powerful counter-cultural strand to his world view. The 'inside', not the 'outside' of society at large, is where the 'truth' lies:

> This world is a slippery place.
>
> Walk carefully; there is darkness (all around you).
>
> Search your inner being (soul) to discover Who dwells there.
>
> Why do the people look for God in the outside? Why don't they search God within themselves?

His antipathy to 'this world' certainly included institutionalized Islam:

> You become a Hafiz [judge] by learning the Quran by heart.
>
> You cleanse your tongue by reading it again and again.
>
> You think of nothing, but dainties.
>
> Your heart becomes like a mad or frenzied dog.

He asks the mullahs, 'Why do you read piles of such books?' continuing, 'You carry the pack of sins, agonies and tortures/Now you look like a hangman.' Even,

> You [the mullahs] say prayers upon prayers.
>
> You scream and yell loudly.
>
> Sitting on the pulpit, you deliver sermons.
>
> Greed has brought disgrace upon you.

For Shah, institutionalized Islam is irredeemably polluted; irredeemably bound up with, whilst cultivating, harmful forms of attachments. In effect, for Shah religion, including those arrangements that encourage vested interests, worldly gain, lust for money, and so forth, is secular; the very opposite to healthcare. It encourages the intolerance of dogmatism; the 'established' blocks the path to the sacred; and so, equally, to health.

Bulleh Shah, himself, sought a realm beyond the turbulent dangers of institutionalized Islam and the imperfect life:

> He who discovers the saint's mystery
> actually carves the passage within himself. He is a
> dweller of the temple of peace, amity where there are
> no ups and downs.
> The irresistible thoughts do not remain suppressed.

He sought 'the River of Unity', what today would be called the sacred. And he sought it with passion:

> I am consumed by the fire of separation and the longing for my Beloved.
> Crazy in Love I am standing and whisking away the crows.

A passion that is not surprising given that the purpose or point of his life was at stake:

> Your lover is being traded for nothing.
> Meet me my Beloved, life is passing without purpose.
> I can't live without You even for a moment.
> I am the nightingale of this garden.

From the perspective of healthcare, the world-rejecting aspect of Bulleh Shah's journey certainly might be perfect for his own health; his own sense of moving away from injurious conflicts, from the clash between his intense yearning for unity and the disunity of so much of life, towards that source of the worthwhile that alone—he 'knew'—would bring the healing of union. Equally, though, he stands as an exemplar for others. Regarded, today, as a highly authoritative 'saint,' his message is that dogmatic, institutionalized Islam is the antithesis to healthcare; his message is that healthcare requires moving away from lust, intolerance, prejudice; and his message is that 'right' values and activities facilitate liberation, and at one and the same time inner-directed healthcare (he is strongly critical of sloth, for example, including overeating and oversleeping).[4] As well as being an exemplar, it can be added, Bulleh Shah serves as a direct healing agency. In the Punjab, as well as many other areas of South Asia, it is irrelevant whether the healing agent, as a person, is alive. Shrines are equally effective. What matters is the power (*baraka*) of the *pir* ('saint') lying with, immanent in, the saint-shrine, with Allah typically falling out of focus. Neither is it of all that great a concern that those attracted are on their own path to inner-healing power. The power of the *pir* is the power of the *pir*, the 'living' saint. Bearing in mind that many *pirs* supplement their 'own' power with those specialized in by the *hakim*, who tend to draw on 'natural' healing forces, and bearing in mind the extent to which the *pir* (and *hakim*) tend to deviate from orthodox, God-on-High Islam, 'alternative' healing of a spiritualities of life, variety is clearly in evidence. Today, what is sometimes called the traditional complementary and alternative medicine (TCAM) of areas like Punjab, is very popular; and, it can be borne in mind, shares a significant amount with many CAM activities of the contemporary west.[5]

Born close to 200 years after Bulleh Shah, in 1861, Rabindranath Tagore's writings resonate strongly with all those of Sufi masters like Bulleh Shah. Tagore draws on the Baul poets of Bengal—who so inspired him—in the most significant chapter of his *The Religion of Man*, namely 'The Man of My Heart'. Here, Tagore refers to a song he had heard from an impoverished Baul worshipper, a song that 'was alive with an emotional sincerity,' which 'spoke of an intense yearning of the heart for the divine which is in Man and not in the temple, or scriptures, in images and symbols'. Addressed to 'Man the ideal', the song runs,

> Temples and mosques obstruct thy path,
> and I fail to hear thy call or to move,
> when the teachers and priest angrily crowd round me.

Writing of the 'God-man', Tagore emphasizes the humanity of what lies within by citing a village poet:

> He is within us, an unfathomable reality. We know him when we unlock our own self and meet in true love with all others.

Or as another village poet puts it, with more force,

> Man seeks the man in me and I love myself and run out.

Songs of this nature cannot but bring to mind Bulleh Shah; looking forwards, one thinks of the outlook encapsulated by the 'I'm spiritual, not religious' refrain of the contemporary West and elsewhere.

For Tagore, 'the Eternal Spirit of human unity', deeper than the 'ever-changing phases of the individual self' of the 'surface of our being',

> ... very often contradicts the trivialities of our daily life, upsets the arrangements made for securing our personal exclusiveness behind the walls of individual habits and superficial conventions. It inspires in us works that are the expressions of a Universal Spirit; it invokes unexpectedly in the midst of a self-centred life a supreme sacrifice. At its call we hasten to dedicate our lives to the cause of truth and beauty, to unrewarded service of others.

Liberation from the realm of being where 'egoism' holds sway, also liberation from the hold of what he calls the 'merely animal', enables people to dwell with the best of two interplaying life-relationships, the relationship with the spirit of perfection within the self, and relationships within the world of the human:

> ... goodness represents the detachment of our spirit from the exclusiveness of our egoism; in goodness we identify ourselves with the universal humanity. Its value is not merely in some benefit for our fellow beings, but in its truth itself through which we realize within us that man is not merely an animal, bound by his individual passions and appetite, but a spirit that has its unfettered perfection. Goodness is the freedom of our self in the world of man, as is love. We have to be true within, not for worldly duties, but for that spiritual fulfilment, which is in harmony with the Perfect, in union with the Eternal.

A great admirer of Zarathustra, Tagore's admiration stems from the fact that Zarathustra proclaimed that 'religion has its truth in its *moral* significance, not in external practices of imaginary value' [emphasis added]. Rather than involving the transmission of some kind of spiritual energy which cares for health by addressing disease, 'spiritual power', for Tagore, is primarily a matter of value-laden human sentiments; of ethically-informed passions—all grounded in the sacred. The sacred transvalues 'love', the primary sentiment—love crosses over from love in secular mode (contaminated, say, by possessiveness) to love in 'true' expression. 'The spirit of love, dwelling in the boundless realm of the surplus, emancipates our consciousness from the illusory bond of the separateness of self; it is ever trying to spread its illumination in the human world'.

Healthcare is for humanity. Healthcare homes in on the erasure of conflict, animosity, and the like. This is healthcare in the fullest—whilst broadest—sense of the term: the dissipation of those imperfections of the secular *order* which generate the afflictions of the mind, body, emotions. And in the process, that greatest of goals—'to increase life', true life—is addressed.[6]

In a key regard, Tagore's life-philosophy is very much in accord with what has emerged as a central orthodoxy of contemporary, academically-respectable healthcare, both in the west and elsewhere. As a slogan, 'health is interpersonal.' Deviations from the 'right' of fruitful health sustaining or enhancing ways of being interpersonal have to be tackled. More or less identical themes are found in Tagore's friend, Mahatma Gandhi ('Mahatma' meaning 'great soul'). Affirming that 'The sum total of all that lives is God', writing of 'the truth within which ever purifies', and stressing the value of 'the permanent element in human nature', Gandhi, too, emphasizes the ethical aspects of healthcare. 'The adjective moral is synonymous with spiritual', he states emphatically. The 'essence of life' or 'the force' that is 'life' is profoundly imbued with the caring humanism of human spirituality. Graphically, 'I am endeavouring to see God through service of humanity, for I know that God is neither in heaven, nor below, but in every one'. Ultimately, healthcare lies with 'knowing' God, not least because until that is achieved, the soul is 'utterly restless'. Furthermore, until that is acquired, the 'force of love,' the 'love of life,' the 'force of the soul' remains dissipated, distorted, perhaps submerged by the impact of the countervailing processes of the secular. For love and similar sentiments—let alone dispositions and value-laden worldviews—to serve the end of healthcare and enhancement by alleviating the diseases of the secular, they have to be 'purified' by way of the 'absolute', essential, 'purity' of the sacred.[7]

Today, there is the Dalai Lama, one of the most respected, and certainly the most widely read, exponents of spiritual humanism-cum-healthcare. Treating 'religion' rather negatively, very negatively when the exclusive comes to the fore to disrupt societies and disturb personal wellbeing, he draws attention to another 'level of spirituality':

> This is what I call *basic spirituality*—'the basic human qualities of goodness, kindness, compassion, caring … as long as we are human beings, as long as we are members of the human family, *all* of us really need these basic spiritual values. Without these, human existence remains hard, very dry. As a result, none of us can be a happy person, our whole family will suffer, and then, eventually, society will be more troubled. So, it becomes clear that cultivating these kinds of basic spiritual values becomes critical.[8]

Critically, healthcare depends on shifting from the goodness, kindness, and caring of the secular condition—where they do not work properly—to the level of the 'basic,' where they are bound up with/infused by the sacred as their perfect exemplification.

Romantic

The greatest of all commentators on western Romanticism, M. H. Abrams, places 'life' at the heart of the movement:

> The ground concept is life. Life is itself the highest good, the residence and measure of other goods, and the generator of the controlling categories of Romantic thought. … Life is the premise and paradigm of what is most innovative and distinctive in Romantic thinkers. Hence their vitalism: the celebration of that which lives, moves, and evolves by an internal energy, over whatever is lifeless, inert, and unchanging.[9]

Like their South Asian counterparts, indeed, sometimes directly influenced by them, Romantics typically favoured what lies within over what lies with institutionalized religion. Some rejected the institutionalized *in toto*; some went further, rejecting the very notion of a Godhead existing over and above anything which the 'life', the 'current of nature', of this world can provide. (That Tagore, for instance, cites Wordsworth—'We live by admiration, hope and love/And ever as these are well and wisely fixed/In dignity of being we ascend'—is, but one indicator of way in which the more recent spiritual humanists of South Asia have, in turn, been influenced by the Romantic sensibility of the West.)

Naturally, when 'life' serves as the ultimate source of the worthwhile-cum-energy, matters to do with cultivation of what it is to be *alive* come to the fore. Strange as it might seem to think of healthcare in connection with poets like Shelly or Wordsworth, concern with health takes its place together with other major themes, the expression of 'life' in the creative arts; the art of life.

For Wordsworth, the spontaneous overflow of powerful feelings is an essential aspect of outstanding poetry. Nature itself, and/or the experience of nature mediated by personal sacrality, serve as a vehicle for healthcare. 'Tintern Abby' makes the point. Wordsworth himself reflected on how memories of the Abby, set by the Wye, provide 'tranquil restoration' in face of the hustle and bustle of urban life. Serving as a moral guardian or teacher, nature contributes to the unification of feelings and the ethicality of the 'good life'. Negative dissipation is circumvented, perhaps transformed. That great neo-Platonic theme—equating the purpose of life with the effort of moving from the differentiated, with all its conflictual features, to the unitary of the sacred, to restore, albeit at a higher level, the non-differentiated state of the womb (in Christian terms, life in the Garden of Eden)—is to the fore.

Shelley is arguably an even greater poet of what lies within, certainly providing a more dark view of the secular world ('grim vale of tears') an edgy, fraught view, if only symbolic, of what god/s above the human can do. His 'Hymn to Intellectual Beauty', with its 'Spirit of Beauty' and 'Awful Loveliness', his 'Queen Mab', with the 'Spirit of Nature' as 'the all-sufficing power' before which false religion falls, his 'Adonais', contrasting the 'One' with the 'Many', his 'Alastor' with its haunting vision of the 'Perfect Being', the 'Ideal Spirit', can be mentioned; or the majestic 'Prometheus Unbound'. Again and again, the theme is of an unseen Power, working from within the world *not* from outside it; working to transform existence in accordance with its own 'radiant' perfection; working as God.

In his unfortunately entitled essay, 'A Defence of Poetry' (unfortunate for it is truly a paean of praise), Shelley writes of 'sacred emotions', emotions that can 'render men more amiable, more generous and wise, and lift them out of the dull vapours of the little world of self'. In today's parlance, here is psychologically-orientated healthcare. In another formulation, which is equally critical of what can be thought of as common diseases of the secular, 'we want the poetry of life; our calculations have outrun conception; we have eaten more than we can digest'. Or again:

> Poetry is something divine … It is that from which all spring, and that which adorns all; and that which, if blighted, denies the fruit and the seed, and withholds from the barren world the nourishment and the succession of the scions of the tree of life. It is the perfect and consummate surface and bloom of all things. … this power [which] arises from within … [this] purity and force.[10]

Poetry as healthcare—not just poetry, another great Romantic poet, Novalis, writing in 1772, 'We touch heaven when we lay our hands on a human body'.[11]

The great Romantic poets emphasized the healing powers of the sacred at work through feelings, sentiments, touch (in the case of Novalis) and, of course, aesthetic sensibilities. The heyday of aesthetic-cum-'philosophical' Romanticism inspired the proliferation of 'applied' activities—Romanticism in action in everyday life. Of all the applications, not least educational, health took prominence. During the nineteenth century, healthcare specialists of inner-life orientation became increasingly numerous, some contributing to, or initiating movements which are very much alive today within the orbit of CAM. (With so many of these developments taking place within Germanic lands, it is not a coincidence that CAM, today, is more popular in Germany than in any other nation.) To mention the best known of the innovative practitioners, homeopathist Samuel Hahnemann (1755–1843) published his 'definitive' edition of the *Organon of Medicine* in 1842. Statements are bold. Operating holistically, the *heilkunst*, the 'art of healing' is informed by 'the life-force itself'; 'In the state of health the spirit-like vital force (dynamis) animating the material human organism reigns supreme'.[12] Then there is Christoph Hufeland (1762–1836), friend and personal physician of Goethe, Herder and Schiller, acquaintance of Hegel and Schelling, who published *The Art of Prolonging Life* (translated into English in 1797) and *Das Makrobiotik* (Kant wrote a commentary). Based on the 'metaphysical spirit' of 'natural laws', the latter emphasizes diet, exercise, lifestyle, fresh air, sunbathing, cleanliness, purification of the body, uplifting travel, and meditation. Turning to northern England, The Retreat in York (now commonly known as York Retreat and serving as a mental healthcare provider) was founded by a Quaker in 1796: the very height of 'elite' Romanticism. Albeit with theistic, supra-this world undertones, the 'inner light', and close integration with nature by way of design, gardening ('the healing garden'), farm labouring and walks, were to the fore, with 'humane' and 'moral' treatments offered from the start. In the Berlin of the time, famous oak trees served as a focal point for life-expression, health.

By the beginning of the First World War, most of the main ingredients of what is now thought of as CAM were securely in place. From the end of the War until the 1980s, the development of CAM in western settings was relatively slow. The counter-cultural sixties, for instance, might have been a time of enhanced interest in spiritualities of life, but as befits the youthfulness of those involved, health, let alone healthcare, was definitely not a top priority. During the last three decades, however, there has been a veritable explosion of things CAM.

Sacred, secular, or something else?

To further understanding, what is it to say that the 'sacred' is brought to bear on healthcare? Could it be the case that much of contemporary CAM operates beyond the sacred? Bearing in mind that many scholars have come to the conclusion that the notion of 'the sacred' is too elusive for academic inquiry, it requires a certain amount of elucidation and justification.

Ultimately, the sacred is the perfect, utopia itself. Being perfect, the sacred spells the death of ideals. For believers, to experience the sacred is not to experience the ideal of true love; it is to experience 'true' love *itself*; 'true' vitality, 'true' health, 'true' freedom, or equality. As the realm of perfect health, it is beyond healing. It is to experience that which cannot be bettered. Comparison with 'the secular' helps make more sense of the nature of the sacred. The secular is the realm of the imperfect. Drawing on a school of thought going back to Kant, then, way before him, to Ecclesiastes, Isaiah Berlin provides the convincing argument that value clash is inevitable. More precisely, and this is what he means when he refers to 'the crooked timber of humanity', to put together sufficient values to inform a way of life, any way of life, inevitably means value-conflict.[13] One does not have to believe in Freud to know that the interior life is prone to emotional turmoil. One does not have to be a Nietzsche to know how easy it is to discredit the exercise of the noblest of virtues by drawing attention to the multi-motivational nature of human action in order to expose the covert operation of the less-than-noble. One does not have to be one of the greatest scientists of the last half of the last century, Richard Feynman, to know that science itself is necessarily imperfect, Feynman himself writing of 'the uncertainty of science'.[14]

From the perspective of those who believe in the sacred, and from the perspective of a great number of thinkers of secular persuasion, the secular is the realm of the irredeemably flawed. However essential the afflictions of the secular for the development of what it is to be human, utopia is incompatible with the secular condition. As the secularist Durkheim quite justifiably states, 'I do not know what an ideal and absolute perfection is'.[15] If it exists at all, the sacred, as the perfect, has to be 'other than' the dystopic; it has to exist in a realm *sui generis*.

Spiritual virtuosi clearly believe in utopia that, from a secular point of view, *is* quite *impossible*. They 'know' perfect health, typically associating this with reference to some kind of immortality, health*care* being entirely irrelevant to the dynamics of the sacred itself. Certain adverts notwithstanding, perfect health is not possible within the secular frame; and it is ill-advised to ignore healthcare. For those confined to the secular sphere, values inevitably clash, with conflict typically generating ill-being. How can values possibly cohere, in perfect harmony, within the sacred? How can perfect health exist without healthcare? And most fundamentally of all, how is it possible for *human* life to be perfect when human life requires the opportunities, challenges, etc., of the flawed, of suffering?

Contemporary complementary and alternative medicine

CAM (and the TCAM of, say, Pakistan) basically has it home in what can be called 'the transformative zone'. This is the zone where people look for, find, engage with, experience, states of affairs or activities, which hold out the promise of transforming what it is to be alive. This is the zone which lies beyond the secular in that the secular is transgressed in crucial regards, *and* which lies beyond the realm of the sacred of traditional, institutionalized God on High, theistic religion in that it, too, is transgressed in crucial manner. To use a Sufi-inspired term, Bulleh Shah 'slants' away from the theistic, transgressing institutionalized Islam, whilst conterminously striving to live in terms of that which lies beyond the secular. Shelley's rejection of Christianity does more than slant away from Christian orthodoxy, and he was profoundly dissatisfied with the mundanities of the secular.

Turning to the contemporary, CAM is not the only incumbent of the transformative zone. Plenty of people draw on the numerous activities and 'meanings' of the zone, including all those who assert 'there *must* be something more'. Although a considerable amount of what is found in the zone probably has little, if anything to do with CAM *per se*, it is almost certainly the most significant occupant.[16]

CAM practitioners, and the great majority of their participants, reject the orthodoxy, and healthcare, of religious tradition. In the felicitous words of David Wulff, 'Life is ordered not in relation to the demands of the Holy spirit or some other divine force, but in reference to the possibilities of the human spirit'.[17] When the 'life-giver' that is the sacred of life-itself is emphasized—a 'life-giver,' which belongs to the person, all of humanity, or nature at large—it differs from, and thereby provides an alternative to, the sacred of God-on-High, over-and-above anything that can exist, as 'complete', in this world. CAM practitioners, with many of their participants, transcend the limitations of the secular. There are those who work beyond what secularists deem scientifically possible with regard to cause and effect; those who work with what secularists deem impossible, as incomprehensible: the sacred. So to the question, 'To what extent is the sacred drawn upon in CAM activities, run, say, in spas, leisure centres, health and fitness clubs, or in people's homes?'

Drawing on research carried out in the Netherlands, Stef Aupers reports that 85% of 'alternative healers' agree that 'everything is energy'; indeed, that 94% believe that 'human energies transcend the human body' [18, p. 191] As a great deal of additional evidence demonstrates, the language of 'energy', 'subtle energy', 'spiritual power' or 'force' lies at the very heart of contemporary CAM, complementary not just alternative. The language of 'energy'—together with evidence provided by other ways in which healers (as 'healthcare providers') and many participants (as 'clients') talk about their involvement, including use of the language of 'spirituality'—appears to indicate that the sacred is at work.

Although the evidence is not conclusive, the fact that CAM people relatively rarely use words like 'sacred', 'pure,' or 'ultimate' suggests that sacred healthcare, of a fully-fledged spiritualities of life nature, is not all that common. (One reason why the evidence is inconclusive in that adventitious influences, on language use, could explain why terms like 'sacred' are not used: they are culturally unpopular, for example.) On the basis of other indicative evidence as well, it is fairly clear that large numbers of those involved with CAM dwell on experienced consequences: not on what has given rise to outcomes. The focus of what can be called *pragmatic CAM* is very much on ameliorating the *back pain* (to give a typical example). What works, works. Even when people experience what they take to be the 'flow' of powerful, subtle energy, even when people experience this as flowing from an 'energy centre', they might well not be interested in the nature of the flow, the energy centre. If the language of spirituality should be used, pragmatic CAM is 'practically' spiritual; when the language is not in use, CAM is probably being treated as 'just' a practical technique. Whatever, emphasis—if any at all—does not rest with the sacred: a fact that is fuelled by the consideration that many practitioners, say yoga teachers in leisure centres, frequently opt to say little, if anything, of the spiritual-as-sacred significance of what they, themselves, believe in. It is likely that most of their participants simply do not consider themselves to be seeking contact with the sacred, let alone experiencing it; they simply do not bother with such matters. Whatever practitioners might believe in, numerous participants treat practices as resources for their secular lives, including their activities as consumers of pleasurable experience.

Nevertheless, pragmatic CAM, with practices 'simply' being practiced—with 'energy'—for outcomes, belongs to the transformative zone beyond. The sacred might not be in evidence, but neither is the secular. In that practices 'evade science' (to use an apt expression from Durkheim, who also uses the term 'supra-experimental'), the secular is transgressed.[19] Energy of a kind that is not open to scientific inquiry is typically involved; and the kinds of outcomes attributed to practices are often of the variety deemed impossible from the scientific perspective. Then there are healthcare and nurturance activities of a *proto-secular* nature, with practitioners and others holding that 'proper' science will one day verify the existence of those currently 'invisible' energies with which they work. When science is able to explain CAM activities (as has recently been claimed for acupuncture), however, activities join the ranks of allotropic medicine, cease to be either alternative or complementary, cease to belong to the transformative zone.

Even among those who are actively seeking the sacred, it is fair to say that *sacred* healthcare is frequently subdued, muted, or muffled; or attenuated. Relatively few have the discipline to practice as the virtuosi do, with commensurate results. Relatively few have the discipline to overcome what are taken to be the formidable lures of the secular, internalized as the 'ego' or 'lower self'. Experience of the sacred is often muffled or muted. *Proto-sacrality* can be in evidence, a *penultimate-sacrality*; or a tentative, hesitant approach, perhaps with scepticism getting in the way. In CAM, the sacred rarely just 'springs out'. In addition, there are those seeking the sacred, for reasons of healthcare, people who focus—in instrumentalized fashion—on what matters to *them*: doing something about their specific complaints. Compared with virtuosi, sacred spirituality is attenuated; narrowed to the flow of energy.

Drawing things together, the healthcare which spiritual virtuosi provide for the secular ('lower self') aspects of their being—as well as for those around them who are more firmly locked into the secular condition—is clearly informed by belief in, and contact with what is taken to be the sacred. At least in the west, at the more popular level it is doubtful that all that many make contact with the sacred in the spirit of a Tagore or Wordsworth. Pragmatic CAM is probably widespread. At the same time, it must be emphasized that sacred CAM is important. Think of Deepak Chopra. Think of those who speak the language of an 'energy' which 'springs from our own immortal unchanging self, that centre of pure consciousness, knowledge and bliss'.[20]

Belief-laden tradition?

Is everything under discussion in the hands of 'tradition'? Whether contemporary CAM, or what belong to the past, practitioners and most participants consider themselves to be beyond the 'hold' of tradition. (At least among participants, TCAM South Asia is often more traditionalized.) For them, 'tradition' carries too many inappropriate meanings. Of particular note, it is associated with the beliefs of religion. Generally speaking, the idea that engagement with the sacred involves believing in beliefs *that* provide information about the nature of sacred agency is regarded with grave suspicion. Religious beliefs almost invariably derive from the past, from the experiences (revelations, etc.) of others. From the spiritualities of life perspective, they are 'second hand'. Unless found to convey the truth of the sacred by way of what really counts—immediate, first hand, personal experience—the working assumption is that beliefs have been contaminated by events occurring over time: the inevitable cultural biases of translators; the ways in which beliefs are put to work to contribute to the malfunctions of political agendas or the secular domain in general. Bulleh Shah did *not* replicate beliefs. Neither did Shelley. Nor, it appears, do believers today. 'Deep' experience is at work, not 'belief that ...' or 'belief about ...,' deep experience generating 'belief in.' So, too, is practice. Although believers might very well agree that they draw on 'traditions' of practice, practices like yoga are pursued when they demonstrably work, in experience, to 'go within.' Believers might very well believe in spiritual virtuosi of the past; in their testimonies, not least their poetry: but only when they ring true in personal experience. At least for believers, the sacred, itself, is believed to replace tradition.

If the sacred exists, it sustains practices, experiences, values-cum-sentiments through time. However, for those who maintain that the sacred does not exist, or that it can be safely ignored on the grounds that even if does exist it does not submit to academic inquiry, attention is directed to the ways in which spiritualities of life—with their healthcare—are 'actually' sustained. One argument is that they are 'actually' embedded in tradition, functioning in 'formative' ways. Without participants realizing it, what they take to come from the sacred 'really' comes from their replicating things learnt from literature; is 'formed' by the influence of their teachers (including reading the texts of spiritual virtuosi of the past); it is derived from all those meanings, values, accounts, diagnoses, promises, portrayals of sentiments, dispositions, capacities, capabilities outlooks, etc., *embedded* in traditions of practice. Socialization—relational, performative, social, historical influences—sustains what amounts to covert tradition. The holistic, 'loving and healing humanism' of the value-laden sentiments and powers of compassionate healthcare, which serves as the hallmark of CAM today, is grounded, informed, accordingly.

Everything appears to hang on whether or not the sacred exists—an irresolvable issue within the framework of academic inquiry. There are ways of making progress, however. For the academic, who adopts an agnostic position, there is plenty to do. For example, arguing that holistic, healthcare spirituality does *not* operate in the same way as strong religious traditions. Participants and 'outside' academics can readily agree on this. To go to a yoga group is not to encounter the kind of creedal, doctrinally-informed moralizing of a great deal of Christianity. Propositional beliefs, even of a covert kind, are rarely encountered within spiritualities of life circles. Resources for living, which plausibly cater for autonomy, are in evidence—not 'the' spelt-out truth-to-be-obeyed proclamation. If 'tradition' is in play, it is of a different variety, with different dynamics, than that typical of traditional religion. To mark the difference, it is perhaps best to think in terms of *paths through time*. Practices, themes, perspectives, values, experientially verified 'truths' *of* the past do not move temporally by virtue of the sheer authority of those of the past who state that *this is what must* be done in the future. Rather than the 'must' being forcefully 'pushed' forward, the emphasis lies with those of the present exercising—of understanding themselves to exercise—their 'personal judgement' to *draw on* what has previously dwelt on the path: as resources to try out, to test by way of personal experience, to adjust, perhaps by combining yoga with tai chi. Paths from the past, together with their 'sign posts', help inform the paths pursued by those dwelling in the present.

Future?

Dwelling on the West, with implications for elsewhere, holistic healthcare of the transformative zone has long been sustained and is growing in significance. It is clear that the trajectories of South Asia and the West have been fuelled by powerful processes.

For many a commentator, the decline of religious tradition generates 'spiritual needs'; a 'vacuum' crying out to be filled, a 'hunger' for spirituality: adding up to a strong motor for the future. When those who are spiritually-orientated speak of 'spiritual needs' in connection with healthcare, namely their need for CAM, social scientific-cum-psychological inquiry has something to attend to: what participants mean by this, why they talk as they do. There is also the consideration that the number of those who report belief in spirituality (a larger number than those who practice CAM activities like yoga), of a transformative zone variety,[21] has considerable implications for how the 'spiritual needs of the patient' can best be attended to. However, for those who do not consider themselves to be on any sort of spiritual path, but are nevertheless involved with CAM, the term 'spiritual needs' is vacuous, non-explanatory, unsupported by evidence.

Turning briefly to another factor bearing on the future, the influential researcher Arthur Kleinman writes, 'in most cases indigenous practitioners must heal.'[22] Those who say that CAM does not work miss the point. CAM works at the level of experience. Generally speaking, CAM is brought to bear on subjective life; and generally speaking participants report improvement in the quality of subjective wellbeing.[23] Without entering the extensive literature explaining the connections between CAM and improvements of this variety, the point is simple. That so many experience CAM as worthwhile—not infrequently to the extent of coming to realize that suffering is worthwhile—omens well for the future.

A related factor is that many are struggling to find the worthwhile: to believe *in* that which is 'truly' worthy. Tolstoy wrote,

> You say you don't know what I believe in. Strange and terrible to say: not in anything that religion teaches us; but at the same time I not only hate and despise unbelief, but I can see no possibility of living, and still less of dying, without faith.[24]

At much the same time as Nietzsche was engaged—albeit differently—with much the same situation, Tolstoy was drawing attention to the major failures, bankruptcies, of two sources of the worthwhile: the sacred of traditional, God-on-High religion and the secular. Bulleh Shah, for example, would not disagree.

Applying this perspective to CAM and healthcare, the argument is that CAM, as an occupant of the transformative zone, has developed as a response to loss of faith in traditional religion (with its healing activities) and by (relative) loss of faith in secular medicine. Failures of these sources direct people to look for the complementary (this alone indicating that secular medicine is inadequate) or the alternative; to look for the different to make a difference. Helping direct people to the zone beyond for healthcare, they are likely to be attracted by activities which chime in with their (culturally generated) concern for improving the quality of their subjective wellbeing; and by activities which frequently chime in with their prior interest, or 'belief in', holistic themes, involving mind-body-spirit, which belong to the transformative zone itself. Providing worthwhile healthcare, for some 'truly' worthwhile, which at the same time emphasizes subjective-life, and is bound up with holistic themes, CAM can readily be seen as just the job.

Reflecting on the significance of the decline of traditional religion, Georg Simmel argued that what he called 'religiousness'—but which today would most likely be called 'spirituality' - '. . . would function as a medium for the direct expression of life'.[25] CAM is 'perfect' for this. Especially in sacred mode, when the sacred is equated with life, CAM practices serve as a 'vehicle' for the *life*-giving, *life*-affirming, *life*-enhancing, dynamics of the '*lived* realities' experienced within. With Simmel again, CAM serves as 'a way of living life itself'.[26] So long as cultural emphasis lies with quality of subjective life and what the depths of life have to offer, CAM is highly likely to continue to expand.

Another advantage for the future concerns the immunity of CAM, in particular in sacred mode, from the assaults of the new atheists. Science, or other secular tools, which are all *imperfect*, can never grasp the *perfect* (if indeed it exists) *perfectly*; the revisable, which science is by definition, cannot grasp that which lies beyond revision. From the secular perspective, the sacred is impossible. It is beyond the intellect of the new atheist; the scientific or logical mind; human comprehension of the secularist; the secular frame of reference in general. It cannot be falsified from within the secular camp; nor, of course, proved. The last depends on having 'inner' experiences that convince.

Acknowledgements

Thanks are due to Judith Everington, Dick Houtman, and David Walton for their suggestions and constructive criticism.

References

1 Catherine, L. (1999). Albanese uses the term kinetic in her illuminating discussion, 'Subtle energies of spirit: explorations in metaphysical and new age spirituality'. *J Am A Religion* **76**(2): 305–25. Nevill Drury (1999) is one of the finest writers on what he calls 'New Spirituality' (*Exploring the Labyrinth. Making Sense of the New Spirituality*. Dublin: Newleaf).

2 Cited by Bendix, R. (1966). *Max Weber*. London: Methuen, p. 464.

3 World Health Organization (1999). *Amendments to the Constitution. Report by the Secretariat*, A 52/24.

4 Extracts are taken from Saeed Ahmad (2003). *Great Sufi Wisdom: Bulleh Shah*. Rawalpindi: Adnan Books, respectively, pp. 67, 28, 27, 11, 66, 22, 70.

5 See Ewing K. (1984). The Sufi as Saint, Curer, and Exorcist in modern Pakistan. *Contrib Asian Stud* **XVIII**: 106–14.

6 Tagore, R. (1961). [1931]. *The Religion of Man*. London: Unwin, respectively, pp. 69, 70, 11–12, 121, 47, 99, 30, 96.

7 Gandhi, M. extracts from Stephen Hay (ed.) (1988). *Sources of Indian Tradition. Volume Two: Modern India and Pakistan*. New Delhi: Penguin, respectively, pp. 253, 250, 256, 271, 250.

8 Lama, D., Culter, H.C. (1998). *The Art of Happiness*. London: Hodder&Stoughton, p. 258.

9 Abrams, M.H. (1973). *Natural Supernaturalism*. London: WW Norton, p. 431.

10 Shelley, P.B. (2009). *A Defence of Poetry and other Essays*. London: Jungle Book, respectively, pp. 9, 11, 12.

11 Novalis (Friedrich von Hardenberg), quoted in McNeil, D. (2000). *Bodywork Therapies for Women*. London: The Women's Press, p. 17.

12 Hahnemann, S. (1982). [1842]. *Organon of Medicine*. Washington DC: Cooper, pp. 14, 76.

13 Berlin, I. (1991). *The Crooked Timber of Humanity*. London: Fontana.

14 Feynman, R.P. (2007). *The Meaning of it All*. Harmondsworth: Penguin.

15 Durkheim, E. (1953). *Sociology and Philosophy*. London: Cohen & West, p. 73.

16 Hughes, B.M. (2006). Regional patterns of religious affiliation and availability of complementary and alternative medicine. *J Religion Hlth*, **45**(4): 549–57.

17 Wulff, D.M. (1997). *Psychology of Religion*. New York: John Wiley, p. 7.

18 Aupers, S. (2005). 'We are all gods'. New Age in the Netherlands 1960–2000. In: E. Sengers, (ed.) *The Dutch and their Gods*. Verlaren: Hilversum, pp.180–201.

19 Durkheim, E. (1971). [1912]. *The Elementary Forms of the Religious Life*. London: George Allen and Unwin, p. 24.

20 Wood, C. (1998). Subtle energy and the vital force in complementary medicine. In: A. Vickers (ed.) *Examining Complementary Medicine*. Cheltenham: Stanley Thornes, pp. 113–23.

21 Heelas, P., Houtman. D. (2009). Research note: RAMP findings and making sense of 'the God within each person, rather than out there.' *J Contemp Religion* **24**(1): 83–98.

22 Kleinman, A. (1980). *Patients and Healers in the Context of Culture*. London: University of California Press, p. 361.

23 Furnham, A., Kirkaalay, B. (1996). The health beliefs and behaviours of orthodox and complementary medicine clients. *Br J Clin Psychol* **35**: 49–61. For the significance of subjectivities in TCAM see Kleinman, [22]. For a summary of efficacy, see Astin, J.A. (1998). Why patients use alternative medicine. *J Am Med Ass* **279**(19): 1548–53; 1552.

24 Rancour-Laferriere, D. (2007). *Tolstoy's Quest for God*. New Brunswick: Transaction, p. 1.

25 Simmel, G. (1968). [1918]. The conflict in modern culture. In: K.P. Etzkorn (ed.) *Conflict in Modern Culture and other Essays*. New York: Teachers College Press, pp. 11–26.

26 Simmel, G. (1997). *Essays on Religion*. New Haven: Yale University Press, p. 21.

CHAPTER 12

Philosophy

Graham Oppy

Introduction

There is a long history of philosophical reflection on connections between human flourishing, health, spirituality and religion. In this chapter, we can do no more than give a brief survey of some of the basic philosophical issues. In turn, we shall discuss human flourishing, health, disease, adverse conditions, spirituality, and religion.

Human flourishing

Aristotle's writings provide one ancient conception of human flourishing. On Aristotle's account, a flourishing human being is a member of a community that aims to bring about the flourishing of its members (*Politics*, Book VII, esp. xiii). Moreover, on Aristotle's account, the flourishing of a member of a community consists in that person's exercise of moral and intellectual virtues: the flourishing person has genuine friendships (*Ethics*, Books VIII and IX), possesses both theoretical and practical wisdom (*Ethics*, Book VI), and acts with courage, self-control, liberality, munificence, magnanimity, patience, amiability, sincerity, wit, and justice in pursuit of worthwhile individual and collective ends (*Ethics*, Books III and IV). Finally, on Aristotle's account, a flourishing human being is not subject to certain kinds of liabilities: a flourishing human being is not impoverished, or unhealthy, or the victim of misfortunes, such as bereavements etc. (*Ethics*, Book I, esp. ix–xi).

Other ancient conceptions of human flourishing are broadly similar to Aristotle's account. Thus, for example, the account that emerges from Confucius' *Analects*, the account that emerges from the teachings of the Buddha, and the account that emerges from the teachings of Hindu sages all run along at least roughly the same kinds of lines. (For discussion of this claim in connection with Buddhist ethics, see, for example, [1,2].) Moreover, even though some modifications emerged in the succeeding centuries—for example, Aquinas added the Christian virtues of hope, faith and charity to the Aristotelian list (*Summa Theologiae* II, II, 1–46)—this account of human flourishing continues to be widely accepted.

However, not everyone agrees. Indeed, some contemporary authors have argued that there is no conception of human flourishing that captures all of the ideal pictures that we might form of human flourishing. So, for example, Strawson [3: 26] says:

> As for the ways of life that may present themselves at different times as each uniquely satisfactory, there can be no doubt about their variety and opposition. The ideas of self-obliterating devotion to duty or to the service of others; of personal honour and magnanimity; of asceticism, contemplation, retreat; of action, dominance and power; of the cultivation of an exquisite sense of the luxurious; or simply human solidarity and cooperative endeavour; of a refined complexity of social existence; of a constantly maintained and renewed sense of affinity with natural things—any of these ideas, and a great many others too, may form the core and substance of a personal ideal.

Similar scepticism about the possibility of a unified conception of human flourishing is evinced in, for example.[4] To some, the possibility of inconsistent yet acceptable ideals of human flourishing may suggest that there is no objective component to conceptions of human flourishing; in the extreme, that one flourishes just in case one supposes that one does. However, it is clearly one thing to suppose that there are objective bounds to what might count as human flourishing, and quite another to suppose that there is a single, objectively required conception of human flourishing.

Moreover, even in ancient times, there were disagreements about details of the Aristotelian account. Some ancient philosophers, e.g. Plato and the Stoics, supposed that flourishing was independent of the vicissitudes of fortune, because primarily a matter of attitudinal and emotional self-control. Other ancient philosophers, e.g. the Epicureans, supposed the flourishing is primarily concerned with the getting of modest pleasure and the avoiding of pain (and only secondarily concerned with knowledge, friendship and virtue as means to these ends). However, in almost any account—ancient or modern—we find the idea that good health is a significant part of normal human flourishing. True enough, some of the ideals mentioned by Strawson are compatible with some kinds of departures from good health, but in general, there are very few ideal pictures of human flourishing that *require* departures from good health; and there are many ideal pictures of human flourishing that are simply incompatible with departures from good health.

(In passing, it is perhaps worth noting that ideal pictures of human flourishing that do require departures from good health often turn out to have religious underpinnings. Some religious ideals of saintliness and piety involve mortification of the flesh, flagellation, extremes of fasting and sleep deprivation, bodily neglect, eschewal of medical care, and so forth. Often these ideals are tied to the notion that humans flourish to the extent that they are good candidates to receive divine favours in the hereafter. Many with commitments to other ideals of human flourishing will suppose that, on the contrary, adoption of this notion—at least when it is tied to further claims about the virtues of self-imposed bodily neglect and the like—is itself a symptom of mental ill-health. Why *would* a perfectly good creator make self-harm an entrance requirement for the next life?)

Health

Conceptions of human health often begin with the idea that at least part of what it takes to be a healthy individual is that your biology functions as it should.

Those who deny that it is part of what it takes to be a healthy individual that your biology functions as it should typically say something like this: that what really matters for health is that you feel comfortable with your biology. Thus, for example, Carel[5] argues that one can be perfectly healthy even if one's biological systems are not functioning as they should, provided only that one feels at home or at ease with one's biological state. While it is not clear exactly what it is at stake here, it seems that one might prefer to say, not that *health* is compatible with malfunctioning biological systems, but rather that *flourishing* is compatible with such malfunctioning. (If one takes this route, then one can say that someone who has a biological liability or disability is flourishing even though they are not perfectly healthy. This sounds less strange to my ear than the suggestion that someone who has a biological liability or disability might nonetheless be in perfect health.)

Those who say that it is only part of what it takes to be a healthy individual that one's biology functions as it should often go on to add that health is also a matter of capacity for goal fulfilment: whether or not one is healthy is also a matter of whether or not one is able to fulfil relevant kinds of goals. Which relevant goals? On one view, the goals in question are biological in nature: goals set by needs that have a biological basis. On another view, the goals in question are related to minimal flourishing: conditions whose satisfaction is necessary and sufficient for a minimal level of happiness. (See [6] for further discussion of these two views.) On yet other views, the goals in question are more demanding: for example, Richman [7] claims that the goals are those that one would choose if one had perfect rationality, and complete knowledge of oneself and one's environment.

One problem for almost any version of the view that includes capacity for goal fulfilment as a condition for health is that it risks undoing the distinction between health and flourishing. It is clear that capacity for goal fulfilment is a condition for flourishing: perhaps, for example, it is true that one could not flourish if one lacked the capacity to fulfil the goals that one would choose if one had perfect rationality and complete knowledge of oneself and one's environment. However, it seems no less clear that one might lack the capacity to fulfil *these* goals for reasons that seem to have nothing to do with health—for example, one might lack the capacity to fulfil these goals simply because one falls at the lower end of the biologically properly functioning end of intelligence (hence, departing further than most from the standards of perfect rationality).

Another problem for almost any version of the view that includes capacity for goal fulfilment as a condition of health is that it leads to apparent misclassifications of enhancements as therapies. While it is agreed on all sides that the distinction between enhancement and therapy is tendentious, it seems fairly clear that something that would merely contribute to capacity for goal fulfilment without impacting on the way that biological systems ought to function would be a case of enhancement. However, surely something only counts as therapy—and hence as making a contribution to improving health—if, in some way, it brings biological systems closer to the functioning that they ought to have.

In the light of these difficulties, one might be tempted to think that we should perhaps rest content with the view that to be a healthy individual is just to have biological systems that function as they should. However, apart from any other difficulties, it is clear that defenders of this view need to say more about the distinction between 'physical' health and 'mental' health. In particular, it is clear that many people will want to contest the idea that 'mental' health is just a matter of having biological systems that function as they should. In order to explore this worry further, we shall turn to a consideration of the notion of illness (or disease).

Disease

Conceptions of illness (or disease) typically begin with the idea that illness and disease involve biological malfunctioning that occasions harm. However, conceptions of illness and disease differ, primarily, in the conception that they offer of the understanding of the biological malfunctioning that is involved.

On the 'naturalist' or 'objectivist' view, the determination that there is biological malfunctioning is simply a matter for biological science. According to this way of seeing things, human beings are composed of biological systems that have natural or normal functions that the systems in question can fail to carry out. Illnesses and diseases are departures from natural or normal biological functioning that are *deemed* to cause harm (where this deeming is most plausibly supposed to depend upon human interests, and perhaps on culturally specific human interests).

On the 'normative' or 'constructivist' view, the determination that there is biological malfunctioning is itself dependent upon human interest, and perhaps even on culturally specific human interests. According to this way of seeing things, judgments that biological systems are not manifesting natural or normal functioning themselves depend upon conceptions of human nature that are grounded in human interests, and most likely culturally specific human interests.

The 'normative' or 'constructivist' view may seem to have some historical support. After all, it is clearly true that there have been cases in which people have been classified as 'ill' or 'diseased' on the basis of culturally specific conceptions of human nature. For example, until recently, the received view was that homosexuality is a mental illness. However, 'naturalists' and 'objectivists' reply that those who classified homosexuality as an illness made that judgment on the basis of culturally specific conceptions of human nature that did not relate in any acceptable way to views about departures from normal or natural functioning of human biological systems. So these kinds of cases do not decisively favour the 'normative' or 'constructivist' view.

'Normative' and 'constructivist' views are subject to at least one serious difficulty. As Murphy [8, p. 8] notes, there is a clear distinction between illness and deviance: pathology and disapproval are not uniformly linked. 'We routinely judge that people are worse off without thinking that they are ill in any way—for example, the ugly, the poor, people with no sense of humour or lousy taste or a propensity for destructive relationships.' Clearly, then, we must suppose that illness involves being badly off on medical grounds. However, we must suppose more than this: for one can be disadvantaged on medical grounds even though one is not sick. For example, one is disadvantaged on medical grounds if one misses out on immunization, or contraception, or a varied diet, and so forth; but one is not *ipso facto* ill if one misses out on these things. It is very hard to see how to specify what it is to be *ill* without having recourse to the idea that illness involves departures from normal functioning in biological systems.

There are some subtleties here. As Murphy [8, p. 5] notes, there have been developments in our concept of illness and disease over time. In the early modern era, diseases were taken to be 'observable suites of symptoms with predictable courses of unfolding.' This notion was displaced by the idea that diseases are 'destructive processes in bodily organs which divert them from their normal functioning.' More recently, the notion has been further refined: certain kinds of elevated risks, e.g. high blood pressure, are also counted as diseases even if there are neither overt symptoms nor destructive pathological processes. So references to 'departures from normal functioning in biological systems' includes cases in which biological systems are in stable, but suboptimal and poorly regulated states.

Even if it is accepted that the 'naturalist' or 'objectivist' view of disease and illness is correct for 'physical' illnesses, it may well be objected that this account is, at best, highly controversial in the case of 'mental' illnesses. Is it really plausible to suppose that 'mental' illnesses are departures from natural or normal biological functioning?

Some people object to the suggestion that 'mental' illnesses are departures from natural or normal biological functioning on metaphysical grounds. For example, *substance dualists* think that human beings are amalgams of two different kinds of stuff: the biological (or physical) and the mental (or spiritual). While substance dualists will typically acknowledge that illnesses in one domain can have causes in the other domain—e.g. mental stress can be a cause of departures from normal biological functioning in bodily organs other than the brain, and genetic inheritance can be a cause of mental disorders—they typically also insist that 'mental' illnesses must be understood as departures from natural or normal mental functioning (where such departures may not be accompanied by any departures from natural or normal biological functioning in the brain or elsewhere). For another—perhaps less dramatic—example, *property dualists* think that human beings have two irreducibly different kinds of properties: biological (or physical) properties and mental (or spiritual) properties. Property dualists also typically suppose that 'mental' illnesses can only be understood as departures from natural or normal mental functioning: there is no way of 'reducing' mental illness to physical illness, no way of explaining mental illness in purely biological or physical terms.

Those who do not have metaphysical grounds for objecting to the claim that 'mental' illnesses are departures from natural or normal biological functioning may have other grounds for objection. In particular, it is worth noting that there are grounds for scepticism about the very distinction between 'physical' and 'mental' illness. As we have already noted, the distinction cannot be drawn in terms of causes of conditions. However, it is equally clear that the distinction cannot be drawn in terms of symptoms—some symptoms are hard to classify (e.g. pain), some characterize both 'physical' and 'mental' illnesses (e.g. fatigue), and some ostensibly 'mental' disorders (e.g. memory loss) can arise from what are clearly physical causes (e.g. a blow to the head). (See Perring [9, p. 4].) In the face of these difficulties, some people have suggested that we should distinguish only between brain-based and non-brain-based disorders, and give up on the pre-theoretical distinction between 'physical' and 'mental' illnesses. However, as things now stand, it is clear that we are not able to think and talk about serious disturbances of thought, experience and emotion—as manifested in schizophrenia, bipolar disorder, borderline personality disorder, and so forth—in purely physical and biological terms. For the foreseeable future, we have no choice, but to continue to make use of such categories as 'thought', 'experience', 'feeling', 'emotion', and so forth in our description, analysis and treatment of mental illnesses.

As things stand, it is clearly not ruled out that the 'naturalist' or 'objectivist' view of diseases is correct. That is, as things stand, it is not ruled out that all illnesses and diseases involve biological malfunctioning that is the proper subject matter of biological science. However, even if the 'naturalist' or 'objectivist' view of diseases is correct, it is clear that, even in the case of paradigmatically physical diseases, we have no choice, but to continue to make use of such categories as 'thought', 'experience', 'feeling', 'emotion', and so forth in our *treatment* of those diseases. Moreover, even if the 'naturalist' or 'objectivist' view of diseases is correct, it is clear that, in a wide range of cases, we also have no choice, but to take into account the relevant metaphysical beliefs of those subject to illness in the treatment of their illnesses. As we noted earlier, freedom from illness and disease is only one dimension of human flourishing, and illness and disease interact in complex ways with other dimensions of flourishing human beings. Since no one could pretend that we can give a 'naturalist' or 'objectivist' account of human flourishing in purely biological or physical terms, there is no option, but to hold commonsense considerations about human flourishing in mind when describing, analyzing, and providing medical treatment.

Adverse conditions

There are many adverse factors and conditions whose negative impact on human flourishing and human health are uncontroversial. Thus, for example, no one disputes that loneliness, stress, low self-esteem, lack of self-control, ignorance, and poverty are all factors that count against human flourishing, and that these are all factors that are linked to poor health, and increased susceptibility to illness and disease. By and large, flourishing people are engaged in worthwhile activities, and they are recognized by other people as being engaged in worthwhile activities. By and large, flourishing people belong to networks of flourishing people, and they have meaningful relationships with people in those networks. By and large, flourishing people have appropriate emotional responses both to themselves and to others. By and large, flourishing people do not have fantastic beliefs about themselves and the world in which they live. By and large, flourishing people do not engage in self-destructive behaviour and excessive risk-taking, etc.

While all of this seems straightforward and unproblematic, there are complicating factors. In particular, there are hard questions that arise if we probe more deeply into the connection between flourishing and the holding of fantastic beliefs about oneself and the world in which one lives. On the one hand, we have the judgment—present in Aristotle—that theoretical and practical wisdom are fundamental components of human flourishing: we do better insofar as we acquire truth and act on the basis of it. On the other hand, we have a large recent literature, going back at least to the 1950s, which suggests that human flourishing may depend upon possession of 'positive cognitive biases', i.e. upon more or less mild self over-estimations of abilities, reputation, importance, and sphere of control (see, e.g. [10]).

Even setting aside considerations about positive cognitive biases, there are hard questions to ask about the connections between true belief and human flourishing. On the one hand, it is fairly uncontroversial that *delusion* is not conducive to human flourishing: most people agree that you are not flourishing if you have too many false beliefs that are firmly sustained despite what everyone else believes (to the contrary) and despite what constitutes incontrovertible and obvious proof or evidence to the contrary (cf. DSM-IV-TR definition of 'delusion'). On the other hand, it is rather less clear how much divergence from beliefs ordinarily accepted by other members of one's culture or subculture is compatible with human flourishing (again, cf. DSM-IV-TR definition of 'delusion').

When we consider the distribution of religious, political, and philosophical beliefs of human beings across the world over history, it is clear that most people have had massively false beliefs in these domains. For, once we move to sufficient level of detail, there are no majority beliefs in these areas—no collections of beliefs about religion, or politics, or philosophy are shared by more than a tiny fraction of human beings across the world over history, and yet each collection of beliefs about religion, or politics, or philosophy is inconsistent with all of the other collections of beliefs about religion, or politics, or philosophy. If we insist that you do not flourish unless you have (largely) true religious and political and philosophical beliefs, then we quickly reach the conclusion that human flourishing is very rare indeed.

Considerations about sharing of beliefs with others in one's culture or subculture interact in interesting ways with some of the other factors that can impact negatively on health. Depending upon the nature of the society to which one belongs, being known as someone who rejects widely shared religious or political or philosophical beliefs may lead to ostracism, abuse, and stress, and perhaps also to lower self-esteem and loneliness. Even in contemporary liberal democracies, it is clear that *some* people suffer in these ways because their beliefs are at odds with the sub-cultures to which they belong. (Similar points can be made about values as well. Given that projects emerge against a background of beliefs and values, it seems equally clear that perceptions of the worth of activities and projects are also linked to factors that can impact negatively on mental and physical health.)

Even if we come to think both that people are unlikely to flourish if their beliefs are widely at variance with the beliefs of the subculture or culture to which they belong and that nearly all people at nearly all times have had massively mistaken religious, political, and philosophical beliefs, we should not move too quickly to the conclusion that truth of beliefs if largely irrelevant to human flourishing. We do not need to move to the extremes of the view evinced in Clifford [11] to suppose that one condition for human flourishing is that one belongs to a sub-culture or culture that accords serious respect to evidential support for belief. Moreover, given the evident frailties involved in the formation of beliefs about religion, politics, and philosophy, there are fairly strong grounds to support the claim that we should be tolerant of those who do respect the demands of reason and evidence, and yet who end up with widely different beliefs from our own.

Of course, there are people who insist on a much more direct connection between belief and flourishing. Some religious believers hold that you do not truly flourish unless you hold a particular set of religious beliefs. Some 'new atheists' hold that you do not truly flourish if you hold any religious or 'spiritual' beliefs. (See, e.g. [12,13].) I think that there are good grounds for rejecting any positions of this kind; but there is hardly space to argue for this contention here. (For further discussion and defence of 'agreeing to disagree', see [14].)

Spirituality

There are various ways in which one might understand the suggestion that 'spirituality' should have a significant role in healthcare. I shall canvass some such ways, in what I take to be a diminishing order of plausibility. It should be noted that the following points are prompted by different ways of understanding the notion of spirituality.

First, as noted in our discussion of illness and disease, it is quite uncontroversial to claim that we need to bear commonsense considerations about human flourishing in mind when describing, analyzing, and providing medical treatment. Health is one of a number of interrelated factors that jointly constitute human flourishing. Medical treatment that is aimed at improving health will often need to take into account some of the other factors that constitute human flourishing. What a person *feels* and what a person *believes* can make a difference to the result of medical treatment. Whether medical intervention disrupts social relationships can make a difference to the outcome of that intervention. Medical treatments that cause or exacerbate stress, or loneliness, or low self-esteem work against themselves (although, of course, in some cases, this kind of self-undermining may be acceptable and even unavoidable). Insofar as 'spiritual' healthcare is defined by contrast with 'merely technical' healthcare, it is surely undeniable that 'spiritual' healthcare will lead to better outcomes in a great range of cases.

Secondly, as noted in our discussion of adverse conditions, it is reasonable to suppose that, insofar as patients have 'spiritual beliefs'—i.e. beliefs about ultimate purposes, immaterial realities, supernatural entities, and the like (cf. [15])—those beliefs should be taken into account in the provision of healthcare. Setting aside hard cases involving religious, or political, or philosophical delusions, it seems clear that it should not be the business of medical practitioners and their supporters to try to *change* the religious, or political, or philosophical beliefs of their clients. On the contrary, if patients belong to sub-cultures that share their religious, political, or philosophical beliefs then—lacking clear legal or medical reasons to the contrary—those patients are entitled to support from within those like-minded sub-cultures. (Some deny that there could be legal reasons that would suffice for denial of such support. Suppose that some conspirators have been injured as part of a failed terrorist action. Should they be allowed to recuperate together, even if there are sufficient grounds to suppose that their recuperating together increases the risk of further terrorist action? Consider, for example, the treatment of the members of the Baader-Meinhoff group by the German state.[16] Many now think that the German state was far too liberal and tolerant in its treatment of the Red Army Faction.) Of course, there are also hard cases where 'spiritual beliefs' come into conflict with the requirements of the best available medical treatment—as can happen, for example, with the beliefs of Christian Scientists, and the like. While this is not the place to pronounce on these hard cases, it is probably worth noting that, while 'spiritual beliefs' should always be taken into account, this hardly means that 'spiritual beliefs' should trump all other considerations concerning the provision of healthcare.

Thirdly, there are people who claim that having of 'spiritual' beliefs, i.e. beliefs in ultimate purposes, immaterial realities, supernatural entities, and the like, is an important component of human flourishing, and perhaps even an important component of human health. Taken in isolation, this claim seems implausible. After all, it would be very surprising if beliefs in evil demons, ghosts, ghouls, and so forth are positively correlated with either human flourishing or good health outcomes. At the very least, one might expect that human flourishing and good health outcomes would correlate only with *positive* 'spiritual' beliefs, i.e. the kinds of 'spiritual' beliefs that are emphasized in the world's major religions— Christianity, Islam, Hinduism, Buddhism, Judaism, and the like—and in similarly patterned systems of belief, e.g. Wicca. Indeed, while the terms 'spiritual' and 'religious' are used widely in the literature on 'spirituality' and healthcare, it seems to me that the distinction that is marked is typically a distinction between holding beliefs that are proper to religion and participating in a religious community. Thus, our focus should really be on those people who claim that having 'religious' beliefs—perhaps in combination with participating in organized religious activities of some kind—is an important component of human flourishing, and perhaps even an important component of human health. This brings us to the final section of this chapter.

Religious belief

There is an enormous new literature on religion and health. Every month, the *Institute for the Biocultural Study of Religion Research Review* brings outlines of dozens of new articles and books on this topic across my desk. Much of this new research is concerned with what are often reported as correlations between 'religiosity' and 'well-being'. Claims are made for connections between 'religiosity' and such diverse things as:

- greater happiness
- life satisfaction
- lower levels of stress
- being better able to cope with life-threatening illness
- lower levels of alcohol consumption
- lower levels of smoking
- lower levels of depression and other mental illness
- higher moral scruples
- lower levels of anxiety
- lower levels of herpes and other STDs
- lower levels of illicit drug use
- more positive attitudes towards marriage, relationships, and attachments
- reduced risks of death and so on.

Taken at face value, these claims offer support for the view that having 'religious' beliefs may make some contribution to human health and flourishing. Of course, even if there are no defeating considerations, these claims are not sufficient to establish that 'religious' belief is a significant, let alone essential, component of human health and human flourishing. At most, the studies claim to show that there is a statistically significant correlation (or, in some cases, that there is a 'positive' statistical correlation that 'approaches significance') between 'religiosity' and human health and flourishing. In any case, there is also a range of defeating considerations that need to be taken into account.

First, the literature is peppered with studies that claim that no definite conclusions can be drawn about relationships between religiosity, and human health and flourishing because of major methodological shortcomings of the studies that have been conducted (for one very recent example, see [17]).

Secondly, evidence that there are methodological problems is not hard to find. For instance, many studies of 'religiosity' and happiness rely on a single self-reported item to measure each of these dimensions: rate your happiness and the intensity of your religious belief on a scale from 1 to 5. While one might have predicted, *a priori*, that there is likely to be some positive correlation between self-assessments of religiosity and happiness, there is plenty of evidence that self-assessments of happiness and flourishing are not reliable measures of either happiness or flourishing. (Of course, this is obvious on the Aristotelian account of flourishing, and, indeed, on any relatively 'objective' account of flourishing.)

Thirdly, the category of 'religiosity' is not a particularly useful one. As some of the more recent studies have noted, it is important to try to draw out the relative significance of such things as: regularity of church attendance, regularity of participation in other religious gatherings, regularity of participation in religious rituals, strength of religious beliefs, nature of religious beliefs, and so forth.

Fourthly, there is some fairly robust counter-evidence that needs to be taken into account. For example, Paul[18] appeals to national census data across the Western world—data of the kind that is contained in the *Britannia Yearbook*—to establish correlations between reported national 'religiosity' and national measures of moral and social dysfunction. On Paul's account, many of these correlations of reported national 'religiosity,' and national measures of moral and social dysfunction contradict the claims that emerge from the literature on religion and health. So, for example, while many US studies report that 'religiosity' is correlated with more positive attitudes towards marriage, relationships, and attachments, the cross-national comparison shows that divorce rates are higher in the United States than they are in Western countries with much lower levels of national 'religiosity' (e.g. Sweden and Australia).

In the light of these and other considerations, it is hard to draw reliable conclusions from the current research on religiosity and happiness. While it is clear that there are significant connections between self-reports of happiness and religiosity, it is unclear what else can be reliably inferred from the data that we have. In particular, it is very important to note that many of the adverse conditions for human flourishing and human health that were discussed previously—e.g. loneliness and low self-esteem—are clearly moderated or removed by some aspects of 'religiosity'—e.g. regular church attendance, regular participation in religious gatherings, and so forth. However, it would plainly take some very cleverly designed studies to find evidence that it is the 'religious' aspect of these activities that are crucially implicated in the alleviation of the adverse conditions. If anything like the Aristotelian account of human flourishing is correct, then one might well suspect that there is only a highly contingent connection between 'religiosity' and health. At the very least, one might wonder whether it is true that, for example, regular church attendance and regular participation in religious gatherings has a higher correlation with good health outcomes than regular attendance and participation in other kinds of human organizations that have no necessary connection to religion—community orchestras, rationalist societies, sporting clubs, and so forth.

Of course, there are other, more dramatic claims that have been made in recent times connecting 'religiosity' and health. So, for example, there have been studies that claim that prayer can be efficacious in securing good health outcomes for those who are prayed about. The very least that needs to be said here is that there are plenty of reasons for scepticism. (See, e.g. [19], for methodological concerns about studies in this area.) However, this is not to say that there could not be any correlations between prayer and good health. I do not think that it would be surprising to learn that prayer has some positive correlation with good health outcomes for those who pray, all other things being equal. There is plenty of evidence that meditation and mindfulness have such correlations, and prayer is often a species of these kinds of activities.

Conclusion

I shall conclude with a final piece of anecdotal evidence. When I first became a philosopher, it was said to me that I had chosen my profession wisely, for philosophers, like priests, are renowned for their long, healthy, and flourishing lives. I do not know whether this piece of folk wisdom is really so. However, if it is so, it is worth noting that, for at least the last 50 years, the majority of philosophers in the West have been non-religious. What priests and philosophers have in common are the things that Aristotle supposed conduce to human flourishing: community, intellectual virtue, lifelong commitment to worthwhile ends, and so forth. Perhaps this is one further sign that, of itself, religiosity has no *unique* significance for health and flourishing: the 'spiritual' dimension of health and flourishing might be much more a matter of 'exercise of virtue in the pursuit of worthwhile individual and collective ends'—or 'solidarity and resistance', or 'social inclusion', or what have you—than it is a matter of *uniquely* religious concerns.

Bibliography

Aquinas (2007). *Summa Theologiae.* Cambridge: Cambridge University Press.

Aristotle (1976). *Ethics*, transl. J. A. K. Thomson; rev transl. H. Tredennick. Harmondsworth: Penguin.

Aristotle (1981). *The Politics*, transl. T. A. Sinclair; rev transl T. J. Saunders. Harmondsworth: Penguin.

Confucius (2010). *Analects*, transl. J. Legge. Available at: http://ebooks.adelaide.edu.au/c/confucius/c748a/index.html

Crisp, R. (2008). Well-Being. *Stanford Encyclopaedia of Philosophy.* Stanford: Stanford University Press.

Green, M., Elliott, M. (2010). Religion, health and psychological well-being. *J Relig Hlth* **49**: 149–63.

Koenig, H., McCullough, M., Larson, D. (2001). *Handbook of Religion and Health*. Oxford: Oxford University Press.

Williams, D., Sternthal, M. (2007). Spirituality, religion and health: evidence and research directions. *Med J Austr* **186**(10 Suppl): S47–S50.

References

1 Keown, D. (1992). *The Nature of Buddhist Ethics.* London: Macmillan.

2 De Silva, P. (2002). *Buddhism, Ethics and Society.* Clayton: Monash Asia Institute.

3 Strawson, P. (1974). Social morality and individual ideal. In his: *Freedom and Resentment and Other Essays.* London: Methuen, 26–44.

4 Wolf, S. (1982). Moral saints. *J Philos* **79**: 419–39.

5 Carel, H. (2008). *Illness: The Cry of the Flesh.* Dublin: Acumen.

6 Nordenfelt, L. (1995). *On the Nature of Health: An Action-Theoretic Perspective*, 2nd edn. Dordrecht: Kluwer.

7 Richman, K. (2004). *Ethics and the Metaphysics of Medicine.* Cambridge: MIT Press.

8 Murphy, D. (2008). Concepts of disease and health. In: E. N. Zalta (ed.) *Stanford Encyclopaedia of Philosophy*

9 Perring, C. (2010). 'Mental Illness' *Stanford Encyclopaedia of Philosophy.* http://plato.stanford.edu/entries/mental-illness/

10 Cummins, R., Nistico, H. (2002.) Maintaining life satisfaction: the role of positive cognitive bias. *J Happiness Stud* **3**: 37–69.

11 Clifford, W. (1879). The ethics of belief. In: S. Pollock (ed.) *Lectures and Essays*, London: Macmillan.

12 Dawkins, R. (2006). *The God Delusion.* London: Bantam.

13 Hitchens, C. (2007). *God is not Great: How Religion Poisons Everything.* New York: Twelve Books.

14 Oppy, G. (2010). Disagreement. *Int J Philos Relig* **68**: 183–99.

15 Sheldrake, P. (2007). *A Brief History of Spirituality.* Malden: Wiley-Blackwell.

16 Aust, S. (1985). *The Baader-Meinhoff Complex*, transl A. Bell. Oxford: Oxford University Press.

17 Visser, A, Garssen, B., Vingerhoets, A. (2010). Spirituality and well-being in cancer patients: a review. *Psycho-Oncol* **19**(6): 565–72.

18 Paul, G. (2005). Cross-national correlations of quantifiable societal health with popular religiosity and secularism in prosperous democracies. *J Relig Soc* **7**: 1–17.

19 Andrade, C., Radhakrishnan, R. (2009). Prayer and healing: a medical and scientific perspective on randomized controlled trials. *Ind J Psychiat* **51**: 4, 247–53.

CHAPTER 13

Secularism

Trevor Stammers and Stephen Bullivant

Introduction

Secularism has two primary meanings, both germane to the subject of healthcare and spirituality.[1] In its first, socio-cultural sense it refers to the lack of religious practice, belief, or interest in a given society. This brand of secularism—or better, *secularity*—is, albeit in differing ways, a characteristic of many modern, western nations.[2,3] Secular societies generate 'secular spiritualities'—forms of spirituality that make no reference to, or perhaps even specifically repudiate, religious, theistic or otherwise supernatural categories.[see 4] Several of these—'Feminist Spirituality', 'Humanistic traditions'—are explored in detail elsewhere in this section. Also important to note in this context is that, even apart from defined traditions, a great many people in western societies view themselves as being a 'spiritual person', and as such presumably believe themselves to have attendant spiritual needs.[5] Furthermore, even those who dislike the term 'spiritual', perhaps for its religious or supernatural overtones, may nevertheless welcome certain aspects of care which typically come under that banner.[6]

In its second and most common meaning, however, secularism is an umbrella term for a cluster of political and philosophical doctrines concerning the status of religious interests in the public sphere. Secularism in this sense defines the legal, financial, and (significantly) ethical contexts in which healthcare is thought about and practiced. Across the world, in very diverse countries and cultures, secularisms—of varying types, as we shall see—set the rules that all the other traditions explored in this section are obliged to follow. Given the overarching import of this to nearly all religious and spiritual concerns in healthcare, this chapter will focus on this highly and increasingly controversial field. In particular, we shall focus on two recent case studies—the question of conscience in medical practice and the state funding of hospital chaplaincies. Although centring on the United Kingdom, these case studies are of far wider significance. Before this, however, it is necessary to distinguish between two basic traditions of philosophical secularism—each of which has significant ramifications for the theory and practice of spirituality and healthcare.

Religion in the public square

Whereas secularity has to do with 'individuals and their social and psychological characteristics' [3, p. 1], secularism relates to the structures and procedures of institutions. Although sometimes referred to as 'political secularism,' its application in fact extends to a range of corporate groupings, including businesses, charities and professional bodies, as well as governmental, public and legal entities.[7,8] From this volume's perspective, one or another version of secularism may be evident in the rules and operation of a national health service, a local healthcare trust, a charity-run hospice, a privately-owned insurance provider, a doctors' union, or a professional association of nurses. This kind of secularism is commonly characterized as 'the separation of church and state', a phrase that betrays the concept's origins (at least in its modern forms) in early-modern Europe after the rise of the nation-state. Though this formulation hints at secularism's true meaning, it obscures both the sheer varieties of secularism manifest in the modern world, and their global and cultural extent. Even confining oneself to national government, evidently the secularisms of (say) the USA, Britain, France, Israel, India, and Turkey will be very different beasts. Note, too, that while there may well be a link between secularity and secularism, the two do not necessarily go together—France is both secularized and secularist; the USA and India are only the latter.

Contemporary secularisms have their roots in European attempts, in the wake of the sixteenth- and seventeenth-century wars of religion, to find a peaceful mediation between confessional groups in 'the public square'.[9] Generally speaking, there have been two basic ways of doing this, although in practice the distinctions may not quite be sharp, especially over time.[9–11] In the first—historically represented, somewhat differently, by Hugo Grotius and Thomas Hobbes—religious reasons and arguments have no place in public life. Different people or groups are, of course, at liberty to hold religiously formulated views in private. However, in order to participate in the shared space of public life, they must translate these into purely secular ones, based on premises that all people, regardless of their own (private) religious persuasions, can, if not accept, then at least reasonably entertain. On at least one reading of this mode of secularism, 'the state'—and one may add here other public bodies too—'upholds no religion, pursues no religious goals, religiously-defined goods have no place in the catalogue of ends it promotes'.[9, p. 35] Such a stance, and others very like, have obvious (potential) ramifications for religious people working in state-funded or state-regulated healthcare provision—most obviously in the case of 'conscience', which we shall explore in detail below.

In the second classic approach, however, an ecumenical 'common ground' is sought, and religious interests and arguments are permitted (and perhaps even strongly encouraged) insofar as they overlap with those of other religious stakeholders in society. For the seventeenth-century philosopher John Locke (to whom this mode of secularism is often traced), this meant that members of Christian 'dissenting' sects, and not merely those in communion with the Established Church of England, could fully participate in public life. This is an attractive solution to the problems generated by increasing pluralism, although how far such a 'common ground' may viably be extended is a vexing issue. For Locke, while the Church of England could share the public square with a discrete number of other Protestant sects, such toleration was not extended to Catholics, atheists, or Muslims.[12] More relevantly to the current situation, the common ground of American 'civic religion' gradually (and not always smoothly) expanded over the centuries from generic Protestantism to a wide 'shared Judeo–Christian heritage' encompassing 'Protestant–Catholic–Jew.' If and how this alleged 'common ground' can expand further to include American Muslims, Hindus, Buddhists, and atheists remains to be seen. Nevertheless, at least in theory, this mode of secularism permits non-secular arguments and convictions to play a role in public deliberations and practice—its 'secularism' consists in not privileging any particular religion, or denomination, over any other. In the United States, for example, most religious groups, Christian or not, qualify for tax exempt, charitable status; in Britain, the state actively funds Anglican schools, but also Catholic, Muslim, Jewish, Hindu and Sikh ones (as well, of course, as a great number of non-faith schools as well). For our purposes, however, it is worth noting that this mode of secularism has clear relevance for the state supporting (whether financially or otherwise) a wide range of different religiously-rooted healthcare initiatives, including hospital chaplaincies, and indeed hospitals, hospices and care-homes themselves. This issue too, with particular reference to chaplaincy funding, will be discussed in detail below. The differing development of secularism in Europe and North America is discussed further in Chapter 64.

Conscience and controversy

The United Kingdom's National Health Service (NHS) is the largest, publicly-funded health service in the world. Serving a population of over sixty million people, every year the NHS receives over £100 billion of tax-payers' money. Furthermore, it employs more than 1.7 million people, including 120,000 hospital doctors, 40,000 GPs, 400,000 nurses, and 25,000 ambulance staff. Given the NHS's social, political, and economic importance, the large numbers of people it both serves and employs, and the gravity of the matters with which it deals, it is not surprising that the role of religious and spiritual concerns within it have been subject to considerable, and often heated, discussion, and argument. Not surprisingly, secularist voices have been prominent here—and nowhere more so, then on the question of conscience in healthcare provision.

There is good evidence that a doctor's religion influences patient care. This is especially true with regard to sexual health and end-of-life issues. A carefully designed study of the influence of doctors' religious beliefs on their care of the dying, for example, showed that 'doctors who described themselves as non-religious were more likely than others to report having given continuous deep sedation until death, having taken decisions they expected or partly intended to end life.'[13, p. 677] Conscience is not, of course, the preserve of religious people—there are a great many doctors who identify with secular spiritual traditions, or who have no religious or spiritual tradition at all, who would equally refuse to authorize or participate in particular (legal) medical procedures on the grounds of conscience. Nevertheless, such objections are indeed frequently influenced and justified on the basis of specifically religious convictions. Although misleading, it is perhaps not surprising that conscientious objection in healthcare is frequently discussed as though this were an exclusively 'religious' issue.

In 2006, the Oxford moral philosopher Professor Julian Savulescu published an article in the *BMJ* (formerly the *British Medical Journal*) on 'Conscientious objection in medicine'. He opens with a tone-setting, though perhaps ironic, quotation from Shakespeare's *Richard III*: 'Conscience is but a word cowards use, devised at first to keep the strong in awe'.[14, p. 294] Savulescu proceeds to argue:

> A doctor's conscience has little place in the delivery of modern medical care. What should be provided to patients is defined by the law and consideration of the just distribution of finite medical resources, which requires a reasonable conception of the patient's good and the patient's informed desires. If people are not prepared to offer legally permitted, efficient, and beneficial care to a patient because it conflicts with their values, they should not be doctors. (14, p. 294)

Furthermore, in a system where 'less than half of doctors whose primary job it is to deal with termination of pregnancy would facilitate a termination at 13 weeks if the woman wants it for career reasons,' [14, p. 295] conscientious objection results in both inefficiency and inequity. While Savulescu is careful not to depict conscientious objection as an *exclusively* religious 'problem', the reader is left in no doubt that it is primarily so. The article's subheading begins 'Deeply held religious beliefs may conflict with some aspects of medical practice,'[p. 294] and at several points 'religious values' are unfavourably contrasted, explicitly and implicitly, with 'secular liberal values'. Moreover, religious values 'corrupt' the delivery of health care and to allow conscientious objection on the basis of them is clearly discriminatory when 'other values can be as closely held and as central to conceptions of the good life as religious values.' [14, p. 295]

This position has clear affinities with the first mode of secularism defined in the previous section. While for Thomas Hobbes, religious reasons or arguments have no place in public life, for Julian Savulescu, they have no place in a publicly-funded health service. Doctors may have private religious convictions, but as public servants they must conform to a shared set of (secular) values and practices, defined and regulated by law and governmental policy. Those unable or unwilling to do this, thereby forfeit the ability to do their job: 'Doctors who compromise the delivery of medical services to patients on conscience grounds must be punished through removal of their license to practice and other legal mechanisms.' [p. 296] Explicitly motivating Savulescu's arguments is a concern for patient care, and the worry that conscientious objection can, at least in some instances, either prevent or delay patients from receiving medical service to which they are legally entitled.

Savulescu's article sparked an avalanche of responses, many of which are available on the *BMJ* website.[15] The vast majority of these—from doctors, patients, and medical ethicists—are strongly negative. The most common criticism is of the suggestion that conscience, however informed, has no legitimate role in medical practice. Without necessarily agreeing with, and perhaps even actively opposing, the specific reasons (and/or their religious or non-religious foundations) put forward by objectors to particular procedures, the idea that such reasons are, in principle, 'out of bounds' was condemned by many respondents. Not only were doctors themselves disquieted by a medical profession that leaves no room for personal moral conviction, several of them raised the important point that patients would likely be so too. Patients do not view doctors as functionaries, devoid of human feeling or conviction. Indeed, one of us (TS) often asks medical students what qualities they would look for in the ideal doctor looking after their elderly mother with a terminal illness. Never yet has technical competence, being an exam prize-winner, or anything remotely 'scientific', been the first item in their list. The replies are usually 'compassion', 'kindness,' 'empathy', 'humanity', and even 'tenderness'. The next question is: 'On balance, is your mother likely to receive better treatment from a doctor who believes that after his or her own death they will have to give account to God of how they have lived their lives, including of how they have practiced medicine?' To this question there is, of course, no right or wrong answer. However, it is arguably a vital part of good medical training to encourage students as well as patients to think about the importance of spiritual values.

Savulescuan secularism is, however, by no means without its supporters.[e.g. 16] Indeed, many of his *BMJ* critics, while upholding the general right to conscientious objection, would presumably themselves disagree strongly with the—in many cases, religiously-informed—objections of their colleagues to specific practices. It is one thing to uphold the value of conscience in medical practice, quite another to believe that an appeal to it is, in every instance, a 'trump card'. Nevertheless, Savulescu's article evidently struck a chord. Even without conflating 'conscience' and 'religion' (another common theme in the *BMJ* responses), the role of religious conviction in a publicly-funded, state-run health service is clearly a significant issue; even those disagreeing with Savulescu may be thankful to him for opening up the debate. In fact, the ongoing debate over conscientious objection can be viewed as just one aspect of a wider controversy concerning religion in the NHS.

This much is clear from a number of recent cases, and the coverage and comment which they have received. In early 2009, Caroline Petrie, an NHS nurse in north Somerset, was suspended by her Primary Healthcare Trust for offering to pray with a patient for healing of her leg ulcer which she was regularly dressing without any rapid signs of improvement. The patient declined, but did not mind nor complain, though she did mention the offer to another nurse, who then reported Mrs Petrie to the Trust. They then suspended her. The story culminated in a *Daily Telegraph* headline on 6 February 2009 that 'NHS staff face sack if they discuss religion.'[17] The subsequent public outrage at the way Mrs Petrie had been treated was such that she was reinstated shortly afterwards, though not without ongoing pressure applied to prevent her from 'reoffending'.

Later that year, the case of another NHS nurse, Anand Rao, also made the papers. He had volunteered to take a postgraduate course in palliative care organized by the Leicestershire and Rutland Organization for the Relief of Suffering (LOROS). During one of the course sessions, Mr Rao was placed in simulated consultation with actors playing the part of married couple. He was told the wife had a serious heart condition and was suffering from stress after a doctor had told her she would not live much longer. Mr Rao 'advised the patient to refrain from smoking, change her lifestyle and try not to dwell on what the doctor had said, because worry in itself can overload and damage the heart further. In addition, I said that she should try to visit a church if possible, because it can sometimes relieve stress.'[18] Unhappy with this suggestion, the course organizers reported him to his employer who subsequently suspended, and later dismissed him. He stated to the press: 'They told me I had breached the [Nursery and Midwifery Council's] code of conduct because I had used the word "God", and that I might use it again in the future and that they would be notifying my employers at the Leicester Royal Infirmary with a view to terminating my post.' Asked whether he wants his job back, he replied: 'Of course, nursing is all I've ever known.'

Both these well-publicized cases attest to a genuine unease about the role of religion—or, more to the point, religious people—in healthcare. As with Savulescu's stance regarding conscientious objection, there are again clear parallels to a version of secularism that would confine religious beliefs and convictions to a purely private sphere. Such things are presumably fine for a doctor or nurse's leisure time, but must not 'interfere' in any way with their professional, secular lives. Such views ought not, however, to be caricatured: in many cases, they arise from a sincere concern for patient care. Behind the disciplinary actions against Petrie and Rao, for instance, is the reasonable desire that vulnerable people not be troubled by unwanted proselytism or religious harassment. This is a worry expressed in the Department of Health's 2008 *Religion or Belief: A Practical Guide for the NHS*: 'Members of some religions [...] are expected to preach and to try to convert other people. In a workplace environment this can cause many problems, as non-religious people and those from other religions or beliefs could feel harassed and intimidated by this behaviour'.[19, p. 22] However, it is difficult to see how the actual actions of Petrie or Rao would count as either proclamation or proselytism. Instead, both cases may be viewed—and were popularly received—as being grave overreactions on the part of the nurses' managers to *any* intimation or expression of a religious commitment. Note too that in neither case was any complaint made by a patient.

Arguably, the attempt to drive all expressions of religious belief, practice, or conviction out of healthcare will itself lead to a sharp decline in patient wellbeing. It ignores the fact that *all* healthcare professionals, regardless of their spiritual tradition or lack of one, possess beliefs and commitments, which in turn influence their actions. This much is recognized in the well-balanced advice of the 2008 General Medical Council (UK) guidelines *Personal Beliefs and Medical Practice: Guidance for Doctors*:

> All doctors have personal beliefs which affect their day-to-day practice. Some doctors' personal beliefs may give rise to concerns about carrying out or recommending particular procedures for patients
>
> Discussing personal beliefs may, when approached sensitively, help you to work in partnership with patients to address their particular treatment needs. You must respect patients' right to hold religious or other beliefs and should take those beliefs into account where they may be relevant to treatment options. However, if patients do not wish to discuss their personal beliefs with you, you must respect their wishes.[20]

This applies just as much to a utilitarian seeking to encourage patients to pursue assisted suicide as a possible option, as it does to the Muslim, Christian, or Jew seeking to dissuade them from it. Both groups could give rise to concerns if undue pressures are exerted, but to try to discriminate against one set of values alone is hardly compatible with any meaningful concepts of equality and diversity—which are, of course, precisely what secularisms set out to safeguard.

Chaplaincy provision and funding

Chaplaincy was recognized as being an integral part of holistic health care right from the foundation of the NHS on 5th July, 1948. Twenty-eight full-time chaplains were appointed employees with five-yearly contracts, although chaplains did not become part of the NHS pension scheme until the mid-1970s. Because of the close connection of the Church of England with the State, originally all NHS-employed chaplains were Anglican. In the 1990s, however, the decline in numbers of practising Anglicans, large numbers of non-Anglican Christians, and the rapid growth of other faiths in an increasingly multi-cultural society, meant that the newly formed NHS Trusts increasingly appointed chaplains of other faiths as well as from churches other than the Church of England.

Given all this, a clear case can be made for the NHS's chaplaincy provision correlating with the second, 'common ground' mode of secularism delineated above. Broadly speaking, this seeks to mediate between competing religious interests in the public square by opening up a shared, ecumenical space to which all may contribute on an equal footing: for example, by outlawing religious tests for public office, and enfranchising members of all religious (and non-religious) groups. The key motivation here is that no one religion or denomination should be unduly privileged over any or all others. The British case is complicated here by various issues, not least the legal establishment of the Church of England. Despite this, with regard to hospital chaplaincy provision (and, indeed, many other sectors of public and social life), there is a widely-held recognition that people of all faiths and none should, if they so desire, receive sufficient pastoral and spiritual care from formally recognized chaplains. To this end, the NHS either funds or otherwise supports (among others) Christian, Jewish, Muslim, Hindu, Buddhist, Sikh, and humanist chaplains of various kinds.

Despite this, critiques are certainly possible from *within* the perspective of the 'common ground' mode of secularism (even if the critics themselves do not explicitly situate themselves in this tradition). It can be argued, for instance, that while the NHS may claim, and indeed genuinely aspire, to be both multi-faith and non-discriminatory in its chaplaincy provision, *in practice* it is far from so. A 2004 study of 72 (out of 100) NHS chaplaincy departments in England and Wales reported that, out of 105 full-time chaplains employed by hospitals, 98 (93.3%) were Christian, as also were 139 out of 152 (91.4%) part-time chaplains. The remaining 7 full-timers were all Muslims, while the remaining 13 part-timers comprised 9 Muslims, two Hindus, a Jew, and a Sikh.[21] Furthermore, respondents from the NHS departments themselves perceived chaplaincy provision to be significantly better for Christians than it was for other groups. The researchers comment:

> This national survey has revealed appreciable differences in reported hospital chaplaincy provision to patients and staff for member of Christian and non-Christian faiths. We have found comparative disadvantage to non-Christians in relation to access to space for worship, chaplaincy staff and quality of chaplaincy care, resulting in poorer spiritual and pastoral care to patients who are not Christians. [21, p. 95.]

It is important to note here that the authors make no suggestion that this instance of 'institutional discrimination in public services' was either an intended or desired one. The predominance of Christian, and indeed specifically Anglican, chaplaincy provision in the NHS reflects several factors, but primarily the historical dominance of Christianity, especially in its Anglican forms, in British society. However, since the NHS's inception in 1945, the United Kingdom's socio-religious profile has shifted dramatically, particularly over the course of the last few decades. At the same time as Christian belief, practice, and self-identification has declined significantly, several waves of immigration have brought many adherents of other religions—especially Islam, Hinduism, and Sikhism—into the country. This fact, and its ramifications for chaplaincy provision, is widely acknowledged. A 2004 Department of Health review of chaplaincy funding, for example, was partly motivated by the fact that: 'the numbers of people who are members of faiths other than Christian or Jewish has grown very substantially since the NHS was first established'.[22, p. 2]

Responding to the problem is not, however, a straightforward task. For a start, the socio-religious profile of a country is notoriously difficult to assess accurately: for example, slight and seemingly insignificant differences in the question asked can yield greatly different results. Furthermore, there is no easy way to translate such statistics into equitable chaplaincy provision. The Church of England, as many otherwise entirely secular people's 'default' option, may well be unfairly privileged if funding is based on a simple 'What is your religion?' type of question. This could deny funds to groups that are numerically smaller, but whose generally more-committed members request and value chaplaincy services a good deal more. Yet feasibly, a more sophisticated measure, based on practice or commitment, could just as easily under-resource the Church of England's chaplains. Arguably, it is its very 'default' status that makes it feel the most approachable to the many people, whether nominally Anglican or not, who value and benefit from spiritual care at their most vulnerable and distressing moments. [e.g. 23]

Issues are further complicated by the fact that, in common with other areas of the NHS, many chaplains are overworked and under-resourced. While under-provisioned religious communities are keen to rectify this, they are apparently unwilling to remove scarce resources from overstretched Anglican or Catholic chaplains. As the author of the 2004 review writes, 'there was reluctance by groups not currently supported to have their needs met at the expense of the existing recipients. I was urged to recommend additional funding'.[22, p. 11] Perhaps not surprisingly, however, this was not an option available to him. Yet while there is clearly much more to be done, the overall picture is not unremittingly bleak. As the authors of a 2010 article in *Mental Health, Religion & Culture* point out:

> However, perceptions of [Anglican] denominational hegemony are challenged by new initiatives such as the Multi-Faith Group for Healthcare Chaplaincy, funded by the Department of Health, seeking to establish a formal scheme of recognition [...] This national development may enable widened participation for a range of faith groups within healthcare chaplaincy. At an operational level joint working between representatives of differing faith communities takes place. [24, p. 598.]

This initiative may well prove crucial to furthering the 'common ground' secularist agenda.

A very different kind of secularist challenge appears in the National Secular Society's *An investigation into the cost of the National Health Service's Chaplaincy provision*, released in April 2009. This puts the chaplaincy service's salary costs, excluding any maintenance to chapels or other facilities, at just over £32 million per annum. The report argues:

> The cost is equivalent to the cost of around 1,500 nurses or over 2,600 cleaners. The money should instead be used to employ front line staff, who are urgently needed [...] We are confident that if patients were asked if they wanted chaplains or thousands more cleaners or nurses, the vast majority would choose the latter.[25, p. 1.]

The National Secular Society sets its critique against three main backgrounds. First of all are the well-documented funding pressures on the NHS, and resulting concerns for the standards of patient care. These are evidenced by the quotation of three news headlines from the previous two months: 'Plan to axe over 700 nursing jobs slammed', 'Hospital hygiene campaign launched', and 'Hygiene failings on NHS wards'. Second is the general decline in religious interest and practice in society, which the report argues leads to lower demand for chaplaincy services:

> While it is undoubtedly true that the chaplaincy services are useful to and valued by some people, for many, if not most, they are an irrelevance.
>
> As Britain becomes a more secular society, clergy are way down on the list of figures that people turn to for advice and support generally, not just in hospitals.[25, p. 3.]

Third is growing religious diversity, which (as we have already seen) demands funding and support of a far broader range of chaplaincy services: 'In trying to accommodate the many religions now extant in Britain, the burden on Hospital Trusts is increasing, at a time when financial pressures are hardest'.[25, p. 2.]

The document is clear that it 'is not seeking to expel religion or religious representatives from hospitals'. Instead, it advocates that all state funding of chaplaincy services be stopped. If patients or their families wish to receive religious support, then their own religious institutions may send someone on an 'as-and-when basis', and at their own cost. Rather than wasting scare resources to 'religious provision', NHS budgets 'should be devoted entirely to the *raison d'etre* of a hospital, which is medical treatment and aftercare'.[25, p. 2.]

The National Secular Society made a strong case, and at a time when NHS chaplaincy services were already being scaled back due to budgetary constraints. Not surprisingly, however, the investigation has been criticized on a number of areas. In the first place, objections may be raised against the accuracy of its portrayal of contemporary healthcare chaplaincy (see also chapter on 'Chaplaincy'). For example, it suggests that 'clerics' (itself an inaccurate term for a great many chaplains) spend 'much wasted time in the hospital'. Yet as one critic notes, 'Idleness and lack of work are not terms normally associated with chaplains'.[26, p. 26] Moreover, while it is indeed true that declining formal religious observance has brought about a change in how chaplains spend their time—most notably, with less formal religious ceremonies (24)—there is strong evidence that chaplains remain highly valued and used by staff and patients alike (21, 23, 26, 27).

Throughout, the NSS' investigation implies that chaplaincy services are only used by people who are otherwise fairly religious: hence its recommendation that patients may receive comfort 'from their own place of worship, which will be able to send people with whom they are familiar and who know more about them'.[25, p. 2] The reality, of course, is very different: the very nature of hospital chaplaincy means they are actively sought out by a large number of patients and families who have hitherto had little, if any, engagement with religious institutions. This includes many who consider themselves to be not at all religious.[28] Finally, it is necessary to put the quoted salary costs of £32 million in some context. While not a small sum in itself, this equates to less than three-hundredths of 1% of the NHS's annual budget of over £100 billion. Given the well-documented evidence base of good 'spiritual care' furthering medical outcomes (see 'Health Outcomes'), a case can certainly be made for the cost-effectiveness of chaplaincy provision specifically in light of 'the *raison d'etre* of a hospital, which is medical treatment and aftercare'. In the words of one critic of the National Secular Society's proposals, while cutting chaplaincy funding might save tens of millions:

> You would, however, find other costs rising to compensate for this, e.g. counselling services, befriending services, staff support services, even drug bills. You could also find patients being less settled in hospital, less responsive, less ready to go home because while their medical condition is treated they are not being treated as whole people with wider needs that impact on their well-being.[26, p. 26.]

Conclusion

Secularism may perhaps have seemed like an odd inclusion in the 'Traditions' section of a textbook such as this. However, first impressions, in this case as in so many others, are deceptive. Secularisms are, on the contrary, of the utmost importance for the proper consideration of spirituality and healthcare. Across the world, in societies as diverse as France, the USA, Canada, Turkey, and India, varieties of secularism set the legal, political, financial, and ethical contexts in which both the theory and practice of healthcare takes place. As strategies for mediating between competing religious interests in the public sphere, the specific relevance of secularism to spirituality and healthcare is undeniable.

In this chapter, we have attempted to do three main things. First, we disentangled the philosophical and political concept of 'secularism proper' from the socio-religious concept of 'secularity', which occasionally also goes by this term. Although the two ideas are by no means unrelated, there is no straightforward correspondence between them. Secularity is indeed significant for the study of spirituality, but since a number of specifically secular spiritual traditions are dealt with elsewhere in this section, these have not been our focus here. Secondly, we explained and explored the distinction between two classic 'modes of secularism'—one seeking to exclude religious interests from public life entirely, and the other attempting to find a public 'common ground' in which they might all share. These are very broad distinctions, and are amenable to a great deal of both theoretical and practical variation. Nevertheless, they are useful lenses for appraising different secularist approaches to religion (and/or spirituality) and healthcare in contemporary societies. Finally, using the United Kingdom's National Health Service as a concrete example, we explored two highly contentious secularist issues: conscientious objection and chaplaincy provision. These case studies, which also drew on other analogous controversies from the past few years, both presented and critiqued recent challenges to how the NHS is funded and run, drawn from both secularist modes. Whatever one's position in these debates—and, it must be admitted, neither of us would regard themselves as purely neutral bystanders—it is clear that secularism is a topic of crucial, and perhaps growing, significance.

References

1 Kosmin, B.A. (2007). Contemporary secularity and secularism. In: B.A. Kosmin, A. Keysar (eds) *Secularism & Secularity: Contemporary International Perspectives*, pp. 1–13. Hartford: Institute for the Study of Secularism in Society and Culture.

2 Bruce, S. (2002). *God is Dead: Secularization in the West.* Oxford: Oxford University Press.

3 Smith, G. (2008). *A Short History of Secularism.* London: I. B. Tauris.

4 Van Ness, P.H. (ed.) (1996). *Spirituality and the Secular Quest.* London: SCM.

5 Heelas, P. (2009). Spiritualities of life. In: P.B. Clarke (ed.) *The Oxford Handbook of the Sociology of Religion*, pp. 758–82. Oxford: Oxford University Press.

6 Hwang, K., Hammer, K., Cragun, R.T. (2011). Extending religion-health research to secular minorities. *J Religion Hlth.* **50**: 608–22.

7 Asad, T. (2003). *Formations of the secular.* Stanford: Stanford University Press.

8 Mahmood, S. (2007). Can secularism be other-wise? In: M. Warner, J. VanAntwerpen, C. Calhoun (eds), *Varieties of Secularism in a Secular Age*, pp. 282–99. Cambridge: Harvard University Press.

9 Taylor, C. (1998). Modes of secularism. In: R. Bhargava (ed.) *Secularism and its Critics*, pp. 31–53. New Delhi: Oxford University Press.

10 Bhargava, R. (1998). What is secularism for? In: R Bhargava R (ed.) *Secularism and its Critics*, pp. 486–542. New Delhi: Oxford University Press.

11 Williams, R. (2008). Secularism, faith and freedom. In: G. Ward, M. Hoelzl (eds) *The New Visibility of Religion: Studies in Religion and Cultural Hermeneutics*, pp. 45–56. London: Continuum.

12 Locke, J. (1689/1955). *A Letter Concerning Toleration*, 2nd edn. Indianapolis: Bobbs-Merrill.

13 Seale, C. (2010). The role of doctors' religious faith and ethnicity in taking ethically controversial decisions during end-of-life care. *J Med Ethics* **36**: 677–82.

14 Savulescu J. (2006). Conscientious objection in medicine. *Br Med J* **332**: 294–7.

15 http://www.bmj.com/content/332/7536/294/reply

16 Cantor, J. (2009). Conscientious objection gone awry—restoring selfless professionalism in medicine. *N Engl J Med* **360**:1484–5.

17 Beckford, M., Gammell, C. (2009). NHS staff face sack if they discuss religion. Available at: http://www.telegraph.co.uk/news/newstopics/religion/4530384/NHS-staff-face-sack-if-they-discuss-religion.html

18 Alderson, A. (2009). Nurse loses job after urging patients to find God during a training course. Available at: http://www.telegraph.co.uk/news/newstopics/religion/5373122/Nurse-loses-job-after-urging-patients-to-find-God-during-a-training-course.html

19 Department of Heath (2008). Religion or belief; a practical guide for the NHS. Available at: www.dh.gov.uk/prod_consum_dh/groups/dh_digitalassets/documents/digitalasset/dh_093132.pdf

20 GMC (2008). Personal beliefs and medical practice: guidance for doctors. Available at: www.gmc-uk.org/guidance/ethical_guidance/personal_beliefs.asp

21 Sheikh, A., Gatrad, A.R., Sheikh, U., Singh Panesar, S., Shafi, S. (2004). The myth of multifaith chaplaincy: a national survey of hospital chaplaincy departments in England and Wales, *Divers Hlth Soc Care* **1**: 93–7.

22 James, J.H. (2004). Report of a review of Department of Health Central Funding of Hospital Chaplaincy. Available at: http://www.dh.gov.uk/en/Publicationsandstatistics/Publications/PublicationsPolicyAndGuidance/DH_4087580

23 Swift, C. (2009). Hospital chaplaincy in the twenty-first century: the crisis of spiritual care on the NHS. Farnham: Ashgate.

24 Merchant, R., Wilson, A. (2010). Mental health chaplaincy in the NHS: current challenges and future practice, *Ment Hlth Relig Cult Hlth.* **13**: 595–604.

25 National Secular Society (2009). An investigation into the cost of the National Health Service's Chaplaincy provision. Available at: http://www.secularism.org.uk/uploads/3549dc90ef8e9eb331062664.pdf

26 Johnston, D. (2009). Chaplaincy in the NHS—a response to the National Secular Society from Northern Ireland. *Scott J Hlthcare Chaplaincy* **12**: 24–7.

27 Sokol, D. (2009). The value of hospital chaplains. Available at: http://news.bbc.co.uk/1/hi/health/7990099.stm

28 Newitt, M. (2009). Chaplaincy services are not only for religious patients. *Br Med J* **338**: 893.

CHAPTER 14

Sikhism

Eleanor Nesbitt

Introduction

For many healthcare professionals the word 'Sikh' conjures up the image of a turbaned Indian man. Awareness of the particular requirements of a Sikh patient may centre on the possible refusal on religious grounds by the patient, or his/her relatives, to allow the removal of hair from the patient's body. However, individual Sikhs' sensitivities and practice on these and other matters vary widely: hence, this chapter's explanatory framework for this wide range of attitudes and behaviour. Cases will illustrate some of the many ways in which religion, culture and health interact, and the issues of which responsible health providers need to be aware.

'Sikh' includes all who (would) enter 'Sikh' as their religion on hospital admission forms. Names indicate Sikh identity: in most cases, a male's second name (whether or not it serves as surname) is Singh (although by no means all Singhs are Sikh) and Kaur is usually a Sikh female's second name. Many (mainly unisex) Sikh forenames end in–deep/dip,

-inder, -jeet/jit, -preet/prit or -pal. Sikhs include the dedicated initiate ('baptized Sikh', *amritdhari*) and individuals, of Punjabi background, who visit a gurdwara (public place of worship) only for marriages. These two descriptions might apply to close relatives, and awareness is needed of the diversity of expectations, sensitivities, and spiritual resources in a patient's immediate (as well as more extended) family, whatever the patient's apparent degree of religiosity. Moreover, Sikhs include individuals whose families have lived outside India for a century and others reared in rural Punjab (in north-west India), or in an Indian city, who have only recently arrived in, say, Vancouver or Southall. Note, too, that in most cases a 'Sikh' is a Punjabi, but that—especially in North America—there are also *gora* (white) Sikhs of European ancestry, whose sensibilities and assumptions may be influenced by their families' Christian and Jewish backgrounds.

This chapter also acknowledges that there are Sikh service-providers, working as nurses and in general practice, and as practitioners in all medical specialisms. Non-Sikhs' affirmative sensitivity to Sikh experience is beneficial to collegial relations, as well as to patient care, and Sikh healthcare professionals should feel confident in drawing upon their cultural, religious and spiritual heritage in meeting client needs and in enriching colleagues' understanding of Sikh patients.

Sikh spirituality has as its focus trying to be one with God. Sikhs acknowledge that there are many paths and that theirs is illuminated by the guidance of the Sikh Gurus (see below). Remembrance of God goes hand in hand with compassionate service (*seva*) and truthful living [1]. It is also inseparable from personal hygiene: Guru Nanak bade followers to bathe before praying, and for a Sikh bathing means washing in running water, i.e. having a shower, if at all possible.(see Hollins 2009, [2, p. 97]

'Sikhism' fits deceptively well the conception of a 'religion', a conception rooted in centuries of European thought. Religions are widely understood to be systems that have:

- a founder
- a scripture
- some distinctive beliefs
- a calendar of annual celebrations
- some characteristic practices such as initiation rites and private and congregational worship.

Unfortunately, this model of 'religion' too easily underpins misleading assumption that religions are freestanding belief systems, with clear-cut lines both between themselves and other religions, and between religion and culture. Also, it is too easily assumed that (at least in communities other than one's own) stated rules equate to the actual behaviour of whole communities, and then to judge and misunderstand individuals who do not fit this stereotype. Apparent contradictions lead to essentializing and polarizing imagined categories such as 'orthodox' and 'unorthodox', 'observant' and 'lapsed', or 'traditional' Sikhs and 'westernized' Sikhs. Instead, this chapter's basis is the understanding that such dichotomies obscure the dynamics at work in Sikh (and other religiously defined) communities, and can distract professionals from engaging effectively with particular individuals and their families.

Contemporary Sikh experience is better understood by reference to three overlapping 'domains' which exert sometimes contrary, and sometimes mutually reinforcing, pulls. Indeed, insofar as each domain involves widely accepted patterns of emotion, each is an 'emotional regime'.[3] The three domains are:

- *sikhi* [living as a Sikh in accordance with the teachings of the Gurus and the requirements of the Khalsa (see below) code of discipline, the Sikh Rahit Maryada]

- *panjabiat* (characteristically Punjabi culture)
- modernity, meaning the norms (opportunities and pressures) of twenty-first century 'westernized' society).

An outline of each domain in relation to spirituality and health precedes discussion of the body in Sikh experience, Sikh understandings of mental and physical illness, and finally, dying, death, and bereavement. This tripartite model is more helpful than presuppositions of 'culture clash', and being torn 'between two cultures',[e.g. 4] although many diaspora Sikhs do describe their experience of internal conflict in this way.

The explication of the three domains applies to the Punjabi Sikh majority, rather than to the much smaller number of *gora* (White) Sikhs. Indeed, as Canadian scholar Verne Dusenbery has pointed out, in his analyses of the differences between (and the relationship between) the *gora* Sikhs and Punjabi Sikhs of North America, the two communities' different socialization results in different assumptions about what being a Sikh means and in different reactions to crisis [5]. *Gora* Sikhs demonstrate strong commitment to the Sikh Code of Conduct (Sikh Rahit Maryada), to vegetarianism and to wearing a turban (regardless of one's gender), but concern with *izzat* (family honour) does not feature in their priorities. By contrast, *izzat* and other aspects of *panjabiat* are at work, to varying degrees, in decision-making and lifestyle choices, as well as psychological and physical illness, of Punjabi Sikhs. The tripartite model [6] corresponds to Kamala Nayar's analysis of the psychosocial experience of Canadian Sikh women [7].

Before examining these three 'domains', we turn to a definition of 'Sikh', a summary outline of 'Sikhism', and some comment on Sikh identity and its outward indicators.

Sikhs and Sikhism

Worldwide, Sikhs number approximately 21 million, so constituting the fifth largest faith community globally. Introductions to Sikhism explain that the faith's 'founder' was Guru Nanak 1469–1539, and attribute the code of discipline for 'baptized,' i.e. *amritdhari* Sikhs to Guru Nanak's ninth and last successor, Guru Gobind Singh. In this connection, they often retell the dramatic events in 1699 on the day of the Spring festival, Vaisakhi, the day that is celebrated annually as the 'birthday' of the Khalsa (the nucleus of *amritdhari* Sikhs) and by extension of the Sikh community more generally. In religious terms a Sikh is any human being who faithfully believes in:

> One immortal Being, Ten Gurus, from Guru Nanak to Guru Gobind Singh, the Guru Granth Sahib [scriptures also known as Adi Granth], the utterances and teachings of the ten Gurus and the baptism [initiation with *amrit* (see below)] bequeathed by the tenth Guru, and who does not owe allegiance to any other religion.[8]

The religion of Sikhs is known as Sikhism, but only because this was the term coined by the British during their colonial rule over India, a period during which other 'isms' were also being coined in Europe. Arising from within the Sikh tradition, Punjabi words for their religious tradition are *sikhi* and *gursikhi*, as well as *gurmat* (the Gurus' doctrine). Underlying these terms are two fundamentals, namely Sikh (the learner, disciple) and Guru (the spiritual guide). The Sikh concept of Guru encompasses 'God' (referred to by many names, including Vahiguru, Satguru, Akal Purakh, Rab, and Hari), as well as the ten human Gurus and the scriptures (Guru Granth Sahib).

The scriptures

The 1430 pages of the Guru Granth Sahib (or Adi Granth) consist of the poetic compositions of six of the ten Gurus, plus selected hymns by religious poets including Muslim and Hindu mystics whose lives predated Guru Nanak's. Devout Sikhs take daily guidance through a *vak/hukamnama* (reading after opening the volume at random). Increasingly, Sikhs tend to access the *hukamnama* from the Harmandir Sahib (Golden Temple, Amritsar) via their mobile phone. The sanctity of the scripture—and the requirements for its maintenance—preclude its being brought to hospital or, indeed, being installed in a hospital chaplaincy or prayer room, although copies of a *gutka* (small scriptural anthology for use in daily prayer) need to be available. The standard 1430-page full volume is arranged according to the *rag* (*raga*, musical mode) in which each passage is sung, and *shabad kirtan* (hearing/singing the scripture) is intrinsically healing.[9,10]

Moreover, Sikhs of whatever educational background draw blessing from simply being in the presence of the Guru Granth Sahib (which has to be appropriately installed and attended). They may organize a continuous, complete reading (a 48-hour-long *akhand path*) or an intermittent reading over a longer period (*sahaj path*) to pray for a successful outcome or to give thanks for healing.

Core teaching

Religiously informed Sikhs draw on the Gurus' emphasis on wholeness, integrity and balance, emphasizing the need to lead a life centred on *nam* (divine reality) in the midst of daily responsibilities. Thus, the Guru-orientated (*gurmukh*) Sikh will, with the Guru's grace, displace ego (*haumai*), and refrain from five tendencies—lust, anger, greed, attachment to temporal things, and pride.[6] Vitally important, in the context of this Handbook, is the Sikh Gurus' insight into the connection between ego and health/disease. The ideal balance is implicit in the principle of *grihasti* (married life, rather than asceticism) and in such pairings as *seva* and *simaran* (voluntary service coupled with remembrance of the divine reality), *miri piri* (temporal and spiritual power) and the ideal of the *sant-sipahi* (warrior saint, the person who combines spirituality with preparedness for courageous action). A motto attributed to Guru Nanak encapsulates Sikh life as *nam japo, kirat karo, vand chhako*, i.e. 'meditate, work and share.'

Meditation (*nam simaran* or sustained remembrance of the *nam* or divine name) may entail repetition of the words 'Satnam Sri Vahiguru', sometimes aided by prayer beads (*mala*). *Nam simaran* is also at the heart of *kirtan* (congregational absorption in the singing of the words of the Guru Granth Sahib). Labun and Emblen note the heart patient recovering through 'several months of developing his spirituality through meditation' and they report the experience that 'pain is taken away during childbirth by praying, 'God is One'' (*ik oankar*).[11, p. 143] The Gurmukh Sikh aspires to living in accordance with *hukam* i.e. in harmony with the divine will. Some patients perceive their sickness as a time for reflection and increasing spirituality with more time to pray.[11, p. 144] They may find that they are praying more sincerely and sense that by so doing they are more likely to recover. Sikhs will pray only after bathing, and—if possible—should not be disturbed while praying. They may bring a *gutka* (see above) into hospital. It is kept wrapped in a clean cloth and should be handled with respect and kept in a clean place.[Hollins 2009, 2, p. 96]

Sikh diversity

Many textbook and online representations of Sikhs are in fact representations not of Sikhs more generally, but of *amritdhari* Sikhs, the minority who have taken initiation into the Khalsa (literally, 'pure' community) in a rite involving *amrit,* empowering water. They observe a code of discipline, the Sikh Rahit Maryada (also transliterated as Rehat Maryada). It is important to ask whether a *keshdhari* patient (i.e. one whose hair appears not to have been cut or trimmed) has in fact 'taken *amrit*', in order to ascertain how strict their observance will be.[12, p. 11] Initiated Sikhs are known too as Gursikhs (Sikhs of the Guru) and Khalsa Sikhs (although the term 'Khalsa' is also sometimes applied more loosely to the *panth,* the Sikh community as a whole). In conversation strictly observant Sikhs are often described as 'proper Sikhs', 'true Sikhs' or 'pure Sikhs'.[13]. Misleadingly, many publications (including those intended for healthcare workers) present religious requirements as if they were (all) Sikhs' actual behaviour. Consequently, an impression is often given that (all) Sikhs (and not only Khalsa initiates) maintain all of the five Ks, i.e. five outward indicators of their religious allegiance, each of which commences with 'k' in Punjabi.

Five Ks

Healthcare professionals need to realize the sanctity of these requirements for *amritdhari* Sikhs and the associated sensitivities for Sikhs more generally. A patient must not be separated from any of the Ks unnecessarily and the Ks may be incorporated in the laying out of a deceased person. The five Ks are: *kesh* (uncut hair), *kara* (bangle—of steel or iron—worn on the right wrist), *kirpan* (sword), *kachhahira* (breeches/underwear), and *kangha* (comb). *Kesh* includes hair on all parts of the body (see 'Understandings of the body'). For devout Sikhs each K carries spiritual significance, as summarized below. Thus the *kesh* signifies respect for the body in its God-given form. The *kara* is usually a thin band of steel, and it is the only K maintained by most non-observant Sikhs. A heavier, rounded iron *kara* often indicates the wearer's strong religious commitment. The *kara* reminds Sikhs to use their hands only for good purposes. As a circle it symbolizes God's infinity, and the *kara* is sometimes described as a 'handcuff to God'. In the case of the *kirpan* many Sikhs are content to wear a miniature (one or two inch) *kirpan,* for example embellishing their *kangha* (comb). However, an *amritdhari* Sikh generally understands his/her baptismal commitment as necessitating the wearing of a sheathed sword, with a blade of about four inches' minimum length, at all times. In spiritual terms the *kirpan* demonstrates defence of the vulnerable and readiness to fight for the unjustly oppressed. Sikhs tend to regard the word *kirpan* as derived from *kirpa* meaning grace or mercy and *an* (honour). For insightful guidance on patients wearing a *kirpan.*[14]

Amritdhari Sikh practice is to only half remove the *kachhahira* before putting the first leg into a clean *kachhahira.* This has implications for childbirth and certain surgery, as one of the patient's legs should be left with the *kachhahira* around it (oral communication from S. Firth, personal communication, 27 July 2010).

Case history

Sikh Chaplain 'F' has been able to advise staff about the importance of Sikh religious symbols and suggest minor adjustments to procedure. He illustrated this with the following scenario:

If it is necessary to remove all the clothing of an unconscious patient in A&E, it is usual practice to place it together with everything they arrive with in a plastic bag. Care is taken that the bag goes to the ward with the patient and that valuables have been listed and stored safely. However, this procedure can be offensive to a Sikh patient because their turban and comb go in the same bag as their pants and shoes ... Kachera are the long smart underwear which makes a Sikh feel well dressed and gives them dignity. However, the Kachera are seen as covering a 'dirty' part of the body. Shoes will be dirty from general use. Chaplain 'F' suggested a relatively simple solution to prevent offence being caused: 'We shouldn't put everything in one bag. To use separate bags is acceptable, especially keeping turban and comb in a separate bag from pants and shoes.'[15, p. 48.]

The turban

The turban, a length of cotton cloth wound skilfully around the head in a number of styles, is one of Sikhism's most potent symbols. While the turban (*pag, pagri, dastar*) is not explicitly a part of Sikh discipline, it is worn not only by *amritdhari* Sikhs, but by hundreds of thousands of uninitiated male Sikhs. It 'is thought of as the crown which covers the Kesh (long hair)'[15, p. 48] and is associated with qualities including courage, honour, responsibility, piety, and friendship. Disrespectful treatment of a Sikh's turban stirs Sikh feelings at a deep level. The colour and style of turban in some cases denotes allegiance to a particular religious grouping. Thus, Sikhs who draw inspiration from the Nihang movement wear a tall blue turban (*dumala*). A white turban wound flat across the brow can indicate adherence to the (strictly vegetarian) Namdhari movement.

An increasing number of *amritdhari* women too wear turbans, in accordance with Sikh Dharma of the Western Hemisphere (whose members tie tall, white turbans) and the Akhand Kirtani Jatha, whose female adherents wear a black or dark blue *keski*—also known as a *dastar.* The Akhand Kirtani Jatha's founder, Bhai Randhir Singh, taught that the *keski,* rather than simply the *kesh* (hair), is one of the five Ks.

In hospital, Sikhs who would otherwise wear a full turban may opt for a head-covering that is easier to manage. Any substitute head covering (e.g. a towel) that a patient adopts in hospital should also be treated with respect

Abstinence and diet

The Sikh Rahit Maryada prohibits the use of tobacco and intoxicants[16] (but see the sections on *panjabiat* and modernity). In practice, it is unusual for a Sikh (whether religiously observant or not) to smoke, and it is much less usual for women than for men to consume alcohol.

Purity is a strong emphasis for devout Sikhs, and should be sought in strict vegetarianism and in life as a whole. It is widely accepted by Sikhs that a vegetarian diet is intrinsic to spirituality, and to the practice of their Sikh faith. Sometimes switching to vegetarianism results from the influence of a respected preacher or *sant* (see 'Protection from harm'). In any case, '[i]t is commonly believed that elderly persons become more spiritual in old age through their actions and thoughts'[11, pp.143–4] and thus, some Sikhs, like some Hindus, may become vegetarian in old age. A vegetarian Sikh usually avoids not only meat, fish, and animal fats, but also eggs, and foods (such as cake) that may include these. At the same time it would be exceedingly unusual for a Sikh to be vegan, as milk and dairy produce are prominent in the Punjabi diet.

If a hospital patient's food arrives tainted by the smell of non-vegetarian food in close proximity, he/she may well refuse it. Menus need to indicate vegetarian dishes that are free of eggs, and such meals need to be delivered separately from non-vegetarian meals.[15, p. 45]

It should be noted that, even among observant Sikhs, dietary practice differs. Many Sikhs are non-vegetarian; they will, however, tend to avoid beef, but this has to do with the Hindu cultural context in which many Sikhs have grown up in India. In fact, the only prohibition in the Sikh Rahit Maryada is of halal (and, by extension, kosher) meat. The Sikh Gurus did not themselves specifically commend vegetarianism: Guru Nanak voiced reservations about brahmins' denunciation of meat-eating, pointing out that vegetarians, too, could be blood-suckers, inasmuch as they 'devour people in the darkness of the night'.[17, p. 1289]

Yet, despite the Guru's criticism of exalting vegetarianism over other principles, subsequent *sant*s have tended to advocate vegetarianism. Baba Nand Singh (of the Nanaksar tradition) insisted that when a Guru hunted, the object was not to eat meat, but to release the *atma* (soul) of the animal from the cycle of birth, death, and rebirth.[18, p. 100] The Namdhari movement in particular emphasizes rigorous vegetarianism. The *gora* Sikhs follow the guidance of their leader, Harbhajan Singh (Yogi Bhajan, 1929–2004), in promoting vegetarianism, and some *amritdhari* members of the Akhand Kirtani Jatha (followers of Bhai Randhir Singh),[19] insist not only on strict vegetarianism, but on only eating from iron utensils and only what has been prepared by other *amritdhari* members of the Jatha. Hospitalization for such patients involves breaching their spiritual discipline.

Protection from harm

In common with many people from South Asia, and from other cultural backgrounds too, many Sikhs regard certain practices as part of their religion, even though their co-religionists would distance themselves from what they see as (merely) superstitious. For example, the physical presence of the scriptures is widely held to be protective. Thus, Labun and Emblen report how some Sikhs:

> talked about having the Holy Book in the house so that no harm will come to them or following religious practice as a magical charm so that they can avoid sickness or misfortune in their life. Generally, the participants who spoke of this kind of belief and practice were less well educated.[11, p. 143.]

Despite the fact that the Sikh Rahit Maryada prohibits keeping water by the Guru Granth Sahib, many Sikhs believe in the healing properties of water from a container that has been kept close to the scriptures during a continuous 48-hour reading (*akhand path*). Such water is felt to have been empowered by the reading of the Gurbani and, in turn, to have acquired an empowering and healing quality.[20,21] Thus, a Sikh might sip a little *amrit* to alleviate a headache, or splash it around the house for protection.

Some *sant*s too advocate the protective and healing power of *amrit*. A *sant* (also known as *baba*, or more respectfully as 'Babaji') is a spiritual master.[22] Many Sikhs attribute a deepening of their spirituality, and of commitment to Sikh discipline, to a *sant*'s blessing and influence, but Sikh views of the *sant* phenomenon in general and of any particular *sant* differ widely. Despite a 'mainstream' Sikh insistence on not showing to a human the reverence due only to the Gurus, devotion to a living guide is consistent with Punjab's (and South Asia's) religious culture, and a *sant*'s blessing will be especially sought for coping with illness.

Panjabiat

Sikhs' spiritual homeland is Punjab. The name Punjab (literally 'five waters') refers to the area of the Indian sub-continent through which the River Indus's five tributaries flow. Since 1947 this 'greater Punjab' has been dissected by the border separating Pakistan and India. In 1966 India's Punjab state was subdivided, with the designation of two new states, Haryana and Himachal Pradesh. Sikhs are now numerically concentrated in India's Punjab, but much of their cultural heritage (language, humour, cuisine, and music) is shared with Punjabis in Pakistan and with Punjabis of other faith communities. Indeed, the 'porousness' of supposed boundaries between 'Sikhism' and other 'religions' attracts scholarly attention, with Ron Geaves,[23] Roger Ballard,[24] Anna Bigelow,[25] and others reporting the lack of separation at certain places of pilgrimage. For example, Roger Ballard [24] usefully identifies dimensions of 'Punjabi religion', including the 'kismetic' dimension i.e. the religious behaviour of the distressed. Harjot Oberoi's work [26,27] provides a historical context for contemporary Sikhs' recorded recourse to traditional healing, including exorcist traditions.[28]

Izzat (family honour) so pervades and motivates Punjabi life that it is vital to take this into account. The 'religious' values enshrined in scripture can be seen as offering a corrective to *izzat*. The *sukh* (peace of mind) of a Guru-focused life that is free from enmity and fear, is far removed from the widespread preoccupation with *izzat*, which draws on pride and fear and feeds competitiveness and factionalism. This social pressure to be seen to succeed contributes to the stress and depression which issue in psychological and physical distress. Thus *izzat* plays a part in the increasing suicides of Sikh farmers in Punjab for whom the sale of their land in order to pay off their debts is too shameful to contemplate, and *izzat* has for generations been implicated in Punjabi expectations of women.[29]

The fact that a family's *izzat* is at risk if a woman's parents give too little as dowry and in wedding expenditure leads to son preference[30] and consequent female foeticide. Clearly, practitioner guidelines which suggest that Sikhs accept abortion only for medical reasons [e.g. 31, p. 33; Hollins 2009, 1, p. 98) or which extrapolate from the Gurus' prohibition of female infanticide (a practice that was prevalent before the rise of the *in utero* sex selection that amniocentesis has made possible), fail to indicate the actual pressures on women. In fact, Punjab (India's only Sikh-majority state) has a high incidence of female foeticide and son preference is evident, too, in Sikh diaspora communities. Healthcare professionals need to be aware that a mother who has given birth to a daughter may feel a sense of failure, which is reinforced by the disappointed or comforting, rather than happy, congratulatory, reactions of visiting relatives.

Izzat militates against disclosure of stigmatized medical conditions. An increasingly familiar scenario in Punjab is for a wife to become HIV positive as a result of her husband's promiscuity. As neither she nor the family can acknowledge the situation, she may (if relatives overseas will sponsor her visit) seek medical attention in (for example) the UK (T. Prashar, personal communication, 23 July 2010). The complex needs of such women cannot be understood if those counselling them are only briefed in the religious, rather than the social values of Sikhs.

Families will often regard illness as a family matter, rather than a primarily individual one, and relatives may oppose certain disclosures being made to the patient. Sensitive discussion involving relatives may well be appropriate. Also:

> Within the family, the mother-in-law or the oldest woman has significant power. This may affect the choices open to younger women in the family.(Hollins 2006 [2, p. 97.]

Unsurprisingly, given the emphasis on family in Sikh society, it is customary—in line with both religious teaching and *panjabiat*—to visit relatives in hospital. On occasion, as Hollins suggests: 'It may be helpful to allow some easing of any regulations limiting the number of people who can visit the bedside at any one time'. [2006, 2, p. 98]

Female modesty is valued, and is inseparable from *izzat* in what is still a patriarchal Punjabi society. In some instances women will prefer to be attended by same-sex practitioners. Sikh women's attitudes vary between generations: modesty in dress and behaviour is one area in which modernity pulls in a contrary direction to both *sikhi* and *panjabiat*.

Modernity

Rather than attempting to define modernity, this section suggests contemporary norms, which variously reinforce and undermine aspects of both *panjabiat* and *sikhi* in individual lives. Among these norms are emphases on individuality, privacy, independence, and autonomy, which are in tension with Punjabi assumptions about family roles and responsibilities, such as elders' involvement in career choice and spouse selection.

In terms of equality, both the rhetoric and the reality of 'western' societies challenges the caste hierarchy that continues to frame much Punjabi interaction and stereotyping. At the same time, modern advocacy of equality fits well with the Gurus' dismissal of caste-based inequality both with regard to spiritual progression towards liberation from rebirths and with regard to serving and eating together in the *langar* (dining area in the gurdwara). Gender equality can find support in feminist readings of Sikh scripture. [32] However, supposedly liberated sexual mores often strain against both *panjabiat* and *sikhi*. The three-way tensions are most acute in the experience of young women—especially with regard to behaviour, appearance, and sexual relationships[7]—but affect to some degree Sikhs of both sexes and all generations.

Conspicuous consumerism, including expenditure on leisure activities and the media, often poses no challenge to families' competition for status (*izzat*), but is at odds with the Gurus' spiritual priorities, and their exhortation to turn from greed and covetousness.

Increasing consumption of alcohol runs counter to both the Gurus' insights and the Khalsa discipline, and the soaring incidence of drug addiction in Punjab is also destroying previously proverbial characteristics of Punjabi culture, which was synonymous with a hardworking rural lifestyle.

The availability of intercontinental travel plus the ongoing communications revolution provides a greater range of media, entertainment and interest groups than any previous generation has enjoyed. For many Sikhs the Internet also strengthens (and indeed introduces) religious and cultural ties that might otherwise have been impracticable. For example, the text of the Guru Granth Sahib is instantly accessible in its original Gurmukhi script, in roman script, in translation, and with commentary. Sikhs are no longer restricted to their family and local congregations for guidance on personal (including medical) dilemmas. Instead, through countless websites and online forums, they can link with Sikhs worldwide. Increasingly, individuals are connecting with diverse groups of politically and/or spiritually bonded Sikhs. 'Tradition' is being shared and re-invented in ways unimaginable to parents and grandparents who struggled for stability and upward mobility as members of a minority in a western environment. Discussion of ethical issues, discovery of Sikhs' martial heritage—as demonstrated in swordplay (*gatka* and *shastar vidya*) - and involvement in devotional music are all facilitated by modern media. So too is access to yoga and alternative medicine via TV Asian networks. [33, p. 84]

Understandings of the body

While Sikhs' understanding of the body is largely shaped by ideas and information available in wider society, there are distinctive emphases relevant to health and healthcare. The image of the *sant sipahi* (warrior saint), and the criteria for being one of the *panj piare* who administer initiation, valorise bodies that are intact, healthy, active and disciplined.[20] (Criteria for being *panj piare* rule out anyone with a missing limb.)

Body and mind are viewed holistically:

> You can't separate mind and body. Our wise man says health is a state of mind and not [just] of body. If you are mentally healthy, you stay fit.[11, p. 144.]

Attitudes to the body do not preclude transfusions or transplants. Indeed these meet with general approval from Sikhs as 'a good example of selfless giving':[33, p. 84]

> A Sikh never hesitates to sacrifice for somebody else. We are happy to donate and to receive. We recognize others' poor quality of life. For example, people have kidney dialysis and this is hard. The better way is a successful kidney transplant. (quoted by [15, p. 56]; and in line with Hollins [2, p. 99])

As already indicated, the ideal of physical intactness relates particularly to the hair, and a Khalsa Sikh's maintenance of *kesh* includes hair on any part of the body. See discussion of Punjabi attitudes to hair by the anthropologist, Paul Hershman [33] and Jasjit Singh's findings on current hair-related Sikh practice.[34] As incidents in Ottawa and New York illustrate, Sikh families and communities are outraged by trimming and shaving carried out without consent by hospital staff:

> The World Sikh Organization of Canada (WSO) is disturbed to learn that... an elderly Sikh patient's beard was cut by a FHA nurse shortly before his death.[36]

> [T]he nurse cut Pyara Singh's beard, eyebrows, and moustache on June 3, 2007, violating his deeply held religious principles. Pyara Singh, who was suffering from Alzheimer's disease, however, passed away on July 18, 2007 ...

The subsequent settlement discussions centered the training of hospital staff to ensure that the same treatment did not happen to other Sikh patients. The final settlement included $20,000 in compensation to Pyara Singh's family, training of Taylor Care Center employees on Sikh patient care, an adoption of United Sikhs' Guidelines for Hospital Admittance and Care/Extended Care for Sikhs as part of nursing department orientation.[37]

While a minority of very devout *amritdhari* Sikhs would rather die than undergo surgery entailing removal of hair from any part of the body, many other Sikhs, male and female, by choice have short hair—although the choice has often been precipitated by peer pressure (including bullying and acts of aggression) and by contemporary fashion. Many males shave or trim their beards, and females visit salons for depilatory procedures. Yet, simultaneously, a growing minority of women are *keshdhari* and wear a turban.

Case of Raj Singh[38, p. 8–9]

Raj Singh, a seventy-two-year-old Sikh from India had been admitted to the hospital after a heart attack. He was scheduled for a heart catheterization ... The procedure involved running a catheter up the femoral artery, located in the groin ... Susan, his nurse, entered Mr Singh's room and explained that she had to shave his groin to prevent infection from the catheterization. As she pulled the razor from her pocket, she was suddenly confronted with the sight of shining metal flashing in front of her. Mr Singh had a short sword in his hand ...

On this case a hospital chaplain, experienced as a radiographer, comments 'When Sikh patients were given good explanations, privacy and time to discuss any concerns, they were always willing to conform to best practice' (Diane Greenwood, personal communication, 27 July 2010).

Understandings of mental and physical illness

Sikh religious writing does not distinguish between mental and physical aspects of *dukh* and *sukh* (suffering and happiness); psychological distress (stress) may be reported as physical dysfunction, such as 'sinking heart'.[39–41]

> People who have a clean soul, will be more healthy in all aspects of their being.[quoted in 11, p. 144.]
>
> [I]n the scriptures, as in Indian tradition more generally, no distinction is made between physical, mental, and spiritual disorder. All *dukh* (suffering) results from *haumai* (ego) and is healed by practising *nam simaran* (remembrance of God).[42]

To quote Arvind Mandair:[33, pp. 83–4]

> The real state of our being is 'dis-ease'... In Sikh scripture, disease is not always 'causally' linked to a bodily misfunction, but to the way in which human beings fundamentally exist in the world – namely the state of ego. Disease occurs when a person asserts 'I am myself' and turns this enunciation of the state of being into a defensive posture resistant to the flows of nature. This Guru Nanak says:
>
> Ego is given to man [sic] as his disease. Disease affects all creatures that arise in the world except those who remain detached. Man is born in sickness, in sickness he wanders through birth after birth. Captive to disease he finds no rest, without the Guru sickness never stops. [17, p. 1140.] For the beneficial physical effects of religious recitation and 'holy dips' see [44–45].

Dying, death and bereavement

The spiritual needs and resources of both the person who is dying and the family call for sensitively informed professional attention.[45] Shirley Firth (in an unpublished paper[46]) emphasises the importance for both patient and family of a 'good death':

> The concept of a good death is also implicit in Sikh teaching. It is a painless, fearless, peaceful death in old age (Adi Granth, 1244, 1254, 793[17]: Cole and Sambhi 1978)... The mind should be in a meditative state or listening to the scriptures, the Guru Granth Sahib, reciting the evening prayer, *Kirtan Sohila*, or The Psalm of Peace, *Sukhmani Sahib*. As the person dies '*Waheguru*' (wonderful Lord), should be repeated peacefully. *Amrit* may be placed in the mouth and on the ears. If a *granthi* is present, prayers (*Ardas*), may be offered.
>
> Looking for the spiritual prepares a person for the soul's change of 'dress' at death. The prayer at death is to 'find shelter at the feet of God' and eventually to be 'absorbed into God'.[11, p. 144]

Sikhs religious teaching of accepting the divine will discourages euthanasia, as:

> [O]ur life' is not 'ours', but a gift from God to be used responsibly. Responsibility is then the key factor that determines Sikh attitudes to euthanasia.[47, p. 163]

Disclosure of the seriousness of a patient's condition can be problematic, as relatives may wish information to be withheld, and to themselves make decisions about what to disclose when. Medical personnel need to be aware that an impromptu interpreter may be close to the patient's family and filter the information (S. Firth, oral communication, 28 July 2010).

After death, in many cases, relatives will wash and lay out the body, where appropriate incorporating the *kachhahira*, *kangha*, *kirpan*, and *kara*. Usually mourners will gather at the close relatives' house to offer condolences (*afsos*). If an infant dies, Sikh custom is to bury, rather than to cremate. Otherwise, cremation is the norm and will, in western countries, take place at the local crematorium, with a short rite in the crematorium chapel, prior to the mourners' recourse to a gurdwara for prayer. Sikh tradition is for the funeral to take place with minimal delay after the death. Often a *sahaj path* takes place at home.

There are no religious objections to a post-mortem, but Sikhs' preference is most certainly for a loved one's body to be left intact. [Hollins 2009, 2, p. 99]

Personnel

Hospital chaplain

Increasingly, hospitals in the UK draw on the services of a Sikh chaplain, a concerned Sikh who has received induction into chaplaincy responsibilities. The hospital chaplain, of whatever faith, has a duty to draw religious sensitivities of any patients to the attention of staff. Thus a chaplain may need to discuss with the Catering Manager ways of transporting and distributing vegetarian meals separately from non-vegetarian ones[15, p. 45] or of treating the Ks and turban with due respect. The chaplain will need especial sensitivity in supporting Sikhs coping with the death of a child, including perinatal death, and may be called on to conduct a hospital funeral.

Verses of the saint, Kabir, from the Guru Granth Sahib, offer patient and professionals solace and perspective:

> Why should we weep at the death of others, when we ourselves are not permanent?
>
> Whoever is born shall pass away; why should we cry out in grief?
>
> We are absorbed into the One from whom we came.[17, p. 337.]

Healthcare professionals

A medical career not only fits the ethical principles of *sikhi*, but it also meets the aspirations of a competitive, upwardly mobile Punjabi community concerned to maintain family honour and to prosper financially. As a result, many young Sikhs (in common with others of South Asian background) are encouraged by their parents from an early age to work towards a career in medicine. To varying degrees they bring to the profession an awareness of Punjabi tradition and competence in spoken Punjabi. However, professional training does not necessarily encourage practitioners to integrate these aspects of their experience in their practice, and some are reluctant (for example) to draw on what may only be very residual 'mother tongue' with Punjabi patients who lack confidence in English.

The centrality of integrity and of balance to Sikh religious teaching, the commitment to *seva* (voluntary service) and the celebrated quality of *chardi kala* (optimism) are supportive to Sikhs engaged in providing healthcare. Sikh teaching affirms *daya* (compassion): a striking exemplar was Bhagat Puran Singh (1904–1992), famed for his life of unflagging devotion to the alleviation of mental and physical illness.[48] Better-known to Sikhs is Bhai Ghanaiya/Kanhaiya who over three centuries ago won praise from Guru Gobind Singh for impartially providing water on the battlefield to the wounded of both sides, and who is increasingly referred to by Sikhs as a precursor of the Red Cross/Red Crescent.

Bibliography

Cole, W.O. (1995). *Teach yourself Sikhism*. London: Hodder and Stoughton.

Cole, W.O. (2004). *Understanding Sikhism*. Edinburgh: Dunedin Press.

Kalsi, S.S. (1999). *Simple guide to Sikhism*. Folkestone: Global Books.

Mann, G.S. (2004). *Sikhism*. Upper Saddle River: Prentice Hall.

Nesbitt, E. (2005). *Sikhism a Very Short Introduction*. Oxford: Oxford University Press.

Shackle, C. (2002). Sikhism. In: L. Woodhead, P. Fletcher, H. Kawanami, D. Smith (eds), *Religions in the Modern World*, pp. 70–85. London: Routledge.

Sikh Rahit Maryada (nd). Available as 'Sikh Reht Maryada' at http://www,sgpc.net/sikhism/sikh-dharma-manual.asp (accessed 17 January 2012).

Singh, C., Ajit, K. (2001). *The Wisdom of Sikhism*. Oxford: Oneworld.

Singh Harinder (2010). *Caring for a Sikh Patient. Sikh Healthcare Chaplaincy Group*. Available at: http://www.sikhchaplaincy.org.uk/Booklet.pdf (accessed 21 July 2010)

Websites

www.srigranth.org

www.sikhnet.com

www.sikhs.org

References

1 Nesbitt, E. (2007) Sikhism. In: P. Morgan , C. Lawton (eds) *Ethical Issues in Six Religious Traditions*, 2nd edn, pp. 118–67. Edinburgh: University of Edinburgh Press.

2 Hollins, S (2009). *Religions, Culture and Healthcare: A Practical Handbook for Use in Healthcare Environments*, 2nd edn. Abingdon: Radcliffe Publishing.

3 Riis, O., Woodhead, L. (2010). *A Sociology of Religious Emotion*. Oxford: Oxford University Press.

4 Ghuman, P.A.S. (2003). *South Asian Adolescents in the West*. Cardiff: University of Wales Press.

5 Dusenbery, V.A. (2008). *Sikhs at Large: Religion, Culture, and Politics in Global Perspective*. New Delhi: Oxford University Press.

6 Nesbitt, E. (2005). *Sikhism a Very Short Introduction*. Oxford: Oxford University Press.

7 Nayar, K. (2010). Sikh women in Vancouver: an analysis of their psychosocial issues. In: D. Jakobsh (ed.) *Sikhism and Women*, pp. 252–75. New Delhi: Oxford University Press.

8 Sikh Rahit Maryada (nd). Available as 'Sikh Reht Maryada' at http://www,sgpc.net/sikhism/sikh-dharma-manual.asp (accessed 17 January 2012).

9 Mansukhani, G.S. (1982). *Indian Classical Music and Sikh Kirtan*. Available at: http://www.esikhs.com/articles/indian_classical_music_&_sikh_kirtan.pdf (accessed 17 January 2012).

10 Kaur, G. (2001). Understanding shabad kirtan in its Sikh context; why is it so important to Sikh religious experience and in what ways does Gurbani convey this? Unpublished MA dissertation, South Asian Area Studies, SOAS, University of London.

11 Labun, E., Emblen, J.D. (2007). Spirituality and health in Punjabi Sikh [sic]. *J Holist Nurs* 25: 141–48. Available at: http://jhn.sagepub.com/content/25/3/141.short (accessed 17 January 2012).

12 Singh Harinder (2010). *Caring for a Sikh Patient. Sikh Healthcare Chaplaincy Group*. Available at: http://www.sikhchaplaincy.org.uk/Booklet.pdf (accessed 21 July 2010).

13 Nesbitt, E. (1999). Sikhs and proper Sikhs: the representation of Sikhism in curriculum books and young British Sikhs' perceptions of their identity. In: P. Singh, N.G. Barrier (eds) *Sikh Identity: Continuity and Change*, pp. 315–34. New Delhi: Oxford University Press.

14 Singh Swaran (2004). Caring for Sikh patients wearing a kirpan (traditional small sword): cultural sensitivity and safety issues. *Psychiat Bull* 28: 93–5.

15 Greenwood, D. (2010). Ethical dilemmas in hospital chaplaincy. Unpublished MA thesis, University of Huddersfield, p. 45.

16 Sambhi, P.S. (1986/1987). A survey of religious attitudes to meat eating. *Sikh Messenger*, Winter/Spring: 27–31.

17 Adi Granth. Available as 'Sri Granth' at: http://www.srigranth.org (accessed 17 January 2012).

18 Doabia, H.S. (rep 1981). (trans) *Life story of Baba Nand Singh Ji of Kaleran*. Amritsar: Singh Brothers, p. 100.

19 Singh Bhai Sahib Randhir (2000). (trans Trilochan Singh). *Autobiography of Bhai Sahib Randhir Singh*. Ludhiana: Bhai Sahib Randhir Singh Trust.

20 Nesbitt, E. (1997). The body in Sikh tradition. In: S. Coakley (ed.) *Religion and the Body*, pp. 289–305. Cambridge: Cambridge University Press, Cambridge.

21 Nesbitt, E. (2004). God and holy water. In: E. Nesbitt (ed.), *Intercultural Education: Ethnographic and Religious Approaches*, pp. 66–80. Brighton: Sussex Academic Press.

22 Tatla, D.S. (1992). Nurturing the faithful: the role of the sant among Britain's Sikhs. *Religion* **22**: 349–74.

23 Geaves, R. (1998). The borders between the religions: a challenge to the world religions approach to religious education. *Br J Relig Educ* **21**(1): 20–31.

24 Ballard, R. (1999). Panth, kismet, dharm te qaum: continuity and change in four dimensions of Punjabi religion. In: P. Singh, S.S. Thandi (eds) *Punjabi Identity in a Global Context*, pp. 7–38. New Delhi: Oxford University Press.

25 Bigelow, A. (2009). *Sharing the Sacred: Practicing Pluralism in Muslim North India*. New York: Oxford University Press.

26 Oberoi, H.S. (1987). The worship of Pir Sakhi Sarvar: illness, healing and popular culture in the Punjab. *Stud Hist* N.S. 3/1, 50–3.

27 Oberoi, H. (1994). *The Construction of Religious Boundaries: Culture, Identity and Diversity*. New Delhi: Oxford University Press.

28 Chohan, S. (2008). The phenomenon of possession and exorcism in North India and amongst the Punjabi diaspora in Wolverhampton. Unpublished MPhil thesis, University of Wolverhampton.

29 Jakobsh, D. (ed.) (2010) *Sikhism and Women: History, Texts, and Experience*. New Delhi: Oxford University Press.

30 Purewal, N. (2010). *Son Preference, Sex Selection, Gender and Culture in South Asia*. London: Macmillan.

31 North Kent Council for Interfaith Relations (nd), p. 33.

32 Singh, N-G.K. (2010). Why did I not light up the pyre? The refeminization of ritual in Sikhism. In: D. Jakobsh (ed.) *Sikhism and Women*, pp. 205–33. New Dehli: Oxford University Press.

33 Mandair, A. (2010). Sikhism. In: S. Sorajjakool, M.F. Carr, J.J. Nam (eds) *World Religions for Health Care Professionals*, pp. 77–94, 84. London: Routledge.

34 Hershman, P. (1974). Hair, sex and dirt. *Man* (N.S.), 9: 274–98.

35 Singh Jasjit (2010). Young British Sikhs, hair, and the turban. *J Contemp Relig* **25**(2): 203–20.

36 Marketwire (2010). Fraser health authority apology to Sikh community not enough. Available at: http://www.marketwire.com/press-release/Fraser-health-Authority-Apology-to-Sikh-Community-Not-Enough-1138290.htm (accessed 20 July 2010).

37 India Post News Service (2009). Healthcare center pays up for cutting Sikh's hair. Available at: http://www.indiapost.com/health-science/3666-healthcare-center-pays-for-cutting-Sikh-hair.html (accessed 20 July 2010).

38 Galanti, G-A. (nd). Cultural diversity in healthcare. Available at: http://www.gagalanti.com/case_studies/cases_by_topic.html (accessed 12 July 2010).

39 Krause, I.B. (1989). Sinking heart: a Punjabi communication of distress. *Soc Sci Med* **29**(4): 563–75.

40 Krause, I.B. (1998). *Therapy Across Culture*. London: Sage.

41 Krause, I.B. (2004). Family therapy and anthropology: a case study for emotions. *J Fam Ther* **15**(1): 35–56.

42 Singh Atamjit (1983). The concept of healing in the Sikh scriptures. *Stud Sikhism Comp Religion*, April, 53–7.

43 Firth, S. (1993). Approaches to death in Hindu and Sikh communities in Britain. In: D. Dickenson, M. Johnson (eds) *Death and Dying*, pp. 26–32. London: Sage.

44 Singh, J., Singh, H., Brar, B.S. (1979). The Sukhmani and high blood pressure. *J Sikh Stud* **6**: 45–62.

45 (1980) Effect of holy dips in treatment of rheumatoid arthritis and osteo arthritis in believers. *J Sikh Stud* **7**: 106–20.

46 Firth, S. Unpublished paper.

47 Holm, J. (1994). *Making Moral Decisions*. London: Continuum.

48 Singh, P., Sekhon, H.K. (2001). *Garland round my neck: the story of Puran Singh of Pingalwara*. New Dehli: BS Publishers.

SECTION II

Concepts

CHAPTER 15

Healthcare spirituality: a question of knowledge

John Swinton

Waterfalls and buckets

A number of years ago I attended a lecture on spirituality and health presented by one of the editors of this book Mark Cobb. He opened his talk with a story:

Imagine yourself walking through a deep, dense wood. You are surrounded by beautiful, luscious foliage; the constantly changing aromas of the rich shrubbery makes your head swirl. Suddenly you reach a clearing. Right in the centre of the clearing is a beautiful stream headed up by a magnificent waterfall. You stand and watch in awe at the mystery and wonder of the waterfall. Multiple rainbows dance across the glistening surface of the water. The sound of the water, the taste of the spray the sight of the magnificence and power of the waterfall touches you in inexpressible places and brings you into contact with a dimension of experience which you can't quite articulate, but which you feel deeply and meaningfully. Eventually, your gaze of wonder begins to change as your curious side clicks into action: 'What is this thing called a waterfall?' 'What is it made of?' 'Why does it have such an effect on me?' So, you pick up a bucket and scoop up some of the water from the falls. You look into the bucket, but something has changed. The water is of course technically the same substance in each setting: H_2O. It remains a vital constituent of your life; you need it to live and without it you will perish. Yet, something has been lost in the movement from waterfall to bucket. In your attempts to break it down, analyse, and explain what it *really* is, the mystery and awe of the waterfall has been left behind. Which is more real? The mystery of the crashing waterfall or the still waters of the bucket?

At the heart of Cobb's story lies the deeply important question: *can we understand the fullness of being human by looking only at the constituent parts of person.* Both the waterfall and the bucket contain truth. Water *is* H_2O and there are clearly potential benefits in knowing and understanding its chemical constitution. However, whether the chemical formulation H_2O-constitutes *all* that the waterfall is, means and signifies is less obvious and more complicated. Is the experience of mystery and wonder that accompanies our perception of the waterfall *really* just a meaningless artefact? Is it only an illusion brought into existence by the random firing of unpatterned neurons within our brains? It could be. However, intuitively many of us recognize the inadequacy of such a proposition, but why is such intuition so difficult to articulate with authority within the healthcare workplace?

In this chapter, I will look at how and why it is that healthcare practices have a tendency to focus on buckets, rather than waterfalls, and why it is that spirituality is required both to bridge and to fill the gap between the two, that is, to offer something new and to affirm the necessity of both. The way that I will approach this task is by beginning with the question of knowledge. The question 'how do we know what we know' sounds like an abstract philosophical argument. However, as will become clear, it is a deeply practical question that is foundational for our understanding of why spirituality in healthcare is not only important, but absolutely necessary. Spirituality is a form of knowledge that reveals important things about how and why we choose to care in the ways we do. It is a form of knowledge that is different from scientific knowledge and yet deeply tied in to it. We need both, in order to care well. The chapter will point out the theoretical and practical significance of spirituality and offer a rationale for its necessary incorporation into contemporary healthcare practices.

The question of knowledge

Before we can begin to understand what spirituality is and how it might fit into healthcare practices, we need first to think through some important questions relating to how we know what we know. I want to suggest that there are basically two forms of knowledge that hold particular relevance current approaches to healthcare. These are *nomothetic* and *ideographic* forms of knowledge.

Nomothetic knowledge

Nomothetic knowledge is knowledge gained through the use of the scientific method. This is the knowledge gained from experiments and randomized control trials. Nomothetic knowledge has three basic criteria on which it bases its validity. To be factual, something must be *falsifiable*, *replicatable* and *generalizable.* (1 p. 41) To be *falsifiable* it must, at least in principle, be possible to show that a particular statement or finding is not true. So, statements such as 'there is a God,' or 'I love you' are not falsifiable (i.e. ultimately they cannot be unquestionably disproved) and are therefore not considered factual according to the criteria of the scientific method. To be *replicable* it must be possible to reproduce an experiment or an experience in contexts other than the original location. This is why there is a methods section at the beginning of all scientific papers.

Anyone anywhere should be able to repeat the experiment and get the same results. Finally, the findings of research must be *generalizable*, that is, they must be applicable to a wide range of people. So, for example, the development of penicillin does not simply apply to the illness of one person, but to all people in all places who require particular bacteria to be destroyed. The findings of any research must be transferable to a wide range of contexts. This then is the essence of the scientific method which has been so influential on our understanding of what evidence based healthcare systems should look like. On this understanding water cannot be proven to be anything other than H_2O and its value can only be gauged by its instrumental functions of quenching thirst and sustaining organisms. The contents of the bucket are all that there is.

This kind of knowledge is convincing, primarily because we have been thoroughly taught its primacy. This is despite the fact that a good deal of our lives are lived according to quite different criteria. Love, relationships, and much of our experience would be classified as invalid on these grounds. The problem is that this perspective on knowledge tends to be quite dependant on the philosophical position of *empiricism*: the belief that only that which falls upon the retina of the eye can be true. However, how do we know that empiricism is true? One has to believe in the primacy of empiricism (which is a philosophical, rather than a scientific position) before one can give it primacy. In other words, there is no empirical evidence for empiricism! By its own premises it cannot be proven. However, perhaps more significant than this obvious philosophical point, is the equally obvious point that while the scientific perspective is extremely useful in some areas of life, it makes much less sense in other areas. An example will help make this point.

Take, for example, the assumptions and practices of a scientist. In the public/professional domain he is tied in to a model of truth that is fundamentally nomothetic. That is the language that makes sense to his profession and to those who fund his profession. So, within his professional life, the scientist defines fact and truth in terms of replicability, falsifiability, and generalizability. However, when he goes home from work, he loves his wife and children, and he believes that love to be real. It is not possible for him to carry out a randomized control trial to test the theory and even if he did, the love he shows for his wife and family would more than probably be quite different from the love a stranger might show towards them, or even the love that he has shown them earlier on in their relationship. So, he finds himself living in two knowledge worlds, one determined by nomothethetic knowledge and the other by a different type of knowledge which he knows intuitively is true, but which fails to fit the verification criteria of his professional/cultural expectations.[1, p. 42]

Ideographic knowledge

This takes us into the realm of our second mode of knowing: *ideographic knowledge*. This form of knowing presumes that meaningful knowledge can be discovered in unique, non-replicable experiences. According to this form of knowledge, no two people experience the same event in the same way; indeed, no individual will experience the same event in the same way twice. Whilst nomothetic knowledge assumes that there is such a thing as a 'typical patient,' for whom generalizable knowledge is necessary and appropriate, ideographic knowledge perceives the uniqueness of people, the particularity of meaning, and the recognition that the general requires the particular before sense can be made of the whole. Ideographic knowledge recognizes that experiences that occur only once, and which are deeply unique to individuals are nonetheless factual and significant even if they can't be replicated or generalized. Ideographic knowledge realises that the meaning of the chemical constituency of H_2O cannot be fully understood apart from mystery and wonder of the waterfall. A good deal of religion and what we have come to describe as spirituality occurs within the realm of ideographic knowledge.

Healthcare spirituality

With these thoughts in mind, we can begin to get a sense for where spirituality might be located and why it may be important. Healthcare spirituality inhabits both domains of knowledge. On the one hand, there are aspects of spirituality which are measurable and generalizable. This is particularly so with regard to religious spirituality wherein certain benefits that are gained from engaging in religious practices can be measured and replicated in line with the scientific method. There are a wide range of scientific studies that show the benefits of spirituality. For example, spirituality has been associated with:

- Extended life expectancy
- Lower blood pressure
- Lower rates of death from coronary artery disease
- Reduction in myocardial infarction
- Increased success in heart transplants
- Reduced serum cholesterol levels
- Reduced levels of pain in cancer sufferers
- Reduced mortality among those who attend church and worship services.
- Increased longevity among the elderly
- Reduced mortality after cardiac surgery.[2–4]

It is, however, important to note that these benefits come from the *structural* aspect of spirituality. In other words, it is not so much the mysterious or transcendent aspects of spirituality or human beings that bring about wellbeing. Rather, it is the more concrete elements of religious practice—community, disciplined spiritual practices, healthy lifestyle—that bring about measurable results. If you don't smoke, drink, or take drugs (and religious people tend not to engage in such risky behaviours), if you eat well, and get lots of exercise you will live longer and have fewer health problems, and will recover more effectively from illness.

However, spirituality also encompasses experiences that are clearly ideographic. Issues of meaning, purpose, hope, love, and God are not observable, replicable, or generalizable. However, they are nonetheless significant for that. It is, of course, possible to reduce them to physical or psychological phenomena. However, one doesn't have to and to, do so is reflective of a faith position (that the material is somehow more convincing than the non-material), rather than a scientific judgement. Illness is not a generalizable experience. There is a very real sense in which each person's illness is very much *their* illness. No two people experience their illness in the same way. If I receive a diagnosis of cancer and I say that 'God is with me,' this is not just a 'by the way.' It is something that is central to my experience of cancer and thus central to what cancer is for *me*. Cancer is not simply a series of pathologically growing cells that requires clinical intervention. For people who are experiencing cancer is a deeply meaningful experience that simply cannot be explained by biological pathology alone. Unique personal experience matters not just in terms of care, but in terms of ontology (i.e. what cancer actually *is*). Cancer *is* a meaningful experience.[5] Biology and experience cannot be separated. True, the biological explanation and the clinical response may have more cultural power than someone's personal story, but as we have seen, that is an illusion. Nomothetic and ideographic knowledge are two sides of the same coin. We need both to see accurately and to care well.

What is healthcare spirituality?

Thus far, we have been speaking about spirituality as if we actually knew what it was. We need now to look and see whether we actually do know what it is. A quick glance at the many and varied definitions of spirituality within the healthcare literature makes it very clear that there is no real consensus as to what spirituality actually is or what it is supposed to do.[6] Part of the confusion relates to the separation between spirituality and religion. For many working within the field of healthcare, the two terms 'religion' and 'spirituality' have come to be perceived as separate although connected entities. This is particularly so with regard to the literature emerging from Europe. It is less so with regard to the United States, which has tended to remain focused more on religion.[7] However, for both contexts the separation of religion and spirituality remains important. In developing an understanding of healthcare spirituality it will be helpful to lay out the similarities, and differences between spirituality and religion.

Religion

Religion is generally accepted as a significant aspect of healthcare spirituality. It is, however, important to note that, like the term 'spirituality,' there is no universally recognized definition of religion. The general tendency within the healthcare literature is to assume that religion is a monolithic term that means the same thing to all people.[2,7,8] However, as Pargament[8] has pointed out, it may actually be the *particulars* of specific religions that have health-bringing capacities, rather than the global properties of any particular religious system. For current purposes we will follow Clifford Geertz in defining religion as:

> (1) a system of symbols which acts to (2) establish powerful, pervasive, and long-lasting moods and motivations in men [sic] by (3) formulating conceptions of a general order of existence and (4) clothing these conceptions with such an aura of factuality that (5) the moods and motivations seem uniquely realistic.[9. p. 4.]

Understood in this way, religion is perceived as a formal system of beliefs held by groups of people who share certain perspectives on the nature of the world. These perspectives are communicated through shared narratives, practices, beliefs, and rituals that, taken together, create particular worldviews, i.e. ways in which people see and interpret the world around them, and make sense of their experiences within that world. Put slightly differently, the structures of belief and systems of practice that form any given religion, shape and form the ways in which those who participate in them see and respond to the world. This shaping and forming aspect of religion impacts on the ways in which illnesses are perceived and responded to by individuals and by communities. As such, religion is a powerful force for shaping a person's understanding of illness. An example will help to make this point. A colleague of mine was recently preaching in a local church. The essence of his message was that God does not inflict suffering, that suffering is a temporary state, which would be ended when this world was ended and that in the interim we should not feel burdened by our experiences of illness as they were neither punishment nor judgement. It was intended as a deeply healing message, designed to relive the burden of suffering. After the service he was approached by two elderly women. They were sisters and it turned out that one of them had terminal breast cancer. They were extremely annoyed at my colleague for the message that he had given. For them it was very important that God *had* inflicted this illness on the sister. If God had done this, so they reasoned, then there was a purpose and a meaning to the illness. If there was purpose and meaning then there was hope. To frame their illness in the way that my colleague had done was to strip away what was, for them, a powerful source of hope. What was intended as a healing sermon turned out to be the opposite. What appears at one level, to be a pathological religious belief turned out to be a significant source of hope. The point is this: *we do not experience our illness in a vacuum*. The things we believe about our illness and the assumptions we have as to how we should behave in the face of it are deeply shaped and formed by what we believe about the world. Religion is a powerful shaper of our worlds. Not to notice this is to fail to see something that is profoundly important for the way in which people cope with their illness. To peer only into the bucket and not to understand the waterfall is to miss the point in a serious way. Spiritual care in its religious mode relates to coming close, slowing down and listening carefully to the unique meanings of a person's experience.

Religion, meaning making, and coping

Religion provides particular ways of making meaning out of the experience of illness and enabling effective coping. Ellison and Levin[10] highlight six possible mechanisms that might be at work with regard to how and why religious spirituality might help patients in times of illness. This structure helps draw out the issues:

1. *Regulation of individual lifestyles and health behaviours.* Most religious systems have prohibitions on certain ways of behaving and living (e.g. the prohibition on alcohol, smoking, etc.), all of which have health benefits for participant

2. *Provision of social resources* (e.g. social ties, formal and informal support).There is a recognized connection between mental health and wellbeing and effective social support structures. Social support can tie people into supportive relational networks which are both protective of mental illness[11,12] and healing of it when it develops.[13] Such support networks can offer meaningful personal relationships that reduce stigma and offer possibilities for recovery which are not available elsewhere.

3. *Promotion of positive self-perceptions.* Religion can promote self-esteem by incorporating people into secure relational networks that are affirming and accepting. It can also engender feelings of personal mastery in ways that can be supportive and health promoting[14]

4. *Provision of specific coping resources* (i.e. particular cognitive or behavioural responses to stress). Adherence to a particular faith tradition realigns a person's thinking and can enable then to cope constructively with trauma and illness. Psychologically, religious

commitment brings with it a cognitive alignment that can have significant implications for coping and health. The signs, symbols, rituals, and narratives of faith communities provide the resources for individuals to re-form their life-worlds in significant ways.[15]

5. *Generation of other positive emotions* (e.g. love, forgiveness) The growing body of literature, for example, within the area of forgiveness research[16] indicates that religion can generate particularly positive emotions which have the potential to be health enhancing.
6. *Additional hypothesized mechanisms, such as the existence of a healing bioenergy.* The literature within the area of prayer studies is indicative of the possibility that there may be supra-empirical dimensions to religion and spirituality that are currently not understood, but which may have healing capacities.[17]

It is fair to say that the reframing and meaning making capacities of religion are not always positive. Positive religious coping such as partnering with God or seeking support and guidance from God brings benefits for psychological wellbeing. However, negative modes of coping, such as feeling abandoned by God or angry with God, leads to a decrease in mental health, depressive symptoms and lower life satisfaction.[18] Likewise, it is possible to ascribe negative religious meanings to illness. However, while the negative effects require recognition, the overall picture that emerges from the literature provides indications that religion has the potential to be of positive benefit for people experiencing a wide variety of illnesses.

However, beyond the structural benefits of religion for health is the crucial fact that meaning is not reducible to biology alone. People *actually* believe that the God they worship is real and it is possible that this is a well-placed belief even if it is not provable within the criteria of nomothetic knowledge. Retaining the possibility of mystery and wonder is not just helpful in terms of empathy with patients, it is epistemologically necessary. One of the problems with the way that the literature functions is that researchers have a tendency to adopt a position of what Peter Berger has described as *methodological atheism.*[19] This term relates to the way in which theologians and historians who study religion as a human creation without declaring whether individual religious beliefs are actually true. The fact that a person may *actually* be experiencing unique experiences that are directly related to their faith tradition is excluded on the basis that it is not measurable. The literature is speckled with scientists and psychologists stating that it is not their task to comment on the authenticity of belief systems *as if* the fact that they are real or unreal did not matter to the research process. It is not possible to follow-up on this point within the confines of this chapter. Suffice to say that there is a tendency towards philosophical materialism (the notion that the ultimate nature of reality is material) even within those religious people who seek to study religion. If my reflections on ideographic knowledge are correct then the possibility of taking seriously claims as to the reality of religious experience must at least remain an open possibility. Within religious spirituality both ideographic and nomothetic knowledge have important roles to play.

Spirituality

When we turn to the literature on spirituality, the first impression is that it is similarly beneficial for health and wellbeing. Spirituality is perceived as a subjective experience that exists both within and outside traditional religious systems. It relates to the way in which people understand and live their lives in view of their sense of ultimate meaning and value. Spirituality in this sense, includes the need to find satisfactory answers to ultimate questions about the meaning of life, illness, and death. It can be seen as comprising elements of meaning, purpose, value, hope, relationships, love, and for some people, a connection to a higher power or something greater than self.

There is a wide range of literature that indicates positive correlations between spirituality and health around similar issues to those raised by religion. Spirituality has been positively associated with quality of life,[20–2] self-esteem,[23] reduced anxiety,[24] meaning-making,[25–6] hope,[27] increased ability to cope,[28] and relationality and social support.[29]

However, there is a problem that is well illustrated in Visser *et al.*'s[30] review of spiritual care and wellbeing in cancer patients. In this study, the researchers reviewed 27 papers that focused on the relationship between spirituality and wellbeing. They concluded that, at least for cross-sectional studies, there was a positive correlation between spirituality and wellbeing. However, a closer analysis of the papers they chose for review reveals that the authors of these studies do not work with any common definition or shared understanding of what spirituality is, other than to state that they are not working with religiosity. This is the problem. While the general thrust of the literature on spirituality seems to indicate a positive correlation, what is actually being measured is not always clear. When spirituality is separated from religion, it becomes unclear what it actually is. Spirituality, particularly in the literature emerging from the United Kingdom, is generally understood as a generic term that may contain, but is not defined by, religion. By focusing on 'spirituality,' the intention is to draw attention to aspects of patient's experiences that are currently overlooked or underplayed in the way health care is delivered.[31]

Within this frame, spirituality is assumed to relate to different combinations of existential needs: the search for meaning, purpose, value hope, love, and transcendence broadly defined. The assumption is that these aspects of human experience have clinical utility, but that within a context that is rapidly secularizing, religion is not the best vehicle for bringing them to the fore. However, the particular combination of existential needs that people choose to bring together to form their definitions of spirituality is wide and diverse. This leads to a situation where understandings of spirituality have become so broad and varied that claims that 'spirituality aids human wellbeing' are difficult to substantiate. In other words, the variety of human experiences that form the content of the term 'spirituality' makes a good deal of sense in terms of ideographic knowledge. Its lack of systemization and the similar lack of reflection on why we would use the term 'spirituality' to describe them is problematic. This is particularly so if the researcher attempts to make nomothetic claims off the back of ideographic experience. This lack of clarity is significant insofar as it tends to weaken the ability of those who advocate for spirituality to convince people that it is an important aspect of the practice of healthcare. If you are not clear what spirituality is and if you are trying to argue that it is a type of knowledge that it is not, then problems will inevitably arise. Without a shared core of meaning, it is difficult to assess what is common to the definitions and why it might be appropriate to compare the various findings. So while the various studies may well indicate positive correlations between spirituality, health, and illness the actual causal factors involved may not be the same across studies.

What does spirituality do?

One way around this is by recognizing the ideographic nature of generic spirituality. Its intention is not to disclose that which is generalizable, replicable, or falsifiable, but rather to help carers to recognize the uniqueness of the illness experience of patients. Religion, of course, seeks to do the same. However, reflection on the contribution of generic spirituality draws out this point very clearly. On reflection, the primary issues that the various generic definitions of spirituality focus on—meaning, purpose, hope, love, transcendence, and relationship—all find their rationale in ideographic knowledge. To find meaning in something is not a generalizable principle. What gives my life meaning is not necessarily what gives your life meaning. What makes me love is not necessarily what makes you love. My understanding of hope might be very different from yours. My sense of the transcendent is probably unique and idiosyncratic. Even if I am in a religion I will interpret that religion in my own way. But our experiences are nonetheless valid for their uniqueness and diversity. You need to come close to understand me. Coming close and understanding is the essence of healthcare spirituality and good spiritual care.

Filling the gaps

Generic forms of spirituality raise a series of questions that are very important within what is often a deeply secular healthcare context: 'what is the role of meaning in healthcare?' 'Why does the language of love sound so odd when it is spoken in the healthcare workplace?' 'What can non-religious persons hope for when they are faced with serious illness?' 'What role do relationships play in the process of caring and curing?' Traditionally, these are the types of question that have been raised by religion. However, in a secular context they need to be raised in a different way and in a different language: the language of 'the spiritual.' These questions are Socratic in their intention and outcome. Socratic questioning occurs when one seeks to ask a series of questions that will enable reflection and change. Socratic questioning seeks to get to the truth of things, to uncover hidden assumptions and to open up problems, and issues for scrutiny and reflection. In this way, the language of spirituality and the questions that it raises bring to light hidden issues that people encounter when they become ill; questions that include, but reach beyond the nomothetic.

Thus, the language of spirituality exposes gaps within current practices. If our practices were meaningful, loving, and hopeful, then we would have no need to 'introduce' the idea of generic spirituality. If the suggestion that for religious people their beliefs profoundly shape their experiences of illness was recognized and accepted, then there would be no real need to try to persuade people of the benefits of religious coping. Our systems would have these dimensions built in to them. The language of spirituality in all of this different definitions and forms reminds us of the importance of the gaps in our knowledge and practice and calls us in different ways to fill them. In other words, spirituality names a series of absences as much as it might reveal the presence of some 'thing' which we might want to define as 'spirituality.'[3]

It is true that the language of spirituality, particularly in its generic forms is personal, ideographic and sometimes vague. However, this is no reason to reject it. Most of our lives are lived like that! It is not what spirituality is or is not that is the key. *It is what it points us towards that matters.* When we look in the direction of where it points us we will be moved into recognizing the gaps and seeking ways of bringing together our perspectives on human beings in a way that holds in tension the need for both waterfalls and buckets.

Conclusion

Spirituality within healthcare in both its religious and non-religious forms can thus be seen to name a series of concerns and absences. Primary amongst these concerns is the wariness that healthcare systems have of taking ideographic knowledge seriously. Naming such concerns and absences is quite a radical step. To ask for spirituality to be considered a significant dimension of healthcare practice is to ask people to change the way that they see the world. In an evidence-based culture so used to prioritizing nomothetic knowledge, convincing people that experience, meaning, hope, love, and the search for God and transcendence should be seen as legitimate clinical categories is never going to be an easy task. Healthcare spirituality calls for a quite profound and perhaps prophetic critique of the priorities, values, and approaches that underlie the practices with which we engage within particular situations and circumstances. We might be tempted to get side-tracked into endless and usually not particularly fruitful conversations around issues of definition, but the issues are too important to allow that to distract us. Not to take cognisance of issues of meaning, hope, love, etc., is to make a very firm statement about what we think is important about human beings. There may be no agreement as to a formal definition, but the general area of human experience that is the focus of spirituality is clearly crucial.

In closing, we can return to the image of the waterfall and the bucket. Reductionism in all of it different forms is inevitably counterproductive. Human beings are always more than their constituent parts. It is true that we can be broken down into pieces. Indeed, one of the things that illness often does is just that. It breaks us down and confines our very being to the boundaries of our ailment. However, such breaking down is illusory. There remains something mysterious and indeed wondrous about human beings that biology and medicine alone cannot fully encapsulate. Healthcare spirituality recognizes the importance of the discrete pieces; it sees the significance of what can be seen when we look into the bucket. However, it also realizes that each piece requires the others in order to be made sense of. There is more to being human than can be explained through the use of one form of knowledge alone, even if, like biology and medicine, that knowledge has great cultural power. Our *experiences* of illness matters. Our relationships matter and, for some, God matters. Spirituality encompasses all of these "hidden" dimensions. If we are truly interested in genuinely person-centred healthcare, then we lose this perspective at our peril.

References

1 Swinton, J., Mowat, H. (2005). *Practical Theology and Qualitative Research.* London: SCM Press.

2 Koenig, H.G., Larson, D.B., McCullough, M.E. (2001). *Handbook of Religion and Health.* New York: Oxford University Press.

3 Swinton, J., Pattison, S. (2010). Moving beyond clarity: towards a thin, vague, and useful understanding of spirituality in nursing care. *Nurs Philos* **11**(4): 226–37.

4 Chatters, L.M. (2000). Religion and health: public health research and practice. *Ann Rev Publ Hlth*, **21**: 335–67.

5 Swinton, J., Bain, V., Ingram, S., Heys, SD. (2011). Moving inwards, moving outwards, moving upwards: the role of spirituality during the early stages of breast cancer. *European Journal of Cancer Care* **20**(5): 640–52.

6 Sessanna, L., Finnell, D.S., Underhill, M., Chang, Y.P., Peng, H.L. (2011). Measures assessing spirituality as more than religiosity: a methodological review of nursing and health-related literature. *J Adv Nurs* **4**: 1365–2648.

7 Swinton, J. (2007). Researching spirituality and mental health: a perspective from the research. In: P. Gilbert (ed.) *Spirituality, Values and Mental Health: Jewels for the Journey*. London: Jessica Kingsley Publishers.

8 Pargament, K.I. (2002). The bitter and the sweet: an evaluation of the costs and benefits of religiousness. *Psychol Inquiry* **13**: 168–81.

9 Geertz, C (1985). *Religion as a Cultural System. Anthropological Approaches to the Study of Religion*. London: M. Banton, Tavistock Press.

10 Ellison, C.G., Levin, J.S. (1998). The religion-health connection: evidence, theory, and future directions. *Hlth Educ Behav* **25**: 700–20.

11 Krause, N. (2010). The social milieu of the Church and religious coping responses: a longitudinal investigation of older Whites and older Blacks. *Int J Psychol Relig* **20**(2): 109–29.

12 Law, R.W., Sbarra, D.A. (2009). The effects of church attendance and marital status on the longitudinal trajectories of depressed mood among older adults. *J Aging Hlth* **21**(6): 803–23.

13 Swinton, J (2001). *Spirituality and Mental Health Care: Rediscovering a 'Forgotten' Dimension*. London: Jessica Kingsley Publishers.

14 Peltzer, K., Koenig, Harold, G. (2005). Religion. Psychology and health. *J Psychol Afr* **15**: 53–64.

15 Pargament, K.I. (1997). *The Psychology of Religion and Coping: Theory, Research, Practice*, New York: Guilford Press.

16 Worthington, E. (2008). *Dimensions of Forgiveness*. Radnor: Templeton Foundation Press.

17 Dossey, L. (1993). *Healing Word*. San Francisco: Harper Collins/Harper.

18 Hebert, R., Zdaniuk, B., Schulz, R., Scheier, M. (2002). Positive and negative religious coping and wellbeing in women with breast cancer. *J Palliat Med* **12**(6): 537–45.

19 Berger, P.L. (1969). *The Sacred Canopy: Elements of a Sociological Theory of Religion*. New York: Anchor Books.

20 Puchalski, C., Ferrell, B., Virani, R., Otis-Green, S., Baird, P., Bull, J., *et al.* (2009). Improving the quality of spiritual care as a dimension of palliative care: the report of the Consensus Conference. *J Palliat Med* **12**: 885–904.

21 Levine, E.G., Targ, E. (2002). Spiritual correlates of functional wellbeing in women with breast cancer. *Integrated Cancer Ther* **1**(2): 166–74.

22 Brady, M.J., Peterman, A.H., Fitchett, G., Mo, M., Cella, D. (1999). A case for including spirituality in quality of life measurement in oncology. *Psycho-oncol* 8(5): 417–28.

23 Ellison, C.G., Flannelly, K.J. (2009). Religious involvement and risk of major depression in a prospective nationwide study of African American adults. *J Nerv Ment Dis* **197**(8): 568–73.

24 Burgess, C., Cornelius, V., Love, S., Graham, J., Richards, M., Ramirez, M. (2005). Depression and anxiety in women with early breast cancer: five year observational cohort study. *Br Med J* 330: 702.

25 Breitbart, W. (2006). Enhancing meaning in palliative care practice: a meaning-centered intervention to promote job satisfaction. *Palliat Support Care* **4**: 333–44.

26 Sorajjakool, S., Seyle, B. (2005). Theological strategies, constructing meaning, and coping with breast cancer: a qualitative study. *Past Psychol* **54**(2): 173–86.

27 Mickley, J.R., Soeken, K., Belcher, A. (1992). Spiritual wellbeing, religiousness and hope among women with breast cancer. *Image J Nurs Scholarship* **24**(4): 267–72.

28 Nairn, R.C., Merluzzi, T.V. (2003). The role of religious coping in adjustment to cancer. *Psycho-oncol* **12**(5): 428–41.

29 Yoon, D.P, Lee, E.K. (2007). The impact of religiousness, spirituality, and social support on psychological wellbeing among older adults in rural areas. *J Gerontol Soc Work*, **48**(3–4): 281–98.

30 Visser, A., Garssen, B., Vingerhoets, A. (2010). Spirituality and wellbeing in cancer patients: a review. *Psycho-oncol* **19**(6): 565–72.

31 Swinton, J., Pattison. S. (2001). Come All Ye Faithful: spirituality and healthcare practices. *The Hlth Serv J* 20 December, pp. 24–25.

CHAPTER 16

Personhood

Rosalie Hudson

Introduction

Spirituality is not an optional extra in a healthcare system that generally describes itself as holistic. Along with the physical, the patient's need for psychological, spiritual, and emotional care form a quadrilateral generally accepted by healthcare professionals. This amalgam of needs is felt and addressed by persons in their unique life narrative; personhood is thus the pivotal point for discussing spirituality.

Although some aspects of personhood are commonly understood within healthcare, differences may be evident in various traditions discussed in Section I of this text. Some overlap will also be noted with other concepts of care addressed in Section II and practice issues covered in Section III.

Personhood in this discussion is distinguished from other person-like terms, such as personality, personal identity, personalism, and individual. It will be argued, first, that personhood can be reduced to 'thinghood', particularly when a person is reduced to component parts, rather than treated as an indivisible unity of body, mind, and spirit. Questions are also raised about patients as persons, and whether or not a human being can be a non-person.

In the second section, the focus is on 'Annie' and her ontological plea. In a culture of autonomous individual rights where rationality is prized above other human qualities and where coherent speech is privileged as the primary means of communication, 'Annie' challenges the notion of personhood. A brief discussion on person-centred care (Section III) will show that, while the term is widely used, there is a dearth of evidence to support its practice and the dialogical character of personhood can be underplayed. In Section IV it will be shown that persons are not isolated monads; personhood therefore is about relations with other persons. In Section V, personhood embodied in practice is described as 'hands on' spirituality. Finally, it will be shown that partnership is the preferred model for promoting personhood within healthcare. A summary of key points is provided at the end of each section.

Personhood defined

Polanyi traces the development of personhood over the millennia from beginnings of a purely vegetative character to successive stages of active, perceptive, and eventually responsible, personhood.[1, p. 395] However, he continues, the full and complete essence of personhood requires principles other than physics and chemistry; personhood can only be fully understood within the purpose for which persons are created (p. 405). His teleology, that persons can ultimately be viewed with awe and wonder—as a mystery—is shared by many other philosophical, religious, and theological traditions.

Personhood, understood theologically, goes beyond the concepts of personal identity, personality, and individual, to the relational aspect of who each person is for the other, in the whole of their humanity. This does not detract from the utter uniqueness and unrepeatable nature of each person. In tracing personhood to its fourth century theological roots Zizioulas says:

> Thus, although the person and 'personal identity' are widely discussed nowadays as a supreme ideal, nobody seems to recognize that *historically* as well as *existentially* the concept of the person is indissolubly bound up with theology.[2, p. 27]

This theological framework for personhood is more fully explored in a recent text, as one approach to spirituality within a variety of traditions.[3]

Personality

'What we usually describe as 'personality' depends on multiple contributions' says Damasio.[4, p. 222] These contributions include 'traits' or 'temperament', and a unique set of interactions that create the foundation for autobiographical memory, the self, and personhood. While some of these traits may be detected soon after birth, they are dependent for their development on unique interactions with others, and with the environment.

The emphasis in this chapter is towards a relational understanding of personhood, rather than regarding each person as a single, autonomous unit. Definitions from various philosophical texts indicate there has never been a univocal concept of person. While one encyclopedia notes persons are defined through the terms 'personalism', 'personal identity', and 'personality'[5, pp. 318–20] Macmurray argues that 'personality' is inadequate for defining a person. He claims that 'personality' has been diverted from its natural meaning—that which defines a person as a person and distinguishes the person from impersonal beings and is shared by all persons. Personality has developed a specialized meaning 'stressing the element of difference between persons instead of what they have in common'.[6, p. 25] It is the commonality of persons, rather than their idiosyncratic personalities, which is the primary focus of this discussion.

Person and individual

It is interesting to note that many databases have no entry under 'person', but refer the researcher to 'individual', a change evident in recent decades. The subtlety of this change exposes a pervasive cultural shift to individualism, particularly in western culture. As the implications of this move can only be briefly mentioned in this discussion one example will suffice.

In the reductionist, bureaucratic world of residential aged care within Australia, each individual is compared with every other individual; their deficits and incapacities calculated according to a sophisticated scoring system. Funding is based on each individual's care needs relative to those of others. Such a departure from the meaning of person can be characterized by the architects of this system who call the residents of the institution neither persons nor individuals, but 'care recipients.' While the intention is certainly not to dehumanize older people it is a far cry from the understanding of person being discussed here. When a person in any healthcare context is regarded merely as a recipient—even of our compassion—it suggests there is neither reciprocity nor mutuality. Furthermore, care recipients are usually regarded as a cost to the community and not a benefit. Defined as individuals they are measured by their independence or lack thereof.

No such calculation is called for in person to person encounters where each is dependent in some measure on the other. Macmurray describes individual independence as an illusion and the isolated self a non-entity.[6, p. 211] Similarly, McGrath says, "'Person' has come to mean 'an individual human being' devoid of any dialogical relationships".[7, pp. 268–9] When persons enter into dialogue, spirituality in healthcare can be transformed; power relations can be converted to partnerships, as the conclusion to this chapter will show.

In contrast to a healthcare system that divides the person's body into parts for specific scrutiny, the following section emphasizes the unity of the human person in the totality of their being.

Person: body/mind/spirit

For Barth, the language that best describes persons is 'embodied souls' and 'besouled bodies'.[8, pp. 350–2] Rather than describing a person as having a soul and a body, Barth's language refuses any such bifurcation. Ramsay takes up this concept in discussing the 'sacredness' of the patient's bodily life, in illness and in dying. 'He [*sic*] is a sacredness in bodily life. He is a person who within the ambience of the flesh claims our care. He is an embodied soul or ensouled body'.[9, p. xiii] A person is more than a collection of component parts. Ramsay applies this framework to his entire medical ethics; notably in relation to the beginning and end of life.[10]

Is the soul a self-contained entity? In a former era, persons were commonly referred to as 'souls' as in 'one hundred souls drowned at sea' or 'she's such a lovely soul'. These descriptions do not connote some disembodied, immaterial entities floating free beyond human grasp; they refer to real, flesh and blood people. Wittgenstein, in what might be described as a meeting of whole persons, said, 'My attitude towards him [*sic*] is an attitude towards a soul'.[11, p. 178]

While Descartes (1586–1650) gave the human body a mechanical description, the only way he could incorporate the soul was to regard it as an anatomical structure, locating it in the pineal gland of the human brain. For Descartes, we are human beings because our rational capacity makes us so. His dictum 'I think, therefore I am' might be given a more communal flavour, 'We are in community, therefore we are.[12, p. 47]

In this very brief excursions into body/soul unity, it is acknowledged that, in some belief systems, the soul is treated as a separate entity with implications for continuity beyond death. For other belief systems, persons are conceived only in their material reality; the spirit or soul is an illusion. Persons, in this discussion, are regarded as an indivisible unity; contrary to Cartesian dualism, spirituality cannot be divorced from bodily reality.

Focus points for Section 1 Personhood defined

- Personhood can be traced through physics and chemistry to theology
- Personality is an inadequate concept to describe the full meaning of person
- Individual and person are not interchangeable, but dialogical in character
- A person is an indivisible unity of body/mind/spirit (or soul).

Who is this person?

With the unity of the human person in mind, we now turn to a real person—'Annie'—who challenges the notion of persons as isolated individuals.

> *In the nursing home it was the evening of our masquerade ball. There was considerable debate as to whether Annie should attend; her behaviour was often inappropriately antisocial, some staff were worried she would become too tired, others were concerned she would become over stimulated. 'She should not miss out' was the opinion that won the day. During a pause in the band's playing and when the wheel chair dancing had stopped, Annie's plaintive cry was heard: 'Where am I? Will somebody please tell me where I am and who I am?'*

Annie's quest would not be solved by the most patient repetition of her name and location. Her plea for identity could not be equated with a missing article, or her search for meaning linked to a deficit of information. Through the plaques and tangles of Alzheimer's disease Annie is asking the question only a person can ask and only a person can answer. This is an ontological cry—and who will respond?

Annie's deficits were not difficult to list; her incapacities were easy to define; her 'behaviour problems' matched the funding criteria. However, neither her remaining capacities nor her considerable personal strengths were ever noted. Her winsome smile, her brisk walk, her sharply focused eyes, and her occasional humorous quip, were considered less remarkable than her 'problems' (perseveration, uninhibited language and actions, 'aimless wandering', etc.). On this understanding of person Annie cannot be known in the unique narrative of her life journey. Qualities, characteristics, and capacities can be calculated: personhood cannot. So, Annie's call goes unanswered.

Patient or person?

Sabat tells the story of Christopher Reeve who considered suicide after an accident left him paralyzed from the neck down. His suicide thoughts ceased when he realized, 'I had to stop being a patient and start being a person'. This conversion entailed devoting the rest of his life to supporting research into spinal cord injuries. Sabat contends that lives seemingly impoverished can flourish, given appropriate support. Beyond the constraints that 'patient' often implies, persons with physical or cognitive impairment can live out their valued social identities. 'It is in the social dynamics of everyday life beyond the neuropathological processes in their brains that people can be supported in, or experience assaults on, their personhood'.[13, p. 298]

Ramsay's ethical framework is 'addressed to patients as persons, to physicians of patients who are persons—in short, to everyone who has had or will have to do with disease or death'.[9, p. xi] The juxtaposition of patient and person is not intended to imply 'patient' is an inappropriate term. Ramsay's inference is that patients and health professionals meet one another as persons in an ethical encounter where the latter is no more worthy of respect than the former.

Cobb contends that medical treatments are commonly considered as techniques in isolation from other dimensions of personhood. 'However, the science of medicine cannot perceive the person, only recognize pathology, and it is with this incomplete knowledge that a doctor as a person has to establish a therapeutic relationship of trust and cooperation with the patient'.[14, p. 85] In the realm of spiritual care Cobb argues that 'spiritual polymaths' are not the answer. He calls for active dialogue between the various healthcare disciplines, incorporating a 'richness of perspectives' (p. 111). He argues that the spiritual dimension:

> ... has less to do with utility and more to do with attending to another human being. This is a hermeneutic that encompasses the enigmatic nature of personhood that is encountered in suffering, dying and death. We can barely understand ourselves, less still another person, and yet we can draw close to another, but know of the remoteness in the encounter.[14, p.119]

Cobb identifies the paradoxical nature of personal encounter, which encourages health professionals to come close to their patients while knowing they can never fully enter their reality. On the other hand, he warns against creating such a distance that the patient is bereft of any attempt at personal engagement, particularly when questions are raised as to the meaning of suffering, illness and death. A 'spiritual agnosticism',[14, p. 122] which focuses primarily on the individual person's right to construct their own meaning can result in missed opportunities for dialogue with the patient as person.

When is a person not a person?

In agreement with the fourth century theological formulation of personhood described above, Singer traces the origins of 'person' to the doctrine of the Trinity. However, he prefers Boethius's sixth century definition of person as 'an individual substance of rational nature'. He follows Locke's (1632–1704) emphasis on the person as one who shows 'elements of awareness of one's own existence at different times and places'.[15, p. 180] Preece argues:

> The views of Singer ... involve a long-discredited (biblically and philosophically) Platonic and Cartesian dualistic view of the self. This view conceives the self or person not as a body/mind-soul unity, but as a core consciousness without which a living, but damaged body is disqualified from personhood and protection.[16, p. 139]

On Singer's understanding persons have no intrinsic value and are therefore expendable if they do not fit the formula.[17, pp. 122] Is a person only a person who can rationally claim to be a person? Swinton argues, 'The inevitable conclusion to this is that some human beings have a right to life and others do not.'[18, p. 189] On this view, Annie has no right to life and it remains a challenge for those who think this way to decide what should be done with her, particularly when she becomes increasingly incapacitated. Having attempted to justify his utilitarian view that it is difficult to see any point to keeping such people alive, Singer confessed when questioned about his mother's increasing dementia: 'Perhaps it is more difficult than I thought before, because it is different when it's your mother.'[19, p. 7]

Is Locke's definition of person as 'a thinking intelligent being that has reason and reflection and can consider itself, the same thinking thing in different times and places,'[20, bk. 2, sec. 9] sufficient for understanding personhood in healthcare? Matthews argues '... there must be something more to being the person I am than simply thinking of myself as that person ... personhood or personal identity cannot be reduced to self-consciousness and its continuity'.[21, p. 170–1] When rationality is prized above all else in a 'hypercognitive society,'[22, p. 128] those whom we may call 'hypocognitive' challenge our belief in a common humanity, particularly when those who have retained their memory forget to care for those who have lost theirs.

MacIntyre is, similarly, concerned that the moral significance of speech and rational thought is overestimated, resulting in a lack of 'just generosity' toward those 'whose extreme disablement is such that they can never be more than passive members of the community, not recognizing, not speaking or not speaking intelligibly, suffering, but not acting'.[23, pp. 127–8] Post contends that such persons cannot become non-persons.

> Our goal, however, must be to remember that the deeply forgetful are neither 'shells' nor 'husks'; they have not become subhuman; they remain part of our shared humanity. About this we must be clear, lest we succumb to the banality of evil'[24, p. 14]

These are strong words, suggesting that a healthcare system which defines, albeit subtly, some patients as less than human, cannot be providing good health. Similarly, Swinton argues, 'A society that is inattentive to the essential interconnectedness of its participants is a society that is open to the possibility of justifying abuse and forms of practice that can be deadly for the weakest and most vulnerable members'.[18, p. 211]

Lewis explores the logical consequences of such a view:

> An object is irreducible and invulnerable, and it does not threaten. However, reduce a human being and one confirms the very personhood which has left him or her open to attack. And when we banish the dependent to a subworld of their own, the guilt and fear they expose in us are proof enough that they belong with us in ours.[25, p. 18]

As Lewis suggests, our own personhood is compromised when we regard the personhood of others as inferior to our own.

Focus points for Section 2

- Annie's quest to know who she is and where she is challenges our view of personhood
- Patients are treated as persons when health professionals enter into dialogue with them
- Personhood can be 'lost' if objective rationality is the main criterion.

Person-centred care

There is no widely accepted view of what person-centred care means or of its efficacy in practice. Haider defines it as 'a philosophical shift from care & protection of the body to support of people in obtaining lives of personal satisfaction ... honouring each person's dignity, rights, self-respect, and independence ...'[26] Others suggest person-centred care is about 'a collaborative and respectful partnership between the service provider and user'.[27, p. 1] These authors found from their literature review 'limited empirical evidence about the effectiveness or otherwise of these approaches'.[27, p. 2] They also found that health professionals from culturally diverse backgrounds whose principles of care might be described differently do not necessarily find this term meaningful.[27, p. 19]

On the understanding of person and personhood being explored here, person-centred care cannot be one-dimensional; it is about relationships and interdependence. Kitwood, whose inspiration for person-centred care came from the work of Martin Buber (referred to below) claims that to care for another person is to know who they are.

> ... to respect their unique qualities and needs; to help protect them from harm and danger; and—above all—to take thoughtful and committed action that will help to nourish their personal being ... No one can flourish in isolation; the well-being of each one is linked to the well-being of all.[28, p. 241]

Without regard for the 'other' a person-centred focus can underplay concepts of reciprocity and mutuality. While not intending to detract from healthcare contexts where person-centred care is achieving stated goals, it is the concept of persons-in-relation which gives personhood its full flavour.

Staff as persons

Person-centred care suggests a culture in which staff are also treated as persons.

> Staff can only give person-centred care to others, in the long-term, if their own personhood is acknowledged and nurtured. Where this is not the case, they will revert to lower aspirations and less committed forms of practice—except for a few lonely heroes who place themselves in grave danger of exhaustion and burn-out'.[28, p. 312]

A discussion on persons in relation indicates the central focus is neither the patient nor the health professional, but both.

Focus points for Section 3 person-centred care

- Person-centred care can be interpreted individually or communally
- More research is needed to demonstrate its effectiveness
- The personhood of staff needs to be included in person-centred care.

Persons in relation

I phoned the nursing home to find out how my mother-in-law was settling in to her new environment. As Flo was no longer able to communicate meaningfully by phone, I was dependent on the senior nurse's account. 'Well, I'm absolutely delighted to tell you that right now she's being accompanied on her third circuit of the unit. I've overheard snatches of the conversation. Flo seems to be telling Margot (the nurse) how she much prefers 'Flo' to her full name. We've all been astonished because we didn't think Flo could walk or talk so well. It's lovely to see her chatting animatedly as though she'd known Margot forever.

I was elated to have this news of Flo, whose path towards nursing home entry had been rocky to say the least. I found when I finished the call that I had made no enquiries nor been given any information about Flo's many and various medical problems. What was conveyed to me was a description of the new relationships Flo was forging; other details could be obtained later.

Macmurray states, 'I can know another person *as a person* only by entering into a personal relation with him [*sic*].[6, p. 28] There can be no person until there are at least two persons in communication. This view is challenged by a humanist anthropology of the self-constructed and self-centred ego, which needs no 'other'. Middleton and Walsh see this notion of self-construction as itself a construct. 'The very notion of the self as an autonomous, self-reliant individual is a modern invention'.[29, p. 50] With these two views in mind, the way health professionals understand personhood will influence their relationship to their patients. If the relationship is one of mutual recognition and open communication then one person will have no hierarchical position over the other. If, on the other hand, each person is viewed as completely self-reliant, the tendency can be for competing egos finding fulfilment in power.

Personhood and power

When personhood is considered not as a self-enclosed entity, but in relation to others, each person is of equal status. When the autonomous self reigns supreme, it is inevitable that some others (usually those with the least capacity for exercising their autonomy) will be regarded as inferior. In other words, the 'autonomous mastery of the heroic individual seems to always result in mastery over other human beings.'[29, p. 49]

Macmurray warns that the pursuit of power may become an end in itself. 'For power of any sort has meaning only in reference to an end beyond itself to which it is the means.'[30, p. 182] This raises the question, to what 'end' are relationships in healthcare directed?

Returning to Annie's questions, Who am I, and where am I? The answer is not to be found in a problem-solving 'end' (for example, by the powerful and knowledgeable health professional conveying facts to the confused, powerless Annie); it is directed to Annie herself in her unique personhood. While Annie's plea is presumed to be a manifestation of Alzheimer's disease her quest is echoed by others of (presumed) sound mind. Middleton and Walsh contend the culture of postmodernity knows little of the unique person; rather a 'multiphrenic person is populated by a plethora of selves.'[29, p. 55] In response to the question, where are we, the answer is 'In a pluralistic world of our own construction.' In response to the question, who are we, the answer is 'We are Legion.'[29, p. 56] We neither know where we are nor who we are for we are 'legion', or many. This post-modern dilemma finds its answer in the notion of persons as interdependent and interrelated. Self-serving autonomous individuals neither make nor receive a compelling call. Annie's call can only be answered by a person who meets her as a person.

Rumbold suggests that understanding power relationships requires self-reflection:

> We will need to face our finitude and impotence as well as our power, our helplessness as well as our hope, to uncover and meditate upon the values by which we live and out of which we offer care. Changed structures have their beginnings in changed people.[31, p. 133]

Encountering the 'other'

Persons emerge when they acknowledge their dependence on others. 'It is only in relation to others that we exist as persons; we are invested with significance by others who have need of us; and borrow our reality from those who care for us.'[6, p. 211] Buber, the quintessential exponent of personhood, says, 'There is no I as such, but only the I of the basic word I-You and the I of the basic word I-It'[32, p. 54] He describes the world of objectification as 'thinghood' when a person is analysed and described rather than addressed as 'You.'[32, p. 68–9] Patients are objectified when referred to in the third person; in Buber's terms they become 'things' or 'its,' rather than persons. Annie's questions can be described, derided, and documented; they will only be answered by an 'other'.

Who is the 'other'? Health professionals readily respond to those who share our language, culture, values, and sense of humour; who can articulate their goals and cooperate with their care planning. However, what of the 'other' who is unlike us, with whom there is no common ground? Reference throughout this discussion to 'Annie' is deliberate. Given the epidemic proportions of dementia, whose numbers worldwide will 'nearly double every 20 years to 65.7 million in 2030 and 115.4 million in 2050,[33, p. 4] serious ethical questions are raised. How do persons with dementia claim care and attention when they cannot articulate their needs? How are they to compete with others for scarce resources, including research dollars? Perhaps MacIntyre's distinction between 'us and us,' and 'them and us' provides a clue.

MacIntyre acknowledges his own failure in his earlier works to adequately treat the subject of vulnerability and dependence on others. He claims the history of Western moral philosophy has also been negligent:

> From Plato to Moore and since there are usually, with some rare exceptions only passing references to human vulnerability and affliction and to the connections between them and our dependence on others ... And when the ill, the injured and the otherwise disabled *are* presented in the pages of moral philosophy books, it is almost always exclusively as possible subjects of benevolence by moral agents who are themselves presented as though they were continuously rational, healthy and untroubled. So we are invited, when we do think of disability, to think of 'the disabled' as 'them,' as other than 'us,' as a separate class, not as ourselves as we have been, sometimes are now and may well be in the future.[23, pp. 1–2]

Persons with dementia and other disabilities which affect cognition and speech raise serious challenges for spirituality in healthcare. While some suggestions are made below, the issue also has implications for policy, organization, and training (Section V).

Focus points for Section 4 Persons in relation

- Persons are interdependent beings
- Power relationships dissolve when all persons are understood as equals
- Each person needs an 'other'—even an 'other' unlike one's self.

Personhood: spirituality in practice

When spirituality is confined to 'an untouchable, ethereal realm' divorced from the everyday realities of bodily life, opportunities for care may be missed.[12, p. 51] When spirituality is located in the private domain of self-sufficient individuals, relationships may be compromised. Swinton's definition emphasizes the communal nature of spirituality. 'Spirituality is an intra, inter and transpersonal experience that is shaped and directed by the experiences of individuals and the communities within which they live out their lives.'[34, p. 20]

When matters of the spirit are reduced to problem solving exercises an alien language emerges. Diagnosis, flow-charts, processes, pathways, goals, measurements, outcomes, engineering terms, such as tools and instruments, and other 'technospeak' purport to profile the profound mystery that is a human person.[12, p. 48] Models of spiritual care and associated assessments clearly have their place (refer Section III of this text). In this chapter, however, the focus is specifically on spiritual care as an encounter of persons. In the seemingly mundane round of daily tasks health professionals—even those who declare they are not 'spiritual'—can 'touch' another's spirit. A firm meeting of hands, a gentle word of encouragement, the sharing of a joke, or simply a smile, can elicit the response, 'Thanks, you've lifted my spirits.'

In an increasingly 'hands off' healthcare culture where technological apparatus replaces human hands, it may be difficult to tap into the human spirit. In his autobiography Cochrane tells of his encounter in a prisoner of war camp with a young Soviet prisoner screaming with pain. With no pain killing drugs and with no common language Cochrane says:

> I finally instinctively sat down on the bed and took him in my arms, and the screaming stopped almost at once. He died peacefully in my arms a few hours later. It was not the pleurisy that caused the screaming, but loneliness. It was a wonderful education about the care of the dying. I was ashamed of my misdiagnosis and kept the story secret. [35, p. 77]

Cochrane surmounted the wall of separation between allopathic practice and spiritual care. His story also recalls Seneca's plea from ancient Rome:

> Here I am—this is me in my nakedness, with my wounds, my secret grief, my despair, my betrayal, my pain which I can't express, my terror, my abandonment. Oh, listen to me for a day, an hour, a moment, lest I expire in my terrible wilderness, my lonely silence. Oh God, is there no one to listen?[36, p. 219]

Another example of listening and responding demonstrates the overcoming of barriers between particular religious and cultural practices.

> Ana's religion was important to her, but her Russian Orthodox priest could only visit on rare occasions and there seemed to be no possible way of getting Ana to the Russian Orthodox Church. The hospital chaplain discussed this with Ana, took her to the chapel and explained the difference between Ana's own ornate, sensual experience of worship involving sights, sounds and smells, and the comparatively plain protestant chapel. The thoughtful chaplain introduced an unfamiliar liturgical practice; a symbolic gesture towards the sharing of meaning. Ana was delighted to report, 'The chaplain lit some candles and I almost felt at home.'

While for many people the locus of their spirituality is the hope which comes from the God of Judaism, Christianity, or other religions, McCurdy reminds us that religious practices are not the sole means of providing hope. Thus, '... connectedness with others and the presence of a supportive community can foster the person's sense of spirituality'.[37, p. 84]

Connectedness can be fostered through 'life story work' where the emphasis is on inclusiveness between the person and their carers.[38, p. 206] Life review is also becoming more common in palliative care, where the person who is dying is encouraged to find meaning in the journey. Their personhood is located in their unique narrative.

Challenges for spiritual care

Challenges in providing spiritual care vary with the context. Some barriers for nurses working in aged care, for example, are identified as:

- Lack of motivation
- Lack of knowledge
- Age differential between nurses and older people
- Lack of confidence
- Feelings of inadequacy
- Unwillingness to enter 'private' domain
- Nurses' own spiritual and cultural beliefs and values
- Uncertainty about criteria for referral.[39, p. 149]

Many of these challenges can be overcome through research leading to best practice guidelines; and through education, which empowers health professionals, giving them confidence to address each person's spirit through person to person care.

The ultimate test of spirituality in health care comes at the point of death. Perhaps Annie's cry is in anticipation of her own life's end. While the concept of hope is addressed elsewhere in this section, Nuland's comment provides an apt conclusion. His hope is that 'our last moments will be guided not by the bioengineers, but by those who know who we are.'[40, p. 95]

Focus points for Section 5 Spirituality in practice

- Spiritual interventions are not confined to problem solving
- Spirituality is practiced in the mundane experiences of everyday life
- A person's spirit can be 'tapped' by entering that person's story
- Challenges can be overcome through education, and dialogue.

Conclusion

Annie's cry, 'Who am I and where am I' came from the dance floor at the nursing home ball. Is she seeking a partner to accompany her on her final journey? Only another person can tell Annie who she is and where she is—not by factual revelation, but by trying to keep in step with her. Partnership takes practice. Personhood is prompted and promoted by persons in relation, where even the seemingly remote 'other' finds a place. In this partnership, persons—health professionals and patients—are not paragons of perfection; they become whole persons not alone, but together. Personhood is nothing less than humanity in its fullness; a worthy aim for all persons concerned with spirituality in healthcare.

Bibliography

Berry, W. (1990). *What Are People For?* New York: North Point Press.

Frankl, V. (1997). *Man's Search for Ultimate Meaning.* Massachusetts: Perseus Books.

Kitwood, T., Bredin, K. (1992). *Person to Person: a Guide to the Care of Those with Failing Mental Powers*, 2nd edn. Loughton: Gale Centre Publications.

Porter, R. (2003). *Flesh in the Age of Reason: the Modern Foundations of Body and Soul.* New York: W.W.Norton & Company.

Vanier, J. (1999). *Becoming Human.* London: Darton, Longman & Todd.

Zeisel, J. (2010). *I'm Still Here: a Breakthrough Approach to Understanding Someone Living with Alzheimer's.* London: Piatkus.

References

1 Polanyi, M. (1962). *Personal Knowledge: Towards a Post-critical Philosophy.* Chicago: University of Chicago Press.

2 Zizioulas, J. (1985). *Being as Communion: Studies in Personhood and the Church.* London: Darton, Longman and Todd.

3 Hudson, R. (2010). Orthodox faith: a lively spirit for older people. In: E. MacKinlay (ed.), *Ageing and Spirituality Across Faiths and Cultures*, pp. 152–66. London: Jessica Kingsley Publishers.

4 Damasio, A. (1999). *The Feeling of What Happens: Body and Emotion in the Making of Consciousness.* New York: Harcourt Brace & Company.

5 Craig, E. (ed). (1998). *Routledge Encyclopedia of Philosophy*, Vol. 7. London: Routledge.

6 Macmurray, J. (1961). *Persons in Relation.* London: Faber and Faber Limited.

7 McGrath, A. (2001). *Christian Theology: an Introduction*, 3rd edn, p. 268–9. Oxford: Blackwell Publishing.

8 Barth, K. (1960). *Church Dogmatics*, II, 1/2. Edinburgh: T&T Clark.

9 Ramsey, P. (1970). *The Patient as Person: Explorations in Medical Ethics.* London: Yale University Press.

10 Ramsey, P. (1978). *Ethics at the Edges of Life: Medical and Legal Intersections.* London: Yale University Press.

11 Wittgenstein, L. (1953). *Philosophical Investigations*, trans. G. E. M. Anscombe. Oxford: Blackwell.

12 Hudson, R. (2006). Disembodied souls or soul-less bodies: spirituality as fragmentation. *J Religion Spiritual Aging* **18**(2/3): 45–57.

13 Sabat, S. (2006). Mind, meaning, and personhood in dementia: the effects of positioning. In: J. Hughes (ed.) *Palliative Care in Severe Dementia in Association With Nursing and Residential Care*, pp. 287–302. London: Quay Books Division, MA Healthcare Ltd.

14 Cobb, M. (2001). *The Dying Soul: Spiritual Care at the End of Life.* Buckingham: Open University Press.

15 Singer, P. (1994). *Rethinking Life and Death: the Collapse of our Traditional Ethics.* Melbourne: Text Publishing Company.

16 Preece, G. (2002). Rethinking Singer on life & death. In: G. Preece (ed.). *Rethinking Peter Singer: a Christian Critique*, pp. 122–77. Downers Grove: InterVarsity Press.

17 Singer, P. (1979). *Practical Ethics*, 1st edn. Cambridge: Cambridge University Press.

18 Swinton, J. (2007). *Raging with Compassion: Pastoral Responses to the Problem of Evil.* Grand Rapids: William B Eerdmans Publishing Company.

19 Campbell, C. (2004). The human face of Alzheimer's. *New Atlantis*, No 6, pp. 3–17.

20 Locke, J. (1894). *Essay Concerning Human Understanding.* Oxford: Clarendon Press.

21 Matthews, E. (2006). Dementia and the identity of the person. In: J. Hughes (ed.). *Palliative Care in Severe Dementia in Association With Nursing and Residential Care*, pp. 163–77. London: Quay Books Division, MA Healthcare Ltd.
22 Post, S. (2000). *The Moral Challenge of Alzheimer Disease*, 2nd edn. Baltimore: Johns Hopkins University Press.
23 MacIntyre, A. (1999). *Dependent Rational Animals: Why Human Beings Need the Virtues.* Chicago: Open Court.
24 Post, S. (2004). Alzheimer's and grace. *First Things*, April 2004, 12–14.
25 Lewis, A. (1982). God as cripple: disability, personhood and the reign of God. *Pacific Theolog Rev* **16**(1): 13–18.
26 Haider, E. *Person-centred Care.* Available at: http://www.personcenteredcare.com/ (accessed 6 January 2012).
27 State Government of Victoria. (2006). *What is Person-centred Healthcare? A Literature Review.* Melbourne: National Ageing Research Institute.
28 Baldwin, C., Capstick, C. 2007. *Tom Kitwood on Dementia: a Reader and Critical Commentary.* McGraw Hill: Open University Press.
29 Middleton, J.R., Walsh, B.J. (1995). *Truth is Stranger than it Used to Be: Biblical Faith in a Postmodern Age.* Illinois: InterVarsity Press.
30 Macmurray, J. (1957). *The Self as Agent.* London: Faber and Faber Limited.
31 Rumbold, B. (1986). *Helplessness and Hope: Pastoral Care in Terminal Illness.* London: SCM Press Ltd.
32 Buber, M. (1970). *I and Thou*, trans. W. Kaufmann, 3rd edn. Edinburgh: T&T Clark.
33 Lyketsos, C. (2009). *Dementia: Facing the Epidemic*, Paper 18. Canberra: Alzheimer's Australia.
34 Swinton, J. (2001) *Spirituality and Mental Healthcare.* London: Jessica Kingsley.
35 Wiffen, P. (2003). The Cochrane Collaboration: pain, palliative and supportive care. *Palliat Med* **17**: 75–7.
36 Saunders, C. (2006). *Cicely Saunders: Selected writings* 1958–2004. Oxford: Oxford University Press.
37 McCurdy, D. (1998). Personhood, spirituality, and hope in the care of human beings with dementia. *J Clin Ethics*, **9**(1): 81–91.
38 McDonald, T. (2010). Integrated support for veterans in aged care homes In: E. MacKinlay (ed.) *Ageing and Spirituality Across Faiths and Cultures*, pp.195–211. London: Jessica Kingsley Publishers.
39 Hudson, R. (2008). Practice development—ageing, spirituality and nursing: application to practice guidelines. *Int J Older People Nurs* **3**: 145–50.
40 Nuland, S. (1994). *How We Die: Reflections on Life's Final Chapter.* New York: Alfred A Knopf.

CHAPTER 17

Belief

Mark Cobb

Introduction

Humanity exists in a rich environment of beliefs that shapes the people we become, evokes and sustains the ways in which we see and experience the world, guides our behaviour and the actions we take, and directs our sense of purpose and meaning. We are all believers, or more specifically we all have a mixture of beliefs and lack of beliefs, and this purposeful human faculty is entangled in the mind as much as in the body, in our thoughts as much as in our actions. Consequently, in considering belief in relation to spirituality and healthcare we have before us a vast field of subjects and disciplines making diligent enquiries into the nature and operation of beliefs. The following chapter aims to provide an overview of some of the ways in which we have come to understand belief and to provide some conceptual spans across discourses and disciplines that customarily do not intermingle. In particular, we will follow a path beginning with ideas about beliefs in general, and moving into the domain of religious and spiritual beliefs. From here we will consider some of the scientific explanations of belief and look specifically at models that describe how beliefs operate in relation to health. This will bring us to one of the more creative and contentious intersections built around the idea of placebos. Finally, we will step behind the professional persona of healthcare professionals, and consider how their sacred and secular beliefs may affect their clinical practice and decision making.

Beliefs in general

Beliefs are part of our everyday lives and such is their ordinariness that they easily go unnoticed. We seldom identify our beliefs explicitly although we manifest them constantly in our thinking, perceiving, speaking, and acting. Beliefs figure in the everyday ways in which we engage with the world: they shape our understanding of this experience and orientate our response. Beliefs therefore help us to navigate the world by functioning as irreducible guiding commitments. To believe something, in the general sense, is to have conviction in the proposition to which it refers: Alex believes that access to healthcare is a basic human right, Jean believes that meditation is good for our mental health, and Matti believes in socialism. It can be expected that these beliefs are manifested in some ways in the lives of Alex, Jean, and Matti, and that even if the circumstances never arise in which their beliefs can be observed they will make a difference to their thoughts and the ways they relate to these aspects of the world.

A distinguishing feature of beliefs is that they relate to things we classify as either true or false. Beliefs carry an implied claim to truth such that what we believe we consider true. When a person says that they believe the water is safe to drink we take it that the person accepts the proposition to be true and will drink it. A simple acknowledgement that something is true is insufficiently strong to be equated with belief. We may hold the idea that smoking causes cancer and continue smoking regardless of this thought, but if we believe this proposition then we are prepared to act as if it is true and quit smoking. This direct causal relationship between beliefs and behaviour is lacking in the state of mind in which we hold ideas without regard to their veracity. Truth is therefore a regulator of beliefs, but it is sometimes a weak regulator, for example, in wishful thinking. This does not mean there are varieties of truth and therefore varieties of correct beliefs, but that the basis of some beliefs may not need to be as substantial because the interests we have in some belief propositions are less significant. For example, a pregnant mother's belief in the ability of her midwife is of critical interest compared with the belief she has in her partner's ability to look after the house plants.

In order to hold a belief a person has to be capable of acquiring relevant information about the object of belief, and therefore a belief is conditional upon what a person can learn or come to know.[1] The acquisition and formation of beliefs is not simply a matter of intentionally inferring a true and warranted conclusion from what we count as evidence. There may be factual, evidential and epistemic grounds for arriving at certain beliefs, but beliefs are also formed through processes of cultural transmission, social interactions and practices, and through other perceptual, emotional, and non-reflective experiences through which we come to know aspects of reality with a high certainty of truth.[2, pp. 47–56] Human beings are believers and do not need to put much effort into developing beliefs, as Steglich-Petersen has commented, 'Many, in fact most, of people's beliefs are formed through subconscious processes of perception and inference which are not in any interesting sense controlled by the intentions of the subjects who have them.'[3]

People hold intuitive beliefs that are grounded in perceptions or inferred from those of others. Mikko sees blood running from his nose and concludes that he has a nose bleed, a belief that motivates him to seek first aid from Eva. Mikko's perception of his epistaxis relies upon his basic senses, prior information about what blood indicates, and knowledge about the sources of blood.[4] We therefore have the cognitive ability to form representations or models of the world without conscious effort, but we also have meta-representational ability. Mikko arrives at the warranted conclusion that he should seek Eva's help because he was informed that Eva is trained in first aid, even though he has never met Eva. Mikko therefore infers from this meta-representation of Eva's first-aid skills that she is likely to help him. Where people infer certainty or creedal attitudes from concepts beyond basic intuition, these are termed reflective beliefs, and these are typical of religions.[5]

Religious and spiritual beliefs

The primary characteristic of religious beliefs is their content or propositional objects referring to non-physical agents, of which a belief in God is a common example. A belief in God refers to an ultimate reality that transcends the natural world and is contingent upon a supernatural premise described variously as the sacred, the holy and their cognates. Some claim that there is substantial evidence that makes probable the existence of God, such as natural laws and the millions of people who have experiences they attribute to God.[6] However, whilst a proposition about God may explain the evidence, a lack of evidence may not be a sufficient reason to disbelieve the existence of God. There are beliefs, such as free will, that cannot be conclusively demonstrated evidentially or through compelling argument alone, but which are not irrational to hold. Similarly, there is an epistemic warrant for a belief in God that does not rely exclusively or substantially upon evidence or argument.[7] A belief in the self does not depend on proof, but it is a necessary presupposition to think and act, and which provides meaning to life and enables individuals to make sense of the world. It is therefore a basic belief that is the source of other beliefs and it is therefore an absolute presupposition that we cannot get behind, test as a hypothesis or empirically verify. Similarly, a belief in the existence of God is a basic or absolute presupposition from which other second-order beliefs are derived and made rational, such as miracles. This is why miracles to an atheist are irrational, but the arguments used by an atheist are unlikely to convince the theist.[8]

Religious beliefs can be informed by propositional knowledge, but more typically they relate to forms of practical knowledge (e.g. gained through participation in rituals) and experiential knowledge (e.g. of the presence of the divine). However, to hold a religious belief requires a conviction beyond a level of ordinary acceptance that is more like a profound trust or allegiance to a truth. This capacity is referred to as faith and Bishop contends that faith involves more than the intentional deliberation of what the evidence shows to be true: 'faith involves *beliefs* which are held 'by faith', in the sense that holding them is an active venture which goes beyond—or even, perhaps, against—what can be established rationally on the basis of evidence and argument.'[9, pp. 471–2] Consequently, beliefs held by faith are never tentatively held or the simple endorsement of propositions, but they are commitments to irrevocable truths that orientate perceptions, thoughts and actions.[10]

In his exploration of the psychology of religion William James considered that, 'Were one asked to characterize the life of religion in the broadest and most general terms possible, one might say that it consists of the belief that there is an unseen order, and that our supreme good lies in harmoniously adjusting ourselves thereto. This belief and this adjustment are the religious attitude in the soul.'[11, p. 41] A belief in God therefore suggests a way of regarding the world that expresses something of how we intend to live in the world.[12] We can contrast the extent and impact of the religious life that James is referring to with the life of the devoted golfer who holds golf to be the most important thing in her life and organizes her life around it as if it were a religion. Golf impacts upon people's lives in terms of commitments, skill, and membership of a group, but it is difficult to see how the commitments required to play golf could extend into a way of regarding the world, or to its possibility as a supreme good. Devoted golf players may risk hitting their ball into a bunker, but golf does not require a doxastic venture of faith about truths that give meaning and value to the whole of life.

Taylor proposes that contemporary religious faith is defined by a double criterion: 'the belief in transcendent reality, on one hand, and the connected aspiration to a transformation which goes beyond ordinary human flourishing on the other.'[13, p. 510] This latter quest refers to the spiritual life and its associated beliefs some of which tend towards immanent concerns. Whereas religious beliefs can be referenced to the official creedal formularies of a faith community and its institutions, it is the personal experience of the self-authenticating subjective life that often validates spiritual beliefs.[14,15] This illustrates something of the contemporary milieu and conditions for beliefs evident in many developed societies that admit a plurality of forms, a wide gamut of content and secularity. In practical terms, this means that beliefs do not necessarily determine a person's religious, or spiritual identity or practices. For example, a person may declare a Christian identity, not attend church, practice meditation, and believe in reincarnation.

Nagel considers whether, leaving aside religious or spiritual beliefs, secular philosophy can provide a satisfactory response to the questions of what it means to be human, how we make sense of our lives, and how we should live our lives within a larger framework of existence and the universe. He recognizes that, 'Existence is something tremendous, and day-to-day life, however indispensable, seems an insufficient response to it, a failure of consciousness' (p. 6). Nagel suggests that one secular response is simply to declare that there is nothing missing, the universe is meaningless and the bigger picture is one adequately described by the sciences. Another response he suggests is one of humanism: that we are part of a universal humanity that collectively is the source of value and meaning beyond the individual. The third response to the cosmic question he considers to be a form of Platonism in which we are conscious of being part of a larger cosmic process that is intelligible and purposeful (though not designed). Nagel concludes that the atheists' position is an evasion of a very real question and that humanism is too limited a response, which means that if the Platonic alternative is rejected we are left with a sense of the absurd.[16]

Scientific explanations of belief

Explanations of beliefs exist in a wide range of scholarly disciplines including philosophy, theology, psychology, neurology, anthropology and sociology. More recently religious beliefs, experiences and expressions appear to have become a compelling subject for the cognitive sciences based upon developments in the theory of mind.[17] Cognitivism is biologically (brain) based and a standard view claims that beliefs are cognitive states that play certain emotional and inferential roles that help guide and explain actions.[18] Neurobiological explanations are partial and, therefore, need integrating with more lived concepts of cognition including the social and cultural dimensions. Baker, for example, rejects the empirical conjecture of neuroscience and the reductive claims of the physicalists arguing instead for an explanation of beliefs derived from how they operate in practice and the effect they have. Beliefs are disclosed in the actions, thoughts, and words of people, which for Baker means that, 'Persons have beliefs; brains have neural states. Having certain neural states is, presumably, necessary for people to have beliefs; but it does not follow that for a person to have a particular belief, there is a neural state that constitutes that belief.'[19, p. 154]

Psychologists propose that beliefs arise from mental processes that give rise to assumptions held to be true about the world we experience and are generative of thoughts and behaviours.[20, p. 110] Similarly religious beliefs are an inevitable result of our ordinary cognitive processes, which is why they are so common. Barrett argues that beliefs in god-concepts and similar religious ideas can be distinguished from other forms of reflective beliefs by a number of distinct characteristics that are supported by the ways our minds make sense of the world:

1. They have a small number of counterintuitive but plausible features which violate the category of the object we have determined by our senses or a property that the object is expected to have. For example a belief in the Virgin Mary is a belief in a person who does not live on earth.
2. They are identified as having agency and attributed with intentionality or motivation, for example people pray to a divinity for help.
3. They possess strategic personal information, for example, moral and social information, which relates typically to survival or reproduction, for example, the parents of a still-born child may ask what they had done wrong for God to let this happen
4. They are capable of acting in the world (such as on objects or events) in detectable ways, for example through miracles
5. They motivate personal and corporate behaviours that reinforce belief, for example, regular congregational prayers in a mosque provide an explicit demonstration of belief and promote resilience to sceptical scrutiny.[21, 22]

Psychological explanations that aim to demonstrate the inevitability of religious beliefs rely upon an understanding of the cognitive functions of human beings. Some take this further and suggest the beliefs are simply and nothing more than manifestations of our cognitive functions. Alper, pursuing this argument under the influence of neo-Darwinian theory, concludes that God is an evolutionary adaptation, in other words God is '... not divine but an organic phenomenon.'[23, p. 227] Similarly, Bering follows an evolutionary argument to explain that human beings have a cognitive predisposition to believing in God, but this is no more than a convincing illusion and adaptive trait implying that in reality the existence of God is improbable.[24] This appears to dismiss the importance and necessity of illusions, symbols, and metaphors as an intermediate psychological space through which we interpret and relate to a reality that we can only partially know and experience.[25] Despite the particular focus on the neural correlates of spirituality the cognitive science of religion is a broader church and has the potential to develop a necessary interdisciplinarity between the natural sciences and other disciplines.[17] However, convincing scientific explanations may come to be, they will always be corrigible and confined by their own methodological and conceptual horizons. Ruthless scepticism or a sense of the absurd in not an inevitable conclusion to the powerful explanatory descriptions of beliefs: 'But the mere fact that a belief cheers us up, or even that it could have helped with survival, does not show that belief is groundless. An alternative possibility is always that it just happens to be true.'[26, p. 113]

Health beliefs

Beliefs about what sustains health, causes illness and brings about healing are part of our beliefs library, and come into play without deliberation or introspection in our thoughts, decisions, and actions when we are making sense of illness experiences, responding to treatment decisions, following advice and seeking help. Health beliefs are commonly used to explain why people do not follow health-maintaining advice and behaviours, vary in their response to symptoms, and adapt or abandon treatment regimens. One of the most prominent theories to explain and predict health-related behaviours is the Health Beliefs Model, a psychosocial model developed from psychological and behavioural theory. The Health Beliefs Model has been used in research into the variance in individual behaviours relating to health prevention and protection behaviours, symptom denial, and treatment compliance. The model includes the following beliefs as contributors to determining health-related behaviour:

- Vulnerability or susceptibility to contracting a condition (including belief in a diagnosis)
- Severity of the illness and its clinical and social consequences
- Benefits or effectiveness of the available action to treat the disease
- Negative consequences of a health action such as side effects, cost, or inconvenience.[27]

The predictive power of these beliefs have been criticize: they are inadequate on their own in explaining health-related behaviours and targeting only beliefs without addressing other determinants is unlikely to provide the basis for an effective intervention strategy.[28] Self-regulation theory is another prominent model accounting for how particular beliefs contribute to the personal representation or model of an illness that, in turn, determines how the individual responds to the threat of an illness.[29] For example, in studies of people with diabetes, beliefs about the seriousness of their condition, complications, and impact on their lives, and beliefs about the effectiveness of the different components of diabetic control were consistent predictors of diabetes self-management.[30]

Shared beliefs are a feature of social groups and may contribute to differences in such things as the utilization of healthcare, the adoption of preventative health behaviours and responses to symptoms of ill-health. A study comparing the beliefs about medicines between undergraduate students from Asian and European backgrounds found that differences were specifically related to beliefs in the capacity of medicines to cause harm and benefit with Asian students having more negative beliefs about medicine.[31] Shared beliefs are also a feature of the groupings of healthcare professionals who are socialized into particular beliefs, values, and behaviours through their training and acceptance as members of a peer group. In clinical practice learnt propositional knowledge, beliefs, experiential knowledge, reasoning, and routines blend as the healthcare professional interacts with the messy world of patient care requiring decisions and actions.[32] Consequently, clinicians do not always practice according to the letter of clinical guidelines, which means that the clinicians' beliefs influence their management of patients which in turn effect the patients' outcomes and the beliefs that patients acquire from their clinicians.[33]

Religious communities promote shared belief systems within lived traditions of practice that address matters of human suffering and wellbeing. They therefore provide people who are ill sources of meaning, practice, experiential knowledge and social support. Idler suggests that one of the pathways connecting religiousness and spirituality to health outcomes is through beliefs: 'Belief in a benevolent God and an afterlife may be key to a generalized expectation of positive outcomes. Moreover, religious beliefs offer individuals cognitive resources beyond these relatively simple or naive beliefs in good outcomes.'[34] A study conducted in a region of the southeastern United States (known for its high levels of religiosity) found that most people (80%) believed that God acted through doctors to cure illness and that God's will is a more important factor than the skill of the doctor in people's recovery from illness.[35] Religious or spiritual beliefs can also mediate illness experience: another study found that, 'Core beliefs were sources that grounded and maintained an interpretative structure through which participants viewed their life events and positively framed their experiences.'[36] These beliefs may contribute to the ways in which people cope with their illness and therefore affect their outcomes, wellbeing and quality of life.[37–39] More specifically health benefits may derive from religious beliefs and practices through the placebo effect.[40]

There is evidence that spiritual and religious beliefs may be a positive factor in health and wellbeing, and as such are tolerated within orthodox healthcare. Spiritual and religious traditions may also challenge biomedical values and beliefs, and promote alternative practices. However, spiritual and religious beliefs may also contribute to problematic ways of coping and maladaptation to the challenges of an illness. For example, a person with a belief in a caring God who suffers from chronic pain may feel abandoned by God or be angry with God if they have no relief from unremitting pain.[41] Religious or spiritual beliefs may therefore be a source of distress or conflict, and cause people to opt for solutions that exacerbate the challenge of the illness. The beliefs a person has in God that were acquired in childhood may, for example, have functioned perfectly well until faced with an illness crisis. In this instance, there is potential for a dissonance between the real-life experience, and the undeveloped beliefs that can lead to negative feelings of despair and abandonment. Similarly, people's beliefs may be poorly integrated with their lives or be rigid, which may be inadequate when a person faces major life challenges or existential uncertainty.[42]

Finally, the beliefs that people hold about health and sources of healing not only have personal implications, but they also have moral, social, and legal consequences. This is most starkly illustrated in people whose beliefs in God's power are absolute and unmediated, such that they turn to their faith and disregard healthcare when they, or those they care for, are at risk of illness or are unwell. This raises philosophical questions about what constitutes reliable ways of knowing and the rationality of belief, but the critical issue here is that religiously motivated health beliefs may have epistemic grounds and yet be inconsistent with morally or legally permissible conduct. In America, there are reported cases where parents of ill children rely upon prayer as treatment and reject medical care on the grounds of their religious beliefs.[43] The suffering and death of children through faith-based medical neglect alerts us to the need to question the ethics of beliefs. An ethical position in relation to health behaviours suggests that legitimate choices resulting from religious beliefs should only be considered preferential where there are no other evidentially decidable options.

Placebos

The relationship between beliefs, healthcare practice and health outcomes have a particular convergence in the use of placebos and the study of the placebo effect. Placebos are substances or techniques that have no active component or known direct therapeutic benefit but are administered with intention of pleasing or bringing comfort to a patient.[44] Placebos are therefore commonly used in trials of drugs where, for example, a control group receives an inert saline injection as a placebo and they are compared with a treatment group that receives an injection of the active drug being studied. More generally, a patient's confidence in a treatment (whether or not it intentionally involves a placebo component) and in the practitioner administering the treatment may give rise to a placebo response. In other words, a fraction of the therapeutic effect may arise from contextual, social, and cognitive factors associated with the treatment and more specifically the development of beliefs in the anticipated benefit of the treatment.[45] Whilst a positive therapeutic effect is referred to as a placebo, a negative effect may result from a disbelief in the treatment or an anticipated worse outcome, known as the nocebo effect. For example, in a study of a new intervention, patients reported more symptoms related to possible side effects mentioned on the consent form they had read and signed compared to patients who used a consent form that had not mentioned these side effects.[46]

That beliefs can result in physiological, behavioural, and subjective effects is not new, however the advent of improved experimental methods and neuroimaging have enabled a better understanding of the mechanisms and mediators of a placebo. In the field of pain, for example, researchers have studied how treatments with no direct pharmacological or physical effects (such as meditation) engage physiological, neurobiological, and psychological mechanisms that can moderate pain through analgesic and hyperanalgesic responses. Placebo analgesia involves the release of endogenous opioids that provide pain relief, whereas nocebo analgesia involves a neurohormone, increased brainstem activity and increased anxiety resulting in increased pain.[47] However, whilst there is a general acceptance of psychosomatic effects there is considerable caution and debate about what can or should be attributed to placebos and their purported therapeutic power.[48] In a Cochrane Review of 202 randomized clinical trials that covered a wide range of clinical conditions comparing a placebo group and a no-treatment group the authors '… did not find that placebo interventions have important clinical effects in general. However, in certain settings placebo interventions may influence patient-reported outcomes, especially pain and nausea, though it is difficult to distinguish patient-reported effects of placebo from response bias.'[49]

Despite the uncertainties about the placebo response and what may cause it there are clinicians who seem willing to some extent to use certain placebo interventions and treatments in the care of patients, although the empirical data on this is limited. The interventions in these cases are typically routine therapeutic treatments but which are known to be ineffective in relation to the condition being treated, for example, prescribing antibiotics for a viral infection, or vitamins against fatigue.[50] Promoting positive expectations in patients through the use of placebos whilst not deceiving them has potential ethical and clinical consequences. The Scientific Advisory Board to the German Medical Association considers that doctors should receive training in the use of placebos and supports their use, '... only when no approved drug is available, the patient has a minor illness or condition, placebo treatment does not raise the risk of harm to the patient, and placebo treatment seems likely to succeed.'[51]

The beliefs of healthcare practitioners

The role of beliefs in healthcare is not just a matter for patients, but for healthcare practitioners. There is often a disregard of personal beliefs as they are deemed a private matter and irrelevant to clinical practice with the limited exception of the conscientious objection in which it is accepted that particular religious beliefs may conflict with certain practices, such as termination of pregnancy. There is a general prohibition of clinicians proselytizing as this is considered to contradict the primary concerns of the patient and the fiduciary relationship of care. In the UK the General Medical Council goes as far as recognizing that, 'Personal beliefs and values, and cultural and religious practices are central to the lives of doctors and patients.'[52] However, it cautions against discussing personal beliefs with patients. Beliefs are therefore typically addressed in relation to ethical values and individual rights leaving the subject in something of a lacuna that is seldom explored or discussed.

Empirical data is beginning to surface about the influence of religious beliefs on practice. In one example, 116 American paediatricians completed a survey about their spiritual and religious identity, beliefs, and practices, and compared their results with a sample of the American public. The paediatricians had weaker religious identities than the public, but a similar spiritual profile. More than half of the paediatricians reported that their beliefs influenced their interactions with patients and colleagues to some extent.[53] In a survey of UK doctors (including general practitioners, neurologists, palliative medicine, and care of the elderly specialists) comparisons were made with the general population and, whilst there was a general similarity in strength of religious faith, there were underlying variations associated with the ethnicity of the doctor. In addition if the respondents reported having attended a patient who had died in the past year they were asked questions about the care of this patient. Variations in reported clinical decisions with the intention of hastening the end of life were associated with religious beliefs—religious doctors were less likely to take such decisions and had lower rates of continuous deep sedation instead.[54]

Variations in clinical practice associated with beliefs (religious or secular) are not widely understood, and there is little evidence that this is addressed in education and supervision. Clinicians must be presumed therefore to be working this out on their own within the minimal guidelines that exist. This is a disservice to the clinicians who hold sincere beliefs, act with integrity and practice ethically, but who are inhibited in exploring and expressing their vocational motivations. Similarly, clinicians may sometimes adopt maladaptive coping strategies with the potential of harmful sequelae. Neutrality in these matters avoids potentially contentious issues, but the beliefs vacuum does not exist. A more open and respectful recognition of the nature and role of beliefs, and those who hold them may enrich the humanity of clinicians, promote more open discussions about the grounds of clinical values and ethical decisions, and minimize the potentially negative effects that may result from incongruence with an idealized 'neutral' professional persona.

Conclusion

Beliefs are central to health and spirituality and are basic to the ways in which people understand and respond to their experiences of the sacred and the human. In considering beliefs in relation to healthcare we should ask questions about the truths by which people navigate their lives, how these beliefs mediate and interpret experiences of being well or ill, and the relationship between particular beliefs and practices of healing. Questions about beliefs exceed traditional biomedical models and remind us of the need to maintain wider perspectives when attempting to understand and care for suffering people. What contributes to a person's health and brings about healing does not simply involve pharmacological agents or clinical interventions but convictions made manifest in the humanity of care and our faith in that which gives our lives meaning and purpose.

References

1 Dretske, F.I. (1983). The epistemology of belief. *Synthese* **55**(1): 3–19.

2 Williams, B.A.O, (2006). Moore AW. *Philosophy as a humanistic discipline*. Princeton: Oxford: Princeton University Press.

3 Steglich-Petersen, A. (2006). No Norm Needed: on the Aim of Belief. *The Philosophical Quarterly*. **56**(225):499–516.

4 Frith, C.D. (2007). *Making up the Mind: How the Brain Creates our Mental World*. Oxford: Blackwell.

5 Sperber, D.A.N. (1997). Intuitive and Reflective Beliefs. *Mind Lang* **12**(1): 67–83.

6 Swinburne, R. (2004). *The Existence of God*, 2nd edn. Oxford: Clarendon.

7 Van Inwagen, P. (2005). Is God an Unnecessary Hypothesis? In: A. Dole, A. Chignell A (eds) *God and the Ethics of Belief*, pp. 131–49. Cambridge: Cambridge University Press.

8 Gilman, J.E. (1988). Rationality and belief in God. *Int J Philos Religion* **24**(3): 143–57.

9 Bishop, J. (2002). Faith as doxastic venture. *Relig Stud* **38**(4): 471–87.

10 Kenny, A. (2007). Knowledge, Belief, and Faith. *Philosophy* **82**(3): 381–97.

11 James, W. (2002). *Varieties of religious experience: a study in human nature*, centenary edn. London: Routledge.

12 Tilghman, B.R. (1998). Isn't belief in God an attitude? *Int J Philos Religion* **43**(1): 17–28.

13 Taylor, C. (2007). *A Secular Age*. Cambridge: Belknap/Harvard University Press.

14 Heelas, P., Woodhead L, (2005). *The Spiritual Revolution: Why Religion is Giving Way to Spirituality*. Oxford: Blackwell.

15 Lynch, G. (2007). *The New Spirituality*. London: I.B.Tauris.

16 Nagel, T. (2010). *Secular Philosophy and the Religious Temperament : Essays 2002–2008*. New York: Oxford University Press.

17 Andresen, J. (2001). *Religion in Mind: Cognitive Perspectives on Religious Belief, Ritual, and Experience*. Cambridge: Cambridge University Press.
18 Zimmerman, A. (2007). The Nature of Belief. *J Consc Stud* **14**(11): 61–82.
19 Baker, L.R. (1995). *Explaining Attitudes:* a Practical Approach to the Mind. Cambridge: Cambridge University Press.
20 Barrett, J.L., Lanman, J.A. (2008). The science of religious beliefs. *Religion* **38**(2):109–24.
21 Barrett, J.L. (2004). *Why Would Anyone Believe in God*? Lanham: AltaMira Press.
22 Barrett, J.L. (2008). Why Santa Claus is not a God. *J Cognit Cult* **8**(1): 149–61.
23 Alper, M. (2006). *The 'God' Part of the Brain: a Scientific Interpretation of Human Spirituality and God*. Naperville: Sourcebooks.
24 Bering, J. (2011). *The Belief Instinct: the Psychology of Souls, Destiny, and the Meaning of Life*, 1st American edn. New York: W.W. Norton & Company.
25 Jacobs, M. (1993). *Living Illusions: a Psychology of Belief*. London: SPCK.
26 Midgley, M. (2010). *The Solitary Self: Darwin and the Selfish Gene*. Durham: Acumen.
27 Janz, N.K., Becker, M.H. (1984). The Health Belief Model: a decade later. *Hlth Educ Behav* **11**(1): 1–47.
28 Harrison, J.A., Mullen, P.D., Green, L.W. (1992). A meta-analysis of studies of the Health Belief Model with adults. *Hlth Educ Res* **7**(1): 107–16.
29 Leventhal, H., Diefenbach, M., Leventhal, E.A. (1992). Illness cognition: using common sense to understand treatment adherence and affect cognition interactions. *Cognit Ther Res* **16**(2): 143–63.
30 Hampson, S.E., Glasgow, R.E., Strycker, L.A. (2000). Beliefs versus feelings: A comparison of personal models and depression for predicting multiple outcomes in diabetes. *Br J Hlth Psychol* **5**(1): 27–40.
31 Horne, R., Graupner, L., Frost, S., Weinman, J., Wright, S.M., Hankins, M. (2004). Medicine in a multi-cultural society: the effect of cultural background on beliefs about medications. *Soc Sci Med* **59**(6): 1307–13.
32 Gabbay, J., Le May, A. (2011). *Practice-based Evidence for Healthcare: Clinical Mindmines*. Abingdon: Routledge.
33 Bishop, A., Thomas, E., Foster, N.E. (2007). Health care practitioners' attitudes and beliefs about low back pain: a systematic search and critical review of available measurement tools. *Pain* **132**(1–2): 91–101.
34 Idler, E.L., Musick, M.A., Ellison, C.G., George, L.K., Krause, N., Ory, M.G., *et al.* (2003). Measuring multiple dimensions of religion and spirituality for health research. *Res Aging* **25**(4): 327–65.
35 Mansfield, C.J., Mitchell, J., King, D.E. (2002). The doctor as God's mechanic? Beliefs in the Southeastern United States. *Soc Sci Med* **54**(3): 399–409.
36 Daaleman, T.P., Cobb, A.K., Frey, B.B. (2001). Spirituality and well-being: an exploratory study of the patient perspective. *Soc Sci Med* **53**(11): 1503–11.
37 Alcorn, S.R., Balboni, M.J., Prigerson, H.G., Reynolds, A., Phelps, A.C., Wright, A.A., *et al.* (2010). If God wanted me yesterday, I wouldn't be here today': religious and spiritual themes in patients: experiences of advanced cancer. *J Palliat Med* **13**(5): 581–8.
38 Koenig, H., King, D., Carson, V.B. (2012). *Handbook of Religion and Health*. New York: Oxford University Press.
39 O'Connell, K.A., Skevington, S.M. (2010). Spiritual, religious, and personal beliefs are important and distinctive to assessing quality of life in health: a comparison of theoretical models. *Br J Hlth Psychol* 15(Pt 4): 729–48.
40 Harrington, A. (2011). The Placebo Effect: What's Interesting For Scholars Of Religion? *Zygon®*. **46**(2): 265–80.
41 Rippentrop, E.A., Altmaier, E.M., Chen, J.J., Found, E.M., Keffala, V.J. (2005). The relationship between religion/spirituality and physical health, mental health, and pain in a chronic pain population. *Pain* **116**(3): 311–21.
42 Pargament, K.I. (2007). *Spiritually Integrated Psychotherapy: Understanding and Addressing the Sacred*. New York: Guilford Press.
43 Hughes, R.A. (2004). The death of children by faith-based medical neglect. *J Law Relig* **20**(1): 247–65.
44 de Craen, A.J., Kaptchuk, T.J., Tijssen, J.G, Kleijnen, J. (1999). Placebos and placebo effects in medicine: historical overview. *J Roy Soc Med* 92: 511–15.
45 Lundh, L.G. (1987). Placebo, belief, and health. A cognitive–emotion model. *Scand J Psychol* **28**(2): 128–43.
46 Myers, M.G., Cairns, J.A., Singer, J. (1987). The consent form as a possible cause of side effects. *Clin Pharmacol Ther* **42**(3): 250–3.
47 Manchikanti, L., Giordano, J., Fellows, B., Hirsch, J.A. (2011). Placebo and nocebo in interventional pain management: a friend or a foe—or simply foes? *Pain Phys* **14**(2): E157–75.
48 Kienle, G.S., Kiene, H. (1997). The powerful placebo effect: fact or fiction? *J Clin Epidemiol* **50**(12): 1311–18.
49 Hróbjartsson, A., Gøtzsche, P.C. (2010). Placebo interventions for all clinical conditions. *Cochrane Database of Systematic Reviews* 2010, Issue 1. Art. No.: CD003974. DOI: 10.1002/14651858.CD003974.pub3.
50 Tilburt, J.C., Emanuel, E.J., Kaptchuk, T.J., Curlin, F.A., Miller, F.G. (2008). Prescribing 'placebo treatments': results of national survey of US internists and rheumatologists. *Br Med J* 337.
51 Stafford, N. (2011). German doctors are told to have an open attitude to placebos. *Br Med J* 342.
52 General Medical Council (2008). *Personal Beliefs and Medical Practice*. London: General Medical Council.
53 Catlin, E.A., Cadge, W., Ecklund, E.H., Gage, E.A., Zollfrank, A.A. (2008). The spiritual and religious identities, beliefs, and practices of academic pediatricians in the United States. *Acad Med* 83(12): 1146–52.
54 Seale, C. (2010). The role of doctors' religious faith and ethnicity in taking ethically controversial decisions during end-of-life care. *J Med Ethics* **36**(11): 677–82.

CHAPTER 18

Hope

Jaklin Eliott

Introduction

From the mid-twentieth century, hope has been a legitimate object of scientific academic enquiry, and transformed from a relatively uncomplicated concept, to a complex construct with multiple elements that may be selectively emphasized.[1] Nonetheless, hope is, for the most part, positively perceived,[2] deemed integral to overall quality of life,[3] essential for well-being,[4] and therefore a legitimate target for assessment and intervention by health professionals.[5] There is, however, marked variation regarding the definition of hope, the origin of hope, and how health professionals can or should attend to the hopes of those in their care.[5–7]

Defining hope

Part of hope's ambiguity rests in its linguistic properties: hope can be a noun (e.g. the/my hope), a verb (e.g. I/we hope), an adverb (e.g. hopefully that's/we're OK), and an adjective (e.g. I'm/we're hopeful).[5] No other word boasts such a rich and flexible linguistic resource (compare, for example, love, want, or know), but this provides potential for discrepancies in how individuals perceive hope, or understand and respond to others' hopes.

Furthermore, differences in emphases or language across time and disparate disciplines (e.g. scientific vs. philosophical vs. theological) means that hope looks different depending on one's point of view. The literary definition of hope provided by Emily Dickinson,[8] defining hope as a bird singing sweetest in the face of a storm, stands in marked contrast to philosopher Marcel's [9, p. 10] version:

> [Hope] is for the soul what breathing is for the living organism. Where hope is lacking the soul dries up and withers.

or the definition given by nurse researchers Dufault and Martocchio:[10, p. 380]

> [Hope is] a multi-dimensional dynamic life force characterized by a confident yet uncertain expectation of achieving a future good which, to the hoping person, is realistically possible and personally significant.

and the psychological operational definition offered by Snyder, Cheavens, and Michael:[11, p. 101]

> [Hope is] the perceived capacity to produce pathways to desired goals… along with the motivation to begin and continue the use of those pathways.

Different representations or definitions of hope capture unique aspects of hope, and collectively exemplify its diversity, complexity, and fluidity (see Table 18.1).

Origins of hope

Hope was once perceived to come from divine beings: some tales of Greek mythology, for example, state that hope was sent by the gods via Pandora to punish humanity,[12] although alternative versions see hope as the one blessing left to console humanity faced with a multitude of evils.[13] Christian theology, past and present, has understood hope as derived from the Christian God, His promise to us, and our relationship with Him.[21]

The psychologist Erikson proposed that hope was part of an innate developmental process within humans,[20] that hope originates in the infant child as a consequence of positive interactions with their carer, but paradoxically, that the infant inspires hope in their adult carer. Erikson further suggested that the successful attainment of hope was vital for successful psycho-social development, implying that hope was relatively stable across the lifespan. Nonetheless, he argued, hope requires ongoing positive social interactions to endure, echoing Marcel's claim that hope does not depend solely on ourselves, and cannot be created or dictated by the individual in isolation.[9]

Others also stress the importance of relationships in the development of hope. Snyder and colleagues, for example, posited that hope is acquired as the infant begins to think about themselves, what they want, and how they can achieve it, but critically, held that these hopeful thoughts arise 'in the context of a dependable, caring 'coach' or caregiver'.[11, p. 110] These theoretical and philosophical claims are supported by numerous studies: for example, Herth[22] observed that a critical finding from studies across diverse clinical populations (including cancer, Alzheimer's disease, HIV-AIDS, Parkinson's disease, spinal cord injury, mental illness, and cardiac problems amongst others) is the importance of the caring relationship.

Certainly, a dominant model of hope within the health literature presupposes that hope can be influenced by others, and this underpins recommendations that health professionals act to sustain, support, enhance, and/or maintain hope in their interactions with patients or clients, and their families.[e.g. 10,23,24] Some clinicians voice

Table 18.1 A selected review of perceptions of hope (adapted and augmented from [1])

Field of enquiry	Source	Hope is defined as...	Understanding of hope: Hope...
Religion	Ancient Greece: e.g.[12,13]	A divine evil	is an evil that encourages foolish over-optimism co-exists with and outlasts woes
	Old/New Testament (the Bible)	A divine gift	comes from God can positively transform the individual
Philosophy	Marcel[9]	A personal attribute gained through connection with others	enables individuals to resist despair derives from connection with the other without hope, life is meaningless
	Frankl[14]	Vital to life	sustains life is morally required without it, we die
	Bloch[15]	Endemic in human activity	drives all positive human endeavours
Medical anthropology	Good, *et al.*[16]	A dominant symbol in American oncology	reflects American beliefs about mind and body shapes physician practices of disclosure justifies funding for scientific, especially medical, research
Medical anthropology	Averill, *et al.*[17]	A culturally determined social practice	consists of rules of practice that vary cross-culturally cannot be understood without consideration of its context reflects and affirms the social mores and values of the community
Bioethics	Simpson [18]	An ethical issue	is an emotional attitude reflects what is important to the individual makes us vulnerable
Nursing	Dufault & Martocchio [10]	Multidimensional and fundamental to healthcare practice	consists of six dimensions: affective, cognitive, behavioural, affiliative, temporal, and contextual manifests within two spheres: generalized and particularized in patients, can and should be monitored, and adjusted by health professionals
Psychiatry	Kubler-Ross[19]	Vital to all, especially the terminally ill	in patients, equals hope of cure endures unto death if appropriately respected by doctors, will foster the clinical relationship
Psychology	Erikson[20]	Part of human development	is acquired in infancy, but sustained throughout life requires supportive interpersonal interaction
Psychology	Snyder *et al.* [11]	A cognitive process	consist of goal setting, pathways, and agency thinking can be systematically and reliably measured through scientific testing has positive associations with psychological health
Critical psychology	Eliott & Olver[5,6]	A linguistic resource	is made real through talk works to maintain engagement with and activity in life, often involving others
Psychology	Jevne[7]	An orientation	is a small voice in our heart that yearns to say 'yes' to life enables individuals to envision a future in which they can participate requires commitment to develop and sustain a science, practice, pedagogy, ethic, and community, of hope

concerns about inadvertently destroying or 'dashing' patients' hopes through ill-timed or inappropriate delivery of bad news, such as a poor prognosis.[e.g. 25,26] Although others have criticized such concerns as based upon an impoverished view of hope, one that limits hope to hope of cure,[27] this conceptualization of hope is dominant in media and medical discourse,[1,26–28] and manifested in patients even during the terminal phase of illness.[29,30]

Hope appears both an enduring and ubiquitous individual characteristic; and, transitory, fluctuating, or changing in response to others' input. Hope's duality was portrayed by Marcel, who spoke of 'transcendent' and 'concrete' hope,[9] and later described in Dufault and Martocchio's seminal study examining hope in patients with serious and life-threatening illnesses.[10] They distinguished between 'generalized hope,' encompassing all aspects of life, providing a relatively enduring positive approach and overall motivation in life—as in 'I don't hope for anything specifically, I just hope'; and, 'particularized hope,' focused on a particular valued outcome, and more transient in nature—as in 'I hope I get the job.' Dying cancer patients similarly distinguished between 'hope' and 'hopes'.[30] The latter, though transient, may reflect and help to define particular stages in life, as what is hoped for, our hopes, determine choices made and subsequent behaviour.[30] Hope, manifested as hopes, may play a pivotal role in establishing and maintaining an identity and sense of self over time. If so, then our expressed hopes are an expression of ourselves, of our needs and wants, and therefore, hope makes us vulnerable, requiring care and consideration on the part of those privileged to hear others' hopes.[18,31]

Somewhat similarly, hope can be something I/we have (a noun/thing) and something I/we do (a verb/process).[5,6] This understanding implies that whilst 'hope' may diminish or vanish, it can be re-created through 'hoping, 'providing opportunity for others to share in the creation of hope: Lynch has argued that 'half of hope is help,'[32] and Weingarten suggested that hope is 'something that people do [together],'[33, p. 289] potentially shifting the locus (and focus) of hope from the individual to their social networks or community. For health professionals, such an understanding acknowledges their capacity to affect others' hopes, but does not hold any one as uniquely responsible for maintaining hope, thereby circumventing attribution of blame when hope is experienced as diminishing or lost.

Characteristics of hope

Characteristics of Hope

Vital for well-being

Dynamic resource

Personalized

Future-oriented

Uncertain

Requires imagination

Requires energy

Relational

Transformative

Transcendent

Despite diversity, there are some constants in hope. Hope is deemed vital for human welfare, and sometimes, for human existence.[e.g. 14,15,20,34] It is consistently viewed as a dynamic resource that assists patients to cope better and find meaning in their experiences.[26,34–37] Hope is thought important enough that health professionals should monitor or measure patients' hopes, intervening where necessary to ensure it manifests appropriately.[5] In early 2011, there were more than 25 English-language scales within the healthcare literature designed to measure hope or hopelessness, the most commonly used being the Trait Hope Scale,[38] Herth's Hope Index,[39] and Beck's Hopelessness Scale.[40]

Some have suggested that hope is prompted by, and inextricably linked with, negative events such as the presence or threat of loss or despair, simultaneously offering the resources to overcome, or at least endure these.[e.g. 3,7,36,37] For example, Farran, Herth, and Popovich depicted hope as

> a delicate balance of experiencing the pain of difficult life experiences, sensing an interconnectedness with others, drawing upon one's spiritual or transcendent nature, [and] maintaining a rational or mindful approach in responding to painful life experiences;[3, p. 7]

whilst Morse and Doberneck described hope as:

> a response to a threat that results in the setting of a desired goal; the awareness of the cost of not achieving the goal; the planning to make the goal a reality; the assessment, selection, and use of all internal and external resources and supports that will assist in achieving the goal; and the re-evaluation and revision of the plan while enduring, working, and striving to reach the desired goal.[37, p. 277].

Many theories or descriptions of hope imply or assert that hope requires, but paradoxically, imparts, energy.[e.g. 41,42] Bloch saw hope as driving humanity to dream of and strive to attain a better life, claiming that hope 'requires people who throw themselves actively into what is becoming'.[15, p. 3] Similarly, Hope Theory proposed that hope provides the motivation and energy needed to move towards an individual's personal goals.[38] Clinically, studies have reported an association between high or uncontrolled pain and reduced hope, implying that continuing and uncontrolled pain can deplete energy reserves, leading to exhaustion which negatively impacts a patient's capacity to hope.[35,43,44] Minimizing pain, even maximizing physical wellbeing, may be critical to fostering hope.

Definitions or descriptions of hope typically reference a possible future, and significantly, posit a personal orientation to that future. The Christian philosopher and theologian Augustine of Hippo wrote that 'Hope ... deals only with the things that are good and which lie only in the future and which have a relevance to him [sic] who is said to entertain it'.[45, pp. 16–17] More recently, hope has been described as 'a confident yet uncertain expectation of achieving a future good which, to the hoping person, is realistically possibly and personally significant',[10, p. 380] or 'a process of anticipation that ... is directed towards a future fulfilment that is personally meaningful'.[34, p. 1459] Definitions referencing goals reveal future and personal significance more implicitly, as goals are inherently something we desire and move towards in the future. For example, Snyder's Hope Theory rests upon 'the goal, or what people want to attain.'[11, p. 105; see also 37] Critically, hopes for the future can reference both short-term (minutes, hours, or days) as well as long-term (months or years) time-frames.[28,46,47]

Hope, however, also draws upon past experiences, and is experienced in and influences the present.[7,10,22,47] Eliott and Olver noted that hope-as-noun (equated with hope of cure) usually functioned in the speech of seriously ill or dying patients to position them as completely helpless to influence future outcomes, with their future deemed limited or negative.[5,6] By contrast, hope-as-verb typically 'positioned patients as actively engaged in their circumstances,'[5, p. 188] working 'to establish and confirm [patients'] agency'[5, p. 143] and to 'facilitate the envisaging of a possible future with positive aspects in it.'[6, p. 144] Hope also featured in the context of leaving a positive legacy to others, affirming the significance of the patient's past and present life now and into the future.[30] The temporal aspect of hope may therefore have therapeutic significance. Larsen and Stege observed that when hope is experienced as diminished or lost, encouraging an individual to reflect on times past when hopes thought unlikely had been realized, may 'open [them] to new possibilities and hope yet to come'[31, p. 301] allowing the experience of hope in the present. Similarly, Eliott and Olver suggested that, when patients ask '"Is there any hope?", [health professionals] respond, "For what are you hoping?"' arguing that this focuses on positive possibilities ahead and enables the patient in the here-and-now 'to express and engage in what is important to them.'[5, p. 188] Others have noted that accessing uplifting memories or experiencing moments of light-heartedness (e.g. playfulness, delight, humour) can renew hope and enrich the present.[7,35,48]

Two other characteristics of hope derive from its future orientation: imagination, and uncertainty.[18] Lynch argued that without an imagined way to overcome difficulties, individuals become hopeless, lose energy, and succumb to apathy.[32] Synder and colleagues' Hope Theory similarly proposed that, to hope, individuals must be able to imagine at least one credible route, and preferably, additional plausible alternate routes to their goals.[11] Some individuals seem better at imagining multiple routes than others, although critically, Hope Theory suggests that hopeful thinking (thus hope) may be taught or encouraged in psychotherapeutic intervention.[11] Indeed, some have asserted that hope (that things can be better) underpins the therapeutic encounter,[see 24 for a review] arguing that hope is 'a central ingredient in overcoming discouragement and producing change'.[24, p. 273]

Nonetheless, as we do not know what the future holds,[14] hope rests on uncertainty, as the hoping person believes that a future desired goal is possible, but not guaranteed.[7,18,49] In hoping for a desired outcome, the hoper intrinsically acknowledges that both positive and negative outcomes are possible in the future, but orientates to the positive.[6,50]

Too much uncertainty, however, may negatively impact hope, so the provision of accurate information about current circumstances and options can play an important role in maintaining hope.[27,35,47,51] Currently, when confronted with the uncertainties attendant on serious illness, individuals are expected to have hope, with the assumption that this hope (usually for cure) is instrumental in fighting against their disease.[5,16,27] Although this hope can work positively to ensure compliance with medical recommendations aimed at attaining cure,[16] it is problematic when cure is deemed unlikely.[18,30] To some, patients' or families' hopes for cure in the face of poor prognoses represents 'denial' or 'false' 'unrealistic' hope, that should be discouraged and redirected,[52] or balanced through encouragement to 'hope for the best, but prepare for the worst'.[53] Others have argued that such activities are misdirected, that this hope for cure (as with other 'unrealistic' hopes) implicitly acknowledges that this outcome may not be possible, and has other vital functions, including to signal the patients' worth to self and others, to keep them actively engaged in life and moving towards positive goals, or even, to provide a moment's respite from an unpleasant 'reality'.[6,30,47,54] Hope for cure, moreover, is continually reinforced by media announcements of imminent medical cures, and this undermines attempts to declare them 'false'.[30] Indeed, hope has been identified as critical to the entire medical and scientific enterprise, as the hope for improvements in health and well-being justifies funding to research institutions, sustains medical workers in the field, and provides the rationale for treatment decisions for clinicians, patients, and families.[16,55,56]

Furthermore, as medical science deals in probabilities not certainties, hope (even of cure) is inherent in the most dire of prognoses,[27,49] and more generally, 'sometimes things do turn out better than we might have expected'.[7, p. 274] Framing an uncertain future through hope, to allow for the possibility (however unlikely) that a good outcome can occur, is a strategy employed by health professionals and patients alike.[16,55,57,58] Certainly, patients and families indicate a preference for clinical interactions that accommodate their hope of cure, even given a terminal prognosis,[6,23,50] providing support for arguments that management of a patient's hope is integral to sound, ethical clinical practice.[18,19,49] Suggested hope-full clinical strategies include conveying the limitations and uncertainties of predictions, providing scenarios describing best and worst case outcomes, presenting data for the best outcomes rather than the worst (e.g. 20% chance of two-year survival, not 80% chance of death),[58] and encouraging patients to focus on important relationships and achievable goals, or finding meaning in their life.[22,23,30,51,59] Jevne has noted, however, that in order to offer hope, the health professional must have hope themselves, and recommended a 'hopeful orientation that allows one to consider possibilities, despite probabilities that are not encouraging'.[7, p. 275]

Many allude to a transcendent or spiritual aspect to hope, sometimes via an explicitly religious belief system.[e.g. 3,29,30,35,42,59] Hope in God, for example, is considered central to both the Christian and Muslim religions.[21,60] Farran *et al.*'s description of Hope Process Framework included an experiential process (the *pain of hope*) that acknowledges the pain of loss and suffering, and, a transcendent or spiritual process (*the soul of hope*) that constituted a connectedness with something greater than the self (possibly including a belief in a higher being/force), and finding meaning and purpose in life.[3, p. 6] Following interviews with terminally ill patients, Herth observed that hope often had a spiritual basis, as a sense of meaning in suffering transcended human explanation and fostered an individual's hopes, whilst reliving positive and meaningful past activities also renewed hopes.[35] Herth concluded that hope was 'an inner power that facilitates the transcendence of the present situation and movement towards new awareness and richness of being',[35, p. 1256] later identifying the facilitation and affirmation of spiritual beliefs or practices as one hope-fostering strategy, and spiritual distress amongst other threats to hope—evident within many studies examining hope in patients and their families across diverse clinical populations[22, p. 191] Feldman and colleagues identified hope as the common component in diverse theories of meaning, concluding that 'hopeful thought may be an important part of what it means to perceive one's life as meaningful'.[61, p. 418] During psychotherapeutic encounters underpinned by hope, examination of meaning emerged as an almost invariant consequence of hope-focused conversation, as individuals spoke of how and who they wanted to be or to become, or of personally meaningful values.[31] Finally, hope and meaning are inextricably linked within two psychotherapeutic therapies targeting the terminally ill: *meaning-centred therapy* designed to counter hopelessness and reframe hope, through exploring 'meaning, spirituality, transcendence, and being connected with something greater than oneself';[59, p. 983] and, *dignity-centred therapy*, an individualized intervention that aims to bolster 'meaning, purpose, and hope,' deeming this integral to 'quality end-of-life care.'[62, p. 975]

Correlates and consequences of hope

The quantification of hope via statistical tools has provided the means to determine its relationship to various psycho-social variables.[1] Hope is consistently reported to be significantly correlated (positively with desirable, and negatively with adverse) with outcomes, behaviours, or psychological variables. For example, a review of several studies examining hope levels in individuals experiencing serious illness and injury (e.g. severe arthritis, major burn injuries, spinal cord injuries, fibromyalgia, and blindness) reported that 'hopeful thinkers' focus on 'ways to minimize the impact of the problem on their lives, adjust better psychologically, and adaptively cope' with their circumstances.[2, p. 123] A study examining the experience and correlates of hope over time similarly concluded that individuals with high levels of hope showed less stress reactivity and more adaptive emotional recovery from stress than those low in hope.[63]

In terms of physical outcomes, higher hope levels are associated with greater capacity to endure pain and a reduced perception of pain, as well as with enhanced athletic performance and superior academic performance in students.[2] Studies examining psycho-social outcomes in both population and clinical studies have reported that higher hope is associated with positive outcomes, such as higher levels of satisfaction with life, feelings of self-worth, and positive social engagement; conversely, those with lower levels of hope exhibit more depressive symptoms, more negative thinking, and tend to be more fearful of interpersonal closeness, lonelier, and less forgiving.[2,64,65] Some studies have suggested that, within families dealing with significant health issues, hope may protect against psychological distress, and could be mobilized to increase familial well-being: for example, lower levels of hope predicted depression in parents of children with intellectual disabilities, whilst higher levels predicted positive affect;[66] and, in mothers of children with Type 1 diabetes, hope was inversely related to anxiety.[67] Few studies have explicitly examined hope and spirituality, with negative,[68] and positive[69] relationships reported, possibly attributable to differences in population characteristics or assessment measures.

As scales to measure hope are translated and validated in new populations, many of the above-cited correlates and consequences of hope appear as reliable associations in diverse cultural groups (for examples, see Table 18.2). Notwithstanding the regularity of positive associations, as hope is a culturally constructed category, with individuals' hope emerging within, shaped by, and varying according to, the characteristics of their social environment,[70,71] it should not be understood without reference to the context within which it is made manifest.

Table 18.2 Selected results of studies of hope in ethnically diverse populations

Ethnic group or country/language (population)	Variables correlated with hope	
	Positively	**Negatively**
Australia/English (Children Age 13–17) [72]	Psychological wellbeing Social wellbeing Satisfaction with life	Depression Anxiety Stress
China/Chinese (breast cancer patients: adult) [73]	Coping styles that are: Optimistic Confrontive Self-reliant Palliative	Coping styles that are: Fatalistic Emotional
Japan/Japanese (chronic mental illness: adult)[74]	Happiness	Depressive tendencies Hopelessness Stress response Trait anxiety
Kuwait/Arabic (college students: adult)[75]	Optimism Satisfaction with life Self-Esteem	Negative affect Anxiety Pessimism
Netherlands/Dutch (adult)[65]	Quality of life Mental health Task-orientated coping	Loneliness
Norway/Norwegian (adult) [76–78]	Quality of life Satisfaction with life	Psychological distress Fatigue severity
Sweden/Swedish (palliative cancer patient and careers: adult)[79]	–	Fatigue Hopelessness
Twain/Chinese (cancer patients: adult][44)	–	Pain severity and interference with daily life

Some have asserted a negative aspect of hope, for example, arguing that (at least in some guises) hope induces apathy and passivity as individuals rely on external forces (e.g. luck, god, someone else) to achieve positive change.[e.g. 80,81] Such assertions may be countered by observations that hope is 'like the crouched tiger which will only jump when the moment for jumping has come,'[71, p. 9] or that the person with hope 'will act in a manner that supports (or minimally does not foreclose) the hope':[18, p. 441]. At least, hope entertains the possibility of, and encourages receptivity to, positive change; at best (and more typically according to many), it encourages movement towards it. Others have argued that hope may foster an unhealthy obsessive focus on attaining a single goal, accompanied by failure to contemplate or pursue other possibilities.[81] Such hopes become problematic, however, when not shared by others: unshared hopes can have negative consequences for interpersonal relationships, potentially causing confusion, conflict, or alienation. [6,18,27,50] Nonetheless, it is significant that during times of stress due to life-threatening emergency, family members reportedly carefully negotiate around hope, acting to respect others' hopes even when they deemed them unrealistic,[47] recognizing the value of that hope to the hoper in that time and place. Indeed, hope's value can be imputed through what happens in its absence: a temporary or permanent lack of hope (hopelessness) is associated with panic, despair, depression, the wish to die, and even suicide;[47,82–84] even 'a day without it [hope] is horrible'.[7, p. 266] Rather than overtly challenging a hope unshared, others (e.g. health professionals) might affirm the values implicit within the hope, and/or facilitate recognition of the possibility that hopes can change in response to changing life circumstances, perhaps encouraging cultivation of a 'portfolio' or 'spectrum' of hopes.[23,30,31]

Conclusion

> Hope is, or can be, positive, negative, divine, secular, interpersonal, individual, social, ideological, inherent, acquired, objective, subjective, a practice, a possession, an emotion, a cognition, true, false, enduring, transitory, measured, defined, inspired, learnt . . . and the list goes on. [1, p. 138]

Despite diversity, hope consistently emerges as a force for good, fundamental to well-being, and inherent in the condition of being human.[see 1] Hope is associated with positive experiences such as connection with others, affirmation of worth, light-heartedness, determination, strength, endurance, inspiration, creative imagination, aspiration, and positive possibilities. Hope is simple and complex: [7] simultaneously grandiose, encouraging us individually and collectively to dare to dream of, aspire and work to attain change in the face of what looks like insurmountable odds. It is also humble, ensuring that we acknowledge the limitations to our knowledge of, and ability to control, what happens next, as well as our dependency on others to achieve much that is worthwhile and good to, and for, us.

References

1 Eliott, J.A. (2005). What have we done with hope? A brief history. In: J.A. Eliott (ed.) *Interdisciplinary Perspectives on Hope*, pp. 3–46. New York: Nova Science, Hauppauge.

2 Cheavens, J.S., Michael, S.T., Snyder, C.R. (2005). The correlates of hope: psychological and physiological benefits. In: J.A. Eliott (ed.) *Interdisciplinary Perspectives on Hope*, pp. 119–32. New York: Nova Science, Hauppauge.

3 Farran, C.J., Herth, K.A., Popovich, J.M. (1995). *Hope and Hopelessness: Critical Clinical Constructs*. London: Sage.

4 Herth, K. (1995). Engendering hope in the chronically and terminally ill: nursing interventions. *Am J Hosp Palliat Care*, **12**(5): 31–9.

5 Eliott, J.A., Olver, I.N. (2002). The discursive properties of 'hope': a qualitative analysis of cancer patients' speech. *Qual Hlth Res* **12**(2): 173–93.

6 Eliott, J.A., Olver, I.N. (2007). Hope and hoping in the talk of dying cancer patients. *Soc Sci Med*, **64**(1): 138–49.

7 Jevne, R.F. (2005). Hope: the simplicity and complexity. In: J.A. Eliott (ed.) *Interdisciplinary Perspectives on Hope*, pp. 259–90. New York: Nova Science, Hauppauge.

8 Dickinson, E. (1976). Hope is the thing with feathers. In: T.H. Johnson (ed.) *The Complete Poems of Emily Dickinson*, p. 254. Boston: Bay Back Books.

9 Marcel, G. (1978). *Homo Viator: Introduction to a Metaphysic of Hope*. Gloucester: Peter Smith.

10 Dufault, K., Martocchio, B.C. (1985). Hope: its spheres and dimensions. Symposium on compassionate care and the dying experience. *Nurs Clin North Am*, **20**(2): 379–91.

11 Snyder, C.R., Cheavens, J.S., Michael, S.T. (2005). Hope theory: history and elaborated model. In: J.A. Eliott (ed.) *Interdisciplinary Perspectives on Hope*, pp. 101–18. New York: Nova Science, Hauppauge.

12 Hesiodus (1914). *Homeric Hymns and Homerica*. London: Heinemann.

13 Aesop (2008). *Fable 526 (from Babrius 58)*. Oxford: Oxford University Press.

14 Frankl, V.E. (1942/1962). *Man's Search for Meaning: an Introduction to Logotherapy*, rev. edn. Boston: Beacon Press.

15 Bloch, E. (1986). *The Principle of Hope*. London: Basil Blackwell.

16 Good, M.G.D., Good, B.J., Schaffer, C., Lind, S.E. (1990). American oncology and the discourse on hope. *Cult Med Psychiat*, **14**(1): 59–79.

17 Averill, J.R., Catlin, G., Chon, K.K. (1990). *Rules of Hope*. New York: Springer-Verlag.

18 Simpson, C. (2004). When hope makes us vulnerable: a discussion of patient-healthcare provider interactions in the context of hope. *Bioethics*, **18**(5): 428–47.

19 Kubler-Ross, E. (1970). *Hope. On Death and Dying*. London: Tavistock.

20 Erikson, E.H. (1964). *Insight and Responsibility: Lectures on the Ethical Implications of Psychoanalytic Insight*. New York: Norton & Co.

21 Dutney, A. (2005). Hoping for the best: Christian theology of hope in the meaner Australia. In: J.A. Eliott (ed.) *Interdisciplinary Perspectives on Hope*, pp. 49–60. New York: Nova Science, Hauppauge.

22 Herth, K. (2005). State of the science of hope in nursing practice: hope, the nurse, and the patient. In: J.A. Eliott (ed.) *Interdisciplinary Perspectives on Hope*, pp. 169–211. New York: Nova Science, Hauppauge.

23 Clayton, J.M., Hancock, K., Parker, S et al. (2007). Sustaining hope when communicating with terminally ill patients and their families: a systematic review. *Psycho-oncol* **17**(7): 641–59.

24 Larsen, D.J., Stege, R. (2010). Hope-focused practices during early psychotherapy sessions. Part 1: implicit approaches. *J Psychother Integr* **20**(3): 271–92.

25 Begley, A., Blackwood, B. (2000). Truth-telling versus hope: A dilemma in practice. *Int J Nurs Pract* **6**: 26–31.

26 Soundy, A., Smith, B., Butler, M., Minns Lowe, C., Helen, D., Winward, C.H. (2010). A qualitative study in neurological physiotherapy and hope: beyond physical improvement. *Physiother Theory Pract*, **26**(2): 79–88.

27 Beste, J. (2005). Instilling hope and respecting patient autonomy: reconciling apparently conflicting duties. *Bioethics*, **19**(3): 215–31.

28 Duggleby, W., Holtslander, L., Steeves, M., Duggleby-Wenzel, S., Cunningham, S. (2010). Discursive meaning of hope for older persons with advanced cancer and their caregivers. *Can J Aging* **29**(3): 361–7.

29 Benzein, E., Norberg, A., Saveman, B.I. (2001). The meaning of the lived experience of hope in patients with cancer in palliative home care. *Palliat Med* **15**(2): 117–26.

30 Eliott, J.A., Olver, I.N. (2009). Hope, life, and death: A qualitative analysis of dying cancer patients' talk about hope. *Death Stud* **3**(7): 609–38.

31 Larsen, D.J., Stege, R. (2010). Hope-focused practices during early psychotherapy sessions: Part II: Explicit approaches. *J Psychother Integr* **20**(3): 293–311.

32 Lynch, W. (1965). *Images of hope*. Notre Dame: Notre Dame University Press.

33 Weingarten, K. (2000). Witnessing, wonder, and hope. *Fam Process* **39**(4): 389–402.

34 Stephenson, C. (1991). The concept of hope revisited for nursing. *J Adv Nurs* **16**(12): 1456–61.

35 Herth, K. (1990). Fostering hope in terminally-ill people. *J Adv Nurs* **15**(11): 1250–9.

36 Lohne, V. (2009). Back to life again—patients' experiences of hope three to four years after a spinal cord injury—a longitudinal study. *Can J Neurosci Nurs* **31**(2): 20–5.

37 Morse, J.M., Doberneck, B (1995). Delineating the concept of hope. *Image J Nurs Sch* **27**(4): 277–85.

38 Snyder, C.R., Harris, C., Anderson, J.R., *et al.* (1991). The will and the ways: development and validation of an individual-differences measure of hope. *J Pers Soc Psychol* **60**(4): 570–85.

39 Herth, K. (1992). Abbreviated instrument to measure hope: development and psychometric evaluation. *J Adv Nurs* **17**(5): 1251–9.

40 Beck, A.T., Weissman, A., Lester, D., Trexler, L. (1974). The measurement of pessimism: the hopelessness scale. *J Consult Clin Psychol* **42**(6): 861–5.

41 Lohne, V., Severinsson, E. (2006). The power of hope: patients' experiences of hope a year after acute spinal cord injury. *J Clin Nurs* **15**(3): 315–23.

42 Owen, D.C. (1989). Nurses' perspectives on the meaning of hope in patients with cancer: A qualitative study. *Oncol Nurs Forum* **16**(1): 75–9.

43 Hagerty, R.G., Butow, P.N., Ellis, P.M., *et al.* (2005). Communicating with realism and hope: incurable cancer patients' views on the disclosure of prognosis. *J Clin Oncol* **23**(6): 1278–88.

44 Lin, C.C., Lai, Y., Ward, S.E. (2003). Effects of cancer pain on performance status, mood states, and level of hope among Taiwanese cancer patients. *J Pain Symptom Manag* **25**(1): 29–37.

45 Augustine (1963). *Faith, Hope and Charity*. Westminster: Newman Press.

46 Ezzy, D. (2000). Illness narratives: time, hope and HIV. *Soc Sci Med* **50**(5): 605–17.

47 Verhaeghe, S.T.L., van Zuuren, F.J., Defloor, T., Duijnstee, M.S.H., Grypdonck, M.H.F. (2007). The process and meaning of hope for family members of traumatic coma patients in intensive care. *Qual Health Res* **17**(6): 730–43.

48 Kim, S.D., Kim, H.S., Schwartz-Barcott, D., Zucker, D. (2006). The nature of hope in hospitalized chronically ill patients. *Int J Nurs Stud* **43**: 547–56.

49 Olver, I.N. Bioethical implications of hope. In: J.A. Eliott (ed.) *Interdisciplinary Perspectives on Hope*, pp. 241–6. New York: Nova Science, Hauppauge.

50 Thorne, S., Oglov, V., Armstrong, E., Hislop, T.G. (2007). Prognosticating futures and the human experience of hope. *Palliat Support Care* **5**: 227–39.

51 Clayton, J.M., Butow, P.N., Arnold, R.M., Tattersall, M.H.N. (2005). Fostering coping and nurturing hope when discussing the future with terminally ill cancer patients and their caregivers. *Cancer* **103**: 1965–75.

52 Kodish, E., Post, S.G. (1995). Oncology and hope. *J Clin Oncol* **13**(7): 1817–22.

53 Back, A.R., Arnold, R., Quill, T. (2003). Hope for the best, and prepare for the worst. *Ann Intern Med* **138**(5): 439–44.

54 Snyder, C.R., Rand, K.L., King, E.A., Feldman, D.B., Woodward, J.T. (2002). 'False' hope. *J Clin Psychol* **58**(9): 1003–22.

55 Miyaji, N.T. (1993). The power of compassion: truth-telling among American doctors in the care of dying patients. *Soc Sci Med* **36**(3): 249–64.

56 Mulkay, M. (1993). Rhetorics of hope and fear in the Great Embryo Debate. *Soc Sci Med* **23**: 721–42.

57 Thorne, S., Hislop, T.G., Kuo, M., Armstrong, E. (2006). Hope and probability: patient perspectives of the meaning of numerical information in cancer communication. *Qual Health Res* **16**(3): 318–36.

58 Kiely, B.E., Tattersal, M.H.N., Stockler, M.R. (2010). Certain death in uncertain time: informing hope by quantifying a best case scenario. *J Clin Oncol* **28**(16): 2082–4.

59 Breitbart, W., Heller, K.S. (2003). Reframing hope: meaning-centred care for patients near the end of life. *J Pall Care* **6**(6): 979–88.

60 Khan FA (2002). Religious teachings and reflections on advance directives: religious values and legal dilemmas in bioethics: an Islamic perspective. *Ford Urb LJ*, **30**(1): 267–75.

61 Feldman, D.B., Snyder, C.R. (2005). Hope and the meaningful life: theoretical and empirical associations between goal-directed thinking and life meaning. *J Soc Clin Psychcol* **24**(3): 401–21.

62 Chochinov, H.M. (2003). Thinking outside the box: depression, hope, and meaning at the end of life. *J Pall Care*, **6**(6): 973–7.

63 Ong, A.D., Edwards, L.M., Bergeman, C.S. (2006). Hope as a source of resilience in later adulthood. *Pers Indiv Differ*, **41**(7): 1263–73.

64 Rideout, E., Montemuro, M. (1986). Hope, morale and adaptation in patients with chronic heart failure. *J Adv Nurs* **11**(4): 429–38.

65 Van Gestel-Timmermans, H., Van Den Bogaard, J., Brouwers, E., Herth, K., Van Nieuwenhuizen, C. (2010). Hope as a determinant of mental health recovery: a psychometric evaluation of the Herth Hope Index-Dutch version. *Scan J Caring Sci* **24**(1): 67–74.

66 Lloyd, T.J., Hastings, R. (2009). Hope as a psychological resilience factor in mothers and fathers of children with intellectual disabilities. *J Intell Disabil Res* **53**(12): 957–68.

67 Mednick, L., Cogen, F., Henderson, C., Rohrbeck, C.A., Kitessa, D., Streisand, R. (2007). Hope more, worry less: hope as a potential resilience factor in mothers of very young children with type 1 diabetes. *Child Health Care*, **36**(4): 385–96.

68 Duggleby, W., Cooper, D., Penz, K. (2009). Hope, self-efficacy, spiritual well-being and job-satisfaction. *J Adv Nurs* **65**(11): 2376–85.

69 Pipe, T.B., Kelly, A., LeBrun, G., Schmidt, D., Atherton, P., Robinson, C. (2008). A prospective descriptive study exploring hope, spiritual well-being, and quality of life in hospitalized patients. *Medsurg Nurs* **17**(4): 247–53, 57.

70 Averill, J.R, Sundararajan, L. (2005). Hope as rhetoric: cultural narratives of wishing and coping. In: J.A. Eliott (ed.) *Interdisciplinary Perspectives on Hope*, pp. 133–65. New York: Nova Science, Hauppauge.

71 Fromm, E. (1968). *The Revolution of Hope: Toward a Humanized Technology*. New York: Harper & Row.

72 Venning, A., Kettler, L., Zajac, I., Wilson, A., Eliott, J. (2009). Is hope or mental illness a stronger predictor of mental health? In: A. Venning (ed.) *Building Mental Health in Young Australian: A Positive Psychological Approach* (thesis), pp. 167–85. Adelaide: University of Adelaide.

73 Zhang, J., Gao, W., Wang, P., Wu, Z.H. (2010). Relationships among hope, coping style and social support for breast cancer patients. *Chin Med J (Engl)* **123**(17): 2331–4.

74 Kato, T., Snyder, C.R. (2005). Relationship between hope and subjective well-being: reliability and validity of the dispositional Hope Scale, Japanese version [Abstract]. *Shinrigaku Kenkyu* **76**(3): 227–34.

75 Abdel-Khalek, A., Snyder, C.R. (2007). Correlates and predictors of an Arabic translation of the Snyder Hope Scale. *J Positive Psychol* **2**(4): 228–35.

76 Rustøen, T., Cooper, B.A., Miaskowski, C. (2010). The importance of hope as a mediator of psychological distress and life satisfaction in a community sample of cancer patients. *Cancer Nurs* **33**(4): 258–67.

77 Rustøen, T., Cooper, B.A., Miaskowski, C. (2010). A longitudinal study of the effects of a hope intervention on levels of hope and psychological distress in a community-based sample of oncology patients. *Eur J Oncol Nurs* **15**(4): 351–7.

78 Wahl, A.K., Rustøen, T., Lerdal, A., Hanestad, B.R., Knudsen, O., Jr, Moum, T. (2004). The Norwegian version of the Herth Hope Index (HHI-N): a psychometric study. *Palliat Support Care* **2**(3): 255–63.

79 Benzein, E.G., Berg, A.C. (2005). The level of and relation between hope, hopelessness and fatigue in patients and family members in palliative care. *Palliat Med* **19**(3): 234–40.

80 Jensen, D (2006). *Endgame, Vol. 1: The Problem of Civilization*. New York: Seven Stories Press.

81 Brooksbank, M.A., Cassell, E.J. (2005). The place of hope in clinical medicine. In: J.A. Eliott (ed.) *Interdisciplinary Perspectives on Hope*, pp. 231–9. New York: Nova Science, Hauppauge.

82 Beck, A.T (1986). Hopelessness as a predictor of eventual suicide. *Ann NY Acad Sci* **487**: 90–6.

83 Breitbart, W., Rosenfeld, B., Pessin, H., et al. (2000). Depression, hopelessness and desire for death in terminally ill patients with cancer. *J Am Med Ass* **284**(22): 2907–15.

84 Chochinov, H.M., Wilson, K.G., Enns, M., Lander, S. (1998). Depression, hopelessness and suicidal ideation in the hopelessly ill. *Psychosomatics* **39**: 366–70.

CHAPTER 19

Meaning making

Laurie A. Burke and Robert A. Neimeyer

Introduction

In the aftermath of the death of her son, Max, in a vehicular accident on his way back to college, Gayle struggled greatly. As a deeply thoughtful young man exploring both Eastern and Western wisdom traditions, Max had been drawn in the months before his death to the music of Cloud Cult, whose songs, like *Journey of the Featherless*, captured in a youthful, modern idiom the cosmic 'flight' of sojourners skyward, beyond social convention, while in related tracks on the same CD, the voices of the performers intoned repeatedly lyrics of love and farewell. When Max alone died in the rollover of the SUV in which he was riding as a passenger, the scorched backpack containing his reflective journal and poetry was one of the few things that escaped the flaming wreckage. As she searched desperately for some meaning in the seemingly senseless death of her son, Gayle took heart in the Cloud Cult music found in Max's CD player in his bedroom, in the philosophic tone of the poetry and prose in his miraculously salvaged journal, and in the survival of Max's girlfriend in the same accident, as the young woman herself was moved to a deep search for significance in the months that followed the tragedy. Together, she and Gayle sought and found some sense in the death through an eclectic spiritual narrative centring on their belief in a compassionate deity, and on their mutual 'soul contracting' with Max, between earthly incarnations, to undergo this trial together in their present lives, so that each might learn what it had to teach them in their respective journeys. Reinforced by a series of memorial services, rituals, and consultations with mediums and various spiritual guides, the new narrative of the meaning of Max's life and death consolidated into a stable resource for not only the two women, but also for an entire community of relevant others, reaching far beyond his friends and immediate family. Ultimately, it made use of social media to mobilize countless people and groups who joined in spontaneous 'strike force philanthropy' in honour of Max, thereby extending the story beyond one of consolation to one fostering social action to mitigate suffering in the world, including a massive medical aid effort to survivors of the earthquake in Haiti.

In the aftermath of life-altering crises, illnesses, or losses, people are commonly precipitated into a *search for meaning* at levels that range from the practical (*How do I adjust to this strange new world?*) through the relational (*Who am I now?*) to the spiritual or existential (*Why did God allow this to happen?*). How, and whether, we engage these questions, and resolve or simply stop asking them, shapes how we accommodate the transition and who we become in light of it. In Gayle's case, anguished and intermittent questioning impelled her forward in her search, ultimately deepening and broadening her existing sense of cosmic purpose, and galvanizing her efforts to live authentically and compassionately in relation to others who shared the same objective loss, or who faced losses and struggles in their own lives. The result was a revised self-narrative that found significance in the *event story* of her son's death, as well as in the *back story* of his life, braided together intimately with her own.[1,2]

As Gayles' story illustrates, existential experiences such as serious illness and the death of a loved one have an uncanny way of stopping us in our tracks, as we pause to reflect on life's most important meanings. For many people, religion provides the frame within which such unwelcome changes are experienced. Spiritual meaning making offers a source of comfort and intelligibility during a difficult passage. Our goal in this chapter is to highlight the important relation between spirituality and health, illustrating this with special attention to bereavement, where the evidence linking a struggle for meaning to mental and physical health outcomes is particularly clear.

Life crises and the quest for meaning

Across cultures and generations, human beings have sought meaning in their life experiences,[3] especially ones that cause distress. Frankl[4] asserted that, 'Once an individual's search for a meaning is successful, it. . .gives him the capability to cope with suffering'.[4, p. 139] By extension, constructivist research has examined the innate human motivation to create and preserve a meaningful self-narrative—the stories that we construct about ourselves and share with others, enabling us to discern a thread of consistency in our lives, especially when those lives have been disrupted by stressful events such as fatal illness or the loss of a loved one.[3,5]

The core themes of our self-narratives consist of fundamental assumptions about the world,[6] which under optimal circumstances include the implicit convictions that we ourselves have value, deserve to have a fulfilling and positive life, are capable of exerting some degree of control over events, and, in general, that the universe is kind and just. Understanding the world in these terms grants one's narrative a reassuring thematic coherence, and an overarching sense of life's meaning that entails faith in the trustworthiness of human intentions and actions, and the solidity of our place in the surrounding world.[7]

The authors gratefully acknowledge the invaluable help of A. Elizabeth Crunk and Natalie L. Davis in this work.

Spiritual coping represents an individual's use of specific religious or spiritual behaviours, actions, deeds, and beliefs to deal with life stressors.[8] Pargament, Smith, Koenig, and Perez[9] measured spiritual coping in distressed individuals by bifurcating the construct into subscales of positive and negative religious coping. Positive religious coping (PRC) was conceptualized as: 'an expression of a sense of spirituality, a secure relationship with God, a belief that there is meaning to be found in life, and a sense of spiritual connectedness with others'.[9, p. 712] Conversely, negative religious coping (NRC) was conceptualized as: 'spiritual discontent, punishing God reappraisals, interpersonal religious discontent, demonic reappraisals (attributing the event to the work of the devil), and reappraisals of God's power'.[9, p. 710] Overall, in their multi-sample study, Pargament *et al.*[9] found that better psychological outcomes and spiritual growth occurred when individuals exercised PRC strategies. Yet, studies show that when facing a variety of life stressors, it is common for people to display both PRC and NRC concomitantly.[10,11] However, those who are characterized by more PRC than NRC manage better overall.[9] The use of religion to manage life's difficulties is a near-universal means of coping that is particularly prevalent in individuals facing medical illness.[9] However, study results are equivocal on the power of religion to affect physical health in the general population.

Physical and psychological health often intersect at depression.[12] Whether poor health predicts low mood or the other way around, the two are often experienced in tandem. Still, research indicates that religiousness may lower depression;[13] in fact, an inverse correlation between faith and low mood is one of the strongest, most consistent findings in studies on spirituality and health.[12] In his review of spirituality and psychopathology, Koenig[14] examined investigations done with AIDS and cancer patients, and found that individuals who were able to find peace and make meaning were less likely to suffer from depression.

Specifically, religious beliefs/instruction appear to promote better decision-making, which in turn helps to lower overall stress levels and the likelihood of poor health. In his review of studies on health-related factors and faith, Koenig[12] reported an inverse relation between religiosity and suicidality. Religious involvement is also associated with lower mortality, but according to Koenig, only in the absence of spiritual struggle. In some studies, religiousness meant better adjustment to illness and more positive emotions, especially for those enduring stressful events. Furthermore, in meeting regularly, religious people often have larger-than-average social circles, potentially providing them with spiritual social support, which can be especially helpful when enduring health difficulties.[12]

Koenig[12] posited that although religion has been implicated in negative outcomes in terms of increasing guilt, fear, and low mood, religious people tend to have a more positive mindset than non-religious people, especially when it is most needed—in the face of medical uncertainty. In McClain, Rosenfeld, and Breitbart's[15] examination of 160 terminally ill cancer patients with less than 3 months to live, they found that spiritual wellbeing was negatively associated with depression and a desire for death. Individuals endorsing low levels of spiritual wellbeing were more likely to express a desire to hasten their own demise; yet, the opposite was true for individuals with high levels of spiritual wellbeing. Thus, spiritual wellbeing may act as a buffer against end-of-life despondency.

Still, not all studies found positive links between spirituality and health. For instance, studies examining disaster victims showed that spirituality frequently is used as a means of coping and healing.[16] However, Koenig[14] reported that the psycho-spiritual foundation of individuals with a solidly religious worldview still can be undermined by unmitigated psychological trauma, where religion no longer acts as a solace in tumultuous times. Likewise, Cohen, Yoon, and Johnstone's[17] study of 168 adults suffering from a variety of medical illnesses found that mental health had a positive association with positive spiritual experiences and positive spiritual support, but had a negative association with NRC and negative spiritual support. Yet, there was no association between psychological health and individual spiritual activities (e.g. prayer). In a variety of distressed samples, Pargament *et al.*[9] discovered that NRC was related to emotional distress (e.g. depression, poorer quality of life, psychological symptoms, and callousness towards others). Moreover, religiousness is sometimes positively related to depression. Research shows that depression is frequently coupled with NRC in distressed individuals, specifically when they are disgruntled with or feel abandoned by God.[13] In fact, spiritual struggle consistently appears in the literature as predicting poor health outcomes, including mortality. Results from Pargament *et al.*'s[11] 2-year prospective study revealed that spiritual crisis was the strongest predictor of the forthcoming death of elderly ill patients. In summary, although it is not inevitably linked with better health and mental health outcomes, spiritual coping and meaning-making tend to function as significant resources in the face of a wide range of life crises.

Spiritual coping in the wake of loss

Because the role of religiosity and meaning in adapting to bereavement has been the focus of a good deal of research in recent years, it provides an especially illuminating example of the link between spirituality and health. Despite the ubiquitous nature of loss, most people are able to accommodate to their changed lives within a few years. However, a substantial subset of mourners struggle with a protracted, debilitating, sometimes life-threatening[18] response to loss known as complicated grief (CG) [19] or prolonged grief disorder (PGD) [20] often requiring professional counselling.[21]

Typically, the distress that follows such loss has been conceptualized in terms of depressive or anxious symptomotology or poor physical health outcomes,[22] but recent studies highlight the prevalence of grief-specific distress, expressed on a continuum. Thus, for some people, bereavement is marked by resilience, with only transitory psychological distress.[23] Others experience significant sorrow (e.g. shock, anguish, sadness) for as long as 1–2 years,[22] during which they adapt gradually to their changed lives. Others suffer from CG—severe, debilitating grief, lasting for many months, years, or even decades. CG signifies a state of persistent grieving, reflected in profound separation distress, psychologically disturbing and intrusive thoughts of the deceased, a sense of emptiness and meaninglessness, trouble accepting the reality of the loss, and difficulty in making a life without the deceased loved one.[24]

Most studies of CG document prevalence rates of 10–20% in general bereaved populations.[25] Yet recent studies suggest that prevalence can be far higher among such groups as bereaved parents,[26] those who have lost loved ones to homicide[27] African

American cancer caregivers[28] and individuals bereaved by terrorism.[29] Moreover, CG has been found to predict a cascade of other serious psychological and physical health problems in bereaved samples, even after depression, posttraumatic stress disorder (PTSD), and anxiety have been taken into account.[30] For instance, CG has been shown to predict cardiovascular illness,[31] insomnia,[32] substance abuse, suicide, immune dysfunction, and impaired quality of life and social functioning.[18,33] Studies show that physical and psychological health is inversely related to levels of CG.[34]

Faith or existential philosophies can be significant coping resources in bereavement,[8] though they also can be affected by bereavement in turn. Spiritual beliefs, practices, and meaning making can support positive religious coping (PRC; e.g. looking to God for strength, support, and guidance), which can act as a buffer against distress. On the other hand, grievers sometimes engage in negative religious coping (NRC; e.g. questioning God's love and power). Whereas one's spirituality can be protective against physical and psychological sickness and disease, in some forms it can also be predictive of overall poorer health.

Meaning-making in bereavement

Like other major life stressors, profound loss can call into question the validity of our core beliefs and the self-narrative they support. In the wake of a loved one's death, the world can instantly appear dangerous, unpredictable, or unspeakably unjust to those who are violently, suddenly, or senselessly bereft.[35] Likewise, the protracted or agonizing death of a loved one due to wasting illness can make the world feel unkind and unsafe, and leave one feeling powerless. Bereavement brings mortality to the forefront, raising questions bearing on life's existential meanings.[36]

From a constructivist perspective, conserving or reestablishing equilibrium requires mourners to employ one of two meaning-making strategies.[37] The first alternative is to assimilate the death into their pre-loss way of construing and being in the world.[35] as when mourners draw upon their prior religious faith to find significance in the loss. This coherence-conserving strategy enables the griever to process the loss, often in terms of spiritual explanations for the death and the deceased's continuing presence in their lives.[35] Assimilation often has a relational component as well, as the griever recruits support from his or her existing social network or faith community, as well as from those with similar losses.[38]

Alternatively, grievers can accommodate the loss by reconstructing their beliefs and self-narrative to accept the loss,[6] which in turn can usher in identity changes and new social relationships. Although initially unwelcome, even disruptive losses can foster personal growth and highlight hidden benefits[39] so that 'restoration-orientated coping' can occur.[40] Whether assimilation or accommodation is employed, studies show that most individuals can psychologically adapt to loss and retain or restore a sense of meaning and purpose in their changed lives. However, an inability to make meaning following loss is more characteristic of the subset of individuals who suffer from CG—whose self-narratives can be splintered by an inability to make sense of their loss.[41]

A growing body of research substantiates grieving as a meaning-making process.[1] Yet, many find that meaning making does not come easily. For example, McIntosh *et al.*'s[42] study of bereaved parents found that only 23% of those who searched for meaning actually found any. Likewise, Lehman*et al.*'s[43] and Keesee *et al.*'s[26] studies found that only 36 and 53%, respectively, of bereaved parents were able to make sense of their loss even years later. Furthermore, such unsuccessful quests for significance pose significant risks for those engaged in them. Coleman and Neimeyer's[44] longitudinal study of widowed spouses found that being thrown into a search for meaning in the early months of loss prospectively predicted the intensity of widows' and widowers' grief over the 4 years that followed. Conversely, those spouses who reported being able to make sense of the loss—often in spiritual terms—enjoyed an enhanced sense of wellbeing characterized by optimism and a sense of accomplishment over this same period.

Spirituality as a resource in bereavement

Spiritual meaning-making

As Baumeister[45] argued, 'Religion is ... uniquely capable of offering high-level meaning to human life. [It] may not always be the best way to make life meaningful, but it is probably the most reliable way' (p. 205). Similarly, Park[46] argued that spirituality/religion provides 'a framework for understanding experience' (p. 304)—it facilitates a cognitive reframing of one's world. Therefore, as in Gayle's experience, what initially appears to be an arbitrary, senseless tragedy, viewed through the lens of faith, can appear purposeful, merciful, or divinely ordained.[38] On the other hand, it is equally arguable that profound loss can, in turn, challenge our spiritual resources, leaving us feeling depleted and directionless. In his description of the 'spiritual pain' experienced when a loved one dies, Attig[47] noted how in our human quest to embrace the best parts of life, these can become secondary losses in the wake of bereavement. 'When we suffer spiritual pain [following loss], we lose that motivation. We feel dispirited . . . . Life seems drained of meaning'.[47, p. 37]

Qualitative research documents this interplay between bereavement and spiritual meaning making. Smith's[48] study of African American women bereaved of their mothers found that faith enabled them to formulate an understanding of life's intangibles, such as belief in an afterlife reunion with their mothers. In another study, women churchgoers typically returned to a near pre-loss way of living as quickly as possible (i.e. going back to work, or quickly giving away the deceased's clothing) and conserved their 'metaphysical beliefs' (such as their belief in an afterlife).[48] Congregants regularly received teachings centering on a specific 'meaning system about death,' including an ongoing four-point directive: in the wake of loss one must go forward with life, because each person has a purpose, all the while preparing for one's own death, as you accept the deaths of those who have gone before you.[49] Thus, as a means of facilitating acceptance, church members frequently reminded each other of their own eventual 'home-going' as an inevitable and natural part of life.

A number of quantitative studies of bereavement also have found correlations between faith and sense making. McIntosh *et al.*[42] found that bereaved parents who professed greater spirituality were more likely to find meaning within as few as three weeks of the loss of their infants. Likewise, Davis and Nolen-Hoeksema's[50] prospective study of older grievers showed that those who endorsed spiritual beliefs prior to the death were three times as likely to find meaning afterward as those who did not.

Spiritual coping has been explored in a variety of bereaved samples, including cancer caregivers,[51] HIV-positive individuals,[52]

Caucasian mothers,[53] and African American homicide survivors.[54] Wortmann and Park's[8] review of over 70 studies on the use of faith in adjustment to loss highlighted how meaning making often mediates or moderates the relation between spirituality and bereavement outcome. Thus, spiritual meaning making appears to be an inherent aspect of spiritual coping following loss,[42] as in Gayle's attribution of intentionality in Max's seemingly accidental death, understood as part of a consensual plan to foster greater wisdom, compassion, and growth on the part of all those most intimately touched by the tragedy.

Psychological health

Most studies on existential adaptation in bereaved samples have examined meaning making or spirituality primarily as a buffer against mental rather than physical health problems, with findings showing mixed evidence in terms of both forms of distress among grievers.[55] Overall, bereaved individuals who report finding meaning fare better than those who do not.[26] In a variety of samples, making sense of loss meant better psychological adaptation, marital satisfaction, and emotional wellbeing,[13] and lower levels of grief.[56] In some bereaved samples, meaning making appeared to mediate the relation between religiousness and positive outcomes.[57] Still, Lichtenthal *et al.*'s[58] study of bereaved parents illustrated that especially when core life assumptions are challenged, as when a child's death precedes the parent's, debilitating grief can challenge a mourning parent's spiritual equilibrium, sense of purpose, and desire to live. For parents in Lichtenthal *et al.*'s study, the most common means of making sense of their loss was the belief that the timing and circumstances of the child's death were shaped by the hands of God, a construction of meaning associated with better bereavement outcome.

One's relationship with God can be a tremendous resource, providing solace and offering the bereaved supernatural love and care that once came from the deceased. Wortmann and Park's[8] review found general religiousness to be related to better bereavement outcome; yet, they also found in some cases that religion was not helpful, and in other cases that religious engagement and outcome were not significantly correlated. For example, Moskowitz *et al.*'s[59] study of bereaved gay men revealed that spiritual beliefs/activities and depression were unrelated at both 1 month and 3 years post-loss.

In relation to grief, bereaved spouses in Brown *et al.*'s[60] study who rated spiritual beliefs as more important after the loss than before experienced lower grief scores at both 18 and 48 months post-loss. However, spirituality was unrelated to depression, anxiety, or general wellbeing. Easterling *et al.*[61] found that positive beliefs about one's relationship with God and God's existence were related to less grief. In another study, belief in an afterlife was associated with less depression, less avoidance of death-related thoughts, increased spiritual wellbeing, and better overall adjustment.[62] Likewise, Brown *et al.*[59] found that widowed persons who assigned greater importance to religious/spiritual beliefs at baseline predicted less grief at 6 and 18 months post-loss. Yet, Kersting *et al.*[63] examined grief severity in women who had aborted their foetuses, and found that those who deemed faith to be more important also experienced more grief. Conversely, in a sample of 195 mourners, the importance of faith was associated with positive mood, but not with grief.[64] These inconsistent results mirror the interpretive discrepancies found in comprehensive reviews of faith-related beliefs and bereavement distress.[8]

Studies show that grievers who attend religious services generally adjust better than those who do not.[8] For instance, using path analyses, church attendance has been modelled through the pathways of self-esteem, familial attachment, prayer, social support, and meaning making, all of which facilitated better outcomes.[42] Unfortunately, members of the faith community do not always reach out to the griever in positive ways following loss. Richardson and Balaswamy[65] found that widowers who attended church-related functions had less positive, but more negative affect, which might reflect grievers' frequently reported sense of isolation and less-than-optimal interactions with others following loss.[66]

Wortmann and Park[8] found that the use of PRC predicted less anxiety and depression in grievers, more so than for non-bereaved, distressed individuals. Likewise, Meert *et al.*[67] found that spiritual coping was negatively associated with both baseline and follow-up grief in parents whose child died in the pediatric intensive care unit. Similarly, Rynearson's[68] study with homicidally bereaved parents revealed that when religious parents sought counseling they subsequently also endorsed less grief, traumatic experiences, and intrusive thoughts than did non-religious parents.

Incongruously, however, use of PRC by bereaved individuals sometimes seems to exacerbate their difficulty in traversing bereavement. In their study of HIV-positive grievers, Tarakeshwar *et al.*[52] found that there was a significant main effect for PRC such that those who used more PRC reported higher levels of grief. Anderson and colleagues[53] found an even more complex relation. They studied 57 mothers whose child had died from homicide, MVA, or other fatalities, and found that neither NRC nor PRC was statistically significant in relation to grief when examined separately. Yet, after controlling for time since loss, an interaction effect emerged between PRC and task-oriented coping (taking charge of the stressful event with a specific goal in mind), such that those who used PRC in combination with task-oriented coping suffered less grief as a result. Such results imply that positive religious engagement may prime other forms of active coping with stressors to mitigate bereavement complications.

Research also links grief and spiritual dissatisfaction—characterized by a sense of discord with God, and feelings of abandonment by God and one's faith community.[13] This less obvious form of bereavement distress has been termed *complicated spiritual grief* (CSG)—a spiritual crisis following loss that includes the collapse or erosion of the bereaved person's sense of relationship to God and the faith community.[69] In their sample of African American bereaved parishioners, Shear's team found that the effects of loss on the bereaved person's faith varied greatly from 'faith stronger than ever' to 'faith seriously shaken,' with 19% of the participants endorsing CSG symptoms. Recent studies with homicide survivors revealed that CH predicted CSG [70], uniquely beyond the effects of PTSD or depression [71]. In Batten and Oltjenbruns's[72] study of adolescents bereaved of their siblings, some reported that their faith had been strengthened in bereavement. Others struggled spiritually, and could not reconcile belief in a just, kind God with their unspeakable despair. Thus, one responded disdainfully: "I don't really care now about sinning … It don't matter to me as much … since [my brother's death]. I guess it is my way of getting back at God" (p. 542).

Physical health

Less is known about the effects of spiritual meaning making on the physical health of bereaved individuals. In fact, faith is associated with both positive and negative outcomes.[73] Bower *et al.*[74] linked higher levels of spirituality to better physical health in their longitudinal study that followed bereaved HIV sufferers for 2–3 years. They found that meaning making was effective in slowing the diminution of CD4 T (antibody-producing lymphocytes) levels, thereby lessening the individual's rapid demise from AIDS. Pearce and colleagues'[75] examination of older grieving adults showed that higher levels of PRC predicted increased physical health. In Krause *et al.*'s[55] study with elderly Japanese adults, they found that individuals who lost a loved one in the 4-year period between baseline and follow-up and who also believed in a pleasurable afterlife at baseline had a lower levels of hypertension at follow-up than those who did not endorse afterlife beliefs.

Paradoxically, however, Richards and Folkman's[76] initial study, conducted 2–4 weeks post-loss, with 125 caregivers grieving the loss of AIDS patients, revealed that higher spirituality meant poorer physical health; and this finding held true in the follow-up study conducted 3–4 years later with 70 members of the original cohort.[77] Likewise, Fry[78] compared 101 widows and 87 widowers, and found that widows adjusted better in terms of mental health and spiritual meaning making. However, even though widowers had fewer spiritual beliefs, participated in fewer religious activities, derived less comfort from religion, and deemed religion to be less important, they also had fewer adverse life events, and fewer physical problems post-loss than did widows. Some studies, like Stroebe and Stroebe's[79] with bereaved spouses, found no link between religiosity and physical health. In light of these discrepancies, further investigation of spirituality's relation to physical outcome is important because research has shown that individuals who suffer from CG have higher rates of suicidality,[18] cancer, heart disease, and sleep disturbances than those who grieve adaptively.[80] Finally, the relation between CSG and physical health is presently unknown, leaving the association between spiritual crisis and somatic complaints in bereaved populations ambiguous.

Conclusions

Our goal was to review aspects of spirituality/religion as they intersect with the health and wellbeing of individuals whose lives have been disrupted by a variety of stressors, including the death of a loved one. Although results are not entirely consistent, numerous studies converge to suggest that religious beliefs/practices can reduce distress in spiritually inclined individuals, and facilitate good decision-making, healthy living, and altruistic behaviours.[12] However, some studies also imply that severe life stressors like traumatic bereavement can severely challenge one's faith in turn.

This review also illuminated how religious coping can be complex to explore, producing findings that are occasionally contradictory and challenging to interpret. Moreover, surprisingly little is known about the antecedents of spiritual crisis. In terms of bereavement, not only is further research needed to explore predictors of CSG, but also to investigate CSG's potential role in predicting physical outcomes following a challenging bereavement.

Studies have coupled doubt about the benevolence and justness of the universe with deleterious psychological and physical outcomes.[81,82] Likewise, an inability to make sense of a loss,[83] and/or a futile search for meaning has been tied to persistent, intense, prolonged distress.[44] Life stressors, in terms of uncertain medical prognosis or anguishing separation distress at the loss of loved one, may undermine the individual's faith or precipitate a spiritual crisis. In the case of severe grief, the loss of secure attachment to a loved one may translate into a compromised relationship with God.[84] Moreover, some individuals find themselves too grief-stricken or frightened by medical diagnosis to receive support, even from members of their faith community. Unfortunately, inability to accept the nurturing support that is offered can alienate distressed individuals from would-be supporters, sometimes resulting in judgmental comments and interactions, from which the distressed individual is likely to further retreat.[66]

Thus, the experience of a compromised relationship with God and/or with one's spiritual community means that the individual is all the more likely to need enhanced professional care. Spiritually sensitive clinicians, physicians, and clergy can serve distressed individuals well by recognizing the importance of attending to their spiritual processes, with the added awareness that strong faith does not render an individual exempt from experiencing spiritual crisis. Periods of tremendous stress, as in bereavement or when facing serious illness, may be accompanied by a substantial crisis of spiritual meaning, where one's usual private and shared involvement in religious activities, scripture reading, worship, prayer, etc., or interactions with members of one's spiritual community prove inadequate in ensuring psychological adjustment or ongoing spiritual growth. As spiritually attuned mental and medical health professionals and spiritual leaders cross-refer and collaborate in an attempt to develop appropriate interventions for religious individuals, the spiritual nature of the human experience will be given the high priority it deserves.

Acknowledgements

The authors gratefully acknowledge the invaluable help of A. Elizabeth Crunk and Natalie L. Davis in this work.

References

1 Neimeyer, R.A., Sands, D.C. (2011).Meaning reconstruction in bereavement: from principles to practice. In: R.A. Neimeyer, H. Winokuer, D. Harris, G. Thornton (eds) *Grief and Bereavement in Contemporary Society: Bridging Research and Practice*. New York: Routledge.

2 Neimeyer, R.A., Burke, L.A. (2012). Complicated grief and the end-of-life: Risk factors and treatment considerations. In: Werth JL, ed. *Counseling Clients Near the End-of-life*. New York: Springer..

3 Neimeyer, R.A. (2009). *Constructivist Psychotherapy*: Distinctive Features. London: Routledge.

4 Frankl, V.E. (1992). *Man's Search for Meaning: An Introduction to Logotherapy*, 4 edn. Boston: Beacon Press.

5 Neimeyer RA. (2004). Fostering posttraumatic growth: a narrative contribution. *Psycholog Inq* **15**: 53–9.

6 Janoff-Bulman, R. (1992). *Shattered Assumptions*. New York: Free Press.

7 McAdams, D.P. (1996). Narrating the self in adulthood. In: J.E. Birren, G.M. Kenyon, J. Ruth, J.J.F. Schroots, T. Svensson (eds) *Aging and Biography:* Explorations in Adult Development, pp. 131–48. New York: Springer.

8 Wortmann, J.H., Park, C.L. (2008). Religion and spirituality in adjustment following bereavement: an integrative review. *Death Stud* **32**: 703–36.

9 Pargament, K., Smith, B., Koenig, H., Perez, L. (1998). Patterns of positive and negative religious coping with major life stressors. *J Scient Study Religion* **37**: 710–24.

10 Hills, J., Paice, J.A., Cameron, J.R., Shott, S. (2005). Spirituality and distress in palliative care consultation. *J Palliat Med* **8**:782–8.

11 Pargament, K.I., Koenig, H.G., Tarakeshwar, N., Hahn, J. (2001). Religious struggle as a predictor of mortality among medically ill elderly patients: A 2-year longitudinal study. *Arch Intern Med* **161**: 1881–5.

12 Koenig, H.G. (2008).*Medicine, Religion, and Health: Where Science and Spirituality Meet.* West Conshohocken: Templeton Foundation Press.

13 Huguelet, P., Koenig, H.G. (2009). *Religion and Spirituality in Psychiatry*. New York: Cambridge University Press.

14 Koenig, H.G. (2005). *Faith and Mental Health: Religious Resources for Healing.* West Conshohocken: Templeton Foundation Press.

15 McClain, C.S., Rosenfeld, B., Breitbart, W. (2003). Effect of spiritual wellbeing on end-of-life despair in terminally-ill cancer patients. *Lancet* **361**: 1603–7.

16 Koenig, H.G. (2006). *In the Wake of Disaster: Religious Responses to Terrorism and Catastrophe.* West Conshohocken: Templeton Foundation Press.

17 Cohen, D., Yoon, D.P., Johnstone, B. (2009). Differentiating the impact of spiritual experiences, religious practices, and congregational support on the mental health of individuals with heterogeneous medical disorders. *Int J Psychol Religion* **19**: 121–38.

18 Latham, A., Prigerson, H. (2004). Suicidality and bereavement: complicated grief as psychiatric disorder presenting greatest risk for suicidality. *Suicide Life Threat Behav* **34**: 350–62.

19 Shear, M.K., Simon, N., Wall, M., Zisook, S., Neimeyer, R., *et al.* (2011). Complicated grief and related bereavement issues for DSM-5. *Depression Anxiety* **28**(2): 103–17.

20 Boelen, P.A., Prigerson, H.G. (2007). The influence of symptoms of prolonged grief disorder, depression, and anxiety on quality of life bereaved adults: a prospective study. *Eur Arch Psychiat Clin Neurosci* **257**: 444–52.

21 Currier, J.M., Neimeyer, R.A., Berman, J.S. (2008).The effectiveness of psychotherapeutic interventions for the bereaved: a comprehensive quantitative review. *Psycholog Bull* **134**: 648–61.

22 Bonanno, G.A., Mancini, A.D. (2006). Bereavement-related depression and PTSD: evaluating interventions. In: L. Barbanel, R.J. Sternberg (eds) *Psychological Interventions in Times of Crisis*, pp. 37–55. New York: Springer.

23 Bonanno, G.A., Kaltman, S. (2001). The varieties of grief experience. *Clin Psychol Rev* **21**: 705–34.

24 Holland, J.M., Neimeyer, R.A., Boelen, P.A., Prigerson, H.G. (2009).The underlying structure of grief: a taxometric investigation of prolonged and normal reactions to loss. *J Psychopathol Behavior Assess* **31**:190–201.

25 Jacobs, S. (1993). *Pathologic Grief.* Washington, DC: American Psychiatric Press.

26 Keesee, N.J., Currier, J.M., Neimeyer, R.A. (2008). Predictors of grief following the death of one's child: the contribution of finding meaning. *J Clin Psychol* **64**: 1145–63.

27 McDevitt-Murphy, M.E., Neimeyer, R.A., Burke, L.A., Williams, J.L. (2011). Assessing the toll of traumatic loss: Psychological symptoms in African Americans bereaved by homicide. Psychological Trauma.: *Theory, Research, Practice, and Policy*, in press.

28 Goldsmith, B., Morrison, R.S., Vanderwerker, L.C., Prigerson, H. (2008). Elevated rates of prolonged grief disorder in African Americans. *Death Stud* **32**: (in press).

29 Shear, M.K., Jackson, C.T., Essock, S.M., Donahue, S.A., Felton, C.J. (2006).Screening for complicated grief among Project Liberty service recipients 18 months after September 11, 2001. *Psychiat Serv* **57**: 1291–7.

30 Lichtenthal, W.G., Cruess, D.G., Prigerson, H.G. (2004). A case for establishing complicated grief as a distinct mental disorder in DSM-V. *Clin Psychol Rev* **24**: 637–62.

31 Prigerson, H.G., Beirhals, A.J., Kasl, S.V., Reynolds, C.F., *et al.* (1997). Traumatic grief as a risk factor for mental and physical morbidity. *Am J Psychiat* **154**: 616–23.

32 Hardison, H.G., Neimeyer, R.A., Lichstein, K.L. (2005). Insomnia and complicated grief symptoms in bereaved college students. *Behav Sleep Med* **3**: 99–111.

33 Prigerson, H.G., Horowitz, M.J., Jacobs, S.C., Parkes, C.M., Aslan, M., Goodkin, K., *et al.* (2009). Prolonged grief disorder: psychometric validation of criteria proposed for DSM-V and ICD-11. *PLoS Med* **6**(8): 1–12.

34 Ott, C.H. (2003). The impact of complicated grief on mental and physical health at various points in the bereavement process. *Death Stud* **27**: 249–72.

35 Park, C.L., Folkman, S. (1997). Meaning in the context of stress and coping. *Rev Gen Psychol* **1**: 115–44.

36 Neimeyer, R.A., Herrero, O., Botella, L. (2006). Chaos to coherence: psychotherapeutic integration of traumatic loss. *J Construct Psychol* **19**: 127–45.

37 Neimeyer, R.A. (2006). Widowhood, grief and the quest for meaning: a narrative perspective on resilience. In: D. Carr, R.M. Nesse, C.B. Wortman (eds) *Spousal Bereavement in Late Life*, pp. 227–52. New York: Springer.

38 Pargament, K.I., Park, C.L. (1997). In times of stress: the religion-coping connection. In: B. Spilka, D.M. McIntosh (eds) *Psychology of Religion:* Theoretical Approaches, pp. 43–53. Boulder: Westview Press.

39 Calhoun, L., Tedeschi, R.G. (eds) (2006). *Handbook of Posttraumatic Growth.* Mahwah: Lawrence Erlbaum.

40 Stroebe, M., Schut, H. (1999). The Dual Process Model of coping with bereavement: rationale and description. *Death Stud* **23**: 197–224.

41 Currier, J.M., Holland, J., Neimeyer, R.A. (2006). Sense making, grief and the experience of violent loss: toward a mediational model. *Death Stud* **30**: 403–28.

42 McIntosh, D.N., Silver, R.C., Wortman, C.B. (1993). Religion's role in adjustment to a negative life event. *J Personal Soc Psychol* **65**: 812–21.

43 Lehman, D.R, Wortman, C.B, Williams, A.F. (1987). Long-term effects of losing a spouse or child in a motor vehicle crash. *J Personal Soc Psychol* **52**:218–31.

44 Coleman, R.A., Neimeyer, R.A. (2010). Measuring meaning: searching for and making sense of spousal loss in later life. *Death Stud* **34**:804–34.

45 Baumeister, R.F. (1991). *Meanings of life*. New York: Guilford Press.

46 Park, C.L. (2005). In: R.F. Paloutzian, C.L. Park (eds) *Handbook of the Psychology of Religion and Spirituality*. New York: Guilford Press.

47 Attig, T. (2001).Relearning the world: making and finding meanings. In: R.A. Neimeyer (ed.) *Meaning Reconstruction and the Experience of Loss*. Washington DC: American Psychological Association.

48 Smith, S.H. (2001). 'Fret no more my child … for I'm all over heaven all day': Religious beliefs in the bereavement of African American, middle-aged daughters coping with the death of an elderly mother *Death Stud* **26**: 309–23.

49 Abrums, M. (2000). Death and meaning in a storefront church. *Public Health Nursing* 17: 132–42.

50 Davis, C.G., Nolen-Hoeksema. (2001). Loss and meaning: how do people make sense of loss? *Am Behav Scient* **44**: 726–41.

51 Fenix, J.B., Cherlin, E.J., Prigerson, H.G., Johnson-Hurzeler, R., Kasl, S.V., Bradley, E.H. (2006). Religiousness and major depression among bereaved family caregivers: a 13-month time 2 study. *J Palliat Care* **22**: 286–92.

52 Tarakeshwar, N., Hansen, N., Kochman, A., Sikkema, K.J. (2005). Gender, ethnicity and spiritual coping among bereaved HIV-positive individuals. *Ment Hlth Religion Cult* **8**:109–25.

53 Anderson, M.J., Marwit, S.J., Vandenberg, B., Chibnall, J.T. (2005). Psychological and religious coping strategies of mothers bereaved by the sudden death of a child. *Death Stud* **29**: 811–26.

54 Thompson, M.P., Vardaman, P.J. (1997). The role of religion in coping with the loss of a family member to homicide. *J Scient Study Religion* **36**: 44–51.

55 Krause, N., Liang, J., Shaw, B.A., Sugisawa, H., Kim, H-K, Sugihara, Y. (2002). Religion, death of a loved one, and hypertension among older adults in Japan. *J Gerontol Series B: Psycholog Sci Soc Sci* **57**: S96-S107.

56 Schwartzberg, S.S., Janoff-Bulman, R. (1991). Grief and the search for meaning. *J Soc Clin Psychol* **10**:270–88.

57 Davis, C.G., Nolen-Hoeksema, S., Larson, J. (1998). Making sense of loss and benefiting from the experience: two construals of meaning. *J Personal Soc Psychol* **75**: 561–74.

58 Lichtenthal, W.G., Currier, J.M., Neimeyer, R.A., Keesee, NJ. (2010). Sense and significance: a mixed methods examination of meaning-making following the loss of one's child. *J Clin Psychol.*

59 Moskowitz, J., Folkman, S., Acree, M. (2003). Do positive psychological states shed light on recovery from bereavement? Findings from a 3-year longitudinal study. *Death Stud* **27**: 471–500.

60 Brown, S.L., Nesse, R.M., House, J.S., Utz, R.L. (2004). Religion and emotional compensation: Results from a prospective study of widowhood. *Soc Personal Soc Psychol* **30**: 1165–74.

61 Easterling, L.W., Gamino, L.A., Sewell, K.W., Stirman, L.S. (2000). Spiritual experience, church attendance, and bereavement. *J Past Care* **54**: 263–75.

62 Smith, P.C., Range, L.M., Ulmer, A. (1992). Belief in afterlife as a buffer in suicidal and other bereavement. *Omega: J Death Dying* **24**: 217–25.

63 Kersting, A., Kroker, K., Steinhard, J., Ludorff, K., Wesselmann, U., Ohrmann, P. (2007). Complicated grief after traumatic loss: a 14-month follow-up study. *Eur Arch Psychiat Clin Neurosci* **257**:437–43.

64 van der Houwen, K., Stroebe, M., Stroebe, W., Schut, H., van den Bout, J., Wijngaards-de Meij, L. (2010). Risk factors for bereavement outcome: a multivariate approach. *Death Stud* **34**: 195–220.

65 Richardson, V.E., Balaswamy, S. (2001). Coping with bereavement among elderly widowers. *Omega:* J Death Dying **43**: 129–44.

66 Burke, L.A., Neimeyer, R.A., McDevitt-Murphy, M.E. (2010). African American homicide bereavement: aspects of social support that predict complicated grief, PTSD and depression. *Omega* **61**: 1–24.

67 Meert, K.L., Thurston, C.S., Thomas, R. (2001). Parental coping and bereavement outcome after the death of a child in the pediatric intensive care unit. *Pediat Crit Care Med* **2**: 324–8.

68 Rynearson, E.K. (1995). Bereavement after homicide: a comparison of treatment seekers and refusers. *Br J Psychiat* **166**: 507–10.

69 Shear, M.K., Dennard, S., Crawford, M., Cruz, M., Gorscak, B., Oliver L. (2006). Developing a two-session intervention for church-based bereavement support: A pilot project. Paper presented at the meeting of the International Society for Traumatic Stress Studies conference; Hollywood, CA. November 2006.

70 Burke, L.A., Neimeyer, R.A., McDevitt-Murphy, M.E., Ippolito, M.R., Roberts, J.M. (2011). In the wake of homicide: Spiritual crisis and bereavement distress in an African American sample. *International Journal Psychology of Religion* 21: 1–19.

71 Neimeyer, R. A., Burke, L. A. (2011). Complicated grief in the aftermath of homicide: Spiritual crisis and distress in an African American sample. *Religions 2* (Invited submission for *Spirituality and Health* special issue): 145–64.

72 Batten, M., Oltjenbruns, K.A. (1999). Adolescent sibling bereavement as a catalyst for spiritual development: a model for understanding. *Death Stud* **23**: 529–46.

73 Hill, P.C., Pargament, K.I. (2008). Advances in the conceptualization and measurement of religion and spirituality: implications for physical and mental health research. *Psychol Religion Spiritual* **1**: 2–17.

74 Bower, J.E., Kemeny, M.E., Taylor, S.E., Fahey, J.L. (1998). Cognitive processing, discovery of meaning, CD4 decline, and AIDS-related mortality among bereaved HIV-seropositive men *J Consult Clin Psychol* **66**: 979–86.

75 Pearce, M.J., Chen, J., Silverman, G.K., Kasl, S.V., Rosenheck, R., Prigerson, H.G. (2002). Religious coping, health, and health service use among bereaved adults. *International Journal of Psychiatry in Medicine.* **32**: 179–99.

76 Richards, T.A., Folkman, S. (1997). Spiritual aspects of loss at the time of a partner's death from AIDS. *Death Stud* **21**: 515–40.

77 Richards, A.T., Acree, M., Folkman, S. (1999). Spiritual aspects of loss among partners of men with AIDS: postbereavement follow-up. *Death Stud* **23**: 105–27.

78 Fry, P.S. (2001). The unique contribution of key existential factors to the prediction of psychological wellbeing of older adults following spousal loss. *Gerontologist* **41**: 69–81.

79 Stroebe, W., Stroebe, M.S. (1993). Determinants of adjustment to bereavement in younger widows and widowers. In: M.S. Stroebe, W. Stroebe, R.O. Hansson (eds) *Handbook of Bereavement Research: Theory, Research, and Intervention*, pp. 208–26. Cambridge: Cambridge University Press.

80 Prigerson, H.G., Bridge, J., Maciejewski, P. Kea. (1997). Traumatic grief as a risk factor for suicidal ideation among young adults. *Am J Psychiat* **156**: 1994–5.

81 Currier, J.M., Holland, J., Neimeyer, R.A. (2009). Assumptive worldviews and problematic reactions to bereavement. *J Loss Trauma* **14**: 181–95.

82 Janoff-Bulman, R., Berger, A.R. (2000). The other side of trauma. In: J.H. Harvey, E.D. Miller (ed.) *Loss and Trauma*. Philadelphia: Brunner Mazel.

83 Neimeyer, R.A., Burke, L., Mackay, M., Stringer, J. (2010). Grief therapy and the reconstruction of meaning: from principles to practice. *J Contemp Psychother* **40**: 73–83.

84 Kirkpatrick LA. (1995). In: R.W. Hood (ed.) *Handbook of Religious Experience*, pp. 446–75. Birmingham: Religious Education Press.

CHAPTER 20

Compassion: luxury or necessity?

Carol Taylor and Susan Walker

Amy Friedman, a physician acquiescing to her physician's gentle insistence that she undergo a colonoscopy after all plausible explanations for her symptoms had been exhausted described herself as 'resigned, cooperative, but with little enthusiasm.'[1] In her short essay she applauds the quality of care she received, but decries the lack of sincere caring:

> I had predominantly felt more like a product on the fast-moving conveyor belt of a health care factory than a human being. …Why do we tolerate an environment in which a reticent, but unafraid patient emerges from an uncomplicated encounter feeling dispassionately processed rather than embraced?

Behaviours of the professional caregivers she encountered, the failure to make sincere eye contact and to ask how she was feeling, and demeanor that was proper, methodical, pleasant, but detached, wrapped her tight within a 'cold, impersonal cocoon.' The one exception was the gastroenterologist who endeared himself with three acts: his battle with the curtains to ensure privacy, his bending to cover her exposed legs with a blanket, and finally his looking directly at her as he asked how she was doing:

> With three such simple acts, the man about to invade the parts of me about which I am most shy and protective endeared himself and earned my deep gratitude. His touch healed.

This chapter will describe efforts to define the compassion undergirding the quality of presence and behaviours demonstrated by the gastroenterologist and explore the question of whether or not compassion is an essential quality for all for all who value spiritual care and the healing it promotes.

Background

Aita,[2] Benner,[3] Cherry,[4] Graber and Mitcham,[5] and Tuckett[6,7] contend that compassionate care, an essential component of holistic in patient care, was suppressed by such factors as the reward system, the time demands, and the organizational culture in the mid to late 20th century. Moreover, during that time American hospitals embraced a culture that extolled rationality, clinical professional skills, and technological advances. The increasingly market-driven and bureaucratic approach to contemporary health care in which measurement and outcome are considered the most important indicators of quality further hinder the moral and emotional work required to care for others.[8]

There are several additional factors that hinder the expression of compassion. One factor is the inability of health care professionals to clearly articulate a meaning of compassion that has been universally accepted within the health care community. Schulz and colleagues[9] and van der Cingel[10] stated that, although suffering and compassion are defining characteristics of human existence, they receive relatively little attention in health and social service policy and in research focused on illness and disability. According to Graber and Mitcham [5], little is known about the nature of an interpersonal relationship between compassionate clinicians and patients. A second factor relates to the failure of health care professionals to consistently explain and model the invisible caring aspects of health care.[11–17] A third factor is that clinicians do not provide compassionate care in a comfortable and relaxed atmosphere, but in highly demanding work settings where they must accomplish multiple tasks while serving numerous patients. Fourth, although compassion has often been identified as a component of caring and caring has been extensively researched,[9,17–24] little research has been directed toward exploring patients' or health care professionals' experiences with compassion. Fifth, compassion is not always easily differentiated from related concepts such as sympathy or empathy. All of these factors highlight the need to more clearly conceptualize that which health care professionals are expected to possess and demonstrate.

Defining compassion

The Latin root of passion, *patior, pati, passus*, is translated as 'suffering something to happen to oneself' or 'to experience with,' to somehow share in the experience of another by putting ourselves in his or her place.[25] In Hebrew, compassion is translated from *racham*, which means to love, pity, or be merciful, and from *rachamim*, which means mercies. Compassion also has its roots in three Greek words: *splagchnizomai* (to suffer with), *metripatheo* (who can bear gently with), and *eleeo* (to show mildness, kindness, pity, or mercy).[26] The New Oxford American Dictionary[27] defines compassion as 'A sympathetic pity and concern for the sufferings or misfortunes of others'.[27, p. 349] According to van der Cingel,[10] compassion is a concept that is inextricably bound up with human relationships. Steffen & Masters[28] defined compassion as 'being moved by the suffering of others and having the desire to alleviate that suffering' and a compassionate personality as one that 'includes altruistic behaviour with a deep sense of empathy for the needs of others'.[28, p. 218]

Many researchers note that people are most likely to engage in altruistic acts when they feel empathy for the person in need. Although the effects of compassion on health have not been directly studied, factors that are related to compassion, such as giving behaviours, providing support to others, and volunteerism have been related to positive mental and physical health outcomes.

What follows is a description of the concept of compassion developed theoretically from a review of nursing, medicine, and psychological literature, and then explored qualitatively with health care professionals and patients.[29]

The use of the concept of compassion in the nursing literature

Sethabouppha and Kane[30] conducted a phenomenological study of 15 Thai Buddhist family caregivers of seriously mentally ill relatives to understand their perspectives about Buddhist caregiving. Analysis of the interviews revealed five major themes of care giving: Buddhist belief, compassion, management, acceptance, and suffering. Sethabouppha and Kane defined compassion as a deep feeling of sharing, giving aid, supporting, or showing mercy. Two categories, caring (*metta*) and support (*karuna*) emerged from the Thai narratives and were conceptualized as compassion.

In Buddhism, caring refers to *metta*, which involves goodwill, universal love, and a feeling of heartfelt concern for all living beings, human or non-human, in all situations. *Metta* is believed to guide caregivers with love, closeness, and sympathy. Feelings of love, missing, thinking of, and worrying were aspects of caring frequently expressed by the caregivers for their seriously mentally ill relatives. The other aspect of compassion that emerged from the interviews was represented by *karuna* or support. *Karuna* is compassion that prompts one to serve others altruistically, expecting not even gratitude in return.

Jormsri and colleagues[31] presented a derivation of moral competence in nursing practice by identifying its attributes as found in Thai culture. Based on a review of the literature (1987–2003) and interviews with nurse educators, nurse practitioners, and patients, the researchers described moral competence as a combination of three dimensions: affective (moral perception), cognitive (moral judgment), and behavioural (moral behaviour). The attributes of moral competence that emerged from the interviews and the review of the literature (loving kindness, compassion, sympathetic joy, and equanimity) are considered to reflect Buddhist ethics in Thai society. Compassion means to have pity for the suffering of others (affective dimension), to have the desire to free sufferers from their pain (cognitive dimension), and to avoid harmful actions and show pity for the human plight (behavioural dimension). Compassion occurs when 'nurses perceive patients' suffering, support their feelings (cognitive dimension), and then perform nursing roles in a spirit of loving kindness (affective dimension), in order to free them from their suffering (behavioral dimension)'.[31, p. 587–8]

According to von Dietze and Orb,[32] 'Compassion involves deliberate participation in another person's suffering, not merely an identification of the suffering, but identification with it'.[32, p. 168] Von Dietze and Orb agree that it is this link with action that differentiates compassion from sympathy and empathy.

In a phenomenological study exploring nurses' and patients' perceptions of expert palliative nursing care and, in particular, the concept of the expert palliative nurse, Johnston and Smith[33] found that dying patients had a desire to maintain independence and remain in control. Patients and nurses agreed that the two most important characteristics of an expert palliative nurse were interpersonal skills and qualities such as kindness, warmth, compassion, and genuineness. 'Connecting' was the key theme for the patients and the central theme from which all other theme categories emerged. Connecting from the patients' perspective was categorized as, 'Someone to talk to,' 'Willing to listen,' and 'Getting to know me'.[33, p. 704] The notion of connecting or connection emerged in several citations in the literature sampled by the researchers and in conversations with nurses. Connection was the term nurses used to describe the basis for a mutually meaningful nurse patient relationship.

In a qualitative study addressing experiences with inpatient end of life care at a faith-based integrated health care system in the Pacific northwest, London and Lundstedt[34] surveyed 2796 families 7–9 weeks after the death of a family member. A total of 354 comments referred to the 'consistent care, dignity, and compassion' that families ($n = 174$), patients ($n = 106$), or 'someone' received during the last hospitalization of the patients.[34, p. 154] Descriptions of consistent care, dignity, and compassion from one wife included 'loving care of my husband and me and our family, provided for all of our comforts, such as places to rest, sleep, bringing food and drinks so we didn't have to leave his room, provided information that I didn't get from his doctors'.[34, p. 156] Behaviours for end-of-life care recommended by family members that the researchers categorized under 'Treat the patient and the family with care dignity, and compassion' included, 'Gather and follow patient and family wishes for end of life care,' and 'Avoid appearing overworked or too busy to meet patient and family needs'.[34, p. 157]

Compassion is often considered an essential component of nursing care. It is not simply a natural response to suffering, but more of a moral choice. Tucker[35] stated that compassion is a moral virtue that gives context and direction to nurses' decisions and actions, and. as such, promotes excellence in nursing practice. Jull[35] stated that compassion is not only a feeling, but also a moral virtue that requires nurses to take action in the presence of suffering. Aita[2,36] and Benner[3] also describe compassion as a response to the distress or suffering of another. The response is not merely a feeling of sorrow or dismay over the other's condition, but involves an action that seeks to alleviate or mitigate the distress or suffering. According to Van der Cingel,[10] compassion is a phenomenon that unites people during times of suffering and distress.

In June 2008 the UK government supported by the Royal College of Nursing stated that nursing care would be measured for compassion. Bradshaw[37] wisely critiqued this approach which she feared would redefine care as a pale imitation, even parody, of the traditional approach of the nurse 'as my brother's keeper.' 'Attempts to measure such parody can only measure artificial techniques and give rise to a McDonald's type nursing care rather than heartfelt care'.[37, p. 465]

The use of the concept of compassion in the medical literature

Clara and colleagues[38] surveyed 253 European vascular surgeons to evaluate ethical attitudes in the resolution of five clinical ethical dilemmas between compassion towards a 'small' or 'very costly' beneficial action versus a reasonable, but more 'pragmatic' allocation of health resources. Specifically, they explored the association between vascular surgeons' compassionate or pragmatic attitudes and professional seniority. Cluster analysis identified two groups of surgeons according to their pattern of answers: Group 1 ($n = 63$) was mainly compassionate whereas Group 2 ($n = 180$) was mainly pragmatic. After adjusting for additional factors such as private practice, on call services, and career status, multivariate analysis disclosed a significant V-shaped relationship between compassionate behaviour and seniority. Surgeons with 8–15 years of experience were the least compassionate. The youngest and senior vascular surgeons were more prone to favour compassionate attitudes when facing clinical ethical dilemmas. The researchers indicated that although both pragmatic and compassionate attitudes may be ethically legitimate, physicians who do not favour compassion may be at risk of leaving the patients without an advocate within the health care system.

Graber and Mitcham[5] interviewed 24 hospital clinicians (multidisciplinary) who were identified by administrators as being exemplary in caring and compassion. Analysis of data indicated that the clinicians did not attempt to distance themselves, but developed warm, empathic relationships with patients. The researchers identified four levels of clinician-patient interaction in three distinct domains: (1) the degree of intimacy between the clinician and the patient, (2) the inner motivational source for the clinicians' interpersonal and affective behaviors, and (3) the comparative amount of personal focus or concern as compared to a focus or concern for the patient in the interaction or relationship. The primary factors that distinguished the four levels were a shift in the nature of motivation and reward factors for the clinician, a gradual diminution of concern for or focus on self, and an increasing concern for the patient or 'other-centered' caring and compassion.

The accounts of patient interactions illustrated some important differences between compassionate care and ordinary care, specifically, the ability of compassionate clinicians to. transcend their personal concerns or issues, which became, if only temporarily, irrelevant. The expression of compassion or empathy appeared to sustain and support the clinicians, rather than tire or weaken them. Graber and Mitcham[5] concluded,

> The clinicians we interviewed did not appear to sacrifice rationality and objectivity in practicing compassionate care, but were able to balance 'the head and the heart.' Compassionate interactions with patients are only one aspect of holistic care. However, in our view, the caring and compassionate clinicians in our study possessed a key quality—the ability to simultaneously care for the body, emotions, and spirit of their patients. Such individuals should be fostered and supported by health care organizations that wish to be valued by their patients and to be recognized for their provision of holistic healthcare (p. 93, with permission from Lippincott Williams and Wilkins).

Wear and Zarconi[16] examined themes derived from 52 fourth year medical students' perspectives on how, where, and by whom they believed the virtues associated with good physicianhood (compassion, altruism, and respect for patients) had been taught to them. Students' thoughts were organized around the idea of influences in three areas:

- Foundational influences (parents, formative years, faith, and experiences preceding medical school)
- Pre-clinical (formal classroom experiences)
- Clinical education (role modeling and clinical environment).

Students' essays drew most heavily on the effects of role modeling (positive and negative) and the conflicting cues between caring and efficiency or personal/professional success. One student reported, '… knowledge to succeed in medical school versus knowledge to help people, battle diseases, and decrease suffering;' another stated, 'personal success is recognized in so many ways as compared to acts of kindness which can easily go unnoticed.'

Characteristics of positive role models included physicians who 'went beyond their prescribed roles and gave freely of themselves, sometimes sacrificing their precious free time and sometimes taking a few seconds to give a few words of encouragement. It felt like water in the desert.' Another student referred to the subtleties of connection that these physicians had with their patients, including holding a patient's hand and being present in a critical moment, such as undergoing anesthesia, taking time to listen to a patient who has just lost a family member, and sitting with a patient who has just had a miscarriage, respectfully answering any questions, and offering consolations.

Use of the concept of compassion in the psychiatric/psychological literature

Hutnick explored the use of the self of the therapist and issues related to boundaries, continuity, ethics, and compassion in psychotherapy. Hutnick defined psychotherapy as 'the compassionate caring for the mental well-being of another person'.[39, p. 399] When therapy is long-term and aimed at achieving a higher level of well-being by deepening self-understanding and acquiring wisdom, Hutnick emphasized that the quality of the therapist's presence in the client's life is one of the most effective predictors of health and happiness. Under such conditions, expert care (empathy, congruence, and unconditional positive regard), not careful expertise goes a long way in ameliorating the alienation and desperate loneliness that many people feel when they initiate therapy.[40,41] According to Hutnick, the clients' experiences of being compassionately or lovingly cared for make for the most effective therapy.

In an observational study involving field notes and narrative interviews, Hem and Heggen[42] examined specific psychiatric nursing practices in the context of compassion and demonstrated how the content of this concept challenges such practices. Several cases that were typical examples of the variety of problems arising in clinical communication between nurses and psychotic patients were selected. The case descriptions illustrated the nurses' experiences in situations in which they took responsibility for patients or ignored patients, as well as situations in which they showed understanding and sympathy or took no notice of and disregarded the patients.

In one case, the patient explicitly confronted the nurses with his suffering; however, there was no response to his appeal (compassion as a value), nor did the appeal lead to understanding and pity, which in turn result in specific actions to help him deal with his distress (compassion in practice). Although appearing to listen, the charge nurse ignored the patient's appeal by 'establishing a framework of "administrative logic" for the meeting and by keeping within it' [42, p.25]. Nor did the other nurses present attempt a solution to the patient's distress, part of which was exacerbated by institutional rules and policies that prevented nurses from authorizing passes for home visits. In fact, the nurses blamed the patient for his lack of insight into his illness and classified him as difficult. They made no attempt to explore the potential in this situation that would have acknowledged and reframed the patient's suffering and distress.

The researchers concluded that while there are many opportunities for compassion within a clinical context, there are also many limitations attached to using compassion as a basis for nursing practice. These depend, to some extent, on the individual nurse, but if the potential inherent in compassion is to be fully utilized, it requires a collective ability and willingness to put the idea of compassion into practice. They agree with Benner,[3] Graber and Mitcham,[5] Schulz and colleagues,[9] and Sturgeon[8] that suffering and compassion receive relatively little attention in health and social service policy, and that the expression of compassion requires institutions that recognize and promote it.

Compassion and suffering

Definitions and examples may provide useful indications of the meaning of a term, but they do not encompass the entire use of that term. The descriptions of compassion on the previous pages indicate that expressions of compassion reflect or require emotions that compel one to act on another's behalf. Ruiz and Vallejos,[43] van der Cingel,[10] von Dietze and Orb,[32] and Nussbaum[44] describe compassion as a feeling mediated or affected by reason. According to von Dietze and Orb, 'compassion is more than an emotion; it revolves around the ways we relate to other people and demands that we act'.[32, p. 168] If, as these sources suggest, compassion requires sharing in the suffering of another person, then an account of compassion may require a definition and a brief account of suffering.

Suffering is distinct from illness and disability in that not all illnesses necessarily entail suffering. Suffering involves an injury or threat of injury to the self, to one's sense of meaning or one's hopes of happiness. Van Hooft[45] states that suffering is a spiritual phenomenon that strikes at the faith one has or the very meaning of one's life. Reich[25] describes it as anguish that may be experienced at one level as a threat to one's composure, one's integrity, and one's fulfillment. On a deeper level, however, Reich, like Van Hooft, describes suffering as a frustration to the very meaning of one's personal existence.

According to van der Cingel[10], compassion expresses the 'knowing' of suffering. 'Compassion may not alleviate suffering, but it gives it an answer by acknowledging it. Acknowledgement of suffering gives us a choice of acting and behaving in such a way that it is evident that we want the suffering to end'.[10, p. 133] To not acknowledge the suffering, verbally or nonverbally, is to ignore it, the loss being of no importance. Compassion shows that a loss is terrible, suffering is visible, and one is not left alone.

Definition of compassion derived from the literature, and from interviews with nurses and older adult patients

The definition derived from these and other sources from the literature indicated that compassion is a quality or character trait that includes an emotional response to and engagement in the suffering or misfortune of another and consistently prompts an individual, willingly and from the heart, to act for the benefit of another. Using this definition to inform interviews with 13 nurses and 10 older adult patients in an acute care setting, Walker[33] derived the following definitions from nurses' and patients' experiences with compassion within a health care setting.

Although the nurses provided practical examples of the attributes of compassion, the definition that emerged from their interviews was very similar to that expressed in the literature. According to the nurses, Compassion is a quality or trait that enables a nurse to recognize the discomfort or suffering of a patient and connect with him or her in such a way that the nurse willingly goes the extra mile to meet a particular need or alleviate the suffering in a way that acknowledges the inherent value of a human being. Interestingly, all of the nurses stated that it generally takes only a few extra minutes to 'connect' with patients and, in so doing, acknowledge both their personhood and their distress or suffering.

Similar to the definitions derived from the literature and interviews with nurses, the patients stated that it is often just a little extra—a touch, a smile, telling and patient when the nurse will be back—that conveys compassion. They also concurred with the literature and the nurses that compassion is a quality or trait, and as the nurses described, a trait that enables a nurse to recognize or discern the need, discomfort, or suffering. The patients, however, stressed that a compassionate nurse did not always have to be told what the patient needed. According to the patients, Compassion is an innate quality or trait that enables a nurse to discern the need, discomfort, or suffering of a patient *without always being told or asked* and provides a level of care for him/her that surpasses basic requirements in such a way that the patient feels cared for, valuable, and safe. According to one patient, 'You can take care of someone without really caring about them; compassion means that you take care of that person as if they were your best friend, mother, or husband. Compassion is caring with care.'

Compassion and spiritual care

Puchalski and colleagues[46] defined spirituality as 'the aspect of humanity that refers to the way individuals seek and express meaning and purpose and the way they experience their connectedness to the moment, to self, to others, to nature, and to the significant or sacred.' Compassion is essential to experiencing the connectedness central to this definition. This can be seen even more strikingly if one reflects on Rahner's[47] definition of spirituality:

> Spirituality is … simply the ultimate depth of everything spiritual creatures do when they realize themselves—when they laugh or cry, accept responsibility, love, live and die, stand up for truth, break out of preoccupation with themselves to help the neighbor, hope against hope, cheerfully refuse to be embittered by the stupidity of daily life, keep silent, not so that evil festers in their hearts, but so that it dies there—when, in a word, they live as they would like to live in opposition to selfishness and to the despair that always assails us.

If one defines spiritual care as ministering to other spiritual creatures 'seeking to realize themselves' one intuitively grasps the need to be able to be able to suffer with others in the often painful stages of realizing their truest self, moving from brokenness to wholeness.

Developmental psychologist Erikson[48] claims that our last developmental challenge is ego identity versus despair. We either live peacefully believing that our lives have meaning and worth or ruminate on our failures and despair. Those who wish to companion the seriously ill and dying who are confronting existential questions about life's ultimate meaning and their personal worth need to be skilled in creating a shared world with the patient. Spiritual care isn't about approaching a patient as a problem to be solved. Rather it entails being consciously in the present moment with another or with others, believing in and affirming their potential for wholeness—no matter what life choices they may regret. A compassionate spiritual caregiver walks with the other into that center deep within where we can all find healing, peace, and the strength to live a new day. The compassionate presence of the spiritual caregiver is a powerful antidote to the loneliness, fear, and despair many feel as they experience their own darkness and vulnerability.

Compassion: essential or elective?

Fish and Shelly[49] identified three universal spiritual needs: meaning and purpose, love and relatedness, and forgiveness. Spiritual care defined most simply is helping others meet these needs. Openness to be moved by the plight of humans struggling to meet these needs, coupled with the will to use one's expertise to support their struggle toward wholeness and integration, in a word, compassion, is spiritual care. Since the quality of one's presence is integral to healing, one cannot provide spiritual care without being compassionately present to the other.

Taylor's[50] model of professional care further illustrates the definitions of compassion that Walker[29] derived from the literature and interviews with practicing nurses and hospitalized patients. Taylor posits that the professional cares only if s/he:

1. Experiences positive regard for the person being cared for (affection)
2. Intellectually grasps what is essential to the well-being of the person being cared for (cognition)
3. Commits expertise and energy to secure the well-being of the person cared for (volition)
4. Is empathically able to enter and share in the world of the one cared for (imagination)
5. Is moved to care primarily because of a commitment to secure the well-being of the person cared for (motivation)
6. Demonstrates caring behaviours which are perceived as such by the one cared for (expression).

Box 20.1 details each of the necessary and sufficient elements of professional care. While compassion is identified as the virtue linked to the affective element, it plays a role in each of the six elements. The model claims that professional caregivers need to possess each quality in a substantial manner and that both deficiencies and excesses of the quality are problematic. Professional caregivers who are deficient in compassion or excessive (prone to burnout)

Box 20.1 Taylor's Model of Professional Caring and related virtues and moral obligations

1. **Affection**: Feeling of positive regard that is experienced as a response to the presence or thought of the one cared for; feelings may range from a simple regard of kinship, which acknowledges another human in need, to feelings of loving and tender regard.

   Continuum: Simple regard to tender solicitude.

   Deficiency and excess: Too little feeling for another can result in the one cared for feeling objectified and depersonalized; too much feeling may overwhelm the recipient of care, incapacitate the caregiver, and make needed therapeutic intervention impossible.

   Virtues: Respect (regard), compassion, therapeutic attentiveness.

   Related moral obligation: To practice in a manner that leaves one open to be moved by the experiences of patients and their significant others.

2. **Cognition**: Intellectual grasp of what is essential to the wellbeing of the one cared for.

   Continuum: General knowledge of essential components of health and wellbeing to very precise knowledge of the same.

   Virtue: Intellectual honesty/humility, practical wisdom (phronesis).

   Related moral obligations:

   - To practice with the knowledge demanded by professional responsibilities
   - To seek assistance when one's competence is unequal to new and changing professional responsibilities
   - To hold other members of the care giving team accountable for responsible practice
   - To critique scientific advances in light of their ability to contribute to human well-being
   - To evaluate treatment regimens, systems of care, and health policy in light of their ability to effect the well-being of particular patients and population aggregates.

3. **Volition**: Commitment to use one's expertise and energy to secure the wellbeing of the one(s) cared for.

   Continuum: Generally meets commitments demanded by role responsibility to full-hearted commitment to patient's wellbeing.

   Virtues: Accountability, trustworthiness.

Related moral obligations:

- To hold oneself accountable for the human well-being of patients assigned to one's care.
- To respond to human need to a degree commensurate with professional responsibilities.

4. **Imagination**: Empathic ability to enter into and share the world of the other sufficiently to understand the other's unique existential situation and needs.

   Continuum: Basic ability to experience patient's life situation and needs to proficient ability to experience patient's life situation and needs.

   Virtue: Empathy.

   Related moral obligations: To empathically share in the experiences of patients and their significant others.

5. **Motivation**: That which influences the will in a manner which predisposes one to act altruistically to promote patient wellbeing; that which explains action.

   Continuum: Wellbeing of patient is not compromised by other professional motivations to wellbeing of patient is the primary professional motivation.

   Virtue: Altruism (subordination of self-interest to patient care).

   Related moral obligation:

   - To make the wellbeing of patients one's primary professional concern
   - To balance appropriate self-care with professional care responsibilities in a manner that does not jeopardize the well-being of patients or colleagues.

6. **Expressiveness of action**: Verbal and non-verbal behaviours used to communicate caring.

   Continuum: Interventions usually communicate caring to interventions consistently are perceived as communicating caring.

   Virtue: Caring.

   Related moral obligation: To interact with patients, their significant others, and colleagues in a manner that is perceived as being respectful and affirming of human dignity.

Taylor's Model of Professional Caring and Related Virtues and Moral Obligations. Reproduced from Taylor C (1997). The Morality Internal to the Practice of Nursing. UMI Dissertation Services, Michigan: Ann Arbor with permission of the author.

should thus be counseled about the need for remediation. This is illustrated in Figure 20.1.

Teaching the art of compassionate presence

Critics of anyone trying to mandate compassion for professional helpers will often claim that compassion is a characteristic like being brown or blue-eyed. Some humans are simply born exquisitely compassionate and others less so, not at all, or worse. There is nothing you can do to change your original condition. While the literature is inconclusive about whether or not being compassionate is essential to being fully human and about whether or not being compassionate confers survival advantages to its bearers, it is true that in moments of vulnerability most humans hunger for a compassionate other who is moved by our plight sufficiently to want to help—even when this means standing silently in solidarity with us, thereby bearing witness to our suffering. To the extent that this is true, those responsible for developing and promoting standards of professionalism for health care professionals need to query if one can be a professional 'X' and not be compassionate. If the answer is 'One must be compassionate to be a professional helper' teaching compassion becomes a critical responsibility of parents, educators, and clinicians. Perhaps more importantly, if compassion is an essential human trait, educating for compassion is a responsibility of all those forming the characters of the next generation.

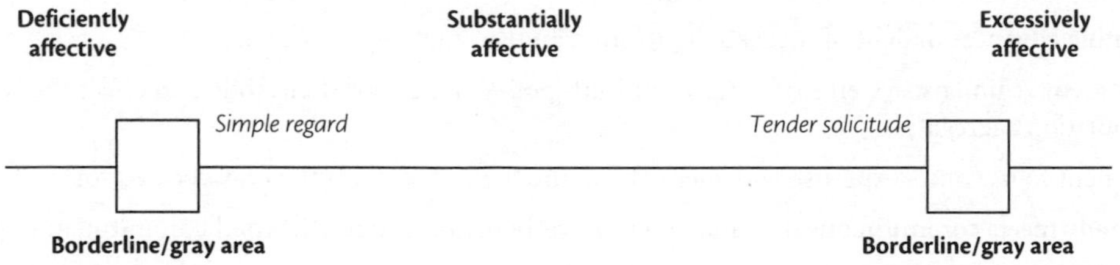

Figure 20.1 Professional caregivers who are deficient in compassion or excessive (prone to burnout) should be counseled about the need for remediation.

In an effort to restore compassion to the center of morality and religion, Armstrong[51] convened a worldwide committee of prominent individuals from all faith communities.

Armstrong counsels that the attempt to become a compassionate human being is a struggle that will last until our dying hour. She recommends putting into practice the following three steps at least once every day:

1. Resolve to act in accordance with the *positive* version of the Golden Rule: 'Treat others as you would wish to be treated yourself.'
2. Resolve to fulfill the *negative* version of the Golden Rule: 'Do not do to others what you would not like them to do to you.'
3. Make an effort to change your thought patterns; if you find yourself indulging in a bout of anger or self-pity, try to channel all that negative energy into a more kindly direction.

While a full exploration of how best to develop compassion is beyond the scope of this chapter we would be remiss not to direct the reader to Armstrong's *Twelve Steps to a Compassionate Life* or to visit the website, http://charterforcompassion.org

The accompanying box illustrates a strategy to teach the art of compassionate presence.

Compassion inventory

When meeting informally with case managers at a comprehensive cancer centre to talk about ethical challenges one young woman surprised the group by saying that her greatest challenge was never knowing when she had 'done enough.' 'We have a real commitment to excellence here ... but my daily caseload is always larger than I can do well. Every day I have to decide whether to stay late to meet the needs of our patients or leave on time and meet my obligations to family and others.' Since the case managers were literally the conduit to resources vitally needed by patients and families to meet valued outcomes the case managers were rightfully troubled by not being able to 'be all things to all people.' A similar challenge presents with compassion. How do any of us know if we are sufficiently compassionate? And when being compassionate exerts a heavy price what trade-offs are appropriate? Given that we have duties to self, to family and to our 'neighbours,' especially the most vulnerable, how can we balance self/family/other care obligations?

Characteristics of compassionate individuals

1. *Tender heart:* routinely moved by the needs of the most vulnerable to the degree that our spirits are afflicted. We talk about the needs and suffering of others, we grieve, we lament; we experience and demonstrate the ability to be moved by the plight of humans in need
2. *Compassion compels us to action:* prayer, donation of time/presence, expertise, money. We go to bed tired each night having tried to 'make a difference'
3. *Authenticity:* you know it when you see it. As one of Walker's patients stated, 'It is hard to describe, but you just know when someone has it.' Do the people who know me well believe that I genuinely care about the most vulnerable? Rephrased, is there enough evidence to convict me if I am on trial for being compassionate ... or if our facilities were on trial for being compassionate? At the very least:

- We should be knowledgeable about and moved by the plight of *some* others in need
- A portion of our interest, time, expertise, money should be invested in redressing local and global injustices.

Compassion fatigue

Halifax[21] describes five challenges in compassionate caregiving: burnout, secondary trauma, moral distress, horizontal hostility, and structural violence. Compassion fatigue is a state of deep physical, emotional, and spiritual exhaustion accompanied by acute emotional pain experienced by those helping people in distress.[52–55] It is an extreme state of tension and preoccupation with the suffering of those being helped to the degree that it is traumatizing for the helper. Symptoms of compassion fatigue include feeling anxious, sad, depressed, or fatigued as a result of sleeplessness.

How would you describe yourself?

Compassion fatigued   Energized to heal
1———-2———-3———-4———-5———-6———-7

How would you describe the colleagues/team with whom you work?

Compassion fatigued   Energized to heal
1———-2———-3———-4———-5———-6———-7

'Standing with'

When it is not possible to alleviate another's distress or suffering, compassion 'stands with' another and thereby recognizes the individual as a valuable human being and the distress s/he is experiencing. A nurse colleague recently recounted a story about her early days as a newly-graduated registered nurse. Invited to work in the office of a general practice physician with a large practice to inner city indigent patients, she routinely encountered patients and families struggling with insurmountable problems linked to poverty, disease, and injury, and violence. As weeks turned to months she was finding it harder and harder to come to work because the weight of problems she couldn't fix and the concomitant heavy burden of human suffering were eroding her vitality and energy. Paradoxically, her physician colleague seemed energized by the very conditions that were draining her. He literally bounded into work each new day and seemed tireless in his efforts to heal. Finally, she confronted him with what she was feeling and asked his secret for not being overwhelmed by the suffering of those he was trying to help. She said he looked directly at me and chided me for appropriating the 'life journeys' of our patients. He said we do them violence when we make their narratives our own. And so she learned to be moved by the plight of the suffering she saw all around her without allowing it to overwhelm her. She used human suffering to call forth her best healing efforts and began to make peace with the truth taught by Buddha and others that life is suffering.

Strategies to prevent compassion fatigue are multiple. Obviously we can't give what we don't have, therefore, cultivating the capacity for compassionate presence begins with excellent self-care. A speaker recently told her audience to think of themselves as a house with four rooms: Physical, mental/emotion, social, and spiritual.

She then counselled everyone to be sure to spend time in each of the four rooms every day:

- *Physical self-care:* diet, exercise, time-outs with deep breathing
- *Mental/emotional self-care:* positive thinking, humour, developing and expressing a spirit of gratitude
- *Social:* supportive relationships both personal and professional
- *Spiritual self-care:* prayer/meditation/contemplation, nature, the arts.

Dunn[56] writes that nurses will grow and thrive if they understand how to self-generate vigour as compassion energy, preventing compassion fatigue or burnout. In addition to good self-care, it's important to seek strategies in the work place to prevent compassion fatigue. The ability to debrief stressful experiences with colleagues is essential as is the need to step back and evaluate work assignments. Sometimes we need a trusted colleague to help us assess how well we are respecting professional boundaries. Sometimes new opportunities for professional development help us to identify strategies to facilitate needed change. Boyle[57] calls for a national agenda to counter compassion fatigue and describes the need to support nurses who witness tragedy and workplace interventions to confront compassion fatigue.

Conclusion

Our research and experience lead us to second the Dalai Lama's[58] assertion, 'Love and compassion are necessities, not luxuries. Without them, humanity cannot survive.'

Spiritual care begins with compassionate healing presence. Since competence in spiritual care is now mandated for all professional caregivers developing the virtue of compassion and the art of compassionate presence are priorities.

References

1 Friedman, A. (2010). Secret shopper. *J Am Med Ass* **304**(19): 2103–4.

2 Aita, V. (2000). Science and compassion: vacillation in nursing ideas 1940's–1960. *Sch Inq Nurs Pract* **14**(2): 115–41.

3 Benner, P. (1998). When health care becomes a commodity: the need for compassionate strangers. In: J. Kilner, R. Orr, J. Shelley (eds) *Changing the Face of Healthcare: A Christian Appraisal of Managed Care, Resource Allocation, and Patient Caregiver Relationships*, pp. 119–35. William B. Erdman's Publishing Co., Grand Rapids.

4 Cherry, M.J. (2001). Foundations of the culture wars: compassion, love, and human dignity. *Christ Bioeth* **7**(3): 299–316.

5 Graber, D.R., Mitcham, M.D. (2004). Compassionate clinicians: take patient care beyond the ordinary. *Holist Nurs Pract* **18**(2): 87–94.

6 Tuckett, A.G. (1998). An ethic of the fitting: a conceptual framework for nursing practice. *Nurs Inq* **5**(4): 220–7.

7 Tuckett, A.G. (1999). Nursing practice: compassionate deception and the Good Samaritan. *Nurs Eth* **6**(5): 383–9.

8 Sturgeon, D. (2010). 'Have a nice day': Consumerism, compassion, and health care. *Br J Nurs* **19**(16): 1052–4.

9 Schulz, R., Hebert, R.S., Dew, M.A., Brown, S.L., Scheier, M.F., Beach, S.R., *et al.* (2007). Patient suffering and caregiver compassion: New opportunities for research, practice, and policy. *Gerontologist* **47**(1): 4–13.

10 Van der Cingel, M. (2009). Compassion and professional care: exploring the domain. *Nurs Philos* **10**: 124–36.

11 Armstrong, A., Parsons, S., Barker, P. (2000). An inquiry into mortal virtues, especially compassion in psychiatric nurses: findings from a Delphi study. *J Psychiatr Ment Health Nurs* **7**(4): 297–305.

12 Georges, J.J., Grypdonck, M., De Casterle, B. (2002). Being a palliative care nurse in an academic hospital: a qualitative study about nurses' perceptions of palliative care nursing. *J Clin Nurs* **11**: 785–93.

13 Morse, J.M. (1991). Approaches to qualitative-quantitative methodological triangulation. *J Nurs Res* **40**: 120–3.

14 Reynolds, W.J., Scott, B. (2000). Do nurses and other professional helpers normally display much empathy? *J Adv Nurs* **31**(1): 226–34.

15 Reynolds, W.J., Scott, B. (1999). Empathy: a crucial component of the helping relationship. *J Psychiatr Ment Hlth Nurs* **6**: 363–70.

16 Wear, D., Zareconi, J. (2007). Can compassion be taught? Let's ask our students. *J Gen Intern Med* **23**(7): 948–53.

17 Young-Mason, J. (2002). Transmuting anger into compassion. *Clin Nurse Spec* **16**(5): 279–80.

18 Apker, J., Propp, K.M., Zabava-Ford, W.S., Hofmeister, N. (2006). Collaboration, credibility, compassion, and coordination: professional nurse communication skill sets in health care team interactions. *J Prof Nurs* **22**(3): 180–9.

19 Forsyth, A. (1998). Compassion. *Geriaction* **16**(1): 17–20.

20 Guinan, P. (2005). The Christian origin of medical compassion. *Natl Cathol Bioeth Q* **5**(2): 243–8.

21 Halifax, J. (2011). The precious necessity of compassion. *J Pain Symptom Manag* **41**(1): 146–52.

22 Jensen, K., Beck-Pettersson, S., Segesten, K. (1995). 'Catching my wavelength:' Perceptions of the excellent nurse. *Nurs Sci Q* **9**(3): 115–30.

23 Sanghavi, D.M. (2006). What makes for a compassionate patient-caregiver relationship? *Jt Comm J Qual Patient Saf* **32**(5): 283–92.

24 Santo-Novak, D. (1997). Older adults' descriptions of their role expectations of nursing. *J Gerontol Nurs* **25**(5): 11–16.

25 Reich, W. (1989). Speaking of suffering: A moral account of compassion. *Soundings*, **72**(1): 83–107.

26 Walker, W. (1996). *International Standard Bible Encyclopedia*. Biblesoft: Electronic Database Copyright. [Internet]. Available from: http://www.biblesoft.com

27 (2011). *The New Oxford American Dictionary*, 3rd edn. Oxford: Oxford University Press.

28 Steffen, P.R., Masters, K.S. (2005). Does compassion mediate the intrinsic religion-health relationship? *Ann Behav Med* **30**(3): 217–24.

29 Walker, M.S. (2009). *Compassion Within the Relationship Between the Nurse and the Older Adult Patient.* Ann Arbor: UMI Dissertation Services

30 Sethabouppha, H., Kane, C. (2005). Caring for the seriously mentally ill in Thailand: Buddhist family caregiving. *Arch Psychiatr Nurs* **19**(2): 44–57.

31 Jormsri, P., Kunaviktikul, W., Ketefian, S., Chaowalit, A. (2005). Moral competence in nursing practice. *Nurs Eth* **12**(6): 582–94.

32 von Dietze, E., Orb, A. (2000). Compassionate care: A moral dimension of nursing. *Nurs Inq* **7**(3): 166–74.

33 Johnston, B., Smith, L.N. (2006). Nurses' and patients' perceptions of expert palliative nursing care. *J Adv Nurs* **54**(6): 700–9.

34 London, M.R., Lundstedt, J. (2007). Families speak about end of life care. *J Nurs Care Qual* **22**(2): 152–8.

35 Jull, A. (2001). Compassion: a concept exploration. *Nurs Prax NZ*, **17**(1): 16–23.

36 Aita, V. (1995). Toward improved practice: formal prescriptions and informal expressions of compassion in American nursing during the 1950's. Doctoral dissertation, University of Nebraska, Dissertation Abstracts International.

37 Bradshaw, A. (2009). Measuring nursing care and compassion: the McDonalised nurse? *J Med Eth* **35**: 465–8.

38 Clara, A., Merina, J., Mateos, E., Ysa, A., Roman, B., Vidal-Barraquer, F. (2006). The vascular surgeon facing clinical ethical dilemmas (the VASCUETHICS Study): 'V'-shaped association between compassionate attitudes and professional seniority. *Eur J Vasc Endovasc Surg* **31**(6): 594–9.

39 Hutnik, N. (2005). Toward holistic, compassionate, professional care: using a cultural lens to examine the practice of contemporary psychotherapy in the west. *Contemp Fam Ther* **27**(3): 383–402.

40 Rogers, C.R. (1951). *Client-centered Therapy*. Boston: Houghton-Mifflin.

41 Rogers, C.R. (1961). *On Becoming a Person*. Boston: Houghton-Mifflin.

42 Hem, M.H., Heggen, K. (2004). Is compassion essential to nursing practice? *Contemp Nurse* **17**(12): 19–31.

43 Ruiz, P.O., Vallejos, R.M. (1999). The role of compassion in moral education. *J Moral Educ* **28**(1): 5–17.

44 Nussbaum, G.B. (2003). Spirituality in critical care: Patient comfort and satisfaction (Review). *Crit Care Nurs Q* **26**(3): 214–20.

45 Van Hooft, S. (1998). The meaning of suffering. *Hastings Cent Rep* **28**(5): 13–19.

46 Puchalski, C., Ferrell, B., Virani, R., Otis-Green, S., Baird, P. et al. (2009). Improving the quality of spiritual care as a dimension of palliative care: The report of the consensus conference. *J Palliat Med* **12**(10): 885–904.

47 Rahner, K. (1971). How to receive a sacrament and mean it. *Theol Dig* **19**: 229.

48 Erikson, E., Erickson, J. (1997). *The Life Cycle Completed*. New York: W. W. Norton,

49 Fish, S., Kelly, J.A. (1978). *Spiritual Care: The Nurse's Role*. Downer's Grove: InterVarsity Press.

50 Taylor, C. (1997). *The Morality Internal to the Practice of Nursing*. Ann Arbor: UMI Dissertation Services.

51 Armstrong, K. (2010). *Twelve Steps to a Compassionate Life*. New York: Knopf.

52 Figley, C. (2002). *Treating Compassion Fatigue*. New York: Brunner-Routledge.

53 Sabo, B.M. (2006). Compassion fatigue and nursing work: can we accurately capture the consequences of caring work? *Int J Nurs Pract* **12**(3): 136–42.

54 Coetzee, S.K., Klopper, H.C. (2009). Compassion fatigue within nursing practice: A concept analysis. *Nurs Health Sci* **12**: 235–43.

55 Lombardo, B. (2011). Compassion fatigue: a nurse's primer. *Online J Issues Nurs* **16**(1): 3.

56 Dunn, D.J. (2009). The intentionality of compassion energy. *Holist Nurs Pract* **23**(4): 222–9.

57 Boyle, D.A. (2011). Countering compassion fatigue: a requisite nursing agenda. *Online J Issues Nurs*, **16**(1): 2.

58 His Holiness the Dalai Lama. (1992). *Mind and Life Meeting*. Presentation in Dharamsala, India.

CHAPTER 21

Dignity: a novel path into the spiritual landscape of the human heart

Shane Sinclair and Harvey M. Chochinov

Introduction

The importance of dignity when facing a serious health issue has been attested to by patients across faith traditions, cultures, and recently, empirical science.[1–5] While understandings of what constitutes dignity vary widely and, in some instances, are diametrically opposed, dignity remains a common thread that weaves across the human tapestry, intertwining the sacred and the secular. The universality of dignity does not only pertain to matters of philosophical debate, but has been identified as an important construct impacting individual health, a commonality that it shares with the spirituality and health literature. While the precise meaning of dignity and spirituality remains elusive, their centrality to human experience and purpose is perhaps most evident in the passion evoked when their importance is challenged. Spirituality and dignity also share the commonality of representing nascent fields of empirical research, both producing an emerging evidence base with compelling results.[6–10] While spirituality and dignity are vital domains across the trajectory of human health, their importance seems to be most evident at the end-of-life, where both are often appealed upon in discourses of dying well.

Dignity: a sacred pillar of spirituality and health

The notion of dignity is of particular interest to the field of spirituality as it is not only within this domain that the concept of dignity was first conceptualized, but where it continues to be an area of relevance. While conjectures of spirituality as an inherent feature of humanity—herein subsuming dignity within this domain—has been criticized as disrespective of individuals who do not identify themselves as spiritual,[11] recent research has demonstrated that when spirituality is broadly understood as relating to human meaning and purpose, it is a term that even atheists find acceptable.[12] The conceptualization of spirituality as a universal facet of humanity was further implied by a recent expert forum, which defined spirituality as, 'the aspect of humanity that refers to the way individuals seek and express meaning and purpose and the way they experience their connectedness to the moment, to self, others, nature, and the significant or sacred.'[13] While many definitions of spirituality do not explicitly mention dignity, as is also the case with other interrelated terms such as hope, peace of mind, and God, its centrality is often implied. Dignity has been defined as the quality or state of being worthy, honoured, or esteemed,[14] and while not an exclusively spiritual term, the reciprocity is difficult to deny, as 'Spirituality has to do with respecting the inherent value and dignity of all persons, regardless of their health status.'[15]

While dignity can be inferred to reside within the definitional spectrum of spirituality, there have been a limited number of empirical studies investigating its specific place within this particular landscape. Chochinov and colleagues reported a positive correlation between spiritual meaning and the conservation of dignity among a sample of patients at the end-of-life.[1] Indian nurses identified spiritual care as the preferred modality in conserving dignity among the terminally ill;[16] and a connection to a spiritual or religious practice or community was identified as positively preserving palliative patients' sense of dignity.[17,18] The importance of dignity within the spiritual domain is underscored by a recent recommendation, that dignity, along with social justice and compassion, be considered a universal construct to unify, codify, and evaluate spirituality-based research.[19] While the specific nature and relationship between spirituality and related constructs, such as dignity, meaning, purpose, quality of life, and existential wellbeing is difficult to discern, this seems less important than recognizing the overlap and reciprocity that exists between them, as an individual's spirituality seems to both inform and be informed by an individual's sense of dignity. In this chapter, dignity is construed as a novel path, among others, to guide health care professionals into the ubiquitous, profound landscape of spirituality.

A history of dignity

Dignity has a long and rich history extending across humanity, traversing cultures, worldviews, ethics, faiths, and politics—in essence, addressing a central feature of what it means to be human. While dignity is variably defined—a feature that is shared with the term spirituality[20,21]—it nonetheless remains a core concept in desire for hastened death (DHD) discussions, statements on human rights, and doctrinal statements of faith.[22,23]

The origins of dignity can be traced back to antiquity, being rooted in the stoic literature and specifically in the biblical account of humanity being created in the image of God.[22,24,25] The notion of humanity being made in the *imago Dei* or image of God is a universal concept within the Jewish tradition, pertaining to every individual, compared to other religions of antiquity, who ascribed dignity exclusively to the kings.[24] The image of God was a holistic concept that encompassed not only the metaphysical, but the psychological, social, and physical domains, including so-called 'lower duties,' such as toileting.[24]

Christianity further expounded the teaching that human dignity was inherently linked to the *imago Dei*, however, with some important variants including:

- A more metaphysical focus
- A specific quality of Jesus Christ, rather than humanity as a whole
- A facet of humanity that was discovered through redemption, rather than an innate quality embedded and active within each individual.[24]

Despite some variations, the *imago Dei* was reinterpreted as a divine spark, which was heavily shrouded in the shadow of original sin.[26] While contemporary Christian theologians construe the *imago Dei*, as it relates to dignity, in a less redemptive and metaphysical tone, it remains a concept that is predominately rooted in the spiritual domain.

Ethics: the dignity of reason

A second significant ontological shift within the discourse of dignity occurred in the field of human ethics at the time of the Enlightenment in the applied ethics of Immanual Kant and his categorical imperative prohibiting the use of persons as a means to an end.[27] According to Kant, dignity was not based on merit, teleology, social, or political status, but in humanity's unique ability to reason between good and evil.[22] Human dignity, according to Kant, was no longer exclusively rooted in the *imago Dei*, but in moral capacity and action.[24] A second important ontological shift related to Kantian thought was ascribing 'dignity' to all rational individuals, a retraction from the universal *imago Dei* notion of dignity pertaining to all individuals, regardless of their rational capacity.[22,28]

Kant's identification of dignity primarily within the loci of reason, rather than *the imago Dei* of humanity perpetuated two distinct divisions of dignity: basic dignity and personal dignity. Basic dignity, while being rooted in humanity's *imago Dei*, evolved into a more secularized form post-Kant, anchored in the fundamental worth of all rational humans regardless of theological belief. While basic dignity expanded beyond a strict religious focus, it remained a fundamental construct of humanity, regardless of worldview. While the metaphysical and ontological starting points vary, the end point remains consistent- worth is a fundamental right by nature of being a human being, a belief that provided the basic building blocks for contemporary statements of human rights.[29] While dignity's centrality to human rights is perhaps most notable in the United Nations Universal Declaration of Human Rights (1948), which is predicated on the 'inherent dignity ... of all members of the human family,' it is also a fundamental concept in the constitutions of Mexico (1917), Ireland (1937), Cuba (1940), the European Convention on Human Rights (1950); UNESCO's Universal Declaration on bioethics and Human Rights (2005), and the Declaration of Helsinki (2008).[22,23]

While basic dignity remains a largely unifying feature of dignity-related discussions, the opposite is evident in discussions related to the concept of personal dignity. Personal dignity has been described as being heavily grounded in individual autonomy and personal choice—an amorphous construct that depends on the social circumstances, personal goals, and issues at hand.[30,31] Whereas the ontological starting point for basic dignity is rooted within in a particular meta-narrative of humanity as a whole, the genesis of personal dignity is rooted within each individual's specific narrative. Personal dignity, which broadly relates to dignity as defined and determined by the individual, is prominent in contemporary western societies,[32] providing the modus operandi of the death with dignity movement, which frequently equates the term with autonomy.[25,29,30] On the one hand, (personal) dignity is invoked as a fundamental principle in the right for a hastened death, while being heralded as a fundamental principle that forbids the provision of a hastened death by its opponents. As Pullman suggests, 'Indeed it is not uncommon to find those on either side of an ethical debate invoking some consideration of human dignity in support of their contrary conclusions.'[29] While contemporary ethical conjectures of dignity are riddled with opacity and complexity—similar to spirituality and its multitude of meanings—it is here that their importance is most pronounced.

The importance of dignity in palliative care

While the importance of dignity across the trajectory of life is of interest to the fields of religion, philosophy, spirituality, and more holistic approaches to human health, empirical research on dignity has focused primarily on end-of-life care, where its importance is vital. While attending to the biomedical needs of dying individuals is critical in achieving quality end-of-life care, the importance of psycho-spiritual issues are increasingly recognized as paramount. Addressing spiritual concerns at the end-of-life, including those related to dignity, have been formerly endorsed by leading health organizations[33,34] and within the standards of practice of various professional organizations, despite the fact that health care professionals typically feel they lack the necessary confidence and training.[35–41] While spiritual concerns have been endorsed at an organizational and professional level, their importance should ultimately be determined by patients themselves. Singer *et al.*, conducted an extensive qualitative study exploring what domains of end-of-life care where most important to cancer patients. These included:

- Receiving adequate pain and symptom management
- Avoiding inappropriate prolongation of dying
- Achieving a sense of spiritual peace
- Relieving burden
- Strengthening relationships with loved ones.[42]

Kuhl's research focusing on self-reported needs of dying patients reported similar findings, as issues of meaning and purpose were as vital as meeting biomedical needs[43]—a conclusion which has been confirmed by others.[15,36,44–50] Likewise, the McGill Quality of Life Questionnaire's existential subscales have been repeatedly shown to be at least as important as any of the other subscales in measuring overall quality of life among palliative care patients.[51] These and other findings caused expert members of a recent consensus project on quality spiritual care at the end-of-life to recommend that spiritual distress be considered a patient vital sign that needs to be routinely screened.[13]

While the concept of dignity, particularly 'personal dignity', is contentiously held by advocates with differing viewpoints regarding physician assisted suicide and euthanasia, its importance in mitigating end-of-life distress is undeniable. In studies that asked physicians the reasons that their patients had selected euthanasia or physician assisted suicide (PAS), loss of dignity represented the most common response, being identified in 50–60% of reported cases.[52–4] The state of Oregon has collected data from patients who ended their life in accordance with the states Death with Dignity Act, which legalized physician assisted suicide in 1997. In 2009, consistent with 11 previous years of reporting, the most frequently identified concerns identified by patients who received PAS were: loss of autonomy (96.6%), loss of dignity (91.5%), and decreasing ability to participate in activities that made life enjoyable (86.4%).[55,56] Based on these and other studies,[57,58] desire for hastened death (DHD) seems to be strongly related to existential and spiritual distress. In a related study, patients who had good social and family supports, and reported modest levels of spiritual wellbeing and were able find meaning in life, were less likely to express DHD.[59] A study of 379 terminally ill cancer patients found that while 62.8% felt that euthanasia or PAS should be legal, only 5.8% of patients indicated that they would ask for it right away, suggesting a difference between anticipatory needs and actual needs.[60] While DHD occurs in 7–9% of patients with advanced disease, this number increases significantly among patients who experience hopelessness, a sense of meaninglessness, and meet criteria for an anxiety or depressive disorder.[61–63] Breitbart *et al*., discovered that DHD was associated with clinical depression and hopelessness in a sample of 92 palliative care patients,[64] while Chochinov found that hopelessness was more highly correlated to suicidal ideation than depression amongst a group of terminally ill patients.[65]

The dignity model: an empirical framework for eliciting patients' spirituality

While disentangling aspects of dignity from other inter-related concepts such as wellbeing, meaning, hope, and quality of life, is conceptually difficult and temporally variable, empirical research has focused on specific items that directly contribute to a sense of dignity. A qualitative study explored fifty dying patients' understanding of dignity,[5] providing a basis for a conceptual model of dignity (Table. 21.1). While 'spirituality specific' factors were identified,[4] when spirituality is broadly conceived as an overarching domain that informs and is affected by the physical, psychological, and social domains of health, the Dignity Model includes various items falling within the purview of personal spirituality. These items or themes include hopefulness, continuity of self, acceptance, resilience,; living 'in the moment', being a burden to others, and care tenor.[8]

This holistic understanding of spirituality, underpinning all dimensions of humanity, has been embraced by contemporary philosophers and various religious traditions.[66] Participants in

Table 21.1 Major dignity categories, themes and sub-themes

Illness related concerns	*Dignity conserving repertoire*	*Social dignity inventory*
Level of independence[1,2]	**Dignity conserving perspectives**	**Privacy boundaries**[20]
Cognitive acuity[9]	Continuity of self[4,11]	
Functional capacity[8]	Role preservation[13]	Social support[21,22]
Symptom distress	Generativity/legacy[15,16]	
Physical distress[3]	Maintenance of pride[12]	Care tenor[25]
Psychological distress[5,6]	Hopefulness[14]	
Medical uncertainty[7]	Autonomy/control[19]	Burden to others[18]
	Acceptance[24]	
	Resilience/fighting spirit[23]	
death anxiety[8]	**Dignity conserving practices**	Aftermath concerns
	Living in the moment[10]	
	Maintaining normalcy[10]	
	Seeking spiritual comfort[17]	

‡Superscripts correspond to the PDI item number that derives from each individual theme and sub-theme.

Reprinted from Chochinov H et al, The patient dignity inventory: A novel way of measuring dignity-related distress in palliative care, *Journal of Pain and Symptom Management*, Volume 36, Issue 6, pp. 559–71, 2008 with permission from Elsevier.

a study of a palliative care interdisciplinary team (n = 20) conceptualized spiritual care as being embedded in all aspects of care, especially the manner in which such care was delivered.[67] While the degree to which specific items relate to spirituality will inevitably vary among patients and practitioners, the Dignity Model is envisioned as a therapeutic map, providing direction for care that encompasses the physical, psychological, social, and spiritual domains. The dignity conserving repertoire, consisting of patients' psychological make-up and spiritual beliefs, is comprised of two major themes—dignity-conserving perspectives and dignity conserving practices. Dignity conserving practices involve 'living in the moment' (being orientated in the present); 'maintain normalcy' (being able to continue, in the face of health-related issues, with regular routines); and 'seeking spiritual comfort' (being able to find solace in ones spiritual beliefs and experiences). Dignity conserving perspectives include [4]:

- Continuity of self: the sense that essence of who one is continues and remains intact.
- Role preservation: an ability to continue functioning in usual roles as a way of maintaining congruence with prior views of oneself
- Generativity/legacy: the sense that one will leave behind something lasting and transcendent of death
- Maintaining pride: the ability to maintain positive self-regard in the face of diminishing independence
- Maintaining hope: an ability to see life as enduring, with sustained meaning or purpose
- Autonomy/control: the sense that one can influence or direct one's life circumstances.
- Acceptance: the internal process of resigning oneself to changing life circumstances, in the attempt to maintain one's sense of dignity

- Resilience/fighting spirit: the mental determination some patients exercise to overcome their illness-related concerns or optimize their quality of life

A cross-sectional study of 213 terminally ill cancer patients, being cared for at home and within a palliative care unit, revealed that loss of dignity was a concern, with 46% of patients indicating they had at least some, or occasional dignity-related concerns.[31] Patients with a fractured sense of dignity were reported as more likely to:

- have a desire for hastened death
- have a loss of will to live
- be depressed
- be hopeless
- be anxious
- have heightened dependency needs.

In a subsequent study of 211 palliative care patients, a cross-sectional quantitative approach was employed to validate 22 items derived from the Dignity Model.[3] Patients were asked to indicate the extent to which each item contributed to their sense of dignity. Nearly 90% indicated that 'not being treated with respect or understanding' and 'feeling a burden to others' negatively influenced their overall sense of dignity. Patients acknowledging a religious affiliation were significantly more likely to identify difficulty with acceptance and not having a meaningful spiritual life as dignity-related concerns, compared with those who did not acknowledge a religious affiliation. It seems that spiritual wellbeing, particularly the meaning-purpose dimension of spirituality, might stave off end-of-life despair, perhaps providing a foundation of basic dignity which reinforces personal dignity.[59] The possibility of religious or spiritual beliefs actuating a sense of basic dignity is further supported by a study investigating the attitudes of 379 palliative cancer patients toward the legalization of PAS or euthanasia. This study found a negative correlation between religious beliefs and requests for hastened death.[62] Another study reported that belief in an afterlife was associated with lower levels of hopelessness, desire for death, and suicidal ideation.[68] As such, the role of spirituality, dignity and the wish to sustain ones personal existence has been empirically articulated.

Conclusion

While what constitutes dignity is individually determined, its centrality in the search for meaning and purpose, especially as it relates to various facets of health, is becoming increasingly apparent. Empirical research on the impact of dignity as it affects various aspects of human health has begun to demonstrate a strong reciprocal relationship between the construct of dignity and the domain of spirituality. Cassel posited that suffering has its source in challenges that threaten the intactness of the self, whether in the form of physical symptoms or psycho-spiritual distress.[69] Whether in relation to suffering or health in general, the interrelated constructs of dignity and spirituality constitute an important salve, which can preserve the human spirit. The pathway to healing will depend upon ones spiritual orientation, and whether achieved through secular means or a connection with a high power or being, is a critical element of human health. The implications and effect of dignity conserving care in clinical practice will be discussed in detail in Chapter 40.

References

1 Chochinov, H., Hassard, T., McClement, S., Hack, T., Kristjanson, L., Harlos, M., *et al.* (2009). The landscape of distress in the terminally ill. *J Pain Sympt Manag* **38**(5): 641–9.

2 Chochinov, H., Hassard, T., McClement, S., Hack, T., Kristjanson, L., Harlos, M., *et al.* (2008). The patient dignity inventory: a novel way of measuring dignity-related distress in palliative care. *J Pain Sympt Manag* **36**(6): 559–71.

3 Chochinov, H., Krisjanson, L., Hack, T., Hassard, T., McClement, S., Harlos, M. (2006). Dignity in the terminally ill: revisited. *J Palliat Med* **9**(3): 666–672.

4 Chochinov, H. (2006). Dying, dignity, and new horizons in palliative end-of-life care. *CA* **56**(2): 84–103.

5 Chochinov, H., Hack, T., McClement, S., Kristjanson, L., Harlos, M. (2002). Dignity in the terminally ill: a developing empirical model. *Soc Sci Med* 54: 433–43.

6 Larson, D. (1993). *The Faith Factor: an Annotated Bibliography of Systematic Reviews and Clinical Research on Spiritual Subjects.* Rockville: National Institute for Healthcare Research.

7 Puchalski, C. (2002). Spirituality and end-of-life care: a time for listening and caring. *J Palliat Med* **5**(2): 289–94.

8 Sinclair, S., Pereira, J., Raffin, S. (2006). A thematic review of the spirituality literature within palliative care. *J Palliat Med* **9**(2): 464–79.

9 Flannelly, K., Weaver, A., Costa, K. (2004). A systematic review of religion and spirituality in three palliative care journals, 1990–1999. *J Palliat Care* **20**(1): 50–6.

10 Chiu, L., Emblen, J., van Hofwegen, L., Sawatzky, R., Meyerhoff, H. (2004). An integrative review of the concept of spirituality in the health sciences. *W J Nurs Res* **26**(4): 405–28.

11 Paley, J. (2008). Spirituality and nursing: a reductionist approach. *Nurs Philos* **9:** 3–18.

12 Smith-Stoner, M. (2007). End of life preferences for atheists. *J Palliat Med* **10**(4): 923–8.

13 Puchalski, C., Ferrell, B., Virani, R., Otis-Green, S., Baird, P., Bull, J., *et al.* (2009). Improving the quality of spiritual care as a dimension of palliative care: the report of the consensus conference. *J Palliat Med* **12**(10): 885–904.

14 Chochinov, H. (2002). Dignity conserving care: a new model for palliative care. *J Am Med Ass* **287**(17): 2253–60.

15 Puchalski, C. (2006). *A Time for Listening and Caring:* Spirituality and the Care of the Chronically Ill and Dying. New York: Oxford University Press.

16 Doorenbos, A., Wilson, S., Coenen, A., Borse, N. (2006). Dignified dying: a phenomenon and actions among nurses in India. *Int Nurs Rev* **53:** 28–33.

17 Daaleman, T.P., VandeCreek, L. (2000). Placing religion and spirituality in end-of-life care. *J Am Med Ass* **284:** 2514–17.

18 Holland, J.C., Passik, S., Kash, K.M., Russak, S.M., Gronert, M.K., Sison, A., *et al.* (1999). The role of religious and spiritual beliefs in coping with malignant melanoma. *Psycho-oncol* **8:** 14–26.

19 Pesut, B., Fowler, M., Reimer-Kirkham, S., Johnson-Taylor, E., Sawatzky, R. (2009). Particularizing spirituality in points of tension: enriching the discourse. *Nurs Inq* **16**(4): 337–46.

20 Rose, S. (2001). Is the term 'spirituality' a word that everyone uses, but nobody knows what anyone means by it? *J Contemp Religion* **16**(2): 193–207.

21 Macklin, R. (2003). Dignity is a useless concept. *Br Med J* **327:**1419–20.

22 Hayry, M. (2004). Another look at dignity. *Cambridge Q Hlth Care Eth* **13:** 7–14.

23 Harmon, S. (2009). Of plants and people. *Eur Mol Biol Org Rep* **10**(9): 946–8.

24 Barilan, Y.M. (2009). From imago dei in the Jewish-Christian traditions to human dignity in contemporary Jewish law. *Kennedy Inst Eth J* **19**(3): 231–59.

25 Pullman, D. (1999). The ethics of autonomy and dignity in long-term care. *Canad J Aging* **18**(1): 26–46.

26 Merton, T. (1994). *Conjectures of a Guilty Bystander*. New York: Bantam.

27 Rothhaar, M. (2010). Human dignity and human rights in bioethics: the Kantian approach. *Med Hlth Care Philos* **13**(3): [Epub ahead of print].

28 Schroeder, D. (2008). Dignity: two riddles and four concepts. *Cambridge Q Healthcare Eth* 17: 230–8.

29 Pullman D. (2004). Death, dignity, and moral nonsense. *J Palliat Care* **20**(3): 171–7.

30 Byock, I. (2010). Dying with Dignity. *Hastings Centre Rep* **40**(2): 3–3.

31 Chochinov, H., Hack, T., Hassard, T., Kristjanson, L., McClement, S., Harlos, M. (2002). Dignity in the terminally ill: a cross-sectional cohort study. *Lancet* **360**: 2026–30.

32 Walters, G. (2004). Is there such a thing as a good death? *Palliat Med* **18**: 404–8.

33 Field, M.J., Cassel, C.K. (1997). *Approaching Death: Improving Care at the End of Life*. Washington DC: National Academy Press, for the Institute of Medicine.

34 World Health Organization. (2007). *Definition of Palliative Care*. Geneva: WHO.

35 Chochinov, H.M., Cann, B.J. (2005). Interventions to enhance spiritual aspects of dying. *J Palliat Med* **8**: 103–15.

36 Daaleman, T., Usher, B., Williams, S., Rawlings, J., Hanson, L. (2008). An exploratory study of spiritual care at the end of life. *Ann Fam Med* **6**(5): 406–11.

37 McEwen, M. (2005). Spiritual nursing care: state of the art. *Holist Nurs Pract* **19**:161–8.

38 Meyer, C.L. (2003). How effectively are nurse educators preparing students to provide spiritual care? *Nurse Educator* **28**:185–90.

39 Nolan, P., Crawford, P. (1997). Towards a rhetoric of spirituality in mental health care. *J Adv Nurs* **26**: 289–94.

40 Pesut, B. (2003). Developing spirituality in the curriculum: worldviews, intrapersonal connectedness, interpersonal connectedness. *Nurs Educ Perspect* **24**: 290–4.

41 Thomsen, R.J. (1998). Spirituality in medical practice. *Arch Dermatol* **134**:1443–6.

42 Singer, P.A., Martin, D.K., Kelner, M. (1999). Quality end-of-life care: patients' perspectives. *J Am Med Ass* **281**: 163–8.

43 Kuhl, D. (2002). *What Dying People Want*. Toronto: Anchor.

44 Bailey, M., Moran, S., Graham, M. (2009). Creating a spiritual tapestry: nurses' experiences of delivering spiritual care to patients in an Irish hospice. *Int J Palliat Nurs* **15**(1): 42–8.

45 Cherlin, E., Schulman-Green, D., McCorkle, R., Johnson-Hurzeler, R., Bradley, E. (2004). Family perceptions of clinicians' outstanding practices in end-of-life care. *J Palliat Care* **20**(2): 113–16.

46 Hinshaw, D. (2005). Spiritual issues in surgical palliative care. *Surg Clin N Am* **85**: 257–72.

47 Kearney, M. (2000). *A Place of Healing*. Oxford: Oxford University Press.

48 Moadel, A., Morgan, C., Fatone, A., Grennan, J., Carter, J., Laruffa, G., *et al.* (1999). Seeking meaning and hope: self-reported spiritual and existential needs among an ethnically-diverse cancer patient population. *Psycho-oncol* **8**: 378–85.

49 Sulmasy, D. (2006). Spiritual issues in the care of dying patients. *J Am Med Ass* **296**(11): 1385–92.

50 White, G. (2000). An inquiry into the concepts of spirituality and spiritual care. *Int J Palliat Nurs* **4**(3): 393–412.

51 Cohen, S.R., Mount, B.M., Tomas, J.J., Mount, L.F. (1996). Existential wellbeing is an important determinant of quality of life. Evidence from the McGill Quality of Life Questionnaire. *Palliat Med* **77**: 576–86.

52 Meier, D.E., Emmons, C.A., Wallenstein, S., Wallenstein, S., Quill, T., Morrison, R.S., *et al.* (1998). A national survey of physician-assisted suicide and euthanasia in the United States. *N Engl J Med* **338**(17): 1193–201.

53 Van der Maas, P.J., van der Wal, G., Haverkate, I., de Graaff, C., Kester, J., Onwuteaka-Philipsen, B., *et al.* (1996). Euthanasia, physician-assisted suicide, and other medical practices involving the end of life in the Netherlands, 1990–1995. *N Engl J Med* **335**: 1699–705.

54 Van der Maas, P.J., Van Delden, J.J.M., Pijnenborg, L., Looman, C.W.N. (1991). Euthansia and other medical decisions concerning the end of life. *Lancet* **338**: 669–74.

55 Department of Human Services. (2009). *Summary of the State of Oregon's Death with Dignity Act. 2009*. Available at: http://public.health.oregon.gov/ProviderPartnerResources/EvaluationResearch/DeathwithDignityAct/Pages/ar-index.aspx (accessed 3 November 2011).

56 Sullivan, A., Hedberg, K., Fleming, D. (2000). Legalized physician-assisted suicide in Oregon: The second year. *N Engl J Med* **342**(8): 598–604.

57 Hudson, P.L., Kristjanson, L.J., Ashby, M., Kelly, B., Schofield, P., Hudson, R., *et al.* (2006). Desire for hastened death in patients with advanced disease and the evidence base of clinical guidelines: a systematic review. *Palliat Med* **20**(7): 693–701.

58 Breitbart, W., Rosenfield, B.D., Passik, S.D. (1996). Interest in physician-assisted suicide among ambulatory HIV-infected patients. *Am J Psychiat* **153**: 238–42.

59 McClain, C., Rosenfeld, B., Breitbart, W. (2003). Effect of spiritual wellbeing on end-of-life despair in terminally-ill cancer patients. *Lancet* **361**:1603–7.

60 Chochinov, H.M., Wilson, K.G., Enns, M., Mowchun, N., Lander, S., Levitt, M., *et al.* (1995). Desire for death in the terminally ill. *Am J Psychiat* **152**(8): 1185–91.

61 Jones, J.M., Huggins, M.A., Rydall, A.C., Rodin, G.M. (2003). Symptomatic distress, hopelessness, and the desire for hastened death in hospitalized cancer patients. *J Psychosom Res* **55**: 411–18.

62 Wilson, K., Chochinov, H., McPherson, C., Kirko, M., Allard, P., Chary, S., *et al.* (2007). Desire for euthanasia or physician-assisted suicide in palliative cancer care. *Hlth Psychol***26**(3): 314–23.

63 Thompson, G., Chochinov,H.M. (2010). Reducing the potential for suffering in older adults with advanced cancer. *Palliat Support Care* **8**:83–93.

64 Breitbart, W., Rosenfeld, B., Pessin, H., Kaim, M., Funesti-Esch, J., Galietta, M., *et al.* (2000). Depression, hopelessness, and desire for hastened death in terminally ill patients with cancer. *J Am Med Ass* **284**(22): 2907–11.

65 Chochinov, H.M., Wilson, K.G., Enns, M., Lander, S. (1998). Depression, hopelessness, and suicidal ideation in the terminally ill. *Psychosomatics* **39**:366–70.

66 Wilber, K. (2006). *Integral Spirituality: A Startling New Role for Religion in the Modern and Postmodern World*. Boston: Shambhala.

67 Sinclair, S., Raffin, S., Pereira, J., Guebert, N. (2006). Collective soul: The spirituality of an interdisciplinary team. *Palliat Support Care* **4**(1): 13–24.

68 McClain, J.C., Rosenfeld, B., Kosinski, A., Pessin, H., Cimino, J.E., Breitbart, W. (2004). Belief in an afterlife, spiritual wellbeing and end-of-life despair in patients with advanced cancer. *Gen Hosp Psychiat* **26**(6): 484–6.

69 Cassell E. (1982). The nature of suffering and the goals of medicine. *N. Engl. J. Med.* **306**:639–45.

CHAPTER 22

Cure and healing

Lodovico Balducci and H. Lee Modditt

Is there a difference between curing and healing: study of two clinical cases?

Case 1: Mary

Mary developed breast cancer at 50, when her last child had left for college and she was ready to go back to teaching. To raise a family she had abandoned her profession in education 22 years earlier. Despite the challenges of ageing she had looked forward to this new time of her life, until a screening mammography had revealed a suspicious mass in the right breast.

At surgery she had a 2-cm ductal carcinoma, positive for hormone receptors and negative for HER2neu; one of 16 axillary lymph nodes was positive for cancer. As per the patient's request, a bilateral mastectomy was performed. She had felt this would give her the best chance for a cure.

At the time of diagnosis Mary tried to reassure her spouse and their three children that the cancer was just a 'nuisance,' and would not interfere with her professional and family goals. However, cytotoxic chemotherapy was associated with an episode of neutropenic infection that led to a 5-day hospitalization. Totally unexpectedly, she developed severe fatigue that kept her from fulfilling her usual social commitments. She grew very angry at her husband because he attended a couple of receptions without her instead of supporting her at home. She also became very annoyed by his clumsy attempts to engage in sex and for his manifestations of hurt at her understandable rejection

Mary grew progressively more intolerant of her husband's presence. Her 25 years of marriage now appeared to her as a form of slavery and exploitation. She had given up her career, and with it her independence, to foster her husband's career. She had been left to take care of the children almost single-handedly. Now the cancer deprived her of a second chance to be her own person. In the meantime, her husband appeared oblivious to her torment. After the chemotherapy was over Mary decided it was time for her to sleep in a different room. Once her husband expressed concerns about the cost of breast reconstruction she told him that he had become so insensitive and ungrateful that she could not tolerate him anymore. To her, marriage had been a tragic mistake and she was ready to move out.

Ten years later, after chemotherapy, 5 years of adjuvant tamoxifen, and a bilateral breast reconstruction that had been complicated by an infected implant, Mary lives with a girlfriend. She has met her spouse again only at the wedding of two of the children and has not attended the christening of her only grandchild. She is supported by alimony and passes her time volunteering in the local chapter of the American Cancer Society and in the local performance art centre. Her husband moved to a different city and lives with his girlfriend.

Mary might have been cured of her cancer, but certainly she has not been healed. The consequences of cancer continue to hover over her and her family. Even if the cancer has been cured, one is hard-pressed to consider the treatment of Mary a medical success. The ultimate treatment goal, to help Mary become whole, had not been reached and appears unreachable. Medical treatment did not prevent and may have even accelerated a process of emotional self-destruction that involved not only the patient, but also her family and arguably the persons that interacted with her family members.

Whether the physicians or the other health care professionals might have prevented or managed Mary's emotional downturn, and whether it was their duty to even confront it is not the issue here. The case of Mary highlights the dissociation between cure and healing, between the control of the disease and the wholeness of the person.

Case 2: Frances

Frances was diagnosed with glioblastoma multiformis 1 year after she had been confirmed in the Catholic faith and had become a very active counsellor in her parish. For 1 year this successful trial lawyer has been on call day and night for the needy of her church—homeless people looking for money, food, and shelter; teenagers problems ranging from parental conflicts, wandering away and unwanted pregnancies; young families in disarray. She sent a form letter to all members of her parish that asked for their prayer, told them about her diagnosis, and informed them that she would be available to them again once her treatment (surgery and 6 weeks of radiation therapy) was over. She was able to do this. Having taken leave from her law firm she had even more time to minister to the parishioners in need. She went to visit her mother on the major holidays, because she wished to mend the broken fences of her youth. During her college years, her mother had disowned her after discovering she was living with two men and doing drugs. Their relationship had remained tense even after Frances had become an established professional and a legitimate spouse. She also took a trip to London with her sister, in part to heal memories of her previous visit when she had been arrested and forcibly repatriated during a manifestation against the US involvement in Vietnam. With her new trip she wished to allow an open emotional wound to close.

Eventually, her disease progressed to the point of paralysis, which kept her from writing the book she had planned about being a patient. The cost of care prevented her from sharing her assets with people in need as freely as she used to. The need for rest, progressively impaired speech, and progressive neurological impairment did not allow her to continue counselling, yet her parishioners kept visiting her until the last days in the hospice house where she had been transferred. They all felt a debt of gratitude, but more than one stated that they felt better after visiting her. Her welcoming smile relieved their fear of disease and death, taught them that death may be lived as deeply as any other life experience, including marriage and childbirth, and that the value of our life can never abandon us as long as we recognize and value the sense of each experience. As part of the wake ritual, the parish organized an ongoing slide show of Frances' life and the whole congregation accompanied her to her final rest.

Six years earlier this childless widow had been spending her weekends binge-drinking alcohol. At the end of one of these binges she finally realized she could not continue to live that way, that she could not get out of her situation without help. After calling Alcoholics Anonymous she was able to face her addiction to alcohol and to recognize it has been responsible of all disorders of her previous life. Through the 12 steps of Alcoholics Anonymous she acknowledged that she could not have overcome her addiction, escape from that emotional prison, without releasing control of her life to a higher power. Eventually, through a friend, she recognized this 'higher power' in the Christian God of the Catholic tradition.

A few months before dying, when she was still able to speak and to type emails, Frances told me, her physician: 'this disease could have not come at a more appropriate time: I learned how precious our time is and how little time we have to make right to the people we have wronged. If I were not dying of cancer I would have never been able to heal the relation with my mother.'

Frances had died, but she was healed: another manifestation of the dissociation between curing and healing: through her disease she had been made whole.

The meaning of healing

Despite quite different outcomes, the cases of Mary and Frances have several common characteristics. For both, cancer unleashed underlying emotional issues. The disease occurs in a person and the effects of the disease involve all the dimensions of the person. This interaction eventually determined the final outcomes here. Health care professionals may not be able to treat the economic, emotional, and social consequences of a disease, but they cannot ignore them either. At the very least they must be aware of these consequences, advise the patient, account for these consequences in the plan of treatment, and ask the help of other professionals qualified to manage such conditions. A competent health professional that ignores the consequences of the disease on domains outside the medical one is comparable to a car maker that designs safe and efficient cars, but ignores the environmental impact of his or her creation.

Although the outcomes were opposite, the human domain that prevented healing in Mary and allowed it in Francis was the same. We'll call this domain spiritual to distinguish it from other well defined domains such as the physical, emotional and intellectual ones. Of course all human domains interact with one another. One may argue that in the case of Mary an underlying depressive mood caused the rejection of her husband and that in the case of Frances a euphoric mood allowed the acceptance of her condition. Yet what determined the presence or absence of healing was the ability/inability to discover the meaning of one's life experiences that is to achieve a sense of transcendence.

As seen is both of these cases, the disease of one person affects other persons. In an aging society the role of the home caregiver for disabled individuals has clearly emerged.[1–2] Caregiving has important medical and social consequences including decreased survival, increased incidence of depression and immune-suppressions, and substance abuse. Mary's husband and children had their lifestyle shattered by Mary's disease. Frances' friends and parishioners were comforted and inspired by the way Frances lived her disease. As a result of her disease Frances had been able to establish a wholesome relationship with her mother.

The treatment of the disease is expected to restore a patient to wholeness. The cure may represent a way to wholeness. Yet the cure is not sufficient to make a person whole and the absence of a cure does not always prevent wholeness. In fact cure is often equated to healing. This finding begs the question: what does it mean to make a person whole? What is the meaning of healing?

Healing, making whole

More than 2500 years ago Plato lamented the incoming trend of 'trusting to different physicians the management of the diseases of the body and of the soul.'[3] In Plato's view, this approach to medicine created an artificial separation among different human domains, and threatened the unity of the human person, that is the wholeness of the person. In Plato's view, to be whole was to be healed. He concluded that only love could bring healing. In this context, love was 'agape,' which involves a personal decision of caring for somebody else, of helping somebody else to gain his/her wholeness.[4] Unlike 'Eros,' that is a sexual passion, or 'philia', the affection of friends, children and parents, and communities, agape is a rational, rather than an instinctive form of love. The foundation of agape is the sacredness of the person. The Latin *sacer* means reserved for a special function. Sacredness implies that each person is unique, reserved for a unique function that only that person can accomplish. Rather than possessing another person, the ultimate form of love, agape consists in helping each person to find his/her unique mission, his/her sacredness, his/her wholeness.

Modern history teaches that Plato's lament was well founded. One of the paradoxes of our time is that the most sophisticated medical advances, including the translation of the human genome, have been uncoupled from healing. Indeed suspicion toward medicine and medical research has reached previously unknown levels. [5,6] A number of causes may explain this phenomenon, including better public information as well as instantaneous and often misleading information through the web. Yet, one may contend that in the 'medicalization' of human life, the privileging of cure over healing is mostly responsible for this dichotomy. The unsubstantiated conviction that an identifiable disease is the root of all human problems, and the blind faith that medical interventions may resolve any human problems, including dissatisfaction with one's own life, underlies the current suspicion toward medical practice and medical science. The public is angry because medicine did not live up to these unwarranted expectations.

In the last 30 years medicine tried to assume a more humanistic face with the assessment of health related quality of life (HRQOL) as a treatment outcome.[7,8] Unfortunately, this effort fell short of its intents. The major shortcoming involves the assessment itself. HRQOL is interpreted in terms of physical and emotional comfort. When assessed by these parameters, the HRQOL of the most consequential persons of our times, from Mother Theresa to Martin Luther King, would appear as very low. In addition, medical scientists cannot agree as to the role of HRQOL in medical decisions. The question whether it is legitimate to deny life-prolonging treatment that may be associated with a deterioration of HRQOL is still unresolved. In other words, HRQOL has not been operationalized. Finally HRQOL elicits important ethical questions. If a decline in HRQOL is understood as a decline in the value of life, as it is implicit in the support of euthanasia and assisted suicide, then the sacrality of the person is denied. The determination of HRQOL indicates the need of a healthcare practitioner to go beyond the pure physical aspect of the disease, but it falls short of establishing how a person might be made whole, how a person might be healed.

The idea of making whole suggests restoration of a pre-existing condition of health, but such a construct is unrealistic. In some situations, such as resection of malignant tumours, cure itself would prevent wholeness, as it implies the permanent removal of a body part. In all serious diseases, as the cases of Mary and Frances illustrated, the disease has long lasting emotional and social consequences that prevent a return to the previous status. However, the most important consideration is the awareness that eventually we are all going to die, and many of us will become disabled before death. This would be the human destiny; to lose one's wholeness. If death and disability are the ultimate enemies, we all are doomed to fail.

The case of Frances demonstrates that there is healing even in presence of disability and death, that wholeness consists in finding a meaning in any human situation, in co-opting disability and death among the valuable and treasured life experiences. Rather than going where one likes, healing consists of liking where one is going. Even in the face of her newly-discovered faith Frances could have found abundant reasons to curse her destiny. For only one year she had been allowed the joy of self-love and self-giving after a lifetime of self-deprecation and self-destruction. I am sure that sometimes she doubted whether her God was playing cat and mouse with human sentiments, as suggested by Saramago in his 'Gospel according to Jesus Christ.'[9] What prevented this last disruption of her life was her new awareness that she had the means to use any human experience, including disability and death, to witness to the ongoing discovery of her authentic sense of life. Rather than a blind trust in God's will, she had direct experience of the power of the means of redemption her God had put in her hand. The redeemer, in ancient Judaism, was the family member that paid the debts of a man and prevented his and his family imprisonment for insolvency. In enduring her disability and her death with the grace of a person that had found a use for each life experience, Frances redeemed death and fear of death for the people who accompanied her to her final journey. She had found wholeness.

How do we find healing?

From the previous discussion one can conclude that healing refers to the personal experience of the disease, unlike cure that refers to its objective physical manifestations.

In differentiating cure and healing, I do not try to dismiss the importance of cure. In highlighting healing in the absence of cure I do not mean to trivialize or ignore the role of cure toward healing. In the majority of cases, healing occurs through cure, and the difficulty of the cure might represent an important opportunity for healing. Had her husband recognized that the breast cancer and its treatment had unearthed a number of interpersonal conflicts, the story of Mary might have been re-written as one of triumphant healing. Her disease had provided an opportunity to review their marriage, to correct its direction, to recognize the wrongs they have done to each other, to ask for and receive forgiveness, to reinvigorate their mutual love with the double ability to forgive and being forgiven. Cure, prolongation of life, symptom management should continue to be the mainstay of medical practice I only want to underscore that it may be necessary to go beyond cure to achieve healing.

Healing occurs in a dimension that comprehends all human dimensions. We may refer to it as conscience or as a spiritual dimension, in that it involves an awareness of the self as a unity, as well as a decision to utilize this unity, in its present status, for a unique function that only that person can perform. In other words, people are made whole when they discover in the present status of health a new meaning for their life, a new opportunity to accomplish their unique mission, to state their 'sacredness.' Frances was healed because she found in her suffering and impending death a unique way to witness her newly-found faith. Yet even in the absence of a religious faith, suffering and death may be experienced as a time of particular closeness with the people one loves or as a time to distillate from life its deeper sense. I often utilize this metaphor for describing the proximity of death: It is like a person who has only a few hours to visit Rome and gains from the Gianicolo hill a vision of the city that allows him or her to decide which monuments are really worth visiting. Impending death may provide a personal Gianicolo hill moment for each person to decide which monuments of life are worthy of attention.

Clearly, there cannot be healing without discovering one's own sacredness, uniqueness. For the people, arguably the majority of people, who spend their life adrift pushed and pulled by waves and winds, a serious disease may appear as threatening as a rock against which one expects to be thrown. Mary did not die of her disease, but breast cancer represented an unexpected obstacle to the life she had planned for herself and her family, and compelled a brisk change of direction to her ride that had been relatively smooth up to then.

To summarize, healing involves a recognition and acceptance of one's unique mission. In medical terms, it means co-opting the disease and its consequences within the scope of this mission and the ability of changing the direction of one's mission accordingly.

When I was diagnosed with bilateral ocular lymphoma, I thought for a while that this had bought an end to my worldwide advocacy for better care of cancer in older people. Instead, my disease represented an opportunity to focus my attention on the care of my grandchild (and the second one on the way) and on heartening my patients affected by similar diseases, according to the best tradition of the 'wounded healer.' Eventually, I learned that my neoplasm was neither life-threatening nor disabling and would not impede my world travels on behalf of the elderly.

The way to healing

While the way to healing is different and unique for each person, some trends are common and can be outlined.

Resolving emotional conflict

Both the cases of Mary and Frances showed that there cannot be healing until one faces the underlying emotional conflicts that are brought to light by the disease. On the way to healing, the patient needs to have the will to overcome these conflicts and to realize that he/she cannot do it alone. That is for two obvious reasons. First, by definition, a conflict involves another entity (another person, another view of oneself, the world, or the deity). Secondly, in the majority if not the totality of cases, a sense of guilt that can only be absolved by another person underlies these conflicts. The intervention of a counsellor or a psychiatrist is beneficial and necessary in most cases. Yet there are situations in which guilt may not simply be resolved by identifying the source of a problem or by medications that quench existential anxiety. I have been inspired by the bravery of Elizabeth Edwards, who endured with grace the ordeal of her husband John Edwards' US presidential campaign and the pain of marital infidelity after her breast cancer relapsed. Her decision to continue being active part of her husband campaign despite the recurrence of her cancer was highlighted in an article I wrote as the testimony of a person aware of her own sacredness.[10] I also admired her candor in revealing her ongoing struggle with God after the death of her 16-year-old child. Yet I cannot help wondering whether that ongoing squabble with the deity might have not prevented her healing. No medication or counselling will relieve the pain of losing a child. The acceptance of the death is ridden with the guilt of letting the child die again. Anger at God or denial of God may appear in these circumstances as the only option for keeping that child alive. This situation was masterfully described by George Bernanos in his 'Diary of a Country Priest.'[11] An imposing countess living in the French countryside had lost a young boy to meningitis. Despite her regular attendance to all religious practices, she had nurtured for 12 years a cold hatred toward God. When she interacts with a young and inexperienced priest, she challenges him by saying, 'If there were a place in this world or in the next where I could subtract myself to God's sight and control, even for a single instant, I would not hesitate to habit that place and to take my child with me.' Eventually, in the course of that debate with the priest she learns that the very hatred she had conceived toward God prevented her from loving the child she had lost, because that hatred kept her in a condition of quiet desperation where not only pain, but even love could not be felt. Only a person able to speak on behalf of her beliefs, a chaplain or a spiritual director could have helped her to get rid of her hatred and her guilt, and helped to heal her.

Another common situation is exemplified in the Greek myth of Orestes[12] that had the religious duty to revenge the death of his father by killing his murderous mother and her lover. Either alternative, to leave his father's death unpunished or to kill his own mother, was ridden with religious guilt. This conflict of family allegiance is particular common today with the disaggregation of the traditional family. It is not uncommon for a physician, and especially for an oncologist, to learn of children unwilling to meet their parents prior to their death. The inability to overcome one's guilt leads to an inability to be healed in these situations.

A third situation in which overcoming guilt is a key to healing was described by Christina Puchalski.[13] A patient dying of pancreatic cancer had terrible pain that was not relieved by high dose of narcotics. Eventually, the physician discovered that the patient, who was homosexual, felt guilt for his lifestyle and felt rejected by the Episcopal congregation that he used to attend and to love. The intervention of a chaplain who assured him of God's love irrespective of his sexual orientation restituted the patient's wholeness and substantially reduced his need of opioids. This is another example of how only a religious or spiritual professional entitled to speak on behalf of the patient's creed could have been able to remove a stumbling block to healing. This form of guilt, related to the transgression of religious commandments is also very common at a time when abortion, divorce and marital infidelity are socially accepted practices although they may be in conflict with a person's religious beliefs.

Thus, the acceptance of one's sacredness in all circumstances, the discovery of the sense of suffering, disability and death in the light of this sacredness, the facing of the emotional conflicts elicited by the disease appear as the ingredients of healing. In my opinion, healing may be effected only by love intended as agape, as the decision to love oneself and the people around us as part of the same human adventure. In recognizing this interconnection between oneself and others, agape also allows one to recognize the redeeming value of suffering. In ministering to thousands of cancer patients I also learned that guilt is the main stumbling block to agape.

Healing: the role of the health care practitioner

In addition to providing the best medical care, physicians and other health care practitioners have a critical role in healing in at least two respects—helping the patient making the decision that is more appropriate for him/her and identifying existential/spiritual problems that may prevent healing.

Helping the patients to take the most appropriate decision

Autonomy is the gauge that indicates the best therapeutic decisions in individual circumstances. To respect the patient's autonomy the provider must be able to take a value history and to provide full information about the possible complications of treatment. A value history includes personal goals and preferences. In situations of life and death for example it may suggest whether to institute respiratory support in the presence of respiratory failure and how long to prolong this form of treatment. In all situations it may favor one form of treatment over another. For example, it is understandable that a professional player of a string instrument or a ballroom dancer may prefer to forgo the extra benefits that the chemotherapeutic class of taxanes confer to the adjuvant treatment of breast cancer in order to avoid a neuropathy that may impair their preferred activities.

Full information in a values history should include the emotional, social, economical, and spiritual consequences of a treatment. Mary's outcome might have been quite different had she and her husband learned that chemotherapy may be associated with loss of libido, fatigue, and depression and had they known about the cost and potential complications of breast reconstruction.

Identifying existential/spiritual issues

Healing, according to the definition I gave, occurs in a spiritual domain. Any conflict in these domains may compromise the ability to heal. I have already referred to a case described by Puchalski where a patient with terminal pancreatic cancer suffered persistent and unrelieved pain until he was assured by a minister of his faith that his god loved him irrespective of his sexual preferences. Cases like this are more common than one suspect as they are a form of response to guilt, a consistent companion of human decisions. In some cases, guilt is due to a misperception of the situation and can be solved by the intervention of a counsellor or a psychiatrist. In others, it is rooted in a dichotomy between one's moral convictions and personal actions, and requires the intervention of a spokesperson for the ruler of the moral standards. In the case of religious faith this is a religious minister. In the absence of a specific religious belief, a spiritual director experienced in the contradiction of the human spirit and human conscience may help. Guilt may be source of a so called spiritual or existential emergency as in the case described by Puchalski. Any health professional should be able to identify these emergencies in the same way he/she should be able to identify a medical or a psychiatric one.

Personally, I also believe that any health care provider should be asked to think about his/her own healing, to confront his/her conscience and spirituality. I believe that, without this insight, nobody can bring real healing, even when he or she practices the highest quality of medicine according to the prevailing guidelines. A modest proposition to this effect involves solutions that have been in part already implemented. Each medical school should have a course on medicine and humanities where the most common current beliefs, as well as the meaning of autonomy and ethics are explored. Medical students should also be instructed in communication techniques in listening to the patients and in learning how to identify keys phrases that suggest underlying spiritual problems, such as unrelieved pain, emotional withdrawal, verbal sparring with spouse or partner. During their training, providers of all specialties should be offered the opportunity to explore their feelings and to review the patient's feeling during regularly scheduled patient centered rounds, such as the Schwartz Rounds. Schwartz Rounds are a grand rounds format where a speaker presents briefly on a topic, a case is presented and the audience participates in a more reflective dialogue about their issues as healthcare professionals in caring for patients. They should also be instructed about the home caregiver as the hidden patient and on the management and support of the caregiver. Last, but not least, discussion of spiritual and existential issues should be encouraged in the course of teaching rounds. These types of educational and clinical interventions will help broaden the understanding of the clinical role of healing in our patients, as well as our own lives.

Bibliography

Hahn, R.A. (1995). *Sickness and Healing: an Anthropological Perspective.* New Haven: Yale University Press.

Kelsey, M.T. (1973). *Healing and Christianity.* London: SCM Press.

Koss-Chiono, J.D., Hefner, P. (eds) (2006). *Spiritual Transformation and Healing: Anthropological, Theological, Neuroscience and Clinical Perspectives.* Lanham: AltaMira Press.

Puchalski, C.M., Ferrell, B. (2010). *Making Health Care Whole.* West Conshohocken: Templeton Press.

References

1 Savundranayagam, M.Y., Montgomery, R.J., Kosloski, K. (2010). A dimensional analysis of caregiver burden among spouses and adult children. *Gerontologist* **51**(3): 3211–31.

2 Palos, G.R., Mendoza, T.R., Liao, K.P., *et al.* (2011). Caregiver symptom burden: the risk of care for an underserved patient with advanced cancer. *Cancer* **117**: 1070–9.

3 Plato. (2005). *Meno and other dialogues: Charmides, Laches, Lysis, Meno,* transl. Robin Waterfield. Oxford; Oxford University Press.

4 Plato. (2008). *Symposium,* transl. Robin Waterfield. Oxford; Oxford University Press.

5 Anonymous. (2002). How medical research has transformed millions of us into human guinea pigs. *Time Magazine,* April 22 47–56.

6 Van Der Weyden, M.B. (2006). Task transfer: another pressure for the evolution of the medical profession. *Med J Aust* **185**(1): 29–31.

7 Bundage, M., Ozoba, D., Bezjak, A., *et al.* (2007). Lessons learned in the assessment of health-related quality of life: selected examples from the National Cancer Institute of Canada Clinical Trials Group. *J Clin Oncol* **10**(25): 5078–81.

8 Lipscomb, J., Reeve, B.B., Clauser, S.B., et al. (2007). Patient-reported outcomes assessment in cancer trials: taking stock, moving forward. *J Clin Oncol* **25**(32): 5133–40

9 Saramago, J. (1994). *The Gospel According to Jesus Christ,* transl. G. Pontiero. Orlando: Harcourt.

10 Balducci, L. (2007). *Elizabeth Edwards Shows How to Treat Cancer.* Available at: http://watchingthewatchers.org/news/1196/doctors-view-edwards-decision (accessed 3 November 2011).

11 Bernanos, G. (2001). *The Diary of a Country Priest.* New York: Carroll and Graf Publishers.

12 Euripides. (1995). *Orestes,* transl. John Peck and Frank Nisetich. New York: Oxford University Press.

13 Puchalski, C.M., Ferrell, B. (2010). *Making Health Care Whole.* West Conshohocken: Templeton Press, p. 7.

14 Silbermann, M., Amal Dweib, Khleif., Balducci, L. (2010). Healing by cancer. *J Clin Oncol* **28:** 1436–7.

CHAPTER 23

Suffering

Betty Ferrell and Catherine Del Ferraro

Suffering and spirituality

At the end of life, the spiritual needs of a patient can transcend physical needs, and unmet spiritual needs can contribute to pain and suffering.[1] Spirituality is most broadly defined as the quest for meaning and purpose in life, while religion provides a means to express spirituality.[2] The spirit is part of our being and religion is viewed as a structured belief system that provides a philosophy and ethical code for living.[3]

Suffering is seen in patients who are confronted with life-threatening diseases for which there is no known cure and who are suddenly forced to face their own mortality. For the purpose of this chapter, the term 'life-threatening and debilitating' encompasses the population of patients of all ages and a broad range of diagnostic categories, who are living with a persistent or recurring condition that adversely affects an individual's daily functioning or will predictably reduce life expectancy. Life-threatening illnesses often cause people to reflect on their lives, and question life's meaning and its purpose. These individuals begin to mourn the life they lived and shared with loved ones.

Spirituality is a word that refers to the many facets of a person's existence, or can be understood as one's relationship to transcendent. For some, spirituality may be centered on God and for others it might be a concept of how they see themselves in the world and in relationship to something outside of themselves.[4] As an expression of spirituality, religious beliefs help the dying make sense of the suffering and uncertainty they experience.[2] A person who is dying may exhibit spiritual pain and suffering through expressions of meaninglessness, worthlessness, loneliness, or emptiness.[1]

In1982, Eric Cassell, MD, published a seminal paper on suffering, which has become an ongoing professional conversation about suffering in the healthcare setting and has challenged healthcare professionals to respond not only to physical injury and disease, but also to human suffering.[5] Cassell, defined suffering as 'an anguish that is experienced, not only as a pressure to change, but as a threat to our composure, our integrity, and the fulfillment of our intentions.'[6, p. 261] Cassell also articulated the relationship between the different facets of a person that makes a person whole, and the relationship of how the physical, psychological, social, and spiritual 'pieces' of a person's being affects each other piece and the relationship of one who suffers. He stated 'In fact, reflecting on suffering should make it possible to see that there is nothing about the body that is not also psychological and social, nothing social that is not physical and psychological and nothing psychological that is not physical or social.'[7] Spirituality helps give meaning to suffering and helps people find hope in time of despair.[4]

Suffering: the four domains of care

Over the past 20 years, our programme of research at the City of Hope Medical Center has been guided by a model of quality of life (QOL) including four domains of physical, psychological, social and spiritual wellbeing (Figure 23.1).[8] As illustrated in this model, the domains of QOL are distinct, yet there is significant interaction between domains. The following case examples are presented in order to illustrate aspects of suffering associated with each domain. The cases also demonstrate how spirituality transcends all domains and influences the experience of suffering.

Physical wellbeing

Clinical experience and significant research has documented the impact of unrelieved symptoms on patient suffering.[6,8–10] This interaction of physical wellbeing and suffering is profoundly apparent in the case of Catherine, an 88-year-old woman diagnosed with stage III Ovarian Cancer 4 years ago. Catherine was born and spent her childhood in Kansas, and at age 17 she entered a convent and became a nun. Catherine's mother died of breast cancer when she was 13 and she explained that her decision to enter the convent was less a matter of spiritual calling and more an attempt to escape from a home life dominated by an abusive father. Catherine remained in the convent until age 35 when she decided to leave the order. She describes the church as being very angry with her decision and that she was left entirely alone with no support to begin her new life.

Over the next 10 years, Catherine worked as a nanny while attending evening courses until she was able to obtain a degree in accounting and secure a position for a non-profit social service agency. Four years ago, Catherine was diagnosed with Stage III ovarian cancer. She underwent surgery followed by chemotherapy. Her life over the past 4 years has been dominated by severe physical symptoms from her disease and from treatment. She has had nausea and vomiting, abdominal pain, and severe peripheral neuropathy post-chemotherapy treatment. She has experienced three

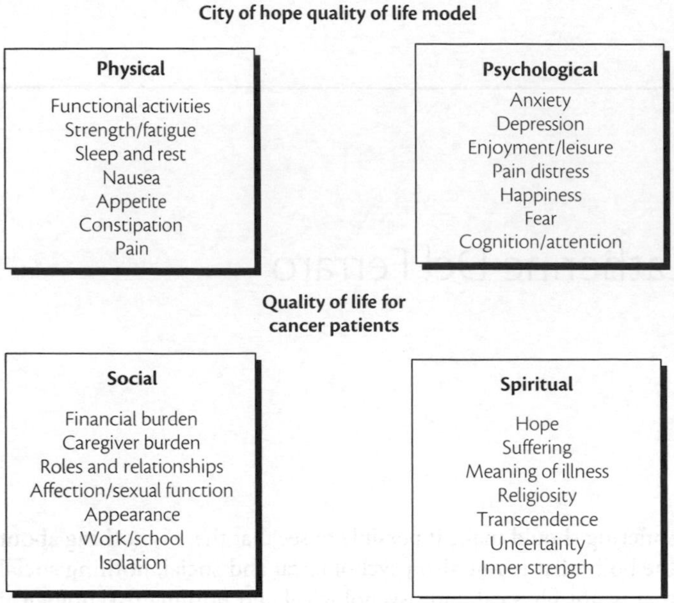

Figure 23.1 City of Hope Quality of Life model.

bowel obstructions. Catherine is very stoic and rarely complains, even when most ill. Her nurse, Josie, has learned to carefully assess her symptoms since she won't complain. Josie arranges to have quiet time with Catherine to discuss her symptoms, as well as her declining status. Catherine confides in Josie that she is terrified of dying and that the symptoms have become unbearable. She also says that she knows her disease and symptoms are punishment for 'abandoning my vows' and that her 'suffering is deserved'.

Psychological wellbeing

Alfred is a 52-year-old chemist and a new patient in a dialysis centre where he has begun treatment for renal failure associated with his diabetes. On initial admission to the centre, the dialysis nurse observed Alfred's obvious depression. He is accompanied to dialysis by his wife, Angie who appears very loving and supportive, but very anxious. The nurse arranged for the wife to meet with the centre's social worker, while Alfred began his first treatment.

Angie told the social worker that both she and Alfred were devastated by his disease and the progression that has led to dialysis. She also said that they had been married for only 1 year and that Alfred suffered from extreme depression after the death of both his parents in his early twenties. The depression improved greatly after they met 2 years ago. Alfred blamed himself for the renal failure, saying that during his 'dark years,' he took terrible care of his health.

Angie also described how both she and Alfred were raised in devout Jewish families, but that Alfred abandoned his faith after the loss of his parents. Angie wept openly, saying that while Alfred had returned to his faith since they met, she had struggled to keep any hope or faith since it was so unfair that Alfred should become so sick after their short time together and they had to suffer so much. She admitted that Alfred's depression was getting worse and she was terrified that he might try to end his life.

Social wellbeing

The domain of social wellbeing as an aspect of QOL depicts the person in relationship to others.[8,11–13] Social wellbeing encompasses issues such as relationships, caregiving, intimacy, and the financial concerns of illness.

Mr. Graedon was a 78-year-old man recently diagnosed with stage IV lung cancer. Despite recommendations from several physicians that he decline chemotherapy and be referred to hospice, Mr. Graedon insisted on being treated and he began a difficult regimen of chemo- and radiation therapy. He seemed to minimize any concerns and was very stoic, and the clinic nurses believed that he was experiencing extreme distress. The nurses arranged to have a chaplain visit during his next treatment and arranged for Mr. Graedon to be placed in one of the few private treatment rooms to provide a confidential space for the chaplain visit.

As the chaplain met with Mr. Graedon, he moved from his usual stoic state and wept openly. He then shared with the chaplain that his decision to opt for chemotherapy was because he hoped to extend his life as long as possible, as he was the only caregiver for his wife who had advanced Alzheimer's disease. He described how he would endure anything himself in order to stay alive, as he promised his wife he would care for her. He told the chaplain that he was a deeply religious man and he trusted God to see him through. It was clear that Mr. Graedon's suffering was deeply rooted in his role as spouse and the commitment he had made to his wife of 60 years.

Spiritual wellbeing

Jolene was a 42-year-old divorced woman who was seen in a major medical centre for the treatment of end-stage heart disease related to previous IV drug use. She had been in recovery for the past 7 years. During her initial recovery years she experienced improved health and made some major life changes, including joining a church, remaining active in AA meetings, and becoming employed as a tram driver at the city zoo. Jolene described the last few years as 'heaven' and said that she never knew such happiness was possible. The joy of positive relationships, a job working around children, and improved physical health were extremely different than her early life of drug abuse, failed marriages, and constant health concerns.

Jolene attended a support group for patients with cardiac disease and became very emotional, expressing her great distress in 'losing my life when I just discovered it'. She expressed her great distress in dying so young and her daily fluctuations of 'trusting God to get me through,' while being so angry at such an unfair God. Jolene said she had not discussed her feelings with her minister, or shared the seriousness of her health with her work or church friends as she feared they would abandon her. The clinic staff and physician had also observed that Jolene was becoming less adherent to her medications and clinic visits, and seemed to increasingly deny the seriousness of her illness.

Tenets of suffering

The above cases describe four very different case scenarios, each revealing a patient with intense suffering and each with important spiritual dimensions. Patients struggle with deriving meaning from their illness experiences and healthcare professionals are intimately involved with patients in their suffering. Box 23.1 presents 10 tenets of suffering derived from an analysis of literature related to suffering.[5] These principles can be seen reflected in these cases and also reveal many opportunities for support.

Box 23.1 Tenets of suffering

1. Suffering is a loss of control that creates insecurity. Suffering people often feel helpless and trapped, unable to escape their circumstances
2. In most instances, suffering is associated with loss. The loss may be of a relationship, of some aspect of the self or of some aspect of the physical body. The loss may be evident only in the mind of the sufferer, but it nonetheless leaves a person diminished and with a sense of brokenness
3. Suffering is an intensely personal experience
4. Suffering is accompanied by a range of intense emotions, including sadness, anguish, fear, abandonment, despair, and myriad other emotions
5. Suffering can be linked deeply to recognition of one's own mortality. When threatened by serious illness, people may fear the end of life. Conversely, for others, living with serious illness may result in a yearning for death
6. Suffering often involves asking the question 'why?' Illness or loss may be seen as untimely and undeserved. Suffering people frequently seek to find meaning and answers for that which is unknowable
7. Suffering often is associated with separation from the world. Individuals may express intense loneliness and yearn for connection with others, while also feeling intense distress about dependency on others
8. Suffering often is accompanied by spiritual distress. Regardless of religious affiliation, individuals experiencing illness may feel a sense of hopelessness. When life is threatened, people may conduct self-evaluation of what has been lived and what remains undone. Becoming weak and vulnerable and facing mortality may cause a person to re-evaluate his or her relationship with a higher being
9. Suffering is not synonymous with pain, but is closely associated with it. Physical pain is closely related to psychological, social, and spiritual distress. Pain that persists without meaning becomes suffering
10. Suffering occurs when an individual feels voiceless. This may occur when a person is unable to give words to his or her experience or when the person's 'screams' are unheard.

Source: Data from Ferrell, B.R., and Coyle, N. (2008). *The Nature of Suffering and the Goals of Nursing*, Oxford University Press, Inc and Kahn, D.L., and R.H. Steeves. (1996). An understanding of suffering grounded in clinical practice and research. In B.R. Ferrell (Ed.), Suffering, pp. 3–28. Sudbury, MA: Jones & Bartlett.

Suffering: witnessed in patients, family caregivers, and healthcare professionals

Suffering is part of a human condition and no human can escape suffering.

All suffering, no matter what kind, touches upon and affects the physical, emotional, mental, spiritual, and social being of a person.[14] To bear witness is to be present to the significant events and the emotions of another's life, good or bad.[15] Suffering that is witnessed in children, adults and geriatric populations have different meaning because of the different stages of growth and development, and life experiences. The five major components of growth and development commonly include: physiological, cognitive, psychosocial, moral, and spiritual.[16] Expanding on Sigmund Freud's theory of development, Erick H. Erickson included the entire life span in his eight stages of development, believing that people continue to develop throughout life.[16] Therefore, since suffering is a part of a human condition that threatens personal wholeness encountered throughout a life span, patient, and family assessment should include attention to developmental stage.

Children, adults, and geriatric populations

When illness or death impacts a child Erikson's development stages from infancy to teenage years (stages 1–5), can be applied.[16] Children are to be born healthy and parents are to nurture their children, watch them grow up to live a long prosperous life. The thought of a child suffering from an illness or dying is emotionally agonizing to discuss and even harder to witness. The avoidance of the prospect of illness, suffering, and death in children is evidenced by the very limited attention given to the topic of paediatric suffering.[5]

However, the Institute of Medicine reports that more than 50,000 children die each year from illness and accidents in the United States.[17] Medically-related suffering has been addressed by many, but little has been written about the suffering of children even though children have the capacity to suffer as much as adults and possibly even more. According to Shapiro,[18] children are more likely than adults to be overwhelmed by their suffering, as their coping skills, defences, and resources are limited. Children experience suffering parallel to their developmental abilities, life experience, and understanding of illness and death. Children struggle in their own way with the existential concerns of essential aloneness, dependence, autonomy, and fears of annihilation. As with adults, identifying the reason that causes a child to suffer is a challenge because they may not easily express these concerns. Causes may be associated with fear and the overwhelming emotions of others in a healthcare environment that is completely unfamiliar to the child, despite the presence or absence of physical pain.

The component of spiritual growth and development refers to individuals' understanding of their relationship with the universe and their perceptions about the direction and meaning of life.[16] In 1971, James W. Fowler investigated and developed a stage theory for the development of religious faith. Fowler believes that faith, or the spiritual dimension is a force that gives meaning to a person's life. Fowler uses the term faith as a form of knowing, a way of being in relationship to an ultimate environment.[19] To Fowler, faith is a relational phenomenon; it is 'an active 'made-of-being-in-relationship' to another or others in which we invest commitment, belief, love, risk and hope' [16, pp. 596, 19,20]. Faith stages, according to Fowler are separate from cognitive stages. Faith stages evolve from a combination of knowledge and values individuals develop throughout life.[16]

Fowler's spiritual theory and development stages were influenced by the works of Piaget, Kohlberg, and Erickson.[16] According to Fowler,[19] the development of faith is an interactive process between the person and the environment. He describes stages of spiritual development of children, as follows:

- *Stage 0:* undifferentiated faith (ages 0–3), infant unable to formulate concepts about self or the environment
- *Stage 1:* intuitive-projective faith (ages 3–7), a combination of images and beliefs given by trusted others, mixed with the child's own experience and imagination
- *Stage 2:* mythic-literal faith (ages 6–12), private world of fantasy and wonder.

In this stage, symbols refer to something specific; dramatic stories and myths are used to communicate spiritual meanings. Fowler continues to describe spiritual development in adolescence, which differ as a person matures and who experience suffering.

Suffering of an ill adolescent may be less associated with fear, but related more to the losses stemming from illness, for example loss of independence, young adulthood, of romance and marriage, and bodily integrity.[5] Fowler describes this in his third stage of spiritual development of an adolescent.

- *Stage: 3*: Is the Synthetic-Conventional faith (ages 12–18), the world and ultimate environment are structured by the expectations and judgments of others, an interpersonal focus. [16,19,20]

To witness suffering in children from pain, illness, or a child's life abruptly come to an end and a life that is short-lived is beyond words. Caring for a child who suffers leaves a devastating impact. Reducing the suffering endured in our children by improving their quality of life and assessing the domains of wellbeing (physical, psychological, social, and spiritual) requires a specialized holistic approach, knowledge, training, and sensitivity to the unique needs of our children and their families.

Erickson describes adulthood in his sixth and seventh stages of development which includes young adulthood (ages 18–25 years) and adulthood (ages of 25–65 years old).[16] In Erickson's stages of development, he reflects both on positive and negative aspects of the critical life periods. Positive indicators, described by Erikson, include creativity, productivity, and concern for others. Negative indicators, include self-indulgence, self-concern, lack of interests, and commitments.[16] Suffering that adults experience is seen in unresolved physical pain, expressions of unresolved anger, guilt, blame, and hatred; absences of joy in life, avoidance of family and friends, and inability to experience comfort in religious participation that previously provided comfort.[21]

Fowler's stages of spiritual development describes two stages of adulthood:

- *Stage 4:* individuating-reflective faith (after 18 years), the sense of identity and outlook on the world are differentiated, and the person develops explicit systems of meaning; high degree of self-consciousness
- *Stage 5:* paradoxical-consolidative faith (after 30 years), awareness of truth from a variety of viewpoints; the person faces up to the paradoxes of experiences and begins to develop universal ideas and becomes more orientated towards other people. [16,19,20]

The suffering of elderly people is unique and for many individuals, physical discomfort is much less a concern than the psychosocial consequences of living a long life.[5] In the eighth stage and final stage of development, Erickson defines maturity at age 65 years to death.[16] During this period, central tasks include integrity versus despair. Indicators of positive resolution include acceptance of worth and uniqueness of one's own life, and the acceptance of death and indicators of negative resolution include sense of loss and contempt for others.[16]

Fowler's final stage of spiritual development is described as:

- *Stage 6:* universalizing faith. This stage may never be achieved by some and is exceedingly rare. The persons best described in this stage have generated faith compositions in which their felt sense of an ultimate environment is inclusive of all being. They have become incarnators and actualizers of the spirit of an inclusive and fulfilled human community; the principles of love and justice.[19,20]

According to Erickson, people who attain ego integrity view life with a sense of wholeness and derive satisfaction from past accomplishments and view death as an acceptable completion of life, by contrast, people who suffer often believe they have made poor choices during life and wish they could live life over.[16] Suffering tests meaning and purpose in life, and suffering of the human spirit can result from confusion about or lack of the meaning of one's life.[14] Suffering, anguish, and despair gives rise to feelings of frustration, discouragement, and a sense that one's life has been worthless.[16]

Family caregivers and suffering

Family is defined as not only biological relatives, but also those people who are identified by the patient as such.[22] Like the patient who suffers, family caregivers suffer as they bear witness to their loved one who is suffering. A family caregiver is identified by the patient and can be described as a significant person in the patient's life who agrees, and who is committed to provide care to enhance quality of life.

Family caregivers feel helpless when they cannot relieve the suffering of their loved one. Patient suffering, whether physical, psychological, social, or spiritual has a major impact on the family caregiver.[23] Those who care for a loved one who is suffering often want to find meaning and understanding, while suffering creates one of the biggest challenges to uncover meaning.[24] Suffering is a personal experience intertwined within the relationship between patient and the individual family caregiver.[25] How a family caregiver deals with observing pain and suffering in a loved one is significantly influenced by the nature of his/her relationship with the ill person.[26]

A life-threatening illness often causes emotional crisis which affects the whole family. A family crisis can be described as a continuous condition of disruptiveness, disorganization, or incapacitation in the family system.[27] A crisis results when a family's current resources and adaptive strategies are not effective in handling the stressor.[27]

Suffering within families is both intense and an individual experience as each, spouse, daughter, or son responds within their own relationship with the patient who suffers, as well as a collective, shared suffering experience of the family.[5] In the midst of suffering, skillful, caring, compassionate healthcare professionals can be a key resource for support in which a patient, family caregiver and family can find solace, meaning, and the strength to move through distress to peace and acceptance.[4]

Healthcare professionals

Caring for people who suffer from incurable illnesses is difficult. Losing patients to diseases with no cure affects the wellbeing of all healthcare providers involved with care. There is often an inseparable relationship between the suffering patient and the suffering of the healthcare professionals who witness suffering while providing care.[5]

Healthcare professionals share the same humanistic qualities as the patient and family caregiver, and are just as vulnerable to emotional suffering. As healthcare professionals provide a continuum of care, they develop a close relationship with the patient and their family caregiver. As disease progresses, healthcare professionals witness the personal and emotional crisis of the patient, family caregiver, and family. In professional practice, healthcare professionals instill hope, empower others, encourage independence, and help improve the wellbeing and quality of life for patients and caregivers. When healthcare professionals have exerted all available treatments, resulting in the inability to achieve even minimal alleviation of suffering for patients, family caregivers, and their families, often a sense of frustration and failure is felt.[28] According to Stark & McGovern [14, p. 28]:

> 'The professional caregiver has the role of facilitating positive outcomes and finding some sense of and the cause of suffering.' 'Suffering has the potential to transform the sufferer and/or family caregiver and/or healthcare professional and offers an opportunity for the sufferer and/or family caregiver and/or healthcare professional to experience discovery and growth and to give and/or receive compassion and love.' 'Thus, those who suffer can find new meaning in life, as can those who care for all who suffers."

Suffering: across the trajectory of a disease

Anxiety and depression is seen in individuals who suffer, and in their family caregivers who care for their loved ones throughout the trajectory of disease. The cause of a life-threatening illness may be an advanced chronic illness, such as diabetes, a progressive debilitating disease, such as multiple-sclerosis, or a disease of short duration yet terminal progressing, such as late stage cancer. Although these diseases vary significantly, they are illnesses for which medicine provides no cure. Specialized care is needed to care for patients with incurable illnesses to increase, enhance, and maintain quality-of-life and their dignity, regardless of the stage in which the illness is in. The need for specialized care to decrease suffering in patients whose life expectancy exceeded 6 months, redefined palliative care with the interest which reflected in international healthcare professional societies.[29]

Acute illness

Acute stress is a common response to the diagnosis of a life-threatening illness, and resurfaces at transitional points in the disease process, which includes the beginning of treatment, recurrence, treatment failure, and disease progression.[30] The response of an acute life-threatening illness is characterized by shock, disbelief, grief, depression, sleep, and appetite disturbances and difficulty performing activities of daily living.[31] A conceptual model of chronic and life-threatening illness, and its impact on families describes five tasks that families must accomplish during the crisis phase of an illness:

- Creating meaning for the illness event that preserves a sense of mastery over their lives
- Grieving for the loss of the family identity before illness
- Moving toward a position of continuity between the past and the future
- Pulling together to undergo short-term crisis reorganization
- Developing family flexibility about future goals.[32,33]

Chronic illness

Chronic illness is irreversible presence, accumulation, or latency of disease states or impairments that involve the total human environment for supportive care and self-care, maintenance of function, and prevention of further disability.[33] Literature supports the emotional impact of a life-threatening chronic illness. Literature also supports positive impact which is dependent upon development of past coping skills of the individual and their families.[31] The process of adaptation to illness, as well as the family's adaptation and coping as a unit has been studied extensively. The adaptation stage is a period when healthcare providers are called to assist families to cope with health stressors.[27]

The family structure describes how the inner dimensions of the family are organized. The four structural inner dimensions are family power and decision-making, role, values, and communications.[27] The presence of a serious, chronic illness in one family member usually has a profound impact on the family system, especially on the family structure. Families are usually the primary caregivers of patients with chronic illness.[34]

Healthcare practitioners play a key role in monitoring and supporting the patient, and their family's psychological, psychosocial, and spiritual needs during adaptation to an illness. Keeping patients informed and involved with their care is also important. Even when a cure is not an option, other hopes and goals to be achieved are. Assisting the patient and family in maintaining comfort helps to facilitate adaptation and improved quality of life. [31] Compassionate care requires skillful attention to the four domains of quality of life, the physical, psychological, social, and spiritual care needs of patients, family caregivers, and their families throughout the trajectory of an illness, especially at the end of life to help ease suffering of grief.

Hospice as end-of-life palliative care

There has been substantial progress in understanding and managing the needs of the terminally ill and their family. Palliative care is defined as the active total care of individuals and their families whose disease is not responsive to curative treatment.[35] Control of pain, other symptoms, and of psychological, social, and spiritual problems, is paramount.[36] Hospice care is considered to be the model for quality, compassionate care at the end of life, believing that each individual should be able to live and die free of pain, with dignity, and that families should receive the necessary support to allow such care.[22] To witness a loved one deteriorate before your eyes over the trajectory of disease is emotionally unbearable. Hospice as end-of-life palliative care is patient and family centred care, which optimizes quality of life by anticipating, preventing, and treating suffering.[22]

Suffering and spirituality are multidimensional with unique meanings to every individual. Understanding the tenants of suffering and the effects suffering has on overall quality of life provides an opportunity to support patients and families. Utilizing the quality of life model (physical, psychological, social, and spiritual) will help healthcare professionals address the special needs of patients, family caregivers, and families. Suffering is part of humanity and seen in patients of all ages. Family caregivers and family members bear witness to suffering of their loved ones. Healthcare professionals involved with caring for these individuals bear witness to human suffering seen in each. In order to reduce and minimize suffering healthcare professionals must work together and provide specialized compassionate care, to minimize the cause and the effects of suffering for our patients. When a cure is not an option, suffering exists, yet spiritual healing is possible. Spiritual healing attends to what makes a person whole and comforts patients, family caregivers, and families throughout the continuum of care, across the trajectory of a disease, and at the end of life.

References

1 Schaffer, M., Norlander, L. (2009). *Being Present: A Nurse's Resource for End-of-Life Communication.* Indianapolis: Sigma Theta Tau International.

2 Puchalski, C.M., Dorff, R.E., Hendi, I.Y. (2004). Spirituality, religion, and healing in palliative care. *Clin Geriatr Med* **20**(4): 689–714, vi–vii.

3 Chochinov, H.M., Cann, B.J. (2005). Interventions to enhance the spiritual aspects of dying. *J Palliat Med* **8**(Suppl. 1), S103–15.

4 Puchalski, C.M., Ferrell, B.R. (2010). *Making Healthcare Whole: Integrating Spirituality into Healthcare.* West Conshohocken: Templeton Press.

5 Ferrell, B.R., Coyle, N. (2008). The nature of suffering and the goals of nursing. *Oncol Nurs Forum* **35**(2): 241–7

6 Cassell, E.J. (1991). *The Nature of suffering and the goals of medicine.* Oxford: Oxford University Press.

7 Cassell, E.J. (1992). The nature of suffering: physical, psychological, social and spiritual aspects. In: P.L. Starck, J.P. McGovern (eds) *The Hidden Dimension of Illness: Human Suffering*, pp. 1–10. New York: National League for Nursing Press.

8 Ferrell, B.R., Cullinane, C.A., Ervine, K., Melancon, C., Uman, G.C., Juarez, G. (2005). Perspectives on the impact of ovarian cancer: women's views of quality of life. *Oncol Nurs Forum* **32**(6): 1143–9.

9 Chochinov, H.M., Hack, T., Hassard, T., Kristjanson, L.J., McClement, S., Harlos, M. (2002). Dignity in the terminally ill: a cross-sectional, cohort study. *Lancet* **360**(9350): 2026–30.

10 Chochinov, H.M. (2006). *Dying, dignity, and new horizons in palliative end-of-life care.* CA: A Cancer J Clin. **56**(2): 84–103; quiz 4–5.

11 Coyle, N. (2006). The hard work of living in the face of death. *J Pain Sympt Manag* **32**(3): 266–74.

12 Daneault, S., Lussier, V., Mongeau, S., Paille, P., Hudon, E., Dion, D., *et al.* (2004). The nature of suffering and its relief in the terminally ill: a qualitative study. *J Palliat Care* **20**(1): 7–11.

13 Williams, B.R. (2004). Dying young, dying poor: a sociological examination of existential suffering among low-socioeconomic status patients. *J Palliat Med* **7**(1): 27–37.

14 Starck, P.L., McGovern, J.P. (1992). The meaning of suffering. In: P.L. Starck, J.P.McGovern (eds) *The Hidden Dimension of Illness: Human Suffering*, pp. 25–42. New York: National League of Nursing Press.

15 Baird, P. (2010). Spiritual care interventions. In: B.R. Ferrell, N. Coyle (eds) *Oxford Textbook of Palliative Nursing*, 3rd edn, pp. 663–71. New York: Oxford University Press.

16 Kozier, B., Erb, G., Olivieri, R. (1991). *Concepts of Growth and Development*, 4th edn. Addison Redwood City: Wesley.

17 Institute of Medicine. (2002). *When Children Die: Improving Palliative and End-of-life Care for Children and their Families.* Washington DC: National Academies Press.

18 Shapiro, B.S. (1996). The suffering of children and their families. In: B. Ferrell (ed.) *Suffering*, pp. 67–93. Sudbury: Jones and Bartlett Publishers.

19 Fowler, J.W. (1981). *Stages of Faith: The Psychology of Human Development and the Quest for Meaning.* New York: Harper and Row.

20 Fowler, J.W., Keen, S. (1978). *Life Maps: Conversations in the Journey of Faith.* Waco: Word Books.

21 Zerwehk, J.V. (2006). *Nursing Care at the End of Life.* Philadelphia: F.A. Davis.

22 City, K.A.E., Labyak, M.J. (2010). Hospice palliative care for the 21st century: a model for quality end-of-life care. In: B.R. Ferrell, N. Coyle (eds) *Oxford Textbook of Palliative Nursing*, 3rd edn, pp. 13–52. New York: Oxford University Press.

23 Hebert, R.S., Arnold, R.M., Schulz, R. (2007). Improving well-being in caregivers of terminally ill patients. Making the case for patient suffering as a focus for intervention research. *J Pain Sympt Manag* **34**(5): 539–46.

24 Borneman, T., Brown-Saltzman, K. (2010). Meaning in illness. In: B.R. Ferrell, N. Coyle (eds) *Oxford Textbook of Palliative Nursing*, 3rd edn, pp. 673–83. New York: Oxford University Press.

25 Ferrell, B.R. (1996). Humanizing the experience of pain and illness. In: B.R. Ferrell (ed.) *Suffering*, pp. 209–21. Sudbury: Jones and Bartlett Publishers International.

26 Ferrell, B.R. (2001). Pain observed: the experience of pain from the family caregiver's perspective. *Clin Geriatr Med* **17**(3): 595–609, viii–ix.

27 Friedman, M.M., Bowden, V.R., Jones, E.G. (2003). *Family Nursing Research, Theory, and Practice*, 5th edn. Upper Saddle River: Prentice Hall.

28 Sherwood, G. (1992). The responses of caregivers to the experiences of suffering. In: P.L. Starck, J.P. McGovern (eds) *The Hidden Dimensions of Illness: Human Suffering*, pp. 25–42. New York: National League for Nursing Press.

29 Grant, M.M., Dean, G.E. (2003). Evolution of quality of life in oncology and oncology nursing. In: C.R. King, P.S. Hinds (eds) *Quality of Life From Nursing and Patient Perspectives Theory Research*, 2nd edn. pp. 3–27. Boston: Jones and Bartlett Publishers.

30 Holland, J. (1989). *Clinical Course of Cancer.* New York: Oxford University Press.

31 Pasacreta, J.V., Minarik, P.A., Nield-Anderson, L. (2010). Anxiety and depression. In: B.R. Ferrell, N. Coyle (eds) *Oxford Textbook of Palliative Nursing*, 3rd edn, pp. 425–48. New York: Oxford University Press.

32 Artinian, N.T. (2001). Family-focused medical-surgical nursing. In: S.M.H. Hanson (ed.) *Family Healthcare Nursing Theory, Practice, and Research*, 2nd edn, pp. 273–99. Philadelphia: F.A. Davis.

33 Rolland, J.S. (1988). A conceptual model of chronic and life-threatening illness and its impact on families. In: C.S. Chilman, E.W. Nunnally, F.M. Cox (eds) *Chronic Illness and Disability:* Families in Trouble Series, vol. 2, pp. 17–66. Thousand Oaks: Sage Publications.

34 Larson, P.D., Lubkin, I.M. (2009). *Chronic Illness: Impact and Intervention,* 7th edn. Sudbury: Jones and Bartlett Publishers.

35 Campbell, T.L. (2000). *Physical Illness: Challenges to Families.* Thousand Oaks: Sage Publications.

36 Hass, M.L. (2010). *Contemporary Issues in Lung Cancer: a Nursing Perspective,* 2nd edn. Sudbury: Jones and Bartlett Publishers.

37 World Health Organization. (2009). *Palliative Care.* Available at: http://www.who.int/cancer/palliative/en/(accessed 1 April 2010).

CHAPTER 24

Ritual

Douglas J. Davies

Introduction

Ritual has found a particular place in the theoretical developments of anthropology as a concept describing shared patterns of behaviour expressing values, evoking emotions, and fostering identity within group contexts.[1,2] Although traditionally associated with liturgical ceremonies of religious movements, ritual covers many aspects of life including healthcare, crises of wellbeing, death, and bereavement. This chapter emphasizes how ritual uses symbols to unite emotions with ideas in generating values that underlie a person's group-based identity. Accordingly, 'ritual' will frequently be synonymous with 'ritual-symbolism'.

Ritual-symbolism

Symbols regularly participate in that which they represent, often due to some appropriate analogy. As we see later for blood, they are rarely arbitrary signs easily replaceable by another sign. However, with time and the power of association, a sign may assume symbolic power. Certain individuals may also gain 'symbolic' status, and their work become ritual-like, especially when they embody life-affirming values. Doctors, nurses, therapeutic staff, alongside the more obvious case of chaplains, all have the potential to be symbolic individuals conducting ritual-like work with significant consequences for healthcare spirituality.

Spirituality as cultural wisdom

Spirituality has, variously, described the mode of life associated with world religions,[3] local healing traditions,[4] New Age,[5] and secular ideologies,[6] and also with medical discourse.[7,8] This chapter's even broader approach identifies spirituality as a form of cultural wisdom generated from folk-insight into life that sustains a sense of meaning, fosters hope, and finds expression through ritual activity. Individuals embody such insight in various ways with each community identifying particular people as sources of succour because of their distinctive talent, inheritance, charisma, sympathetic nature, or special training. These individuals make 'wisdom' explicit in religious, philosophical, musical, dramatic, or literary performance. In some traditional societies, the old were often reckoned to have accumulated wisdom, while modern societies often approach 'wisdom' as acquired and practised in ritual-like ways through major professions of law, medicine, religion, education, science and drama, each governed by their ethical codes. Such ethics acknowledge professional responsibility and the emotional trust vested in qualified practitioners who serve as access points to a certain power-source fostering wellbeing.

Hope, ritualizing optimism

In healthcare terms, ritual would seem to help promote wellbeing through celebrations of birthdays and anniversaries amongst kith and kin and wider social celebrations of seasonal festivals, sporting success or celebrity events that affirm community membership and individual identity: fear is assuaged and hope fostered.[9–12] This basis of wellbeing is often intensified at times of life-crisis when responsive ritual events increase in number and frequency.

While ritual is often associated with tradition, and a sense of identity with familiar activity, moments sometimes occur when 'invention of tradition' occurs,[13] as with the multiplication of road-side accident shrines from the 1990s in the UK. Created by bereaved families and friends these rapidly gained social recognition as expressions of grief. Theoretically, we might interpret them anthropologically as converting a 'non-place' into a place of significance.[14] Few locations are more devoid of significance than some nondescript stretch of roadway, and few would wish death there to be framed by 'nothingness'. Such ritualization of place prompts the question of how healthcare sites provide significant locations for illness, recovery, death, or bereavement. The invention of ritual tradition is especially relevant, where different traditions meet during times of social change, not least in terms of medical centres, hospital, hospice, retirement home, or domestic scene, each prompting challenges for healthcare spirituality.

Although ritual is frequently embedded in familiar theological narratives of deep comfort to traditionally religious devotees, especially in times of crisis, there are some patients whose beliefs change over time, a factor reminding healthcare contexts to avoid any simple tick-box of religious identity. Moreover, it suggests that the taking of a narrative-history of patients might valuably complement their medical history in mapping their ideological-religious reference points and indicating their preferred ritual expression.

Healthcare contexts of ritual power

So, ritual not only embraces 'healthy' life, fostering identity-wellbeing in general, but also periods when life-crises challenge and constrain erstwhile meaningful lives. The diagnosis of serious illness, experience of serious pain in self or relatives,[15] anticipation of death, support of dying people, and the experience of bereavement, can all prompt anxiety over identity that may be partly ameliorated through responsive ritual behaviour. Such life-circumstances recall Aquili and Laughlin's claim that, 'ritual behaviour is one of the few mechanisms at man's disposal that can solve the ultimate problems and paradoxes of human existence'.[16] Although, at first, appearing excessive, this claim begins to make sense once we appreciate that 'meaning' derives both from rational thought and the emotional dynamics of hope generated by the supportive presence of others.[17]

One key theoretical issue on this sense of ritual power is the question of whether ritual is a coded scheme -like a language- whose message can be understood once its code is cracked, or is it something else?[18,19] While religious professionals are often trained to assume the former, stressing the doctrinal-historical significance of rituals, many ordinary devotees may well not engage with ritual in that way at all, but gain their 'meaning', often an emotion-focused meaning, from the sheer act and comfort of traditional observance. Rodney Needham's anthropological mind saw ritual as something that 'can be self-sufficient, self-sustaining, and self-justifying. Considered in its most characteristic features, it is a kind of activity -like speech or dancing- that man as a 'ceremonial animal' happens naturally to perform.'[20] Resembling Aquili and Laughlin, Needham indicates the predisposition of human nature to practice patterns of behaviour that confer a sense of meaning through performance. English expressions of 'doing things properly' typify this capacity of convention to provide satisfaction.

Rites of intensification

The ritual-force accompanying collective behaviour is reflected in the idea of the 'flow' of ritual, a sensed unity of the self, action, goal and context, that generates its own deep satisfaction.[21] Though often associated with sport and being 'in the zone', a sense of 'flow' can give participants in other ritual events a remarkable sense of unity, group power, and strength. The emotional tone of 'flow' varies according to skill of leadership, as well as context, e.g. from the joy at the birth of a much anticipated child to the calm waiting at a deathbed. It is important to think of such varied arousals alongside the core values often invoked or assumed in context.

Here, the anthropological idea of rites of intensification is valuable when identifying events that highlight, express, and embrace anew core group values,[22] whether at the personal level in birthdays and anniversaries, or in religious contexts of prayer and worship in daily, weekly, or calendrical festivals, such as a New Year. Similarly, with Christmas in Christianity, *Diwali* in Hinduism, or *Id al-Fitr* at the conclusion of Islam's Ramadan fasting. These give pride of place to core doctrines and encourage devotees in their commitments as community, congregation, or family gather and wish each other well, often by giving presents and by eating, drinking, and singing.

Blessing

These celebratory acts constitute a kind of 'blessing', a common ritual form and of great significance in healthcare spirituality as a group summons its energies in the desire to foster positive outcomes. Here, we find 'hope' emerging in a ritualized fashion to enhance a sense of meaning and wellbeing in participants.[23,24] That food and drink, as basic elements of life, play significant roles in many rites of intensification underscores the nature of ritual as a life-sustaining behaviour pattern. Singing, music, and movement are also important media of emotional stimulation, and their distinctive form in specific cases shows how groups, especially religious traditions, are often typified by preferred moods and their management. These media typically allow people to express themselves without fear of contradiction since songs are not discussions. Music in therapeutic contexts also creates a ritual-like context by adding its own dimension to the otherwise functional relationship of patient and professional.

Intensification ritual also underlies memorial events commemorating the life of deceased individuals or group with many now referring to 'life-centred' funeral rites in which eulogy—on the life of the deceased, replaces homily—on the religious nature of afterlife identity.[25] Increasingly popular in the later decades of twentieth century Britain and beyond such events seem to intensify individual emotions of loss within a group context and may compensate for an increasing dislike for extended formal social mourning behaviour. Periodic commemorative rites are common the world over, reflecting how people understand psychological and emotional shifts associated with the passing of time, and often including blessings as people speak well of the dead and express their concern for surviving kin. Blessing is usually associated with formal religious acts in which the authoritative power of a tradition is directed towards devotees through a designated officiant. As previously indicated, this has been important in Catholic traditions of the 'last rites' when the dying is anointed with oil, blessed, and may take the Holy Communion as the strengthening *viaticum* or provision for the journey to the afterlife.

Whether in religious or more general forms, blessing uses a social force to foster wellbeing by enhancing hope in contexts aligned with moods of harmony and good will. This suggests why blessing can play an important role in the spirituality of healthcare, not least of end of life care. One of its associated features concerns a sense of completion and unity of life-work and endeavour captured in the difficult popular concept of 'closure'. Blessing is, then, a rite whose end is in itself, whether for the dead and for the living.

Power and hope: authority and wellbeing

Words are frequently integral to blessing or, indeed, to cursing, as to ritual at large. Cannon's early work, for example, argued for the power of the community to curse one of its members and for death to ensue.[26,27] Later, Austin's philosophical idea of a performative utterance described statements that achieve what they state—'I name this ship': to say it is to do it. Austin also identified a certain 'force' inherent in performatives, and which we can identify as derived from individuals invested with social power.[28,29] Healthcare workers often own degrees of such power and this makes their words important,[30] and some of their relationships ritual-like, as when a doctor 'breaks the news' of chronic or terminal illness to patient or family member. For such an event easily becomes a ritual context involving performative force for good or ill.

These issues of power in healthcare contexts of spirituality highlight human awareness of certain people, events, and circumstances as strengthening of one's sense of identity and wellbeing, while others contribute to its depletion. Theoretically, this 'power' reflects notions of social force or energy field that constitutes the medium within which individuals gain or lose identity as group members. It is closely aligned with the emotions of hope or despair,[31] themes familiar to many million children through J. K. Rowling's *Harry Potter* books whose 'dementors ... drain peace, hope and happiness'[32] from people, and from Dan Smith's hero, Robert Langdon, whose ultimate discovery was 'an emotion he had never felt this profoundly in his entire life. *Hope.*'[33] More technically speaking, two anthropological concepts elaborate this 'power-perspective' for healthcare and spirituality: one concerning the interplay of jural and mystical forms of authority, the other dealing with moral-somatic relationships.[34]

Jural and mystical authority in moral somatic relationships

Everyday life depends both upon jural or legal authority to organise and control society and mystical forms of authority to foster human flourishing.[35] The judiciary, police, military, family, school, employers, and professional healthcare bodies all exercise some form of authorized power as evident in laws and codes of professional conduct that embrace medical ethics. Yet, in a different, but often complementary fashion, mystical forms of authority are also exercised by some of these figures, although priests and ritual performers seem the obvious examples. These bless, ritualize goodwill and human optimism, often in contexts of sacred places. However, if either jural or mystical authority are abused there ensue important negative consequences for wellbeing and, consequently, for healthcare. If police are corrupt, a doctor intentionally kills a patient, or priests abuse those in their care, it is no accident that the expression 'it makes you sick' is often used, with the media enhancing this response. This phrase easily introduces our second expression of social power in the 'moral-somatic relationship' between the values of a group and the wellbeing of its constituent individuals. Here, 'moral-somatic' extends the familiar notion of 'psycho-somatic' to link individuals with their social-moral environment.[17, pp.186–211]

Both in terms of jural-mystical and moral-somatic dynamics healthcare personnel often stand as key players in the relationship between individuals and 'society', serving as 'power-points' to 'society', offering hope in times of crisis through procedures that amount to rituals.

While there is an obvious sense in which medical diagnosis is grounded in scientific knowledge, doctors also deal with human wellbeing that involves a person's destiny. Loosely speaking, there is an element of mystical 'knowing' or *gnosis* in 'diagnosis' with the surgery holding an element of sacred space within itself. Healthcare encompasses a wide band of responsible activity influencing the moral-somatic interplay of social support and sense of personal wellbeing. To be well looked after by those in positions of social power is therapeutic to an ailing self. This is why medical ethics is of paramount significance as the ground-base of medical practice as a form of ritual practice. The proverbial 'bedside-manner' reflects the allied mystical authority of a doctor that may cause a patient to flourish as a complementary action to any technical therapy deployed as treatment, this may offer a sociological complement to the placebo effect.

Mystical authority also makes healthcare chaplains of interest since, traditionally speaking, they are a source of explicit mystical authority with rites of blessing to offer succour in times of crisis. While increasingly more complex in contexts of mixed religious and secular traditions there remains a need for an interplay of healthcare staff, chaplains, family and friends to encourage, support, and give appropriate hope to failing individuals through appropriate forms of identity intensification.[36]

Rites of passage

This enhancement of an individual's social identity is related to van Gennep's notion of rites of passage. This Dutch anthropologist identified a process by which a person passes from one social status to another by crossing specific boundaries.[37] Taking the Latin *limen* or threshold, he described transitions such as those from child to adult, single to married person, lay to priestly status, from living to ancestor, in terms of a shift from a preliminal through a liminal to a post-liminal stage. Separation from an original status inaugurates a period apart, prior to reincorporation into society in a new status. He noted the potential danger and anxiety associated with such changes and the way 'society' takes us by the hand and conducts us from one position to another often involving blessings. Depending upon the goal of the ritual, he argued that one of these three elements—separation (pre-liminal), apartness (liminal), or reincorporation (post-liminal)—would predominate, e.g. a wedding's goal might be that of the incorporation of a woman into a new kinship group, or a funeral the separation of the dead from the living. Being made a monk, for example, could be interpreted as entering a permanently liminal stage of separation from others.

Later, Victor Turner focused on the liminal stage and emphasized its emotional or existential sense of *communitas,* a shared togetherness experienced by people undergoing hardship, especially in traditional societies where isolation and some potential trauma underpinned initiation.[38] This idea has been applied to hospital contexts in terms of 'ward-liminality' and 'ward-communitas,' as individual patients 'learn to function together in this powerfully charged emotional atmosphere.'[39] More recently, two further anthropologists proposed ritual ideas grounded in dynamic schemes of experience.

Life-force: conquest and trauma

First, Maurice Bloch argued that changes of status involved experiential change within identity through a process of 'rebounding conquest' or 'rebounding violence.'[40] For example, through initiation the 'man' who is no longer a 'boy', enacts his transforming experience by now seeking to conquer phenomena that symbolize boyish things, or when religious converts might seek to change others just as they have been changed. Wider examples might include those having undergone a near-death-experience who now wish to bring their new worldview, free of any fear of death, to 'conquer' that fear of death in others.

Secondly, Harvey Whitehouse developed ideas of ritual effect in his 'two modes' theory of religion. The 'doctrinal mode', familiar to many, is taught in classroom-style settings, easily understood and spread by missionaries.[41] The 'imagistic mode' is different, originating in traumatic ritual and involving flashbulb 'image' memories. Occurring in some very tradition-based, small-scale tribes, individuals are initiated together and form strong bonds, but tend not to speak of what occurred. While having little cognitive explanation of things they may have 'learned', and no discursive information to teach others, they do possess shared knowledge of having endured hardship together. While this strongly united, small-group, and ritual-derived experience, does not lead to evangelism, its *communitas* helps provide core leadership groups for their societies. While some analogy with soldiers' or disaster survivors' trauma, might apply here, one difference is that returnees or survivors are more likely to be socially marginalized than to be acknowledged as those who have endured and 'know' certain things that qualify them as community leaders. Major questions arise here over 'spirituality' as the quality of life-experience, and of the nature of therapy provided by those professionally trained in a didactic -almost doctrinal- mode of knowledge, but devoid of personal trauma. Does the ritual-like nature of the trauma resonate with the ritual-like nature of later therapy or not?

Symbols and symbolic selves

That question cannot be answered here, but we can ask how individuals appropriate or create ideas and emotions within ritual contexts?[42] Having already argued for ideas and emotions combining as values symbolically deployed in ritual behaviour we find Turner depicting symbols as possessing both an ideological pole embracing abstract notions and a sensory pole dealing with the variety of bodily senses. He described symbols as multivocal or polysemic, bearing numerous meanings open to mutual influence during ritual performance.[43] Here ritual symbolism, engendering its own form of embodied awareness, becomes relevant to healthcare contexts where medical personnel carry a symbolic significance as those embodying potentially life-enhancing values. Some patients and families, for example, even comment on how uniformed nurses convey a sense of competence and support for the sick. So it is, too, with chaplaincy staff and their distinctive embodiment of mystical authority. Within healthcare it is important to stress this embodiment[44] of values in personnel who become 'symbols' of potential wellbeing. To emphasize the notion that a symbol participates in what it represents[45] may also partly explain why some healthcare professionals might find it difficult when they become ill and their embodied-identity of 'health' conflicts with 'sickness'. A contrasting form of embodied values may be found in lay volunteers in health-care contexts who stand as 'normal' people, bringing a sense of the ongoing nature of 'ordinary life' into what, for many, is the extraordinary ritual-like world of healthcare, including end of life care.

Ritualizing relationships: gifts and wellbeing

Another healthcare perspective on ritual, identity, and wellbeing lies in gift-exchange rituals first formulated in Mauss's anthropology of reciprocity and subsequently developed by scholars such as Godelier.[46,47] Mauss described both a 'threefold obligation'—to give, receive, and repay alienable gifts that carry a market-value, and a 'fourth obligation'—expressed in inalienable 'gifts' whose sentimental significance transcended mere cost. Inalienable gifts tend to be passed on, rather than returned, they link people to the core values of prime kin, ancestors, or gods, and help establish a sense of identity. Even get-well cards received during short illnesses, sympathy cards at bereavement, and small gifts taken to people in hospital, reflect something of this fourth obligation, all rooted in the ultimate desire for life's flourishing and not for death. For many, objects like wedding rings typify inalienable gifts of the 'fourth obligation', symbolizing values of relationship associated with the ritual act of giving and receiving rings, often the last symbolic object to remain with a person at the end of their life. Ritually speaking, acts of blessing also belong to and accompany this 'fourth' dimension. If we also consider healing-outcomes in this way interesting questions arise over payment for healthcare, and of the nature of the relationship between individuals and their society, and of health-providers as symbols of that relationship.

Habitus and spirituality

Moving from these general observations to one example of a symbolic object used ritually in healthcare we pinpoint how some hospice contexts offer a small, smoothly fashioned, 'holding-cross', to a dying patient. This object, easily hand-held even by one so ill, offers sensory stimulation with a capacity for being a profound symbol for those with a Christian background.

That case exemplifies another sociological concept valuable when considering healthcare spirituality, viz., *habitus.* This describes the character, customary disposition, or embodied mode of knowing and perceiving the world that comes to underlie the identity someone develops over time within a particular group.[48–50] Etymologically related to 'habit' as dress, as in monk's habit or riding habit, *habitus* aptly applies to spirituality understood as the quality of identity inherent in people's lives and relationships. It encompasses one's daily life-style and material culture of home and possessions.[51] Contexts of illness, life-crisis, and bereavement, however, easily shift people from such familiarity into strangely alien spheres of incapacity and loss of control. Such events bring new challenges to previous spiritual resources, identity and *habitus*, making the availability of assistance from professionals possessing jural and mystical capacities all the more vital. Then, the ritual-symbolism of healthcare, in both personnel and facilities, become newly familiar territory.

Ritual space

Irrespective of philosophical or theological ideas, the pragmatic facts of embodied life and illness bring people into contexts of healthcare spirituality set in time and place. Waiting, consulting and treatment rooms, wards, and the tellingly named operating theatre, all intimate aspects of life, illness and death explored in routines experienced as ritual-like events, all subject to traditional expectations of professional-patient privacy and ethics. Visually speaking, the decoration of hospital and hospice contexts often seeks some aesthetic-symbolic benefit to people through artwork, flowers, plants, windows onto scenes of nature, gardens, fields, or water features. The variety of interpretation of these is extensive, e.g. the use of stones to bring 'echoes of childhood' as well as 'of permanence' in a world now changing for patients. The provision of a 'family room' may furnish its own symbolic refuge where some respite may be found from watching with seriously ill relatives. Many hospital and hospice contexts also provide spaces devoted to prayer, meditation, or rituals of patients' own traditions. While wards and individual rooms are, to a degree, public places they, too, are often managed in semi-formal and even ritualized fashion. Individual rooms may also become more directly ritual places when housing patients close to death, especially if prayers or some particular ritual is requested or required. If these differ from those familiar to the dominant hospital or regional culture then some difficulties can ensue though in hospices such arrangements may be easier, with a facility for the patient to have personally chosen music played, material read, or with deepening silence and quiet as life moves towards its close. The relatively quiet speech or whispers of relatives, a sense of silence that may surround them and their dying kin, or the formal recitation of scriptures, all highlight patterns of spirituality with its emotion-pervaded ideas of the end of life.

Blood's ritual symbolism: an example

To conclude this general chapter, and to exemplify many of the technical points already discussed, we focus on the specific topic of blood, a substance whose symbolic significance and ritual use is effectively universal. Understood in many societies as symbolic of 'life' itself, blood participates in that which it represents. To 'give blood' is to foster life, and for heroes or martyrs to shed blood in self-sacrifice is to express life's deepest values, while to take blood in murder is to deny them.[52] Here 'life' stands as its own end-value, an idea highly charged with emotional affect and often embedded within clusters of complex religious, philosophical and scientific ideas.

Singling out the Jewish-Christian tradition, life's complexity is evident in the double notion that the 'life is in the blood'- (Leviticus 17: 11), and that there is a life-force associated with a divinely sourced breath of life (Genesis 2: 7). Aligned with the creative wind or spirit of God this breath gives dynamism to the human being, while the symbolic 'life-blood' of the individual resonates with bodily life and human kinship. Blood also sealed covenant relationships between divine and human parties and in sacrificial ritual made atonement between aggrieved parties.[53,54] In Christianity, Jesus' crucifixion became interpreted as a blood sacrifice for sin, an idea ritualized in the Eucharist whose ritual bread and wine gained various interpretations. In catholic traditions following the concept of transubstantiation they 'become' the very body and blood of Jesus through divine power and the ritual of consecration at the hands of authorized priests. In protestant versions these elements aid the believer's memory of Christ's life-giving self-sacrifice and strengthens faith. The religious power of these sacred ritual-symbols, associated with their capacity to enhance earthly life, is believed by some to contribute to a believer's journey to a heavenly domain, hence their use in the 'last rites'.

Moreover, human rootedness in ritual-symbolism and meaning-making has extended these blood-related themes with the idea of blood shed to 'save' others within Jewish-Christian perspectives probably influencing blood-donation practice[55] more as an inalienable gift of the fourth obligation than as an alienable commodity—blood should be 'given' not 'sold'. Likewise, the purchase of organs for human transplantation also triggers the ethics of healthcare spirituality while the Jehovah Witness objection to blood transfusion, based on its interpretation of the Leviticus text cited above, has caused periodic medical-ethical problems. Finally, the issue of menstrual blood has also played an important symbolic-ethical role in some societies where menstruating women are not allowed to be in contact with core ritual-symbols of their society[56,57] and probably played a part in restricting priesthood to men.

Times change, however, and bring new ritual symbolic matters to light, even in terms of blood. Medical advances now make it no longer possible to restrict ideas of 'life' to that of 'blood': blood transfusions may sustain life yet even its full complement will not offset 'brain-death'. Mechanical means of supporting organic life have introduced acts, such as the ending of life-support, that raise new questions of ritualizing such a key point in a patient's legal identity and in the life-experience of relatives.

Although usually discussed in terms of ritual purity and impurity the blood-related issues of menstruation and transfusion, and in some sense, the capacity to end a life, all raise the general rule that a person must be in a certain state before being fit to engage in key rituals and the key cultural symbols and values they enshrine.[58] In an extended application to healthcare we might say that proper training, acquired qualifications, and an engaged *habitus* constitute a form of ritual purity conferring the capacity to practice. Abuse of skill or patient renders the practitioner ritually impure for a designated period. In this sense ritual-practice exemplifies that spirituality which is the professional cultural wisdom of healthcare.

Bibliography

Corrigan, J. (ed) (2004). *Oxford Handbook of Religion and Emotion.* Oxford: Oxford University Press.

Cottingham, J. (2005). *The Spiritual Dimension, Religion, Philosophy and Human Value.* Cambridge: Cambridge University Press.

Davies, D.J. (ed.) (1986). *Studies in Pastoral Theology and Social Anthropology.* Birmingham: Birmingham University: Institute for the Study of Worship and Religious Architecture.

Girard, R. (1977). *Violence and the Sacred.* London: Johns Hopkins University Press.

Lévi-Strauss, C. (1963). *Structural Anthropology.* London: Allen Lane.

McCauley, R.N., Lawson, E.T. (2002). *Bringing Ritual to Mind: Psychological Foundations of Cultural Forms.* Cambridge: Cambridge University Press.

Stanner, W.E.H. (1960). On aboriginal religion 1: The lineaments of sacrifice, mime, song, dance, and stylized movements. *Oceania* **30**(1): 108–27.

Toulis, N.R. (1997). *Believing Identity: Pentecostalism and the Mediation of Jamaican Ethnicity and Gender.* Oxford: Berg.

Young, A. (1997). Suffering and the origins of traumatic memory. In: A. Kleinman, V. Das, M. Lock (eds) *Social Suffering.* pp. 245–60. Berkeley: University of California Press.

References

1 Rappaport, R. (1999). *Ritual and Religion in the Making of Humanity.* Cambridge: Cambridge University Press.

2 Grimes, R.L. (2000). *Deeply into the Bone. Re-inventing Rites of Passage.* Berkeley: University of California Press.

3 McNeill, J.T. (1951). *A History of the Cure of Souls.* New York: Harper and Row.

4 Ohnuki-Tierney, E. (1981). *Illness and Healing among the Sakhalin Ainu.* Cambridge: Cambridge University Press.

5 Wood, M. (2007). *Possession, Power and the New Age, Ambiguities of Authority in Neoliberal Societies.* Aldershot: Ashgate.

6 Comte-Sponville, A. (2007). *The Book of Atheist Spirituality*, transl. Nancy Huston. London: Bantam Books.

7 Cook, C., Powell, A., Sims, A. (2009). *Spirituality and Psychiatry.* London: RCPsych Publications.

8 Stålhandske, M.L. (2005). *Ritual Invention, a Play Perspective on Existential Ritual and Mental Health in Late Modern Sweden.* Uppsala: University of Uppsala.

9 Smith, W.R. (1894). *The Religion of the Semites (1880).* Edinburgh: A & C Black.

10 Durkheim, E. (1976). *The Elementary Forms of the Religious Life (1912)*. London: Allan Lane.

11 Hocart, A.M. (1952). *The Life-giving Myth (1935)*. London: Tavistock.

12 Malinowski, B. (1974). *Magic, Science and Religion (1948)*. London: Souvenir Press.

13 Hobsbawm, E., Ranger, T. (eds) (1983). *The Invention of Tradition*. Cambridge: Cambridge University Press.

14 Augé, M. (1995). *Non-places*. London, New York: Verso.

15 Good, M-J.D., Brodwin, P.E., Good, B.J., Kleinman, A. (eds) (1992). *Pain as Human Experience: an Anthropological Perspective*. Berkeley: University of California Press.

16 D'Aquili, E.G., Laughlin, Jr. C.D. (1979). The neurobiology of myth and ritual. In: E.G. d'Aquili, C.D. Laughlin, Jr, J. McManus (eds) *The Spectrum of Ritual, a Biogenetic Structural Analysis*, pp. 152–82. New York: Columbia University Press.

17 Davies, D.J. (2011). *Emotions, Identity and Religion: Hope, Reciprocity and Otherness*. Oxford: Oxford University Press.

18 Davies, D.J. (2002). *Anthropology and Theology*. Oxford: Berg.

19 Lewis, G. (1970). *The Day of Shining Red*. Cambridge: Cambridge Academic Press.

20 Needham, R. (1980). *Reconnaissances*. Toronto: University of Toronto Press.

21 Csikszentmihalyi, M. (1991). *Flow: the Psychology of Optimal Experience (1974)*. New York: Harper Perennial.

22 Chapple, E., Coon, C.S. (1947). *Principles of Anthropology*. London: Cape.

23 Bloch, E. (1986). *The Principle of Hope (1959)*, transl. Neville Plaice, Stephen Plaice and Paul Knight. Oxford: Basil Blackwell.

24 Default, K., Martocchio, R.N. (1985). Hope: its fears and dimensions, *Nurs Clin N Am* **20**(2): 379–91.

25 Quartier, T. (2007). *Bridging the Gaps, an Empirical Study of Catholic Funeral Rites*. Berlin: Lit Verlag.

26 Cannon,W.B. (1929). *Bodily Changes in Fear, Hunger and Rage*, 2nd edn. New York: Appleton and Co.

27 Cannon, W.B. (1942). 'Voodoo' death. *Am Anthropolog* n.s. XLIV.

28 Austin, J.L. (1961). *Philosophical Papers*. Oxford: Clarendon Press.

29 Schechner, R. (1988). *Performance Theory*, rev edn. New York: Routledge.

30 Galanter, M. (2005). *Spirituality and the Healthy Mind*. Oxford: Oxford University Press.

31 Rolls, E. (2005). *Emotion Explained*. Oxford: Oxford University Press.

32 Rowling, J.K. (1999). *Harry Potter and the Prisoner of Azkaban*. London: Bloomsbury.

33 Brown, D. (2009). *The Da Vinci Code*. London: Corgi.

34 [18]

35 [20]

36 Pugh, E.J., Smith, S. Salter, P. (2010). Offering Spiritual Support to Dying Patients and their Families through a Chaplaincy Service. *Nurs Times* **106**(28): 18–20.

37 Gennep, A. van (1960). *The Rites of Passage*, transl. M.K. Vizedom, G. Caffee. London: Routledge and Kegan Paul.

38 Turner, V. (1969). *The Ritual Process*. London: Routledge and Kegan Paul.

39 Oliver, L. (1986). Liminality and the hospital ward: unity through adversity. In: D.J. Davies (ed.) *Studies in Pastoral Theology and Social Anthropology*, pp. 70–81. Birmingham: Institute for the Study of Worship and Religious Architecture.

40 Bloch, M. (1992). *Prey into Hunter*. Cambridge: Cambridge University Press.

41 Whitehouse, H. (2004). *Modes of Religiosity*. New York: Altamira Press.

42 Obeyesekere, G. (1981). *Medusa's Hair, an Essay on Personal Symbols and Religious Experience*. Chicago: University of Chicago Press.

43 Turner, V. (1989). *From Ritual to Theatre*. New York: PAJ Publications.

44 Csordas, T.J. (2002). *Body/Meaning/Healing*. New York: Palgrave-Macmillan.

45 Tillich, P. (1953). *Systematic Theology*, 3 vols. London: Nisbet & Co.

46 Mauss, M. (1954). *The Gift: Forms and Functions of Exchange in Archaic Societies (1925)*, transl. I. Cunnison. London: Cohen and West.

47 Godelier, M. (1999). *The Enigma of the Gift*. Oxford: Blackwell.

48 Weber, M. (1963). *The Sociology of Religion (1922)*. London: Routledge.

49 Mauss, M. (1979). *Sociology and Psychology (1936)*, transl. Ben Brewster. London: Routledge and Kegan Paul.

50 Bourdieu, P. (1977). *Outline of Theory of Practice (1972)*. Cambridge: Cambridge University Press.

51 Miller, D. (2008). *The Comfort of Things*. Cambridge: Polity.

52 Marvin, C., Ingle, D. (1999). *Blood Sacrifice and the Nation, Totem Rituals and the American Flag*. Cambridge: Cambridge University Press.

53 Glick, L.B. (2005). *Marked in Your Flesh*. Oxford: Oxford University Press.

54 Lienhardt, G. (1961). *Divinity and Experience*. Oxford: Clarendon Press.

55 Titmuss, R.M. (1970). *The Gift Relationship: From Human Blood to Social Policy*. London: Allen and Unwin.

56 Delaney, C. (1988). Mortal flow: menstruation in Turkish village society. In: T. Buckley, A. Gottlieb (eds) *Blood Magic, the Anthropology of Menstruation*, pp. 74–93. Berkeley: University of California Press.

57 Buckley, T., Gottlieb, A. (1988). *Blood Magic, the Anthropology of Menstruation*. Berkeley: University of California Press.

58 Douglas, M. (1966). *Purity and Danger*. London: Routledge and Kegan Paul.

CHAPTER 25

Culture and religion

Peter van der Veer

Introduction

The nineteenth century witnessed the emergence of a great interest in spirits and spirituality. This interest also entered the anthropology of religion when the evolutionist thinker Edward Tylor (1832–1917) defined religion as the 'belief in spiritual beings'. Spirituality and the belief in spirits are certainly not the same, but the difference is not always clearly demarcated and this leads to (sometimes creative) confusion. For example, in Christianity one has the Holy Spirit descending on the Apostles and making them speak in tongues at Pentecost. However, nineteenth-century Pentecostalism describes this oneness with the Holy Spirit as a spiritual experience. Another nineteenth-century phenomenon was a sudden interest in communicating with the spirits of fallen soldiers after the American Civil War. Colonel Olcott who had fought in the Civil War had initially a great interest in such forms of communication, but together with Madame Blavatsky developed it in something quite different by founding the Theosophical Society, a spiritual movement led by 'masters of the universe' with whom Madame Blavatsky had privileged communications. Since Madame Blavatsky claimed to have been to Tibet and was under the influence of 'Eastern Spirituality,' they sought to connect the Theosophical Society to India and Sri Lanka.

Origins of modern spirituality

The origins of *modern* spirituality are, in my view, to be found in the nineteenth century and in the West. One can, obviously, find deep histories of spirituality in mysticism, gnosis, hermeticism, and in a whole range of traditions from Antiquity, but modern spirituality is something, indeed, modern. It is part of modernity and thus of a wide-ranging nineteenth-century transformation, a historical rupture. Spirituality is notoriously hard to define and I want to suggest that its very vagueness as the opposite of materiality, as distinctive from the body, as distinctive from both the religious and the secular, has made it productive as a concept that bridges various discursive traditions across the globe. I want to suggest that the spiritual and the secular are produced simultaneously as two connected alternatives to institutionalized religion in Euro-American modernity. A central contradiction in the concept of spirituality is that it is at the same time seen as universal and as tied to conceptions of national identity. Moreover, while the concept travels globally, its trajectory differs from place to place as it is inserted in different historical developments. To provide that specificity I will focus later on India and to some extent China, because the cultures and societies of the Orient are a privileged site for spirituality. I want to show that oriental spirituality is not a straightforward product of the traditions of the East, but a product of interactions with imperial modernity. [1] That this spirituality is directly related to discourses on health and medicine can be readily seen by looking at the traditions of yoga in India and Qi Gong in China. In most places in the world one can follow courses in Yoga and Qi Gong. These forms of Indian and Chinese spirituality have gone global, but are still connected to national identities. There is no contradiction between the global and the national, since the national is directly connected to a global system of nation-states. They are often described in the literature that accompanies such training courses as the Indian or Chinese 'gifts to the world', but that does not mean that the givers have lost them. They are complex products of the national construction of 'civilization' and are, at the same time, aspects of cosmopolitan modernity. However transcendent they claim to be as forms of spirituality, they are deeply embedded in political and economic history. Historically, yoga is an ancient system of breathing and body exercises that was re-formulated at the end of the nineteenth century as part of Hindu nationalism, but simultaneously as a form of Eastern spirituality that was an alternative to Western, colonial materialism. Today, it is embedded in global ideas of health and good living, but also in modern management practices and corporate culture. Historically, in China there are several forms of exercise, including breathing, that are called qi gong, and that develop skills (gong) to use the vital energy (qi) present in the body and connect it to the natural world of which the body is a part. Like yoga, they are part of ancient systems of thought and practice, but have been reformulated in recent history and made part of national heritage. Whatever the connections of these exercises in yoga or qigong with theologies, cosmologies and broader discursive traditions the central issue for those who participate in them is to learn what the exact practice is and what the benefits of that practice are. Much of the study of such practices, like Eliade's classical treatise, is therefore devoted to their phenomenology and historical connection to textual traditions.[2] The differences between breathing techniques and their mental and physical effects are also the subject of much debate among the different schools that propagate certain styles. What I want to suggest, however, is that religious movements, dealing with spiritual matters and body exercises, in short with spiritual transcendence attained through the body, are a central part of modern political and economic history.

The spiritual as a modern category emerges in the second half of the nineteenth century as part of the Great Transformation. As such, it is part of nineteenth-century globalization, a thoroughgoing political, economic, and cultural integration of the world. As Prasenjit Duara has convincingly argued, this integration is uneven in time and place, and occurs at different levels of society, integrating markets and political systems in a differential process. In this paper, we are dealing with what an instance of what Duara calls 'cognitive globalization,' which produces ´unique´ national formations of spirituality within a global capitalist system.[3] The emergence of spirituality is tied to the better-known ascendancy of the secular. Again, like spirituality, the concept of the secular also has deep histories, as in the separation of worldly and transcendent orders or in that of transcendence and immanence, but modern secularism is, indeed, modern and yet another aspect of the Great Transformation.[4] Much sociological attention and imagination has gone into first the development of the secularization thesis as part of the modernization paradigm and more recently in its dismantling. Jose Casanova has been in the forefront of this dismantling with his important book Public Religions.[5] He has argued that the three propositions of the secularization thesis, namely the decline of religious beliefs, the privatization of religion, and the differentiation of secular spheres and their emancipation from religion should be looked at separately in a comparative analysis. He comes to the conclusion that comparative historical analysis allows one to get away from the dominant stereotypes about the US and Europe, and to open a space for further sociological enquiry into multiple patterns of fusion and differentiation of the religious and the secular across societies and religions. This means the moving away from teleological understandings of modernization. Or perhaps better, it means a questioning of that telos by recognizing its multiplicity and its contradictions. Casanova's intervention can be understood as building on the Weberian project of comparative and historical sociology, but going beyond it by avoiding to reduce civilizations to essences that can be compared and by avoiding a Hegelian evaluation in terms of 'lack' or 'deficit' in the world-historical process of modernization and rationalization. Eizenstadt's proposal to speak about multiple modernities similarly creates space for such a post-Weberian project, but the question has to be asked what the role of secularity and secularism is in the production of these multiple modernities.[6]

Understanding European spirituality

Casanova's post-Weberian perspective is entirely acceptable, but I want to make a few observations. The first is that the project of European modernity should be understood as part of what I have called 'interactional history'.[7] That is to say that the project of modernity with all its revolutionary ideas of nation, equality, citizenship, democracy, rights is developed not only in Atlantic interactions between the US and Europe, but also in interactions with Asian and African societies that are coming within the orbit of imperial expansion. Instead of the oft-assumed universalism of the Enlightenment, I would propose to look at the universalization of ideas that emerge from a history of interactions. Enlightened notions of rationality and progress are not simply invented in Europe and accepted elsewhere, but are both produced and universally spread in the expansion of European power. This entails a close attention to the pathways of imperial universalization. Examining India and China uncovers some of the peculiarities of this universalization by showing how it is inserted in different historical trajectories in these societies.

The second is that with all the attention to secularization as a historical *process* there is not enough attention to secularism as historical *project*. Casanova has rightly drawn attention to the importance in Europe of secularism as an ideological critique of religion, carried out by a number of social movements.[8] Secularism as an ideology offers a teleology of religious decline and can function as a self-fulfilling prophecy. It is important to examine the role of intellectuals in furthering this understanding of history, but also their relation to sources of power: state apparatuses and social movements. Secularism is a forceful ideology when carried by political movements that capture both the imagination and the means to mobilize social energies. It is important to attend to the utopian and, indeed, religious elements in secularist projects in order to understand why many of these movements seem to tap into traditional and modern sources of witchcraft, millenarianism, and charisma, while at the same time being avowedly anti-traditionalist. Much of this remains outside of the framework of discussions of secularization, but the cases of India and China show us how essential this is for understanding the dynamics of religion and the secular.

Thirdly, I would like to point out that the spiritual and the secular are produced simultaneously and in mutual interaction. As many scholars have been arguing, religion as a universal category is a modern construction with a genealogy in universalist Deism and in sixteenth and seventeenth century European expansion.[9] One needs therefore to analyse how the categories of 'religion', 'secularism,' and 'spirituality' are universalized. This is also true for the category of the secular that has a genealogy in Church–World relations in European history, but is transformed in modernity both in Europe and elsewhere. The modern origins of 'the secular' are already clear when we look at the first use of the term secularism in England by George Holyoake in 1846. Holyoake attacked Christianity as an 'irrelevant speculation' and his attack was carried forward by Secular Societies that were formed in the early 1850s. One of the interesting aspects of these societies is that they combined radical anti-Church attitudes, anti-establishment socialism, and freethinking with spiritual experimentation. Secular Societies had a membership that was hugely interested in connecting to the other world by do-it-yourself science. These practices were not considered to be anti-rational, but rather to constitute experiments that were scientific though different from what was going on in the universities. They did not need (or want) to be legitimated by a scientific establishment that was considered to be intimately intertwined with high society and the established church, as indeed Oxford and Cambridge were in this period.

A good example of the combination of socialist radicalism, secularism, and spirituality is the prominent feminist Annie Besant. In the 1870s Annie Besant became a member of the Secular Society of London and began to collaborate with Charles Bradlaugh, a prominent socialist and President of the National Secular Society, in promoting birth-control and other feminist issues. She combined her radical socialist views and her scientific training as the first woman graduating in science at University College in London with a great interest in spiritual matters. After meeting Madame Blavatsky she became a leading Theosophist and after going to India she even became for a short moment President of the Indian National Congress.[10]

Science and scientific rationality are fundamental to the secular age and scientific progress is often seen to depend on the secularization of the mind.[11] From our contemporary viewpoint it seems strange that spirituality and secular science were not seen as at odds with each other in the nineteenth century. A common view of the history of science is that science purifies itself from unwarranted speculation. So, for instance, while the contribution of Alfred Russell Wallace in developing evolutionary theory concurrently with that of Darwin is generally acknowledged, Wallace's spiritual experiments are generally seen as an aberration from which science has purified itself.[12] What falls outside of this teleological perspective on science as a process of progressive purification is the social and political embedded nature of both the elements from which science is purified and of purified science itself. Spiritualism was seen as a secular truth-seeking, experimental in nature, and opposed to religious obscurantism and hierarchy. This was a truth-seeking that was hindered by both the State and the Church, in England two intertwined institutions. It is within the context of spiritualism, spirituality, and the antinomian traditions of Britain that an anti-colonial universalism was born.

Spirituality as an alternative to religion

An important element in the emergence of spirituality was that it offered an alternative to religion. This was first and foremost institutionalized religion. In the West spirituality formed an alternative to Church Christianity. Together with the so-called secularization of the mind in nineteenth-century liberalism, socialism, as well as in science (especially Darwin's evolution theory), one can find widespread movements in different parts of the world that search for a universal spirituality that is not bound to any specific tradition. Good examples in the United States are the transcendentalists from Emerson to Whitman, as well as Mary Baker's Christian Science. Theosophy is another product of spirit-searching America. In fact, not only America is full of spirituality as Catherine Albanese has shown,[13] but there is a huge proliferation of this kind of movement that parallels the spread of secularist ideologies around the world.

However, it is important to highlight that spirituality should not be relegated to the fringes of modernity, as often happens, but that it is located at the heart of Western modernity. The extent to which spirituality emerged as a sign of Western modernity can be best shown by its direct connection to abstract art. In December 1911 Wassily Kandinsky published his *Über das Geistige in der Kunst* ('On the Spiritual in Art'), one of the most influential texts by an artist in the twentieth century, and stated that the book had as its main purpose to arouse a capacity to experience the spiritual in material and abstract things. It was this capacity that enabled experiences that were in the future absolutely necessary and unending. Kandinsky emphasized that he was not creating a rational theory, but that as an artist he was interested in experiences that were partially unconscious.

Art and European modernity

Abstract art is one of the most distinctive signs of European modernity. One can study its gradual development from the impressionism of Monet and others through symbolism, but it is hard to escape the sense of drastic rupture with representational art. Kandinsky, one of the pioneers of abstract art, connects abstraction with the spiritual. He is certainly not exceptional, since other leading abstract pioneers as Frantizek Kupka, Piet Mondrian, and Kazimir Malevich, similarly saw themselves as inspired by spirituality, either through the influence of Theosophy and Anthroposophy or otherwise.[14] This may be somewhat unexpected for those who see the modern transformation of European life in the nineteenth and early twentieth century in Weberian terms as demystification. In one of the most pregnant expressions of modernity, namely in modern art, the spiritual stages a come-back as the return of the repressed. The connection between art and spirituality points at the way in which art comes to stand for the transcendental interpretation of experience that is no longer the exclusive province of institutional religion. While some of the theories one encounters in this area seem to be of the crackpot variety (especially Mondrian tends to be incredibly confused and confusing in his writings) one should be careful not to dismiss them too quickly as irrelevant. Artists are groping for a radically new way of expressing transcendental truth and are often better in doing that in their chosen medium than in words. The transcendental and moral significance of modern art, enshrined in museums and galleries, makes ideological attacks on art seem inevitable. Such attacks acquire the status of blasphemy and iconoclastic sacrilege, as in the Nazi burning of Entartete Kunst. One could legitimately argue that the spirituality of Western modernity is enshrined in Art.

Modernity and Spirituality

In Christianity, the religion of the colonial powers, we find in the second half of the nineteenth century attempts not so much to convert people to Christianity, but to find a universal morality or spirituality in other religious traditions and, thus, a kind of Hegelian Aufhebung of all traditions. This is exemplified in the Unitarian organization of the World Parliament of Religions in 1893 at Chicago, where representatives of World religions were invited to speak on a common platform, as well as in the newly-developed discipline of the Science of Religion that went beyond Christian theology. The term 'world religions' has been coined in this period to designate religious traditions of a high morality that could be treated as relatively equal. Buddhism was a perfect candidate to be included in this category, while Islam, despite its clear global presence and similarity to Christianity, was excluded at first.[15]

Spirituality as a concept emerged to enable the inclusion of a variety of traditions under the rubric of universal morality without the baggage of competing religious institutions and their authoritative boundary maintenance. Missionary work and conversion have certainly continued full blast until today and are still, in my view, the most important religious aspect of modern globalization in its current phase. The so-called decline of religion is limited to Western Europe, but the globalization of Christianity and other religions is continuing.[16] However, the importance of the globalization of spirituality as an alternative to both institutionalized religion and secularism should not be underestimated.

While modernity and spirituality are conceived to be universal, Asia is thought to have a special connection to spirituality .There is no term equivalent to 'spirituality' in Sanskrit or Mandarin Chinese (although there are words for 'spirit'), but this term is increasingly used to connect discursive traditions that have come to be called Hinduism or Confucianism or Daoism, none of which are 'isms' before the imperial encounter. Following I.A. Richards's explorations of the translation of Chinese thought I would propose that an embracing, vague term like spirituality has been adopted precisely to make peaceful communication between different conceptual universes possible.[17]

Nineteenth century discovery of the East

At the end of the nineteenth century the discovery of the traditions of the East engendered great interest in the West. The concept of spirituality played a crucial role continuously throughout contemporary history in the nationalist defence of Hindu civilization. In taking this up, the nationalists adopted the Orientalist perspective of European Romanticism in which Hindu civilization is highly appreciated for its spiritual qualities. Schopenhauer was deeply influenced by the Upanishads, while Goethe adopted specific theatre techniques from Sanskrit theatre in his writing of the Faust. Hindu civilization and its offshoot Buddhism are central to what Raymond Schwab has called the Oriental Renaissance. Indian religious movements in the second half of the nineteenth century re-appropriated Western discourse on 'Eastern spirituality'. The translation of Hindu discursive traditions into 'spirituality' meant a significant transformation of these traditions. This process can be closely followed by examining the way in which one of the most important reformers Vivekananda (1863–1902) made a modern, sanitized version of the religious ideas and practices of his guru Ramakrishna (a practitioner of tantric yoga) for a modernizing, middle class in Calcutta.

Vivekanada

Vivekananda's translation of Ramakrishna's message in terms of 'spirituality' was literally transferred to the West during his trip to the USA after Ramakrishna's death. He visited the World Parliament of Religions in Chicago in 1893, a side-show of the Columbian Exposition, celebrating the four-hundredth anniversary of Columbus voyage to the New World, but perhaps more importantly Chicago's recovery from the Great Fire of 1871. Religions represented in this show of religious universalism included Hinduism, Buddhism, Judaism. Roman Catholicism, Eastern Orthodoxy, Protestantism, Islam, Shinto, Confucianism, Taoism, Jainism, and various others.[18] However, the show was stolen by the representative of Hinduism, Swami Vivekananda. In his speech to the Parliament Vivekananda claimed that 'he was proud to belong to a religion which had taught the world both tolerance and universal acceptance.'[19] Vivekananda's spirituality was not modest or meek; it was forceful, polemical, and proud. As the response in the Parliament and in his further lecture tours in the United States indicates this was a message that resonated powerfully among American audiences. His writings in English often compare the lack of spirituality in the West with the abundance of it in India. Vivekananda is probably the first major Indian advocate of a 'Hindu spirituality' and his Ramakrishna Mission, the first Hindu missionary movement, following principles set out in modern Protestant evangelism.[20]

Vivekananda's construction of 'spirituality' has had a major impact on Hindu nationalism of all forms, but also on global understandings of 'spirituality'. Two major figures in the history of Modern India have been deeply influenced by Vivekananda's ideas about spirituality: the great Indian political leader Mohandas K. Gandhi and the Noble Prize winning poet Rabindranath Tagore. The first has developed the nationalist strand in the idea of spirituality while the second has developed the international strand, both showing the extent to which the national and transnational are actually interwoven. They argued that the materialism of the West created warfare and colonial exploitation, while the spirituality of the East provided an alternative that would lead to world peace and equal prosperity for all. After the Second World War some of these ideas entered into the ideology of the Third Way, especially exemplified by the Bandung Conference of 1955 and the Non-aligned Movement.

Gandhi

As in the West, Indian spirituality transcends institutionalized religion. It uses and transforms existing traditions, but goes beyond the authority of priestly lineages and monastic institutions. Gandhi used the ideas of Tolstoy, Ruskin, and Nordau about civilization, spirituality, and industry to transform the Hindu traditions in which he had been socialized. His political actions against the British colonial state were meant to pose a spiritual alternative to materialist exploitation. Since one of the biggest problems in the Indian subcontinent till today is the relation between Hindus and Muslims a transcendence of religious difference in universal, all-embracing spirituality is of the utmost political significance. Interestingly, Gandhi found a way to tie this universalist spirituality to the nationalist project by arguing that since one was born in a particular tradition and civilization one should not proselytise or convert. Instead, each person had to find the Truth in their own traditions. In this way, Gandhi could argue for a spiritual nation that transcended internal religious differences. India was seen to be very rich in its spiritual resources and should develop them, rather than imitate the materialism of the West. It is clear that Gandhi's brand of spirituality found as many supporters as opponents. Within his own Hindu community his assassins, inspired by a radical form of Hindu nationalism, argued that his spirituality was 'foreign' and meant to emasculate the Hindu nation by bending over backwards in allowing privileges to Muslims.

Tagore

Besides Gandhi it is the Bengali poet Rabindranath Tagore (1861–1941) whose understanding of spirituality has been very influential both within India and outside of it. Tagore was, however, deeply ambivalent, if not hostile towards 'the fierce self-idolatry of nation-worship'.[21] However, as the irony of history has it, today both India and Bangladesh use his poems as national anthems. Tagore was convinced that a unique spirituality unified Asia and in a series of lecture tours in Japan and China tried to persuade Chinese and Japanese intellectuals to create a pan-Asian movement towards a common Asian civilization. Crucial for the Pan-Asian turn that Tagore's Bengali spirituality took is his encounter with Kakuzo Okakura (1862–1913), a leading figure in the Japanese art scene, who in 1901 stayed a year with the Tagore family in Calcutta. In Japan Okakura had established a national art school combining traditional art with modern techniques. Rabindranath was very interested in Okakura's educational experiences, since he himself was starting an educational experiment in Shantiniketan ('Abode of Peace') outside of Calcutta.

After receiving the Noble Prize in 1913 and the outbreak of the First World War in Europe, Rabindranath Tagore felt that Asia should assume a role of spiritual leadership in the world. Three years after Okakura's death he visited Japan and was received by huge crowds with unbridled enthusiasm. At Tokyo Imperial University he delivered a speech on 11 June, 1916, entitled: 'The Message of India to Japan.' His major theme was the unity of Asia and the spiritual mission of Asia in the World. While Europe's achievements are not denied Tagore points at its great materialistic pursuit of self-interest and the need for the spiritual resources of a regenerated Asia. Japan had at that time already made the most successful transition to modernity and certainly not by rejecting material civilization. Not being colonized by Western powers, but acutely feeling their backwardness the Japanese Meiji reformers had embarked on a very ambitious adoption of Western science and technology, while creating a religious nationalism centering on the Emperor. All Asian nations looked with awe at the Japanese model and especially the Chinese nationalists tried to adopt important elements from it. The Japanese also saw themselves very much as the leaders of Asia. What, then, did the Japanese make of Tagore's claim of an Asian spirituality that transcended national boundaries?

While Japanese intellectuals accepted that there was a spiritual element in Japanese civilization they tended to see it as a part of their national heritage in a way very similar to followers of Vivekananda in India who interpreted Hindu spirituality as a part of religious nationalism. They also definitely liked Tagore's denunciation of Western imperialism, but rejected Tagore's denunciation of Japanese fledging imperialism. Tagore's attitude towards Japanese militant nationalism was explained as a sign of his membership of a defeated, colonized nation. His critics rightly saw that there was a contradiction between his rejection of Japanese militancy and his praise of Japanese spirituality of which that militancy was part and parcel. Tagore's and Gandhi's interpretation of Eastern spirituality as non-violent ignored or rejected the militant aspects of Asia's religious traditions. In India, this rejection led to an antagonism between Gandhi's pacifistic nationalism and the militant nationalism of Hindu radicals who ultimately murdered him. In Japan militancy was even more pronounced in the samurai traditions that became foundational to Japan's nationalism.

In 1924 Tagore went to China. His reception in China resembles the one in Japan. At first there is great interest in this great poet from unknown India and, in general, he draws large audiences. However, quite quickly his message of Pan-Asian spirituality and the revival of ancient religious traditions in China met with strong criticism especially in Beijing where there is considerable student activism. Tagore was received by Liang Qichao (1873–1929), one of China's most prominent nationalist intellectuals who supported Tagore throughout his visit, as well as by younger leading literary and intellectual figures like Hu Shih (1891–1962) who had studied at Columbia with John Dewey. Much of the opposition against Tagore was organized by Communist activists who painted Tagore as a traditionalist from a weak and defeated colonized nation. However, more generally, the poet's visit was a failure because Chinese intellectuals had been leading a revolution against the Qing Empire and the traditions that supported the ancient regime. They were too much inclined to reject the past in building a modern society to be able to accept Tagore's praise of ancient traditions.

After the great Taiping and Boxer rebellions of the nineteenth century Chinese nationalists had in majority decided that Chinese traditions were to be blamed for the backwardness of Chinese society and that in order to progress China had to adopt Western materialism, based as it on science and secularism. In Chinese modern fiction of the first part of the twentieth century there is a strong sense that China is a society not so much endowed with a spiritual heritage, but afflicted with a spiritual disease.[22] Nevertheless, there are important currents of thought in China that attempt to recuperate some of the spiritual resources of the past and especially those of Buddhism and Confucianism.

It is only after the development of Deng Xiaoping's socialism with Chinese characteristics and especially under Jiang Zemin in the early nineties that Chinese intellectuals can again develop Neo-Confucian spirituality both as the spirit of the nation and as a Chinese contribution to global humanism.[23]

The success of spirituality in the East

The relative success of 'spirituality' in India and its relative failure in China cannot merely be explained by the rise of communism in China. More deeply it is the conviction that Chinese traditions had to be replaced by Western science that has characterized Chinese modernity long before the Communist take-over, while in India traditions were made into resources in the anti-imperialist struggle against a material modernization that culturally and politically subjected India to Western power. The distrust of material civilization was shared by both metropolitan and Indian intellectuals criticizing imperialism in a dialogue that was fed by the use of a common English language.

The wide span of world views and traditions that are bridged by the word spirituality ranges from American transcendentalists like Emerson, Thoreau, and Whitman, to European abstract painters like Kandinsky and Mondriaan, to Neo-Confucian thinkers like Tu Wei-Ming, to political leaders like Gandhi. Walt Whitman's funeral with its readings of the words of Confucius, Jesus Christ, and Gautama Buddha, as well as Gandhi's hunger strikes are instances of interventions in society and culture on behalf of 'spirituality'. Boycotts and satyagraha can be seen as attempts to create bridges between radically different conceptual universes in order to create possibilities for non-violence. At the same time it is important to realize that spirituality can also be harnessed to a narrow vision of the spirit of the nation, as Tagore was well aware.

Spirituality is not quite the opposite of secularity or materiality. The aggressive secularism in China that attacked religion, destroyed temples and their priests, simultaneously promised a transcendence of bodily limits and the coming of a socialist paradise. The charisma of Mao Zedong seemed hardly secular, but on the contrary rather close to that of the Son of Heaven. In India it was colonial rule that brought the legal and constitutional fiction of secular neutrality, but it was Gandhi who made that secular neutrality of the state into a feature of Indian spirituality. Today, it is with the opening up of Indian and Chinese production and consumption that not only materialist consumption is enabled and grows, but also the marketing of spirituality by entrepreneurs in yoga, taiji quan, qi gong, shaolin wushu.

Perhaps the most interesting part of the alignment with neo-liberal capitalism are global business practices, in which spirituality is part of the training for more success in the market-place as well as better living. A number of Indian spiritual leaders today have a following in secular business schools and IT companies. Their mediation techniques and emphasis on spiritual experience seems to fit well with the lifestyle and case study orientated intellectual style of young urban professionals. Training experiential styles of spiritual life is central to what is presented as both an alternative to empty secular and religious life. From an outside perspective, however, it seems to allow people to pursue their secular goals in career and life within deeply disciplining institutions without being too stressed or depressed. Instead of challenging the nature of one's life it leads to feeling comfortable with it from an experience of spirituality, however produced. In the postcolonial period it is really the liberalization of the Indian and Chinese economies under the impact of global capitalism that frees the energies of spiritual movements to organize civil society. This is very clear in the Chinese case where liberalization first gives space to a spontaneous 'qi gong fever' and later to the rise of movements like Falun Gong that connect qigong to older ideas of a moral and political nature. In India one can see this especially in the rise of a Hindu nationalism that rejects an earlier secular and multicultural project of the state by emphasizing Hindu traditions as the basis of Indian civilization, thereby excluding other contributions by religious minorities. It is especially a new-fangled urban religiosity that is both interested in yoga and in a strong nation that supports this kind of politics.

Conclusion

As we have seen, Indian spirituality has been formulated by Vivekananda during a trip to Chicago and has been further developed in constant interaction with the rest of the world. A political figure like Mahatma Gandhi fits seamlessly in this history. When in the 1970s and 1980s till the present day highly educated members of the Indian middle class migrate to the USA for medical and engineering jobs they are confronted with a quite aggressive marketing of Indian spirituality in a market for health, for exercise, and for management practices. This, in turn, is brought back to India where especially successful new movements like the Bangalore-based Art of Living with Guru Ravi Ravi Shankar cater for a mobile, transnational class of business entrepreneurs. China's isolation between 1950 and 1980 has ensured a belated entry of Chinese spirituality on this market, but nevertheless it is quickly catching up with products like taiji quan and qigong. In the Chinese case there is a stronger connection with sports and especially martial arts, which are also promoted by Hong Kong and mainland movies. In both India and China one finds a similar appropriation of spiritual traditions to cater for the newly emerging middle classes. These newly manufactured spiritualities have a tenuous relationship with textual traditions, guarded by centers of learning and spiritual masters. They are creative in their response to new opportunities and anxieties produced by globalization and are, as such, comparable with Pentecostal and charismatic varieties of Christianity.

This new political deployment of spirituality is what is now considered to be 'new age' or indeed a form of de-politicization. I hope I have shown, however, that these understandings of spirituality as a-political or even anti-political obscure the fact that spirituality, as much as secularity, can be and has been deployed in radical struggles both in the East and in the West.

References

1 van der Veer, P. (2001). *Imperial Encounters. Religion and Modernity in India and Britain.* Princeton: Princeton University Press.
2 Eliade, M. (1958). *Yoga. Immortality and Freedom.* Princeton: Princeton University Press.
3 Duara, P. (2009). *The Global and Regional in China`s Nation-Formation.* London: Routledge.
4 For an intellectual history of the Western concept of the `secular,` see Taylor, C. (2008). *A Secular Age.* Cambridge: Harvard University Press.
5 Casanova, J. (1994). *Public Religions in the Modern World.* Chicago: University of Chicago Press.
6 Eizenstadt, S. (ed). (2002). *Multiple Modernities. Edison.* Piscataway: Transaction Publishers.
7 van der Veer, P. (2001). *Imperial Encounters: Nation and Religion in India and Britain.* Princeton: Princeton University Press.
8 Casanova, J. (2004). Religion, Secular Identities, and European Integration. *Transit* **27**, 1–14.
9 Asad, T. (1993). *Genealogies of Religion.* Baltimore: Johns Hopkins University.
10 Nethercot, A.H. (1961). *The First Five Lives of Annie Besant* London: Hart-Davis.
11 Nethercot, A.H. (1963). *The Last Four Lives of Annie Besant.* London: Hart-Davis.
12 Chadwick, O. (1990). *The Secularization of the European mind in the Nineteenth Century.* Cambridge: Cambridge University Press.
13 Pels, P. (2003). Spirits of Modernity Alfred Wallace, Edward Tylor, and the visual politics of fact. In: Birgit Meyer and Peter Pels (eds) *Magic and Modernity.* Stanford: Stanford University Press.
14 Albanese, C. (2007). *A Republic of Mind and Spirit: A Cultural History of American Metaphysical Religion.* New Haven: Yale University Press.
15 Tuchmann, M. (1986). *The Spiritual in Art: Abstract Painting 1890–1985*, Exhibition catalogue. New York: Abbeville Press.
16 Masuzawa,T. *The Invention of World Religions.* Chicago: University of Chicago Press,
17 Jenkins, P. (2002). *The Next Christendom. The Coming of Global Christianity.* New York: Oxford University Press.
18 Richards, I.A. (1932). *Mencius on the Mind. Experiments in Multiple Definition.* Kila: Kessinger Publication.
19 Ziolkowski, E. (ed.) (1993). *A Museum of Faiths.* Histories and Legagies of the 1893 World's Parliament of Religions. Atlanta: Schlars Press.
20 Mullick, S. (1993). Protap Chandra Majumdar and Swami Vivekananda at the Parliament of Religions. Two Interpretations of Hinduism and Universal Religion. In: E. Ziolkowski (ed.) *A Museum of Faiths. Histories and Legacies of the 1893 World's Parliament of Religions*, p. 221. Atlanta: Scholars Press.
21 See van der Veer, P. (1994). *Religious Nationalism: Hindus and Muslims in India.* Berkeley: University of California Press.
22 Tagore, R. (1916). *Nationalism.* New York: MacMillan.
23 Goldman, M., Ou-Fan Lee, L. (eds) (2002). *An Intellectual History of Modern China.* Cambridge: Cambridge University Press.
24 Tu Wei-ming. (2005). Cultural China: The Periphery as the Center. *Daedalus*, Fall Issue, 145–67. Tu Wei-ming and Tucker M.E. (eds) (2003–2004) *Confucian Spirituality*, vols 1 and 2. New York: Crossroads.

SECTION III

Practice

CHAPTER 26

Models of spiritual care

Bruce Rumbold

Introduction

We use models intentionally to simplify complex situations in an attempt to grasp them more clearly and respond more appropriately. Sometimes modelling simplifies by choosing out of many possibilities to focus on one dimension or one set of priorities alone. Sometimes complementary models are used (in physics the wave-particle duality is the classic example) to highlight the utilitarian aspect of using models. A 'horses for courses' approach is taken; we choose the model that best fits the questions we wish to ask and the answers we wish to obtain.

The use of models

Models are to be taken seriously, but not literally.[1] This is less a problem in areas of human endeavour where model making is intentional and overt, more so in areas where it is not. Physics' mathematical representation of fundamental atomic processes is an example of the former; religion can be a prime example of the latter. Theological statements and even doctrinal propositions are models intended to allow us to represent and discuss a spiritual domain that transcends us and clearly cannot be captured in its entirety by human thought forms and in human language. Statements and propositions need to be revised to ensure that they continue to speak to new situations. Yet there are many, believers and non-believers, who regard these statements as 'truth' or 'fact', and see attempts to negotiate or reformulate them as a rejection of faith, rather than an attempt to develop a better representation of complexity.

Models are developed both within and across paradigms. Paradigms are perspectives characterized by a distinctive ontology and epistemology, which is, in turn, expressed in particular methodologies and axiologies.[2] To translate these terms, a paradigm offers a particular understanding of what reality is and what can be known about it (ontology), of the nature of the relationship between the knower and what can be known (epistemology), of strategies for finding out what can, according to this paradigm, be known (methodology) and ideas about what's worth knowing (axiology). Guba and Lincoln, in a research context, identify five paradigms: positivist, post-positivist, critical theory, constructionist and participatory, each distinguished from the other by substantial differences in several of these characteristics.

Paradigms may be regarded as incommensurable, but may be linked by models that find common ground in a set of observations and statements on which they can concur.[3] The power of such models is their capacity to transcend at a practical level the conceptual difficulties that underlie them. At their best they can lead to re-conceptualization of the issues they address; at their worst they simply confound the issue.

Turning more specifically to the topic of this chapter, models for spiritual care must thus relate not only to ways of understanding spirituality, but also to ways of implementing those understandings in particular practice domains. A spiritual care model that is appropriate in, say, a religious community may not be appropriate for a secular institution. A different practice model will be required, even if it draws upon similar understandings of spirituality.

In this chapter I will explore both conceptual and practice models, with particular attention paid to different models of spiritual care that relate to different models of health. This approach will I hope provide some insight into the multiple variations of perspective and language concerning spiritual care. These variations arise from the conceptual differences between paradigms, driven in part by research studies that commit themselves to paradigmatic purity, and from practice models that negotiate paradigmatic truces in pursuit of good patient care.

Models of health

In any public conversation between spirituality and healthcare today, certainly in any policy making conversation, healthcare has the dominant voice. Thus, spiritual care models need to be expressed in terms commensurate with the model or models of health on which healthcare provision is based.

Three basic models of health inform contemporary discussions. These models are complementary, as we shall see, although in most societies a version of the biomedical model remains most prominent. I'll first outline the three models, then discuss in more detail how spirituality might engage each of them and what this might imply for practice. Rather than continually qualify my statements I'll simply remind you at the start that these are models: the actual construction and implementation of each perspective is more complex than can readily be represented in the schematic way I'm attempting here. In practice most health systems incorporate at least aspects of all three.

The Biomedical model: healthcare as a science

A biomedical understanding of health is at the core of most contemporary health systems. This model is, however, much clearer and more knowledgeable about disease and illness than it is about health. In essence, it treats health as the absence of disease and sees the goal of healthcare as the cure of illness.

The language that characterizes this model reflects this knowledge and aim. Diagnosis, prognostication, treatment, referral to specialists, clinical management, quality assurance, discharge are all key strategies, and the stories that are told by healthcare providers in particular—but also by recipients of care—are about assessing, referring, diagnosing, prognosticating, treating, managing.

The model assigns particular roles to those who participate within it. The identity of the sick individual is that of a patient. As in Parson's classic description of the sick role,[4] people who believe themselves to be sick are obliged to consult experts for diagnosis and treatment, and to accept those experts' opinions and recommendations. Through this process a person becomes a patient; his or her illness is legitimated, and the person is provided with certain benefits (care, time off work to recover, reimbursement for at least some of the costs incurred). Having followed correct procedures the person is then expected to recover and resume his or her social responsibilities. The health professionals' role, legitimated and regulated by society, is seen to serve the interests of both individual and society.

The biomedical model is based upon knowledge developed in the nineteenth century, particularly the anatomical and the biological sciences. The key practice disciplines are those with the greatest expertise in this core knowledge. Doctors are central in allocating resources, and other disciplines (nursing, allied health) co-operate in addressing priorities determined primarily by medical practitioners.

The strength of the model is of course its capacity to treat disease. The understanding of physiological processes that is at its core continues to deliver solutions for infectious disease in particular, but also for many of the conditions that in previous generations brought to an end the lives of otherwise active individuals. Stents and statins have substantially reduced mortality in later mid-life, while other previously fatal illnesses have become in effect chronic conditions.

A weakness of the model is its narrow focus upon pathology as the explanation for and cause of disease, and the instrumental relationships it encourages. People who are caregivers are professionals trained to relate in terms of their expertise. People who are cared for are patients, a role that focuses around receiving care. The model treats isolated individuals, on the one hand depriving them of agency while on the other ignoring structural constraints that shape their capacities to respond and decide. The ambivalence and ambiguity inherent in the model can be seen from Parson's description. People must have sufficient knowledge and autonomy to identify that their symptoms require attention, but thereafter as patients relinquish their care to experts. The experts are assumed to be motivated solely by altruism and to be unlikely to misuse the power they have over others.

The biomedical model works best for acute illness where medical expertise is essential to resolving the problem and patients are willing to relinquish control for the period it takes to do so. It does not work well for chronic illness, disability or mental health conditions where the questions are not so much about resolution as living with the condition. Yet the biomedical model continues its cultural dominance, reinforced by the medical soaps and reality shows that focus on medical triumphs, but seldom convey the continuing erosion of compassionate care that characterizes health systems today.

The Biopsychosocial model: healthcare as a practice

In 1977 George Engel put forward what he called a biopsychosocial model intended to broaden the horizons of the biomedical model. [5] As a psychiatrist, Engel saw the need for medical practice to take account of factors that influence whether people present themselves for biomedical care in the first place, whether they comply with treatment, and whether they have adequate support to change their behaviour. That is, the focus remains essentially upon the individual, but attention is given to determinants that address health behaviours and thus influence the physiological processes that are the core interest of a biomedical approach.

In contrast with the biomedical model, which is a theory-driven model constructed around a scientific understanding of human biology, the biopsychosocial model is a practice model of particular relevance to clinicians. It deals not only with the science of disease, but also with the issues that present in clinical relationships. Not surprisingly, this approach is now reflected in all major medical association journals and most health service provision.

The strength of the model obviously is its inclusion of perspectives relevant to clinical encounters with individuals, not just the disease process within them. The model remains however a variant of the biomedical model. It continues to be based in a positivist scientific paradigm, where biological explanations and solutions are preferred to the 'softer' science of psychology and its explanations of behaviour. While 'social' is included in the title, it is 'social' as psychologists tend to use the term, referring to personal relationships, not the social determinants that are structural constraints upon individual agency.

Nevertheless, the biopsychosocial model is one that begins to cross the borders of conceptual paradigms. It begins to open up the positivist biomedical framework to questions and insights that are not directly suggested by, or answerable within, that paradigm. By focusing more upon the realities of practice and less upon scientific purity, it also lays a foundation for the evidence-based medicine movement of the next decade where outcomes, not scientific orthodoxy, become the arbiter of practice.

Spirituality in the biomedical and biopsychosocial model

The biomedical model in its days of dominance had no place for spirituality. There was thought to be no biological basis for taking spirituality into account, and it was seen as a private matter for individual patients, not something to be taken into account in their treatment. The expanded framework of the biopsychosocial model provided room for this assumption to be questioned. It became clear that people's religious or spiritual commitments had significant effects upon lifestyle and decision-making, and that this in turn had clinical relevance.

Discussion of the impact spiritual belief and practice has upon illness, and debates about healthcare professionals' potential role in spiritual care, began to appear regularly in healthcare literature around the end of the 1980s. These discussions, as this book evidences, have both established common ground and identified key points that continue to be disputed.

One prime example of common ground is the way spirituality has been incorporated in healthcare discourse in ways consistent with the biopsychosocial model. Swinton refers to this as a generic approach.[6] Spirituality is identified as a universal human characteristic, stripped of any particularities of content, class, culture, and religion. Just as psychological and social needs should be attended to in healthcare, so should spiritual needs be included. Spiritual care becomes something that should be available for all, for people of all faiths or none. As with 'psychosocial needs', spiritual needs are of interest because of their effect: they can shape patients' response to care, their decision-making, even perhaps the outcome of their treatment.

Generic spirituality opens up fresh possibilities of attending to aspects of experience that have been marginalized or neglected in the healthcare models of the twentieth century. However, we need also to remember that this generic spirituality is a model adapted to healthcare thinking. It may bear little resemblance to the thinking of patients and families, or the religious traditions to which many still belong.

We will return to this discussion later in the chapter in considering Sulmasy's biopsychosocio-spiritual model which, as the name suggests, is an intentional amplification of the biopsychosocial model.[7,8]

Social models of health

The focus of the biomedical model and its biopyschosocial extension is primarily upon what can be controlled and delivered by the health system. The boundaries of the conversation about health are the boundaries of that health system. A social model extends the horizons of the discussion to include not only the health system, but also other social institutions that influence the health status of individuals, communities and whole populations.

The social model sees health in terms of participation—having a place in your community. The goal of care is to support a person's capacity to participate as fully as possible in society, thus maintaining their social identity as a citizen. The language of social care reflects this—policies and mission statements talk about belonging, participation, and support. The key strategies are supporting, normalizing, educating, resourcing, and the core stories are about networking, negotiating, allocating, prioritizing, mediating, and counselling.

Social models are supported by social science disciplines, particularly psychology and sociology, and the central healthcare practitioners are social workers and health promoters.

Social models are particularly important for people living with chronic illness or disability. Caplan puts it succinctly:

> To argue that we need more medical specialists in chronic illness or disability, more hospitals and long-term care facilities for the chronically-ill and disabled … is to miss the point. What many of those with chronic illnesses or disabilities need is equal opportunity, not … charity. The acutely ill or those facing catastrophic health care emergencies require our beneficence and charity, but those with chronic illnesses and disabilities who are not facing an acute medical crisis deserve something radically different - the right to equality of opportunity. [Reprinted from Caplan H (1992). If I were a rich man could I buy a pancreas? And other essays on the ethics of health care. Courtesy of Indiana University Press.]

In recent years, Caplan's point concerning the structural injustice that can result from treating illness rather than attending to the rights of the person has been radically extended and deepened. The work of the WHO Commission on the Social Determinants of Health has consolidated a huge volume of epidemiological data at a global level to show the health gradient that exists within every society, as well as between societies.[10] The steepness of the gradient is a function of social inequality—the more unequal the society, the worse the health of those of lower socio-economic status. Increasing healthcare expenditure and providing further health services may benefit some individuals of higher status; however, improving the health of populations depends upon a just and reasonable distribution of the nation's wealth, fair work, affordable housing, and opportunity for all citizens to realize their capabilities—even if they choose not to take up that opportunity.[11]

A major strength of the social approach is that it represents health as something that can be pursued even in the midst of illness and disability. In this respect, the situation of 'nothing more to do' that occurs in a curative model at the point when treatment options run out does not occur, or occurs much later, in a participation model. A weakness of the model until recently was its inability to produce hard data in support of the social theory that informed it. That problem has largely been overcome but, in so doing, the model itself becomes a problem to society at large. Pursuing health in a social framework requires fundamental change that few seem willing to contemplate. Not only do health systems (that is, systems for dealing with illness) need to be overhauled, but also all other social systems must be reviewed in terms of equity and justice. Health is to be created outside, and in some respects in spite of, our current health systems.

While the social model expresses health through a different paradigm it is interested in relativizing, not replacing or opposing, a biomedical perspective. The biomedical model is embedded within the social model. Thus, the social model still incorporates the conversation of biomedicine, but adds a further relativizing dimension of social and cultural realities. These bring personal and cultural variation and colour to biomedical evidence, showing that there is more to health than is revealed through the study of illness.

Spirituality in the social model

Spirituality finds a place within this model in at least two ways. One is functional, in that spirituality, at least in its organized forms, fosters social support and participation that improves health. Spirituality can contribute to the social goal of this approach. The other is substantive. Spirituality is seen as an integral aspect of culture, at least of cultures that distinguish themselves from the mainstream of western culture. Such spiritualities are to be respected and included in care because they are an integral part of cultural identity.

This model operates more readily in critical theory or constructionist paradigms. It notes how knowledge is selected to protect the interests of powerful social groups, or constructed to reflect and legitimate the experience of particular communities. What matters is the opportunity to participate in society and live out one's citizenship. If spirituality can contribute, that contribution is welcomed.

The value of participation is primary and with it the social model bypasses the truth claims of spirituality or religion, treating these more as cultural artefacts. Belief—any belief—can be treated as a social fact and evaluated in terms of its social utility. The meaning of a belief may be of vital concern to a patient, but for a healthcare provider what matters is the way it contributes to clinical or social goals.

Interestingly, while social constructionism most often relativizes the truth claims of spiritual and religious discourses, thus reflecting a post-Enlightenment secular analysis, the process has been turned neatly on its head in the work of Hay and Nye[12] on children's spirituality. They argue that a child's biologically-innate spirituality is compromised or eliminated through the training received from the contemporary education system. As Swinton[6] points out, from their perspective it is secularism, not spirituality, which is socially constructed.

Holistic/ecological models

Holistic and ecological models of health further expand the boundaries of the health conversation to include not only the social system, and the health system within that, but also the wider systems of the environment and of cultural worlds. Health is seen as a quest for humanness, for wholeness. The goal of healing is becoming one's self. As with previous models, language reflects this: quest, meaning, companionship are key terms. The core stories are about healing, sustaining, guiding, reconciling, nurturing, liberating and empowering, and a primary strategy is companionship in the search for meaning. To the enquiry disciplines that have supported the previous models, the holistic model adds the arts—literature, philosophy, religion, fine arts. The healthcare practitioners most closely aligned with this perspective tend to be pastoral carers, arts therapists, transpersonal psychologists. They operate at the margins of the health system, linking patients with resources that have nurtured them in the past, or introducing them to fresh sources that will nurture their essential humanity.

Ecological models are now attracting global attention as a consequence of climate science predictions concerning the fate of the planet and the survival struggles that are likely to ensue within decades as resources (water, energy, food) become scarce, and more and more populations find themselves under pressure from an increase in unpredictable climate events and climate shifts that town planning and infrastructure development of the past had never envisaged. Implications for health systems are enormous, but are only now beginning to be explored.[13]

The new public health also engages with these models.[14] At the core of this expansive understanding of health is a commitment to values concerning what society should be like, what global justice requires, how health for all should be pursued. The perspective of the new public health is thoroughly holistic, although for the most part its debates with the clinical and social models of health are conducted on their territory and in their language rather than in terms of underlying values and assumptions about the world.

The strength of the holistic and ecological models is their inclusiveness. A variety of voices that have been systematically marginalized in the other models can now contribute. The weakness of the models is also their inclusiveness. The narratives of health that emerge are varied, complex, products of synthesis and negotiation. The variety that can offer a place to many perspectives can also find it difficult to influence, convince or persuade. Recent public debate on climate change, for example, demonstrates little understanding of how models of complex situations work, in particular that a few variant findings do not invalidate an increasingly-solid predictive model with profound implications for current action.

Spirituality in holistic/ecological models of healthcare

Authority in these models is located in the realm of human experience, beyond the domain of the biological and social sciences alone. Spirituality can contribute 'in its own right' to the multiple conversations that take place. Rather than be constrained by the utilitarian perspectives of the previous models, where health draws upon spirituality primarily for its own purposes, spirituality is free to comment upon health. This commentary ranges from fundamentalist voices railing against the use of healthcare resources for procedures such as abortion, to more liberal voices calling for just and equitable provision of care, through to prophetic eco-spiritual voices drawing attention to the unsustainable nature of our current health systems and the need to prepare for a different future.[15] Behind this diversity is a common theme: spirituality demands that values be overt in healthcare conversations. The implications of any healthcare policy should be evaluated in terms of inclusion and equity, the use and abuse of power implicit in 'clinical judgement' should be explored, the medical industry should be called to account for the ways in which, through public funding of research, private donation, and covert influence, it shapes evidence, practice and policy. The health of the planet, not just of populations, should be of concern, because the latter depends on the former.

Spirituality calls for social transformation, even if the different voices cannot agree on what this transformation should be. The fact, if not the current content, of today's spiritual revival is a sign of hope that transformation is possible. Two decades ago social theorist Anthony Giddens suggested that integral to a new social order will be a new spirituality, a shared way of affirming particular values that will support the new institutions and put bounds on the utter openness of modernity.[16] That new spirituality is needed now.

The tradition of spiritual care

The previous section indicates the capacity for spirituality to lead the healthcare discussion, but health systems are as yet reluctant to engage with these broader issues, just as they struggle to respond to mounting evidence of the profound effects of social determinants of health. The conversation spirituality is able to have with today's health systems is about the contribution spirituality might make to health as healthcare conceptualizes this.

Healthcare became an autonomous institution in modernity and correspondingly less inclined to remember its pre-clinical past. Traditional healing practices, although still surviving, are very much at the margins of today's healthcare. Religious spirituality however continues to live with a consciousness of its past, one consequence of which is that spiritual traditions provide options from which to respond to healthcare. Another is that understandings of spirituality from other eras can continue to confound contemporary conversations within healthcare.

Spirituality and social organization

Western society has experienced two major patterns of social organization, traditional society and modern society, and is currently undergoing a further transition to a post-modern era.[17] Contemporary society is not yet post-modern, but significant changes to social organization foreshadow a different future. Institutions serve different purposes in different social eras. Similarly core beliefs and values, even when the same names are retained, undergo shifts in their meaning. This has been the case with spirituality.

In traditional western society the principal authority was religion. Belief was held in common and spiritual practices involved rituals intended to anchor that belief in everyday life. Exemplary spiritual lives were lived in community by religious specialists on behalf of the whole society. A spiritual life was characterized by right practice, not necessarily by any capacity to articulate belief—that was the role of the experts. Spirituality was a response to the God who had created the whole social order.

In modern society the principal authority was that of the sciences that catalysed massive technological change leading to new patterns of social organization. In this new social order belief became private and individual, and spirituality was identified with the private piety of religious individuals. Spiritual practices came to involve principally the mind rather than the body—right belief became more important than right practice. Spirituality was concerned with individual salvation.

In today's contemporary society the principal authority increasingly is the self. Belief is each individual's choice, and spirituality focuses on the human spirit: spirituality has a complex relationship with religion. Spiritual practices involve both mind and body, expressing personal preferences and seeking control of one's own life. Individual spirituality focuses on right fit—is it right for me? There is no authoritative institution or discourse that can dictate spirituality's meaning as did religion in traditional society or science/medicine in modern society.

Spiritual care and its changing relationships with health care

Walter outlines, using the hospice movement as an example, how all three of these understanding of spirituality have engaged successively with healthcare to produce different models of spiritual care.

1. A religious community provides total care according to its particular beliefs and practices
2. Only some people are religious, and their needs can be met by referral to the appropriate religious practitioner
3. All people are spiritual, and all staff members are involved in some fashion in spiritual care.

All three of these approaches to spiritual care are still active within contemporary healthcare systems. The first is now a minor presence, associated with religious healthcare institutions that to varying degrees shape care according to their beliefs. The second continues to have a major influence. Despite a growing literature of spiritual care and training in spiritual care there remains at the practice level a default understanding of spirituality as expressed in religious affiliation and therefore the business of the chaplaincy department. No matter that most chaplaincy departments operate out of the third approach: many staff still see this approach as imposing further responsibilities on an overloaded workforce.

Walter expresses reservations about all three models.[18] His conclusion is:

> In all three approaches, the question of vulnerability is crucial. Committed Christians can hide behind creeds and dogmas, busy nurses can protect themselves from patients' unanswerable questions by calling in the chaplain, and the new holistic practitioner can use listening skills to disengage from the pain of 'having no answer'. Whether spiritual care can be organized on a large scale, and still be worthy of the name, has yet to be demonstrated.

Walter's warning is worth noting, but even more worthy of note is his contention that spiritual care depends upon the quality of relationship offered rather than ways in which spiritual care may be organized.

Models of spiritual care

It is clear from the previous discussion that developing a model for spiritual care involves both articulating an understanding of spirituality and choosing a context for practice. It is also clear that it is unusual for a contemporary healthcare institution to embrace religious understandings of spirituality, except insofar as these are assimilated within cultural needs. For spirituality to be included within contemporary healthcare systems it must adopt a generic form, that is, one applicable to all. Lartey (see also Chapter 41) provides a useful example of this. He suggests that spirituality involves relationships:

- With places and things (spatial)
- With self (intra-personal)
- With others (inter-personal)
- Among people (corporate)
- With transcendence ('God', 'Something There').[19]

Obviously any model based on such a description will be both interdisciplinary and inter-paradigmatic, for the disciplines needed to understand and address all these aspects come from across the span of human enquiry. Further, the description provides not only a general guide for spiritual enquiry (which relationships matter, which have been disrupted, which might be renewed? …), but it also identifies a framework into which relational content unique to each person can be mapped. The capacity to provide both a general framework and specific attention to individual needs, resources and possibilities is an essential feature in meeting the demands of a health service and respecting the uniqueness of an individual's spiritual path.

Most screening and assessment tools (see chapters 44–46) are derived from a description of spirituality, which is in turn frequently developed from enquiries into the views and patients and caregivers. Lartey's description too has been used as the basis for a Relational Web model of spiritual screening.[20]

Operational models of spiritual care

Spiritual care models predominantly need to address a health services context where care provision is organized according to a biopsychosocial model. Spirituality is introduced as a further dimension or domain of care alongside physical, psychological and social domains, and spiritual needs assessments are carried out alongside psychosocial assessments. Usually these spiritual assessments are adapted to the style of other assessments carried out in the psychosocial domains. That is, the assessment of spiritual needs and resources adopts a form readily recognisable to the host system with a view to acceptance, and ideally participation, by all healthcare staff.

Frequently, this spiritual domain of care is simply juxtaposed with other domains: little attention is given to the effects of expanding the system of care in this way or the compromises involved in adapting spiritual care to the host model. Some of these conceptual compromises have already been outlined in the 'spirituality in the biomedical and biopsychosocial models' discussion above. A further risk is one endemic to health systems: that spiritual care strategies will become stereotyped and that workforce substitution will put initial spiritual screening in unskilled or unsympathetic hands.

The biopsychosocial-spiritual model, by including spiritual care within an integrated model, attempts to reduce these risks by addressing them directly. Sulmasy's comprehensive discussion that introduces the model[8] identifies such compromises and calls attention to conditions that are essential to maintaining spiritual care as spiritual, not pop-psychological, care.[18] These include an awareness of the richness and diversity of spirituality beyond the functional approach taken in healthcare settings, and the need for healthcare practitioners to be formed in spiritual care, not merely trained in using the assessment tools. This in turn has implications for the way spiritual care participates and cooperates in the whole enterprise of care. Further discussion of this can be found in Sulmasy's book[8] and in contemporary applications to spirituality in end of life care.[21,22] In practice the biopsychosocial-spiritual model finds natural allies in the patient centred care model and further developments of this approach.[23–26] These are models that cross between or combine conceptual paradigms with the aim of creating unity of practice. All are examples of the participatory enquiry paradigm[2,27] that integrates the insights of a range of conceptual frameworks through collaborative practice.

Sulmasy's own account identifies the importance of moving spirituality beyond health systems models. The spirituality of health systems remains individualistic and spiritual care professionalized. Broader spiritual concerns, such as social inclusion and justice, are not addressed. While health systems aim for, and struggle to achieve, some degree of equity in treating illness they cannot address equity in health. Health is created and maintained in places beyond the control of the health system, where people are born and brought up and live their lives.

Narrative development within and beyond healthcare

Spiritual journeys may well begin, or be revived, within the health system, but they should not end upon discharge from the system. Spiritual care models within healthcare must point to wider horizons. One description of a process by which this can take place is Bury's account of chronic illness narratives.[28] He identifies three categories or storylines. Each storyline incorporates, but transcends the previous one. They are not inevitably progressive, but are potentially so. They correlate with the storylines of the expanding horizons of health outlined at the beginning of this chapter.

The initial stories people tell are about the origins, onset, symptoms and effects of illness. Bury calls these contingent narratives, and they are located within a health services (biomedical) framework. People recount how they recognized the illness, how they presented for diagnosis and treatment, how their career as a patient is developing.

In the midst of these contingent narratives another storyline usually begins to appear. Bury calls this moral narratives, and these are stories that explore and evaluate altered relationships with body, self and society. People begin to reflect upon how their engagement with everyday life is changed as a consequence of their illness. These narratives are located in a social framework. While contingent stories are still told, they are told now within the wider horizon of social participation, which gives a meaning to illness experience beyond that provided by the diagnostic and prognostic interpretations of a health services perspective.

As contingent and moral narratives are developed further, another storyline begins to appear. These stories are about people's changes in identity and self-presentation. Bury calls them core narratives, and they represent a further expansion of the horizon to include reflection upon meaning and purpose in life. These narratives are located in a holistic model of care.

Bury thus sketches an illness journey that takes its participants through experiences that, to be assimilated into a person's life, require expanding the horizons of that person's understanding of health. Transitions between storylines are not always easy—Frank[29] names as chaos the first transition that occurs when biomedical perspectives no longer work and meaning must be found elsewhere—but the process outlined is that of a spiritual journey.

Conclusion

Current conversations between spirituality and healthcare are conducted largely on healthcare terms. Within the biomedical model interest is in whether providing spiritual services will serve its goals, decreasing the length of admissions, improving patient compliance, and increasing responsiveness to treatments. Within the social model interest is in whether spirituality will increase social cohesiveness and social support, and promote resilience.

From the viewpoint of those with spirituality as a primary interest, contemporary models of spiritual care must avoid assimilation to health service models even while accepting that a cost of incorporating spiritual care in healthcare is a degree of conceptual narrowing and functional application of spiritual insights. One safeguard is to ensure that there is a robust and expansive spiritual discussion beyond the boundaries of the health system so that healthcare spirituality models can never be seen as comprehending the richness and diversity of human spirituality. The wider discussion must move beyond the interiority of modern spirituality to engage with issues of human destiny and human possibility that currently confront us as the unsustainability of modern culture becomes increasingly apparent. It should also stand as a constant reminder that spiritual care takes place within genuine human encounters, and requires both skill and humility of its practitioners; it is not something that can be delivered simply as a professional service.

A further suggestion here is that encounters within health services can catalyse a spiritual journey. For many people in western societies it is a change in health status that provides the challenge to view life in a different way. For this challenge to invite a spiritual journey we need health practitioners that can respond to patient' experiences of disruption and health services that are open to them doing so. However, for the journey to continue, and for health practitioners to be resourced themselves, we need communities that nurture lively spiritual enquiry.

In the chapters that follow in this section many of these issues are worked out in accordance with differing disciplinary stances and contexts of practice.

References

1 Barbour, I.G. (1974). *Myths, Models and Paradigms: the Nature of Scientific and Religious Language.* London: SCM Press. p. 6

2 Lincoln, Y., Guba, E. (2005). Paradigmatic controversies, contradictions and emerging confluences. In: N. Denzin, Y. Lincoln (eds) *The Sage Handbook of Qualitative Research*, 3rd edn, pp. 191–215. Thousand Oaks: Sage.

3 [1]. p. 9
4 Parsons, T. (1951). *The Social System*. New York: Free Press.
5 Engel, G. (1977). The need for a new medical model: a challenge for biomedicine. *Science*, **196**(4286): 129–36.
6 Swinton, J. (2010). The meanings of spirituality: a multiperspective approach to 'the spiritual.' In: W. McSherry, L. Ross (eds) *Spiritual Assessment in Healthcare Practice*, pp. 17–35. Keswick: M&K Publishing.
7 Sulmasy, D.P. (2002). A biopsychosocial–spiritual model for the care of patients at the end of life. *Gerontologist* 42: Oct, 24–37.
8 Sulmasy, D.P. (2007). *The Rebirth of the Clinic: an Introduction to Spirituality in Health Care*. Washington DC: Georgetown University Press.
9 Caplan, H. (1992). *If I Were a Rich Man Could I Buy a Pancreas? And Other Essays on the Ethics of Health Care*, p. 235. Bloomington: Indiana University Press.
10 WHO Commission on the Social Determinants of Health (2008). *Closing the Gap in a Generation*: Health Equity Through Action on the Social Determinants of Health, final report of the Commission on Social Determinants of Health. Geneva: World Health Organization.
11 Nussbaum, M.C. (2011). *Creating Capabilities: the Human Development Approach*. Cambridge: Harvard University Press.
12 Hay, D. (2006). *The Spirit of the Child*. London: Jessica Kingsley.
13 McMichael, A.J., Campbell-Lendrum, D.H., Corvalan, C.F., Ebi, K.L., Githeko, A., Scheraga, J.D., *et al.* (2003). *Climate Change and Human Health: Risks and Responses*. Geneva: WHO.
14 Baum, F. (2008). *The New Public Health*, 3rd edn. Melbourne: Oxford University Press.
15 Flannery, T. (2010). *Here on Earth: an Argument for Hope*. Melbourne: Text Publishing.
16 Giddens, A. (1990). *The Consequences of Modernity*. Cambridge: Polity.
17 Walter, T. (1994). *The Revival of Death*. London: Routledge.
18 Walter, T. (1997). The ideology and organization of spiritual care: three approaches. *Palliat Med* **11***:* 21–30.
19 Lartey, E. (1997). *In Living Colour: an Intercultural Approach to Pastoral Care and Counselling*, p. 113. London: Cassell.
20 Rumbold, B. (2007). A review of spiritual assessment in health care practice. *Med J Aust* **186:** S60–2.
21 Puchalski, C., Ferrell, B, Virani, R. *et al.* (2009). Improving the quality of spiritual care as a dimension of palliative care: The report of the consensus conference. *J Palliat Med* **12**(10): 885–904.
22 Puchalski, C., Ferrell, B. (2010). *Making Health Care Whole: Integrating Spirituality into Patient Care*, pp. 55–73. West Conshohocken: Templeton Press.
23 Tresolini, C.P., Pew-Fetzer Task Force (1994). *Health Professions Education and Relationship-centered Care*. San Francisco: Pew Health Professions Commission.
24 World Health Organization Noncommunicable Diseases and Mental Health Cluster, Chronic Disease and Health Promotion Department (2005). *Preparing a Health Care Workforce for the 21st Century: the Challenge of Chronic Conditions*. Paris: WHO.
25 World Health Organization Regional Office for the Western Pacific (2007). *People at the Centre of Healthcare: a Policy Framework*. Manila: WHO.
26 Johansson, I.L. (2010). *Patient Centred Care*. Bradford: Emerald Group.
27 Heron, J., Reason, P. (1997). A participatory inquiry paradigm. *Qual Inq* **3**(3): 274–95.
28 Bury, M. (2001). Illness narratives: fact or fiction? *Soc Hlth Illness* **23**(3): 263–85.
29 Frank, A. (1995). *The Wounded Storyteller*. Chicago: University of Chicago Press.

CHAPTER 27

Healthcare chaplaincy

Chris Swift, George Handzo, and Jeffrey Cohen

Introduction

This chapter concerns the role of the chaplain as the person explicitly in charge of the provision of religious and spiritual care in healthcare. What we offer here will help all health professionals understand the part played by the chaplain in healthcare. This is important because the ability of a chaplain to work effectively is dependent on the full integration of the chaplain into the healthcare team. To achieve this chaplains have accelerated their professional development in order that other healthcare staff encounter them as competent, qualified, and vocationally focused members of the team. From personal experience as well as published research we know that when spiritual care is well integrated and effective the patient's ability to cope; find meaning; and be supported during a crisis, is enhanced.[1] Despite some unevenness in the emerging body of evidence for spiritual care, and the inevitable difficulty in applying such research findings from one culture to another, the overall conclusion is clearly that effectively supported spirituality makes a beneficial difference to the experience and progress of illness.[2]

A significant characteristic of Westernized countries from the mid-twentieth century onwards has been the move away from religious affiliation and authority towards a less defined and more individual expression of religion and spirituality.[3] One consequence of this change is that many people who need spiritual support when they are ill do not have a faith community to supply it. The response of professional chaplains has been to become more skilled at ministering to people of a wide variety of spiritualities and religions. It may be helpful at this point to say that when we talk about 'religious care' we mean pastoral, ethical, and ritual support that recognizably belongs to an established religion (Sikhism, Judaism, Islam, Christianity, etc.). When we use the term 'spiritual care' we are referring both to aspects of religious care and also to actions taken in situations where there is no formal religious identification, but many of the issues usually associated with religion are present, such as existential considerations, concerns about hope, anxieties about isolation, and the need for contemplative silence. When we refer to 'chaplaincy care', we are addressing that part of spiritual care specifically reserved for professional chaplains.

The response to spiritual need is shaped significantly by its context, including the healthcare system in which it is set. For this reason, we give a brief synopsis of the health environments where we operate before focusing on three episodes of chaplaincy care. These, in turn, will form the basis for a wider discussion of spiritual care practice from the perspective of the chaplains' participation in the care team. With reference to the growing literature underpinning chaplaincy, both of research and professional guidance, this section will link the case studies to a broader view of the unique contribution the chaplain makes to spiritual care.

Spiritual care in the UK

The UK is made up of four home countries that all operate versions of the National Health Service (NHS). Since the creation of the NHS in 1948 chaplains have continued to be funded by the health provider (e.g. hospital), although a significant body of voluntary chaplaincy has also co-existed with the paid provision. While this ownership of chaplaincy by the NHS produced some uniformity (for example, in pay and conditions) it has allowed for considerable diversity in the expression of spiritual care in each hospital.[4] Within the UK there are some differences in the approach to spiritual care. For example, in Scotland there is a strong emphasis on generic spiritual care[5] while in England there is a formula linking chaplaincy staffing very closely with the religious demographics of the inpatient population of local hospitals.[6] Chaplaincy departments contain a mix of faith representatives who share a common path of training and are expected to work together in a corporate way to meet both the religious and spiritual needs of patients, staff and visitors. The total number of whole-time funded chaplains in England in 2009 was 503.[7]

To inform the practice development of chaplaincy, the use of data has become more important in recent years. An independent survey of 73 health providers in England showed that approximately 15.2% of recently discharged acute hospital patients had wished to practice their faith while in hospital.[8] Of these 16.5% had said they had been unable to do this in the way they would wish. Extrapolated across the NHS in England in one year this could mean that between 260,000 and 385,000 patients wished to practice their faith, but were unable to do so properly. In short, even in a society popularly understood to be secular, the scale of religious need continues to be striking within healthcare due to many factors, not least the questions which illness raises and the demographic characteristics of the sick. Consideration also needs to be given to the evidence that as traditional religious affiliation changes there is a growing interest in spirituality and new forms of spiritual expression. Reflecting this development chaplains are contributing to an increasing literature exploring the identification of spiritual needs and the kind of care that is required to assess and meet those needs in the context of illness.[9]

Spiritual care in Australia

Since healthcare is a state responsibility, spiritual care is driven through the prism of regionalism. Often there is an established body whose role is to represent faith communities to state agencies (prisons, health, and mental health). It is only in the last decade that non-Christian faiths have been included. In the century since Australia became a Federation in 1901, those identifying as Christian in the census has fallen from 96.1 to 63.9% in 2006.

In general, chaplaincy is done on a faith-based basis in each state. Funding for some chaplains is allocated by the State's Health budget. Some funding comes directly from the faith communities and it is not unusual for pastoral care to be provided by the local church, synagogue, mosque, or temple. This may be by the minister or some lay visitors. Large teaching hospitals are those which tend to receive state funding, but through the faith communities.

Those hospitals which are faith based believe Pastoral and Spiritual Care is a base value of the institution and employ people more in a 'discipline' based care with chaplains assigned to clinical units with the inherent skills development and relationship to a particular unit and its staff.

The one exception is the state of Victoria where the government which has supported Healthcare Chaplaincy Council of Victoria Inc. HCCVI is moving more and more to discipline specific pastoral care. They are involved in the selection process for many institutions as they develop their Spiritual Care. HCCVI has the dual role in its mission of education and training as well as the development of chaplaincy and pastoral care services across the State of Victoria. Perhaps their most important contribution has been the development of a Capabilities framework.[10]

For a period, one hospital appointed a Humanist Chaplain. Recognizing that people can be spiritual without being committed to any faith is becoming more and more common

Spiritual care in the United States

In the US, most patients and families want their religious and spiritual beliefs and practice taken into account by their healthcare providers.[11] However, many patients are unaffiliated with religious communities, which can support them when they are suffering.[12]

Over time, the responsibility for health ministry has shifted from the religious community to the healthcare institution itself. Services provided by religious communities are increasingly confined to ritual and sacramental ministries. In the last decade in particular, chaplaincy is becoming a professional discipline which increasingly operates as a multifaith, referral service. Generally, it is no longer the case that particular chaplains visit only the patients of their faith tradition. In current best practice, chaplains visit patients of all faiths selected according to specific protocols and are assigned to specific locations or service lines, generally selected for their strategic importance to the institution.[13,14]

In 2004, the major chaplaincy membership associations in North America adopted common standards for certification of chaplains which require 1600 hours of clinical pastoral education, graduate theological education and demonstration of 29 competencies.[15] In 2009, the Association of Professional Chaplains promulgated the first standards of practice for professional chaplains[16] These standards specify that the chaplain will assess, document, and have a plan for interventions and expected outcomes. Professional board-certified chaplains are beginning to be required in consensus standards particularly in palliative care and cancer[17,18] and increasingly considered the spiritual care lead on the healthcare team. Increasingly, patients admitted to hospital are screened for spiritual distress and spiritual belief and practice is a part of a complete history taken by the primary care giver. Patients with demonstrated spiritual need are then referred to a professional chaplain.

Case study: England, UK

The on-call chaplain is paged by the hospital switchboard to attend the wife (Mrs M) of a patient who has died. Within 10 minutes the chaplain arrives and meets the nurse in charge, who provides a basic outline of the situation and why the chaplain has been called. A Muslim patient has died who has not been practicing his faith for many years. He had married a Christian who has no Church connection. The couple had been together for nearly 20 years and the man's wife knows that he wished to be buried as a Muslim. As she has no idea how to go about this, the staff suggested calling a chaplain. On meeting Mrs M, the nurse's account is confirmed: she wishes to respect his wishes, but has no idea how to achieve this. The chaplain explains that a Muslim colleague is on the team and would be happy to speak with her. Mrs M agrees to this while asking for the support of the present chaplain to continue. After spending some time hearing about the deceased at the patient's bedside, offering pastoral support by listening and empathy, the chaplain makes a brief entry of his involvement in the patient's medical notes and goes to speak with his Muslim colleague. Following this conversation the chaplain begins an electronic record on the hospital's chaplaincy database including the core elements of his visit and subsequent action. When both chaplains go to the ward together they begin to discuss how the funeral might be managed. It emerges that one disparity of expectation centres around Mrs M's presence at the funeral. Muslim women in this community do not go to the graveside—but that would be alien to the practice of this widow. Through careful and sensitive discussion, eventually including the local Muslim leadership, it is agreed how the funeral will be conducted and a place is identified near the grave where Mrs M can stand to see the burial take place.

In the UK it is normal for acute hospitals to provide a 24/7 on-call chaplaincy service. In this case the call came during normal working hours, but it could equally have arisen late at night. Either way, the response is prompt and begins with a briefing from the clinical staff. It is important that the chaplain does not proceed solely on the information provided by the nurse. In difficult situations a briefing is important, but needs to be checked out directly with the relative. A lot can get lost in transmission and the patient or relative's narrative may undergo subtle changes depending on their listener. While evaluating the needs of the relative the chaplain is also providing pastoral support, giving space and respect to the personal crisis of the widow. When the situation is understood, and the conversation has reached a natural point of change, the chaplain leaves to explore in discussion with a qualified colleague how the spiritual and religious needs might best be addressed. The chaplain does not simply 'pass the buck' to his Muslim colleague, but seeing the need for ongoing pastoral support at a stressful time, returns to the wards with the Muslim chaplain. It could well be that in making her request about a husband who has both not practiced his faith and also married outside his religion, the widow is anxious about being judged. The ability of both chaplains to work together enables a compromise to be found about the burial. This is felt to honour the integrity of all involved and highlights the way a multi-faith chaplaincy team can negotiate complex spiritual needs with the local community. This approach is not only helpful to the family, but also shows how spiritual expertise can reduce the anxieties of nursing staff who may feel out of their depth in the face of such situations. In pluralist societies like the UK situations such as this are likely to increase in the coming years.

Case study: Australia

The catholic chaplain/priest is called to the post-natal area of the Women's Hospital to meet with a couple. They introduce themselves as members of a catholic church in the local diocese. They do attend the parish services about once a month. They inform the chaplain that the wife has just had an abortion. This would have been their first child. The mother is in her mid-thirties and thus feels the biological clock ticking loudly! They know that their own priest would only castigate them for breaking the rules of the Church. What they want from the chaplain is some prayers for both themselves and the child which will not be the fulfilment of their dreams.

Parts, if not all of this scenario would be familiar to anyone working in Obstetrics. The priest knows that had they consulted him prior to the event he would have needed to explain the Church's position to the couple, but ultimately it would always be the couple's decision. The priest is only too well aware that the language of the church, especially in relation to all matters sexual, is largely irrelevant to the faithful, for the model was never designed for an educated, thinking middle class laity. The Bishop is seen as an authoritarian reactionary, who could make an issue of any action the priest takes if the bishop ever learns of anything differing from the established values of the church. Only weeks before, Bishops in another part of the world had taken a position that individuals who divorced (secularly) should be denied communion and that some local bishops desired to take a similar position.

The Chaplain believed in Ministry of Presence. He was not interested in reducing any psychological dissonance. What he wanted to offer to the couple was to be non-judgemental. He knew that in this situation he needed to bring the Creator's presence to this couple at a time when they clearly were struggling, both psychologically and existentially, of whether they had made the correct decision. He realized that the couple had not sought guidance of the Church in this matter prior to the procedure. Rather what they sought was two things. First, was the baptism of the foetus, and second to have prayers for both the foetus and themselves. He had no problem with either request. First, the foetus should not be judged by any action of the parents and that, had it been a spontaneous abortion, rather than induced, a baptism would have been given. Second was the more complex issue about the parents. The chaplain saw what was necessary was Prayers of Reconciliation. These needed to be offered on two levels. The couple needed to be reconciled to each other and their action so that neither would have recriminations over their actions. Just as important was that they be reconciled to their faith and church. Faith is as much a cultural and ethnic issue as it was about belief. They felt most comfortable attending a Roman Catholic church and his offering such reconciliation would be appropriate.

On the following Sunday, the family gathered with the chaplain where a special liturgy of reconciliation was offered.

Case study: USA

Mrs S is a 65-year-old woman with chronic obstructive pulmonary disease admitted to the hospital for difficulty breathing for the fourth time in the last 3 months. The emergency room physician referred her to the hospital's palliative care team. On initial screening, it was noted that religion was very important to Mrs S, but she had not been able to attend church recently because of her health. The spiritual history noted that Mrs S was Jewish and considered herself to be a righteous woman of deep faith, but her physical suffering was causing her to doubt whether God really cared about her. The palliative care referral had automatically triggered a referral to the palliative care chaplain in the hospital, Fr. Jones, an Episcopal priest. The chaplain's assessment confirmed the findings of the history. The chaplain's spiritual care plan included a request to the hospital rabbi to visit regularly for prayer. The chaplain worked with Mrs S. to help her examine her beliefs about how God was present in her life and rediscover the ways God was supporting her even in her suffering. The chaplain's plan was documented in the patient's medical record. On discharge, the chaplain, with Mrs S's consent, called her synagogue to request regular home visits from the congregations' Bikur Cholim members and to help monitor Mrs S's physical condition with the goal of receiving outpatient treatment before emergency care and hospitalization was required.

While this is a composite case, it is consistent with best practice in spiritual care and chaplain care in the USA, especially in palliative and end-of-life care. As a person with a chronic illness where anxiety and spiritual distress can clearly exacerbate symptoms, research suggests that Mrs S is a prime candidate for intervention by the chaplain.[19] Her spiritual and religious needs were considered both on her initial screening and on her full history. The screening would probably have been a question or two, which would determine whether she is religious and whether that religious belief and practice is helping her at this time. The inclusion of questions on religion and spirituality in the full history are again to gather data on the impact of spirituality on the patient's coping and to help the primary caregiver (i.e. doctor or nurse practitioner) have a better direct appreciation of the patient's spiritual like. The chaplain referral was automatic with her referral to palliative care. Other conditions that often trigger such an automatic referral include death, respiratory arrest, referral to hospice, request for organ donation, and referral for an ethics committee consult. Again, according to best practice, the responding chaplain was the chaplain assigned to Mrs S's medical team, even though he was not of her faith group. Because of his training and particular knowledge of the spiritual issues of patients like Mrs S, Fr. Jones was especially able to help Mrs S. address her spiritual concerns while accessing hospital and community religious resources appropriately. Since Fr. Jones rounds regularly with the palliative care team, he is able to coordinate Mrs S's spiritual needs. Although Mrs S. belongs to a formal religious group, the chaplain's intervention around her spiritual distress would have been roughly the same if Mrs S's spirituality were rooted in a love of nature or a devotion to social causes.

Professional chaplaincy care

What we have described so far indicates some of the skills and knowledge that chaplains bring to the situations they face in healthcare on a daily basis. Across our different contexts we see many common themes, such as essential information recording and sharing, that illustrate the determination of the chaplain to work with colleagues to provide the best possible support for the patient. That approach is one of the reasons why in each of our countries chaplains have moved outside any exclusive sense of a narrow denominational role. The response of chaplains is shaped by the human reality they encounter, requiring them to deliver bespoke spiritual care services, which recognize the uniqueness of every situation. In the community a *minister* is associated with the life and vitality of a church, synagogue, or mosque, maintaining and developing a particular theology and spirituality. In a hospital the *chaplain* is tasked with discerning spiritual needs as they are encountered and shaping with the patient a response that may not sit within a single tradition. As our case study from the USA demonstrates, both the chaplain and synagogue carers work together in different ways to a common end: to relieve suffering and enhance the patient's capacity to cope positively with their experience. It remains important that chaplains are rooted and formed in a spiritual tradition, enabling them to work in the territory of existential concerns even when they do not share the specific beliefs of those they attend. In recent years this has been supplemented by a growing body of literature defining the professional character of the chaplain, including new policies that connect the chaplain to particular duties and a consensus of practice. This not only enables a shared focus on the challenges and dilemmas of chaplaincy, but also communicates to other health professionals the nature and scope of the chaplain's responsibilities.

In the US these developments include the standards for distress management in cancer from the Consensus Conference on Spiritual Care in Palliative Care. These require Board Certified Chaplains (BCC) to be the spiritual care leads on palliative care teams. The National Comprehensive Cancer Network lays a similar obligation on the role of chaplains within oncology services. In the UK there has also been a focus on the chaplain's involvement in clinical guidance on supportive and palliative care (NICE, 2004) and further clarification of role is expected in new guidance for end of life care. At the same time chaplains have produced a new *Code of Practice* and the UK Board of Healthcare Chaplaincy has set out standards for the profession.[20] The *Code* provides profession-specific guidance on topics that have particular impact within the practice of chaplaincy. Examples of this include the use of touch (alongside prayer; anointing, etc.), as well as a description of spiritual abuse and safeguards against proselytizing.

All these publications evidence the development of chaplains as a profession and provide a detailed understanding of how chaplaincy spiritual care is integrated into clinical practice. As we have seen in the three case studies, chaplains require the skill, knowledge and experience to provide spiritual care that crosses the limits of particular faith boundaries. While in many instances chaplains will work to meet religious need in partnership with ministers of a particular faith, on other occasions chaplains encounter less defined expressions of spiritual need. To do this safely and responsibly it is important for the chaplains concerned, and also for the organization providing the care, that a shared body of knowledge is available and understood. Chaplains must be skilled brokers of spiritual care, enabling responses well beyond the limits of their own faith formation. The reality of that experience means that chaplains must be literate in the beliefs and practices of their hospital population, knowledgably shaping spiritual care to meet the needs of each patient. In turn this approach has led to the growth in all our countries of schemes and resources for continuing professional development. In the USA the long tradition of Clinical Pastoral Education provides a comprehensive framework for chaplains of all faiths to reflect and improve practice together. While in the UK the emphasis has been on masters' level training informed by critical reflection on many different aspects of the chaplain's context and pastoral responsibilities. As the strategic provider the NHS and four national departments of health have also led aspects of policy review, research appraisal, and educational resourcing.[21]

In addition to their own training and development it is important to note that chaplains are frequently required to teach the spiritual care elements of training for a host of other health professions. While nursing may be the largest of these groups the chaplain as a CPD provider resources physiotherapists, medics, psychologists, pathologists and midwives—to name, but a few.

In each of the case studies other hospital staff were supported by the chaplain's involvement. When faced with specific or complex spiritual needs the clinical team has the means to make a referral to the chaplain as a colleague. Like the nursing and medical staff the chaplain is trained and appraised as a competent member of the care team. This can include mandatory training about infection control, information governance, the care of vulnerable people, the spiritual dimensions of dying, and major incident response. Unlike the visiting minister from the community, who has a distinct and important role to play, the chaplain is embedded within the hospital as a trained and supervised professional colleague of the staff. Alongside the on-the-spot support for colleagues that can arise when the chaplain is involved in a traumatic or difficult case, chaplains are also available for debriefing after such situations, even when they have not been directly involved in the episode itself. This can include a wide range of stressful events, from a patient death that has affected a nurse, to anxieties about job security, a risk of burnout, or work related tensions in a team. While the chaplain is a loyal member of the hospital organization this does not prevent her from reflecting 'shop floor' anxieties when these appear to stem from particular institutional practices or approaches to change. A unique feature of a chaplaincy team is its wide-ranging presence throughout the organization, including attendance during the night and on holidays, leading to a potentially impressive level of awareness about how the hospital is functioning. This supplies an important narrative to accompany performance data and broaden the management's understanding of the organization as a whole.

It is increasingly common to find chaplains achieving accreditation for their work from professional bodies and boards. In the USA this system is well established while in the UK it is an emerging phenomenon. One consequence of this development is a growing practice for healthcare chaplaincy to be referred to as a profession in its own right alongside groups such as social work and nursing. With the Internet there is also a wider international forum for chaplaincy, including publications such as *Plain Views* that are read by a multinational group of subscribers numbering over one thousand. As chaplaincy develops in this way, drawing in a more diverse group of spiritual carers, there is a gradual process of refinement in our understanding of the unique contribution the chaplain makes to the care of patients.

One widely recognized aspect of the chaplains' practice relates to ethical debate. As scientific and technical advances enable ever more treatment choices in care the importance of ethical frameworks is emphasized. The values that inform decisions are often in question, and in some cases religious beliefs impact on the willingness of clinicians to take part in certain activities. The UK's General Medical Council has issued guidance for doctors on the role of their beliefs in relation to the care they are expected to provide.[22] Yet even when such guidance exists it does not imply that doctors and nurses always feel at ease with what they are doing. The role of chaplains is one of understanding and supporting these staff concerns, exploring together a spiritual tradition or beliefs in relation to the practices of healthcare. Such concerns extend well beyond longstanding issues such as abortion, and can include staff uniforms and religious modesty; signing cremation certificates; and providing advice or a referral seen to be at odds with faith convictions. As a pastor embedded in the hospital environment the chaplain is ideally placed to perform a role supporting the dignity of the clinicians' personal belief as they seek to bring about healing. At other times, the chaplain relates to ward staff when spiritual, religious, and ethical difficulties arise for patients and their relatives. The complex identity of the chaplain (a community figure, as well as a hospital employee) becomes a useful resource when patients find that their beliefs become difficult to honour in the context of healthcare. Situations can range from the need for a religious diet, to the discussion of withdrawing life-support, to the provision of accessible prayer and chapel facilities. As someone seen to provide an independent ear for such situations the chaplain can bridge differences of understanding to enable positive solutions. In our case studies this role can be seen, where further distress is averted by the chaplain's ability to use a network of internal and external resources to develop effective responses to spiritual and religious need.

Conclusion

In this chapter we have set out a dynamic picture of religious and spiritual care with reference to a growing literature and three brief case studies. We have noted the persistence of needs arising in healthcare not only from those with clear religious affiliations, but increasingly from those whose spirituality is not defined by traditional boundaries. The chaplain's leading role in spiritual care is characterized by a detailed knowledge of personal beliefs and the relationship of these to health and illness. Through the chaplain's expertise patients are supported during some of the most difficult experiences any of us ever faces. The care that is provided enables the patient to cope and make sense while often engaging a network of support that benefits the patient long after discharge. In an era when medicine has excelled in its ability to treat ever smaller and discrete aspects of illness the care provided by the chaplain is essential for keeping the complete person in view. As chaplains work alongside other staff, and transect the organization as a whole, they are embodied reminders of the way in which spirituality is connected to the ancient and sacred tasks of healing and caring for the sick.

When critics have drawn attention to the enormous breadth of how the term 'spirituality' has been employed in healthcare literature,[23] they have ignored the personal beliefs and experiences, which define us. Since the modern professional chaplain works with the patient's sense of what is spirituality significant for *them*, there is indeed a flexibility in the use of the term, which is wholly appropriate. There is no exclusion list of items, which may not, under any circumstances, be considered to be spiritual. Where experiences link us to sacred themes,[24] or become contextualized by broader relationships to creation, human, or divine communities, the description of spirituality is both accurate and meaningful. It follows that the delineation of a spiritual experience for someone is the framing that leads their passage through healthcare to be seen with deeper significance. In hospitals, that framing may be the illness itself, the relationships and beliefs it changes, or the sense of transcendence arising from a more imminent sense of our aging and mortality. Above all else, as sickness can change a person's fundamental outlook, the process of spiritual support and exploration cannot be an isolated endeavour. All healthcare staff play a part by providing care which recognizes the overall impact of illness on patients, their values, and relationships. The spirituality of care chaplains promote within healthcare recognizes that what may be routine to healthcare workers is not routine to patients. Some patients will enter new and difficult territory, and the need for those who are highly trained and skilled in handling spiritual matters will continue, both as a resource to staff and as direct care to patients.

References

1 Faigin, C.A., Pargament, K.I. (2010). Strengthened by the Spirit: Religion, Spirituality, and Resilience Through Adulthood and Aging. In: R. Resnick, L. Gwyther, K. Roberto (eds) *Resilience in Aging*, pp. 163–80. New York: Springer.

2 Wachholtz, A.B., Pearce, M.J., Koenig, H. (2007). Exploring the relationship between spirituality, coping, and pain. *Journal of behavioral medicine* **30**(4): 311–18.

3 Hay, D (2002). The spirituality of adults in Britain—recent research. *Scott J Healthcare Chaplaincy*. **5**(1): 4–10.

4 Orchard, H. (2000). *Hospital Chaplaincy Modern, Dependable?* Sheffield: Lincoln Theological Institute for the Study of Religion and Society.

5 HDL, NHS. 76 (2002). *Spiritual Care in NHS Scotland: Guidelines on Chaplaincy and Spiritual Care in the NHS in Scotland*. Edinburgh: Scottish Executive Health Department.

6 NHS. (2003). *NHS Chaplaincy: Meeting the Religious and Spiritual Needs of Staff and Patients*. London: Department of Health.

7 Data produced by the UK's National Secular Society. Available at http://www.secularism.org.uk/uploads/chaplaincy-costs.pdf. The figure derived in this report excludes those chaplains employed by Primary Care and Mental Health Trusts.

8 Clayton, A. (2010). *Religious Need in the NHS in England: The Contribution of the Picker*, Inpatient Surveys. Leeds: Leeds Teaching Hospitals NHS Trust.

9 McSherry, W., Ross, L. (2010). *Spiritual Assessment in Healthcare Practice*. Keswick: M&K Update Ltd.

10 Healthcare Chaplaincy Council of Victoria (2009). *Capabilities Framework for Pastoral Care and Chaplaincy*. Abbotsford: HCCCV Inc.

11 Astro, A.B., Wexler, A., Texeira, K., He, M.K., Sulmasy, D.P. (2007). Is failure to meet spiritual needs associated with cancer patients' perceptions of quality of care and their satisfaction with care? *J Clin Oncol* **25**(36): 5723–57.

12 Balboni, T.A., Vanderwerker, L.C., Block, S.D., Paulk, E., Lathan, C.S., Peteet, J.R., *et al.* (2007). Religiousness and spiritual support among advanced cancer patients and associations with end-of-life treatment preferences and quality of life. *J Clin Oncol* **25**(5): 555–60.

13 Handzo, G. (2006). Best practices in professional pastoral care. *Sthn Med J* **99**(6): 663–4.

14 LaRocca-Pitts, M., Batchelor, G., Connelly, L., Duvall, R.W., Green, B.K., *et al.* (2008). A collegial process for developing better practices. *Chaplaincy Today: J Ass Profess Chaplains.* **24**(1): 3–15.

15 Association of Professional Chaplains. Common Standards for Professional Chaplains. Available at: http://www.professionalchaplains.org/uploadedFiles/pdf/common-standards-professional-chaplaincy.pdf

16 Association of Professional Chaplains. (2010). *Preamble: Standards of Practice for Professional Chaplains in Acute Care Settings.* Available at: http://www.professionalchaplains.org/uploadedFiles/pdf/Standards%20of%20Practice%20Draft%20Document%20021109.pdf

17 Puchalski, C.M., Ferrell, B., Virani, R., Otis-Green, S., Baird, P., Bull, J. *et al.* (2009). Improving the quality of spiritual care as a dimension of palliative care: the report of the consensus conference. *J Palliat Med* **12**(10): 885–904.

18 National Comprehensive Cancer Network. (2010). *NCCN clinical practical guidelines in oncology*. Available at: http://www.nccn.org/professionals/physician_gls/f_guidelines.asp

19 Iler, W.L., Camac, M., Obershain, D. (2001). The impact of daily visits from chaplains on patients with chronic obstructive pulmonary disease (COPD): A pilot study. *Chaplaincy Today* **17**(1): 5–11.

20 Cobb M, (2005). *The Hospital Chaplain's Handbook: a Guide for Good Practice.* Norwich: Canterbury Press.

21 Examples include: 'Caring for the Spirit: A strategy for the chaplaincy and spiritual care workforce', South Yorkshire Workforce Development Confederation, England, (2003); 'Standards for Spiritual Care in the NHS in Wales', Welsh Assembly Government (2010); 'Guidance on Spiritual Care in the NHS in Scotland', The Scottish Government (2009).

22 Dyer, C. (2008). News: Doctors must put patients' needs ahead of their personal beliefs. *Br Med J* **336** (7646): 685.

23 Paley, J. (2008). Spirituality and nursing: a reductionist approach. *Nurs Philos* **9**(1): 3–18.

24 Pargament, K.I. (2007). *Spiritually integrated psychotherapy*. New York: Guilford.

CHAPTER 28

Complementary, alternative, and integrative medicine

Margaret L. Stuber and Brandon Horn

The essence of medicine is the prevention or alleviation of suffering. Whether we are looking at ancient or modern times, the ultimate goal has always been the same. Historically, Western allopathic medicine departed from the spiritual component of its more ancient predecessors primarily as a result of conflicts between science and religion.[1] While this was an arguably necessary departure for scientific and medical advancement, it had the unfortunate consequence of creating an artificial compartmentalization that split the body and mind from the spirit.

In contrast, until recently, 'Eastern' medical models, such as traditional Chinese medicine have continued to evolve over thousands of years without separating physical, mental and spiritual aspects of the person.[2] This continuity was easier to maintain in China because the major religions in China had large overlaps in their belief systems.[3] It was not until the Cultural Revolution in the mid-20th century that Chinese medicine was stripped of its spiritual origins. In hindsight this had some important consequences. The first is that, without its religious and spiritual context, Chinese medicine could be widely accepted and practiced in places with religious heterogeneity. The second is that the ancient traditions were preserved in places that were not subject to China's laws. This preservation has allowed us to understand some of the advantages of utilizing a system that does not separate the mind, body and spirit.[3]

In the United States, systems of medicine, such as traditional Chinese medicine and its non-religious components (e.g. acupuncture, herbs, Tai chi, and qigong) have been widely adopted. These are considered to be 'complementary' or 'alternative' approaches to allopathic medicine, and referred to as complementary and alternative medicine (CAM). A nationwide study in the United States in 1998 examined the reasons people gave for using CAM. Dissatisfaction with conventional medicine was not the primary reason for most people. Rather, these people found the CAM approaches to be more congruent with their own beliefs, values, and philosophy of life.[4] A recent editorial comments that CAM approaches appeal to a young generation of people who consider themselves to be spiritual, but not necessarily affiliated with an established religion. CAM approaches are more appealing to these people because they incorporate a variety of faith traditions, rather than seeing spiritual healing as specific to only one set of religious (and, often, political) beliefs.[5]

The purpose of this chapter is to explore the intersection of spirituality and religion with CAM or integrative medicine (IM). In this chapter we will examine:

- The definition of complementary, alternative and integrative medicine
- Some religious or spiritual groups which have what are considered to be alternative medical beliefs and practices
- How specific modalities which are considered complementary to allopathic medicine are interpreted in the context of different religious traditions.

What is complementary and alternative medicine or integrative medicine?

The National Center of Complementary and Alternative Medicine (NCCAM) is the organization within the National Institutes of Health in the United States, which coordinates and funds research into complementary and alternative medicine. NCCAM defines CAM as a 'group of diverse medical and health care systems, practices, and products that are not generally considered part of conventional medicine.' In this approach, complementary treatments are those which are used *with* conventional medicine, often to deal with side-effects of treatment or for pain or fatigue related to the underlying diagnosis. Alternative therapies would be those used *instead of* conventional medical approaches.[6]

However, defining CAM by what it is *not* (i.e. conventional medicine) creates two types of problems. First is that some interventions offered by CAM practitioners, such as advice about diet, exercise and lifestyle change, are also a part of conventional medicine. Are those, therefore, not CAM? Secondly, once an approach formerly conceptualized as CAM is researched, found to be 'effective', and then adopted in Western practice, that practice is no longer a CAM treatment. This leaves CAM therapies to be, by definition, those approaches for which there is no evidence base.

To deal with this problem, the term 'integrative medicine' has been adopted by the academic community and many physicians practicing in this field. As defined by NCCAM, integrative medicine 'combines mainstream medical therapies and CAM therapies for which there is some high-quality scientific evidence of safety and effectiveness.'[6] Integrative medicine physicians assist patients in choosing from a broad array of therapies, ranging from the very alternative to the conventional.

NCCAM groups the various CAM approaches into five broad domains: alternative or whole medical systems, biologically based therapies, mind-body interventions, manipulative and body-based therapies and energy therapies. *Whole medical systems* are based on a different philosophical approach to health care and conceptualization of illness than current Western or allopathic medicine, and are often based on religious or cultural beliefs. The therapies within each system are consistent with the philosophy and are often personalized to the patient. Examples include Traditional Chinese Medicine and Ayurvedic Medicine. Some of the components, such as yoga, herbs, massage, or acupuncture, may also be used independently of the whole approach. They would then be classified within one of the other domains.

Biologically-based therapies are usually naturally occurring materials that can be ingested or used topically. These include herbs, minerals, vitamins, and other dietary supplements. Many of the elements of Traditional Chinese Medicine or Ayurvedic Medicine are included in this category. These approaches are of great interest and the topic of significant research as components separate from any spiritual meaning.[7] They will be primarily addressed for the purposes of this chapter within the context of the whole medical systems of which they are a part, as the spiritual significance of biological interventions can only be understood in this way.

Mind-body interventions are based on the interaction between cognitive and physical aspects of the body. Yoga and the various forms of meditation are included in this category, as is biofeedback. These are very familiar interventions to most in the United States, where they have been adapted to fit with a variety of philosophical approaches. We will consider the origins and some of these adaptations in the chapter.

Manipulative and body-based systems focus on direct touch and/or movement of the body designed to correct structure or posture, or to relieve tension or strain. Chiropractic and osteopathic medicine are included in this category, as are massage, Trager and Feldenkrais techniques. Since these are generally not conceptualized as spiritual interventions, these will not be addressed in this chapter.

Energetic therapies are based on the modification of an energetic field around the body or a flow of energy within the body. Examples include therapeutic or healing touch, acupuncture, and Reiki healing. Intercessory (distance) prayer is sometimes included within this category, as is the use of the Holy Spirit to heal. We will consider these at the end of this chapter.

We will start with consideration of three whole systems of medicine that can be seen as based in beliefs about the relationship between health and spirituality. Traditional Chinese Medicine and Ayurveda are based on spiritual beliefs, but are more associated with a specific culture than one religion. Christian Science, on the other hand, is viewed as and views itself as a denomination within Christianity. All stress the natural capacity of the body to heal itself, and are based on maintaining or restoring spiritual wholeness as a means of maintaining or restoring physical and psychological health and wellness.

Whole systems of medicine within the context of religion and spirituality

Traditional Chinese medicine has its origins in Chinese philosophy. Emphasizing this, the seminal medical text in China, the *Inner Classic*, begins with a discussion of how one's health is a direct result of one's outlook on life. According to the author, it is our dissatisfaction with our present situation that leads to our constant need to change the natural cycles, leading to extremes. As a result, we are unable to fulfil our physical potential (of a lifespan of 120 years) and we go through our relatively shorter lives in a constant state of dissatisfaction.[8]

When looking at overall mortality and morbidity, Chinese medicine feels that a significant portion of the underlying susceptibility to illness is psycho/spiritual. The practice of Chinese medicine, therefore, does not differentiate between a physical illness and a psychological illness. Each will either begin with or transform into the other. This is part of the cycles used in Chinese medical theory of what are termed 'yin and yang.'[2]

Chinese medical theory is based on the idea that the universe is holographic. Matter and energy are interchangeable and transform into each other (mathematical derivation of $E = mc^2$ from the taiji symbol).[9] Therefore, the ideas of life and death have to do simply with the embodiment of the spirit. Death is seen as a shift from a denser form (more matter than energy) to a less dense form (more energy than matter). Because of this, the Chinese believed that our ancestors or other creatures that were once 'alive' in this world continue to live in the afterlife. Unfortunately, death purges our physical bodies, but not our psycho-spiritual hang-ups. Therefore, a person who dies can become a spirit that continues to try to interact with the physical world, and not always in a way that is beneficial for those still alive.[3] Therefore, to the ancient Chinese, our world was not limited to what we can see. This allowed them to develop a complex understanding of illness that took into account a myriad of illnesses caused by things that could not be seen.

To understand this development, it is helpful first to understand the context of Chinese medical language. Ancient China was an agrarian society. As such, their language was largely developed around things that would be present in such a culture. Diseases, aetiologies, and treatments, therefore, had to be communicated within the language they had available to them. Understandably, they developed descriptions for diseases that were based on climactic factors, such as heat, cold, wind, damp, and so forth. In describing a microbial invasion, such as a virus characterized by chills, headache, and cough, they may refer to it as 'wind-cold'. In this case, the first factor ('wind') describes the origin and the second ('cold') describes its behaviour. So it originated in the wind (acquired through the air) and it behaves by inducing 'cold' in the body, meaning it causes constriction. Therefore, even though they did not have microscopes, they knew that the wind carried many diseases. They could tell that some of these diseases behaved in one way, and others behaved in a different way. Without having ever seen a microbe, they set up classes of these 'unseen pathogens traveling in the wind' that are very similar to the major classes we have today (viral, bacterial, fungal, etc.).[3]

These spiritual entities (which we would call microorganisms) could not be seen by the naked eye, and had an agenda in conflict with that of the host. Physicians, therefore, had to become adept at treating the unseen or the unknown. There were also detailed classifications of various 'entities' that could control the mind to make people do things they wouldn't normally do. While there is variation depending on the tradition, most traditions had a classification of mental illnesses caused by worms (i.e. parasites). This has interesting parallels to current understanding of various microorganism infections that are known to release chemicals (cytokines) that alter our behaviour to help the organism infect other organisms.[10]

There was another equally important aspect to the ancient focus on the spirit and philosophy in medicine. When someone is ill, they look to physicians to provide basic answers. These answers relate to the past (aetiology), present (treatment), and future (prognosis) of things that impact our wellbeing. The problem is the answers to these questions are often outside of how modern medicine defines its boundaries. Why does a child get cancer or have to suffer so much? What will happen in the immediate future? What will happen when we die? These are the ultimate questions people want to know when confronted with medical problems. To the ancient Chinese, these would all be answered by the physician.[2] In fact, in many cases, the monks or priests were also physicians. Because the doctor could provide a context for life, and answer questions about death, it relieved an enormous psychological burden from the patients and the families.

Traditional Chinese Medicine interventions are used in a holistic and individualized way, based on the symptoms and needs of each patient. Specific methods will be discussed in more detail below. They include the use of herbs and supplements (biological), acupuncture (energy based), and qigong or tai chi (body therapies).

Ayurveda

Another ancient holistic view of medicine is Ayurveda, which originated in India several thousand years ago.[11] The name is based on the Sanskrit words 'ayur', meaning life, and 'veda', meaning knowledge or science.[12] Like traditional Chinese medicine, the fundamental understanding of the human body in Ayurvedic medicine is one based on nature. The universe (and the body) is seen as made up of five elements: earth, water, fire, air, and ether (space). There are also three kinds of energy (dosha), Vat, Pitta, and Kapha, each of which is comprised of two of the five elements. Human illness is seen as an excess or insufficiency of one of these three types of energy. Recommendations for diet, exercise, and specific tastes (bitter, pungent, sour, salty, sweet, astringent) are based on the specific energy or dosha, which needs to be enhanced or offset.[12] Two texts, written in Sanskrit over 2000 years ago, serve as the basis for the practice of Ayurveda, the Caraka Samhita, and Sushruta Samhita.

The focus of Ayurveda is on 'disease prevention and promotion of good health by proper lifestyle and adopting therapeutic measures that will rejuvenate the body,'[13] by:

1. *Eliminating impurities* through the digestive tract and the respiratory system, using enemas, massage, medical oils administered in a nasal spray, and other methods.
2. *Reducing symptoms* through physical exercises, stretching, breathing exercises, meditation, massage, lying in the sun, changing the diet, or taking herbs, metals, or minerals.
3. *Increasing resistance to disease* through herbs, proteins, minerals, and vitamins in tonics to improve digestion and increase appetite and immunity.
4. *Reducing worry and increasing harmony* using techniques that promote release of negative emotions.

Christian Science

Christian Science is a much more recently developed conceptual model of healthcare than traditional Chinese Medicine or Ayurveda. The Church of Christ, Scientist was founded in 1879 by Mary Baker Eddy as a drugless healing method. There are over 2000 branch churches in over 70 countries around the world.[14] The Church is based on the belief that God created humans as spiritual beings. The natural state when one is in communion with God is health. Disease is a disruption in communion with God, and is thus a mental attitude, which can be countered by disciplined prayer. 'To take a medical analogy, a Christian Scientist regards all forms of disease as symptomatic of an underlying condition that needs to be healed.'[15] Christian Science practitioners are not trained to diagnose illness, but to 'assist the sick person to access God's healing love through prayer and spiritual communications with God in order to correct the error in thought.'[16] Some of the states have recognized these beliefs by allowing exemptions from required immunizations, premarital, and prenatal blood tests, metabolic testing of newborn babies, and use of silver nitrate drops.[17] Members of the Church are actively discouraged from receiving concurrent care from a Christian Science practitioner and a medical doctor or nurse, but are encouraged to choose one or the other when ill.[15]

Mind–body interventions

As is mentioned above, most traditional and some modern healing systems conceptualize the mind, body and spirit as interconnected. Yoga, tai chi, and meditation are viewed within the Chinese medicine and Ayurvedic systems as interventions designed to facilitate health and healing in mind, body and spirit. They are therefore categorized by NCCAM as mind-body interventions. However, in the United States these approaches are often taught and used in ways which are separated from their spiritual origins. Yoga and tai chi are presented as physical interventions to improve posture, balance, flexibility and strength, and are offered at health clubs and senior centres.[18] The benefit to psychological wellbeing of yoga and tai chi are often seen to be a result of diminished pain or physical tension,[18] although there are increasing numbers of studies examining the utility of yoga for depression.[19] Meditation, on the other hand, is conceptualized in many Western adaptations primarily as a way to deal with anxiety and stress. Although meditation is believed to have physical benefits, these are understood to result from the reduction of stress and the subsequent reduction of the impact of stress on the body. Without the spiritual component of Chinese medicine or Ayurveda these approaches are more acceptable to those with Western religious beliefs, as well as to those with a non-spiritual understanding of the body and psyche.

Traditional Buddhist meditation has been practiced for 2500 years.[20] Over the years there have been many adaptations for different purposes. The common theme of the various forms of meditation is focused attention, although the point of focus (called a *drishti*) differs. For example, the focus may be on one's breath, a chanted or thought mantra, a sacred object, or on specific thoughts or sensations. Meditation may be used to achieve spiritual enlightenment, physical relaxation, and/or psychological calm.[21]

The meditation practices commonly used (and studied) medically in the United States are not associated with any specific religious or spiritual beliefs. For example, meditation was specifically adapted as a stress reduction intervention, called mindfulness-based stress reduction, by Jon Kabat-Zinn. He described this 'mindfulness meditation' as 'paying attention in a particular way; on purpose, in the present moment, and non-judgmentally.'[22] Mindfulness meditation, mindful awareness, and mindfulness-based cognitive therapy have all been used to reduce depression, anxiety and psychological distress in people with chronic medical illness, and to reduce stress, ruminative thinking, and anxiety in healthy people.[23]

Similarly, yoga has evolved over the past 4000 years. The word *yoga* derives from the Sanskrit word *yuj*, meaning 'to yoke, or unite.' The physical postures with which we are familiar are only a small part of what yoga means within the Hindi tradition. Initially, the emphasis was on reuniting the physical and spiritual worlds, and was considered to be a path to enlightenment. Later, the 'Bhagavad Gita', written between 500 and 200 BCE, became a guide to the path to transcendent understanding through action, devotion, and wisdom. Yoga then became much more formalized, with eight major 'limbs': ethical controls, ethical observances, postures, control of vital energy, sense-withdrawal, concentration, meditation, and enlightenment. It was not until *hatha yoga* in the first century that yoga began to look like the physical exercise practiced today. Since then many styles of yoga have developed. Some are intensely physical (e.g. Bikram yoga), while others include a significant amount of meditation and chanting (e.g. Integral Yoga). These meditations may include traditional Buddhist meditation techniques, such as *metta* (loving kindness) and *vipassana* (insight) meditations.[24] Thus, yoga may mix a variety of religious traditions as it brings mind, body, and spirit together, as was the original intent.

Biofield therapies and energy healing

The concept of energy as a vital component of human health has been a part of medical or healing practice for thousands of years. The Chinese term ch'i, Indian term prana and the Japanese term qi are all used to refer to an invisible or powerful force which can be used to stimulate a natural healing process.[25] As mentioned above, energy or spirit is a part of commonly used interventions such as yoga, tai chi and meditation. However, the use of energy is most evident in what NCCAM calls the *biofield therapies*. These include proximal direction of energy, such as laying on of hands, as well as distance practices, such as intercessory prayer.

There are a number of proximal energy interventions. *Reiki* originated in Japan and was introduced by Mikou Usai in the 1840s. [26] The word Reiki means universal life energy and involves the practitioner placing his or her hands gently on or just above the person receiving treatment, to access and direct the flow of energy to facilitate healing. *Therapeutic touch* is the name used for one adaptation of this and other religious traditions of the laying on of hands for healing. It was founded in the 1970s by Kreiger and Van Gelder Kunz.[27] *Healing touch* is another adaptation, developed by Janet Mentgen in the 1980s, drawing on the methods of therapeutic touch and Reiki.[28] Some types of massage would also be considered to be energy or biofield therapies, although deep tissue massage is usually administered as a physical rather than spiritual intervention.

Each of the energy approaches requires the use of trained practitioners who are following specific protocols for an identified problem, based on a theoretical understanding of how and where energy flows, and how it can be facilitated. Although none of these is affiliated with a religious organization or belief system, all are based on a non-allopathic medicine conceptualization of the body.

There have been some randomized controlled studies of these approaches, using sham or mock touch as a control. Outcome variables assessed included subjective measures of pain, function, worry, and emotional state, as well as objective measure of respiratory rate, heart rate, and blood pressure. There has been some evidence for the potential clinical effectiveness of Healing Touch in improving health-related quality of life.[29] A review of the literature on Reiki, therapeutic touch, and healing touch between 1980 and 2008 found that the average therapeutic intervention took place over 5–10 minutes, and was generally associated with a decrease in the amount of pain medications used, or with increased time between dosages of narcotic pain medications. Anxiety was not consistently reduced in these studies.[26]

Proximal prayer, meaning prayer in the presence of the patient, and intercessory prayer, meaning prayer at some distance from the patient, are both used in the Church of Christ, Scientist, as mentioned above. Both are also part of practice of many evangelical and charismatic Christian churches around the world.[30] When prayer is included in surveys of the use of CAM, it is the most frequently used modality. In a 2002 study of 31,044 people over 18 years of age in the United States, 43% said they had prayed for their own health (43.0%), and 24.4% had prayed for another's health in the previous 12 months.[31] Studies of the efficacy of this clearly spiritual intervention have had mixed results. A 2009 Cochrane systematic review of ten studies of distant intercessory prayer to God by believers found that the majority of the studies did not strongly support the utility of this intervention.[32] A recent study of proximal intercessory prayer with a charismatic context in rural Mozambique found a significant improvement in auditory and visual acuity in the patients.[31]

Acupuncture is a key component of Traditional Chinese Medicine. According to TCM theory, energy is distributed throughout the body via a network of channels termed 'meridians'. These meridians supply all cells with the energy to function. If the energy supply to a particular area is inadequate, one will experience a variety of hypo-function induced pathologies. Likewise, if the energy supply to an area is overabundant, pathologies due to hyper-function ensue. Chinese medicine developed a number of modalities to address these energetic imbalances and help return the body to homeostasis. While there are many techniques to manipulate energy, acupuncture has been found to be one of the most effective.

As practiced in modern times, acupuncture is the insertion of fine, metallic needles in areas of the body where energy is believed to gather. Because metals conduct energy, a practitioner can use the needles to direct the energy to places that don't have enough, and away from places that have too much. The ensuing balance of energy allows the body to function optimally and subsequently heal itself. While meridian theory is controversial, the efficacy of acupuncture is not. To date, there are over 17,000 peer reviewed studies that have been done on acupuncture, demonstrating various degrees of efficacy.[33] The main issue with studying acupuncture is that each acupuncture point has a different physiological effect. With over 2000 acupuncture points, a typical treatment of 10 needles would lead to more than 3e + 26 possible combinations (calculated using the following formula: $n!/r!(n - r)!$ where $n = 2000$ and $r = 10$). The vast majority of studies only look at the efficacy of one combination. Therefore, research conclusions can only relate to the exact combination used and cannot be imputed to acupuncture as a whole.[34]

The World Health Organization lists a number of conditions where acupuncture has been proven in controlled trials to be effective. These include a wide variety of pain conditions, depression, allergic rhinitis, leucopenia, nausea and vomiting, rheumatoid arthritis, stroke, and infertility.[35]

Conclusion

What is now regarded as CAM emerged from ancient faith traditions, primarily in India and China. They are deeply spiritual approaches to health, and to the integration of the body, mind, and spirit. Western allopathic medicine has adopted and adapted some of the practices (often separated from the underlying philosophy). The current public interest in the use of yoga, acupuncture, and meditation suggests that there may be a wish for the spiritual component to be reunited with the physical and mental. This is a challenge to physicians, already under time pressure, and dependent on technology. However, the need to teach medical students about mind–body connections (at least) has been recognized by the Institute of Medicine, the medical advisory group to the federal government and Congress.[36] As medicine becomes more interdisciplinary, a new and more powerful type of integrated medicine may once again be possible, as it was four thousand years ago.

References

1 Koenig, H.G. (2000). Religion and medicine I: historical background and reasons for separation. *Int J Psychiat Med* **30**(4): 385–98.

2 Moyers, B. (1995). *Healing the Mind*, p. 297. St Boswells: Main Street Books.

3 Horn, B. (2006). *Taoist Priest and Chinese Medicine Educator, Jeffrey C. Yuen*, Unpublished interview.

4 Astin, J.A. (1998).Why patients use alternative medicine: results of a national study. *J Am Med Ass* **279**(19): 1548–53.

5 Dossey, L. (2011). CAM, religion, and Schrödinger's one mind. *Explore* **7**(1): 1–7.

6 National Center on Complementary and Alternative Medicine (2011). Available at http://nccam.nih.gov/ (accessed 10 April, 2011).

7 Ven Murthy, M.R., Ranjekar, P.K., Ramassamy, C., Deshpande, M. (2010). Scientific basis for the use of Indian ayurvedic medicinal plants in the treatment of neurodegenerative disorders: ashwagandha. *Cent Nerv Syst Agents Med Chem* **10**(3): 238–46.

8 Lu, Henry. (1978). *A Complete Translation of the Yellow Emperor's Classic of Internal Medicine and the Difficult Classic.* Vancouver: International College of Traditional Chinese Medicine.

9 Horn, B. (2007). *Deriving Classical Five Element Theory: How Insights from Contemporary Physics Help us Understand the Mysteries of the Five Elements.* Los Angeles: AUCM Press.

10 Moalem, S., Prince, J. (2008). *Survival of the Sickest: the Surprising Connections Between Disease and Longevity*. Hammersmith: Harper Perennial.

11 Singh, R.H. (2010). Exploring larger evidence-base for contemporary Ayurveda. *Int J Ayurveda Res* **1**(2): 65–6.

12 Meduri, K., Mullin, G. (2010). Ayurvedic diets for wellness and disease intervention. *Nutr Clin Pract* **25**(6): 685–6.

13 Baliga, M.S. (2010) Triphala, Ayurvedic formulation for treating and preventing cancer: a review. *J Altern Complement Med* **16**(12): 1301–8.

14 Cadwell, V. (1995). Christian Science and emergency care: a case of reconciling conflicting beliefs. *J Emerg Nurs* **21**(6): 489–90.

15 Talbot, N.A. (1983). The position of the Christian Science church. *N Engl J Med.* **309**(26): 1641–4.

16 Gazelle, G., Glover, C., Stricklin, S.L. (2004). Care of the Christian Science patient. *J Palliat Med* **7**(4): 585–8.

17 Swan, R. (1983). Faith healing, Christian Science, and the medical care of children. *N Engl J Med* **309** (26): 1639–41.

18 Jahnke, R., Larkey, L., Rogers, C., Etnier, J., Lin, F. (2010). A comprehensive review of health benefits of qigong and tai chi. *Am J Hlth Promot* **24**(6): e1–e25.

19 Uebelacker, L.A., Epstein-Lubow, G., Gaudiano, B.A., Tremont, G., Battle, C.L., Miller, I.W. (2010). Hatha yoga for depression: critical review of the evidence for efficacy, plausible mechanisms of action, and directions for future research. *J Psychiat Pract* **16**(1): 22–33.

20 Young, S.N. (2011). Biologic effects of mindfulness meditation: growing insights into neurobiologic aspects of the prevention of depression. *J Psychiat Neurosci* **36**(2): 75–7.

21 Hayes, M., Chase, S (2010). Prescribing yoga. *Prim Care* **37**(1): 31–47.

22 Kabat-Zinn, J. (1994). *Wherever You Go, There You Are: Mindfulness Meditation in Everyday Life.* New York: Hyperion.

23 Chiesa, A., Serretti, A. (2009). Mindfulness-based stress reduction for stress management in healthy people: a review and meta-analysis. *J Altern Complement Med* **15**: 593–600.

24 Feuerstein, G. (2001). *The Yoga Tradition: its History, Literature, Philosophy and Practice.* Arizona: Hohm Press Prescott.

25 Jain, S., Mills, P.J. (2010). Biofield therapies: helpful or full of hype? A best evidence synthesis. *Int J Behav Med* **17**(1): 1–16.

26 Fazzino, D.L., Griffin, M.T., McNulty, R.S., Fitzpatrick, J.J. (2010). Energy healing and pain: a review of the literature. *Holist Nurs Pract* **24**(2): 79–88.

27 Macrae, J. (1987). *Therapeutic Touch: A Practical Guide.* New York: Knopf.

28 Winstead-Fry, P., Kijek, J. (1999). An integrative review and meta-analysis of therapeutic touch research. *Altern Ther Hlth Med* **5**(6): 58–67.

29 Anderson, J.G., Taylor, A.G. (2011). Effects of healing touch in clinical practice: a systematic review of randomized clinical trials. *J Holist Nurs.* Published online ahead of print Jan 12.

30 Brown, C.G., Mory, S.C., Williams, R., McClymond, M.J. (2010). Study of the therapeutic effects of proximal intercessory prayer (STEPP) on auditory and visual impairments in rural Mozambique. *Sth Med J* **103**(9): 864–9.

31 Barnes, P.M., Powell-Griner, E., McFann, K., Nahin, R.L. (2004). Complementary and alternative medicine use among adults: United States. *Adv Data* (343): 1–19.

32 Roberts, L., Ahmed, I., Hall, S., Davison, A. (2009). Intercessory prayer for the alleviation of ill health. *Cochrane Database Syst Rev* (2): CD000368.

33 National Center on Biotechnology Information search term 'Acupuncture' as of 1/6/2012.

34 Balk, J.(2008). Why we should change the course of acupuncture research. *J Chin Med* **87:** 54–9.

35 World Health Organization (2011). acupuncture: review and analysis of reports on controlled clinical trials. Available at: http://apps.who.int/medicinedocs/en/d/Js4926e/5.html#Js4926e (accessed 24 April 2011).

36 Institute of Medicine (2009). Available at: http://www.iom.edu/Activities/Quality/IntegrativeMed/2009-FEB-25/Agenda.aspx (accessed 27 April 2011).

CHAPTER 29

Restorative medicine

Christina M. Puchalski

Introduction

Spirituality, broadly defined, is increasingly recognized as an essential element of care. Spirituality helps people find hope in the midst of despair, find meaning in suffering and increase resiliency against the negative effects of stress. Spirituality is intrinsically linked to the way people find coherence and a sense of authenticity in life. Spirituality goes beyond religion and culture, though it can be an element of both. It is sometimes referred to as inner life, or what gives people their authenticity. As one of my medical students noted, 'without the soul, people are just their outer shell and are incomplete ... we don't just treat the shell of people.' Spirituality is foundational to many models of care including whole-patient care, patient-centred and relationship-centred care.

Spirituality encompasses the realm of how individuals finds hope and healing in the midst of serious illness, stress, or loss, but also how individuals find resiliency in the face of stress. Spiritual therefore encompasses all of care and not only palliative care. Spirituality also forms the basis of relationships between the patient/family and the clinician. Compassion can be thought of as spirituality in action. Spirituality in this context is the aspect of a healing relationship between the patient and the clinician. Spirituality forms the glue that binds what is referred to as the mind–body–spirit aspects or the biopsychosocial–spiritual aspects of caring for the patient. Spirituality is what can lead to restoration of health for the patient and restoration of professional call for the clinician.

Healthcare systems throughout the world present challenges to treatment of the whole person. They continue to become more technical, with attention focused on evidence-based medicine, technology and the physical aspect of care. There are also more complicated treatment choices for patients and families, as well as for the clinicians who treat them. Increased life expectancy has resulted in people living longer with chronic illness or conditions that limit their abilities. Thus, the need for coping with suffering, disability, illness, and for finding meaning, hope, coherence, and authenticity becomes a critical element of healing. In addition, lack of attention to meaning and purpose in one's life can lead to demoralization, less resilience, and possibly further illnesses such as depression, so it is important that spirituality be screened for in preventive medicine as well.

Historical roots

Spirituality and health has a number of historical roots. In the United States as in many other countries, healthcare was started and/or by religious organizations, which emphasized the role of service, compassion and holistic care. In the United States in the early 1900s there was a move away from integration of spirituality and a more humanistic component in medical education to a more science-based focus.[1] There was resurgence in the 1980s of patients requesting religious and other healing practices to be integrated into their care. In addition, there was interest by the lay pubic in a more holistic care model in which beliefs, as well as complementary and alternative medicine, would be more integrated into their care. In a 1977, psychiatrist George Engel proposed the need for a 'new medical model,' which he came to call the biopsychosocial model.[2] Since 1980s, an increased number of papers were published describing the mind-body connection[3,4] and the importance of the healing relationship within the clinical encounter, which was integrated into courses on bioethics, and professional development of physicians.[5]

Scientific advances in the 1960s influenced a more specialized focus in medicine until the 1990s with the advent of managed care models in which generalist care was re-emphasized. In this model, mother physicians and nurses advocated for the importance of interdisciplinary teamwork, and whole-patient care. In this time two important theoretical models, patient-centred[6] and relationship-centred[7] began to influence changes in the medical model. These models both support a whole-patient approach to care.

In the last quarter-century, medical educators who have recognized the often-dehumanizing effects of the medical system and medical education have created guidelines to expose students to more humanistic care. The resultant curricular changes include narrative medicine, spirituality and health, and culturally sensitive care. Competencies have been developed in cultural competence as well as spirituality and health. In 1992, the first curriculum in spirituality and health was offered at George Washington University School of Medicine. Since then, required curricula on spirituality and health are found in the majority of schools in the United States and beginning to be taught in the United Kingdom, Australia and other countries (see chapter 56 for more information).

Models of care

Spiritual care is grounded in two fundamentally important theoretical frameworks: the biopsychosocial-spiritual model of care[8] and the Patient-centred care model.[6] Integral to both of these models of care is the recognition that there is more to the care of the patient than the physical. The biopsychosocial-spiritual model assumes that all dimensions of a person impact their presentation of symptoms, as well as their treatment. Saunders wrote of 'total pain' where patients' pain may be physical, emotional, social, or spiritual.[9] The model emphasizes the totality of a patient's experience in the context of their illness and/or dying. Thus, the clinician's assessment and treatment of that patient includes the physical signs and symptoms of the patient's illness as well as the patient's emotional response to the illness, the social ramifications of the illness on the patient and his or her family and friends, and the spiritual issues that may be present as a result of the illness. Integrating all dimensions of a patient's experience with illness is key to patient-centred or whole-patient care. When healthcare professionals do not invite patients to discuss their spiritual needs, they are unable to understand how patients define wellness and quality of life—critical information for effective, individualized diagnosis and treatment. A Picker Institute study showed that when the treatment plan is individualized to include a patient's values and beliefs, healthcare outcomes improve, including shorter average lengths of hospital stays, lower costs per case, and higher overall patient satisfaction scores.[10]

In the patient-centred model of care, there is evidence that patient health outcomes are improved by engaging in shared decision-making. Thus, the physician in encouraged to view his or her relationship with the patient as a partnership where decisions are made together and where the physician supports the patient throughout the professional relationships—i.e. 'we will get through this together.' In order to be able to have shared decision-making, physicians must know the values and beliefs of the patient. This is fundamental to treating the patient with respect and dignity. Finally, involvement of a larger community of caregivers is recognized as essential in the patient-centred care model. In this sense, the interdisciplinary team becomes one community, but there are other communities, such as faith-based communities, families, or other communities of individuals that participate in the care of patients. To practice truly patient-centred care based on transparency, individualization, recognition, respect, dignity, and choice in all matters important to each person, and his/her circumstances and relationships, the patient's spirituality must be given equal weight when conducting the patient assessment to identify health strengths and risks. The spiritual history focuses on the person's values, unique needs, preferences, and life priorities. The healthcare team uses this information to attend to the patient's whole experience of health or illness.

Empirical and ethical principles

Spirituality is supported by ethical as well as empirical literature.[11–14] Spirituality has been shown to influence a patient's coping skills, pain and suffering, healthcare decision making[15,16] and healthcare outcomes, including quality of life.[17–20] Many studies have indicated that patients want their spiritual issues addressed.[21–24] One study asked patients if they wanted their physicians to ask about their spirituality; 83% said yes, at least in some circumstances. Patients responded that they believe information concerning their spiritual beliefs affects physicians' ability to encourage realistic hope (67%), give medical advice (66%), and change medical treatment (62%). Of those patients who wanted to discuss their spirituality with their physician or clinician, 85% said the reason for doing so was the desire for physician-patient understanding (87%).[25] Patients also say they have more trust in their healthcare team when the physician or clinician has asked about their spirituality. They feel more listened to, and more respected—all requirements of patient-centred care. In Australia a study showed that the majority of patients reported spirituality to be important with greater than 50% saying therapists should consider spiritual beliefs in the management of 'child problems'.[26] In a hospital setting, whether spiritual needs of patients are attended to is the strongest predictor of patient satisfaction with care and with patient perception of quality of care.[27] Studies have also indicated that spiritual or religious beliefs can impact end-of-life decision-making.[28] The Picker Institute has noted that respecting patients' beliefs and values may improve patients' healthcare outcomes and is critical to the practice of patient-centred care.[6]

Increased spiritual or existential distress can in turn exacerbate the presentation of other symptoms such as pain, agitation, anxiety and depression. Some studies suggest that existential and spiritual issues may be of greater concern to patients than pain and physical symptoms.[29,30] Surveys and other studies suggest that spiritual and religious beliefs and practices are associated with better health outcomes, including better coping skills, better quality of life, and less anxiety and depression.[31–37] Fitchett and others have shown that spiritual struggles are associated with poor physical outcome and higher rates of morbidity.[38] Research validates the relationship of spirituality to a higher quality of life,[39,40] increased hardiness in persons with HIV/AIDS,[41] reduced loneliness in chronically ill and healthy adults,[42] and reduced anxiety for hospice patients.[43] Spiritual wellbeing has also been positively correlated with decreased perception of pain.[35] These studies demonstrate that patients may utilize their spiritual or religious beliefs and values as a way to understand their illness, find meaning in the midst of their suffering, find hope in the of grief, loss and distress, and find inner peace. The Institute of Medicine has identified overall quality of life and achieving a sense of spiritual peace and wellbeing among the key domains of quality end-of-life care.[44]

Policy and guidelines

Several organizations have cited in their definition of palliative care that spiritual care is essential to good palliative care: NHS Education for Scotland's Spiritual and Religious Care Capabilities and Competences for Healthcare Chaplains,[45] the Clinical Standards for Specialist Palliative Care,[46] National Institutes for Clinical Excellence (NICE) Guidelines,[47] The National Consensus Project, and National Quality Forum[48] and the revised World Health Organization (WHO).[49,50] To provide excellent palliative care, physicians, and other healthcare professionals must be able to address all dimensions of care, including the spiritual. Palliative care is defined as starting from diagnosis and thus includes a wide range of people from diagnosis of any illness, those coping with chronic illness including, for example, cancer survivors, as well as others who do well. Many clinicians feel palliative care is a good model of care in general and that the precepts could be applied to care across all of life.

In 1996 the World Health Organization adopted a revised definition of health to include spiritual wellbeing. 'Health is a dynamic state of complete physical, mental, spiritual and social wellbeing, and not merely the absence of disease or infirmity.'[51] Thus, according to this definition, spirituality is relevant across life. The American Academy of Family Physicians (AAFP) made the case for including patients' spirituality in a medical history over 10 years ago, acknowledging that patients understand the meaning of their illness in the context of their spirituality and rely on their spirituality to cope with their illness and stress.[52] The Joint Commission on Accreditation of Healthcare Organizations has a policy that states: 'Pastoral counseling and other spiritual services are often an integral part of the patient's daily life. When requested, the hospital provides, or provides for, pastoral counseling services.'[53] More recently, the Joint Commission mandated a spiritual 'assessment.'[54] Since spiritual health is part of overall health, it would be important to assess for spiritual risk. People who lack meaning in life may well be at risk of demoralization and depression, or may in fact have impaired resistance to the negative effects of stress. Conversely, those people who are able to find meaning, hope, and purpose may find a restoration to wholeness.

The role of the physician

In 1998, the Association of American Medical Colleges (AAMC), responding to concerns by the medical professional community that young doctors lacked these humanitarian skills, undertook a major initiative—The Medical School Objectives Project (MSOP)—to assist medical schools in their efforts to respond to these concerns. The report notes that 'Physicians must be compassionate and empathetic in caring for patients ... they must act with integrity, honesty, respect for patients' privacy and respect for the dignity of patients as persons. In all of their interactions with patients they must seek to understand the meaning of the patients' stories in the context of the patients', and family and cultural values.'[55] In recognition of the importance of teaching students how to respect patients' beliefs, AAMC has supported the development of courses in spirituality and medicine in medical schools.[56,57] Today the majority of medical schools have required courses in spirituality and health; it is increasing becoming a field of study within medicine.

The American College of Physicians convened an end-of-life consensus panel, which concluded that physicians should extend their care for those with serious medical illness by attentiveness to psychosocial, existential, or spiritual suffering.[58] The American Medical Association in its Code of Medical Ethics states that 'The physician shall be dedicated to providing competent medical care with compassion and respect for human dignity and rights.'[59] Spiritual care supports the dignity of each patient by honoring the inherent value of that person, their beliefs and values that support them, and the practices that enable them to find meaning and hope in the midst of suffering. By being attentive to the spiritual dimension of peoples' lives, care becomes compassionate and whole. Other national organizations such as American Academy of Hospice and Palliative Medicine, American Psychiatric Association, Society of Teachers and Family Medicine, Association of American Medical Colleges, American Association of Nursing Colleges, to cite a few, have also supported the inclusion of spirituality in the clinical setting. Organizations outside the US also support the integration of spirituality including most international Palliative Care associations.[55,60–63]

Physicians and other clinicians who diagnose and develop treatment plans should address spirituality with patients because it can affect how a person understands their illness, how they make treatment decisions, and how they cope with suffering, illness, disability, and/or stress. Patients have also noted that they feel increased trust with their clinicians in the context of being asked about their spirituality.[64] Building trust is crucial in creating an environment where patients feel they can share all their concerns. Being able to hear all the concerns will enable physicians and other clinicians to have all the information needed to make the correct diagnosis. In difficult clinical situations, such as breaking bad news, or working with a dying patient, addressing spiritual needs of the patient can be crucial to providing the best patient-centred care possible. It can help physicians communicate more sensitively and effectively with patients, families, and staff about these difficult situations.[65]

There is also anecdotal evidence that healthcare providers whose clinical practices are consistent with their call, are happier, are more intentional in their work and make fewer errors. Hospital settings that have piloted spirituality interventions show increased patient satisfaction, as well as greater healthcare team coherence.[66] Thus, attention to patients' and healthcare professionals' spirituality can improve overall delivery of care.

Spirituality in clinical care

While spirituality is recognized as an essential element of care, there have been challenges in implementing spiritual care due to lack of models or practical tools, as well as lack of diagnostic criteria for spiritual distress and tested interventions for this distress. In 2009, George Washington Institute for Spirituality and Health (GWish) and City of Hope convened The National Consensus Project for Quality Palliative Care (NCC), funded by the Archstone Foundation. Forty interdisciplinary experts in palliative care and spiritual care convened, including physicians, nurses, social workers, chaplains, theologians, spiritual directors, counsellors, faith community nurses, psychologists, a medical anthropologist, as well as individuals who worked with organizations such as the National Consensus Project for Quality Palliative Care (NCP), the National Quality Forum (NQF), and the National Comprehensive Cancer Network (NCCN). The group identified points of agreement about spiritual care as it applies to healthcare, and developed a consensus-based definition of spirituality.

> Spirituality is the aspect of humanity that refers to the way individuals seek and express meaning and purpose and the way they experience their connectedness to the moment, to self, to others, to nature, and to the significant or sacred.[62]

To create resources for implementation, they developed guidelines and tools for healthcare professionals and institutions to ensure that spirituality is fully integrated into the care of patients nationally. Palliative care was chosen as the field because of the well-established requirement to include spirituality into the care of patients. Palliative care is defined as being applicable to patient care from the moment of diagnosis of a chronic, serious or life threatening illness and by this definition, applicable to most hospitalized patients, and all patients with a chronic illness. However, as described above, the model and recommendations from this conference can be applied to care across life. While this model was developed in the US, it is gaining interest from other countries. For example, the European Association for Palliative Care (EAPC) Task Force was formed to support spiritual care of patients in palliative care utilizing the NCC as a basis for their work.[61] We would suggest that it form the basis of work internationally, with modifications as appropriate for different cultural contexts.

Five literature-based categories of spiritual care (spiritual assessment, models of care and care plans, interprofessional team training, quality improvement, and personal and professional development) were identified and provided the framework for the Consensus Conference. The resulting document and conference recommendations build upon prior literature, the NCP Guidelines[67] and National Quality Forum (NQF) Preferred Practices[48] and Conference proceedings.[62,68]

Spiritual care models are based in dignity, respect and providing whole-patient care as described above. The key recommendations are that spiritual distress be treated as any other type of distress, that spirituality should be a vital sign, that all patients should receive a spiritual screening, history and assessment, and that resources of patient's spiritual strength as well as spiritual distress should be documented in and attended to in the treatment plan. The implementation model (see Figure 29.1) describes the process by which patients spiritual issues would be addressed in the clinical setting.

Figure 29.2 describes how this would occur in an outpatient setting. Central to this model is the concept of a generalist-specialist model in which the physicians, nurses, and social workers are the generalists with regard to spiritual care; the board certified chaplains are the specialists.

The NCC produced guidelines for taking a spiritual history and for the formulation of spiritual treatment or care plans,[62] including:

- All healthcare professionals should be trained in doing a spiritual screening or history as part of their routine history and evaluation
- Spiritual screenings, histories, and assessments should be communicated and documented in patient records (e.g. charts, computerized databases, and shared with the interprofessional healthcare team)
- Follow-up spiritual histories or assessments should be conducted for all patients whose medical, psychosocial, or spiritual condition changes, and as part of routine follow-up in a medical history
- A spiritual issue becomes a diagnosis if the following criteria are met:
  - the spiritual issue leads to distress or suffering (e.g. lack of meaning, conflicted religious beliefs, inability to forgive);

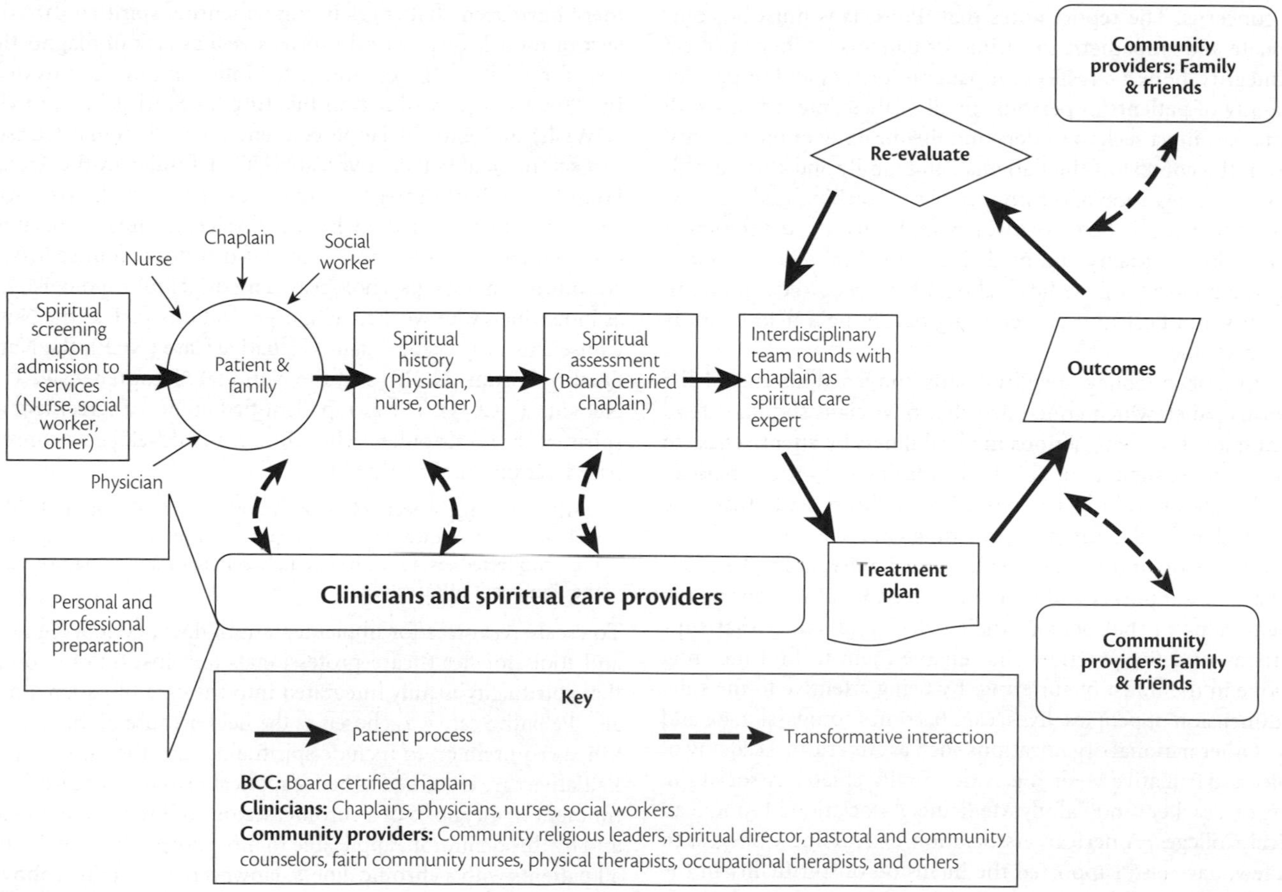

Figure 29.1 Implementation model.

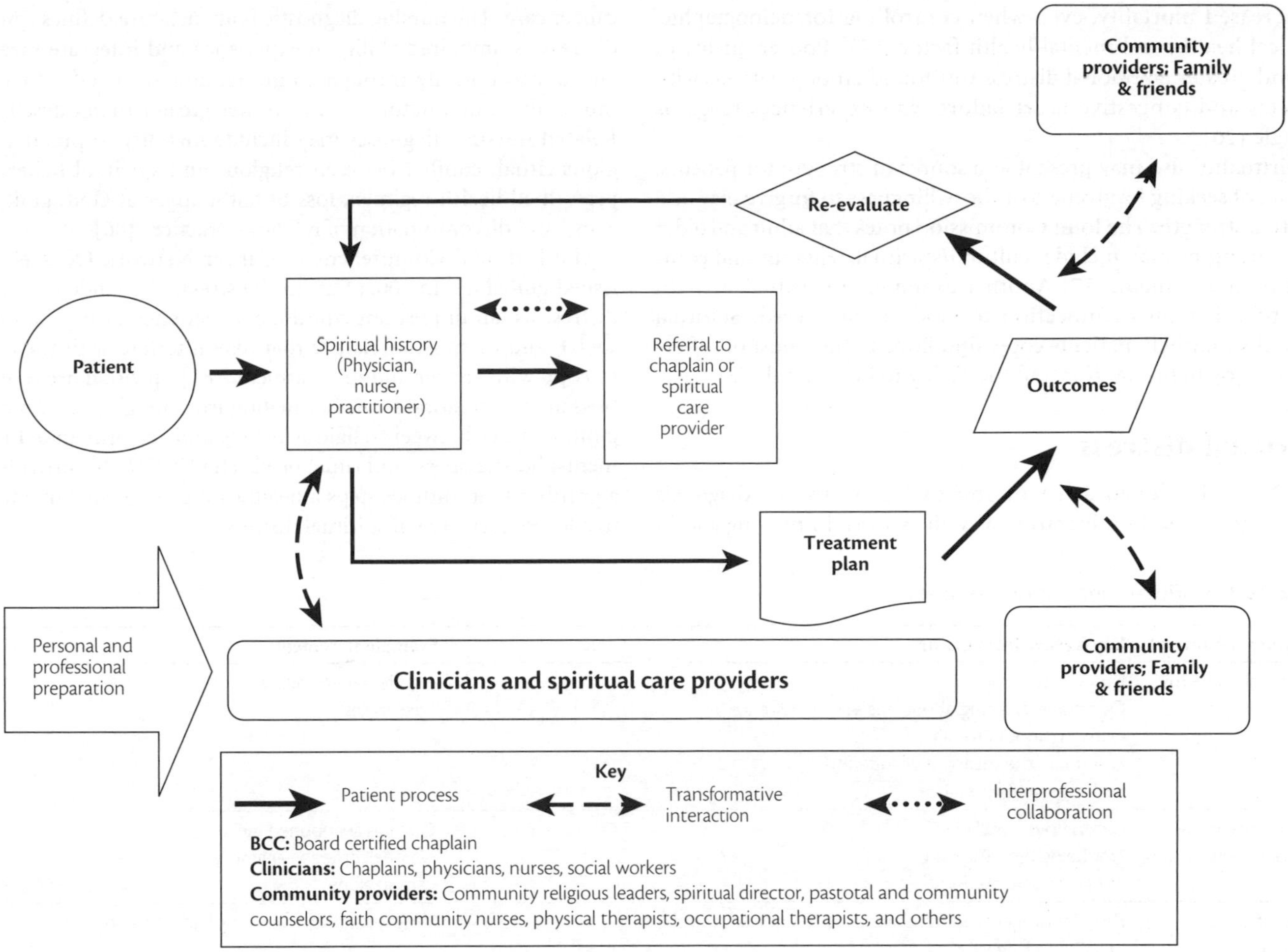

Figure 29.2 Outpatient spiritual care implementation model. Reprinted with permission from *Journal of Palliative Medicine* 12 October, 2009, published by Mary Ann Liebert, Inc., New Rochelle, NY.

- the spiritual issue is the cause of a psychological or physical diagnosis such as depression, anxiety, or acute or chronic pain (e.g. severe meaninglessness that leads to depression or suicidality, guilt that leads to chronic physical pain);
- the spiritual issue is a secondary cause or affects the presenting psychological or physical diagnosis (e.g. hypertension is difficult to control because the patient refuses to take medications because of his or her religious beliefs).

◆ Treatment or care plans should include, but not be limited to referral to chaplains, spiritual directors, pastoral counsellors, and other spiritual care providers including clergy or faith-community healers for spiritual counselling; development of spiritual goals; meaning-orientated therapy; mind–body interventions; rituals, spiritual practices; and contemplative interventions.

What is key to these models is the important role of relationship and the opportunity for personal transformation of both patient and clinician. In these relational models, patients and their healthcare professionals work together in the process of discovery, collaborative dialogue, treatment, and ongoing evaluation and follow-up. The model is based on the biopsychosocial-spiritual care model and implementation steps adhere to the patient-centred care models[11] requirement that healthcare professionals be attentive to patients' spiritual needs, treat patients with respect and dignity, and view the healthcare professional–patient relationship as a partnership in which decisions are made with the patient. Examples in the literature[69–71] and discussions at the NCC further contributed to the models' design.

Spiritual diagnosis and resources of strength

The diagnosis of chronic or life-threatening illness and other adverse life events can lead to spiritual struggles for patients. The turmoil may be short for some patients and protracted for others as individuals attempt to integrate the reality of their diagnosis with their spiritual beliefs. The journey may result in growth and transformation for some people, and to distress and despair for others.[72]

Studies have found patients with spiritual or religious struggles had poorer physical health, worse quality of life, and greater depression;[73] those with chronic spiritual or religious struggles also had increased disability[72] and higher indices of pain and fatigue, and more difficulties with daily physical functioning.[74] Religious struggle also has been found to be a significant predictor of increased mortality, even when controlling for demographic, physical health, and mental health factors.[75] Poorer quality of life and greater emotional distress was found among patients with diabetes and congestive heart failure who experiences religious struggle.[76]

Spirituality also may present as a source of strength for patients. The act of seeking forgiveness or the willingness to forgive may be a spiritual strength. The Joint Commission notes that adult and older adult strengths may include 'cultural/spiritual/religious and community involvement.'[77] Another example of spiritual strength may be a patient's connection to God or the sacred. Spiritual strengths may help patients cope, find hope in the midst of suffering, find joy in life, and/or find the ability to be grateful.[78]

Spiritual distress

The NCC developed a list of spiritual concerns or diagnosis (Table 29.1) based on literature as well as work in nursing and in cancer care. The nursing diagnostic nomenclature defines spiritual distress as 'impaired ability to experience and integrate meaning and purpose in life through connectedness with self, other, art, music, literature, nature, and/or power greater than oneself.'[79] Related nursing diagnoses may include inability to practice religious ritual, conflict between religious and spiritual beliefs and prescribed health regimen, loss of faith, anger at God, guilt over 'sins,' and discontinuation of religious practices.[80]

The National Comprehensive Cancer Network (NCCN) first issued guidelines in 2003. Entitled 'Distress,' the guidelines define distress as 'an unpleasant emotional experience of psychological, social, and/or spiritual nature that may interfere with the ability to cope with cancer and its treatment.'[81] Spiritual areas of distress include pastoral services, isolation from religious community, guilt, conflict between religious beliefs and recommended treatments, hopelessness, and ritual need. The NCCN also provided an algorithm that outlines steps a healthcare professional might take to address each area of spiritual distress.

Table 29.1 Spiritual concerns or diagnoses

Diagnoses (Primary)	Key feature from history	Example statements
Existential concerns	Lack of meaning Questions meaning about one's own existence Concern about afterlife Questions the meaning of suffering Seeks spiritual assistance	'My life is meaningless' 'I feel useless'
Abandonment by God or others	Lack of love, loneliness Not being remembered No sense of relatedness	'God has abandoned me' 'No one comes by anymore' 'I am so alone'
Anger at God or others	Displaces anger toward religious representatives or others Inability to forgive	'Why would God take my child ... it's not fair'
Concerns about relationship with deity	Desires closeness to God, deepening relationship	'I want to have a deeper relationship with God' 'I want to understand my spirituality more'
Conflicted or challenged belief systems	Verbalizes inner conflicts or questions about beliefs of faith Conflicts between religious beliefs and recommended treatments Questions moral or ethical implications of therapeutic regimen Expresses concern with life/death or belief system	'I am not sure if God is with me anymore' 'I question all that I used to hold as meaningful'
Despair/ hopelessness	Hopelessness about future health, life Despair as absolute hopelessness No hope for value of life	'Life is being cut short' 'There is nothing left for me to live for'
Grief/loss	The feeling and process associated with the loss of a person, health, relationship	'I miss my loved one so much' 'I wish I could run again'
Guilt/shame	Feeling that one has done something wrong or evil Feeling that one is bad or evil	'I do not deserve to die pain fee'
Reconciliation	Need for forgiveness or reconciliation from self or others	'I need to be forgiven for what I did' 'I would like my wife to forgive me'
Isolation	Separated from religious community or other community	'Since moving to the assisted living, I am not able to go to my church anymore' 'I have moved and no longer can go to my usual 12-step meeting'
Religious specific	Ritual needs Unable to perform usual religious practices	'I just can't pray anymore'
Religious/ spiritual struggle	Loss of faith or meaning Religious or spiritual beliefs or community not helping with coping	'What if all that I believe is not true?'

Reprinted with permission from *Journal of Palliative Medicine* 12/10, 2009, published by Mary Ann Liebert, Inc., New Rochelle, NY.

The National Comprehensive Cancer Network (NCCN) Practice Guidelines in Oncology describe the following spiritual diagnostic codes:[82]

- Grief
- Concerns about afterlife
- Conflicted or challenged belief systems
- Loss of faith
- Concerns with meaning and purpose of life
- Concerns with relationship with deity
- Isolation from religious community
- Guilt
- Hopelessness
- Conflict between religious beliefs and recommended treatments
- Ritual needs.

A patient may present the above with other symptoms such as mood alterations, nightmares, and lack of trust, uncontrollable pain for example whose cause is spiritual distress. These symptoms (see Figure 29.3) are secondary diagnosis if the primary is spiritual. For example, a patient may have despair, which presents as uncontrollable pain or anger or lashing out.

A clinician may identify spiritual distress that is a spiritual diagnosis or identify a spiritual issue or resource of strength that does not meet the criteria for a spiritual diagnosis. In general, a spiritual issue becomes a diagnosis if the follow criteria are met:

1. The spiritual issue leads to distress or suffering (e.g. lack of meaning, conflicted religious beliefs, inability to forgive)
2. The spiritual issue is the cause of psychological or physical diagnosis such as depression, anxiety, or acute or chronic pain (e.g. severe meaninglessness that leads to depression or suicidality, guilt that leads to chronic physical pain)
3. The spiritual issue is a secondary cause or affects the presenting psychological or physical diagnosis (e.g. hypertension is difficult to control because the patient refuses to take medications because of his or her religious beliefs).[83]

Figure 29.4 is a decision tree algorithm that may aid in the development of a treatment or care plan.[84] In this decision tree, the clinician first recognizes the patient's spiritual distress and the determination is made about whether the distress is physical, emotional, spiritual, or social. Often there will be elements of each dimension.

(A primary spiritual diagnosis must be present to be considered spiritual) (NCCN Guidelines)

Secondary
Behavior/mood alterations as evidenced by anger, crying, withdrawal, etc.
Pain
Feeling out of control
Uses gallows humor
Anger
Nightmares/sleep disturbances
Feelings of abandonment
Lack of trust

Figure 29.3 Secondary spiritual diagnosis. Reprinted with permission from *Journal of Palliative Medicine* 12 October, 2009, published by Mary Ann Liebert, Inc., New Rochelle, NY.

There is some debate over the word 'diagnosis' when referring to spiritual issues, and particularly when referring to suffering. Some are concerned about the over-medicalization of spirituality. Spirituality is often deemed too private or interior. However, in fact, data supports patients desire to have their spirituality addressed in clinical settings. So much of what physicians discuss with patients is private (e.g. sexuality, abuse). Suffering underlies most of what patients experience in the context of illness. To neglect to address suffering would be unethical. The NCC members felt that the lack of diagnostic criteria may be the reason spiritual distress has been overlooked as an essential element of patient care.

Communicating with patients about spiritual issues

The goal of communicating with patients about their spirituality is to get to know the whole of the patient, not just their physical of psychosocial issues. While one can of course never know a person in his or her fullness, one can respect what offers deep meaning to a person, find out how people cope with their illness and their stress, and what communities or beliefs are supportive to them. All of these have been shown to impact health and wellness. It is also critical for healthcare professionals to identify and treat spiritual distress. Treatments may range from compassionate presence to chaplain referral. In addition, spiritual resources of strength can be identified.

The first step in communicating about spiritual issues is to listen to spiritual themes such as meaning, hope, connection, religious rituals, beliefs, and values. Distress, as listed above, includes despair, demoralization, grief, isolation from religious or other community, hopelessness, lack of love and connection. Once the physician or other healthcare professional hears these themes, they can ask open-ended questions to find out from the patient what the themes mean to them and what relationship the patient's spirituality has on his or her illness or perception of health.

More formal ways of inquiry include a spiritual screening or history for the non-chaplain clinicians and a full spiritual assessment which the chaplain undertakes. These are described more fully below.

Spiritual screening

A spiritual screening, history, and assessment are formal tools of the medical history during which patients are asked about their spiritual (including religious) beliefs. Clinicians do a spiritual screening or history; chaplains do a spiritual assessment.

Usually, a nurse or social worker does a spiritual screening upon triage or admission in settings such as hospitals, nursing homes, or hospices. Spiritual screenings might not be performed in outpatient settings. If the clinician senses spiritual distress, the screening may be done in conversation with the patient. Spiritual screenings have two primary objectives:

1. Assess for spiritual emergencies that may require the immediate need for a chaplain
2. Identify patients who may benefit from an in-depth spiritual assessment from a chaplain.

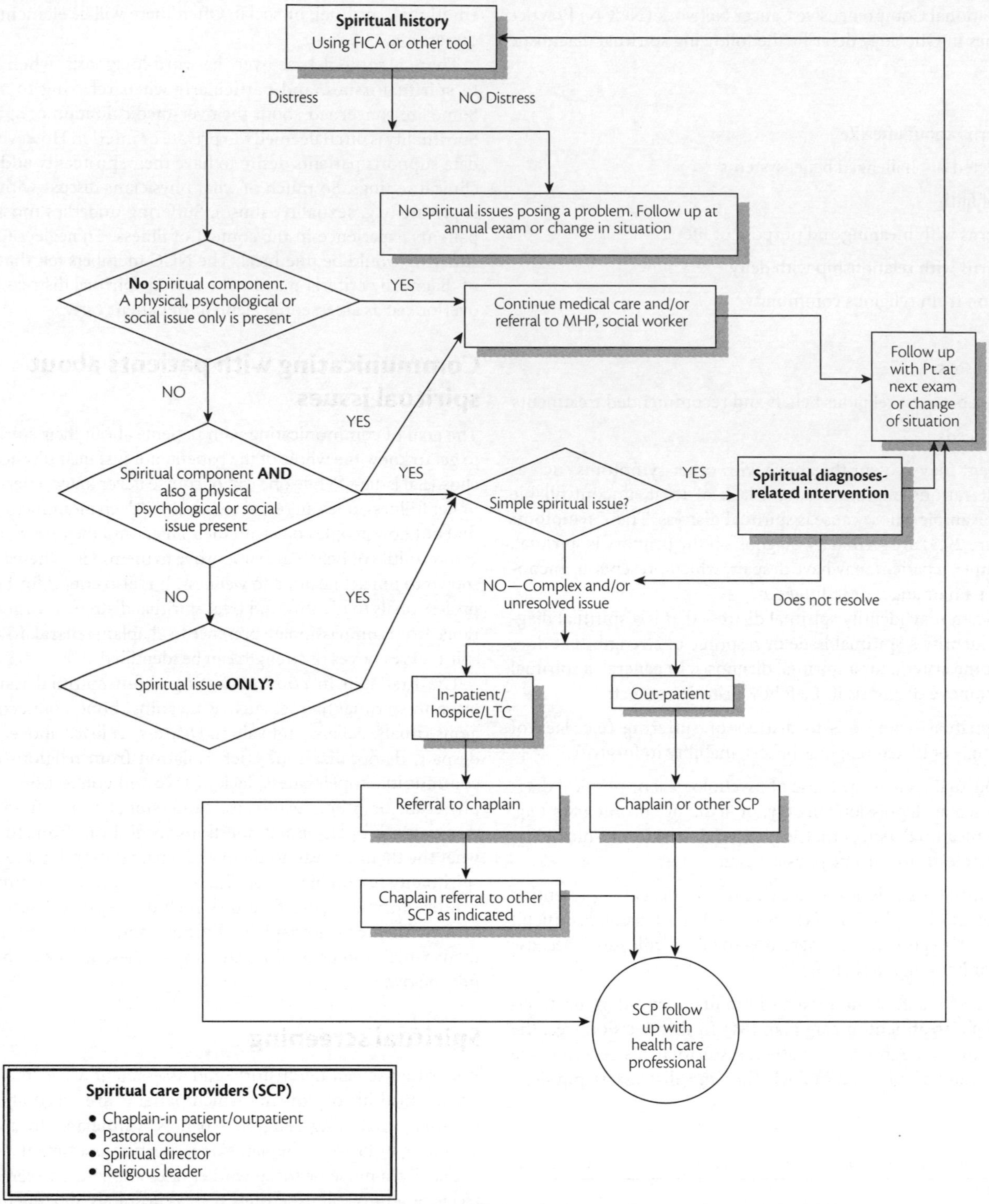

Figure 29.4 Spiritual diagnosis decision pathways. Reprinted with permission from *Journal of Palliative Medicine* 12 October, 2009, published by Mary Ann Liebert, Inc., New Rochelle, NY.
(Source: Puchalski C., Handzo G., Wintz S., and Bull J., 2009)

Effective spiritual screening models use a few simple questions any healthcare professional can ask as part of the initial screening. Two examples of questions are:[85]

1. Are there any spiritual beliefs that you want to have discussed in your care with us here?

Or:

2. One can use the two-item screening below, a yes/no combination of answers to these questions should trigger a chaplain referral:
    - 'How important is religion and spirituality in your coping?'
    - 'How well are those resources working for you at this time?'

Spiritual history

A spiritual history is an interview in which the patient is asked a broader set of questions about his or her life so the clinician and team members can better understand how a patient's spiritual needs and resources may complement or complicate the patient's overall care. These questions are usually part of a comprehensive examination by a clinician responsible for providing direct care or referrals to specialists, including professional chaplains. A spiritual history typically is asked in the context of the social history.

A spiritual history is a set of targeted questions that invite the patient to share his or her spiritual and/or religious beliefs, and that guide the patient to delve into the meaning of life events. The questions are not meant as checklists, but as guides to help the clinician create a caring environment that encourages the patient to share his or her beliefs, hopes, fears, and concerns. The spiritual history is the process of interviewing patients, asking them questions about their lives in order to come to a better understanding of their needs and resources. The history questions are usually asked in the context of a comprehensive examination by the clinician who is primarily responsible for providing direct care or referrals to specialists, such as professional chaplains.

The goals of the spiritual history are to:[86]

- Invite patients to define what spirituality is for them and their spiritual goals
- Learn about the patient's beliefs and values
- Assess for spiritual distress (meaninglessness, hopelessness) and spiritual resources of strength (hope, meaning and purpose, resiliency, spiritual community)
- Provide an opportunity for compassionate care whereby the healthcare professional connects to the patient in a deep and profound way
- Empower the patient to find inner resources of healing and acceptance
- Identify spiritual and religious beliefs that might affect healthcare decision-making
- Identify spiritual practices or rituals that might be helpful to incorporate into the treatment or care plan

The spiritual history is done as part of the social history for a new patient, yearly, or intake visits, or can be done within the context of an acute visit, for example when breaking bad news. Organizations from the Association of American Medical Colleges (AAMC) to the 2009 National Consensus Conference for Spiritual Care in Palliative Care (NCC) recommend that clinicians be able to take a spiritual history.[55,62] There are several studies that have found that the majority of patients would like their physicians to address the patients' spiritual issues in the clinical setting.[21,64,87]

In addition to being fully present and caring with our patients, physicians should specifically address spiritual issues in the clinical interview and follow-up in subsequent visits as appropriate. The spiritual history is patient-centred. One should always respect patients' wishes and understand appropriate boundaries. Physicians and other health care providers must respect patients' privacy regarding matters of spirituality and religion and should avoid imposing their own beliefs on the patient.[88]

The FICA Spiritual History Tool is a validated tool for taking patients' spiritual history.[71,88,90] The format of the tool follows:

- *F—Faith and Belief* 'Do you consider yourself spiritual or religious?' or 'Do you have spiritual beliefs that help you cope with stress?' If the patient responds 'No,' the physician might ask, 'What gives your life meaning?' Sometimes patients respond with answers such as family, career, or nature
- *I—Importance* 'What importance does your faith or belief have in our life? Have your beliefs influenced how you take care of yourself in this illness? What role do your beliefs play in regaining your health?'
- *C—Community* 'Are you part of a spiritual or religious community? Is this of support to you and how? Is there a group of people you really love or who are important to you?' Communities such as churches, temples, and mosques, or a group of like-minded friends can serve as strong support systems for some patients
- *A—Address in Care* 'How would you like me, your healthcare provider, to address these issues in your healthcare?'

Other spiritual history tools include Hope[69] and Spirit;[70] however, these have not been validated for clinical use. FICA was also used as a basis of a tool in Germany called, SPIR.[91]

Too often medical clinicians are uncomfortable using screening and/or history tools that focus on patients' spiritual concerns. Because the spiritual history uses a set of questions that are not meant to be a checklist, but to guide a discussion with the patient, training on the use of the FICA Spiritual History Tool and other spiritual history tools is recommended.

Spiritual assessment

A spiritual assessment is an in-depth, extensive, ongoing conversation in which a chaplain listens to a patient's story to understand the patient's needs and resources.[92] Models for spiritual assessments are not built on a set of interview questions, but on interpretative frameworks that require extensive training to use effectively. Spiritual assessments are done with patients from many different religious or spiritual traditions and belief systems. Clinical Pastoral Education is the educational training board certified chaplains receive that enables them to do an assessment and to treat spiritual distress (see Chapter 56).

A spiritual assessment has these primary objectives:

1. Develop a relationship with the patient in a clinical setting
2. Identify spiritual issues and confirm, elaborate, or make a spiritual diagnosis
3. Develop a spiritual care plan that can be shared with the treatment team
4. Document in the chart.

Formulating a spiritual treatment plan

Information from the spiritual history should be documented in the patient's chart and discussed by the healthcare team responsible for caring for and developing a treatment plan with the patient. Understanding all of the patient's needs allows for the development of a comprehensive patient-centred treatment plan that is congruent with the patient's beliefs and values, and that integrates spiritual practices, as appropriate, and if those practices are identified by the patient as important. Addressing only patents' physical and/or mental health may compound patients' stress and suffering.

In Figures 29.1 and 29.2 we reference simple versus complex spiritual issues. Complex spiritual issues would need a chaplain referral. These include religious specific issues, despair, meaningless or hopelessness that is moderate to severe. However, many issues can resolve with continued presence and dialogue with the clinician. A patient may express a sense of meaninglessness that is not causing that person distress, but the patient would like to discuss it further with the clinician. Even in distress, sometimes talking with the clinician may help the patient sort out the meaning issues on their own. If however, the patient cannot do that, then the simple intervention, i.e. talking with the clinician becomes complex and needs to be referred to a board certified chaplain. When patients want to learn about yoga, meditation, or art or music therapy, healthcare professionals may make the appropriate referral or implement a course of action. Once the clinician finds out about the patient's spiritual beliefs, their issues, and their resources for coping, he or she can then address any spiritual practices that are important to the patient. These might be prayer, meditation, listening to certain music, enjoying solitude, or writing poetry, or journeying. One can then incorporate these practices as appropriate.

For complex issues, a board-certified or board-eligible chaplain, as the expert in spiritual care, should provide input and guidance as to the diagnosis and treatment or care plan with respect to spirituality.[93] If simple interventions do not resolve the spiritual distress or meet the patient's needs, then a referral to chaplain should be made.

The ultimate goal of spiritual interventions is to promote a patient's spiritual wellbeing. Therefore, there are many possible interventions, such as encouraging patients to:

- Visit with a chaplain or other spiritual care professionals (e.g. spiritual director, pastoral counsellor)
- Continue with their established spiritual practices (e.g. prayer, meditation) provided the patient identifies these as important to them or referral to practices the patient expresses interest in such as yoga
- Participate in faith or spiritual communities; though religious interventions should only be suggested when the clinician knows the intervention is acceptable to the patient
- Participate, as referred, in meaning-centred therapy, dignity therapy groups
- Visit, as referred, an art or music therapist
- Participate in journaling, reflection, narrative approaches
- Visit, as referred, mind-body medicine clinics
- Continue to discuss needs with primary clinician.

A number of spiritual therapeutic models have been studied, as described below.

- Dignity-Conserving Practices Model[94–96] encompasses techniques patients can use to increase or maintain their sense of dignity, including:
  - living in the moment (focusing on immediate issues in the service or not worrying about the future)
  - maintaining normalcy (continuous or routine behaviours that help people manage day-to-day challenges
  - Seeking spiritual comfort (turning toward or finding solace in one's religious or spiritual belief system)
- Meaning-centred psychotherapy[97] in which patients participate in group therapy sessions facilitated by spiritual directors focused on helping the patients find meaning in the midst of their illness.
- Mind–body interventions, such as prayer, meditation, yoga, tai chi, and others that have been shown to reduce the effects of chronic stress, to rebalance autonomic nervous systems, and as effective modalities to medical management of chronic conditions, such as pain and high blood pressure.[98,99] The growing body of evidence shows that these interventions can help patients tap into their own ability to heal and cope, to find meaning and purpose and hope and to live well within the experience of their illness. These interventions offer healthcare professionals the opportunity to treat the whole person by recognizing patients' ability to transcend suffering.[100]
- Spiritual counselling, conducted by board-certified or board-eligible chaplains, clergy, or pastoral counsellors, is a 'step forward out of the immediate moment of the situation and ideally build on the pastoral or spiritual care' a patient has already received.[100] The goal is to promote positive coping rather than meaning that conforms to the patent's 'generally accepted belief system.'[101]
- Spiritual practices and rituals that promote wellbeing, coping, growth, and relationships, such as religious practices and attending religious services to prayer, meditation, visualization, sacred or inspirational reading, journaling, reflection, intentional appreciation of beauty, or finding peace in nature.[102] Rituals may be from the patient's religious practices or personal rituals people create themselves that are expressions of their spiritual beliefs, longings, or values.[103]

Table 29.2 provides examples of spiritual health interventions.[104] Some of these may be done by the primary clinician; others need referral to specialists such as chaplains, mind-body specialists, meaning-oriented group therapy, etc.

Documentation

Treatment plans should be documented and framed in a biopsychosocial-spiritual framework. An example is shown below in Table 29.3. An 80-year-old man dying of end-stage colon cancer with well controlled pain, some anxiety, unresolved family issues, and fear about dying.

Barriers to spiritual care

Some of the barriers to practicing spiritual care that physicians often cite include not having adequate time to address spiritual issues and fear that raising the question about spirituality will open the door to uncomfortable conversations about the physician's own spiritual beliefs and practices. However, the spiritual assessment as described above is meant as a screening tool, similar to other items in the history, such as personal history, exercise history, brief depression inventory, occupational history, etc. Each of these additional items is not time consuming in and of themselves and each is included in the history because they are important to a patient-centred approach to care. It is true that some issues may

Table 29.2 Examples of spiritual health interventions

Therapeutic communication techniques	1. Compassionate presence
	2. Reflective listening, query about important life events
	3. Support patient's sources of spiritual strength
	4. Open-ended questions to illicit feelings, inner life issues
	5. Inquiry about spiritual beliefs, values, and practices
	6. Life review, listening to the patient's story
	7. Continued presence and follow-up
Therapy	8. Guided visualization for 'meaningless pain'
	9. Progressive relaxation
	10. Breathing practice or contemplation
	11. Meaning-orientated therapy
	12. Referral to chaplain or spiritual care provider
	13. Use of story telling
	14. Dignity-conserving therapy
Self-care	15. Massage
	16. Reconciliation with self or others
	17. Spiritual support groups
	18. Meditation
	19. Sacred/spiritual readings or rituals
	20. Yoga, tai chi
	21. Exercise
	22. Referral to art or music therapist
	23. Journaling

Reprinted with permission from *Journal of Palliative Medicine* 12/10, 2009, published by Mary Ann Liebert, Inc., New Rochelle, NY.

arise in the assessment that may take more time. However, the goal of the history is recognition of the issues and appropriate referral. Thus, the physician need not be responsible for solving all the issues for the patient; he or she can rely on the interdisciplinary team for assistance. Even in the outpatient setting, the physician can utilize chaplains, spiritual directors, clergy and other spiritual care professionals to help patients with spiritual issues that arise in the clinical context.

Physicians need not engage in conversations about their own beliefs any more than they need to share other aspects of their personal lives in the clinical context. Appropriate boundaries of sharing should be followed so that patients do not feel coerced by physicians to share more than they are comfortable or to feel they need to adopt their physicians' beliefs and practices simply because the physician is in a position of power. It is critical that physicians be aware of that power differential and in all their interactions with their patients is respectful of the patient and do what is in the best interest of the patient.

Compassionate presence

A key recommendation from the NCC was that spirituality should be part of the personal and professional development of the physician and other clinicians.[62] This is particularly important in helping clinicians practice compassionate care, and engage in deep relationships with patients. As shown in Figure 29.1, an important element of the clinician patient relationship is the transformation that can occur in both patient and clinician as a result of the encounter. In order to be open to this transformation, but also to be able to handle the stresses associated with caring for seriously ill patients, clinicians need to have opportunities for reflection, self-care, and practice. Thus, physicians should consider their call to medicine and align their practice patterns to be congruent to the call. They should have training in reflective practice, as well as attend to self-care as part of their professional work. In addition, having a spiritual or personal practice such as meditation, appreciation of beauty, journaling, and creative arts could support physicians in their abilities to provide more compassionate care for their patients.[63]

Conclusion

The goal of medicine is the identification and relief of suffering, as well as the promotion of health. As seen in health outcomes research as well as policy, spirituality is a key element of health and wellbeing, as well as a way people cope with suffering. It is also the basis of compassionate relationships. Dr Francis Peabody wrote in his 1927 medical classic, *The Care of the Patient*, 'One of the essential qualities of the clinician is interest in humanity, for the

Table 29.3 Case example: assessment and treatment plan

Dimension	Assessment	Plan
Physical	Well-controlled pain Nausea and vomiting, likely secondary to partial small bowel obstruction.	Continue current medication regimen. Evaluate treatment options to relieve nausea associated with bowel obstruction.
Emotional	Anxiety about dyspnea that may be associated with dying Anxiety affecting sleep at night	Refer to counsellor for anxiety management and exploration of issues about fear of dying. Consult with Palliative Care Service for treatment of dyspnea and anxiety.
Social	Unresolved issues with family members as well as questions about funeral planning and costs	Refer to social worker for possible family intervention as well as assistance with end-of-life planning.
Spiritual	Expresses fear about dying; seeks forgiveness from son for being a 'distant dad.'	Refer to chaplain for spiritual counseling, consider forgiveness intervention, encourage discussion about fear of death. Continue presence and support.

Reprinted with permission from *Journal of Palliative Medicine* 12/10, 2009, published by Mary Ann Liebert, Inc., New Rochelle, NY.

secret care of the patient is in caring for the patient.'[105] Since healing springs from the therapeutic relationship, spiritual care is grounded in relationship-centred care. Spiritual care begins from the moment the healthcare professional enters the patient's room. This means that the clinician brings his or her whole being to the encounter and places full attention on the patient, not allowing distractions to interfere with that attention. Integral to this is the ability to listen and to be attentive to all dimensions of patients' and their family's lives. Spiritual care is the foundation of whole person, patient-centred care. The principles and practices of inter-professional spiritual care will help restore medicine and healthcare to its roots of compassion and service.

References

1 Flexner, A. (1910). *Medical Education in the United States and Canada:* A Report to the Carnegie Foundation for the Advancement of Teaching, Bulletin No. *4*. New York City: Carnegie Foundation for the Advancement of Teaching.

2 Engel, G.L. (1977). The need for a new medical model: a challenge for biomedicine. *Science* **196:** 129–36.

3 Siegel, B.S. (1990). *Peace, Love and Healing: Body Mind Communication and the Path to Self-Healing An Exploration*. New York: Perennial Library.

4 Benson, H. (1979). *The Mind/Body Effect: How Behavioural Medicine can Show You the Way to Better Health*. New York: Simon and Schuster.

5 Pellegrino, E.D., Thomasma, D.C. (1996). Virtue-based ethics: natural and theological. In: Pellegrino ED, Thomasma DC (eds) *The Christian Virtues in Medical Practice*, pp. 6–28. Washington:Georgetown University Press.

6 Picker Institute (2004). *Patient-centred Care 2015:* Scenarios, Visions, Goals & Next Steps. Alexandria: Institute for Alternative Futures on Behalf of the Picker Institute.

7 Pew-Fetzer Task Force on Advancing Psychosocial Health Education (1994). *Health Professions Education and Relationship-Centred Care*. San Francisco: Pew Health Professions Commission.

8 Sulmasy, D.P. (2002). A biopsychosocial-spiritual model for the care of patients at the end of life. *Gerontologist* 42(Spec No 3): 34–9.

9 Saunders, C. (1964). Care of patients suffering from terminal illness at St. Joseph's Hospice Hackney, London. *Nurs Mirror* 14: vii–x.

10 Stone, S. (2008). A Retrospective Evaluation of the Impact of the Planetree Patient Centred Model of Care Program on Inpatient Quality Outcomes. *HERD* **1**(4): 55–69.

11 Astrow, A.B., Puchalski, C.M., Sulmasy, D.P. (2001). Religion, spirituality, and healthcare: social, ethical, and practical considerations. *Am J Med* **110:** 283–7.

12 Sulmasy, D.P. (1999). Is medicine a spiritual practice? *Acad Med* **74**: 1002–5.

13 Puchalski, C.M., Lunsford, B., Harris, M.H., Miller, R.T. (2006). Interdisciplinary spiritual care for seriously ill and dying patients: a collaborative model. *Cancer J* **12**(5): 398–416.

14 Ferrell, B.R., Coyle, N. (2008). The nature of suffering and the goals of nursing. *Oncol Nurs Forum* **35**(2): 241–7.

15 Phelps, A.C., Maciejewski, P.K., Nilsson, M. et al. (2009). Religious coping and use of intensive life-prolonging care near death in patients with advanced cancer. *J Am Med Ass* **301**: 1140–7.

16 Silvestri, G.A., Knittig, S., Zoller, J.S., Nietert, P.J .(2003). Importance of faith on medical decisions regarding cancer care. *J Clin Oncol* **21**(7): 1379–82.

17 Burgener, S.C. (1999). Predicting quality of life in caregivers of Alzheimer's patients: The role of support from and involvement with the religious community. *J Pastoral Care* **53**(4): 433–46.

18 Koenig, H.G., McCullough, M.E., Larson, D.B. (2001). *Handbook of Religion and Health*. New York: Oxford University Press.

19 Roberts, J.A., Brown, D., Elkins, T., Larson, D.B. (1997). Factors influencing views of patients with gynecologic cancer about end-of-life decisions. *Am J Obstet Gynaecol* **176**(1): 166–72.

20 Tsevat, J., Sherman, S.N., McElwee, J.A. et al. (1999). The will to live among HIV-infected patients. *Ann Intern Med* **131**(3): 194–8.

21 Ehman, J.W., Ott, B.B., Short, T.H., Ciampa, R.C., Hansen-Flaschen, J. (1999). Do patients want physicians to inquire about their spiritual or religious beliefs if they become gravely ill? *Arch Intern Med* **159**(15): 1803–6.

22 Puchalski, C.M., McSkimming, S. (2006). Creating healing environments. *Hlth Progr* **87**(3): 30–5.

23 Balboni, T.A., Vanderwerker, L.C., Block, S.D. *et al.* (2007). Religiousness and spiritual support among advanced cancer patients and associations with end-of-life treatment preferences and quality of life. *J Clin Oncol* **25**(5): 555–60.

24 Frick, E., Riedner, C., Fegg, M.J., Hauf, S., Borasio, G.D. (2006). A clinical interview assessing cancer patients' spiritual needs and preferences. *Eur J Cancer Care (Engl)* **15**(3): 238–43.

25 McCord, G., Gilchrist, V.J., Grossman, S.D. *et al.* (2004). Discussing spirituality with patients: A rational and ethical approach. *Ann Fam Med* **2:** 356–61.

26 Mathai, J. (2003). Spiritual history of parents of children attending a child and adolescent mental health service. Austral Psychiat **11**(2): 172–4.

27 Astrow, A.B., Wexler, A., Teixeira, K., Kai He, M., Sulmasy, D.P (2007). Is failure to meet spiritual needs associated with cancer patients' perceptions of quality of care and their satisfaction with care? *J Clin Oncol* **25**(36): 5753–7.

28 Phelps, A.C., Maciejewski, P.K., Nilsson, M., *et al.* (2009). Religious coping and use of intensive lifeprolonging care near death in patients with advanced cancer. *J Am Med Ass* **301:** 1140–7.

29 Field, M.J., Cassel, C.K. (1997). *Approaching Death: Improving Care at the End of Life*. Committee on Care at the End of Life, Division of Health Care Services. Washington: Institute of Medicine, National Academy Press.

30 Breitbart, W., Rosenfeld, B., Passik, S. (1996). Interest in physician-assisted suicide among ambulatory HIV-infected patients. *Am J Psychiat* **153:** 238–42.

31 Townsend, M., Kladder, V., Ayele, H. (2002). Systematic review of clinical trials examining the effects of religion on health. *Sthn Med J* **95**(12): 1429–34.

32 Mueller, P.S., Plevak, D.J., Rumans, T.A. (2001). Religious involvement, spirituality and medicine: implications for clinical practice. *Mayo Clin Proc* **76:** 1225–35.

33 McClain, C.S., Rosenfeld, B., Breitbart, W. (2003). Effect of spiritual wellbeing on end-of-life despair in terminally ill cancer patients. *Lancet* **361**(9369): 1603–7.

34 Puchalski, C.M. (2006). The role of spirituality in the care of seriously ill. In: C.M. Puchalski (ed.) *Chronically and Dying Patients in a Time for Listening and Caring*, pp. 10–21. New York: Oxford University Press.

35 Yates, J.W., Chalmer, B.J., St. James, P., Follansbee, M., McKegney, F.P. (1981). Religion in patients with advanced cancer. *Med Pediat Oncol* **9**(2): 121–8.

36 Puchalski, C.M. (2002). Spirituality. In: A. Berger, R. Portenoy, D. Weissman (eds) *Principles and Practice of Palliative Care and Supportive Oncology*, 2nd edn. Philadelphia: Lippincott Williams & Wilkins.

37 Pargament, K., Smith, B., Koenig, H.G., Perez, L. (1998). Patterns of positive and negative religious coping with major life stresses. *J Scient Study Religion* **37**(4): 710–24.

38 Fitchett, G., Rybarczyk, B.D., DeMarco, G.A., Nicholas, J.J. (1999). The role of religion in medical rehabilitation outcomes: a longitudinal study. *Rehabil Psychol* **44**(4): 333–53.

39 Cotton, S.P., Levine, E.G., Fitzpatrick, C.M., Dold, K.H., Targ, E. (1999). Exploring the relationships among spiritual wellbeing. *Psychooncol* **8**(5): 429–38.

40 Fehring, R.J., Miller, J.F., Shaw, C. (1997). Spiritual wellbeing, religiosity, hope, depression, and other moral states in elderly people coping with cancer. *Oncol Nurs Forum* **24**(4): 663–71.

41 Carson, V.B., Green, H. (1992). Spiritual wellbeing: a predictor of hardiness in patients with acquired immunodeficiency syndrome. *J Profess Nurs* **8**(4): 209–20.

42 Miller, J.F. (1985). Assessment of loneliness and spiritual wellbeing in chronically ill and healthy adults. *J Profess Nurs* **1**(2): 79–85.

43 Kaczorowski, J.M. (1989). Spiritual wellbeing and anxiety in adults diagnosed with cancer. *Hospice J* **5**(3–4): 105–16.

44 Field, M.J., Cassel, C.K. (1997). *Approaching Death: Improving Care at the End of Life.* Committee on Care at the End of Life, Division of Health Care Services, Institute of Medicine. Washington: National Academy Press.

45 NHS Education for Scotland (NES) (2008). *The Spiritual and Religious Care Capabilities and Competences for Healthcare Chaplains.* Available at: http://www.nes.scot.nhs.uk/media/206594/010308capabilities_and_competences_for_healthcare_chaplains.pdf (accessed 6 Feb 2012).

46 Clinical Standards Board for Scotland (2002). *Clinical Standards for Specialist Palliative Care* http://www.healthcareimprovementscotland.org/previous_resources/standards/specialist_palliative_care.aspx (accessed 27 July 2011)

47 National Institute for Health and Clinical Excellence (NICE) (2004). *NICE clinical guidance on supportive and palliative care (CSG).* Available at: http://guidance.nice.org.uk/CSGSP (accessed 26 July 2011).

48 National Quality Forum (2006). *A National Framework and Preferred Practices for Palliative and Hospice Care Quality: A Consensus Report.* Washington: NQF.

49 World Health Organization. (2001). *WHO Definition of Palliative Care.* Available at: http://www.who.int/cancer/palliative/definition/en/ (accessed 20 July 2011).

50 Gordon, T., Mitchell, D. (2004). A competency model for the assessment and delivery of spiritual care. *Palliat Med* **18**(7): 646–51.

51 World Health Organization. (2006). *Constitution of the World Health Organization. Basic Documents,* 45th edn, Supplement, p.1. Geneva: WHO.

52 Dent, S.D. (2011). *Spirituality: Don't Make Patients Check it at the Door*, FP Report. Available at: http://www.aafp.org/fpr/990700fr/2.html (accessed 20 July2011).

53 Joint Commission on Accreditation of Healthcare Organizations (1996). *Implementation Section of the 1996 Standards for Hospitals.* Oakbrook Terrace: JCAHO.

54 Joint Commission on Accreditation of Healthcare Organizations (2008). *Provision of Care, Treatment, and Services (CAMH/Hospitals): Spiritual Assessment.* Available at: http://www.jointcommission.org/standards_information/jcfaqdetails.aspx?StandardsFAQId = 290&StandardsFAQChapterId = 78 (accessed 20 July 2011).

55 Association of American Medical Colleges (1999). *Contemporary Issues in Medicine: Communication in Medicine. Medical School Objectives Project (MSOP) Report III.* Washington: AAMC.

56 Puchalski, C.M., Larson, D. (1998). Developing curricula in spirituality and medicine. *Acad Med* **73**(9): 970–4.

57 Puchalski, C.M. (2006). Spirituality and medicine: curricula in medical education. *J Cancer Educ* **21**(1). 14–18.

58 Lo, B., Quill, T., Tulsky, J. for the ACP-ASIM End-of-Life Care Consensus Panel. (1999). Discussing palliative care with patients. *Ann Intern Med* **130**(9):744–9.

59 American Medical Association. (2011). *Principles of Medical Ethics.* Available at: http://www.ama-assn.org/ama/pub/physician-resources/medical-ethics/code-medical-ethics/principles-medical-ethics.page? (accessed 20 July 2011).

60 Puchalski, C.M., Larson, D.B., Lu, F.G. (2001). Spirituality in psychiatry residency training programs. *Int Rev Psychiat* **13**(2): 131–8.

61 Nolan, S., Saltmarsh, P., Leget, C. (2011). Spiritual care in palliative care: working towards an EAPC Task Force. *Eur J Palliat Care* **18**(2): 86–9.

62 Puchalski, C.M., Ferrell, B., Virani, R. *et al.* (2009). Improving the quality of spiritual care as a dimension of palliative care: The Report of the Consensus Conference. *J Palliat Med* **12**(10): 885–904.

63 Puchalski, C., Lunsford, B. (2008). *The Relationship of Spirituality and Compassion in Health Care* (White Paper). Kalamazoo: Fetzer Institute.

64 McCord, G., Gilchrist, V.J., Grossman, S.D. *et al.* (2004). Discussing spirituality with patients: A rational and ethical approach. *Ann Fam Med* **2**: 356–61.

65 Sulmasy, D.P., Snyder, L. (2010). Substituted interests and best judgments: an integrated model of surrogate decision making. *J Am Med Ass* **304**(17): 1946–7.

66 Puchalski, C.M., McSkimming, S. (2006). Creating healing environments. *Hlth Progr* **87**(3): 30–5.

67 National Consensus Project for Quality Palliative Care. (2009). *Clinical Practice Guidelines for Quality Palliative Care,* 2nd edn. Pittsburgh: NCPQPC.

68 Puchalski, C.M., Ferrell, B. (2010). *Making Health Care Whole: Integrating Spirituality into Patient Care.* West Conshohocken: Templeton Press.

69 Anandarajah, G., Hight, E. (2001). Spirituality and medical practice: using the HOPE questions as a practical tool for spiritual assessment. *Am Fam Physician* **63**(1): 81–9.

70 Maugans, T.A. (1996). The SPIRITual history. *Arch Fam Med* **5**: 11–16.

71 Puchalski, C.M. (2006). Spiritual assessment in clinical practice. *Psychiat Ann* **36**(3): 150–5.

72 Pargament, K.I., Koenig, H.G., Tarakeshwar, N., Hahn, J. (2004). Religious coping methods as predictors of psychological, physical and spiritual outcomes among medically ill elderly patients: a two-year longitudinal study. *J Hlth Psychol* **9**(6): 713–30.

73 Koenig, H.G., Pargament, K.I., Nelson, J. (1998). Religious coping and health status in medically ill hospitalized older adults. *J Nerv Ment Dis* **186**(9): 513–21.

74 Sherman, A.C., Simonton, S., Latif, U., Spohn, R., Tricot, G. (2005). Religious struggle and religious comfort in response to illness: health outcomes among stem cell transplant patients. *J Behavior Med* **28**(4): 359–67.

75 Pargament, K.I., Koenig, H.G., Tarakeshwar, N., Hahn, J. (2001). Religious struggle as a predictor of mortality among medically ill elderly patients: a two-year longitudinal study. *Arch Intern Med* **161**(15): 1881–5.

76 Fitchett, G., Murphy, P.E., Kim, J., Gibbons, J.L., Cameron, J.R., Davis, J.A. (2004). Religious struggle: Prevalence, correlates and mental health risks in diabetic, congestive heart failure, and oncology patients. *Int J Psychiat Med* **34**(2): 179–96.

77 Joint Commission. (2010). *Specifications Manual for Joint Commission National Quality Core Measures* Available at: http://manual.jointcommission.org/releases/TJC2011A/(accessed 20 July 2011).

78 Puchalski, C.M., Ferrell, B. (2010). *Making Health Care Whole: Integrating Spirituality into Patient Care,* pp. 76–7. West Conshohocken: Templeton Press.

79 Puchalski, C.M., Ferrell, B. (2010). *Making Health Care Whole: Integrating Spirituality into Patient Care,* p.125. West Conshohocken: Templeton Press.

80 North American Nursing Diagnosis Association (2007). *NANDA-1-nursing diagnosis: Definitions and classification, 2007–2008.* Philadelphia: NANDA International.

81 Kuebler, K.K., Davis, M.P., Moore, C. (2005). *Palliative Practices: an Interdisciplinary Approach.* St. Louis, MO: Mosby.

82 National Comprehensive Cancer Network Inc. (2010). *NCCN Clinical Practice Guidelines in Oncology (NCCN Guidelines™). Guidelines for Supportive Care: Distress Management.* Available at: http://www.nccn.org/professionals/physician_gls/pdf/distress.pdf (accessed 25 July 2011).

83 Puchalski, C.M., Ferrell, B. (2010). *Making Health Care Whole: Integrating Spirituality into Patient Care*, pp. 126–7. West Conshohocken: Templeton Press.

84 Puchalski, C.M., Ferrell, B. (2010). *Making Health Care Whole: Integrating Spirituality into Patient Care*, pp. 128–9. West Conshohocken: Templeton Press.

85 Fitchett, G., Risk, J.L. (2009). Screening for spiritual struggle. *J Past Care Counsel* **63**(1,2): 1–12.

86 Puchalski, C.M., Ferrell, B. (2010). *Making Health Care Whole: Integrating Spirituality into Patient Care*, pp. 99–100. West Conshohocken: Templeton Press.

87 Corbett, J.M. (1990). *Religion in America*. Englewood Cliffs: Prentice-Hall.

88 Post, S.G., Puchalski, C.M., Larson, D.B. (2000). Physicians and patient spirituality: professional boundaries, competency, and ethics. *Ann Intern Med* **132**(7): 578–83.

89 Puchalski, C., Romer, A.L (2000). Taking a spiritual history allows clinicians to understand patients more fully. *J Palliat Med* **3**(1): 129–37.

90 Borneman, T., Ferrell, B., Otis-Green, S., Baird, P., Puchalski, C. (2010). Evaluation of the FICA tool for spiritual assessment. *J Pain Sympt Manag* **40**(2): 163–73.

91 Frick, E., Riedner, C., Fegg, M., Hauf, S., Borasio, G.D. (2006). A clinical interview assessing cancer patients' spiritual needs and preferences. *Eur J Cancer Care* **15:** 238–43.

92 Fitchett, G., Canada, A.L. (2010). The role of religion/spirituality in coping with cancer: evidence, assessment, and intervention. In: J.C. Holland, W.S. Breitbart, P.B. Jacobsen, M.S. Lederberg, M.J. Loscalzo, R. McCorkle (eds) *Psycho-oncology*, 2nd edn. New York: Oxford University Press.

93 Puchalski, C.M., Ferrell, B. (2010). *Making Health Care Whole: Integrating Spirituality into Patient Care*, p. 127. West Conshohocken: Templeton Press.

94 Chochinov, H.M. (2002). Dignity-conserving care—a new model for palliative care: Helping the patient feel valued. *J Am Med Ass* **287**(17): 2253–60.

95 Chochinov, H.M. (2006). Dying, dignity, and new horizons in palliative end-of-life care. *CA: Cancer J Clinic* **56**(2): 84–103.

96 Chochinov, H.M., Hack, T., Hassard, T., Kristjanson, L.J., McClement, S., Harlos, M. (2004). Dignity and psychotherapeutic considerations in end-of-life care. *J Palliat Care* **20**(3): 134–42.

97 Chochinov, H.M., Breitbart, W. (2009). *Handbook of Psychiatry in Palliative Medicine*. New York: Oxford University Press.

98 Schneider, R.H., Alexander, C.N., Staggers, F. *et al.* (2005). Long-term effects of stress reduction on mortality in persons > or = 55 years of age with systemic hypertension. *Am J Cardiol* **95**(9): 1060–4.

99 Puchalski, C. (2006). Spirituality and medicine: curricula in medical education. *J Cancer Educ* **21**(1): 14–8.

100 Puchalski, C.M., Ferrell, B. (2010). *Making Health Care Whole: Integrating Spirituality into Patient Care*, p. 114. West Conshohocken: Templeton Press.

101 Puchalski, C.M., Ferrell, B. (2010). *Making Health Care Whole: Integrating Spirituality into Patient Care*, p. 117. West Conshohocken: Templeton Press.

102 Puchalski, C.M., Ferrell, B. (2010). *Making Health Care Whole: Integrating Spirituality into Patient Care*, p. 120. West Conshohocken: Templeton Press.

103 Puchalski, C.M., Ferrell, B. (2010). *Making Health Care Whole: Integrating Spirituality into Patient Care*, p. 121. West Conshohocken: Templeton Press.

104 Puchalski, C.M., Ferrell, B., Virani, R. *et al* . (2009). Improving the quality of spiritual care as a dimension of palliative care: the report of the Consensus Conference. *J Palliat Med* **12**(10): 885–904.

105 Peabody, F.W. (1927). The care of the patient. *J Am Med Ass* **88**(12): 877–82.

CHAPTER 30

Nursing

Wilfred McSherry and Linda Ross

Introduction

This chapter presents an overview of the historical and contemporary development of spirituality and spiritual care within nursing. The chapter commences with a historical perspective of nursing care drawing attention to the medical and holistic models that have existed. This is followed by an analysis of the key arguments that provide a basis for spiritual care within nursing. This section reviews some of the primary drivers; political, professional and societal, resulting in nursing engaging with spiritual aspects of the person. It is acknowledged that the concepts and debates outlined in this chapter have a relevance to nursing globally. There is an increasing recognition of the importance that the spiritual part of an individual's life may make to health, wellbeing, and recovery. A significant evidence base to support this is emerging, for example the pioneering work of Koenig *et al.*[1] The importance of nurses addressing the spiritual dimension is also reflected in some of the healthcare guidance at world, European, and national levels. These issues are discussed in more detail in Ross.[2]

Historical perspective

Historically, in the West the sick were looked after in religious orders. The body and spirit were cared for together, signifying the practice of truly holistic care at that time, i.e. care of the body, mind, and spirit, where the whole is more than the sum of the parts. There then followed the 'period of enlightenment', with all that brought with it, including an escalation in medical research, and knowledge and prevalence of a medical model of treatment which focused on disease processes and cures, rather than the spirit. This medical model still prevails today within many health care services across the world. However, it could be said that, until recently, nursing has never lost sight of the holistic concept of care, which has remained at the heart of the profession right through to the current day. This unswerving focus on the whole person is a constant core and founding principle shaping and influencing how nursing is defined, practised and taught as shown in the next section. Nursing is also in the process of developing its own evidence base for spiritual care.

Above we implied that nursing has maintained its focus on the holistic concept of care. However, in the United Kingdom (UK) at present, there is concern that nursing may be in danger of losing sight of this focus moving away from the founding principles on which it is based. The need to refocus on these core values of nursing, such as care, compassion, dignity, respect is evident in a number of reports where the quality and standard of nursing care are criticized.[3–8] In these reports nurses are accused of treating individuals without dignity and respect. Claire Rayner (the late President of The Patients Association in the UK) wrote:

> For far too long now, the Patients Association has been receiving calls on our Helpline from people wanting to talk about the dreadful, neglectful, demeaning, painful and sometimes downright cruel treatment their elderly relatives had experienced at the hands of NHS nurses.[4, p. 3]

For nurses to be described in such derogatory terms is of great concern, since it implies that the core principles, beliefs, and values that underpin nursing have been eroded, lost and misplaced within contemporary nursing practice. While these reports have been published within the UK the ramifications and lessons to be learnt are of international relevance, since they bring into question the public's image of the nursing profession, and the need for nurses to re-establish the fundamental principles of care and caring.

Basis for spiritual care within nursing

Definitions of nursing

The International Council of Nursing[9] defines nursing as:

> Nursing encompasses autonomous and collaborative care of individuals of all ages, families, groups and communities, sick or well and in all settings. Nursing includes the promotion of health, prevention of illness, and the care of ill, disabled and dying people. Advocacy, promotion of a safe environment, research, participation in shaping health policy and in patient and health systems management, and education are also key nursing roles.

This definition emphasizes the importance of nurses working collaboratively with the individual to establish their needs. The definition underlines and reinforces the importance of nursing adopting a holistic and patient centred approach to care which is at the heart of the American Holistic Nurses Association mission statement.[10]

Florence Nightingale considered that 'the sick body … is something more than a reservoir for storing medicines'.[11, p. 36] This sentiment is still evident in the Royal College of Nursing's (RCN) most recent definition of nursing, where nursing is defined in terms of its key functions. These are concerned with promoting, improving and maintaining health and healing, helping people to cope with health problems, and to achieve the best possible quality of life. The nurse's focus is on the whole person and their response to health, illness, disability which includes their spiritual response. Spiritual support is identified by the RCN as a key part of the nurse's role.[12] In addition the first of the 8 new principles of nursing practice is concerned with dignity, respect, individual need and compassion.[13]

Models of nursing

In an early model of nursing, Virginia Henderson said it was the duty of the nurse to assist the patient to 'worship according to his faith' (p. 13) and to 'practice his religion or conform to his concept of right and wrong.'[14, p. 19] More recent nursing models also incorporate the spiritual. For example, Jean Watson talks about the caring presence of the nurse and focuses on transcendence and the quest for meaning in life in her model.[15] One of the most commonly used models of nursing, the Activities of Daily Living (ADL) model[16] considers spirituality as a factor influencing ADL's and spirituality features specifically under the 'death and dying' ADL. Yet other models address the spiritual through their focus on meaning, wholeness and/or transcendence.

Oldnall[17,18] suggested that the assertion that most nursing models have a holistic approach to care is inaccurate. This is because, up until recently, some nursing models and theories, while espousing and embracing the mantra of holistic care, do not explicitly address the spiritual dimension. McSherry[19, p. 79] offers a possible explanation for this:

> Models should not be solely developed in the 'ivory towers of academia' and then be expected to work in practice. This top-down approach to theory development may overlook and fail to incorporate many issues that are being faced by nurses working on the front line. This approach may have prevented the spiritual dimension from being incorporated within contemporary nursing theories and models.'

Martsolf & Mickley[20] undertook a detailed review of some modern nurse theorists' ideas concerning spirituality. Their review sheds light on two key areas:

1. The contribution to nursing knowledge made by some of the contemporary nurse theorists
2. The position that spirituality has within those ideas; whether implicit or explicit.

It is beyond the scope of this chapter to provide a full critique of the place spirituality holds within each model. It is sufficient to say that, within nursing models and theories, the importance of the spiritual dimension for individual health and wellbeing is now recognized.

Codes of ethics and education guidelines

Spiritual care is central to nursing Codes of Ethics, both internationally and within the United Kingdom (UK). The International Council of Nurses (ICN) Code of Ethics for Nurses states:[21, p. 2]

> In providing care, the nurse promotes an environment in which the human rights, values, customs and spiritual beliefs of the individual, family and community are respected.

The Australian Nursing & Midwifery Council[22] accepts and builds upon the ICN Code.

In the UK, the Nursing and Midwifery Code of Professional Conduct states that: 'You must treat people as individuals and respect their dignity.'[23]

Unlike the ICN code[21] the spiritual dimension is not explicit, but implicit within the NMC (2008) code (and its associated publications) through the use of the words 'individual' and 'respect for dignity.' Therefore, failure to include a spiritual dimension within nursing and recognizing the importance of this for some individuals, may lead to a violation of an individual's fundamental human rights. The NMC further expects that at point of registration newly qualified graduate nurses should be able to:

> 'Carry out comprehensive, systematic nursing assessments that take account of relevant physical, social, cultural, psychological, spiritual, genetic and environmental factors …'.[24, p. 18.]

The Essential Skills Clusters for pre-registration nursing programmes identifies 'skills that are essential' in order to be 'a proficient nurse.' Included under the 'Care, compassion and communication' cluster is the expectation that the nurse will 'demonstrate an understanding of how culture, religion, spiritual beliefs … can impact upon illness and disability.'[24, p. 108]

This is a similar expectation of the Quality Assurance Agency for Higher Education which expects nurses to be educated to:

- Undertake a comprehensive systematic assessment using the tools/frameworks appropriate to the patient/client taking into account relevant… spiritual needs
- Plan care delivery to meet identified needs
- Demonstrate an understanding of issues related to spirituality. [25, pp. 10, 12]

Despite the above guidance, there is great variation in the amount and nature of the spirituality component within nurse education programmes. Despite these inconsistencies, there is evidence that spiritual care teaching is gaining more attention as evidenced by the increasing numbers of papers debating the many issues and dilemmas raised. Currently, a great deal of work has[26–28] and is being done (a current doctoral level study is in progress) to establish competencies in spiritual care for nurses and midwives at point of registration. This is a much needed development.

Spiritual care: what is it and what does it look like?

If one looks at the evolution of spirituality and spiritual care in nursing then there is a noticeable shift in emphasis and direction. Much of the early pioneering work sought to elucidate and define the concept at a macro level. Macro in this instance, means applying generally and universally to the nursing profession. This early work was concerned with understanding the meaning and perception of spirituality, and the practice of spiritual care and much of it was American.[29–31] The emphasis now is not so much on elucidation of the concept, but about practical relevance and application. Nurses are now engaging with the concept at a micro-level. Micro- meaning they are trying to apply the general principles of spirituality and spiritual care and developing knowledge and understanding specific to their own sphere of practice be this mental health, orthopaedic or critical care nursing. This micro approach has seen nursing focus on spiritual assessment within the different branches of nursing.

Spirituality

The spiritual dimension is deeply subjective and there is no authoritative definition of spirituality.[32] Swinton and Pattison[33, p. 236] affirm that it is probably more beneficial for nursing not to have a definitive definition when they write:

> 'As a matter of fact, it is probably important that spirituality remains a contested and functional concept rather than becoming consolidated if it is usefully to denote the kinds of contextual absences that need to continue to be recognized and worked with.'

However, when one looks at the range of definitions of spirituality across disciplines involving diverse groups of people with differing worldviews, there seem to be common attributes, namely: hope and strength; trust; meaning and purpose; forgiveness; belief and faith in self, others, and for some a belief in God/deity/higher power; values; love and relationships; morality; creativity and self-expression.

Given this broad concept of spirituality, what then does spiritual care look like? And how can it be given?

Recent criticisms

The concept of spirituality and its place within nursing has been the subject of recent debate and criticism. The spirituality-in-nursing debate has been accused of insularity; that is it has not drawn sufficiently on the established body knowledge of other academic disciplines, meaning it has lacked the external scrutiny or peer review from groups of people from outside of nursing such as theology, psychology, philosophy, sociology and religious studies. This is an important point since many of these disciplines have engaged with the concept of spirituality over many centuries and they have a wealth of knowledge and skills that shed valuable light enabling a deeper understanding of the concept. However, while nursing must and should draw upon the wealth of knowledge generated by such disciplines it must not be held ransom by them, in that they are not the sole avenues of knowledge and understanding. Nursing must continue to plough its own furrows with regards to spirituality and its application to nursing, however being mindful of the important contribution other disciplines can make to helping nursing understand and expedite this field of enquiry.

A further criticism of the spirituality-in-nursing debate has been the perpetuation of concepts theory and definitions that have not been developed within the context of empirical study. One example of this is the uncritical and almost universal adoption of a definition of spirituality first presented by Murray and Zentner.[34] This definition was used uncritically and unchallenged by nursing scholars and academics, especially within the UK. A further concern raised has been the relationship of spirituality with other humanistic aspects of the individual, such as psychosocial care. Clarke[35] proposes that nurses have always addressed the spiritual concerns of individuals which were accommodated within the psychosocial domain. Clarke[35, p. 1672] suggests that the reason for the inability to distinguish between the spiritual and psychological domains is that the model of spiritual care developed by nursing is '... too large, too existential and too inclusive to be manageable in practice without being indistinguishable from psychosocial care.'

For nursing research into spirituality to be more representative then it must seek to be more heterogeneous.[36] This point is made because, if one reviews the many studies undertaken in this area, the samples are often homogenous, lacking religious, ethnic, and cultural diversity, primarily reflect a Judeo-Christian perspective and often only focus on key groups, such as nurses, chaplains, and patients. There is a need for the nursing profession to be more inclusive, ensuring that study samples reflect the diversity of people, cultures, and groups within contemporary societies.

One of the positive outcomes of the recent debates associated with spirituality is that nursing scholars, researchers, and practitioners are more cautious and aware of the need to be analytical and critical, if concepts are to be developed in a meaningful and rigorous manner. Therefore, as Swinton[37] points out, nurses do need enemies, not to be confrontational, but to assist in the development and refinement of concepts so that these will be better constructed and understood.

Some of the contemporary criticism raised within the nursing literature related to spirituality and spiritual care have been summarized in a recent article written by Swinton and Pattison.[33] This article offers a positive way forward for nursing in understanding and applying the concepts of spirituality and spiritual care within nursing practice. The following quotation presents succinctly the outcome of recent controversy and where a solution may be found outlining the direction for future activity:

> 'We suggest that instead of arguing about whether or not spirituality can exist in any realist, essential sense—a line of argument that has proven to be somewhat circular, controversial, and unhelpful—it is more useful to develop a thin, vague, and functional understanding of what this word and its cognates might connote and do in the world of health care.' (p. 227)

Spiritual care

For some people, the experience of illness, the uncertainties about diagnosis and the possibility of disability or even death may trigger spiritual distress. It has been said by Granstrom that:

> 'Many individuals do not seriously search for meaning and purpose of life, but live as if life will go on forever. Often it is not until crisis, illness ... or suffering occurs that the illusion (of security) is shattered ... Therefore illness, suffering ... and ultimately death by their very nature become spiritual encounters as well as physical and emotional experiences.'[38, p. 26]

Karl Jaspers[39] calls such encounters 'limit situations,' i.e. situations that we cannot change and cause us to think about what is really important in life. Questions like 'Why is this happening to me?', 'Am I going to die?', 'What lies after death?' may be triggered, and cause existential, spiritual distress. Nurses are often the first point of contact for people facing such challenges. It is important, therefore, that they are equipped to be able to respond appropriately in such circumstances.

Spiritual care has been defined as:

> 'That care which recognizes and responds to the needs of the human spirit when faced with trauma, ill health or sadness and can include the need for meaning, for self-worth, to express oneself, for faith support, perhaps for rites or prayer or sacrament, or simply for a sensitive listener. Spiritual care begins with encouraging human contact in compassionate relationship, and moves in whatever direction need requires.'[40, p. 6]

Giving spiritual care

The practice of spiritual care is about meeting people at the point of deepest need. Some pointers are given in Box 30.1 and have been adapted from the RCN Pocket Guide which the authors helped to produce.[41]

Box 30.1 Some pointers for giving spiritual care

Spiritual care is about:

- Not just 'doing to', but 'being with' the person
- The nurse's attitudes, behaviours and personal qualities i.e. how he/she relates to the person
- Treating spiritual needs with the same level of attention as physical needs.

Skills that are useful include (from the research on nurses and patients):

- Adopting a caring attitude and disposition. Showing empathy. Watson (15) referred to this as the 'caring presence of the nurse'.
- Being respectful
- Recognizing and responding appropriately to people's needs
- Being sensitive
- Giving time to listen and attend to individual need. Good communication skills
- Being aware of when it is appropriate to refer to another source of support e.g. chaplain, counsellor, another staff member, family or friend
- Ability to remain fully present in the face of suffering
- Being personally hope-filled, believing that what one does and what one is always of some value. Knowing that it is never too late to do good.

Assessing spiritual needs

Just as a nurse would assess patients' physical needs, so an initial assessment of patients' spiritual/religious concerns is also important. Assessment may take different forms. It may involve, for example:

- Using observation to identify clues that may be indicative of underlying spiritual need, e.g. peoples' disposition (sad/withdrawn), personal artefacts (photographs, religious/meditational books and symbols)
- Using questions to open the area up for discussion. The following are examples:
  - Do you have a way of making sense of the things that happen to you?
  - What sources of support/help do you look to when life is difficult? (Would you like to see someone who can help you?)
  - Would you like to see someone who can help you talk or think through the impact of this illness/life event? (You don't have to be religious to talk to them)
- It will usually involve some form of documentation within the nursing notes and care plan as part of the wider nursing process.

Knowing when to seek further help:

It is important to know your strengths, limitations and when to seek help (42). There is nothing wrong with referring to someone else, e.g. colleague, mentor/preceptor, chaplaincy team (who are there for staff and patients of all faiths and none), counsellor, psychologist.

Of course our own values and beliefs are very dear and personal to each one of us. This can cause conflict for nurses in their dealings with patients, clients and families, particularly if the latter's life view differs from that of the nurse. When this happens we often hear about it in the media. Some examples of recent UK headlines and their knock-on effect are given in Box 30.2.

This media interest resulted in two of the biggest ever surveys of nurses by the Nursing Times[42] (which attracted more comments and views than any other story to date) and the Royal College of Nursing[43] whose survey had the 2nd largest response to a survey by its members. These response rates underline the importance nurses place on spiritual aspects of care and on the general interest nurses have in these concepts.

The overwhelming message from both surveys was that nurses recognize the importance of spiritual care, but want more guidance on spiritual care practice, particularly in relation to the conflict between their own personal beliefs/values and their professional practice. Here, are some key findings from the RCN survey.[44] Of the 4054 members who responded:

- 83.4% agreed that spirituality and spiritual care are fundamental aspects of nursing care
- 90% believed that providing spiritual care enhances the overall quality of nursing care
- Only 4.3% felt that it was not the nurses role to identify patients spiritual needs
- 79.3% agreed nurses do not receive sufficient education and training in spirituality
- 79.8% felt that spirituality and spiritual care should be addressed within programmes of education
- 78.8% felt the provision of guidance and support should come from the NMC. While 78.1% felt that the RCN also have a responsibility in this area.

The RCN commissioned a Task and Finish group (which the authors were part of) to produce guidance for nurses tackling some of the key concerns raised above by participants in the survey about this important part of care. This guidance is in the form of a 'Pocket Guide' and on-line resource.[45] A checklist of things to think about before responding to patient/client spiritual need is given in these resources.

Evidence base

Nursing practice today should be based upon research evidence. The evidence base for spiritual care within nursing is fairly new,

Box 30.2 Some recent media headlines

- 'Nurse suspended for prayer offer'[48]
- 'Nurse sacked 'for advising patient to go to church' (News, 26 May 2009)[49]
- 'Muslim nurses CAN cover up, but Christian colleagues can't wear crucifixes' (Mail Online, 19 Oct 2010)[50]
- 'British Medical Association to debate religion and prayer in the NHS' (News 29 June 2009)[51].

but has escalated in recent years. For instance a literature review conducted by LR in the late 1980s/early 1990s showed that there was very little published research on spirituality by nurses at that time, with only one American published study.[46,47] Most unpublished Masters work was also American in origin. When this review was repeated in 2006, 45 original research papers were identified for the period 1983–2005. Whilst much of this research was still American, the number of countries had expanded to include the UK, other European countries, Scandinavia, Australia and Japan. The full review is published,[45] but in brief showed that on the whole nurses consider spiritual care to be an important part of their role, but they feel unprepared for it, feeling in need of further education and training. They also tend to focus on the more obvious religious part of care which in many ways is easier to deal with than the broader aspects of spiritual care.

Integrating personal belief and professional responsibility

The nurse's own personal spirituality seems to have a bearing on how spiritual care is delivered. This can be illustrated by referring to two cases that gained considerable media attention in the UK: one involved the suspension of a nurse who offered to pray for a patient. The nurse had been caring for a woman in the community and as she left asked if the lady would like her to pray for her. The women said 'no'. Subsequently, the lady complained to the Trust and the nurse was suspended pending an investigation. Her suspension was on the grounds that she had not followed her code of professional practice specifically around the use of professional status; promoting causes that are not related to health. The nurse was later reinstated, after public outcry that political correctness has been taken to extremes with her suspension.[for more details see 48]

The other case concerned a nurse who refused to remove a crucifix which she claimed she had worn from a necklace for over 30 years whilst on duty. She was asked to remove the crucifix to comply with the hospital's dress code and health and safety policy. The case actually ended up in an industrial tribunal and court of appeal. The tribunal claimed that the wearing of a crucifix is not a mandatory requirement of the Christian faith.[50]

These cases bring into question the relationship that exists between the nurse's own personal beliefs and professional practice. It is clear that there is a professional duty for all nurses to practice in accordance with their professional codes of ethics which guide conduct. Ultimately, these situations highlight the importance of nurses developing self-awareness of their own spirituality and not using their privileged position to peruse their own goals or purposes. One of the biggest challenges nurses face is the integration of personal belief and professional practice. Spiritual care is not about imposing your own beliefs and values on another or using your position of trust to convert or proselytize. Therefore, nurses must always be guided by the person for whom they are caring; spiritual care like any other nursing intervention requires consent, and this must always be obtained prior to performing any task or intervention. Furthermore, the nurse must always act in accordance with their professional and employers code of practice. Crucially, the nurse must have the prerequisite knowledge, skills, and support to carry out any task competently and safely[41].

Assumptions and expectations

Nursing cannot make assumptions about what spirituality may mean for diverse groups of patient. A significant finding from McSherry's,[19] investigation was that some of the patients interviewed had very little expectation regarding the provision of spiritual care. Furthermore, the investigation stressed the importance of nursing not making assumptions that patients and the general public, share the same understanding of spirituality as that constructed within nursing. However, this is not to say that just because some nurses and patients do not share the same understanding that the spiritual dimension is unimportant or, indeed, obsolete. On the contrary, for some patients, the spiritual part of their life is important to them, particularly when faced with illness and all the uncertainties that come with that, providing them with strength, hope, meaning, and wellbeing. For those with a faith, being able to continue to practice that faith is important. For those with no faith issues surrounding meaning, hope, love and belonging, forgiveness, peace, direction, and guidance can become important. Many patients, however, feel they are given little help with these sorts of concerns and that hospital staff are too busy dealing with the physical part of care to be concerned with the metaphysical. However, there is evidence that when spiritual care is offered it is valued.[52,53,54]

Practice

McSherry[54, p. 66] provides a useful framework for considering four major challenges that require deliberation by the nursing profession if the practical application of spirituality is to be fully realized. The four broad challenges are:

- *Conceptual:* consideration must be given to the diverse ways people define, perceive and understand the nature of spirituality. Assumptions and generalizations cannot be made by nurses with regards to this personal dimension of human existence. If concepts and theories of spirituality and spiritual care are to be developed that have meaning and relevance to practice then flexibility will be required so that the needs of diverse groups and individuals can be accommodated.
- *Organizational:* all institutions and organizations that are involved in the provision of nursing care, in whatever context, community, hospital, residential facility, must acknowledge the importance of people, places, and processes when seeking to offer or provide any form of spiritual care. Unless these organizations acknowledge the importance of this dimension for the health and wellbeing of those receiving and providing care, then the provision of spiritual care will be *ad hoc*, uncoordinated, and fragmented.
- *Practical:* this is a broad term that spans any of the practical implications for the delivery of spiritual care. This may include attention to areas such as spiritual assessment, the resources to support nurses in the delivery of spiritual care and the educational preparedness of nurses to be involved in the spiritual dimension of people's lives. The nursing profession has made excellent progress in some of these areas. The emerging literature reveals that nursing scholars and practitioners are engaged in a broad range of debates and activities that will develop nursing practice in this area such as the development of educational competences and the construction of spiritual assessment

tools for use in specific clinical settings. More importantly there is a real desire to ensure that these developments are informed by the voice of patients and those who require nursing care.

- *Ethical:* the nursing profession must start to engage in a more meaningful way and consider the ethical issues and potential dilemmas raised and encountered when supporting people with the spiritual aspects of human existence. The spiritual dimension of people's lives is influenced by a number of factors, personal, social, cultural, political. Therefore, the spiritual dimension by its very nature is 'ethically laden'. Until recently little attention has been paid to the ethical issues inherent when supporting patients with spiritual aspects of their lives. For example is it correct to routinely assess all patients for spiritual needs only to find that there are inadequate resources to support both the individual and staff involved in this activity. A further consideration may be educational preparedness that is do nurses have the requisite knowledge and understanding to support patients with these deeply personal aspects of human existence?

A way forward for nursing is to review and evaluate the evidence base developed to date mapping this activity against the four challenges outlined. This exercise would provide a benchmark for where the nursing profession has come and more importantly the direction it needs to go in the future. It would be fair to say that the nursing profession has pioneered understanding and developments in spiritual care. Recent debates highlight that the nursing profession is not closed and rigid, but flexible and willing to engage in dialogue and further debate in order to advance this important dimension of holistic care.

Conclusion

This chapter has offered a brief synopsis of the nursing profession's involvement in the spiritual dimension of care. It is by no means a definitive account of all the pioneering research and scholarly activity that has been undertaken by nurses internationally, over several decades and indeed since its historical inception and evolution in the twentieth and twenty-first centuries. The chapter has highlighted that the spiritual dimension of care is perceived by the nursing profession to be a legitimate and fundamental aspect of nursing practice. The spiritual dimension is recognized as one of the core founding principles of nursing that is enshrined in many codes of ethics and practice. The research evidence demonstrates that spirituality and spiritual care are considered by nurses to be intricately linked to the quality of nursing care and in maintaining the general health and wellbeing of patients.

The chapter affirms that the nursing profession's liaison with the spiritual dimension is not some attempt at professionalization, or some fleeting interest, but a sustained and sincere attempt to ensure that the spiritual aspects of holistic care are understood, realized and integrated within nursing practice. This will ensure that spiritual care is available for all individuals who require support with this dimension of their lives.

References

1 Koenig, H.G., McCullough, M.E., Larson, D.B. (2001). *Handbook of Religion and Health*. Oxford: Oxford University Press.

2 Ross, L. (2010). Why the increasing interest in spirituality within healthcare? In: W. McSherry, L. Ross (eds) *Spiritual Assessment in Health Care Practice*. Keswick: M&K Publishing.

3 Health Care Commission. (2009). *Investigation into Mid Staffordshire Foundation Trust Commission for Healthcare Audit and Inspection*. London: HCC.

4 The Patients Association. (2009). *Patients… Not numbers, People … Not statistics*. Available at: http://www.patients-association.com/Portals/0/Public/Files/Research%20Publications/Patients%20not%20numbers,%20people%20not%20statistics.pdf (Accessed 17-1-2012).

5 The Patients Association. (2010). *Listen to Patients Speak Up for Change*. Available at: http://www.patients-association.com/Portals/0/Public/Files/Research%20Publications/Listen%20to%20patients,%20Speak%20up%20for%20change.pdf (Accessed 17-1-2012).

6 The Mid Staffordshire NHS Foundation Trust Inquiry. (2010). *The Independent Inquiry into Care Provided by Mid Staffordshire NHS Foundation Trust January 2005—March 2009*, Volume I. Available at: http://www.dh.gov.uk/prod_consum_dh/groups/dh_digitalassets/@dh/@en/@ps/documents/digitalasset/dh_113447.pdf (Accessed 2 May 2011).

7 The Mid Staffordshire NHS Foundation Trust Inquiry. (2010). *Independent Inquiry into Care Provided by Mid Staffordshire NHS Foundation Trust January 2005—March 2009*, Volume 2 Available at: http://www.dh.gov.uk/prod_consum_dh/groups/dh_digitalassets/@dh/@en/@ps/documents/digitalasset/dh_113069.pdf (accessed 2 May 2011).

8 Parliamentary and Health Service Ombudsman. (2011). *Care and Compassion? Report of the Health Service Ombudsman on Ten Investigations into NHS Care of Older People*. London: PHSO. Available at: http://www.ombudsman.org.uk/__data/assets/pdf_file/0016/7216/Care-and-Compassion-PHSO-0114web.pdf (accessed 17/1/12).

9 International Council of Nurses. (2010). *Definition of Nursing*. Available at: http://www.icn.ch/about-icn/icn-definition-of-nursing/(accessed 2 May 2011).

10 American Holistic Nurses Association. *Mission Statement*. Available at: http://www.ahna.org/AboutUs/MissionStatement/tabid/1931/Default.aspx (accessed 5 July 2011).

11 Kramer, P. (1957). *A survey to determine the attitudes and knowledge of a selected group of professional nurses concerning spiritual care of the patient*, Unpublished Master's thesis. Oregeon: University of Oregeon.

12 Royal College of Nursing. (2003). *Defining Nursing: Nursing is …* London: RCN.

13 Royal College of Nursing. (2010). *The Principles*. Available at: www.rcn.org.uk/nursingprinciples (accessed 13 December 2010).

14 Henderson, V. (1973). *Basic Principles of Nursing Care*. Geneva: ICN.

15 Riehl-Sisca, J. (1989). *Conceptual Models for Nursing Practice*. Connecticut: Appleton and Lange.

16 Roper, N., Logan, W., Tierney, A. (2000). *The Roper–Logan–Tierney Model of Nursing: Based on Activities of Living*. London: Churchill Livingstone.

17 Oldnall, A.S. (1995). On the absence of spirituality in nursing theories and models. *J Adv Nurs* **21:** 417–18.

18 Oldnall, A. (1996). A critical analysis of nursing: meeting the spiritual needs of patients. *J Adv Nurs* **23:** 138–44.

19 McSherry, W. (2004). *The meaning of spirituality and spiritual care: an investigation of health care professionals', patients' and publics' perceptions*, Unpublished PhD thesis. Leeds: Leeds Metropolitan University.

20 Martsolf, D.S., Mickley, J.R. (1998). The concept of spirituality in nursing theories: differing world-views and extent of focus. *J Adv Nurs* **27:** 294–303.

21 International Council of Nurses. (2006). *The ICN Code of Ethics for Nurses*. Geneva: ICN.

22 Australian Nursing & Midwifery Council. (2008). *Code of Ethics for Nurses in Australia*. Canberra: Australian Nursing and Midwifery Council, Royal College of Nursing, Australia and the Australian Nursing Federation.

23 Nursing & Midwifery Council. (2008). *The Code*. London: NMC.
24 Nursing & Midwifery Council. (2010). *Standards for Pre-registration Nursing Education*. London: NMC.
25 Quality Assurance Agency for Higher Education. (2001). *Benchmark Statement: Healthcare Programmes*. Gloucester: QAAHE.
26 Baldacchino, D. (2006). Nursing competencies for spiritual care. *J Clin Nurs* **15:** 885–96.
27 Van Leeuwen, R., Cusveller, B. (2004). Nursing competencies for spiritual care. *J Adv Nurs* **48**(3): 234–46.
28 Van Leeuwen, R., Tiesinga, L.J., Middel, B., Post, D., Jochemsen, H. (2009). The validity and reliability of an instrument to assess nursing competencies in spiritual care. *J Clin Nurs* **18:** 1–13.
29 Carson, V.B. (1989). *Spiritual Dimensions of Nursing Practice*. Philadelphia: WB Saunders.
30 Stoll, R.I. (1979). Guidelines for spiritual assessment. *Am J Nurs* **79:** 1574–7.
31 Fish, S., Shelly, J.A. (1978). *Spiritual Care: the Nurse's Role*. Illinois: Intervarsity Press.
32 Narayanasamy, A. (2001). *Spiritual Care: A Practical Guide for Nurses and Health Care Practitioners*. Salisbury: Quay Books.
33 Swinton, J., Pattison, S. (2010). Moving beyond clarity: towards a thin, vague, and useful understanding of spirituality in nursing care. *Nurs Philos* **11:** 226–37.
34 Murray, R.B. Zentner, J.B. (1989). *Nursing Concepts for Health Promotion*. London: Prentice Hall.
35 Clarke, J. (2009). A critical view of how nursing has defined spirituality *J Clin Nurs* **18:** 1666–73.
36 McSherry, W. (2007). *The Meaning of Spirituality and Spiritual Care within Nursing and Health Care Practice*. Salisbury: Quay Books.
37 Swinton, J. (2006). Identity and resistance: Why spiritual care needs 'enemies'. *J Clin Nurs* **15**(7): 918–28.
38 Hitchens, E.W. (1988). *Stages of faith and values development and their implications for dealing with spiritual care in the student nurse-patient relationship*, Unpublished EdD thesis. Seattle: University of Seattle.
39 Wallraff Charles, F. (1970). *Karl Jaspers: an Introduction to His Philosophy*. Princeton: Princeton University Press.
40 NHS Education for Scotland. (2009). *Spiritual Care Matters. An Introductory Resource for All NHS Scotland Staff*. Edinburgh: NES.
41 Royal College of Nursing. (2011). *Spirituality in Nursing Care: a Pocket Guide*. London: RCN.
42 Ross, L.A. (1997). *Nurses' Perceptions of Spiritual Care*. Aldershot: Avebury.
43 Mooney, H. (2009). Can the NHS cope with God? *Nurs Times* **105**(7): 8–10.
44 RCN. (2011). *RCN spirituality survey 2010*. London: RCN.
45 Royal College of Nursing. (2011). *Spirituality in nursing care on-line resource*. London, RCN. http://www.rcn.org.uk/development/practice/spirituality/about_spirituality_in_nursing_care (accessed 17/1/12).
46 Waugh, L. (1992). *Spiritual aspects of nursing: a descriptive study of nurses' perceptions*, Unpublished PhD thesis. Edinburgh: Queen Margaret College.
47 Ross, L.A. (2006). Spiritual care in nursing: an overview of the research to date. *J Clin Nurs* **15**(7): 852–62.
48 BBC (1 February 2009). Nurse suspended for prayer offer. Available at: http://news.bbc.co.uk/1/hi/england/somerset/7863699.stm (accessed 7 November 2011).
49 Nursing Times (2009). 'Nurse sacked for advising patient to go to church'. Available at: http://www.nursingtimes.net/whats-new-in-nursing/management/nurse-sacked-for-advising-patient-to-go-to-church/5001982.article (accessed 16 January 2012).
50 BBC news (2009). Row over nurse wearing crucifix. Available at: http://news.bbc.co.uk/1/hi/england/devon/8265321.stm (accessed 7 November 2011).
51 Nursing Times (2009). 'British Medical Association to debate religion and prayer in the NHS'. Available at: http://www.nursingtimes.net/whats-new-in-nursing/management/bma-to-debate-religion-and-prayer-in-the-nhs/5003339.article (accessed 16 January 2012).
52 Murray, S.A., Kendall, M., Boyd, K., Worth, A., Benton, T.F. (2004). Exploring the spiritual needs of people dying of lung cancer or heart failure: a prospective qualitative interview study of patients and their carers. *Palliat Med* **18:** 39–45.
53 Ross, L.A. (1997). Elderly patients' perceptions of their spiritual needs and care: a pilot study. *J Adv Nurs* **26:** 710–15.
54 Ross, L., Austin, J. (2012). Spiritual needs and spiritual support preferences of people with end stage heart failure and their carers. Paper presented at the 12th Annual Spring Meeting on Cardiovascular Nursing, 16-17 March 2012, Copenhagen, Denmark.
55 McSherry, W. (2010). Spiritual Assessment: definition, categorization and features. In: W. McSherry, L. Ross (eds) *Spiritual Assessment in Health Care Practice*. Keswick: M&K Publishing.

CHAPTER 31

Faith community (parish) nursing

Antonia M. van Loon

Introduction

Faith community nursing (also known as parish nursing, pastoral nursing, congregational/church nursing) is a specialist nursing practice distinguished by its endorsement of a faith-based perspective of the person, which focuses nursing care on integration, nurture, and restoration of the whole person in all their dimensions (physical, mental, spiritual and socio-cultural).[1] Faith community nurses (FCNs) help people with existing diseases or complex conditions to manage their condition enabling the person to maximize their potential and their quality of life. However, the FCN's primary focus is on preventing disease and illness, and promoting the preconditions for personal and community health.[2] This is largely undertaken by nurturing healthy relationships within the person, between the person and God, between the person and the environment, and between people by addressing social justice issues, providing education and support regarding faith and health issues.[3] All these activities are undertaken in the context of, and with the support of, an auspicing faith community. The FCN's clients are not restricted to that faith community, thus all activities and programs conducted by FCNs have the capacity to reach into the wider geographic and/or the cultural community which that faith community seeks to serve.[4]

Faith-based healthcare

This chapter focuses on the development and outworking of faith community nursing within Christian faith communities. This faith has embraced the FCN role and this group are most frequently represented in the published literature internationally. There is limited information as to how faith-based healthcare and particularly the FCN role is enacted in groups from other faiths, but information is becoming available as nurses from other faiths (such as Islam and Judaism) share spiritual and religious aspects that impact healthcare delivery in the published literature.[5–7] Many religions have a philosophical worldview that enables them to positively influence values formation and human behaviour which promotes health and wellbeing.[8] Many Christian denominations are embracing the FCN health ministry as a vital and contemporary ministry that enables a tangible outworking of their mission.[9–11] Health ministry provides compassionate care activities related to health needs, as well as health promotion and disease/injury prevention and healing activities that are conducted as a part of the church's overall calling.[12]

The amount of faith-based healthcare varies within and between countries. Policy and perspectives differ as to the amount and type of services religious groups can offer. People continue to debate the role that organized religion should play in the delivery of healthcare; however, there are 1.3 billion people lacking healthcare worldwide, so the World Health Organization (WHO) states there will continue to be room for faith- based organizations to make a contribution alongside, and in tandem with, government and private sectors.[13] In the developing world faith-based organizations already provide a significant percentage of health care.[14] For example, in Sub-Saharan Africa, faith-based groups provide up to 70% of the region's HIV/AIDS health services, and up to 40% of other health care.[13,15]. As the cost of healthcare escalates and the populations of the developed world continue to age, the health systems of many western countries are under strain as the cost burden of current healthcare is difficult to maintain. The governments of many countries are looking for innovative and sustainable ways to care for people within the community. Some gaps have become apparent which are readily addressed by faith-based health ministries such as aged care, community mental health, primary healthcare, community health.[10,14,16–18] Large denominational health ministry networks exist in most western countries and these can be brought together to effectively meet the needs of many people in culturally competent, accessible, affordable, and socially acceptable ways.[11,19]

Background to faith community nursing

Faith community nursing is a renewal of the Deaconess role, which is where contemporary nursing has its historical roots.[20] Nursing in western countries today is commonly based on the Nightingale model that developed in Christian churches in Europe, particularly the Deaconess Institute at Kaiserswerth, Germany. Lutheran pastor, Theodor Fliedner, commenced a hospital to train young women to care for the sick and needy using a Deaconess model. [21] Florence Nightingale chose to obtain her nursing education at Kaiserswerth, graduating in 1851.[22] The 'Nightingale model' she implemented at St Thomas's hospital in London was characterized by a focus on sanitation, hygiene, client education, and benevolent support of the client, as well as the personal, moral, and spiritual discipline of the nurse who was trained in theology and nursing skills.[22] Nightingale nursing viewed nursing work as a vocational call, where, in return for a simple salary, nurses were housed, fed, trained, cared for, and provided with spiritual oversight.[23] Graduates trained in this model travelled to countries across the globe, therefore this model became the template for much western healthcare after the mid-1800s.[21]

The past century has seen an increased emphasis on biomedical, disease-centred approaches to healthcare with improved body care, which is the practice domain of medicine, nursing and the allied health professions. The care of the mind has become the practice domain of psychiatrists, pyschologists, and counsellors, and the care of the human spirit has been relegated to pastors/priests/chaplains/imams/rabbis, etc., and faith community-based volunteers. However, the 1970s called into question the scientific reductionist view of the 'body as machine,' claiming it was a narrow perspective that did not attend to the needs of the whole person. Arguments for a more holistic perspective of the person focused more attention on disease prevention, health promotion, and illness management.

American churches responded to the holistic health movement in the 1970s/1980s by trialling holistic models of health service delivery by faith communities.[24] Rev. Granger Westberg, a Lutheran pastor, was involved in trialling holistic health centres that used a team approach to service delivery by clergy, doctors, nurses, and social workers, but Westberg noted that nurses were the vital link between all aspects of the health system and the faith community.[25] Consequently, he launched the first 'parish nurse' programme aiming for more economically viable models to provide holistic programmes within the faith community.[26] From these trials came the revitalization of nurses working with/in churches known as 'parish nursing'[27] and later as 'faith community nursing' because this name encompassed a broader ecumenical and interfaith movement.[4] The FCN role has many names that are adapted to fit the local culture and the language of the faith community and the country in which the role is enacted [e.g. parish nursing (Catholic and some protestant denominations) congregational nursing (Jewish), church nursing and pastoral nursing (some protestant denominations), crescent nursing (Muslim)]. Today there are approximately 12,000 FCNs in the United States[28] and networks have commenced in Australia, the Bahamas, Canada, United Kingdom, Fiji, Korea, Madagascar, Malaysia, New Zealand, Palestine, Scotland, Singapore, South Africa, Swaziland, Wales, and Zimbabwe.[29]

Describing health ministry

Health ministry is the deliberate organization and resourcing of appropriately qualified and gifted people to facilitate the pastoral health, healing, and care of people within the church, and the community it serves. The contemporary movement of health ministry includes specific worship rituals and liturgy, such as healing services, anointing of the sick, prayer, and sacraments.[30] However, there is more to health ministry and it includes education for healthy living, good stewardship of the person, as well as communal health and wellbeing.[12] It includes activities that promote social justice, and reduce and prevent violence, oppression and poverty.[8] Activities that provide advocacy, support, direct assistance, and healthcare for those who are sick or in need are central to health ministry, as are actions that prevent injury and disease, promote healing and health, and improve the social determinants impacting an individual's or community's health and wellbeing.[31–33]

The faith community and the healthcare continuum

Christian churches have long seen the need to provide care to the sick in response to the gospel directives of Jesus Christ to follow his example and become actively concerned about the physical, mental and spiritual health of people. Consequently, faith communities have provided acute care hospitals, secondary health services and community health services. In fact, in Australia the largest district nursing services were all commenced in the 1800s by Christians compelled to enact their ethos and send out trained women and religious nuns to work amongst the sick, poor and needy within the community.[34] Faith communities recognize the importance of a social perspective of health and seek to provide food, clothing, medicines and care to those most in need within the community, aiming to prevent hospitalization and promote wellbeing.[22]

Christian denominations today continue to play an important part in healthcare provision within most western countries. However, healthcare is becoming secularized and concurrently faith communities have lost their capacity to meaningfully connect with people in their time of need, which is an important part of their mission and mandate. When sickness occurs people often have questions about life, hope, meaning, purpose, suffering and transcendence, but aside from appointed healthcare chaplains/spiritual care workers, most personnel working in modern healthcare organizations have little time, or perhaps inclination, (and at times they have no permission) to discuss such important issues with the sick person.[35]

The Christian faith community is largely absent from the primary healthcare aspect of the healthcare continuum except for the FCN and health ministry programs (see Figure 31.1). Faith communities are key service providers in secondary and tertiary healthcare, but have little input into primary healthcare (PHC). PHC is gaining importance as countries search for sustainable ways to develop their communities and improve the health of their population.

The PHC movement was endorsed by the World Health Organization[36] in 1978 as a solution to the escalating cost of high tech healthcare, which was viewed as unsustainable and a contributing factor in increasing inequity between the developed and developing world.[37,38] PHC seeks to reorganize healthcare by developing strategies to promote sustainable health services using a philosophical framework that includes analysis, planning, action, and awareness that health requires inter-sectoral collaboration, community engagement, and sound political governance if it is to be available, affordable, acceptable, accessible, and sustainable to all.[39,40] In recent times, PHC has recognized that wellbeing depends on a range of social, cultural, political, economic, and environmental factors that need to be configured effectively if they are to promote health.[37,41] This has become known as 'the new public health' which focuses planning on ten social determinants of health,[37,42] which include one's earliest life experiences, social status, presence of stress, level of social inclusion, level of work, level and type of employment, level of social support, presence of addiction, presence and availability of food and water,

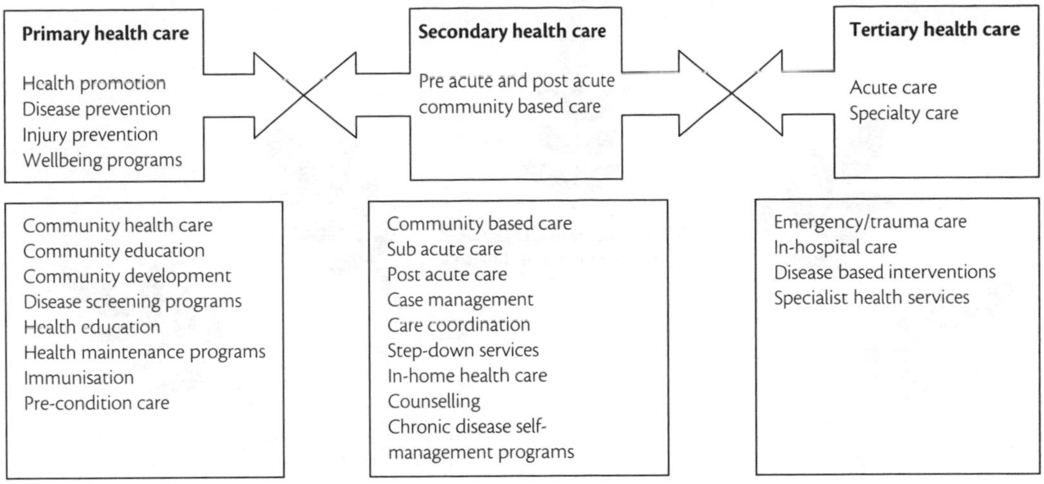

Figure 31.1 Continuum of healthcare with examples of services/programmes.

and availability and accessibility of transport.[43] Faith communities can contribute positively to these determinants in the activities they conduct in their local community and as global entities.

Nurses as leaders of health ministry teams

The office most often associated with health ministry historically is that of deacon/deaconess and the religious orders. However, today health ministry includes lay people with specific gifts in pastoral health and care who work alongside qualified and educated health professionals as a team. In the FCN model (Figure 31.2) the health ministry team is often led by a registered nurse. Some reasons FCN leadership was recommended by Westberg[44, p. 2] include, 'The nurse has the sensitivity—the peripheral vision ... to see beyond the patient's problems and verbal statements. She can hear things left unsaid. And she is the best listener.' Westberg asserted nurses have scientific expertise, special gifts in caring, and excellent people skills, which are essential requirements for effective health ministry. He noted nurses command respect from the community and are trusted by people enabling them to open up to a nurse. For example, every year in Australia, an annual 'Image of Professions' survey is undertaken by a reputable national polling group, nurses have consistently topped that poll for 16 consecutive years, as the most ethical and honest professional group, surpassing both the medical profession and ministers of religion.[45] Westberg[27] notes that nurses use their 'peripheral vision' to identify people who they know need to be visited quickly leading him to recommend nurses as the profession of choice to lead a faith community-based health ministry. Nurses today are well educated in primary healthcare and community health, and have a broad knowledge that crosses multiple discipline boundaries, making them ideal 'navigators' of an increasingly complex health system, and an excellent resource people to promote health within the faith community.

A health ministry model using faith community nurses

In the late 1990s a group of five South Australian Christian faith communities came together to develop a research-based model of health ministry which could be adapted across Christian faith communities, employing faith community nurses.[1] This model has been successfully adapted by faith communities in Australia and overseas. The themes and concepts are briefly summarized in this chapter. (Box 31.1)

The overarching goal of all FCN functions is transformation that leads to healing and restoration in all the dimensions of the person (body, mind, spirit, socio-cultural).[1] This includes transforming the individual's and the community's conceptualization of health and healing, empowering people to act in ways that enable them to respond positively to life and improve their well-being. This transformative process is a dynamic, life-long journey, which enables people to grow closer to Jesus Christ and to find their healing and wholeness in Him.

How this model works to facilitate transformation and promote health and healing is best understood by examining the dimensions of the person (keeping in mind that in reality there is no distinction between these dimensions). Humans are inseparable wholes, but the prevailing western perspective of the person in contemporary healthcare continues to reduce the person to component parts. The reductionist worldview of most medical care focuses attention on parts of the body and still smaller parts that give rise to sub-specialties within medical specialties.

In the FCN model there are four dimensions to the person. For simplicity these are termed physical (body), mental (mind), socio-cultural (relational), and spiritual (spirit). Each of these dimensions is governed by unifying principle/s. For healing to occur people need to undertake certain activities to reconstitute or nurture health within each dimension. FCN care is directed toward unifying activities aiming for outcomes that change thoughts, behaviours, and actions and lead to healing, restoration, and health.

The physical dimension is governed by the principle of homeostasis. Reconstituting activities revolve around adaptation, aiming to restore or maintain equilibrium, wellness, and promote healthy growth. Nursing care is focused on prevention of diseases, curative regimes, and/or management of the condition/disease, and the promotion of healthy growth and development.

The mental dimension is governed by the principle of creative balancing. Reconstituting activities involve enlightenment and creative activities aiming to bring contented thinking, inner

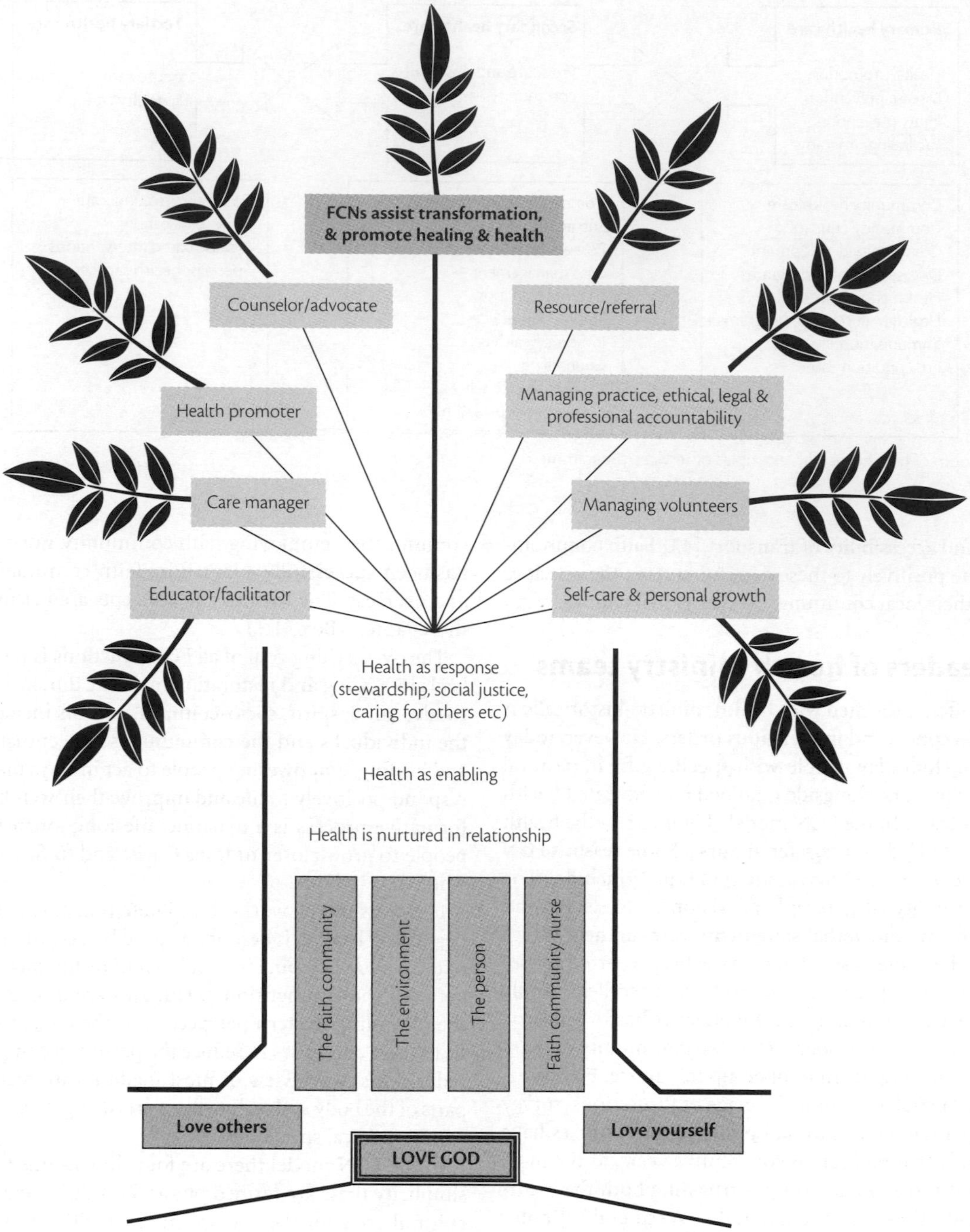

'And the leaves of the tree are for the healing of the nations'.
Revelation 22:2b NIV *Holy* Bible

Figure 31.2 Faith Community Nursing Model.[4] (NB. revised 2010 for this edition.)

harmony, stable identity, creativity and mental growth. Nursing care is focused on emotional and intellectual support, stimulation, and/or rest.

The socio-cultural dimension is governed by the principle of connection. The reconstituting activities pivot around unifying activities that seek to facilitate identity and values formation, connection, and community growth. Nursing care is focused on promoting developmental health and strengthening interpersonal relationships.

The spiritual dimension is governed by the principle of restoration, healing and salvation. Reconstituting activities encompass transformative activities that seek to provide spiritual growth,

Box 31.1 Health ministry model using faith community nurses

The model represents health ministry as a life giving tree that yields fruit all year that brings forth healing transformation, health and life for individuals and the community. The tree is grounded and rooted in love for God and from God, love for other people and from other people, and love for one's self and from one's self.

The tree trunk represents the major model concepts that give the model cohesion. The model's applicability and utility depend on how these concepts interrelate, because when they work together they sustain the life-giving capacity of the health ministry.

- The Person is understood as a whole unity of body, mind and spirit; made in the image of God and sanctified by God to live in relationship. Those relationships include a relationship with God, the natural environment and with other people.
- The Faith Community is a gathering of people who share a common religious belief, and commune together for the purpose of worshipping God, fellowship, witness, teaching, encouragement, service and healing. The faith community is built in and on love.
- The **FCN** is called by God to focus her/his unique gifts, talents and professional nursing knowledge to the goal of promoting health, transformation, and healing, and the compassionate care of people. The religious faith of the FCN motivates her/him to a life of service, stewardship, and whole person care that intentionally integrates the FCN's faith with their professional nursing practice.
- The Environment is understood as the circumstances and conditions (e.g. natural, physical, socio-cultural) in which a person or community live, relate, grow and develop. All of life is an endowment from God and humans have been made stewards of the environment, which brings both accountabilities and responsibilities.

How these four concepts relate and interrelate impacts healing capacity and health. Health is nurtured in life-affirming relationships within one's self (body, mind, spirit, socio-cultural), between the self and others, between the self and the environment, and between the self and God. Health enables people to fulfil many purposes in life, but it is not the be all and end all of living. Relationships that promote harmonious interconnectedness facilitate transformation, growth, healing and health. Health can be promoted by responsible stewardship of one's body, one's relationships and one's environment. It is promoted and dependent upon social justice and the capacity to provide compassionate care to others in their time of need.

Disease and illness are the person's reaction to internal and/or external stressors which can act in/on any human dimension, but the impact is experienced by the whole person. The act of living requires responses to change, stressors, and perceived stressors that may originate within or external to the person. Stressors can vary from tangible microbes to environmental pollutants, substance misuse, or mystical spiritual issues. All individuals must adapt to stressors, remove them, ameliorate their effect, or build up inner resources to prevent stressor impact. Certain life changes are in the person's control, such as some relational and lifestyle stressors, but other stressors are outside the person's control, such as developmental changes, war and natural disasters. The whole person must respond by finding new ways to live and be in the world. The FCN can assist the person/community to respond to their changing conditions by developing new and alternate patterns of living.

healing, wholeness and shalom (Table 31.1). Nursing care is focused on nurturing relationships within self, with others, with the environment, and with God.

The functions of the faith community nurse

The branches of the tree represent the key functions of the FCN that enable the health ministry to meet its goals. These functions include:

Educator and facilitator

The FCN uses various methods to educate individuals and facilitate small groups in the community regarding such issues as lifestyle factors, relationships, faith and health enhancement activities, illness/injury/disease prevention or risk reduction, disease management for those with chronic conditions, environmental awareness, social justice issues, and other health and wellbeing issues that are pertinent to the specific community of people that the FCN serves.

Care manager

The FCN may assist clients with existing illnesses, complex conditions, and/or disabilities to manage their condition, aiming to prevent exacerbation of illness and/or limit complications. The FCN's holistic approach to care management considers the client (body, mind, spirit, relational), their family, the client's environment and the faith community, when developing care management *with* the client and their family.

Health promoter

The FCN seeks to promote health by facilitating the transformative growth that enables a person/community to respond positively to life's changes, empowering them to act in ways that improve their well-being. Much FCN work focuses on creating and fostering positive relationships as the foundation for the personal growth and transformation that nurtures health. This can be enacted via specific programmes and activities targeted at lifestyle choices, e.g. physical fitness programmes, immunization, mental health awareness, suicide prevention activities, sexual health programmes, courses that develop interpersonal skills etc.

Table 31.1 The process of healing and transformation in the human dimensions

Dimension	Unifying principle	Personal reconstituting activities	FCNs focus	Anticipate client outcomes
Physical	Principle of homeostasis	Adaptation activities	Care focused on: prevention of condition, disease cure and/or management of condition, disease promotion of healthy growth development	Equilibrium Wellness Body growth
Mental	Principle of creative balancing	Enlightenment and creative activities	Care focused on emotional and intellectual support, stimulation and rest	Contentment Inner harmony Creativity Mind growth
Socio-cultural	Principle of connection	Unifying activities	Care focused on developmental health and strengthening interpersonal relationships	Value formation Connection Community growth
Spiritual	Principle of restoration and healing	Transformative activities	Care focused on relationships within self, with others, with the environment, and God. Communicating God's love in word and deed.	Shalom Spiritual growth Wholeness

Counsellor and advocate

Personal and small group counselling is an important aspect of the role. The focus of such counselling is brief, aiming to help people with issues impacting their health, listening and advising as required, supporting and recommending referral when needed, in addition to home visits and monitoring progress. The focus of this function is to empower people to make an informed choice within a supportive milieu, which can include offering knowledge of viable options to assist the individual in the decision making process.

FCNs may be called upon to publicly support, uphold, advocate, or defend a particular position/person. This may involve interpreting a point of view or helping someone to 'see' another perspective. Advocacy often occurs on behalf of the client with the broader health system, but it is always undertaken with the client's permission. Advocacy can include mediation to bring about agreement and/or reconciliation between people. It also includes prayer with and for the client and their family.

Resource and referral

The FCN liaises between the individual and the faith community, and the individual and other health and community services. The FCN is able to negotiate access and assist entry into health services and local community support networks of which the person may be unaware. This resource and referral activity occurs within the faith community and beyond, aiming to better manage and coordinate care for the individual, the family/group and the community.

Managing practice

The FCN role is an advanced practice registered nurse role that is supported by other health ministry team members. As a regulated profession, nurses must manage their practice in ways that can demonstrate the use of moral reasoning and ethical decision making. The nurse must be able to document and authenticate her/his practice, and demonstrate that she/he is practicing accountably and legally by adhering to professional standards of practice and the laws governing healthcare. To that end accountability and governance processes must be in place before the FCN commences and the FCN should report against these and be held accountable for the stated standard of practice. Further to this, all faith communities must have in place adequate public liability and professional indemnity insurance for the FCN and their health ministry team to cover all their salaried and voluntary activities.

Managing volunteers

Health ministry is a corporate ministry of the church therefore it is useful to have a team of people working from their knowledge, life experience, gifts, and strengths. This will help to assure the viability of the ministry for the long-term and provide corporate support to the FCN. The FCN may need to coordinate, educate, equip, and support lay volunteers and health ministry workers to ensure the health ministry is practising to its full capacity in an accountable manner.

Self-care and personal growth

The FCN role can become overwhelming as the ministry grows. When people know there is a trustworthy, helpful and compassionate ministry to meet their needs they start using it and referring others to it. Many FCNs have said that they have felt burdened, overwhelmed, and at risk of burn-out within a few years of commencement.[46] This is particularly true for those in volunteer FCN roles and those who do not have the support of a team. Therefore, it is important that, as part of the FCN function, the nurse practices good stewardship of her/his personal boundaries, health, growth, and development.[47] To that end, the health ministry team needs to enable the FCN to factor activities such as professional development, retreats, mentoring, spiritual direction, professional association memberships, conferences, journals/books, study opportunities, etc.[48]

The challenges and opportunities of health ministry

In most western countries there is no organization other than the faith community, which regularly and voluntarily congregates people of all ages and facilitates the development of long-term relationships across the life span.[35] It brings people of diverse backgrounds and ages together into meaningful relationships, where they have the freedom to share and have a share, to give and participate. People may think that relationships need to be perfect to be beneficial, but life lived in a community enables us to learn from each other's victories and mistakes.[49] Relationships can grow in the midst of trial and testing. The key to growth lies in the connection and common grounding that enable people to transcend difference and move on. This makes the faith community a fertile ground for the development of social connectedness and consequently social capital, which is known to benefit community health. Putnam[50, p. 327] notes that 'social connectedness matters to our lives in the most profound way', yet we know participation and affiliation to long-term groups is declining throughout the western world, but group affiliation and volunteering is still present within religious contexts.

The challenge for many of today's faith communities in western countries is the need to rediscover the health giving value of communing with each other and God, learning how to be a community, rather than a weekly gathering place. Health ministry enables the provision of people to listen, accompany and care, so that everyone experiences a sense of connection to the faith community.[51] Health ministry mobilizes the resources of the congregation to supplement and compliment those already available in the community from the health and social welfare systems.[52] The entire faith community has the opportunity to support the health ministry, by using their gifts, talents, professional expertise and networks of contacts, thus building the social capacity of that community.[53]

We are living in a time of unprecedented challenge to healthcare as governments around the world face spiralling healthcare costs perpetuated by advancing health technologies, pharmaceuticals, and treatments that come at a price. There is a huge demographic shift and altered disease patterns in most western countries with ageing populations and the growing burden of chronic disease.[38] Many countries are experiencing shortages in their health workforce, which is unevenly distributed across countries, leaving rural, remote, Indigenous and developing communities underserved, and concerned about the quality and safety of their health services.[19] There is a growing recognition that many current healthcare systems around the world are unsustainable.[38] In this challenging context faith communities have an opportunity to provide a viable ministry that promotes health, healing and wellbeing, prevents disease and illness, develops personal and social capacity, and provides many of the preconditions for good community health.[33] The questions is, are faith communities ready and willing to re-embrace this ministry and respond to these contemporary challenges by recommencing health and healing ministries that can serve their community?

References

1 Van Loon, A.M. (2000). *A conceptual model of faith community nursing in Australia.* Unpublished Doctor of Philosophy thesis. Adelaide: South Australia Flinders University, Adelaide.

2 Solari-Twadell, P., McDermott, M.A. (2006). *Parish Nursing: Development, Education, and Administration.* St Louis: Elsevier Mosby.

3 Van Loon, A.M. (2006). *Faith Community Nursing.* Available at: http://www.ahwo.gov.au/n3et_Projectsview.asp?ID=32 (accessed 7 Feb 2012).

4 Van Loon, A.M. (1999). The Australian concept of faith community nursing. In: P. A. Solari-Twadell, M.A. McDermott (eds) *Parish Nursing: Promoting Whole Person Health Within Faith Communities*, pp. 287–96. Thousand Oaks: Sage Publications.

5 Frank, K. (2010). *Bringing Caring to the Synagogue with Jewish Congregational Nursing.* Available at: http://www.ncjh.org/downloads/seraf-BringingCaring.pdf (accessed 1 October 2010).

6 Hussein Rassool, G. (2008). The crescent and Islam: healing, nursing and the spiritual dimension. Some considerations towards an understanding of the Islamic perspectives on caring. *J Adv Nurs* **32**(6): 1476–84.

7 Salman, K., Zoucha, R. (2010). Considering faith within culture when caring for the terminally ill Muslim patient and family. *J Hospice Palliat Nurs* **12**(3): 156–63.

8 Evans, A.R. (2008). *Redeeming Marketplace Medicine: a Theology of Health Care.* Cleveland: Pilgrim Press.

9 Baptist Union of Great Britain. (2008). *What Is Health Ministry?* Available at: www.baptist.org.uk (accessed 1 November 2010).

10 McCabe, J. and Somers, S. (2009). Faith community nursing: meeting the needs of seniors. *J Christ Nurs* **26**(2): 104–9.

11 Lindner, E.W. Welty, M.A., National Council of the Churches of Christ in the USA (2007). *Congregational Health Ministry Survey Report.* (New York: National Council of the Churches of Christ in the USA, and the Office of Research and Planning, Roberts Wood Johnson Foundation)

12 WHO. (2007). *Towards Primary Health Care: Renewing Partnerships with Faith-Based Communities and Services*, Available at: http://www.chagghana.org/chag/assets/files/FBO%20Meeting%20report%20_2_.pdf (accessed 10 October 2010).

13 Chand, S., Patterson, J. (2007). *Faith-based Models for Improving Maternal and Newborn Health.* Available at: http://pdf.usaid.gov/pdf_docs/PNADK571.pdf (accessed 10 October 2010).

14 WHO. (2007). *Faith-based Organizations Play a Major Role in HIV/AIDS Care and Treatment in Sub-Saharan Africa.* Available at: www.who.int/hiv/mediacentre/news66/en (accessed 10 October 2010).

15 Francis, S., Liverpool, J. (2009). A review of faith-based HIV prevention programs. *J Religion Hlth* **48**(1): 6–15.

16 Mayernik, D. Resick, L.K. Skomo, M.L., Mandock, K. (2010). Parish nurse–initiated Interdisciplinary Mobile Health Care Delivery Project. *J Obstet Gynecol Neonat Nurs* **39**(2): 227–34.

17 Tyrell, C. Klein, S. Gieryic, S. Devore, B. Cooper, J., Tesoriero, J. (2008). Results of a statewide initiative to involve faith communities in HIV prevention. *Publ Hlth Manag Pract* **14**(5): 429–36.

18 Anderson, E.T., McFarlane, J. M. (2010). *Community as Partner: Theory and Practice in Nursing.* New York: Lippincott Williams & Wilkins.

19 Olson, J.E. (1992). *One Ministry, Many Roles: Deacons and Deaconesses Throughout the Centuries.* St Louis: Concordia.

20 Donahue, M. (1985). *Nursing the Finest Art: an Illustrated History.* St Louis: Mosby.

21 Calder, J. (1971). *The Story of Nursing*, 5th edn. London: Methuen.

22 Godden, J. (2003). Matching the ideal? The first generation of Nightingale nursing probationers, Sydney Hospital, 1868–84. *Hlth Hist* **5**(1): 22–41.

23 Tubesing, D.A. (1976). *An Idea in Evolution: History of the Wholistic Health Centers Project 1970–1976.* Illinois: Wholistic Health Centers.

24 Westberg, G.E. (1984). Churches are joining the health care team. *J Urb Hlth* **60**: 34–6.

25 Westberg, G.E. (1990a). A historical perspective: wholistic health and the parish nurse. In: P. A. Solari-Twadell, A. Djupe, M. McDermott (Eds) *Parish Nursing: the Developing Practice.* Park Ridge: Lutheran General Health System.

26 Westberg, G.E., Westberg McNamara, J. (1990). *The Parish Nurse: Providing a Minister of Health for Your Congregation.* Minneapolis: Augsburg Books.

27 International Parish Nurse Resource Center. (2009). *Parish Nursing Fact Sheet*. Available at: http://www.parishnurses.org/DocumentLibrary/Parish%20Nursing%20Fact%20Sheet.pdf (accessed 1 October 2010).

28 Solari-Twadell, P.A., McDermott, M.A. (1999). *Parish Nursing: Promoting Whole Person Health Within Faith Communities*. Thousand Oaks: Sage Publications.

29 Catanzaro, A.M., Meador, K.G., Koenig, H.G., Kuchibhatla, M., Clipp, E.C.G. (2007). Congregational health ministries: A national study of Pastors' views. *Publ Hlth Nurs* **24**(1): 6–17.

30 King, M.A., Tessaro, I. (2009). Parish nursing: promoting healthy lifestyles in the church. *J Christ Nurs* **26**(1): 22–4.

31 Trinitapolia, J. Ellison, C.G., Boardman, J.D. (2009). US religious congregations and the sponsorship of health-related programs. *Soc Sci Med* **68**(12): 2231–9.

32 Van Loon, A.M. (2011). Community nursing in Australia: past present and future. In: D. Kralik, A.M. Van Loon (eds) *Community Nursing in Australia*. Brisbane: Wiley Blackwell.

33 Linn, R. (1993). *Angels of Mercy: District Nursing in South Australia 1894–1994*. Norwood: Royal District Nursing Society of South Australia Inc.

34 Van Loon, A.M. (2005). *Engaging Faith Communities in Health Care. International Conference on Engaging Communities*, Brisbane Convention Centre. Brisbane: United Nations and Queensland Government.

35 WHO. (1978). *Primary Health Care*, report on the International Conference on Primary Health Care, Alma-Ata, USSR September 6–12, Vol. 2010. Geneva: World Health Organization.

36 Talbot, L., Verrinder, G. (2010). *Promoting Health: the Primary Health Care Approach*, 4th edn. Sydney: Elsevier.

37 WHO. (2008). *Closing the Gap in a Generation: Health Equity Through Action on the Social Determinants of Health*. Geneva: World Health Organization.

38 Keleher, H. (2009). Public health and primary health care. In: H. Keleher & C. MacDougall (eds) *Understanding Health: a Determinants Approach*, 2nd edn, pp. 17–41. South Melbourne: Oxford University Press.

39 McMurray, A. (2007). *Community Health and Wellness: a Socioecological Approach*, 3rd edn. Sydney: Mosby.

40 Vaughan, C. (2009). Determinants of health: case studies from Asia and the Pacific. In: H. Keleher, B. Murphy (eds) *Understanding Health: a Determinants Approach*, pp. 97–112. South Melbourne: Oxford University Press.

41 Baum, F. (2008). *The New Public Health: an Australian Perspective*. South Melbourne: Oxford University Press.

42 Marmot, M., Wilkinson, R. (2006). *Social Determinants of Health*, 2nd edn. Oxford: Oxford University Press.

43 Westberg, G. E. (1989). Parish nursing's pioneer. *J Christ Nurs* **6**(1): 26–9.

44 Morgan Gallup Polls. (2010). Nurses Most ethical profession for the 16th year in a row, Australia. *Med News Today*. Available at: http://www.medicalnewstoday.com/articles/193220.php (accessed 1 November 2010).

45 Thomas, S. (2002). Spiritual formation for parish nurses. In: L. VandeCreek, S. Mooney (eds) *Parish Nurses, Health Care Chaplains, and Community Clergy: Navigating the Maze of Professional Relationships*. Birmingham: Haworth Press.

46 Hickman, J.S. (2006). *Faith Community Nursing*. Philadelphia: Lippincott, Williams & Wilkins.

47 Matzo, M., Gothberg, S. (2004). Parish nursing: promoting whole person health within faith communities. *Geriat Nurs* **25**(1): 62–3.

48 Gunderson, G. (1997). *Deeply Woven Roots: Improving the Quality of Life in your Community*. Minneapolis: Fortress.

49 Putnam, R. (2000). *Bowling Alone: the Collapse and Revival of American Community*. New York: Simon & Schuster.

50 Chase-Ziolek, M., Iris, M. (2002). Nurses' perceptions on the distinctive aspects of providing nursing care in a congregational setting. *J Commun Hlth Nurs* **19**(3): 173–86.

51 Van Loon, A.M. (2011). Contexts of community nursing in Australia. In: D. Kralik, A.M. Van Loon (eds) *Community Nursing in Australia*. Brisbane: Wiley Blackwell.

52 Chase-Ziolek, M. and Gruca, J. (2000). Clients' perceptions of distinctive aspects in nursing care received within a congregational setting. *J Commun Hlth Nurs* **17**(3): 171–83.

CHAPTER 32

Psychiatry and mental health treatment

James L. Griffith

Introduction

Religion and spirituality in patients' lives have presented a long-standing conundrum for psychiatry and mental health professionals. On the one hand, the great majority of Americans profess to be actively religious.[1] Specifically, most patients with serious mental illnesses indicate that they use religion to cope.[2,3] These observations argue for the importance in treatment that should be afforded patients' religious and spiritual resources for supporting hope, buffering stress, providing communities of support, and possibly activating psychosomatic processes that promote health.[3–7] They point to a need for mental health professionals to regard patients' spiritualities and religious lives as clinical resources.

Yet concerns about potential deleterious effects of religion and spirituality also have been raised. Harmful effects from religious coping are noted periodically in the lives of ill patients, whether by exacerbating guilt or despair, contributing to refusal of needed psychiatric treatment, or, in rare cases, justifying self-neglect, suicide, or violence towards others.[8,9] Moreover, psychopathology can be expressed in religious experiences, thoughts and behaviours, and emotions.[8–11] Religious involvement also sometimes activates mood, psychotic, or anxiety symptoms that are misdiagnosed as serious mental illnesses.[4,8,12] The challenge then is how to harness the therapeutic potential of religion and spirituality, but while countering any adverse effects upon mental health. These concerns point to several questions that need answers:

1. How can a mental health professional draw upon a patient's spirituality and religious life as a therapeutic resource, notwithstanding the secular context of healthcare and an absence of shared religious faith between clinician and patient?
2. How can effects of spirituality and religious life that promote mental health be distinguished from deleterious ones?
3. How can unusual or idiosyncratic, but normal, expressions of religious experience be distinguished from psychopathology?

Meeting a patient's religious identity respectfully: a cultural handshake

Treating a patient's spirituality and religious life as a therapeutic resource must begin with a clinical conversation that learns about his or her religious experience, and its relevance for illness and health. Initiating such a conversation, however, may require more than sincerity and good intentions due to commonly-held fears by patients that their religious lives may be stigmatized by clinicians. Mutual distrust and stigmatizing judgments kept distance between religion and the professional disciplines of psychiatry and psychology throughout most of the twentieth century. Sigmund Freud's attitude towards religion long-held sway in keeping religion at an intellectual distance from the mental health disciplines. Due to this long history of stigmatization, a clinician often must express an active interest in a patient's religious life. Specific invitation may be required in order for a patient to reveal comfortably his or her religious life during psychiatric treatment or psychotherapy.[13]

Erving Goffman described how all forms of stigma—race, ethnicity, gender, physical disability, as well as religion—tend to evoke in targeted persons a heightened vigilance for potentially disdainful or humiliating responses from others.[14] A mental health clinician seeking to learn about a patient's religious or spiritual must anticipate that the patient may:[7,8,13]

- Feel vulnerable or exposed when questions about religious faith or spirituality are asked
- Watch vigilantly for subtle signs of acceptance or rejection
- Edit responses to questions in order to avoid risk of ridicule
- When unsure, interpret by default that silence or ambiguous communications indicate disdain, contempt, scorn, or belittlement.

In order for open dialogue to begin, safety and respect must be conveyed by courtesy and etiquette coupled with sincere expression of interest. The FICA interviewing tool has become widely used by primary care clinicians interested in incorporating spirituality into patient care.[15,16]

- F—*Faith and belief* (Do you consider yourself to be spiritual or religious? Do you have spiritual beliefs that help you cope with stress?)
- I—*Importance* (What importance does your faith or belief have in your life?)
- C—*Community* (Are you part of a spiritual or religious community?)
- A—*Address in care* (How would you like me, your healthcare provider, to address these issues in your healthcare?)

Case history: Mr Winton

For example, Mr Winston was a 67-year-old man admitted to the hospital for subacute bacterial endocarditis. Psychiatry had been consulted due to concerns that the emotional distress of his illness had precipitated depression. During his interview, the psychiatric consultant asked: 'Do you consider yourself to be a religious or spiritual person? Are there any important beliefs or religious practices that you would want us to know about?' Mr Winston told how their church was the centre of their family life, a setting where they attended Sunday School and worship services on Sundays, and formed enduring personal friendships. A son now coached a sports team in the church league. 'A lot of people will be praying for me while I'm here,' Mr Winston commented. 'Sometimes they will come here to be with me. I hope you are comfortable with that.' The psychiatrist's questions opened a conversation in which Mr Winston could make clear how important it was that his religious identity be acknowledged and respected.

The FICA questions or similar ones, invite a patient to reveal his or her social identity as a religious or spiritual person. The patient states how this identity ought to be regarded during treatment. The clinician conveys acknowledgement and respect. Such an interchange is a 'cultural handshake' that helps build a collaborative and egalitarian therapeutic alliance.[8] It can be regarded as a routine component of humanistic care. Further, it facilitates collaboration with chaplains or clergy as a natural juncture for asking: 'Would you like for the chaplain to stop by your room?' In the clinician–patient relationship, it also helps put aside any felt aversion towards expressions of religious language, dress, beliefs, or practices that are off-putting for the clinician.[13] Contrary to common assumptions, discovering differences in beliefs and worldview often advances mutual respect to a greater extent than does emphasizing commonalities, provided that inquiry is conducted out of authentic interest and discovered differences are treated with respect.[17]

Meeting a patient's personal spirituality: an existential inquiry

Personal spirituality is religion for the person. Personal spirituality is shaped by the lived experiences of an individual person as a moral agent relating to other people and the Divine, more so than by compliance with prescribed beliefs and practices of a religious group. Utilizing a patient's spirituality in psychotherapy or psychiatric care thus extends beyond simple acknowledgment and respect for a patient's social identity as a religious person. It actively incorporates elements of a patient's personal religious experience in treatment. Opening treatment to a patient's personal spirituality means learning from the patient how his or her spirituality has made a difference in coping with life's adversities. Existential questions provide a clinical tool for this kind of inquiry.[8]

Existential questions inquire how a person responds to the struggles and sorrows of everyday existence.[8,18,19] They focus upon lived experience, rather than social identity. Existential questions usually are experienced as normalizing, rather than pathologizing, since they ask about dismal and threatening circumstances through which all people, including the clinician, eventually journey:

- What has sustained you through hard times? From where do you draw strength?
- Where do you find peace?
- Who truly understands your situation?
- When you are afraid or in pain, how do you find comfort?
- For what are you deeply grateful?
- What is your clearest sense of the meaning of your life at this time?
- Why is it important that you are alive?
- To whom or what are you most devoted?
- To whom do you freely express love?

Case history: Mr Miller

Mr Miller was a 64-year-old man who sought psychiatric consultation because he feared that his despair would lead him to take his own life. He lived alone with no close friends or family. His social world appeared to exist solely in his workplace, where he had been employed for 28 years, but from where he was now facing mandatory retirement at age 65. He so feared the loneliness of retirement that he preferred death, rather than witnessing his 65th birthday. He found comfort in fantasies of suicide. Although adjustment of antidepressant and anxiolytic medications could relieve specific sleep and anxiety symptoms, the greater challenge was how to help him discover a life worth living beyond his working years.

As Mr Miller told his story, it became evident that his impending retirement was not his first encounter with adversity. His father had bullied his son. His mother had a long series of psychiatric hospitalizations for depression. Mr Miller succinctly summarized his childhood as 'alone, lost, and helpless,' a recollection now echoed in the waves of anxiety that brought him again back to psychiatric treatment. His marriage had ended in divorce. Over the years, his intellect and work ethic brought him success in his profession, but no close friends with whom he could confide. 'Most of my life has been a struggle,' he said. He struggled with loneliness.

Against this bleak sketch of his life, I asked: 'What kept you from giving up? When life is so hard and you are so alone—as a child and now as an adult—what has kept you from giving up?' Mr Miller responded with a story that he initially had not mentioned. In the Presbyterian Church of his youth, he found a community that noticed and responded to him. 'I saw in them another way of living I didn't see in my family,' he commented. He recollected vividly a day when one of the adult church leaders put his arm around him. As a teenager, he immersed himself in church youth activities and for a time toyed with the idea of becoming a minister. Throughout his adult life, he always maintained some level of participation in a local church. There seemed to have been no consistent pattern of doctrinal belief among the churches he had attended, whether theologically liberal or conservative fundamentalist. 'My church is the only social place I have,' he reflected. The relationships he had with other church members and his priest, albeit limited in scope, nevertheless kept alive some sense that life can be worthwhile.

Despite his dread of it, Mr Miller successfully managed the transition to retirement. Critical to this success was his locating a larger church with a well-developed programme of weekly small groups that met in members' homes, together with an array of community ministries in which Mr Miller could volunteer. Although he embraced daily personal prayer, specific theological beliefs and ecclesiastical practices of either his childhood church or his current one, this played little role in his religious experience. The essence of his personal spirituality was his finding communion with others in open and compassionate relationships, despite his social awkwardness. Out of this communion, hope and purpose in living emerged.

Personal spirituality often stands as a major strategy for coping with adversity. If a person has a meaningful religious life, the conversation usually turns there after an existential question has been posed. The types of questions posed to Mr Miller: 'What kept you from giving up? What kept alive a sense that life could be good?' were not intrinsically religious questions, yet immediately brought forth a rich account of his religious life. As anthropologist Arthur Kleinman (p 14) has noted, 'Failure and catastrophe empower religion; religion, in turn, empowers people faced with adversity to overcome self-doubt and fear of failing, and to act in the world.'[20] Existential questions provide a safe and reliable path for learning about personal spirituality. Facing illness and hardship, they provide narrative accounts for how spirituality can strengthen the patient as a person.

When a patient has already made explicit the importance of his or her religious life, existential questions can be asked that elicit details for how specific religious beliefs, practices, or community support resilience:[8,18,19]

- What does God know about your experience that other people don't understand?
- Do you sense that God sees a purpose in your suffering?
- What does God expect of your life in days to come?
- How do your beliefs help you prevail through this illness?
- How do your spiritual practices help during a time like this?

Existential questions elicit a dual description of a patient's encounter with adversity—How did this affect you? How did you respond? They refer not only to suffering, but also to how one stands against it. The two sides are in fact inseparable. As H. J. Blackham (p. 52) put it, a person 'may learn to accept them [death, suffering, conflict, fault] as definitive and at the same time find that they are not dead-ends, but frontiers where being-in-itself is to be encountered.'[21] Each person's life narrative can be mapped across such existential themes.

To guide the crafting of interview questions, existential postures of vulnerability and resilience can be displayed as in 32.1.[8,18] Existential postures in the left column of Table 32.1 collectively make up the features of demoralization as a human condition. Demoralization refers to the 'various degrees of helplessness, hopelessness, confusion, and subjective incompetence' that people feel when sensing that they are failing their own or other's expectations for coping with life's challenges.[22, p. 14] Rather than coping, they struggle to survive. It is apt that 'dispirited' is a synonym for demoralization, which feels so much like the disappearance of one's spirit. For many, religion and spirituality serve an important role in supporting hope and countering demoralization.[19]

As a patient tells how personal spirituality has mattered, it is important to hear its manifold expressions—as metaphors, stories, beliefs, prayers, spiritual practices, community, or ethical commitments.[7] Which of these are most salient differs among persons and among religious traditions. Mr Miller's recollection of his Presbyterian Church was a narrative of religious experience expressed as community. For others, prayer or doctrinal beliefs or spiritual practices might have been more central. Listening for the specific forms through which a particular patient's spirituality is expressed opens conversations that support resilience by clarifying meaning, purpose, and connection.

Table 32.1 Existential postures of vulnerability and resilience

Vulnerability	Resilience
Confusion	Coherence
Isolation	Communion
Despair	Hope
Helplessness	Agency
Meaninglessness	Purpose
Indifference	Commitment
Cowardice	Courage
Resentment	Gratitude

Reprinted from *Psychosomatics*, Volume 46, Issue 2, James L. Griffith and L Gaby, Brief psychotherapy at the bedside: Countering demoralization from medical illness, 2005, pp. 109-16, with permission of Elsevier.

Distinguishing health-promoting from deleterious effects of religious coping

Religious faith for many patients provides the bulwark upon which they survive and prevail against hardships, uncertainties, and sorrows of illness. Yet religious beliefs, practices, or communities sometimes diminish, rather than strengthen, coping; or intensify, rather than attenuate, suffering.

Some examples of dichotomous effects that religion can bear upon mental health include:[3,8,23,24]

Health behaviours

- *Protective*: Religious adherence promotes healthy diet, exercise, and avoidance of excessive alcohol or recreational drugs, with improved mood as a consequence.
- *Harmful*: Reliance upon religious faith for healing motivates patients to refuse needed antidepressant, mood-stabilizing, or antipsychotic medications.

Exposure to stressors and life events

Protective

Physical and emotional support by a religious community protects vulnerable group members from financial stress or social isolation, thereby reducing anxiety and depression.

Harmful

- Excessive emotional stimulation during the fervour of worship or ritual observances activates psychosis in patients with chronic schizophrenia or bipolar disorder
- Religiously-induced shame and guilt contributes to emotional suppression that activates an internalizing psychiatric illness, such as conversion disorder, anxiety disorder, or depression.

Perceived stress and coping

Protective: Religious beliefs, practices, and community promote coherency, hope, purpose, gratitude, commitment, and community, thereby strengthening morale.

Harmful

- Religious faith blames illness or misfortune upon personal sinfulness or abandonment by God, inducing profound demoralization
- Religious beliefs justify domestic abuse or parental neglect or provide the rationale for accepting an exploitive or abusive relationship

The tools of sociobiology and evolutionary psychology help distinguish personal spirituality from religiousness as a member of a religious group.[8] Personal spirituality is most associated with social processes that operate in intimate 'whole person to whole person' relatedness, whether that relatedness is expressed with other persons, with a personal deity, or reflexively with oneself. Such relatedness has been explicated by existentialist philosophers in terms of 'I-Thou'[25] or 'face-to-face' relations.[17] Personal spirituality is characterized by social processes of dialogue, empathy, compassion, and expression of primary (i.e. authentic, unguarded, non-instrumental) emotional responses. By contrast, life in religious groups is organized by sociobiological processes of social identity, group role, hierarchical status, in-group/out-group distinctions, reciprocal altruism, and related group-based behaviours. In order to strengthen the group, social processes of religious groups typically prioritize the monitoring and regulation of personal emotions, hence constraining, rather than encouraging individual spontaneity. Religious groups often rely upon social emotions such as shame, guilt, and honour to maintain social roles and group cohesion. Primary emotions are often suppressed, with secondary (reactive) emotions, edited for social acceptability, displayed instead. For example, joy may be publicly expressed even though anguish may be felt privately. While these distinctions between personal spirituality and religious group life have been noted in sociological studies of populations,[26] advances in social neuroscience have clarified how much their differences also reflect different brain circuitry that each utilizes to process social information.[8]

Both religious groups and personal spirituality impact physical and mental health, but in different ways and by different mechanisms. For mental health, they each have their strengths and vulnerabilities. In a meta-analysis of eleven studies, Powell *et al.*[27] found committed church attendance to produce a 25% reduction in mortality compared with non-attenders, even after confounding factors and medical risk factors were accounted for. These salutatory effects upon health seem to arise from a general protection that tightly-knit social groups confer on human beings, rather than the depth of personal religious experience. That is, a similar level of commitment and participation in an Elks Club, a sewing circle, or a hunting club might improve health as much as church attendance. By contrast, there is little empirical evidence that personal spirituality reduces mortality risks.[23,27] Personal spirituality, however, does provide powerful protection for mental health by promoting individual creativity and a robust sense of a personal self. Its generation of hope, purpose, and communion with others strengthens resilience against suffering. Optimally, group religion and personal spirituality complement each other in their support of mental health. The monastic life, for example, provides monks with both a highly-organized social group, as well as facilitation of personal spirituality.

As a general rule, religion that does harm, damages lives, and exacerbates suffering, is religion in which religious group life with its roles, beliefs, and practices has hypertrophied and personal spirituality has dissipated. Distinguishing between group-based religion and personal spirituality is thus critical for understanding instances when religious adherence propels suffering. Therapeutic efforts that counter such religion-fostered suffering often must operate at dual levels by nurturing a reawakening of personal spirituality while simultaneously attenuating the influence of shame- or fear-based religious group authority.[8]

Case history: Mary

Mary was a 23-year-old woman who struggled with depression and suicidal impulses. She had a hidden aspiration that she would someday open a school to help children from troubled families. However, she felt too shame-ridden with inadequencies to openly embrace this vision for her future.

Mary's family had been an integral part of a fundamentalist Christian church that also served as a hub for family social life and a primary source of values. The church taught that children arrive on earth as unsaved heathen until they are redeemed as young adults by Christ's salvation and Christian parenting. Mary's father had ruled her family with iron discipline, tightly controlling every aspect of the lives of Mary and her three siblings well into adolescence. Her memories of home life were replete with regular and harsh punishments, whether whippings or, worse, standing in the winter cold on a back porch shunned by other family members until a time of penance had passed. Her father, and their preacher's sermons, justified this harshness with Biblical quotes that still rang in her memory:[28] 'Children, obey your parents in the Lord, for this is right' (Ephesians 6: 1); 'He who spares the rod hates his son,' (Proverbs 13: 24); 'Do not withhold discipline from a child; if you beat him with a rod, he will not die. If you beat him with the rod you will save his life from hell.' (Proverbs 23: 13–14). Her mother stood by silently, submissive to Mary's father in accordance with the injunction that 'Wives, be submit to your husbands, as to the Lord' (Ephesians 5: 22). During her childhood, Mary internalized the moral voices of her father and church that continued their critical scrutiny long after she had left her family home.

As an adult, Mary spurned any wish to marry and have a family that would bring children into a world of suffering. As a school teacher, she laboured through daily life, feeling numb and empty. She had abandoned her childhood religious beliefs in a cloud of doubt, yet felt deeply unworthy and shame-ridden. In recollecting her childhood, she blamed herself in part for her misery. 'It was always the case that I had done something wrong when I was punished, even if it was too harsh.' Images from her childhood church's teachings circulated in her thoughts even as she wanted to disbelieve them.

Psychotherapy with Mary proceeded on two fronts—first an effort to re-discover her own spontaneous moral impulses. 'You were abused, but you do not abuse others. From the stories you have told me, no student, co-worker, or even a stranger in your life has been treated cruelly, abusively, or by lacking compassion. From where does that commitment come?' 'Suppose that God were to be no more good than you are good. If God were to possess at least the level of goodness that you show daily in your life, how would that be for you?'

The second front was to deconstruct and challenge the authority of her fundamentalist family and church that, now internalized, continued to conduct its surveillance. 'As a teacher in your

classroom, do you ever catch glimpses of your students' lives that might call into question your church's teaching that all children are heathen?' 'If you were God looking down upon this earth, how do you suppose God might have experienced your father's conduct as a parent?' 'What might God have experienced as he watched your father justify his actions by quoting the Bible?' 'If God were to witness how you extend generosity and compassion, what might be God's experience of that?' 'To which of you—you or your father—would the old expression be best applied 'he/she walks with God?' These questions did not bring forth simple answers, but opened long, reflective conversations that extended over multiple psychotherapy sessions. Their ultimate effect was to re-open her personal curiosity about human goodness and the place of God in human affairs, but without the interpretive framework of her childhood church.

As a practical exercise, I further suggested that she examine positions taken by different major religious traditions—Christian, Muslim, Jewish, Buddhist—as they had struggled to understand how divine revelation applied to family life, particularly a parent's responsibility towards his or her child. How would have these traditions have critiqued her father's claimed authority for his interpretations of scripture?

After 24 psychotherapy sessions, Mary began attending a Unitarian Church that had active ministries of service to its surrounding community. She was still unsure about her theological beliefs: 'I'm not sure I believe in God, but I do believe in Good.' With church members, she began discussing her dream of a school for children whose childhoods had been emotionally-deprived.

Distinguishing unusual or idiosyncratic, but normal, expressions of religious life from psychopathology

It is sometimes daunting to tell the difference between mental illness, and unusual or idiosyncratic forms of 'normal' religious experience. Psychopathology can use religious themes to fill in the content of hallucinations, delusions, or aberrant mood states. Hallucinations of God's voice are a common auditory hallucination in schizophrenia. Over a quarter of patients with schizophrenia in the United States, and a fifth of patients with bipolar disorder, have religious delusions.[11] Patients with psychotic depression can exaggerate religious guilt to delusional degrees, sometimes even justifying suicide as moral penance for personal sin.[8,11] However, nearly any symptom of psychopathology—hallucinations, delusional thinking, dissociation, dramatic shifts in mood— can also be evoked within religious groups among persons not otherwise mentally-ill.[12,29,30] In other cases, persons who carry particular vulnerabilities to mental illnesses can have their illnesses activated by intense religious experiences. In addition, patients with chronic mental illnesses can have religious lives that are not only normal, but also buffer the severity of their psychiatric symptoms. In any particular instance, it can be confusing which of these four patterns holds sway.

How to distinguish symptoms of psychiatric disorders from the breadth of religious thoughts, emotions, and behaviours that can be expressed by a non-ill religious person has no simple answer. There are some general guidelines, but no fool-proof algorithm or set of criteria for making the distinction. Importantly, there is no specific psychiatric symptom whose presence is a sure marker for psychiatric illness. Hallucinations, delusional fears, dissociative trance states, panic anxiety, and erratic mood states each can occur among otherwise normal people during intense religious experiences.[29,30]

Some clues do exist for what lies within the range of normality and what is psychopathological. In general, behaviours due to the distorted information-processing of a psychiatric illness are outside the range of normality in terms of activation threshold, duration, or intensity.[31] Ecstasy, anguished guilt, fearful premonitions of doom can occur among many religious people who participate in certain rituals, observances of worship, or systems of beliefs. However, someone who becomes ecstatic too easily, too long, or too intensely also have a mental illness as well. Often other members of a person's religious group are better able than clinicians to distinguish psychiatric illness from normative religious experience for that group.[29,30]

Thoughts that are bizarre or abnormally organized may point to a psychotic disorder. The key is not so much the specific religious content of a patient's thoughts, but how the thinking is constructed. Such abnormalities include disjunctures of logic in the flow of thoughts, or an absence of awareness for other people's thoughts or feelings, or non-modulated thoughts or emotions that dominate a patient's mental life to excess. For example, a patient with schizophrenia often cannot sustain a smooth, logical flow of ideas. The associative links between the words of schizophrenic thought are often odd, bizarre, or illogical (loose associations). Similarly, the rapid flow ideas of someone with mania shows consecutive ideas each veering off in a new direction so that the point of the conversation is lost (flight of ideas). Commonly, psychotic thought is characterized by paranoia, meaning that emotional appraisal and logic are unable to determine who is trustworthy, so the person retreats to a defensive posture of pervasive suspiciousness and excessive vigilance for potential threats. Severe mental illnesses are commonly characterized by impaired perspective-taking, so that a patient is unable to imagine with accuracy how other people think or feel in a situation and has lost access to common wisdom for what makes emotional sense. Major depression and mania are usually associated with disturbances in sleep, energy, hedonia, appetite, and libido, in addition to the elevated or depressed mood that may be the presenting concern. Schizophrenia and other psychoses are usually associated with disorganized thinking, apathy, impaired sociality, and difficulties with such executive functions as planning, organizing, and multi-tasking.

It is generally the case that authentic religious experiences, regardless how strange or uncanny, stimulate creativity, personal growth, and a deepening of compassion for others.[30] A person's life mission can take a new direction, but new growth in work and relationships is a usual consequence. Psychiatric illness, on the other hand, typically causes stagnation in productivity and withdrawal from relationships.

Finally, disturbing behaviours that are largely shaped by psychiatric illness often remit to dramatic degrees when treated with appropriate psychiatric medications.

Case history: Ms Baci

Ms Baci was admitted by her family to a psychiatric unit after her employer reported that she was irrationally accusing co-workers in her office of plotting against her. Ms Baci said that her manager at work was out to do her harm, and others in her office were conspiring as well. She perceived a message from God, 'Mess with me and I will mess with you!' that she delivered to her co-workers. She aggressively began giving orders to everyone in the office, until her family arrived to take her to the hospital. When interviewed by the psychiatrist, Ms Baci revealed that she had not slept for two nights, up and down, pacing through the night. Through this, she heard God's voice audibly speaking to her about his intent to protect her. Although she regarded herself as a 'spiritual person,' she had not previously followed any particular religious tradition. She had never before heard God's voice speaking. Ms Baci was diagnosed with a brief reactive psychosis, or possibly schizophrenia. After a week of hospitalization and antipsychotic medications, Ms Baci's sense of external threat and entrapment had largely diminished. The audible voice of God disappeared. She continued to feel God's presence, however, which transmuted from its earlier defensive, belligerent character to one of comfort and reassurance.

Disturbing behaviours generated via normal sociobiological systems rarely respond to psychiatric medications. Normal grief, demoralization, or stigma-induced humiliation, although productive of great suffering, are not improved by antidepressant medications. Mood-stabilizing and antipsychotic medications have no benefits for the up and down mood shifts or frazzled thinking that life stresses produce among people without underlying psychiatric illnesses. Even so, response to medication itself is not a perfect test for psychiatric illness. Benzodiazepines (diazepam, alprazolam, lorazepam, clonazepam) and alcohol help anyone feel more relaxed, not just those with anxiety disorders. Psychostimulants, such as methylphenidate or amphetamine, will sharpen any person's concentration, not just those with attention deficit disorder. Despite these limitations, a clear-cut response to medication is an additional piece of evidence that can be weighed when combined with other dimensions of assessment.

Clinical assessment for distinguishing idiosyncratic, but normal religious behaviour from psychiatric illness must thus consider a number of questions:

- Is the onset, intensity, and duration of the behaviour typical or unusual compared to other members of patient's religious group?
- Do associated symptoms of a psychiatric disorder co-occur? That is, are there loose associations of schizophrenia, flight of ideas of mania, or abnormal sleep, energy, hedonia, and appetite of major depressive disorder?
- Does the behaviour represent creativity and growth in work and relationships, or does it represent stagnation and withdrawal from work and relationships?
- Are there identifiable biological (e.g. history of substance abuse, family history of mental illness) or psychosocial (traumatic stress, losses, stigmatization) risk factors that make occurrence of a psychiatric disorder more likely?
- Is there a past history of a psychiatric disorder? If so, has it shown a pattern of relapse and recurrence?
- Is there a robust response to a psychiatric medication? If not, can the failure of response be attributed to psychological or social stressors that are so overwhelming that any beneficial effects of medication might have been over-ridden?

Answering the above list of questions often requires more than a routine examination in an office setting. Collateral information about a patient's spontaneous, unstructured interactions with family members, church elders, or neighbors in community settings often is vital for assessment. Functional impairments are often more evident in daily life than in structured office or hospital examinations. In daily life, a well-functioning prefrontal cortex is needed to manage ambiguity and uncertainty, to make moment to moment shifts from one social context to another, to show discretion by checking emotional impulses, and to gauge how intensely to express feelings. Most major psychiatric disorders, whether mood, anxiety, psychotic, or dissociative, show these kinds of impairments in daily life settings. Access to such collateral information requires a therapeutic alliance that includes not only the patient, but also the patient's family or other close relationships.

In the end, distinguishing a psychiatric disorder from unusual or idiosyncratic religious behaviour requires a clinical judgment that is based upon the preponderance of evidence. Even when the gathering of evidence is conducted systematically and completely, there still can remain uncertainty as to role of psychiatric illness in disturbing religious behaviours. Yet this distinction matters greatly for practical reasons. Diagnosis of a psychiatric disorder points towards symptoms best treated by evidence-based pharmacological or psychosocial interventions. However, it also confers the label of 'illness,' prescribes a sick role, incurs risks for stigmatization, and reframes the meaning of religious behaviour as a symptom that perhaps should not be regarded as valid religious experience.[8] Behaviours generated by normal sociobiological responses to stress should elicit from a clinician a normalizing message that 'most anyone would feel what you are experiencing, given what you are going through.' Interventions that appropriately follow do not treat illness, but unload stressors, strengthen personal coping, access family and social relational support, and mobilize spiritual and religious resources.[18]

Conclusion

Assessment of mental health effects of a person's religious beliefs and practices can be incorporated into the usual diagnostic evaluations that clinicians conduct. Such an assessment can guide interventions that maximize salutatory effects and minimize harmful ones, while respecting the person's religious identity and cultural traditions. This clinical role differs from the faith-based roles of clergy and chaplains by its primary reliance upon the human sciences in understanding how religion and health interact. It makes best use of a clinician's 'outsider' role as one who does not have a faith-based stake in how a patient conducts religious life, but does wish to reduce suffering and promote health. From this outsider position, a clinician can ask questions with concern, respect, and authenticity. A clinician without dictating or prescribing how to be religious nevertheless can help a patient to become a more capable and effective moral agent in his or her religious life.

References

1 Hoge, D.R. (1996). Religion in America: the demographics of belief and affiliation. In: E.P. Shafranske, H.M.E. Maloney (eds) *Religion and the Clinical Practice of Psychology*, pp. 22–41. Washington, DC: American Psychological Association.

2 Tepper, L., Rogers, S.A., Coleman, E.M., Malony, H.N. (2001). The prevalence of religious coping among patients with persistent mental illnesses. *Psychiat Serv* **52**: 660–5.

3 Pargament, K.I. (1997). *The Psychology of Religion and Coping: Theory, Research, Practice.* New York: Guilford Press.
4 Galanter, M. (2005). *Spirituality and the Healthy Mind: Science, Therapy, and the Need for Personal Meaning.* New York: Oxford University Press.
5 Josephson, A.M., Peteet, J.R. (eds). (2004). *Handbook of Spirituality and Worldview in Clinical Practice.* Arlington: American Psychiatric Publishing.
6 Koenig, H.G. (ed.). (1998). *Handbook of Religion and Mental Health.* Boston: Academic Press.
7 Griffith, J.L., Griffith, M.E. (2002). *Encountering the Sacred in Psychotherapy: How to Talk with People About Their Spiritual Lives.* New York: Guilford Press.
8 Griffith, J.L. (2010). *Religion That Heals, Religion That Harms: A Guide for Clinical Practice.* New York: Guilford Press.
9 Pargament, K.I., Koenig, H.G., Tarakeshwar, N., Hahn, J. (2004). Religious coping methods as predictors of psychological, physical and spiritual outcomes among medically-ill elderly patients: A longitudinal study. *J Hlth Psychol* **9**: 1713–30.
10 Clarke, I. (ed.). *Psychosis and Spirituality: Exploring the New Frontier.* London: Whurt.
11 Peteet, J.R., Lu, F.G., Narrow, W.E. (2011). *Religious and Spiritual Issues in Psychiatric Diagnosis: a Research Agenda for DSM-V.* Arlington: American Psychiatric Association.
12 Linden, S.C., Harris, M., Whitaker, C., Healy, D. (2010). Religion and psychosis: the effects of the Welsh religious revival in 1904–1905. *Psycholog Med* **40**: 1317–23.
13 Griffith, J.L. (2006). Managing religion countertransference in clinical settings. *Psychiat Ann* **36**: 196–204.
14 Goffman, E. (1963). *Stigma: Notes on the Management of Spoiled Identity.* New York: Simon & Schuster.
15 George Washington University Institute for Spirituality and Health. *Spiritual Assessment: FICA Spiritual Assessment Tool.* Available at http://www.gwumc.edu/gwish/clinical/fica.cfm (accessed 14 January 2012).
16 Puchalski, C.M., Ferrell, B. (2010). *Making Health Care Whole: Integrating Spirituality into Patient Care.* West Conshohocken: Templeton Press.
17 Levinas, E. (1961). *Totality and Infinity*, transl. A. Lingis. Pittsburgh: Duquesne University Press.
18 Griffith, J.L., Gaby, L. (2005). Brief psychotherapy at the bedside: Countering demoralization from medical illness. *Psychosomatics* **46**: 109–16.
19 Griffith, J.L., Dsouza, A. (2012). Demoralization and hope: their role in clinical psychiatry and psychotherapy. In: R.D. Alarcon, J.B. Frank (eds) *The Psychotherapy of Hope: the Legacy of Persuasion and Healing.* Baltimore: Johns Hopkins University Press.
20 Kleinman, A. (2006). *What Really Matters: Living a Moral Life Amidst Uncertainty and Danger.* New York: Oxford University Press.
21 Blackham, H.J. (1952). *Six Existentialist Thinkers.* New York: Harper Torchbooks.
22 Frank, J.D., Frank, J.B. (1991). *Persuasion and Healing: a Comparative Study of Psychotherapy*, 3rd edn. Baltimore: Johns Hopkins University Press.
23 Baumeister, R.F. (2005). *The Cultural Animal: Human Nature, Meaning, and Social Life.* New York: Oxford University Press.
24 Pargament, K.I. (2007). *Spiritually Integrated Psychotherapy.* New York: Guilford Press.
25 Buber, M. (1958). *I and Thou*, 2nd edn. New York: MacMillan.
26 Hood, R.W. Jr, Hill, P.C., Spilka, B. (2009). *Psychology of Religion: an Empirical Approach*, 4th edn. New York: Guilford Press.
27 Powell, L.H., Shahabi, L., Thoresen, C.E. (2003). Religion and spirituality: Linkages to physical health. *Am Psycholog* **58**: 36–52.
28 *Holy Bible*, rev standard version. (1952). New York: Thomas Nelson.
29 Galanter, M. (1999). *Cults: Faith, Healing, and Coercion*, 2nd edn. New York: Oxford University Press.
30 Menezes, A., Jr, Moreira-Almeida, A. (2009). Differential diagnosis between spiritual experiences and mental disorders of religious content. *Rev Psiq Clin* **36**: 75–82.
31 Horwitz, A.V., Wakefield, J.C., Spitzer, R.L. (2007). *Loss Of Sadness: How Psychiatry Transformed Normal Sorrow into Depressive Disorder.* New York: Oxford University Press.

CHAPTER 33

Social work

Margaret Holloway

Introduction

The last 20 years have seen some interesting developments in the relationship between social work and spirituality in healthcare. First, there are signs that after a history of suspicion, social work as a profession is cautiously engaging with spirituality, both as something to be taken account of in their interactions with individuals, families, and communities, and as something which potentially should be a focus for social work interventions. An increasingly widespread acceptance of the significance of spirituality is a major step forward for a profession that, for a long time, viewed anything to do with religion as inappropriate for social work intervention and was, if anything, inclined towards the view that religion, for many service users, particularly those with long-term mental health problems, was often part of the problem. A second important development is social work's rediscovery of the importance of health, including physical health, to overall wellbeing.[1,2] Social work since the 1970s has operated from a social structural theoretical foundation, which sees problems as socially situated, if not created, and itself as the guardian of social explanations, fiercely opposed to 'the medical model,' which it characterized as unfavourably pathologizing the individual, placing the responsibility to 'cope' or to change, squarely in the court of the individual and family. However, the once rather entrenched positions adopted by medical and social model proponents have seen a welcome and increasing integration of perspectives in pursuit of quality health and social care.

It may be that the reader does not recognize the picture painted above. In its crudest form, it relates primarily to social work in northern Europe, and countries such as Hong Kong and Australia, where the British influence was strong in the early development of social work practice. In the USA, the influence of faith-based social work organizations, as well as a markedly more religious society, has produced a different approach, although a tendency to draw the boundaries sharply between professional and client also led to sensitivity about charges of proselytizing when it came to religion. In the countries of central Europe, many of whom have set up social work services much more recently, the old hang-ups have not held the same sway.

In order to look at social work practice and spiritual care, therefore, it is important to review its historical development, as well as to examine the current picture.

Social work's developing engagement with spiritual care

Taking that fundamental caution about religion as our starting point, we see that most of the early literature from social work, written in the last decades of the twentieth century when the contemporary spirituality discourse emerges in the 'caring professions', is concerned to establish two things. First, that in contemporary discourse, 'spirituality' implies something that is much broader, more diffuse, and less prescribed than 'religion'; thus, considerable attention is paid to defining and elaborating the concept of spirituality and distinguishing it from religion, for which various definitions are also offered. Secondly, and as a consequence of the way in which spirituality is defined, arguments are put forward as to why social workers should pay attention to spirituality, particularly in their assessments. Increasingly, such arguments are put forward on the basis of small scale empirical (qualitative) research studies.

The search for an acceptable definition of spirituality

To take first the attempts to define a broader concept of spirituality, which might be more acceptable in a fundamentally secular profession, we see a number of common themes emerging in social work:

- Spirituality is concerned with meaning and purpose, in particular, the *search* for meaning
- Spirituality is experienced through relationships, and those relationships may be with an external or 'higher' source, or they may be proximate, for example, sources of spiritual strength may be experienced through families, friends or communities
- Spirituality promotes certain behaviours and practices, within oneself and also towards the other person.

So, for example, in one of the earliest definitions offered for social work by Patel *et al.* spirituality is defined as:

> ... the human search for personal meaning and mutually fulfilling relationships between people, between people and the natural environment and between religious people and God ... Social work practice can be described as a spiritual voyage which involves promoting the growth and fulfillment of user, professional helper, and the wider community.[3]

In another early definition, Canda and Furman were explicit about breaking the automatic link with religion when they said that this cluster of concepts could be understood, '... in terms which are theistic, atheistic, nontheistic, or any combination of these.'[4]

It might seem surprising that there has been such a struggle to get spirituality on the social work agenda, when we realize that in defining spirituality in this way, social work writers are locating it squarely within the underpinning value base for all social work practice: that is, social work is concerned with that which has meaning and value for the service user; the relationship between the social worker and service user is of prime importance; and social work adheres to a clear code of conduct that stems from the fact that it is essentially a moral activity (although there are sensitivities about this in terms of distinguishing between the ability and requirement to make *moral judgments*, and the need to avoid being *judgmental* or moralistic). In fact, there are also arguments to be made that the origins of social work are rooted in strong religious (Judeo-Christian) traditions and values.[5–7] Bringing this firmly upfront in terms of current debate about the core role and tasks of social work, Graham declaims:

> To those colleagues who state that ours is a flash in the pan, that ours is a new and ephemeral way of looking at social work ... (which) should not unduly influence mainstream social work, I think we should respond ... that ours is the continuation of a long history within social work.[8]

There is, however, one problem in defining spirituality in this way and representing its inclusion in social work practice as no more than what the profession has always adhered to. I have argued previously that to characterize spirituality and its importance for social work in such a way as might also be described as the best of 'traditional' social work practice runs the risk of alienating those who wish to nurture those values, but remain firmly secular in their outlook and do not buy into this new 'secular spirituality.' At the same time, calls for social work to return to its Judeo-Christian roots may suggest a retreat into forms of practice that have been challenged by certain groups of service users as culturally oppressive.[9] Yet it is from many of those same groups of service users that the growing insistence has come for social work to recognize the importance of both religion and spirituality in the lives of many of the people with whom we work [10–13]. This is not so much of a contradiction as it may at first appear. The implications are that there are aspects of this way of engaging with service users that are distinct to spirituality (and also religion) and move social work practice into a realm which is not so familiar, or comfortable, for the established western paradigm. Social work writers who have taken up this challenge also suggest that herein lies the greatest contribution of contemporary understandings of spirituality for social work practice as a whole.

Unusually amongst the earlier work, my own study of spiritual and philosophical issues in death, dying, and bereavement, took a different angle in defining spirituality as '... a dimension which brings together attitudes, beliefs, thoughts, feelings and practices reaching beyond the ... material.'[10] Individual faith, meanwhile, was defined as 'Humanistic or religious beliefs which guide the way an individual seeks to live.'[10]

It is interesting that there are rarely attempts to define *faith as held by individuals* in contemporary discussions of spirituality, although *faith communities* are increasingly a focus for attention, principally as spiritual and community resources. This distracts from the fact that faith communities are built around shared beliefs, and an individual's 'faith' is derived from adherence to a belief system. It is the arena of belief with which, I suggest, social work, is most ill at ease. On the one hand, social workers tend to feel that a person's beliefs are not their concern, but on the other, there may be a perceived conflict between social work's commitment to address inequalities and challenge oppression, and religious systems that adhere to beliefs which appear to establish social inequalities. A less obvious tension, is over a concept that is not always explicit in the definition of humanistic spirituality, but which emerges in discussions of spiritual care, particularly in the more recent literature. This is the notion of *transcendence*, and it is a process which my own early definition offered as distinctive to spirituality.

Transcendence

Although the term is used by all the world religions, little of the spirituality literature from the secular helping professions deals directly with transcendence as a concept for spiritual care, nor is it necessarily implied by the extensive literature dealing with existential questions and sources of meaning and support. Yet arguably, it is the inclusion or not of transcendence which divides contemporary understandings of spirituality.[7,14] Kellehear's short-hand definition of transcendence as 'making the most of' hardship and suffering[14] may not sit well with social workers if they see this as helping the service user to accept conditions in their life (whether material or relationships) which are unjust and oppressive where social work would see its role as working alongside the person to empower them to challenge discrimination and oppression and change the circumstances of their lives. However, transcendence should be seen as a powerful tool in those situations which cannot be changed in essence—such as the person who has an incurable illness—but can be fundamentally changed in the way in which they impact on the person's experience. Thus, if the person can be helped to *transcend* the problem or pain, even though its source cannot be removed, such that the problematic or painful impact no longer has the power to control their whole being, an experience of powerlessness is changed into an empowering and liberating process.

Transformation

Linked to transcendence is transformation. The work of Canda and Furman in the US has been particularly influential in developing the notion of social work practice as transformative practice when it embraces spirituality.[4,15] This strand builds on another core value and theme in social work—that social work is about bringing about change. Historically, it has always been understood that a whole other branch of social work activity has to do with maintenance—supporting people and situations where fundamental change for the better is not possible, but social work's job is to delay as long as possible the situation becoming worse. However, since the 1990s, social work has been increasingly concerned with improving the quality of life of all service users and if we couple this with an understanding of transcendence as discussed above, we see that both change-orientated practice and supportive practice have the potential to transform people's lives. For Canda and Furman, this is what 'spiritually sensitive' social work practice is all about since it,

> ... includes, but is more than problem solving. It includes, but is more than promoting coping, adapting, or recovery ... When change is transformational it moves people forward on their life paths.[16]

In their first edition, Canda and Furman[4] refer to life paths as 'spiritual' paths.

Social justice

Social work can be credited with introducing another strand to the contemporary spirituality debate—the link with social justice. The earliest explorations of this emerge in the writings of social workers challenged by the injustices heaped on the indigenous peoples of Australia and New Zealand, where the Maori influence in particular raised the question of the total neglect of the spiritual dimension in social work interventions. The inextricable link with social justice and social responsibility is a direct consequence of this way of understanding spirituality and spiritual care:[7]

> What makes for a holistic spirituality is the recognition that we are all interdependent, that we need to see the divine spark in one another and respect that, and that we need to specifically protect the most vulnerable, the poorest and the most powerless.[17]

Holloway and Moss[7] further argue that two strands—celebrating diversity and championing social justice—come together in spiritually-aware social work practice. In other words, it is our awareness of what it means to be human, including our spiritual essence, which drives both of those underpinning values for social work practice. We both celebrate and respect our different spiritual and cultural heritages and promote the common human rights which stem from recognition of our shared humanity.

Thinking outside of the western paradigm

The last 20 years or so has shown an increasing awareness of how the core underpinning principles and values which mark out social work as a profession are identifiable across the global stage, but equally, how social work internationally may espouse markedly different 'worldviews'. At the heart of these different worldviews is the whole issue of contemporary understandings of spirituality and their implications for social work practice.[7] Indeed, it was social work in Africa, India, the Pacific Rim, and practitioners from and in the indigenous communities of North America, Australia, and New Zealand, which together have been most vocal in their protest about the exclusion of a spiritual dimension in western-imposed models of social work practice.[18–21] These arguments are further refined along lines that have particular significance for social work and healthcare. They stem from an eco-spiritual worldview which differs from western models in two particular ways. First, greater emphasis is placed on relatedness and community than on the rights and needs of the individual. Second, the relationship between the individual and the environment is conceptualized radically differently, as:

> the starting point for rethinking social work's commitment to *person in environment:* what does it mean to live well in this place? We may never get to the profound spiritual dimensions of that question if we continue to constrain spirituality within the narrow boundaries of a person-centred approach.[22]

To return to the first of these differences, the different starting points of those western cultures that are orientated towards individualism and autonomy, and those, for example, Asian and eastern societies, which privilege communitarian values, and social and familial duty, can be seen to have profound significance for healthcare and to exert significant imperatives in dying and bereavement in particular.[23,24] Social work has always cherished its family-centred models of practice, but a perennial dilemma in social work practice is how to manage conflicting rights and needs between the service user at the centre of the intervention, and other family members. Yet when we come to the topic of spirituality, this may be a false dilemma. A dominant theme in the spirituality discourse is that spirituality is a *relational* concept.[25] Thus, a person experiences their spirituality through relationships, which may be transcendent, with a (sometimes Divine) 'other', but very frequently are focused on, or at least include, family, friends, and their immediate community.

When an individual experiences ill-health and, most especially, when they are dying, we know that to be surrounded by family and friends, and to be reconciled with estranged loved ones, is an important contributor to wellbeing and a peaceful death. This is a priority that shows remarkable consistency across cultures.[26,27] When family problems are evident in healthcare settings and adversely affecting the patient's treatment and care, it is frequently the social worker who is called upon.[28,29] Such interventions are rarely conceptualized as 'spiritual care' yet there are arguments that when viewed within a holistic model of health and wellbeing, they should be.[9,30–32] This relational understanding of spiritual wellbeing and the significance of incorporating this for successful social work intervention is embedded in the literature emerging from social work practice with aboriginal communities, which argues for the mobilizing of the spiritual energy bound up in a sense of community and community responsibility, to heal relationships.[20,33]

The second critical overturning of the established social work mind-set concerns a re-evaluation of how we understand the individual in their social and environmental context, and the importance of 'place' for health and wellbeing. Social work has long recognized these elements to be crucially bound up with an integrated sense of self and identity. Social work has contributed significantly to the highlighting of the importance of 'place' for health in its championing of ageing and dying 'in place.'[34–36] However, the explicit linking of this with promoting spiritual wellbeing suggests a number of new approaches for social work. For example, it illuminates still further why many frail older people rapidly decline when removed from their home into a more intensive care environment, and suggests that attending to their spiritual needs and ensuring that these are met, at least in part, *through their new environment*, may be a relatively untapped, but potentially important resource in preventing unnecessary decline. Likewise, interventions that foster a sense of connectedness and oneness with their environment in people who demonstrate profound social and emotional alienation—both of which contribute to spiritual distress—may also be seen as spiritual care.[7] This notion of place embedded in the person is the foundation of eco models of spirituality, which do not distinguish between the sacred and the secular or humankind and the natural environment: 'I'm not in the place, but the place is in me'; 'Here nature knows us.'[37]

Social work and healthcare

The second development that I highlighted at the outset is social work's rediscovery of the importance of health in the lives of service users and hence the relevance of health issues for social work interventions. In fact, hospital social work was one of the earliest specialisms to develop despite the more recent neglect of the health dimension to which Bywaters points.[1,2] Alongside this, the hospice multidisciplinary team as originally envisaged by Cicely Saunders included social work from the start. Recent developments in social work's engagement with health and with spirituality both point to a convergence along particular lines. The significance of health inequalities for overall wellbeing and increasing evidence of the role that poor health and unequal access to good healthcare play in further disadvantaging people who are already disadvantaged in socio-economic terms, alongside the demographic trend that sees more and more users of social work services in need of continuing healthcare, has focused social work's attention on those with poor and declining health.

Social work's contribution to holistic care at the end of life

Work in the UK under the auspices of the government's National End of Life Care Programme is re-asserting the importance of social work and social care for quality end-of-life care, which, despite its early prominence in the hospice movement, has remained a relatively marginalized role in the UK, both within end-of-life care services and also in relation to mainstream social care services. A similar process can be seen in all the countries of the developed world which adopted care management as the major vehicle for delivering social care services, although the UK has lagged some way behind others in highlighting and supporting the contribution of social work to holistic care at the end of life.[38] Consideration of the key elements in good care for people who are dying and their families, makes clear the essential overlap, not only with the fundamental values and established practice of social work, but also with current key thrusts in all social care services. Importantly for our discussion here, these same themes are reflected in what is increasingly recognized as good spiritual care. These can be summarized as:

- *Personalization*—an approach that respects and keeps central the wishes and perspectives of the service user and their family and tailors the response from professionals and services accordingly
- *Empowerment*—a way of working which seeks to enhance the dignity and control of the service user
- *Partnership*—a mode of engagement with the service user, which respects the knowledge and expertise of both s/he and the worker and seeks to integrate these for maximum effectiveness
- *Holistic assessment*—an approach to assessment which looks at the whole person and seeks to understand the needs, problems and resources of the individual in their wider social and cultural context;
- *Personal narrative*—a framework for listening, understanding, and intervening in the lives of service users, which recognizes the unique journey that each person undertakes, the importance of the past to where they are now and the potential in the present to influence their future course.

What is distinctive to this particular professional approach is that no one element can stand alone—the self-same values are embedded in each and contribute to the effectiveness of each. For example, it may be through employing their professional knowledge and skills in a partnership model of assessment, which takes account of the life they have lived, that the social worker is able to empower the person who is dying to make and achieve those choices which are essential to *who they are*—and hence their wellbeing—in death. I myself have developed a model for spiritual care based on these essential elements, which I now term 'The Fellow Traveller' (Figure 33.1).[7] This can be applied in the context of any health and social care worker's role, and was originally developed for pastoral care workers.[39] However, it derives much from the core principles of social work practice.

A recent review of the literature on spiritual care at the end of life[25] found that there is a marked tendency amongst practitioners, particularly in the UK, to favour 'companioning' and narrative models.

The social worker as companion

Palliative care nurses tend to talk about the importance of simply 'being there'—reflected in the increasing tendency to couple palliative care with 'supportive care'—but social work has always seen its supportive functions as complemented by its role as an agent of change.[40] The 'fellow traveller' is a companion who *assists* with the journey, and it brings into play roles of listening, sharing, guiding, and sustaining.

Thus, the worker must first engage with the person at the point that they are at, including being aware of their spiritual needs. As they listen and gather a picture of what the issues may be for this person, in this situation and at this point in time, and also

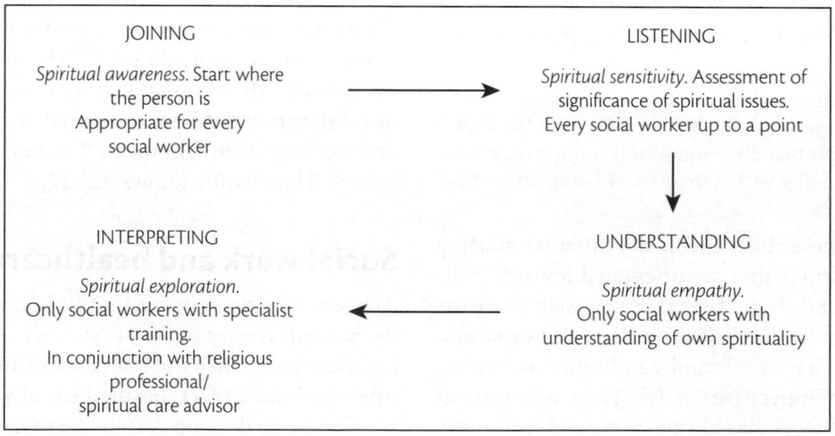

Figure 33.1 The Fellow Traveller Model for spiritual care.

the resources on which they draw or might potentially draw, the *relative significance* of spiritual problems and resources becomes clearer. Some social workers will be feeling out of their depth at this point. They do not understand enough about the other person's 'worldview' to understand where they are going or what the obstacles are to their progress. This point in the journey, as much as any, also requires understanding of where the other person *is coming from,* their spiritual biography and cultural context. It may be that the worker needs to consult with another colleague in order to be able to continue to engage meaningfully with the other person, or they may suggest that another professional may be better able to help with the spiritual aspect. Only someone who is able to empathize and understand the spiritual needs of the other person will be able to go further with them in their spiritual journey. The final stage involves interpreting both needs and problems and helping the other person to understand and get in touch with those spiritual resources which will heal and sustain them as death approaches. It is worth noting here that the dying person and those closest to them may follow separate pathways, but an important role for the professional is to enable those paths to come together at critical points. Spirituality is also experienced in relationship and one source of spiritual distress at the end of life is repeatedly identified as fractured relationships and the absence of forgiveness or reconciliation.[41,42]

See Chapter 5, Holloway and Moss.[7]

Case study: The social worker as Fellow Traveller

Laura is a social worker in a children's hospital. She had only been qualified for two years when she moved to this post where she has been for six months. She finds the work emotionally challenging, but also very satisfying. One of the problems is that her training had not really prepared her for the type of encounter where she feels she has nothing to offer the family, but herself, and this is particularly the case when people raise existential sorts of questions—which she finds they do quite frequently in this work. For example, how does she deal with grandparents who cannot come to terms with the fact that their young grandchild is dying while they are still alive and comparatively well, yet standing helplessly by, unable to comfort the parents or themselves?

One busy afternoon she was asked to go up to the ward to see a young mother—Samantha—whose 9-year-old daughter Maddy had just died during an operation. Laura knew Sam as Maddy used to come in quite regularly for treatment and Sam had asked for help with bus fares on a number of occasions. Sam was about the same age as Laura and seemed to choose her to confide in when she was anxious. The last time Maddy was in, Sam had seemed angry, asking why her baby should have been condemned to a life of suffering in this way, but she snapped out of it when Laura pointed out how well Maddy was doing and what a happy child she was. This operation was supposed to be routine and low risk. Laura felt a sense of dread and horribly inadequate as she approached the ward. As it turned out, Sam was quiet and withdrawn, but nodded apathetically when Laura suggested that she should visit her at home next week.

Over the next few weeks, Laura visited Samantha once a week. Sam talked freely about her feelings of loss and pain, and the fact that she felt she could not get too upset with her friends as they couldn't cope with it. They especially couldn't cope with her questions. Laura asked her what particular questions and Sam said that she has to know what has happened to Maddy 'on the other side'. She asked Laura whether she had lost anyone close and if so did she wonder where they are? Laura said she was very close to her gran and still felt a connection to her, but she didn't have any firm beliefs about life after death. She suggested that Sam might like to talk to the chaplain, but Sam dismissed this idea, saying that she 'feels sorry for him' because he didn't have any answers.

Feeling out of her depth, Laura approached Tim, the hospital chaplain for advice. Tim remembered Sam being very hostile to him when he offered to pray with her after Maddy's death, but said that he thought she had had a Christian upbringing. Laura remembered that Sam had said to her once that it was probably God's punishment that Maddy had been born with this disorder because she had been a bit wild. Laura hadn't known how to respond and had laughed it off. Tim suggested that Laura help Sam to focus on those things that give her a sense of peace about and connection with Maddy. Laura could identify with this because this was what she did at times when she missed her gran most. Laura tried this approach the next time she saw Sam. They seemed to be making some progress, but Sam returned to the difficult questions about an After Life and whether God was punishing her. Laura said that didn't seem to make sense to her since Maddy had brought so much joy to Sam, as well as many other people. However, she said honestly that she didn't think she could help Sam with those particular questions, but that she had found the chaplain very friendly and open when she had talked to him herself about some of the things she was struggling with about Maddy's death. Sam was struck by this and said she would like to talk to Tim. She had been shocked and angry when he spoke to her at the hospital, but she had, nevertheless, appreciated his concern for her.

Social work's use of narrative

Crucial to understanding where someone is at in their journey, is the dying person's 'story' of where they have been and how they experience their journey. Social work has made important contributions to the use of narrative in spiritual care. David Hodge built his model for spiritual intervention around an interpretive narrative approach. Hodge's 'interpretive framework' identifies six psycho-social-moral domains—*affect, behaviour, cognition, communion, conscience*, and *intuition*—which are explored in order to illuminate the individual's personal narrative, identifying strengths and coping strategies, but also counter-productive or damaging beliefs and behaviours.([30] Other social work writers have suggested that the task in the latter instance is to work together to 'co-construct' a new story, one that redefines the problem without reinforcing the damaging narrative, but in a manner which is, 'different enough from their situation, yet not too different, to further the conversation.'[43] This last point is important. Social work has been in the forefront of ensuring that spiritual care must work with the other person's tradition, respecting diversity, but without the sort of cultural reductionism, which fails to see the subjective needs of the individual within their cultural context—which may, of course be one fraught with cross-cultural issues.[44]

There are many situations in healthcare, including, but not limited to work with users of mental health services, where the 'script' which the person has followed, including those derived from religious beliefs and understandings, is at the root of their ill health or preventing their recovery or healing. This applies as much to an acute problem open to 'cure', as to chronic conditions and those which ultimately end in death. It is crucial that exploration of the other person's story, and how they tell it, is a jointly undertaken activity in which worker and service user together identify spiritual resources which have served in the past, and how they could be called into play now, at the same time as contradictory and harmful scripts are gently challenged and reframed. For example, beliefs in illness as punishment from God are set alongside what spiritual traditions have to say about suffering and being sustained through suffering; death is seen not as a fearful encounter with an avenging deity, but as the culmination of a life in which preparation for death involves acts of love, reconciliation, and forgiveness. This process, at any point in the life, often hinges around 'making sense' of the life so far, and that may involve both 'laying to rest' those painful memories that we cannot change and, often coincidentally, discovering joys and fulfillments previously overshadowed by the hurt. Elsewhere in social work, Parton and O'Byrne[45] have talked of the need for service users to 'reclaim' their own narrative, and we can apply this to spirituality using the concepts of transcendence and transformation discussed earlier.

Conclusion

Transcendence, transformation, engendering, and maintaining hope, engaging with the whole person in their biographical and cultural richness, seeing spiritual care as intrinsic to the pursuit of social justice, understanding the embodied relationship between personal wellbeing and the social and environmental context—these are all aspects of a humanistic understanding of spiritual care that contemporary social work can relate to its core agenda. Indeed, social work writers have contributed significantly to the development of these concepts and approaches, and to an understanding of spiritual care in contemporary healthcare, which has the potential to go way beyond western-dominated individualistic treatment models. Social work has maintained a critical focus on spiritual care, which refuses to embrace as social work those distinctly religious and spiritual practices which belong outside the realm of a secular profession, but which increasingly recognizes the importance of a spiritual *and* religious dimension[46] as intrinsically embedded in the lives of many service users. Moreover, in refining the ways in which social workers may incorporate broader humanistic understandings of spirituality into their assessments and interventions, social work has opened up for itself new ways of engaging with service users that have the potential to enhance social work practice as a whole.

References

1 Bywaters, P. (2000). Critical commentary. Talking about inequality: accounts of ill health. *Br J Soc Work* **30**: 873–78.

2 Bywaters, P., Napier, l. (2009). Revising social work's international policy statement on health: Process, outcomes and implications. *Int Soc Work* **52**: 447–57.

3 Patel, N., Naik, D., Humphries, B. (1998). *Visions of Reality: Religion and Ethnicity in Social Work*, p. 11. London: CCETSW.

4 Canda, E., Furman, L. (1999). *Spiritual Diversity in Social Work Practice: the Heart of Helping*, pp. 43–4. New York: Free Press.

5 Goldstein, H. (1990). The knowledge base of social work practice: wisdom, analogue or art?. *Fam Soc J Contemp Hum Serv* **71**(1): 32–43.

6 Bowpitt, G. (1998). Evangelical Christianity, secular humanism, and the genesis of British social work. *Br J Soc Work* **28**: 675–93.

7 Holloway, M., Moss, B. (2010). *Spirituality and Social Work*. London: Palgrave Macmillan.

8 Graham, J (2008). Who am I? An essay on inclusion and spiritual growth through community and mutual appreciation. *J Religion Spiritual Soc Work* **27**(1–2): 1–24, p. 14.

9 Holloway, M. (2007). Spiritual need and the core business of social work'. *Br J Soc Work* **37**(2): 265–80.

10 Lloyd, M. [M Holloway] .(1997). Dying and bereavement, spirituality and social work in a market economy of welfare. *Br J Soc Work* **27**(2): 175–90.

11 Nash, M., Stewart, B. (eds) (2002). *Spirituality and Social Care: Contributing to Personal and Community Wellbeing*. London: Jessica Kingsley.

12 Coyte, M.E., Gilbert, P., Nicholls, V. (2007). *Spirituality, Values and Mental Health: Jewels for the Journey*. London: Jessica Kingsley.

13 Harrison, P. (2007). Holistic thinking and integrated care: working with black and minority ethnic individuals and communities in health and social care. *J Integ Care* **15**(3): 3–6.

14 Kellehear, A. (2000). Spirituality and palliative care: a model of needs. *Palliat Med* **14**: 149–55.

15 Canda, E., Furman, L. (2010). *Spiritual Diversity in Social Work Practice: the Heart of Helping*, 2nd edn. New York: Free Press.

16 Canda, E., Furman, L. (2010). *Spiritual Diversity in Social Work Practice: the Heart of Helping*, 2nd edn, p. 315. New York: Free Press.

17 Consedine, J. (2002). Spirituality and social justice. In: M. Nash, B. Stewart (eds) *Spirituality and Social Care: Contributing to Personal and Community Wellbeing*, p. 45. London: Jessica Kingsley.

18 Sacco, T. (1994). Spirituality and social work students in their first year of study at a South African university. *J Soc Develop Afr* **11**(2): 43–56.

19 Sermabeikian, P. (1994). Our clients, ourselves: the spiritual perspective and social work practice. *Soc Work* **39**(2): 178–83.

20 Lynn, R. (2001). Learning from a 'Murri Way'. *Br J Soc Work* **31**: 903–16.

21 Yip, K. (2005). A dynamic Asian response to globalization in cross-cultural social work. *Int Soc Work* **48**(5): 593–607.

22 Zapf, M.K. (2005). The spiritual dimension of person and environment: perspectives from social work and traditional knowledge. *Int Soc Work* **48**(5): 633–42.

23 Holloway, M. (2007). *Negotiating Death in Contemporary Health and Social Care*. Bristol: Policy Press.

24 Hsu, M.T., Kahn, D., Yee, D.H., Lee, W.L. (2004). Recovery through reconnection: a cultural design for family bereavement in Taiwan. *Death Stud* **28**: 761–86.

25 Holloway, M., Adamson, S., McSherry, W., Swinton, J. (2011). *Spiritual Care at the End of Life: a Systematic Review of the Literature*. Crown/Department of Health. Available at: http://www.dh.gov.uk/en/Publicationsandstatistics/Publications/PublicationsPolicyAndGuidance/DH_123812

26 Seymour, J., Payne, S., Chapman, A., Holloway, M. (2008). Hospice or home? Expectations of end-of-life care among white and Chinese older people in the UK. *Sociol Hlth Illness* **29**(6): 872–90.

27 Holloway, M. (2006). Death the great leveller? Towards a transcultural spirituality of dying and bereavement. *J Clin Nurs* (Special Issue Spirituality) **15**(7): 833–9.

28 Sheldon, F. (1997). *Psychosocial Palliative Care: Good Practice in the Care of the Dying and Bereaved*. Cheltenham: Stanley Thornes.

29 Beresford, P., Adshead, L., Croft, S. (2007). *Palliative Care, Social Work and Service Users: Making Life Possible*. London: Jessica Kingsley.

30 Hodge, D. (2008). Constructing spiritually modified interventions: cognitive therapy with diverse populations. *Int Soc Work* **51**(2): 178–92.

31 Callahan, A.M. (2009). Spiritually sensitive care in hospice social work. *J Soc Work End of Life Palliat Care* **5**(3): 169–85.

32 Crunkilton, D.D., Rubins, V.D. (2009). Psychological distress in end of life care: a review of issues in assessment and treatment. *J Soc Work End of Life Palliat Care* **5**(1): 75-93.

33 Cheers, B., Binell, M., Coleman, H., Gentle, I., Miller, G., Taylor, J., *et al.* (2006). Family violence: an Australian indigenous community tells its story. *Int Soc Work* **49**(1): 51–63.

34 O'Connor, M., Pearson, A. (2004-5). Ageing in place—dying in place: competing discourses for care of the dying in aged care policy. *Aust J Adv Nurs* **22**(2): 32-8.

35 Berkman, B. (ed) (2006). *Handbook of Social Work in Health and Ageing.* New York: Oxford University Press.

36 Chui, E. (2008). Introduction to special issue on ageing in place. *Ageing Int* **32**: 165-6.

37 Zapf, M.K. (2005). The spiritual dimension of person and environment: perspectives from social work and traditional knowledge. *Int Soc Work* **48**(5): 633–42, p. 637.

38 Holloway, M. (2009). Dying old in the twenty-first century. *Int Soc Work* **53**(5): 1–13.

39 Lloyd, M. [M Holloway]. (1995). *Embracing the Paradox: Pastoral Care with Dying and Bereaved People,* Contact Pastoral Monographs No 5. Edinburgh: Contact Pastoral Limited Trust.

40 Roberts, R.W., Nee, R.H. (eds) (1970). *Theories of Social Casework.* Chicago: University of Chicago Press.

41 Hinshaw, D.B. (2002). The spiritual needs of the dying patient. *J Am Coll Surg* **195**(4): 565–8.

42 Burton, R. (2004). Spiritual pain: origins, nature and management. *Contact* **143**: 3–13.

43 Greene, G., Jensen, C., Harper, D. (1996). A constructivist perspective on clinical social work practice with ethnically diverse clients. *Soc Work* **41**(2): 172–80, p. 174.

44 Altilio, T., Otis-Green, S., Dahlin, C.M. (2008). Applying the national quality forum for palliative and hospice care: a social work perspective. *J Soc Work End Life Palliat Care* **4**(1): 3–16.

45 Parton, N., O'Byrne, P. (2000). *Constructive Social Work: Towards a New Practice.* London: Macmillan.

46 Furness, S., Gilligan, P. (2010). *Religion, Belief and Social Work: Making a Difference.* Bristol: Policy Press.

CHAPTER 34

Care of children

Patricia Fosarelli

Benjy looked at his mother and began to cry. 'I don't want to stay in the hospital,' he cried. 'It's scary.' His mother hugged him and said, 'I'll stay with you, honey. I won't let them hurt you.' 'But they hurt me already,' Benjy insisted. Caressing his hair, his mother said, 'Want to say a prayer that you get well real soon?' He looked frightened. 'Suppose God is too busy to hear my prayer? Does God even know I'm here?'

Introduction—the world of ill children and their siblings

The illness of a child is distressing to parents; the greater the severity of the illness, the more distress it evokes. This is especially true when children are so ill that they must be hospitalized. Although this distress can be expected to decrease (at least somewhat) when the child is finally on the road to recovery, when a child is terminally ill, and there is diminishing hope for recovery, the distress experienced by child and parent can be profound, regardless of socio-economic factors and aspects of family dynamics and structure. No loving parent is at ease with a seriously or terminally ill child, not even the most religious of parents. Faith in God does not eradicate the feeling of protection parents have for their children and the sense of helplessness they feel when they are ill. For that reason, care for ill children also includes supportive care for their parents and siblings.

Many adults in health professions, ministry, or chaplaincy find it difficult to care for or minister to seriously and terminally ill children and adolescents, often because they identify ill children with their own children or grandchildren. Questions about God's justice in permitting a young person to suffer are often voiced, not only by these professionals, but often by his or her relatives as well. Often complicating the emotional and spiritual difficulties that these professionals have is the lack of knowledge of how to best minister to patients of varying developmental abilities.

Development in physical, emotional, cognitive, and social realms (to name a few) is a natural, ongoing process from infancy through adolescence, but it is not always an easy one, especially in a health-care setting. For example, the lack of development in speech means that a child cannot express what hurts him and probably cannot understand why he must endure seemingly endless tests and physical exams. The lack of development in social adaptability, as another example, means that a child will be frightened by the many unfamiliar people coming into her room, especially if they expect her to speak to them.

This lack of development extends to the siblings of the ill child, who might be both frightened for their sibling and frightened for their own wellbeing. Young children in an ego-centric phase of development may fret over why the parents leave them to be with their ill sibling; do the parents love the sibling more? Will the parents ever return or will they abandon the other children in order to remain with the ill sibling? Although many healthy siblings are troupers at this time in a family's life, others act out, socially or in school. Depending on their age, they might also abandon their belief in God or refuse to pray because God has not answered a prayer for the ill sibling's healing.

Siblings may feel guilty because they had argued with the ill child, even wishing he were dead. Now that the sibling is so ill, they feel remorse and guilt. In addition, they might be afraid that what happened to the ill child will also happen to them. Furthermore, if a sibling had prayed for God to 'punish' the ill child for something he had done to her, she might be afraid of her own power or that God will now 'punish' her.

For ill children and their siblings, particularly children who are old enough to express a belief in God, illness brings about some difficult questions about God. After all, if God can do anything, why can't God make Johnny better? A child asks, 'If God loves me, why doesn't he make my cancer go away so I won't be so sick?' It is important to understand the spiritual development of children and adolescents, and how its normal expression is disrupted by illness. Because spiritual development is often affected by development in other aspects of the child's life, a holistic approach must be embraced.

What is spirituality?

One of the best definitions of spirituality was offered by Yust *et al.* in their work on nurturing the spirituality of young people from the perspectives of various world religions. Although the majority of patients in the United States are, at least nominally, Christian, those caring for ill children and adolescents often encounter individuals who espouse other religions (or no religion at all). Hence, the Yust *et al.* definition is particularly apropos here.

> Spirituality is the intrinsic human capacity for self-transcendence in which the individual participates in the sacred – something greater than the self. It propels the search for connectedness, meaning, purpose, and ethical responsibility. It is experienced, formed, shaped, and expressed through a wide range of religious narratives, beliefs, and

practices, and is shaped by many influences in family, community, society, culture, and nature.[1]

While spirituality seeks to connect to that which is often beyond easy human understanding, it is affected by common experiences and relationships. Many people have had the experience of seeing something exquisitely beautiful and being held in silent awe. That is a spiritual moment evoked by nature. Many people have had relationships that demonstrated pure love. That is a spiritual moment evoked by another person. These experiences are important for human beings of all ages. Individuals often do not often have words for these real, but hard-to-describe, experiences, yet they are aware that something profound has taken place, an awareness that is more intuitive than cognitive.

Complicating this discussion is the distinction that some individuals make between non-religious spirituality and religious spirituality. In describing *non-religious spirituality*, Allen quotes two views, Lewis' relational understanding ('an orientation toward ourselves and our relations with all other things') and Willard's interiority view ('a kind of 'interiority'—the idea that there is an inside to the human being, and that this is the place where contact is made with the transcendental').[2] British researchers Hay and Nye view such spirituality in this way: 'Each of us has the potential to be much more deeply aware both of ourselves and of our intimate relationship with everything that is not ourselves.'[3] In addition to relationships and transcendence, *religious spirituality* intentionally includes references to the Ultimate (however the Ultimate is named and understood), especially being open to a relationship with the Ultimate. Many persons of faith understand the Ultimate as God, known by a multitude of names.

Development can be expected to play a role (but not necessarily *the* role) in spiritual awakening and maturing, especially in the ability to be in relationship and to enter into transcendence. At one period of our lives, we might describe a numinous (i.e. a highly spiritual) experience in one way, but at another period, we describe the same kind of experience in another way, based on our relationships, experiences, and ability to reflect on what has taken place. One might be an atheist at one period in her life, but a believer at the next; the interpretation of numinous experiences would be expected to differ at the two different stages of life, even if the experiences are similar. Numinous experiences do not just happen to believers in God, but to all who are open to them.

Children's spirituality

In the immediacy in which young children encounter the world, experiences and relationships play a very large role in how they make sense of what they encounter. Young children do not learn about their world primarily through cognitive processes. Children's own experiences with what they can see help them think about what they cannot see. Children's relationships—with parents, siblings, friends, and teachers—help them think about relationships with those whom they cannot directly experience with their senses, such as God.

Developmental approaches

Initially, much of the work on children's spirituality was largely based on developmental theorists, such as Jean Piaget (how children learn);[4] Erik Erikson (how human beings form relationships);[5] and James Fowler (how human beings come to religious faith).[6]

Swiss psychologist Jean Piaget (1896–1980) was interested in how children learn. By observing children, he came to the conclusion that there were four stages. Each successive age brings about greater sophistication in learning, culminating in an adult style:

- sensorimotor (infants and toddlers)
- pre-operations (preschoolers)
- concrete operations (elementary school-age children)
- formal operations (adolescents and adults).

Erik Erikson (1902–1994) was a Danish-German psychologist and psychoanalyst, who was interested in how human beings form relationships across the lifespan. He described eight stages, each of which has a developmental task that must be mastered in order to optimally move on to the next stage. Paediatric stages are:

- trust vs. mistrust (infants);
- autonomy vs. shame and doubt (toddlers);
- initiative vs. guilt (preschoolers);
- industry versus inferiority (elementary school-age children);
- identity vs. role diffusion (adolescents).

Finally, James Fowler (1940–) is an American developmental psychologist and Methodist minister. His interest was in how individuals came to faith. His work made no claim to address spirituality, although one's spirituality can certainly be influenced by one's faith tradition, and vice versa. Fowler identified a pre-stage of undifferentiated faith in infants and toddlers, and six stages across the remainder of the lifespan. Fowler relied heavily on the stages of Piaget and Erikson in formulating his own. Given the subject of this chapter, Fowler's stages will be explained in greater detail than those of his predecessors.

(1) Intuitive-projective is the preschoolers' stage. At this stage children learn through their experience with the world, projecting on to new persons, situations, places, or things, their previous experience with similar persons, situations, places or things. Many times, they project onto God the attributes (and flaws) of those adults who are significant in their lives. Yet, preschoolers are very intuitive about faith, having ideas that are not necessarily wrong, but certainly different from that of adults.

(2) Mythic-literal is the elementary school-age children's stage. At this stage, children are attracted to stories in which good defeats evil and to superheroes and super-heroines; many of these are found in Scripture. In addition, they can be very literal because literality is what is rewarded in early grades of school.

(3) Synthetic-conventional is the pre-teens' and early adolescents' stage. At this stage, children have an affiliation to their faith tradition of their younger years, while being exposed to and trying to make sense of different ways of thinking about God (or not thinking about God).

(4) Individuative-reflective is the older adolescents' and young adults' stage. At this stage, young people are grappling with what they believe. To come to an understanding of their beliefs, they must do much interior work which can only be done by them.

Sole reliance on strict stages of development is inappropriate for spirituality, for it would imply that the ability to encounter the Ultimate is merely a developmental one. Furthermore, although many children and teens progress through developmental stages at predictable times, the presence of a chronic, serious, or terminal illness might retard progress in one or more realms of development, even as young patients often transcend their illnesses to become more spiritually aware.

Experiential approaches

In 1983, Robinson described the religious experiences in childhood, as recalled by 4000 adult interviewees.[7] Such religious experiences were not uncommon, but there was a common theme that ran through many of the accounts, namely, that the individuals had not spoken very much about the episodes, as they had not been believed when they first reported them. This was surprising, since many of the respondents noted that their ideas about God clearly came from their parents or other significant adults in their lives. The difficulty seemed to be in the fact that the respondents' experiences were not overtly religious; there were no obvious religious persons, images, or symbols. For example, many of Robinson's subjects reported feeling oneness with all that is, a particular affinity with nature, and that there was more than could be experienced with the senses. Two examples follow:

> When I was about 10, I had a strange experience … I was walking back from school and suddenly stood still as the realization [sic] came over me, 'My body is now that of a child – but it's not ME. Soon I shall have the body of a young girl and later of a woman – but it still won't be ME; I am apart from my body and always will be'[8]
>
> When I was about five … [s]itting in the garden one day, I suddenly became conscious of a colony of ants in the grass, running rapidly and purposefully about their business … [I wondered] how much of their own pattern they were able to see for themselves. All at once I knew that I was so large that, to them, I was invisible—except, perhaps, as a shadow over their lives. I was gigantic, huge—able at one glance to comprehend … the whole colony. I had the power to destroy or scatter it, and I was completely outside the sphere of their knowledge and understanding. They were part of the body of the earth. However, they knew nothing of the earth except the tiny part of it which was their home …
>
> [compared with the larger world] I was tiny—so little and weak and insignificant that it really didn't matter at all whether I existed or not. And yet, as insignificant as I was, my mind was capable of understanding that the limitless world I could see was beyond my comprehension. [However,] I could know myself to be a minute part of it …
>
> A watcher would have to be incredibly big to see me and the world around me as I could see the ants and their world … Would he think me to be as unaware of his existence as I knew the ants were of mine? ... I *was* aware of him, in spite of my limitations. At the same time he was, and he was not, beyond my understanding …
>
> Every single person was a part of a Body, the purpose of which was as much beyond my comprehension now as I was beyond the comprehension of the ants. I was enchanted … No one [else] understood, but that was unimportant. I knew what I knew.[9]

Cognisant of this work, and following the lead of Rizzuto (see below), investigators such as Nye, Hay, and Coles sought a different way to approach children's spirituality. Although they acknowledged the influence of development on some aspects of spirituality, they recognized the limitations of a strict developmental model and trying to fit children into certain stages. These investigators started with the children who were permitted to express themselves through conversations (employing open-ended questions), drawing, and play. This has the advantage of permitting a young person to express what is on his mind, especially when describing God. Additionally, this would be in keeping with the views of most religions, i.e. human beings all are different and cannot be neatly categorized.

Rizzuto studied twenty young people and found that their images of God were drawn from a variety of sources (especially significant persons in their lives) and that their views affected their views of self, others, and the world.[10] Hay and Nye noted that four relationships were important in understanding spirituality from a non-religious view: a child's relationship to (1) self, (2) the world, (3) other people, and (4) God (this being the closest to traditional religious spirituality).[11] Coles interviewed a number of children in a very free, open-ended manner and found that many spontaneously included God in the conversation.[12]

Much interest (often tied to trying to encourage better religious pedagogy) has been expressed in the *Christian* spirituality of children and adolescents. For reasons of space, only three will be mentioned here, and all three firmly believe in the spiritual awareness of the child. In her work with young children, Sofia Cavalletti observed that even those from atheistic backgrounds could speak of insights about God and that they appreciated a transcendental reality independent of cognitive processes.[13] She wrote that children have 'the capacity to grasp the Mystery in its essentiality and to move within the world of Mystery with ease and spontaneity.'[14] Furthermore, '... the particular nature of the child's relationship with God could be problematic for the adult ... [can God] be so poor that there could be only one pathway—that of the adult—for establishing and maintaining a viable relationship with him.'[15] Donald Ratcliff echoed Cavalletti's beliefs: 'Children are just as much spiritual beings as are the adults in their lives.'[16] Furthermore, he was concerned about the over-reliance of developmental stages in interpreting a child's spirituality: 'While certain aspects of spirituality are influenced by development in other area, other aspects may be distinct from development ... While some features of stage theories may be questioned, there *are* systematic differences corresponding with age that can be identified ...'[17] Stonehouse noted:

> '... spiritual formation during childhood is seldom mentioned … From infancy, the personality is forming; children are developing the elements of their personhood with which they will relate to God. They are becoming persons who will be inclined toward faith or persons who will find it hard to trust, persons who take the initiative, can stick with a task and are ready to serve others, or persons who do not believe that they can make a difference in their own lives or the lives of anyone else … The spiritual life of the child is forming at a deep level … To not be concerned about spiritual formation during childhood is to ignore the very foundation of the spiritual life.'[18]

The experiences of ill children and adolescents

Children who have chronic, serious, or terminal illness have very different experiences than do their healthy peers, and such experiences can be expected to play a role in their spirituality, as can their relationships with members of the medical team.

An investigator who has done work in this area is Pendleton, a physician with an interest in how children cope with the stress of illness. In writing about her work, she quotes Coles: 'Children try to understand not only what is happening to them, but why; and in doing that, they call upon the religious life they have experienced, the spiritual values they have received, as well as other sources of potential explanation.'[19] Pendleton found that children approach an experience of illness by appraising it and then deciding upon a strategy with which to cope with it; coping strategies are influenced by the child's family and their coping styles, as well as the child's community. In terms of their religious/spiritual coping, in one study, she and her colleagues found that children either deferred to God (i.e. they understood God is in complete control, needing no input from them) or collaborated with God (i.e. they worked with God).[20] In a second study, she and her colleagues interviewed children with cystic fibrosis (for which there is no cure) to determine how their faith helped them cope with their illness. Eleven sets of religious coping strategies were identified:

> *Declarative* [child announces something to happen and God is thought to automatically do it], *Petitionary* [child appeals to God to intercede], *Collaborative* [child and God both take the responsibility for dealing with the stressor], *Divine Support* [God is viewed as assisting, benefitting, protecting, and comforting the child], *Divine Intervention* [God intercedes without direction or appeal from child], *Divine is Irrelevant* [child does not rely on God at all], *Benevolent Religious/Spiritual Reframing, Negative Religious/Spiritual Reframing, Spiritual Social Support, Discontent with God or Congregation,* and *Ritual Response* [use of ritual in an effort to cope with the stressor]. Interestingly, some of the strategies identified (e.g. *Divine is Irrelevant*) were not similar to adult religious coping strategies – highlighting the uniqueness of the child's experience ... Also unique to children, most reported that coping strategies were helpful to their physical, mental religious/spiritual, and social adjustment'.[21, with permission of Wiph and Stock publishers.]

Yet, ill children and teens have deeply spiritual experiences as well, experiences that just seem to be given to them. Diane Komp, a pediatric oncologist has described some of their insights in her book *A Window to Heaven*.[22] Several of her examples follow

> [Mary Beth, a six-year-old with cancer] told her mother that Jesus came to her in a dream with one of her grandfathers who had died before she was born. Together, Jesus and her grandfather told her of her impending death and encouraged her not to be afraid. She awoke with the peace and reassurance that she would soon be with Jesus and her grandfather ... It was her absolute peace that baffled her mother.[23]

> [A four-year-old Asian boy] whose family did not practice a Christian faith, had a vision of an angel visiting him and then summoned members of the hospital staff into his room. He thanked each of them for helping him and then said goodbye. Then he laid [sic] down and died ... He was not upset, not at all.[24]

> [A 19-year-old patient, whose spinal cord tumour left him a quadriplegic, spoke of a vision while he was meditating.] Tom saw himself in a beautiful garden and saw a man there, seated on a bench ... The man touched him, and Tom reported that he moved in his bed for the first time in months. He did not want to leave the garden or the man's presence, but his companion went ahead and told him that he could not come with him yet. I asked Tom if he knew who the man was. He said, 'I *know* it was Jesus.'[25]

> [Tony was a child with leukaemia.] Out of the blue, Tony said [to his mother], 'He wants me.' His mother was frightened, but found the courage to ask, 'Do you mean God?' When he answered in the affirmative, his mother asked him if God spoke to him in a dream. 'No. He speaks to me when I pray.' 'What do you mean, when you pray?' 'I start praying and then I listen.' 'Is it scary?' 'No. It's peaceful.'[26]

How do these theories and stories relate to working with an ill child or adolescent? For the remainder of this chapter, each age group will be approached both developmentally and 'super-developmentally' (i.e. beyond that which is strictly development). Each section will open with a vignette; identify several key features of the age, noting how illness can impact development; and demonstrate how to approach the age group beyond strictly developmental bounds, in the context of illness. Emphasis will be on ill children and adolescents.

Infants (0–12 months of age) and Toddlers (12 months to about 2 ½ years of age)

Lenny is a 14-month-old boy with repeated infections requiring hospitalizations. During these hospitalizations, Lenny usually needs an IV and has to undergo many procedures. He clings to his mother, but when he must be taken from her for a particular procedure, he screams and holds his arms out to her.

Developmental considerations

Because these children engage their world by looking at and touching objects, and listening to them (if they make a sound), this developmental stage is curtailed when an ill child is restrained or not permitted to take anything by mouth (NPO) and cannot relate to the world freely.

Either a very young child learns to trust his caregivers and his environment, or he does not. Infants and toddlers with multiple hospitalizations, often accompanied by painful procedures and encounters with strangers, experience much mistrust of their world, especially when two developmentally appropriate anxieties (stranger anxiety and separation anxiety) are also present. Since children who experience acute, chronic, or terminal illness are often approached by strangers in a healthcare facility, they are often distraught.

Because very young children do not have the language to express their ideas about God, it is difficult to know what those ideas are. We do know that they often take their lead from those closest to them. Children older than 6–8 months of age can often imitate religious gestures made by their family members. With repeated observation and modelling, they can use a gesture at the appropriate time (e.g. folding hands before eating or sleeping). Although it is not clear what the child really understands about the gesture, it is clear that when a parent says to a 12-month-old infant, 'Let's pray,' a child who has seen parents fold their hands when they say, 'Let's pray,' will do so herself.

In terms of relationships, children learn to have a rudimentary faith in others and their environment. When those persons are trustworthy and speak about God in a reverent way, children learn to associate God with good things, something that does not happen if God's name is used profanely or sloppily.

Super-developmental considerations

Because infants and toddlers cannot speak, it is impossible to know if children are having any numinous experiences. Because nearly every world religion believes that children have a special place in God's eyes, the wisest course of action is to assume that such young children *are* having highly spiritual experiences and to treat them gently and with great respect, permitting a familiar person to stay with them.

Preschoolers (3–5 years of age)

Becky is a 4-year-old girl who is being treated for leukaemia; her prognosis is uncertain. She has already been hospitalized 7 times in the last year. Becky becomes angry when people need to touch her or perform procedures. She is often demanding and whiney. Her mother usually stays with her, and when her mother gets upset, Becky becomes even more demanding. Becky's mother is very religious and is often praying in Becky's room.

Developmental considerations

Healthy preschoolers are in love with life, active, playful, and talkative. Instead of using adult logic to make sense of the world, they use their own 'logic,' which can be fanciful and ego-centric (e.g. when asked why the sun is shining, a preschooler might respond, 'It's my birthday'). Preschoolers have vivid imaginations, which can be used to have fun, but can also cause fear when they imagine scary things. Chronically and seriously ill children have often had a great deal of medically inflicted pain (in the name of making them better), and they can demonstrate anticipatory fear, because pain is scary. Chronically and seriously ill children often believe that their illness and pain are punishments for something they have done (an example of their ego-centricity).

Preschoolers also fear being abandoned by their parents, and every time a parent leaves, it can cause even many ill children to become distressed. Since relationships are so important, emotionally and spiritually, efforts should be made to permit a familiar person to be present. These children do not understand the permanence of death, so regardless of how ill they are, they cannot understand that they might die (and never return) from their illness.

Even though young children take their lead from parents and other significant adults in their lives *vis-à-vis* God, they have many intuitive ideas about God that are not necessarily wrong, but are different from adult ideas. For example, a 5-year-old might draw a picture of God that contains all colours because 'everyone is in God and God is in everyone. So, God has to be the colour of everyone.' At the same time, a child can project onto God the experiences that she has had with her parents or other significant adults. If parents are punitive, then God is presumed to be also. If parents are kind, so is God. Children whose parents threaten them with God's wrath are particularly likely to have negative images of God, while the opposite is true for children whose parents reassure them of God's love. The experience of a chronic or serious illness causes the ego-centric preschooler to conclude that God is mad and punishing her, often for reasons that have no basis in reality, but make sense to her. Being ill seems like punishment, as one can't go out and play, and one often can't eat what one chooses.

Super-developmental considerations

Children, healthy or ill, can be asked open-ended questions about what they think of the world or how they feel about various situations. Many will spontaneously mention God. As has been noted earlier, healthy preschoolers can have numinous experiences, as can children who are seriously or terminally ill. Ill children might describe seeing Jesus, an angel, or another religious figure when children are not Christian; a deceased relative or friend might also be seen. These experiences should *never* be attributed to an overactive imagination without further questioning, and no attempt should be made to lead them to answer in a certain fashion. Such children should be invited to speak about the experience and the way it made them feel, using open-ended questions, such as 'What did you see? How did that make you feel? How did you know who the person was? What did she or he say to you?' Many times, children of this age like to draw what they have seen or experienced, and that should be encouraged.

Elementary school-aged children (5–10 years of age)

Eddie is an 8-year-old boy with severe asthma. He has been hospitalized many times in his young life. He has also had admissions to the intensive care unit, and he has needed to be on a ventilator twice. Eddie hates what asthma is doing to his life, because it limits his activities, especially during seasons when his asthma symptoms are worse. He says, 'Did I make God mad at me? Why am I so sick and all my friends are OK? I wish I knew what I did to make God so mad. Maybe God doesn't love me.'

Developmental considerations

Children of this age use concrete objects to learn new skills or concepts, and are highly concrete in their approach to the world; in school, they quickly learn that there is often only one right answer, but many incorrect ones. Hence, they see the entire world with a 'black or white' lens, unable to detect any shades of grey. This has its drawbacks, because in seeing the world as one way or the other, the child becomes concerned when things do not fit neatly into a category. This is especially heightened during illness, when we often do not have the results of a test immediately or the results are inconclusive. The inability to give a clear answer to questions about his health increases a child's anxiety, potentially harming his relationships with others. Terminally ill children of this age generally understand the irreversibility of death, but they do not always make the connection between their own dying and the fact that they will not go to college or get married, for example.

School is the centre of the social lives of children in this age group; hence, chronic or serious illness that disrupts a child's school attendance or participation in school activities is very difficult for an ill child. Children are often urged to work hard in school in order to succeed, but chronically and seriously ill children often miss many days of school. Not only do they miss peer interactions, but they also miss a part of their education. Even when ill children are tutored at home, they still miss the experience of class learning. This can make susceptible children feel different and inferior, even though—academically—they know the material. The unfairness of life really hurts these children who prefer a predictable, cut-and-dried world.

Children's experience with schooling affects the way they think about God, which tends to be literal. Faced with a world that seems out of control, these children enjoy hearing, seeing, and reading about situations in which good people or situations overcome their bad counterparts. This is especially true for ill children. Children of this age love to hear stories from their faith tradition's scripture, and the 'bigger' the story, the better it is. The younger children in this stage tend to accept such stories wholeheartedly, but with time, they begin to question how certain stories (especially miraculous events) could possibly be true.

Children of this age who believe in God usually adopt the beliefs of parents and other significant adults. Like adults, they are often confused and distressed by unanswered prayers. Because they think in such 'black and white' terms, they often believe that *they* have done something to make God mad (so that God won't grant their prayer), God doesn't love them, God is punishing them, or God is too busy for them. For ill children, whose prayers poignantly beg for release from their illnesses, unanswered prayers are particularly painful.

Super-developmental considerations

Children, healthy or ill, can be asked open-ended questions about what they think of the world or how they feel about various situations. Many will spontaneously mention God. When they do, additional open-ended questions include: 'Of all the people that you know, who do you think knows God best? When you think about God, how do you feel? Do you talk to God (prayer)? What sort of things do you talk to God about? Have you ever been somewhere and thought God was nearby?'[27]

As has been noted earlier, children of this age (healthy or ill) can have numinous experiences and, if encouraged, they will talk about them. Often, it is their fear that they will not be believed that keeps them from sharing their experiences. In these experiences, they often see a religious figure from their faith tradition or a deceased relative. In both cases, the person whom they encounter often encourages them to not be afraid or tells them something that will happen. In general, these experiences bring great comfort and peace to the children, although the adults in their lives might be frightened by them. Although some presume that such experiences are the result of lack of oxygen or the effects of certain medications, there have been many occasions in which such experiences have occurred in children not receiving any medications or not obviously experiencing a lack of oxygen. A non-judgmental approach to these young people is important, permitting them to tell of their experiences in their own ways, especially by using open-ended questions, such as the ones above, and listening carefully to their responses. Drawing a picture of the experience is also helpful.

Pre-teens and young adolescents (10–14years of age)

Felicia is tired of the constraints that her illness places on her activities. At a time when she wants to be with her friends and do what they do, she must watch her diet. In addition, she is not permitted to engage in certain activities because they will tire her out. 'I hate my life,' she says. 'Why can't I be like everyone else? Where is God when I need him? Maybe we're all just fooling ourselves. Maybe there is no God to whom prayers go. Maybe it's all made up.'

Developmental considerations

Young people at this age are beginning the process of thinking and reasoning in an adult manner, and they can imagine themselves in situations or places of which they have no actual previous experience. They understand that death is irreversible, and terminally ill young people can express deep hurt that they will not become adults, with all that entails. They might quietly grieve inwardly or express grief outwardly, either in a traditional 'sad' way or in an 'acting out' stage.

Young people of this age prefer to be with their peers more than with other individuals. They can spend hours conversing in-person, by phone, and texting. Their peers help them to better understand themselves and where they fit in. When they were younger, they took their identity largely from their parents. As they become older, they want their own identity to be separate from their parents, no matter how much they love them. So, they often try different 'roles' to see which fit, to see who they really are. Obviously, an emotionally healthy peer group is one of the best influences a young person can have in his life, because they model good behaviour and normalize it. Chronically, seriously, or terminally ill young people often miss out on much of the 'give-and-take' of peer groups. Because their development might be delayed and they have many medications to take, procedures to undergo, or medical appointments to keep, they might not be able to spend as much time with their friends in ways that they would like. They especially feel left out if friends don't keep in touch by phone, e-mails, or texting.

Although, in the past, young people have often adopted the ideas of their parents, now they consider new ideas, either because they are encountering them for the first time, or because they are rebelling (to some extent) against the wholesale acceptance of their parents' ideas. Because they have just emerged from a period of literalness about their faith, they have many questions, especially in light of their formal operational level of thinking, as they try to make sense of various other ways of thinking about God. Does God exist? Is there more than one God (and do I believe in the 'right' God)? Why does God permit innocent people to suffer? Does God really care about people? Chronic and serious illness precipitate questions about God's existence, love, and concern for those who are suffering. Ill young people might express anger at the God who permits them to be ill, blaming God for it all. Other ill young people might abandon belief in God altogether.

Super-developmental considerations

Young adolescents, healthy or ill, can be asked open-ended questions about what they think of the world or how they feel about various situations. Many will spontaneously mention God. When they do, additional open-ended questions include: What is the difference between someone who *knows* about God and someone who knows God? How do you think someone gets to know God? Do you think you know God?' Have you ever felt God close to you?'[28]

Still other young people have numinous experiences that actually draw them closer to God, even in the midst of their pain and suffering. These numinous experiences are as varied as the young people themselves and might not contain 'overt' religious images or symbols. The common denominator is that they help the young person receiving it to be less fearful and experience something of the divine. When we hear of such experiences, they should always be taken seriously and treated sensitively, especially if they bring greater peace and comfort to an ill young person. Attentive listening is one of the best gifts such a young person can receive.

Older adolescents (15–19 years of age)

18-year-old Josh has cystic fibrosis. As he has gotten older, he needs oxygen continuously, and this makes it go to places that he would like to go. Although he had more friends when he was younger and his lungs were healthier, few of the guys come around to see him now because they don't know what to say. Josh has resigned himself to never getting married ('What girl would want me?'). Although he was very religious when he was younger, he now often wonders if there really is a God. 'If there's a God, why did he let things like cystic fibrosis come into existence?'

Developmental considerations

Older adolescents are still working out their identity and trying out various roles, including interpersonal relationships, future career, or college, etc. Naturally, terminally ill and many chronically ill adolescents might not be able to think about a future, because their own is so unsettled.

Older adolescents are also increasingly interested in romantic relationships, usually with a person of the opposite gender. Although there is still great interest in peer groups, many adolescents prefer the company of a best friend or girlfriend/boyfriend. Chronically, seriously, and terminally ill adolescents might not have the opportunities for romantic relationships, often because of rejection by those in whom they are interested. In addition, opportunities for close friendships might also be limited, depending on the severity of the illness. Like younger teens, they especially feel left out if friends don't keep in touch by phone, e-mails, or texting.

Older adolescents often question what they themselves believe. For most of their lives, they have been heavily influenced (positively or negatively) by the beliefs of parents, guardians, and peers. Now they must come to a better self-understanding of what they truly believe. For chronically, seriously, and terminally ill adolescents (especially the latter), what they believe is often tied to their experience of being ill. As they grapple with issues of limitation and mortality, these individuals cannot necessarily rely on the opinions of those who may not share their condition.

Super-developmental considerations

The same approach can be taken that was described for younger adolescents. Although some of the older adolescents' numinous experiences might not be obviously religious, they might be profound nonetheless, as she gains insight that she would not have had without the illness or that healthy peers do not appreciate.

For these individuals—as for all children and adolescents—nonjudgmental listening, patience, respect, and openness will encourage growth in self-awareness and growth in spirituality.

Conclusion

In the area of paediatrics, one must have a healthy respect for a given patient's developmental level and the ways that parents and other significant adults have shaped his or her views. Yet, one must also be aware that children and adolescents often have deeply spiritual experiences that are not necessarily limited by what they 'should' be thinking or experiencing at their age or stage, experiences that might even be unfathomable to those closest to them. Hence, one must be open to hearing about such experiences without judgment, encouraging young patients to tell their stories in their own ways. Although understanding a patient's development *is* highly important in order to provide age-appropriate physical, emotional, and spiritual care, the essence of spirituality is that it transcends neat categories. Appreciating a patient's spirituality—whether it seems to have a developmental basis or a super-developmental basis—can encourage health professionals to grow in their own spiritual lives.

References

1 Yust, K., Johnson, A., Sasso, S., Roehlkepartain, E. (2006). *Nurturing Child and Adolescent Spirituality: Perspectives from the World's Religious Traditions*, p. 8. Lanham: Rowman & Littlefield Publishers.

2 Allen, H. (2008). Exploring children's spirituality from a christian perspective. In: H. Allen (ed.) *Nurturing Children's Spirituality: Christian Perspectives and Best Practices*, p. 7. Eugene: Cascade Books.

3 Hay, D., Nye, R. (2006). *The Spirit of the Child*, rev. edn, pp. 21–2. London: Jessica Kingsley Publishers.

4 Singer, D., Revenson, T. (1978). *A Piaget Primer: How a Child Thinks*. New York: New American Library.

5 Erikson, E. (1997). *The Life Cycle Completed*. New York: W.W. Norton & Co.

6 Fowler, J. (1981). *Stages of Faith: the Psychology of Human Development and the Quest for Meaning*. New York: HarperSan Francisco.

7 Robinson, E. 1983). *The Original Vision: a Study of the Religious Experience of Childhood*. New York: Seabury Press.

8 [7], pp. 114–15.

9 [7], pp. 12–13.

10 Rizzuto A.M. (1979). *The Birth of the Living God*. Chicago: University of Chicago Press.

11 [3], pp. 115–18.

12 Coles, R. (1990). *The Spiritual Life of Children*. Boston: Haughlin-Mifflin Co.

13 Cavalletti, S. (1992). *The Religious Potential of the Child*. Chicago: Liturgy Training Publications.

14 Cavalletti, S. (2002). *The Religious Potential of the Child: 6–12 Years Old*, p. x. Oak Park: Catechesis of the Good Shepherd Publications.

15 [14], p. xiii.

16 Ratcliff, D., May, S. (2007). Identifying children's spirituality. In: D. Ratcliff (ed.) *Children's Spirituality: Christian Perspectives, Research, and Applications*, p. 7. Eugene: Cascade Books.

17 Ratcliff, D. (2008). The spirit of the child past: a century of children's spirituality research. In: H. Allen H (ed.) *Nurturing Children's Spirituality: Christian Perspectives and Best Practices*, p. 37. Eugene: Cascade Books.

18 Stonehouse, C. (1998). *Joining Children on the Spiritual Journey: Nurturing a Life of Faith*, p. 21. Grand Rapids: Baker Books.

19 Pendleton, S., Benore, E., Jonas, K., Norwood, W., Hermann, C. (2004). Spiritual Influences in Helping Children to Cope with Life Stressors. In: D. Ratcliff (ed.) *Children's Spirituality: Christian Perspectives, Research, and Applications*, p. 361. Eugene: Cascade Books.

20 [19], pp. 370.

21 [19], pp. 371.

22 Komp, D. (1992). *A Window to Heaven: When Children See Life in Death*. Grand Rapids, MI: ZondervanPublishingHouse.

23 [22], pp. 35–36.

24 [22], pp. 41.

25 [22], pp. 43.

26 [22], pp. 73.

27 Allen, H., Oschwald, H. (2008). God across the generations: the spiritual influence of grandparents. In: H. Allen (ed.) *Nurturing Children's Spirituality: Christian Perspectives and Best Practices*, pp. 284–5. Eugene: Cascade Books.

28 [27], pp. 284–5.

CHAPTER 35

Care of elderly people

Elizabeth MacKinlay

Introduction

Increasing longevity and an increasing number of older people living with multiple chronic diseases are two main factors that have changed the face of ageing and care of the ageing, particularly in western countries in recent decades. In the past, the focus has been on acute healthcare episodes; but this has changed to the need to care for more people living with chronic conditions that need interventions from time to time, where often cure is not possible and the focus has moved largely to maintenance of health and wellbeing in later life.

The majority of older people continue to live in the community, either independently, or with the assistance of some services. In most western societies, approximately 5% of older people live in residential aged care, with that percentage increasing in those over 85 years of age.

More recently, a growing emphasis has been given to positive and successful ageing,[1] especially to active physical and psychosocial ageing. This was an important development in addressing issues of ageing, but the focus on physical and psychosocial aspects was not enough. The question of meaning is being raised as an important component of the quality of the life for elderly people. Do more years of life result in greater enjoyment, happiness, and health, or simply the experience of a longer time to wait until death? Put more simply, do added years of life mean *life* is added to those years? These questions introduce yet another perspective to ageing, that of meaning and the spiritual dimension of ageing. As the baby boomers join the ranks of older adults, these issues of life meaning can be expected to gain greater importance.

The possibility of the spiritual journey continuing into later life was neglected until recently. The journey of later life is not only about vulnerability, frailty, mental health, illness, and dying, but also about resilience and flourishing. Sometimes the journey can be surprising to those who watch and care, as some older people with multiple diseases and little capacity for independent living seem to live with hope and tenacity in the face of even death itself. This chapter addresses both the possibilities for continued spiritual growth in ageing and for care of spiritual needs of older people.

Mental health and growing older

Many authors have written of ubiquitous feelings of sadness and loneliness experienced by older people, and in part this can be attributed to loss of loved ones through death or perhaps separation from others through admission to residential aged care facilities. Depression has sometimes been attributed simply to growing older, and it has been said that being old is enough to make one depressed. However, how much is this part of the ageing process and how much of this is disease process, somc of which can be treatable? Issues of mental health have increasingly gained attention; dementia and depression have been identified as the cause of significant morbidity in later life. Yet according to Butler,[2] depression is the most treatable of all mental health problems of later life. A large prospective study of people moving into later life[3] found that depressive symptoms independently predicted the development of limitations of activities of daily living and that these people may be at greater risk of losing functional ability than people who were not depressed as they grow older. Blazer[4] has linked spirituality, depression and older people, as he brings a wealth of research and practice to reflect on depression in later life, noting 'finding meaning in one's life at the end of life is critical to avoiding a prolonged and terminal dark night of the soul.'[4, p. 1178]

Dementia is another condition that adversely affects the mental health of older adults, with forecasts of increasing numbers of people living with dementia, in coming decades. In 2008 in Australia, the third leading cause of death was dementia.[5] According to one source, from 2000 to 2050 the number of Australians with dementia is predicted to increase by 327%;[6] Jorm *et al.*[7] give a slightly more conservative estimate of 241%. When cognitive capacity diminishes in the process of dementia, connecting with these people becomes increasingly challenging, but a number of studies now have shown that it is still possible to communicate with people who have dementia, spiritually and emotionally. Engaging with the person and recognizing individuality and spiritual wellbeing may be fostered and encouraged.[8] Strategies identified by Ryan *et al.*[8] to affirm personhood and encourage spirituality include communication, sharing life stories (reminiscence), and assisting with participation in religious life.

The spiritual dimension in later life: meaning in life

In recent decades there has been an increased awareness of the importance of the spiritual dimension in later life. Research has mapped the spiritual dimension of ageing, the importance of the spiritual dimension to the process of ageing,[9–11] and spiritual care in frail older people.[12] Scholarship in the area of spirituality, theology and ageing is growing.[13] Swinton particularly has addressed issues of disability, dementia, and spirituality in later life,[14,15] and has further explored the spiritual and theological ramifications of dementia in relation to notions of persons, personhood, and dementia; concepts vital for understanding spiritual and pastoral needs and care with older people. Even so, more remains to be achieved in this field in developing research that can guide evidence-based practice of spiritual care.

A model for spiritual growth and care in later life

What are the possibilities for spiritual growth and care in later life? Like the psychological dimension, changes can still occur in the spiritual dimension in later life. In fact some important changes are possible. Just as Erikson's[16] eighth stage of psychosocial development, integrity versus despair, described an outcome of wisdom where this stage was successfully negotiated; changes within the spiritual dimension can also occur in later life. Like Erikson's model, not all people achieve these changes; some may become locked in despair, while others find peace and joy.

The later years of life are the years when physical decline may stimulate questions of life meaning with greater urgency than earlier in life.[2,10,12] A growing awareness of impending mortality, as the time left to live grows shorter will often help to focus the ageing person's thoughts and reflections on meaning.

Many definitions of spirituality have been presented over the past few decades. For all the variations, almost all contain a focus on meaning and relationship. MacKinlay's model of spiritual tasks and process of ageing,[10] based on data from older people, recognizes a total of six themes; first, a central core of ultimate meaning, and secondly, response to life, based on the person's sense of ultimate meaning. There are four other spiritual themes; transcendence (or transformation), searching for final life meanings, finding new relationships or intimacies, and finding hope. The model is dynamic with close interrelationships with each of the themes. It is based on the assumption that all humans have a spiritual dimension, although not all will choose to practice a religion. Religion is seen as a part of spirituality, in those who practice religion. There are aspects of religion, however, such as ritual and symbol that all humans respond to, even in secular societies.

Spiritual growth and living independently

Ideally, we would continue to develop our spiritual dimension into later life, building spiritual strategies to enable flourishing and resilience, in the same way as we become conscious of the need to exercise the body to gain and retain physical fitness in late life. Health in the latter part of life requires physical, social, psychological, and spiritual care. It has long been recognized that people begin to become more introspective from mid-life onwards,[17] and as people become more aware of this new quest, this is an ideal time to begin consciously doing life review, through reminiscence and spiritual autobiography.

The current cohort of older people in western societies is more likely to be living in their own homes for much longer. However, even those who are in residential aged care need a focus on holistic health and wellbeing that includes spiritual wellbeing. Not only is this vital for personal flourishing, but it is likely to have the added effect of reducing costs of care for older people. It is likely that those who show evidence of resilience will need fewer care services, but showing this through research is challenging as there are many variables to take into account.

Spiritual assessment and older people

The first important aspect of spiritual care for older people is to discover how the particular person addresses issues of the spiritual dimension in their own lives. It is not possible to prescribe processes of spiritual care for all older people. There are many differences between older people; their birth cohort, life experiences, education, family relationships, spiritual, and/or religious orientation and work history, all of which need to be considered when spiritual care and needs are addressed.

Furthermore, a score of spiritual health/wellbeing will not be particularly helpful in deciding appropriate spiritual care. Taking a spiritual history and listening to the person's story will be valuable. Even people with dementia have a story, although this story is often ignored or brushed over in the busyness of residential aged care. It is vital to connect with the person at their point of need for spiritual growth or spiritual care.

Spiritual tasks and process of ageing

Spirituality is more than a set of leisure skills, as it is sometimes described. Spirituality is about core meaning and relationship. There is the potential for continuing spiritual growth and development in the latter part of life. Yet, there are enormous variations between different people as they grow older. Some people experience blockages in their spiritual growth; sometimes traumatic experiences from earlier life may impede spiritual growth and healing. Sometimes these experiences and memories present as serious problems preventing the older person coming to a sense of peace, joy, and fulfilment in their final years of life. Yet some older people are able to process these issues, and come to a sense of wholeness and wellbeing in these last years. Issues of guilt, lack of forgiveness and the need for reconciliation are examples of common factors that may impede spiritual growth and dilute hope. Recent studies have illuminated the process of spiritual changes in later life.[12] The aim for older people is to meet their potential for flourishing, even in the face of losses and disabilities that so frequently accompany growing older.

Spiritual tasks and process of ageing

The model of spiritual tasks and process of ageing, developed by MacKinlay[10] is used in this chapter as a framework for spiritual assessment and growth in later life. Five of these six tasks are outlined in the next section.

Relationship and connectedness

Relationship is a vitally important aspect of human need. Often relationship is considered from a psychological perspective. However, there is an important spiritual component to the spiritual dimension that is played out in the very depths of relationships. The need for relationship is at the core of what it means to be human. Consider the fact that societies use solitary confinement as punishment for people. It is hard to be separated from other human contact, yet many older people do live alone. While many do so from choice, others have no choice. Older people who are able to maintain social activities often enjoy the freedoms of living alone, but this often changes when they lose their ability to drive or to use public transport due to increased disability. People can become 'house-bound'. Older people are more likely to have lost the closest relationships in their lives; the need to develop new relationships is as important in later life as it is at any point across the life-span.

This need for depth of relationship, and for intimacy with another, is at its core, spiritual. Carroll and Dyckman[18, p. 123] write that 'At the deepest core of my being I need to be known and loved as I am'. Older people also need this sense of intimacy; too often these needs are forgotten in the busyness of aged care facilities. We[19] found in one study with people with dementia that the need for connection with others was almost synonymous with meaning in people with dementia, even if they were unable to articulate the exact nature of the relationship.

The intimacy of sexuality in later life is often removed for older people due either to physical ailments, or as they lose their partners through death and physical separation. As people live longer there will be times where new relationships may be formed among those in their 70s or even into their 90s. Current residential aged care facilities are too often not welcoming to any kind of sexual expression, even within marriage, and would find it even harder to look favourably upon sexuality within homosexual relationships or outside marriage, despite community attitudes in so many places changing towards greater acceptance of gay and lesbian relationships, and non-married partnerships.

Transcendence and transformation in older people

There is often an assumption that older people can't change; yet, in some ways, older people have to make some of the biggest changes of their lives as they adjust to losses and disabilities that they experience. It is this very experience of loss that may assist the older person to begin a journey into transcendence. Transcendence can mean self-transcendence, moving beyond the focus on self. Frankl[20] disputes the belief that this state can be arrived at merely by striving ones-self, maintaining that people can't 'self-actualize'. Rather, this state of transcendence is one of grace. Frankl has described transcendence as 'self-forgetting.'[21, p. 138] Tornstam[22] coined the term 'gerotranscendence,' which means a sense of cosmic transcendence, a need for solitude that seems to occur with a number of older people. MacKinlay[12] found that self-transcendence was sometimes stimulated by increasing losses, frailty, and disabilities of ageing. This is similar to gerotranscendence in some aspects, but different in that it might also have a spiritual aspect.

Searching for final life meanings

Humans naturally respond to story. The major faiths all have story at their core. For the Abrahamic faiths, the stories carries the sense of relationship with God, and hence with community and family, and ultimately, with each individual person. As we go through life we attach meaning to life experiences, at some times more consciously than at others. When confronted by a terminal illness or simply realising the nearness of our own death, as in extreme old age, we may begin to revisit our story, to search out the ultimate meanings of our journeys. Questions arise such as: 'Why am I here?' 'What has been the purpose of my life?' It is then that feelings of guilt and the need for forgiveness and reconciliation may become evident. This is more likely in older people.

Doing life review or spiritual reminiscence

Kenyan has written that 'we are story,'[23, p. 30] meaning that story is so central to our identity as individual human beings that it is not possible to strip our stories from us. An important aspect of growing older is the possibility of being able to tell our whole story for the first time. Through our life journey we are often conscious of having a life story, but our consciousness of our story increases in importance as we become more aware of our own mortality. Being able to tell the story requires a story teller and a story listener.[24] The story is never complete until the end of a person's life, but each time it is told there is the possibility to add or subtract, or to edit it as new meanings are perceived. To be authentic, the story must ring true, but it is always necessary to acknowledge that each story is told from the story teller's perspective, and each person's story may differ in some aspects from others' accounts, even others in their own families. In recent years with the work of Butler[2] and others, reminiscence work has become common. Often groups will work on telling their life story, perhaps recording it, printing, and illustrating it. Activity groups in residential aged care use reminiscence in various ways, as activities, to draw on memories of times long-gone. However, there is also the possibility of enriching the lives of older adults by engaging in spiritual reminiscence in which the participants use various strategies to tell their stories, including life lines and metaphors, and then linking events of their stories with God's story and the story of their community of faith. In doing this, they seek to ask the question, of both highlights of their lives, and the low points and tragedies, where was God? It is often the act of reflecting on the connecting points that these earlier life events can be celebrated, or in the case of difficult times, brought to a sense of healing, reconciliation, and wholeness. Such groups may be conducted over a 6–12-week period, with small groups of people working together and sharing of their life stories. Birren and Cochran[24] have produced a valuable guide for guided autobiography groups. Burnside's Working with Older Adults[25] and Morgan's[26] remembering your story, on spiritual autobiography are other valuable resources in this area. Spiritual reminiscence can also be effective with people who have no explicit faith, adapting the guidelines by focusing on life meaning, rather than relationship with God.

Hope

Hope is difficult to define; it can be easier to identify hopelessness than hope. Yet Moltmann[27] sees hope in Christian perspective, 'forward looking and forward moving, and therefore also revolutionizing and transforming the present.'[27, p. 16] He describes hope as 'the glow that suffuses everything here in the dawn of an expected new day.'[27, p. 16] It is this glow that lights up the elderly people who have identified hope in their lives; people who now flourished in spite of all the losses, all the disabilities—people who find there is still hope. *Hopelessness* is an important component in the decision to take one's own life through suicide. Gulbinat, cited in De Leo.[28, p. 2] noted that when the 15–24 age group is compared with the 75+ age group, suicide is up to seven times more likely among the 75+ group, taking the medians for suicide in four continents Yet, there is a clear difference in community perceptions of the meaning of suicide, based on the age of the person dying, in most western societies. When young people take their own lives it is widely regarded as a tragedy; when a person over 75 years of age does it is often regarded as being sad, but it may also be said: 'he/she had lived a good life and didn't suffer,' based on the assumption that there is no meaning left in life for older people. On the contrary, living into old age has the potential to bring the life story to completion, with renewed sense of meaning and purpose. Suicide at any point of life is to be prevented if possible. One of the complicating factors among older people who suicide is the difficulty of identifying those at risk due to the fact that, unlike younger people, older adults do not usually have a history of suicide attempts.[28]

What is the reality of hope among older people themselves? In a study[29] evaluating the effectiveness of small group pastoral care and prayer and meditation for older people with dementia, group members readily discussed their sources of hope; main sources were prayer and friends, some spoke of God. People with dementia do not often get the opportunity to speak and share on meaningful topics, and these excerpts from session transcripts (using pseudonyms) clearly show their engagement with issues of hope: 'Beverly: ... it's all God for me now because I'm in the old, old age now, yes, no, I think it's necessary for some people, it helps them very much, nice to know that that help is there.'

In another session, the facilitator used the image of seasons of life to open discussion with the group, around the topic of hope:

Facilitator 4: It sounds as if you have a pattern in a day. You seem to find that helpful.

Adeline: Yeah.

Facilitator 4: How is that helpful?

Adeline: It is not because you want to do these things, you have to, it's a must, you've got to, no matter how much you might be hurting you can also ... you're also thinking, well if I'm hurt I can't go on, but I'm not hurting anymore, because I asked Jesus to help me and he has.

Others in the groups did not show a sense of hope in any religious sense, but more in the kindness of others. Hope for frail older people and people with dementia can be as simple as knowing that someone cares about them:

Facilitator 4: What is it in your life that has given you hope, Rhoda?

Rhoda: I'm just very happy here. And all the friends and ladies are very nice and if you need something you can speak to them, things like that. I find everyone is really nice and no one sort of puts you back."

Response to meaning

Humans respond to the meaning that they find in their lives, sometimes in formal ways, and at other times informally.

Rituals, symbols, and liturgies

Meaning is conveyed through symbols and rituals. For those who practise a religion, the liturgies or services of worship play an important part in spiritual and religious wellbeing and care. All humans respond to meaningful symbols and rituals.[12] The key is to find, and sometimes to develop, with the person, through the use of symbols and simple rituals, rituals that will be meaningful. These can be powerful in expressing meanings that are hard to put into words for families facing, for example, the death of a loved one. Rituals and symbols can connect loved ones together.

A symbol is something that is seen to represent something, perhaps unseen. It might be the reminder of something from the past; it might be something as simple as a photo. It might be a flower, it might be working tools, or a book, it might even be a pet; a dog or cat, or even a horse. The key is that the symbol needs to carry meaning for the person or persons involved. For an elderly person who is dying, it may need to carry the meaning of a lifetime, as they attempt to say goodbye to their family, and their family attempts to say goodbye to the dying person. Sometimes, only the person and their family will know what those symbols are. Symbols can sometimes just happen; for example, I had taken some of the first camellias of the season when I visited a friend who was dying. Later that week, on the day she died, a camellia bloom dropped off its stem and my friend said to the nurse, 'that flower has died, but look, there is another bud coming out—see, new life.' In this case, the flower became the symbol of the cycle of life and death by which we are surrounded; it connected with the dying woman's sense of peace and hope. Symbols can have a spiritual nature, such as a candle, stone, flower, picture, or carry a religious meaning, such as a cross, an icon, or a prayer mat.

The natural environment also provides symbols, the beautiful sunrise or sunset that brings a sense of awe. The beauty of nature, of mountains, of the sea, all can connect people with something larger than themselves, and can connect to the Creator.

Niven[30] writes that *rituals* have important functions in both historical continuity and in providing indicative character (meaning). Historical continuity involves connections between past present and future, for a frail older person, it may mean the regular visits of a friend, or even the arrival of a favourite magazine. Ritual can be religious or non-religious. Niven has described the effects of non-religious rituals for a frail elderly woman who was joyful at the arrival of her favourite magazine and her friend, who would help her by writing in the words of the crossword, saying 'I'm not enjoying the treatment at the moment, but Jean and my crossword get me through.'[30, p. 222] Rituals can be understood as orientating anchors, connecting the community with meaning. Friedman[31] describes the functions of rituals as anchors or grounding in times of crisis, connecting with a sense of 'otherness' and the environment, reducing isolation and building community, affirming and reaffirming meaning, (rituals can be repeated and this is often the power of religious rituals), rituals can provide security in times of uncertainty and mark milestones in the life journey.[32, p. 135] The indicative character of ritual is to become a 'symbol that points beyond itself, expresses something different and invites us to remembrance, to hope, or to a new page in life.'[31, p. 263]

Times to use rituals and/or symbols

Rituals and symbols can be used at any time. Some examples include celebrating milestones in life, significant birthdays, closures and thanksgivings, leaving a family home and the moving into residential aged care settings. Funerals are obvious examples of rituals. Memorial services are often used in residential aged care to acknowledge the deaths of residents and to assist the residents, staff, and families to grieve, by making the connections between them. Rituals give people the opportunity to experience, engage in, and talk about death and grief and loss.

Finding the right ritual or symbol

Questions that might be asked are:

- How have you celebrated special events in the past?
- Are there any special symbols that carry meaning for *you*, for example, is there something that has been important in your life, either personal, about relationships, or about work or special life interests? Or, important life events may need a symbol to represent them; the question becomes—what can represent that meaning for that event? Are there important symbols for those you love and wish to honour?

It may be necessary to connect with the person's story to gain entry into what symbols may be important for them.

The arts: art, music, poetry, drama

The arts may provide vital connecting points for older people seeking meaning in their lives. For instance, art may focus as a way into the divine. The arts may form aspects of rituals and provide symbols. Music may facilitate the person's entry into meditation and prayer. The arts are valuable for cognitively competent older adults, and no less so for people with dementia. A recent study looking at participation in choir by people with dementia[33] found that depression levels of choir members were lowered during the 20-week programme, although with the small numbers it was not possible to demonstrate statistically significant changes. Often the arts can be means of mediating spiritual matters. The arts can be used creatively as ways of entry into meditation and prayer.

Issues of care

Spiritual care is part of holistic care and it is important to develop evidence-based strategies that chaplains, pastoral carers, and other health professionals can incorporate into their practice. Too often activities that are offered to older people, especially those in residential aged care, may not engage the older person either in making new friends or in any meaningful activity. The question must be asked is: at what level does this activity benefit the resident? Often the activity focuses on enjoyment or distraction. The spiritual dimension requires nurturing at a deeper level, to touch the depths of being for that person. Certain activities do aim to do this; meditation, for instance. Moody[34] has written of ageing as a natural monastery, where older people gradually become more introspective and less active, moving from a focus of human doing to human being.[10] Spiritual reminiscence and spiritual autobiography are also means of assisting the older person to search their life story, to find the connecting points, the unity of narrative across their lives. Spiritual reminiscence in small groups can have the added benefit of helping people to know each other better; make new friends, and deepen the friendships with people who have known each other for a long time. It is a way of overcoming loneliness and isolation, both within the community and within residential care.

Aged care environments

Much has been achieved in improving the physical environment within aged care facilities in recent decades, but the environment requires social planning as well to facilitate interaction between frail elderly people. The Eden Alternative[35] has been introduced into a large number of residential aged care facilities, with the result of making these places more friendly and less institutional. Their goals are to make a difference to the wellbeing of older people across seven domains of identity, growth, meaning, autonomy, connectedness, security, and joy. These goals fit into a broad canvas that could be called spirituality. The programme has a strong focus of empowerment of older people, and the introduction of plants, pets, and other environmental changes, moving the focus of care from a medical model toward a pleasant environment with greater emphasis on psychosocial elements of care for older people. An enhancement of this model might include explicit attention to spiritual needs and spiritual possibilities of residents.

Conclusion

With increasing longevity comes increasing diversity of this latter part of the life cycle. Increased life-span has come for most people, with better physical health, but perhaps a lack of sense of purpose and meaning in societies that devalue older people. Mental health issues assume enormous importance in gauging the ability of older people to continue to live independently and to flourish. The ability to continue to live independently, even when living alone is important for wellbeing. Entry to residential aged care is often due to issues related to dementia, such as agitation, incontinence, or increasing functional decline. Palliative care for older people who are dying from any cause, including those who have dementia and are frail, should be readily available; spiritual care has the potential to enhance the final life journey and needs to be an intrinsic component of palliative care.

Recognizing the spiritual dimension and fostering continuing spiritual growth in later life become important aspects of achieving wellbeing. This chapter has addressed major challenges of growing older in early twenty-first-century western countries. We suggest that by focusing on spiritual growth and spiritual care of elderly people, some of the challenges of growing older can be mitigated with enhanced focus on strategies that support and strengthen spiritual well-bring.

References

1 Rowe, J., Kahn, R. (1999). *Successful Aging*. New York: Random House.
2 Butler, R. (1995). Foreword. In: B.K. Haight, J.D. Webster (eds) *The Art and Science of Reminiscence: Theory, Research, Methods, and Application*. Washington, DC: Taylor & Francis.
3 Covinsky, K.E., Yaffe, K., Lindquist, K., Cherkasova, E., Yelin, E., Blazer, D.G. (2010). Depressive symptoms in middle age and the development of later-life functional limitations: the long-term effect of depressive symptoms. *J Am Geriat Soc* **58**(3): 551–6.
4 Blazer, D.G. (2006). Spirituality, depression and the elderly. *Sthn Med J* **99**(10): 1178–9.
5 Australian Bureau of Statistics. (2010). *Causes of Death, Australia, 2008*. Canberra: Australian Bureau of Statistics.
6 Alzheimer's Australia. (2008). *Dementia Facts and Statistics*. Available at: http://203.17.29.161/upload/StatisticsMar08.pdf
7 Jorm, A.F., Dear, K.B.G., Burgess, N.M. (2005). Projections of future numbers of dementia cases in Australia with and without prevention. *Aust NZ J Psychiat* **39**: 959–63.
8 Ryan, E., Schindel, M.L., Beaman, A. (2005). Communication strategies to promote spiritual wellbeing among people with dementia. *J Past Care Counsel* **59**(1–2): 43–55.

9 Atchley, R.C. (2009). *Spirituality and Aging.* Baltimore: John Hopkins University Press.
10 MacKinlay, E.B. (2001). *The Spiritual Dimension of Ageing.* London: Jessica Kingsley Publishers.
11 MacKinlay, E.B., Trevitt, C. (2007). Spiritual care and ageing in a secular society. *Med J Aust* **186**(10): S74–6.
12 MacKinlay, E.B. (2006). *Spiritual Growth and Care in the Fourth Age of Life.* London: Jessica Kingsley Publishers.
13 Hauerwas, S.M., Stoneking, C.B., Meador, K.G., Cloutier, D. (eds) (2003). *Growing Old in Christ.* Grand Rapids: William B. Eerdmans Publishing Company.
14 Swinton, J. (2001). *Spirituality and Mental Healthcare: Rediscovering a 'Forgotten' Dimension.* London: Jessica Kingsley Publishers.
15 Swinton, J. (2007). Forgetting whose we are: theological reflections on personhood, faith and dementia. *J Religion, Disabil Hlth* **11**(1): 37–62.
16 Erikson, E.H., Erikson, J.M., Kivnick, H.Q. (1986). *Vital Involvement in Old Age.* New York: W.W. Norton & Co.
17 Neugarten, B.L. (1968). Adult personality: toward a psychology of the life cycle. In: B.L. Neugarten (ed.) *Middle Age and Aging: A Reader in Social Psychology*, pp. 137–47. Chicago: University of Chicago Press.
18 Carroll, L.P., Dyckman, K.M. (1986). *Chaos or Creation: Spirituality in Mid-life.* New York: Paulist Press.
19 Trevitt, C., MacKinlay, E. (2006). 'I am just an ordinary person ...:' spiritual reminiscence in older people with memory loss. *J Relig Spiritual Aging* **18**(2/3): 77–89.
20 Frankl, V.E. (1984). *Man's Search for Meaning.* New York: Washington Square Press.
21 Frankl, V.E. (1997). *Man's Search for Ultimate Meaning.* Reading: Perseus Books.
22 Tornstam, L. (2005). *Gerotranscendence: A Developmental Theory of Positive Aging.* New York: Springer Publishing Company.
23 Kenyon, G.M. (2003). Telling and listening to stories: creating a wisdom environment for older people. *Generations* **xxvii**(3): 30–3.
24 Birren, J.E., Cochran, K.N. (2001). *Telling the Stories of Life Through Guided Autobiography Groups.* Baltimore: John Hopkins University Press.
25 Haight, B., Gibson, F. (2005). *Burnside's Working with Older Adults: Group Process and Techniques.* Sudbury: Jones & Bartlett.
26 Morgan, R.L. (2002). *Remembering Your Story: Creating Your Own Spiritual Autobiography.* Nashville: Upper Room Books.
27 Moltmann, J. (1993). *Theology of Hope.* Minneapolis: Fortress Press.
28 De Leo, D., Hickey, P.A., Neulinger, K., Cantor, C.H. (2001). *Ageing and Suicide*, Australian Institute for Suicide Research and Prevention. Canberra: Commonwealth of Australia.
29 MacKinlay, E., McDonald, T., Niven, A., Russell, F., Seidel Hooke, D. (2011). *Minimizing the Impact of Depression and Dementia for Elders in Residential Care*, Project supported by grant: ANZ Charitable foundation, JO & JR Wicking Trust Grant (2008–2010) Unpublished
30 Niven, A. (2008). Pastoral rituals, ageing and new paths into meaning. In: E.B. MacKinlay (ed.) *Ageing, Disability & Spirituality: Addressing the Challenge of Disability in Later Life*, pp. 217–32. London: Jessica Kingsley Publishers.
31 Moltmann, J. (1977). *The Church in the Power of the Spirit.* London: SCM Press.
32 Friedman, D.A. (2003). An anchor amidst anomie: ritual and aging. In: M.A. Kimble, S.H. McFadden (eds) *Aging, Spirituality and Religion: A Handbook*, vol. 2. Minneapolis: Fortress Press.
33 Robertson-Gillam, K. (2008). Hearing the voice of the elderly: the potential for choir work to reduce depression and meet spiritual needs. In: E.B. MacKinlay (ed.) *Ageing, Disability & Spirituality: Addressing the Challenge of Disability in Later Life*, pp. 182–99. London: Jessica Kingsley Publishers.
34 Moody, H.R. (1995). Mysticism. In: M.A. Kimble, S.H. McFadden, J.W. Ellor, J.J. Seeber (eds) *Aging, Spirituality, and Religion: A Handbook.* Minneapolis: Augsburg Fortress Press.
35 Thomas, W. *The Eden Alternative.* Available at www.edenalt.org. (accessed 26 October 2010).

CHAPTER 36

Palliative care

Jackie Ellis and Mari Lloyd-Williams

Introduction

Modern hospice and palliative care expects clinicians to provide 'total' care to patients and their families. Such care incorporates not only physical, emotional, and psychosocial care, but spiritual care as well. Spirituality is an important part of the lives of many people and may be particularly significant for people with advanced disease who are facing death and there is no talk of hope or meaning.[1–4] Spiritual care is increasingly identified as an integral part of health-care systems across the world. This is particularly so in palliative and end of life care where a holistic approach is established as both a philosophy and a model of care. The goal of spiritual care today is to relieve spiritual distress and promote personal growth.[5]

Spiritual care has risen in visibility in health services over the last two decades, from a position where it was equated with religious care and regarded as the sole province of chaplains to one where a broad concept of spirituality is employed and spiritual care is recognized as having relevance for all sectors and to lie potentially within the remit of all health and social care workers. However, this perceptual shift has not necessarily occurred at the level of practice, and there is anecdotal and other evidence of continuing uncertainty and ambiguity over how, when, and where spiritual need should be addressed.[6] In this chapter, using exemplifiers from policy, practice and research, we look at how spiritual issues are addressed and explore the practice of spiritually within palliative care and identify the challenges to its implementation. First, however, we define the concept of palliative care and locate it in its historical context.

Defining palliative care

'The goal of palliative care is to prevent and relive suffering and to support the best possible quality of life for patients and their families regardless of the stage of the disease or the need for other therapies.'[7] Palliative care is viewed as applying to patients from the time of diagnosis of serious illness to death. From this perspective, 'the principles of spiritual care can be applicable across all phases and setting for the seriously ill, without regard to culture, religious traditions or spiritual frames of reference.'[4] Palliative care guidance emphasises the importance of a holistic assessment and advocate the need to integrate physical, psychosocial and spiritual aspects within palliative care.[7,8] Over recent years palliative care has become more expansive in its goals and has sought to move its influence upstream to earlier stages in the disease progression.[9]

The most recent definition from the WHO defines palliative care as 'an approach that improves the quality of life of patients and their families with life-threatening illness, through the prevention and relief of suffering by means of early identification, assessment and treatment of pain and other problems, physical, psychosocial and spiritual.'[10] Embedded within the WHO definition is a commitment to relieving pain and other distressing symptoms, the affirmation of life while regarding dying as a normal process, an intention either hasten nor postpone death, an integration of psychological and spiritual aspects of patient care, the provision of support to help patients live as actively as possible until their death, with support being provided to help families cope during their loved ones' illnesses and into their own bereavement. Whenever possible, palliative care endeavours to enhance the quality of life of patients as they move toward death. Palliative care can be applied at all stages of life-threatening disease and should intensify once cure is no longer deemed possible.[4]

The concept of modern palliative care is recognized as starting with St Christopher's Hospice in London (1967). At that time professional and public interest in cancer mainly focused on the potential for curative treatment and patients dying from cancer were abandoned by physicians and told to go home as there was nothing more that could be done.[9] Dame Cicely Saunders, the central pioneer to the foundation of the St Christopher Hospice, recognized, along with her colleagues, that the care of the dying was suboptimal on hospital wards,[11] and that a new philosophy of care of the dying was needed. Saunders was to become instrumental in defining this new knowledge base of care for those dying from malignancies. She advocated that we are invisible, physical and spiritual beings.[12] Clark[9] notes that her articulation of the relationship between physical and mental suffering outlined in her research papers, was seen in almost dialectical terms, each capable of affecting the other. Clark[13] also notes that Saunders description of this relationship reached full expression in her idea of total pain which was taken to include physical symptoms, mental distress social problems and emotional difficulties and was captured so comprehensively by the patient who told her 'all of me is wrong.' [13, p. 431] St Christopher's Hospice served as a template for a developing a model of multidisciplinary clinical care, teaching, and research. From the 1980s pioneers of modern hospices and palliative care worked to promote their goals in many countries.

Defining spiritually

The basic concept of spirituality is the notion that human beings need to seek and find a meaning beyond their current suffering which allows them to make sense of that situation.[14] There appears to be consensus that spirituality is not limited to religion or faith and that all people are spiritual beings.[15–17] Spirituality can be defined as a person search for existential meaning and purpose in life within a given life experience, which may or may not be related to religion.[18,19]

There has been growing separation of the concepts of spirituality and religion.[19] Religion is more about systems, a social institution that is joined or organized by individuals who share the same belief, traditions, and rituals[20,21] and characterized in many ways by its boundaries and spirituality by a difficulty in defining its boundaries. 'Spirituality' may be used by those who wish to move beyond institutional religion.[22]

There are many individuals who are both spiritual and religious and who discover meaning, strength and support in particular symbols, beliefs, forms of worship and ritual that they share with their religious community. The events of a person's life shape a person's spiritually. Thus, individuals express their spirituality not only different faiths and religious practices, but also in relation to gender, culture, and ethnicity. Spirituality also changes during the course of a person's life.[23] Spirituality is inherently relational, including relationships with self, others, nature, and God.[24,25] The focus on relationships and connections with family and significant others, rather than being just on meaning-making, appears for Edward and colleagues, to be the most important dimension of spirituality. In fact, these authors found that patients most often found meaning in relationships.

Surveys have demonstrated that spirituality is a need and affects patient decision making and healthcare outcomes, including quality of life.[4] A meta-analysis of data from 42 published mortality studies involving approximately 126,000 participants demonstrated that persons who reported frequent religious involvements were significantly more likely to live longer compared to persons who were involved infrequently.[26] Another study of almost 600 older, severely ill, patients, found that those seeking a connection with a benevolent God, as well as support from clergy and faith group members, were less depressed and rated their quality of life as higher, even after taking into account the severity of their illness.[27] In a study of 1600 cancer patients, the contribution of patient reported spiritual wellbeing to quality of life was similar to that associated with physical wellbeing. Among patients with significant symptoms such as fatigue and pain, those with higher levels of spiritual wellbeing had a significantly higher quality of life.[28]

Some initial contemporary efforts have been made to define spirituality from the perspective of dying patients.[6] Chao and colleagues[2] asked six Buddhist and Christian terminally ill cancer patients in Taiwan what the essence of spirituality was to them. Ten themes in four broad categories emerged:

- communion with self (self-identity, wholeness, inner peace)
- communion with others (love, reconciliation)
- communion with nature (inspiration, creativity)
- communion with a higher being (faithfulness, hope, gratitude).

Hermann[29] notes as in-depth interviews with 19 hospice patients progressed, many whose initial definitions of spirituality related to God or other religious terms, later identified terms associated with meaning and purpose or nature, and acknowledged that spirituality was part of their total existence. McGrath[30] interviewed 14 people living at home in Australia with a prognosis of less than 6 months. He found that most did not seek explicitly religious comfort in response to their illness and that there was a degree of eclecticism in the religio-spiritual concepts expressed by participants. In a comparative study of cancer survivors and hospice patients, McGrath concluded that maintaining an intimate connection with life through family, friends, leisure, home, and work was just as important to individuals as transcendent meaning-making, religious or otherwise.[31]

Some studies report that religious involvement and spirituality may have negative health outcomes[29,32] and it can create distress and increase the burden of illness,[33,34] as people find that their life has been so altered by illness that previous landmarks make no sense and their future is deeply uncertain.[23] Nevertheless, there appear to be widespread agreement that human beings are spiritual and need spiritual support at the end-stage of life.[17] Inquiry by those caring for patients about the experience of patients provides not only an opportunity for greater understanding of the experience of those for whom they care, but also the potential for relieving spiritual distress either by simple discussion or, as appropriate, referral to others with the training and expertise to explore some of these issues.

Spiritual pain/suffering

Spiritual suffering or pain may manifest itself within various domains of the patient's experience, be it physical (e.g. intractable pain), psychological (e.g. anxiety, depression, hopelessness), religious (e.g. crisis of faith), or social (e.g. disintegration of human relationships).[5] However, McGarth[35] maintains that it is not possible to recognize spiritual pain on basis of symptoms alone. Rather, spiritual pain is the combination of the aforementioned symptoms and characteristic behaviours. These behaviours often evoke descriptions such as 'suffering' or 'anguish,' which may help to identify this form of pain.

In a study of caregivers, hospital chaplains, palliative care physicians, and pain specialists,[36] definitions of existential pain ranged from those that stressed issues of guilt and religion (chaplains) to those that related to annihilation and impending separation (palliative care physicians). While some pain specialists emphasized that living is painful, they concluded that existential pain is most often used as a metaphor for suffering. Carroll[37] found hospice nurses identified spiritual distress as arising from the loneliness of dying. Callahan[38] similarly suggests that spiritual pain arises from the dying person's struggle to accept the dying process. Musi[39] prefers the term 'spiritual suffering' arising from threat to the integrity of the self which may occur as identity and personal resources are changed or diminished through the dying process.

In an article which questions whether spiritual need should be assumed in everyone and also whether all staff in palliative care should assume responsibility for spiritual care Hinshaw[40] agrees that threats to personal meaning and purpose creates spiritual suffering in the dying. However, this (US) study also identifies specific spiritual concerns identified by Americans about death: not being forgiven by God; not being reconciled with others; dying while cut off from God or some higher power; not being forgiven by others for a past offence including not having the blessing of family or clergy; concerns about after death. Walter[22] suggests that spiritual pain is really biographical pain: life has not gone as the person wished and for those in palliative care it is too late to do anything about that. According to McGrath[35] who developed a paradigm of spiritual pain from a qualitative study of 12 survivors of haematological malignancies, the notion of spiritual pain or suffering includes: a sense of diffuse emotional/existential/intellectual pain directly related to the meaninglessness created as a result of a break with the expected/normal network of relationships that function to connect one to life. A key ingredient in that pain is the sense that the experience with life is failing to meet the individual's needs, and thus the expected satisfaction and meaning-making from life are not forth-coming.'

Spiritual need

Unlike in the USA where studies tend to describe spiritual needs in more religious terms than those originating from USA the UK literature takes a broadly 'common humanity' approach to spiritual need.[6] These authors cite a study conducted in Northern Ireland[41] whereby 92% of participants self-identified a faith in God or Higher Being, and highlighted their top six spiritual needs as:

- to have time to think
- to have hope
- to deal with unresolved issues
- to prepare for death
- to express true feelings without being judged
- to speak of important relationships.

Edwards *et al.*[24] identified similar themes which included life review and reminiscence, involvement and control, a positive outlook, a need to talk about 'regular' things, death and dying and a need for ordinariness and normality.

A survey comparing chaplaincy services in hospices and hospitals across England and Wales[42] found patients were not concerned with issues of transcendence or forgiveness, but rather the spiritual needs arising from suffering and concern for relatives; interestingly, religious needs (such as desire for communion featured more in hospitals than in hospices). However, Murray *et al.*[43] found that patients and their carers sometimes expressed the need for transcendence, alongside love, meaning, and purpose. This study also distinguished the separate spiritual needs of patients and carers. Specific issues identified were problems with the language of spiritual care for both patients and workers, where terms such as meaning, purpose, forgiveness, hope, and compassion may more easily facilitate engagement with spiritual need.[44] Walter[22] suggests that this is a particular form of contemporary western discourse in which broadening spirituality to a 'personal and psychological' search for meaning allows all staff to engage with this dimension.

Practice issues

Studies have noted that patients themselves may not recognize the concept of spirituality as defined by healthcare professionals[22,45,46] and may not understand the term 'spirituality'.[47,48] Moreover, what professionals assume to be spiritual care might not correspond to patients' understandings and needs.[47,48] It is important therefore to clarify the meaning of spirituality in relation to healthcare in order to enhance communication, practice, education, and research and to reduce the gap between policy and patient expectations. Furthermore, patients are often reluctant to raise such issues or might prefer to discuss their spiritual needs with competent persons other than their professional caregivers.[43] Studies have also reported that patients find it difficult to express their spiritual needs and distress, which were overlooked when hidden or disguised with a brave face, humour, silence of physical and emotional symptoms).[49–51] Ehman *et al.*[52] identified that a majority of patients would like their physician to ask about spiritual or religious beliefs if they become gravely ill. More recent studies found that more attention to spiritual issues was needed from their professional caregivers.[29,53,54]

The (UK) Standards for Hospice and Palliative Care Chaplaincy Association[55] affirms that the assessment of spiritual and religious need should be available to all patients and carers, including those of no faith, defining spiritual needs as:

- exploring the individual's sense of meaning and purpose in life;
- exploring attitudes, beliefs, ideas, values and concerns around life and death issues;
- affirming life and worth by encouraging reminiscence about the past;
- exploring the individual's hopes and fears regarding the present and future for themselves, and their families/carers; exploring the why questions in relation to life death and suffering.

In 2008 the UK Government launched its End of Life Care Strategy for England, which advocates the need for holistic assessment that covers physical, psychological, social, cultural environmental, spiritual, and financial needs. This document acknowledges that people at the end of the life frequently have highly complex and wide ranging needs, and states that effective processes for holistic assessment are particularly important in this context in order to minimize repeated unnecessary assessments in the final phase of life. It also emphasizes the importance of treating people as individuals, assessing their needs, preferences and priorities, supporting them in making choices about care and agreeing a care plan that reflect these.

US studies indicate that most patients would like their spiritual needs to be addressed, but for the majority they are not.[56] The US 2009 Consensus Conference produced clear recommendations for spiritual care practice in palliative care, most of which are focused on the assessment of spiritual need and distress, routinely for all patients and operationalized by all types and levels of staff at screening and referral stages, followed up by more structured and detailed assessment carried out by chaplains (who should respond within 24 hours).[4]

The model of spiritual care outlined in these recommendations is grounded in important theoretical frameworks, one of which is the Biopsychosocial–Spiritual Model of Care,[57,58] which builds on the Biopsychosocial Model for care proposed by Engel[59] and White.[60] Another is a patient-centred care model in which the focus of care is on the patient and his or her experience of illness as opposed to a focus on the disease.[4] Integral to both these models is the recognition that there is more to the care of the patient than the physical.[61] The spiritual care model that underpinned the work of the Consensus Conference (2009) is a relational model in which the patient and clinicians work together to process of discovery, collaborative dialogue, treatment, and ongoing evaluation and follow-up.

Despite the increasing emphasis on assessing spiritual needs it appears they are not being meet through a lack of spiritual awareness in the workforce generally, together with lack of confidence to broach spiritual issues, with at the same time a reluctance to refer to chaplains.[8] There is also often a reluctance on the part of caregiver to consider spiritual issues or discuss them with patients.[23] This is attributed to factors such as lack of time, uncertainly about how to ask questions or how to respond to what patients tell them about their spiritual experience or concern about the appropriateness of discussing such issues in a clinical context. Nurses who consider spiritual needs as their responsibility maintain that spiritual needs are neglected because of time constraints, lack of confidence in dealing with such concerns and role uncertainty.[62] Studies indicate that physicians feel unskilled and uncomfortable discussing their patients' spiritual and religious concerns.[43,54] Other studies which report nurses' concerns stress that raising the subject of spirituality might cause distress to patients.[63]

The spiritual need (and spiritual distress) of the care-giving professionals is also highlighted and often linked to their ability to relate the spiritual needs of patients.[64] A study of palliative care workers in Flanders Belgium,[65] advocates greater awareness and assertiveness amongst workers of their own spiritual experiences to address the 'hidden spiritual agenda' of the palliative care team as a necessary forerunner to responding to the spiritual needs of patients. Sheehan[23] calls for this issue to be addressed amongst physicians caring for people of the end of life. Hegarty[66] argues that workers need to be aware of their own vulnerabilities, describing them as 'wounded healers'. It is also suggested[8] that health and social care professionals in the UK tend to feel awkward about discussing their own spiritual needs

Chaplains, occupy integral roles within palliative care teams[67] and their role has expanded to include responsibilities such as education and bereavement care,[42] and are still expected to offer an appropriate religious ministry to those who remain in membership of faith communities. They are also called upon to give spiritual care to the majority of patients, carers, and staff who have no association whatsoever with any religious group.[68] Even among chaplains, there seems to be a lack of clarity about their role, which has implications for their wellbeing.[42] Studies have highlighted the need for chaplains to feel adequately supported and valued within palliative care.[69]

Simply referring a patient with spiritual distress to clergy may be unwise for at least two reasons. First, not all spiritual distress is religious and is not best addressed by a religious figure like a priest, minister, rabbi, or imam. Secondly, being ordained in a religious tradition does not mean that the individual will necessarily have any expertise in dealing with people who are facing life-threatening illness.[23] However, Sheehan acknowledges that this does not mean that one might not have excellent, skilled, and compassionate resources among local clergy.

Various practice guidance together with research studies highlight the need for all staff to have basic training in understanding spiritual needs and assessing spiritual care, as well as formal supervision, which addresses the spirituality and spiritual needs of healthcare workers themselves.[8,65,70] In a wide ranging analysis of spiritual care at the end of life Cobb[71] calls more training, more consistency, and a more integrated approach to spiritual care-giving.

Spiritual care also includes spiritual 'practices,' which patients and family members are encouraged to utilize such as prayer, meditation, massage and relaxation techniques.[72] In some hospices patients are offered aromatherapy, acupressure hypnotherapy and music therapy, which focuses on harmonizing as vibrational energy. Wasner *et al.*[73, p. 100] suggest that hospice staff be trained in the use of 'non-denominational' spiritual practices such as contemplation and meditation. These practices are offered as 'spiritual not religious' with little recognition of their specific cultural roots, most often in Buddhism or New Age religions,[5,74] As ritual studies scholar Ronald Grimes[75, p. 150] asserts there is little awareness of the way in which spirituality 'underwrites the expropriation of other people's beliefs, stories and practices.'

Much practice guidance is concerned with identifying the religious beliefs and spiritual practices of the dying patient and relatives in order that healthcare practice does not offend or contravene important tenets of faith or religious practice and staff are aware of the implications of specific treatments for particular religious groups.[6] These authors point out that this includes actions which should be taken by healthcare staff to facilitate religious practice and create the necessary environment for a patient of a particular religious persuasion to die in the manner prescribed by their religion[8,76,77] However, as Holloway *et al.* [6] assert, the practice guidance literature does not address broader spiritual needs at the point of death other than relational needs: that is, the presence of family and friends although the belief of many religions that dying is an opportunity for spiritual insight is highlighted.[76]

A number of empirical studies and commentaries focus on broader spiritual need and distress in suffering at the very end of life and suggest the main approaches as companionship—'being there'—and helping the patient to find sources of strength and meaning, not necessarily in the suffering itself, but in their life more generally.[6] The issue of clinical presence, in the form of being there or being fully present for patients in need has been explored by way of 'nursing present,'[78] 'caring presence,' and 'healing presence' [79–81] in the palliative care literature. Presence carries significant development, spiritual, and existential meaning for patients as they face end of life issues. The process of being present unites the listener and the speaker in a spirit of compassion.[82]

Other sources refer to a 'supportive presence,' which affords the patient a safe space to ask questions;[38] new ways of being in which spiritual care involves being rather than doing[83] 'sharing the journey' of the dying person,[22,42] the importance of attentive listening and silence;[44] 'focused discussion' rather than formal assessment.[84] Edwards *et al.*[24] asserts that having more time to listen and get to know patients and develop relationships, enabled sensitivity to individual needs and help facilitate spiritual discussions, as was allowing more time for caregivers to reflect on their own spiritually and belief systems.

Patients may have their own inner spiritual strengths and resources, regardless of whether an overt faith is present.[85,86] The aim of spiritual care is to try and identify and support these. [87] Other writers have demonstrated the value of developing relationships, which may in themselves be therapeutic.[19,88] Mako *et al.*[81] found that while some patients requested prayer and other religious rituals the most frequently requested intervention was to spend time with a healthcare professional who would listen to the patient's story. However, few requested sacramental presence (7%), which these authors maintained would indicate that what is being sought is not so much religious intervention, but human compassion.

Breitbart and colleagues[89,90] have explored the spiritual and existential dimensions of meaning in advanced stage cancer and end-of-life care and have developed meaning-centred group and individual psychotherapeutic interventions for advanced stage cancer patients to help enhance their sense of meaning and purpose in their life as they face uncertainty of illness. Such an approach is largely based on Frankl's[91–93] existential work, and seeks to enhance patients spiritual wellbeing by teaching them ways to tap into sources of meaning in order to cope with the spiritual and existential pain of living in the face of death.

More detailed assessment of specific spiritual needs does not feature in these approaches).[6] In fact, Gysels *et al.*[94] assert that there is a body of opinion which opposes the 'medicalizing' of spiritual need through an over-emphasis on assessment through standardized scales, and is particularly a concern amongst chaplains.[95] Set against these concerns others suggest core transferable concepts of spiritual need, such as the search for meaning and purpose, across cultures,[96] and patient groups.[97,98]

Conclusion

Spiritual care is central to healthcare, particularly in palliative and end-of-life care, where a holistic approach is established as both a philosophy and model of care. However, the practice of spiritual care at the end of life is challenging and complex, and there is still significant work to be done. The fact that spiritual care may be by provided by all professionals is both strength and a challenge. Not only does the perception of what exactly constitutes spiritual care vary between individuals (and disciplines), but at an institutional level there is often blurring off boundaries, roles and expectations within the team, which appears to be complicated by factors, such as lack of time and limited resources.

The evidence suggests that there a great deal of confusion, ambiguity, uncertainty, and lack of confidence in addressing spiritual need, and offering spiritual care or support in the workforce. At one level this may be understood in terms of the differing approaches to the assessment of need, and the provision and management of spiritual care. In addition, particular sensitivities, ethical concerns, and practice skills required in work with people at the end of life and their families, raise issues for spiritual care in both its theoretical underpinning and practice delivery, which are unique to this environment.

Whilst various practice guidance and research studies highlight the need all staff to have basic training in understanding spiritual assessment as well as formal supervision which addresses spirituality and spiritual needs of the healthcare workers themselves this clearly is insufficient We need to ensure that training and education in spiritual care is incorporated into the teaching curricula of the health professionals This needs to be supplemented with ongoing training and support and should be available to all those involved in the delivery of spiritual care, at all levels. This to some extent will help to build knowledge and understanding (and by implication, confidence) in spiritual care.

References

1 Koenig, H.G. (2009). Research on religion, spirituality, and mental health: a review. *Can J Psychiat* **54**(5): 283–91.

2 Chao, C., Chen C., Yen M, (2002). The essence of spirituality of terminally ill patients. *J Nurs Res* **10**: 637–46.

3 McClain, C.S., Rosenfeld, B., Breitbart, W. (2003). Effect of spiritual wellbeing on end-of-life despair in terminally-ill cancer patients. *Lancet* **361**(9369): 1603–7.

4 Puchalski, C., Ferrell, B., Virani, R., Otis-Green, S., Baird, P., Bull, J., et al. (2009). Improving the quality of spiritual care as a dimension of palliative care: the report of the consensus conference. *J Palliat Med* **12**(10): 885–904.

5 Garces-Foley, K. (2006). Hospice and the politics of Spirituality. *OMEGA*—J Death Dying **53**(1): 117–36.

6 Holloway, M., Adamson, S., McSherry, W., Swinton, J. (2010). *Spirtual Care at the End of Life: a Systematic Review of the Literature*. Hull: University of Hull.

7 National Consensus Project for Quality Palliative Care. (2009). *Clinical Practice Guidelines for Quality Palliative Care*, 2nd edn. Available from: http://www.nationalconsensusproject.org.

8 National Institute for Clinical Excellence, (2004). *Improving Supporting and Palliative Care for Adults*. London: NICE.

9 Clark, D. (2007). From margins to centre: a review of the history of palliative care in cancer. *Lancet Oncol* **8**(5): 430–8.

10 World Health Organization. *WHO Definition of Palliative Care 2007*; Available from: http://www.who.int/cancer/palliative/definition/en/ (accessed 24 January 2011).

11 Saunders, C. (1983). Living with dying. *Radiogr* **49**(580): 79.

12 Saunders, C. (1996). A personal therapeutic journey. *Br Med J* **313**(7072): 1599.

13 Clark, D. (1999). 'Total Pain', disciplinary power and the body in the work of Cicley Saunders, 1958–1967. *Soc Sci Med* **49**(6): 727–36.

14 Kellehear, A. (2000). Spirituality and palliative care: a model of needs. *Palliat Med* **14**(2): 149.

15 Bartel, M. (2004). What is spiritual? What is spiritual suffering? *J Past Care Counsel* **58**(3): 187.

16 Cassidy, J.P., Davies, D.J. (2004). Cultural and spiritual aspects of palliative medicine. *Oxford Textbook of Palliative Medicine*. 3rd ed. Oxford University Press, Oxford, 2004: pp. 951–7.

17 Wright, M.C. (2002). The essence of spiritual care: a phenomenological enquiry. *Palliat Med* **16**(2): 125.

18 Byrne, M. (2002). Spirituality in palliative care: what language do we need? *Int J Palliat Nurs* **8**(2): 67.

19 Tanyi, R.A. (2002). Towards clarification of the meaning of spirituality. *J Adv Nurs* **39**(5): 500–9.

20 Dyson, J., Cobb, M., Forman, D. (1997). The meaning of spirituality: a literature review. *J Adv Nurs* **26**(6): 1183–8.

21 Strang, S., Strang, P., Ternestedt, B.M. (2002). Spiritual needs as defined by Swedish nursing staff. *Journal of Clinical Nursing* **11**(1): 48–57.

22 Walter, T. (2002). Spirituality in palliative care: opportunity or burden? *Palliat Med* **16**(2): 133.

23 Sheehan, M.N. (2005). Spirituality and the care of people with life-threatening illnesses. *Techn Region Anaesth Pain Manag* **9**(3): 109–13.

24 Edwards, A., Pang, N., Shiu, V., Chan, C. (2010). The understanding of spirituality and the potential role of spiritual care in end-of-life and palliative care: a meta-study of qualitative research. *Palliat Med* 24(8): 753–70.

25 Reed, P.G. (1992). An emerging paradigm for the investigation of spirituality in nursing. *Res Nurs Hlth* **15**(5): 349–57.

26 McCullough, M.E., Hoyt, W.T., Larson, D.B., Koenig, H.G., Thoresen, C. (2000). Religious involvement and mortality: a meta-analytic review. *Hlth Psychol* **19**(3): 211–22.

27 Koenig, H.G., Pargament, K.I., Nielsen, J. (1998). Religious coping and health status in medically ill hospitalized older adults. *J Nerv Ment Dis* **186**(9): 513.

28 Brady M J, Peterman, A.H., Fitchett, G., Mo, M., Cella, D. (1999). A case for including spirituality inequality of life measurement in oncology. *Psycho-oncol* **8**: 417–28.

29 Hermann, C.P. (2001). Spiritual needs of dying patients: a qualitative study. *Oncol Nurs Forum* **28**(28): 67–72.

30 McGrath, P. (2003). Religiosity and the challenge of terminal illness. *Death Stud* **27**(10): 881–99.

31 McGrath, P. (2003). Spiritual pain: a comparison of findings from survivors and hospice patients. *Am J Hospice Palliat Med* **20**(1): 23.

32 King, M., Speck, P., Thomas, A. (1999). The effect of spiritual beliefs on outcome from illness. *Soc Sci Med* **48**(9): 1291–300.

33 Fitchett, G., Murphy, P.E., Kim, J., Gibbons, J.L., Cameron, J.R., Davis, J.A. (2004). Religious struggle: Prevalence, correlates and mental health risks in diabetic, congestive heart failure, and oncology patients. *Int J Psychiat Med* **34**(2): 179–96.

34 Pargament, K.I., Koenig, H.G., Tarakeshwar, N., Hahn, J. (2001). Religious struggle as a predictor of mortality among medically ill elderly patients: a 2-year longitudinal study. *Arch Intern Med* **161**(15): 1881.

35 McGrath, P. (2002). Creating a language for 'spiritual pain' through research: a beginning. *Support Care Cancer* **10**(8): 637–46.

36 Strang, P., Strang, S., Hultborn, R., Arnér, S. (2004). Existential pain—an entity, a provocation, or a challenge? *J Pain Sympt Manag* **27**(3): 241–50.

37 Carroll, B. (2001). A phenomenological exploration of the nature of spirituality and spiritual care. *Mortality* **6**(1): 81–98.

38 Callahan, A.M. (2009). Spiritually-sensitive care in hospice social work. *J Soc Work End-of-Life Palliat Care* 5(3): 169–85.

39 Musi, M. (2003). Creating a language for spiritual pain: why not to speak and thing in terms of spiritual suffering? *Support Care Cancer* 10: 637–46.

40 Hinshaw, D.B. (2002). The spiritual needs of the dying patient. *J Am Coll Surgeons* **195**: 565–8.

41 Kernohan, W.G., Waldron, M., McAfee, C., Cochrane, B., Hasson, F. (2007). An evidence base for a palliative care chaplaincy service in Northern Ireland. *Palliat Med* **21**(6): 519.

42 Wright, M.C. (2001). Chaplaincy in hospice and hospital: findings from a survey in England and Wales. *Palliat Med* **15**(3): 229.

43 Murray, S.A., Kendall, M., Boyd, K., Worth, A., Benton, T.F. (2003). General practitioners and their possible role in providing spiritual care: a qualitative study. *Br J Gen Pract* **53**(497): 957.

44 Byrne, M. (2007). Spirituality in palliative care: what language do we need? Learning from pastoral care. *Int J Palliat Nurs* **13**(3): 118.

45 Bradshaw, A. (1996). The spiritual dimension of hospice: the secularization of an ideal. *Soc Sci Med* **43**(3): 409–19.

46 Thomas, J., Retsas, A. (1999). Transacting self-preservation: a grounded theory of the spiritual dimensions of people with terminal cancer. *Int J Nurs Stud* **36**(3): 191–201.

47 McSherry, W., Cash, K., Ross, L. (2004). Meaning of spirituality: implications for nursing practice. *J Clin Nurs* **13**(8): 934–41.

48 Ross, L. (2006). Spiritual care in nursing: an overview of the research to date. *J Clin Nurs* **15**(7): 852–62.

49 Tan, H.M., Braunack-Mayer, A., Beilby, J. (2005). The impact of the hospice environment on patient spiritual expression. *Oncol Nurs Soc* 32(5): 1049–55.

50 Grant, E., Murray, S.A., Kendall, M., Boyd, K., Tilley, S., Ryan, D. (2004). Spiritual issues and needs: perspectives from patients with advanced cancer and nonmalignant disease. A qualitative study. *Palliat Support Care* **2**(4): 371–8.

51 Kawa, M., Kayama, M., Maeyama, E., Iba, N., Murata, H., Imamura, Y., et al. (2003). Distress of inpatients with terminal cancer in Japanese palliative care units: from the viewpoint of spirituality. *Support Care Cancer* **11**(7): 481–90.

52 Ehman, J.W., Ott, B.B., Short, T.H., Ciampa, R.C., Hansen-Flaschen, J. (1999). Do patients want physicians to inquire about their spiritual or religious beliefs if they become gravely ill? *Arch Intern Med* **159**(15): 1803.

53 Farber, N.J., Urban, S.Y., Collier, V.U., Metzger, M., Weiner, J., Boyer, E.G. (2004). Frequency and perceived competence in providing palliative care to terminally ill patients: a survey of primary care physicians. *J Pain Sympt Manag* **28**(4): 364–72.

54 Lo, B., Ruston, D, Kates, L.W., Arnold, R.M., Cohen, C.B., Faber-Langendoen, K., et al. (2002). Discussing religious and spiritual issues at the end of life: a practical guide for physicians. *J Am Med Soc* **287**(6): 749.

55 Association of Hospice & Palliative Care Chaplains. (2006). *Standards for Hospice & Palliative Care Chaplaincy*, 2nd edn. Milton Keynes: AHPCC.

56 Puchalski, C.M. (2007). Spirituality and the care of patients at the end-of-life: an essential component of care. *OMEGA*—J Death Dying **56**(1): 33–46.

57 Barnum, B.S. (2006). *Spirituality in Nursing: From Traditional to New Age*. Springer Pub Co.

58 Sulmasy, D.P. (2002). A biopsychosocial-spiritual model for the care of patients at the end of life. *Gerontologist* **42**(Suppl 3): 24.

59 Engel, G.L. (1977). The need for a new medical model: a challenge for biomedicine. *Science* **196**: 129–36.

60 White, K.L., Williams, T.F., Greenberg, B.G. (1996). The ecology of medical care. *Acad Med* **73**: 187–205.

61 Puchalski, C.M. (2009). Ethical concerns and boundaries in spirituality and health. *Virt Mentor* **11**: 804–6.

62 Kristeller, J.L., Sheedy Zumbrun, C., Schilling, R.F. (1999). *'I would if I could': how oncologists and oncology nurses address spiritual distress in cancer patients. Psycho-Oncol* **8**(5): 451–8.

63 Hunt, J., Cobb, M., Keeley, V.L., Ahmedzai, S.H. (2003).The quality of spiritual care—developing a standard. *Int J Palliat Nurs* **9**(5): 208.

64 Brown, D. (2001). A leap of faith: enabling hospice staff to meet the spiritual needs of patients. *Scott J Hlthcare Chaplaincy* **4**(1): 21–5.

65 Cornette, K. (2005). For whenever I am weak, I am strong. *Int J Palliat Nurs* 6–13.

66 Hegarty, M. (2007). Care of the spirit that transcends religious, ideological and philosophical boundaries. *Ind J Palliat Care* **13**(2): 42.

67 Lloyd-Williams, M., Friedman, T., Rudd, N. (1999). A survey of antidepressant prescribing in the terminally ill. *Palliat Med* **13**(3): 243.

68 Scottish Executive Heath Department (SEHD). (2002). *Guidelines on Chaplaincy and Spiritual Care in the NHS in Scotland SEHD*, Glasgow: SEHD.

69 Lloyd-Williams, M., Cobb, M., Shiels, C., Taylor, F. (2006). How well trained are clergy in care of the dying patient and bereavement support? *J Pain Sympt Manag* **32**(1): 44–51.

70 Gordon, T., Mitchell, D. (2004). A competency model for the assessment and delivery of spiritual care. *Palliat Med* **18**(7): 646.

71 Cobb, M. (2001). Dying well: a guide to enable a good death. *Mortality* **5**(2): 221.

72 Smith, S.A. (2000). *Hospice Concepts: A Guide to Palliative Care in Terminal Illness*. Campaign: Research Press Publications.

73 Wasner, M., Longaker, C., Fegg, M.J., Borasio, G.D. (2005). Effects of spiritual care training for palliative care professionals. *Palliat Med* **19**(2): 99.

74 Walter, T. (1996). Developments in spiritual care of the dying. *Religion* **26**(4): 353–63.

75 Grimes, R.L. (1999). Contribution to 'Forum on Spirituality.' *J Religion Am Cult* Summer: 145–52.

76 Department of Health, (2009). *Religion or Belief: a Practical Guide for the NHS*. London: DH Publications.

77 Bauer-Wu, S., Barrett, R., Yeager, K. (2007). Spiritual perspectives and practices at the end-of-life: A review of the major world religions and application to palliative care. *Ind J Palliat Care* **13**(2): 53.

78 Doona, M.E., Haggerty, L.A., Chase, S.K. (1997). Nursing presence: an existential exploration of the concept. *Res Theory Nurs Pract* **11**(1): 3–16.

79 McDonough-Means, S.I., Kreitzer, M.J., Bell, I.R. (2004). Fostering a healing presence and investigating its mediators. *J Altern Complement Med* **10**(Supplement 1). 25–41.

80 Godkin, J. (2001). Healing presence. *J Holistic Nurs Offic J Am Holistic Nurses' Ass* **19**(1): 5.

81 Cimino, J.E. (2000). *Humanizing Hospitals: Total Care. The Humanization of Care in the Age of Advanced Technology*, pp. 123–7. publication of the Universita of Campus Bio-Medical, Roma, Italy, editors Pier Giovanni Palla, Stefano Grossi Gondi.

82 Mako, C., Galek, K., Poppito, S.R. (2006). Spiritual pain among patients with advanced cancer in palliative care. *J Palliat Med* **9**(5): 1106–13.

83 Mowat, H., Swinton, J. (2005). *What Do Chaplain Do? A Report on a Two Year Investigation into the Nature of Chaplaincy in the NHS in Scotland*. Edinburgh: Scottish Executive.

84 Johnson, L.S. (2003). Facilitating spiritual meaning-making for the individual with a diagnosis of a terminal illness. *Counsel Values* **47**(3): 230–41.

85 Dominian, J. (1983). Doctor as prophet. *Br Med J (Clin Res Ed)* **287**(6409): 1925–7.

86 Lipsman, N., Skanda, A., Kimmelman, J., Bernstein, M. (2007). The attitudes of brain cancer patients and their caregivers towards death and dying: a qualitative study. *Br Med Coun Palliat Care* **6**(1): 7.

87 Cortis, J.D., Williams, A. (2007). Palliative and supportive needs of older adults with heart failure. *Int Nurs Rev* **54**(3): 263–70.

88 Anderson, J.H. (2007). The impact of using nursing presence in a community heart failure program. *J Cardiovasc Nurs* **22**(2): 89.

89 Breitbart, W., Gibson, C., Poppito, S.R. (2004). Psychotherapeutic interventions at the end of life: A focus on meaning and spirituality. *Can J Psychiat* **49**: 366–72.

90 Breitbart, W. (2002). Spirituality and meaning in supportive care: spirituality-and meaning-centered group psychotherapy interventions in advanced cancer. *Support Care Cancer* **10**(4): 272–80.

91 Frankl, V.E. (1959). *Man's Search for Meaning*. Boston: Beacon Press.

92 Frankl, V.E (1967). *Psychotherapy and Existentialism: Selected Papers on Logotherapy*. London: Simon Schuster.

93 Frankl, V.E., Frank, V.E.(1969). *The Will to Meaning: Foundations and Applications of Logotherapy*. New York: New American Library.

94 Gysels, M., Higginson, I.J., Rajasekaran, M., Davies, E., Harding, R. (2004). Improving Supportive and Palliative Care for Adults with Cancer. Research Evidence Manual. London: National Institute of Clinical Excellence.

95 MacConville, U.N.A. (2006). Mapping religion and spirituality in an Irish palliative care setting. *OMEGA*—J Death Dying **53**(1): 137–52.

96 Narayanasamy, A. (2007). Palliative care and spirituality. *Ind J Palliat Care* **13**(2): 32.

97 Narayanasamy, A., Clissett, P., Parumal, L., Thompson, D., Annasamy, S., Edge, R. (2004). Responses to the spiritual needs of older people. *J Adv Nurs* **48**(1): 6–16.

98 Tanyi, R.A., Werner, J.S. (2008). Women's experience of spirituality within end-stage renal disease and hemodialysis. *Clin Nurs Res* **17**(1): 32.

CHAPTER 37

Spirituality and the arts: discovering what really matters

Nigel Hartley

Introduction

The arts—music, painting, sketching, poetry, storytelling, drama—allow us to access and represent aspects of our experience that may otherwise elude recognition and articulation. This can, in turn, reinforce resilience and enhance understanding of our selves, other people, and our world. A growing body of evidence shows that the arts and humanities can help patients to manage pain and the side effects of some treatments, to alleviate stress and anxiety, and to come to terms with what can be major and distressing episodes in their lives.[1] Not surprisingly, the arts have for many years been used for therapeutic support and intervention in serious illness,[2] and end-of-life care.[3] Similarly, arts-based programmes that promote collective action have been used to improve health knowledge and practice and develop community resilience.[4] The arts and humanities encourage us to value ways of knowing, particularly experiential and presentational knowing[5] that in healthcare contexts can be marginalized by the clinical sciences' focus on propositional and practical knowing.[6] Arts-based enquiries explore how individuals and communities construct meaning by representing and reflecting upon experiences that challenge prior understandings of the world and our place in it. Arts-based enquiry is thus a natural ally of spiritual growth and care.[7,8] Creative arts methods are also increasingly being used in research enquiries in which spirituality is an integral, albeit at times more an implicit than explicit, part.[6,9,10]

This chapter outlines possibilities opened up by arts-based enquiries carried out in the particular setting of St Christopher's Hospice, London, and the context of end-of-life care. Following an orientation to the setting and its approach to care, three stories illustrate the development of spiritual insight through creative arts enquiry, and in doing so demonstrate the potential for arts-based approaches to offer support in critical life transitions in general.

St Christopher's Hospice, London

St Christopher's Hospice is based in Sydenham, South London. It was opened in 1967 and is often described as the first modern hospice. The inspiration of Dame Cicely Saunders who had worked in the new National Health Service of the 1940s and 1950s where dying was not part of the vision,[11] it aspired to be a place where dying could be accepted as a normal experience and managed well. A unified mix of care, education, and research was at the core of the provision and utilization of hospice care from the outset and the success of Saunders early research into pain and symptom management both challenged and inspired the world of medicine to change its focus.[12] In order to address all the needs of those who were dying, Saunders created the concept of 'total pain',[13] which brought together in an integrated way the physical, emotional, social, and spiritual pain of those who are dying. The inclusion of the needs of patients' families and carers was also an essential part of her 'total pain' model. The promotion and formulation of multidisciplinary working was key to Saunders' vision and continues to remain at the heart of end-of-life care.[14]

Despite the realization of Cicely Saunders' vision with almost 300 hospices in the UK and end-of-life care programmes in over 115 countries across the world, we are still left with some considerable and pressing challenges. More people will come to the end of their lives in care homes due to a growing ageing population and ways will need to be found to care for the many people who will live longer with multiple, chronic illnesses. Single person households will put additional pressure on formal health and social care providers, and those who belong to 'excluded' groups, such as black and minority ethnic people, those living with deprivation and those living with the 'wrong disease' will need to access good care in the places they need it, at the time they need it.

Spiritual care and the multidisciplinary team

> *... the necessity for, and utility of, multidisciplinary teams in palliative care has become an almost automatic assumption. The assumption stems from an understanding of the need to integrate and co-ordinate the multiple skills and complex knowledge base required to deliver the holistic care to which palliative care aspires ...'[15]*

One of the strengths of the development of modern hospices has been the formulation of a broad range of health and social care professionals into multidisciplinary teams in order to meet the complex needs of those that they care for at the end of life. The strengths and benefits of multidisciplinary working, such as good communication, sharing knowledge, the preparation of detailed care plans and the enactment of those plans are obvious and well documented.[16] However, the complexities and downsides of working in close relationship with a range of different healthcare professionals are rarely addressed. These include, for example, the difficulties of an increasing part-time work force, which can lead to gaps in communication and knowledge. Also the struggle to comprehend a plethora of uniquely specialized professional languages can sometimes cause confusion and uncertainty.

The reality of the task of providing a multi-faceted web of 'total' care to the dying, their families and carers raises challenges for multi-disciplinary team members.[16] It is not as straightforward as doctors providing medical care and nurses providing physical care, with psychologists, social workers, therapists and artists providing psychological and emotional care and the chaplain providing spiritual care. In reality there are a myriad of grey areas. Many members of the team will address and offer a variable blend of the four segments of the 'total pain' quadrant which provides the team as a whole with a complex and demanding task. Spirituality and spiritual care perhaps provide the biggest challenge of all. This may be because of the apparent difficulties in defining what spirituality is and how it is addressed, and also how health and social care providers struggle together to share a common understanding of a definition and its meaning. This is evident in a recent book where Aldridge cites seventeen different definitions of the word 'spirituality';[17] the world of 'new age' theory offers innumerable other possibilities.[18]

St Christopher's and spiritual care

Background

St Christopher's Hospice was originally opened as a Christian Foundation, with the large chapel on the ground floor of the building supporting the care of those who were looked after on the in-patient wards above. The chapel also provided an important personal place for Saunders herself, together with the staff that she employed, to congregate and worship regularly.[19] In order to support her own calling and the wider practice of the multi-disciplinary team, Saunders appointed a Church of England chaplain. It is well documented that the establishment of St Christopher's Hospice was strongly based on Cicely Saunders' personal Christian calling.[20] A St Christopher's Hospice Foundation group was formed in 1961, well before the opening of the building, articulated Saunders' vision in an early document:

> *St Christopher's Hospice is based on the full Christian faith in God, through Christ. Its aim is to express the love of God to all who come, in every possible way; in skilled nursing and medical care, in the use of every scientific means of relieving suffering and distress, in understanding personal sympathy, with respect for the dignity of each person as a human being, precious to God and man. There are no barriers of race, colour, class or creed.*[21]

This is further supported in a letter written in the same year where Saunders writes to the Lord Bishop of Stepney setting out her Christian vision for the work and asking for the support of the church to realize this:

> *13 January 1961. The plans for St. Christopher's Hospice are going along slowly … I am enclosing a draft of the Memorandum and also of the précis, because I would like you to see … the parts which refer to the spiritual side of the work … he (Lord Taylor) suggested to me that it was really time for me to see the Bishop of Southwark … also suggested that I should see the Dean of Westminster … but I would like to see them to discuss the vision … Could I … say that I am having your help and blessing?*[20]

Current changes and challenges

The community of St Christopher's services has experienced enormous changes since the hospice opened in 1967. In 2010, South East London incorporates a diverse population of people from a range of different cultures with a variety of belief systems and none. With regard to the latter, it is true that many people who are cared for by St Christopher's today will have no religious belief or will carry negative impressions because of their past associations and experiences with, and of, organized religion. This diversity presents the modern day multi-disciplinary team with a number of challenges and dilemmas. Rather than being placed within a specific tradition, it is evident that spiritual care must now cover and address a broader range of need driven by the expectations of service users who represent a range of religious beliefs together with a large group of people who do not have any religious belief system at all. However, experience shows that just because people do not enact their lives within a formal religious framework, does not mean that their spiritual needs as they come to die are not vastly important. Human beings carry with them a wealth of important experiences. We are told that these include things such as falling in love, experiencing joy and laughter, as well as feeling compassion and seeking justice.[22] We also know that these experiences include knowing what it is like to be sick and vulnerable, and what it is like to lose and to be hurt. It is evident that when people come to die such experiences need to be explored and understood. Doing so can offer a wealth of valuable material which can then be utilized in order to give people's lives a context within which to explore both meaning and worth. Of course, those who have a religious belief might call upon that belief to support them and St Christopher's employs a full time Chaplain to support the needs of such people and also to guide the staff who care for them and to provide contact with a range of community faith leaders. The Chaplain's role extends beyond just supporting, to include engaging and educating both the staff and faith leaders within the local community about the needs of the users that the organization supports. However, the increasingly large number of users who will not have such belief systems to call upon demands something different. Indeed, they may not know what they need and a range of possibilities will be required to enable them to see what is possible. It is therefore important for an organization providing good end-of-life care to think seriously about what kinds of services may be useful in supporting the spiritual needs of users, particularly beyond the confines of a specific religious belief.

Spiritual care: a shared definition

During 2010 the National Council for Palliative Care (UK) brought together a working party in order to explore spiritual care provision for those facing the end of life. The results of the working party, which consisted of key end-of-life care practitioners from across the UK, were published in a document outlining current thinking and practice.[23] Three questions were recognized as being a significant part of a useful framework to be used when asking people to explore meaning at the end of life:

1. How do people understand what is currently happening to them?
2. When life has been difficult in the past, what kind of things have helped?
3. Would any of these things, or anything else they can think of, be helpful to them now?

Using these questions with people facing the end of life offers both potential and possibility. The uniqueness and singularity of each person's responses removes the mystery and magic which can sometimes be associated with the spiritual. Answers range from 'playing bingo' to 'watching the sunset,' from 'holding my grandchild in my arms' to 'listening to Louis Armstrong singing '*What a wonderful world.*' These answers may be more straightforward than we might anticipate, but with them comes the potential for motivation and change. The questions also offer the possibility for spirituality to be explored in an uncomplicated way.

Spirituality and the arts: three stories

It is not unusual for the arts to be related to spirituality.[17] Iris Murdoch, the British novelist writes that all serious art, in an unreligious age, provides for many people their clearest experience of something grasped as separate, precious, and beneficial.[24] There are many examples of people coming to the end of their life being able to access both their past experiences and also new possibilities with art forms, such as music, painting, and poetry when all else might seem lost. James, an elderly gentleman with advanced dementia, had lost all speech and did not communicate. A chance playing one day on the care home radio of Frank Sinatra singing 'Fly me to the moon' saw him not just singing along complete with perfect lyrics, but *performing* to other residents. Anita, a young mother, coming to the end of her life in a hospice, decorated her room with a number of paintings created by herself some years previously. Her ambition had been to train as an artist, but an early pregnancy had prevented this and was quickly followed by a diagnosis of cancer. Her paintings were deeply important to her, and introduced a part of her to both her friends and the hospice staff, which they might never have known. Finally, Harry had been a long haul trucker and lived alone. During the last weeks of his life, living with advanced chronic obstructive pulmonary disease (COPD) he was visited at home by an artist from the local hospice. After he died, his children discovered a series of tender, moving poems in his bedroom that articulated things he had never been able to say to them.

The arts offer a range of possibilities, a set of atypical structures, languages, and contexts for things to be explored and understood. The arts also move us, not just emotionally, but physically.[3] It is this motivation that can draw out of us an unusual energy that impels us to respond, create, and make sense of the situation in which we find ourselves.[25]

The following three stories give examples of the arts being used in different ways. However, it is the use of different art forms as part of each person's story which offers the possibility and potential for the person to discover meaning and to gain a unique and deeper understanding of what is happening to them.

Story one: Danny

Danny is 38 and is spending the last days of his life in the hospice in-patient unit. He has primary cancer of the oesophagus with liver metastases. He has been admitted to the unit as an emergency due to difficulties in managing pain and the complexities of his lifestyle. On admission, Danny's problems were assessed as follows:

- Continuous abdominal pain
- No appetite, nausea, and vomiting
- Low mood and little motivation
- Lack of willingness to mobilize.

Although it appeared that Danny was aware of his diagnosis, he was prone to aggressive verbal outbursts when approached directly, and constantly sobbed and cried with different degrees of intensity. His eyes were almost permanently closed tight. Over 2 days, the medical consultant and the nursing team worked as best they could to reduce his pain, and make him comfortable. A syringe driver was set up consisting of a combination of:

- Diamorphine—pain
- Metoclopramide—nausea
- Dexamethasone—pain, appetite, mood.

It was difficult to assess the success of the drug combinations as Danny always appeared to be in agony due to his constant crying and holding himself in a foetal position. Mostly, when any member of the team approached Danny he was verbally aggressive towards them.

A couple of months before Danny's admission, he was visited at his hostel by a community nurse specialist, together with a social worker. During this visit, although wary and distrusting, Danny opened up and told them part of his life story. The social worker fed back the content of the interview with Danny to the multidisciplinary team when he was admitted to the hospice ward some weeks later.

Danny was homeless and had spent a number of years living on the streets of the city, staying in hostels when he was able to collect enough money through busking with his guitar in order to buy himself a night's accommodation. He told them that he sang Simon and Garfunkel, and Beatles songs, as he could relate many of them to his own life. Over the past two years, Danny had been admitted to the Accident and Emergency Unit of the city hospital on a number of occasions. He was also admitted to the hospital for cancer treatment, but the pattern evolved that when Danny felt strong enough, he discharged himself from the hospital and returned to the streets. Danny was a veteran of the first Gulf War of the early 1990s. He was a member of the coalition ground forces which invaded Iraq in 1991 as part of Operation Desert Storm. He was reluctant to talk about his war experiences in detail, and when asked directly about anything he became verbally aggressive and defensive. He said that, following his time in the army, he had been discharged on 'medical grounds,' and admitted that recurring images in his head had turned him into a 'loner' and a 'freak'. He described himself as 'crazy' and said that he expected nothing from anyone, and chose and deserved to live the life he did. Danny also disclosed that he had spent periods of time in prison, and when people 'wound him up', he became 'out of control' and physically aggressive. His medical records from his previous admissions into hospital showed that there was a history of alcohol abuse.

During a multidisciplinary team meeting, frustration was aired due to the teams' inability to allay Danny's distress through any pharmaceutical or physical means and there was also a growing request to draw the line as to what was acceptable in terms of the aggressive behaviour displayed by Danny towards staff. The nursing team was concerned for other patients, as Danny's cries could be heard across the unit, especially during the night when they appeared to be at their worst. It was agreed that gaining an understanding of Danny's psychological and emotional state would be key to successfully managing the situation.

The physiotherapist had spent some time massaging Danny's hands for short periods, during which his distressing vocalizing had calmed for brief moments. She visited him two or three times during the day. The team agreed that it was important for her to continue seeing him and I agreed to visit with her, responding to the team's request to improvise some 'gentle music' in order to support her work to see if this might help calm Danny.

The first time that I met Danny, I accompanied the physiotherapist for one of the massage sessions. I took with me a simple stringed instrument resembling a small harp. Danny lay on the bed in a foetal position with his eyes tightly closed. He was restless and he intermittently vocalized harsh sounds and rude words. The physiotherapist introduced me to him, but there was little observable response. It is interesting to point out that there was no noticeable aggressive verbal outburst either to the physiotherapist or myself. The physiotherapist began to gently massage his hands and I began to play softly in the background. His vocal sounds were gruff and musically based around a minor 2nd interval. Occasionally, I picked out the minor second on the strings, and when I did this, his vocalizing became stronger and more intense. Although I had agreed to gently support the physiotherapist's work with my playing, my instinct was to meet his vocal sounds head on. However, I decided to continue to play gently in the background during this first meeting. It was clear that the massage comforted him as he was noticeably more relaxed when we left him.

Following this first meeting, the physiotherapist, social worker, medical consultant, nurse, and myself talked together about what had happened and discussed our future plans. The physiotherapist and social worker agreed with the instinct to meet Danny's crying head on; however, the doctor was anxious about increasing his distress and disturbing other patients. We decided that, in order to remove him from the ward, it would be possible to take Danny to the music room in his bed. I asked that the physiotherapist came with him and carry on massaging him in a similar way. We planned this meeting for the afternoon of the following day.

The nurse, physiotherapist, and myself took Danny in his bed to the music room and made him as comfortable as possible. His vocalizing was still very distressing and his body cramped with pain. As the physiotherapist began to massage his hands and arms, I began to accompany Danny's vocal sounds from the piano. I used a Spanish style of music, based around a tonality of F. This not only provided a basis to meet the minor 2nd interval of Danny's vocal sounds, but also a capacity to extend the structure of the vocalizing into more 'declamatory' bursts of sound. I used the piano to provide a basis for our musical improvisation and began to match Danny's voice with my own. Initially, I reflected the minor second non-verbally. I then moved on to singing his name intermittently. Each time I sang his name, his vocalizing stopped for a brief moment. A few moments into the improvisation, there was a noticeable change in Danny's posture. This was verbalized by the physiotherapist when she said gently, 'You're relaxing Danny, that's it ...' His head turned towards where I was situated at the piano, although his eyes still remained shut. He began to speak very slowly over the music, occasionally slipping into melody created within a minor 3rd. The verbal content of Danny's song follows:

'Why you tryin'? Why you tryin'?

Don't, don't, don' you please ...

It's all dark, all gone, gone, gone,

I'm alone without her smilin', is she smilin'?

Was she ever there, there, there?

I'm waitin' in the dark, waitin', waitin',

Take my hand, reach my hand toward the silence,

Sound o' silence, the hauntin' sound o' silence.

Mmmmm (humming)

My ol' friend, yeah, my ol' friend,

I know she's comin', comin', comin',

I see her now all clothed in light,

She understands me, does she? doesn't she?,

Takes my hands, does she? doesn't she?

Does she know I did it all for her?

Does she know it? Does she know?

Mmmm (humming)

Imagine it could be OK? OK?

Imagine she could understand?

We're almost there, almost, almost,

I see a yellow ribbon in ya' hair, ya' hair,

Ya' welcome me, Ya' welcome me

It's fair, I care, you cut my hair,

Ya' dare... to cut my hair...

It's OK, OK,

I'm there ... take my hand ... take it ... take it ...

Mmmm (humming)[27]

At the end, Danny's voice slows and he exhales long, heavy breaths. He is calm and relaxed. The physiotherapist, having gently massaged his arms during the entire musical improvisation, speaks gently, 'thank you Danny, thank you'. Following a period of silence we take him back to his room.

Danny remained quiet and relaxed for the following two days with only intermittent periods of unrest. He died peacefully with the nursing staff present.

As Danny had no money and there was no knowledge of any living relatives, the local council provided assistance for a basic cremation. He was cremated at the city crematorium and his ashes were scattered there in the Garden of Remembrance. There was no formal funeral service.

About two years after Danny's death, the hospice was contacted by an elderly couple who had been searching for their missing son. They had not seen him for over eight years, and thought that he had moved to the area following his discharge from the armed forces. Their searching had led them to contact hospitals in the area and they had come to the end of their search at the hospice. They asked to see Danny's multidisciplinary notes, and the social worker and myself met with them. They told us of Danny's childhood and how proud they were of him when he joined the army. Some months before he was called up to Iraq, he was married to his childhood sweetheart. While he was there, she had been killed in a tragic road accident. When Danny was discharged from the army, he disappeared and they never saw or heard from him again, apart from a couple of brief phone calls. We told them of Danny's last days in the hospice and of his calm and peaceful death. I also told them about his song, which felt relevant as the story they told helped us to understand it. They were obviously moved by the experience, but were not surprised by Danny's creativity as they told us he had spent most of his childhood writing and improvising songs using his guitar. Danny's parents left us with the intention of visiting the crematorium where their son's ashes had been scattered. They gave us permission, and indeed encouraged us, to tell Danny's story as part of our work. It has taken a number of years to do so.

Story two: Christopher

Christopher lived in a care home in South East London. He was living with a muscle wasting disease and had lost all use in his limbs. His career had been in the parachute regiment, and he had recently finished a long-term relationship. He had a young son, who lived with his ex-partner some distance away and he was becoming increasingly anxious that his ex-partner would never let him see his son again. During a conversation with his community nurse, Christopher articulated some of these fears. The nurse described a feeling of hopelessness and desperation when she recounted her meeting to the multidisciplinary team with which she worked. When she asked what might be of help to him, he said that he would like to make a DVD recording, so that he could leave behind something of himself for his son so that he would have an 'accurate record' of his father's life.

Following a discussion back with the team back at the hospice, a community artist visited him. During the first meeting Christopher told her that he wanted to record himself speaking into a video camera. She set it up and during a number of visits, Christopher recorded his life story, recounting his pride of being in the parachute regiment. During one session, Christopher said to the artist that one of the things other people constantly asked him was how he coped with his increasing disability and isolation. He told her that he would like to write a poem for his son, answering this question 'head on', so that when his son saw the recording of his father, he would not feel sorry for him, but be proud of the way he had coped. Together, Christopher and the artist wrote the following poem which was then recorded on camera as part of the DVD. Although Christopher never saw his son again before he died, the DVD was given to him, and the son now has it, not only as a memory, but as a testament to his fathers' living and dying.

I long for the day to become night, for the clouds to come down.
I long to sleep at night, because then my dreams start.
Quiet solitude, noises of the night, time goes by.
It's true, I look forward to my nightly dream,
Once my dreams are here I exit my body
I'm running on air, I'm walking on air.
I run up the road with my face all aglow with the breeze,
I'm skiing down the ski slope, surfing the waves of the sea
I'm standing in the door of a Hercules with my parachute hooked up
I'm waiting for the doors to open—'Red on, Green on, Go!'.
I have the feeling of space between me and the ground
Like I used to do when I was able bodied.
I'm with you and time goes by.
At night I open the window, I hear the sea roar,
I listen to the wind howling, time goes by.
I can't use my arms and legs, all that is functional is my head
I escape my body through my mind.
While I'm awake I feel like a prisoner.
I stimulate my mind, it stops me from cracking up, time goes by.
Warmth on my back, I lay in fields of wheat waving in the Summer breeze,
Lying down looking up at the sky.
I walk to the beach, there's not a soul around,
I have a beach but which gives me shelter and security,
I watch the sun set skimming over the water gently down to the sea.
All of a sudden there is darkness and time goes by.[27]

Story three: Francesca

I first met Francesca in the garden of St Christopher's Hospice one afternoon. On my way back from a meeting, I was met by one of our nurses. She told me that Francesca had arrived that morning as a new day patient, but had been too afraid to come into the building. She had spent most of the day sitting in the garden intermittently joined by a variety of multi-disciplinary team members, including volunteers. The nurse asked me if I would mind sitting with Francesca for while until her friend arrived in order to give her a lift home. Francesca was 42 years old with advanced chronic obstructive pulmonary disease. She used a wheelchair and was on constant oxygen. When I met Francesca, she was smoking and her eyes were red from crying. I introduced myself and she immediately began to sob. She asked questions, such as: 'What will it be like when I die?' 'Have you ever been with anyone when they died?' 'What will it be like when I stop breathing?' 'Why is this happening to me?' 'How can I leave my 8-year-old son behind?' In my helplessness and not knowing, I found my mind racing and I struggled to know how to respond. It seemed clear to me that Francesca would have asked these questions a number times that day, probably to each person who had sat with her in the garden. In a moment I reached out and touched her hand and said 'Do you mind if I stop you?' She stopped immediately and appeared shocked. My next question was 'What makes you laugh?' I had no idea where this question came from, it was certainly not thought out or planned. For a moment I was shocked too and was convinced I had made a mistake. Quick as a flash, Francesca answered my question—'Orang-utans of course!' She was animated and her eyes flashed. I responded 'Orang-utans? What do they look like? Monkeys, chimpanzees, gorillas, they're all the same to me!' 'No' she said, 'Orangu-tans are really funny! They're orange and full of mischief. My son and I love them so much, we have adopted one at the local zoo and pay some money regularly so it can be looked after. We've had some great trips there to see him, he's called Seamus'. There was then a sudden pause. 'Many orang-utans abandon their children. How can anyone leave a child behind?' She began to cry again. Her friend came to collect her and she left.

On reflection, I never thought that I would see Francesca again and the memory of our conversation faded after a couple of days. Some days later, one of the hospice nurses told me that one of the patients wanted to see me. I went up to the day care centre and saw Francesca sitting in her chair drinking a gin and tonic. She waved me over, and when I did so she presented me with a large envelope. She said it was for me and asked me to open it. When I did so, I discovered a painting of an orang-utan. She told me that her son had painted it the night before and they wanted me to have it, so that I really knew what an orang-utan looked like. I thanked her and asked her to thank her son. She concluded our conversation:

> As he (her son) was painting, choosing the colours and different brushes, I realized something. That even though orang-utans abandon their children, they do survive!

Francesca died at home about a week later. I still have the painting of the orang-utan. It continues to remind me of the powerful nature of the arts and how the simplicity of a brush stroke, the structure of a repeated group of words or the configuration of a basic musical chord progression can sometimes enable a profound realization, as unique and individual as the person who creates them.

Conclusion

It is regularly commented upon that the spiritual needs of those coming to the end of life are articulated through asking the 'big questions,'[22] such as 'Why is this happening to me?' and 'What have I done in my life to deserve this?' Where we might fail those people who we care for is when we leave them alone with their questions, helpless and afraid. Although such questions may never be answered, we need to commit ourselves into a relationship which must remain full of potential and possibility, both exceptional and dynamic. Without the arts, we lack one of the most important vocabularies with which to engage with these 'big questions', a vocabulary to articulate the unconscious which includes, for example, myths, symbols, poetry and music.

Whilst good pain management is vital and widely thought to lie at the heart of palliative care, in reality, it is only the tip of the iceberg. Cicely Saunders coined the phrase 'spiritual pain,' a pain that for many is deeply related to fear and anger and the search for understanding and value. Such fears can never be met by medication alone; such fears can never be met by religious belief and ritual alone; such fears can never be met by the arts alone. The concept of 'total care' commits all of us, whatever our professional role or part or personal belief, to engage with the unique needs of each dying individual and those close to them. Understanding and meaning will be found in different ways for each person. However, we must not forget the usefulness of the arts. At the end of life a previously undiscovered significance might be found in that song which was played at a wedding, in that painting that hung above a fireplace in a favourite hotel, or in that dance in the street during the declaration of peace in 1945.

St Christopher's sits within a changing community, which incorporates many different religious beliefs and spiritual practices. In response to this, St Christopher's no longer exists within a single or rigid religious frame, and it is within an increasingly eclectic mix of religious and spiritual need that current spiritual care and practice should be set. The Pilgrim Room, which provides a space within the hospice building for users to reflect, contemplate, and remember was designed around users' requests for a place where they could light candles and write messages and memories within a large book. A large contemporary stained glass window, together with an installation of mosaics, made by a group of patients, help to bring a stature and ambiance to the space, which users regularly comment on. With regard to the provision of spiritual support to present day hospice patients and their carers, we are currently encouraging the entire multidisciplinary workforce to recognize their part in addressing the spiritual needs of those that they care for. Spiritual care should not be seen as a separate specialism. Most dying people will not compartmentalize their care needs. When needing to ask the 'big questions', it is more than likely it will be in the context of their everyday care. These questions will be asked of the nurse, the doctor and the social worker, of the cleaner and the volunteer. St Christopher's is creating training and education programmes so that all members of the multidisciplinary team feel as competent and confident as possible in addressing the spiritual needs of patients. This competence and confidence should also include knowledge of when and how to signpost the user to a more appropriate person when it is needed. This may well be the chaplain, but also the physiotherapist, the social worker, artist or other practitioner. As more people come to the end of their life within the places that they live, a real challenge will be how we equip both health and social care workers together with community faith leaders to realize their responsibility in responding to, and supplying people with appropriate and realistic spiritual support. At St Christopher's we believe that the hospice has a responsibility to act as a 'hub' and to work together with community groups in order to educate and facilitate good spiritual care provision for people whoever they are, wherever they might be. This is part of a current ongoing development programme.

There is a 'bigness' about the arts. They provide infinite room and space for a myriad of stories and experiences to be created, shared and witnessed. If spirituality is about anything, it is about 'bigness' too. When it comes to the end of life, size does matter. Marianne Williamson writes that our deepest fear is not that we are inadequate and small, but that our deepest fear is that we are powerful and big beyond measure.[26] Most people coming to the end of their life are likely to question what it has all meant and ask, usually from a place of smallness and fear, if they have really made a difference. Our job is to be as open and flexible as possible so that those placed in our care at the end of their life can die knowing that they too have lived a life which has been not only powerful and big, but also full of meaning and purpose.

References

1 Starikof, R. (2004). *Arts in Health: a Review of the Medical Literature*, Research Report 36, London: Arts Council England.

2 Waller, D., Sibbett, C. (eds) (2005). *Art Therapy and Cancer Care*. Maidenhead: Open University Press,

3 Hartley, N., Payne, M. (2008). *The Creative Arts in Palliative Care*. London: Jessica Kingsley Publications.

4 White, M (2009). *Arts Development in Community Health: a Social Tonic*. Oxford: Radcliffe.

5 Heron, J., Reason, P. (1997). A participatory inquiry paradigm. *Qual Inq* **3**(3): 274–95.

6 Liamputtong, P., Rumbold, J. (eds) (2008). *Knowing Differently: Arts-based and Collaborative Research Methods*. New York: Nova Science Press.

7 McNiff, S. (2004). *Art Heals: How Creativity Cures the Soul*. Boston: Shambhala.

8 Stanworth, R. (2003). *Recognizing Spiritual Needs in People Who are Dying*. Oxford: Oxford University Press.

9 McNiff, S. (1998). *Art-based Research*. London: Jessica Kingsley.

10 Knowles, G., Cole, A. (eds) (2008). *Handbook of the Arts in Qualitative Research*. Thousand Oaks: Sage.

11 Monroe, B., Oliviere, D. (2003). *Patient Participation in Palliative Care: A Voice for the Voiceless*. Oxford: Oxford University Press.

12 Watson, M.S., Lucas, C.F., Hoy, A.M., Back, I.N. (1993). *The Oxford Handbook of Palliative Care*, Oxford Handbooks Series. Oxford: Oxford University Press.

13 Saunders, C. (1978). The philosophy of terminal care. In: C. Saunders (ed.) *The Management of Terminal Disease*, pp. 193–202. London: Edward Arnold.

14 Hartley, N. (2008). The arts in health and social care—is music therapy fit for purpose? *Br J Music Ther* **22**(2): 88–96.

15 Monroe, B. (2006). Team effectiveness—a reflection. In: P. Speck, (ed.) *Teamwork in Palliative Care: Fulfilling or Frustrating?* Oxford: Oxford University Press.

16 Speck, P. (2006). *Teamwork in Palliative Care: Fulfilling or Frustrating?* Oxford: Oxford University Press.

17 Aldridge, D. (2000). *Spirituality, Healing and Medicine*. London: Jessica Kingsley Publications.

18 Mayne, M. (1998). *Pray, Love, Remember*. London: Darton, Longman and Todd.

19 Saunders, C. (1967). Cited in: Clark D (2002). *Cicely Saunders—Founder of the Hospice Movement Selected Letters* 1959–1999. Oxford: Oxford University Press.

20 Saunders, C. (1961). *St Christopher's Hospice Aims and Objectives.* Unpublished

21 Clark, D. (2002). *Cicely Saunders—Founder of the Hospice Movement Selected Letters* 1959–1999. Oxford: Oxford University Press.

22 Mayne, M. (2002). *Learning to Dance*. London: Darton, Longman and Todd.

23 National Council for Palliative Care. (2010). *Finding the Missing Piece—the Results of a Working Party*. London: NCPC.

24 Whibley, M.E.L. (1998). The redemption of Art. *Br J Aesthet* **38**(4): 375–83.

25 Ansdell, G. (1995). *Music for Life—Aspects of Creative Music Therapy with Adult Clients*. London: Jessica Kingsley Publications.

26 Williamson, M. (1992). *A Return to Love—Reflections on the principles of 'A Course in Miracles'*. London: Harper Collins.

CHAPTER 38

Care of the soul

Michael Kearney and Radhule Weininger

Healing is about relationships. The healing process is one of establishing, tending, and deepening relationships, and may be experienced as a sense of connectedness and meaning. Fear of change, which is, in essence, the existential fear of the unknown and of death as the ultimate unknown, can impede or even prevent this process. While there is something in us that is inherently afraid of death, there is also something in us that is not afraid of death. As clinicians we continuously make choices about to how to prioritize our therapeutic interventions. In this context, we might ask ourselves: do we begin by trying to contain and lessen our patients' fear or by attending to that in our patients that is unafraid? This matters, hugely, because as psychologist William James reminds us, 'What we attend to becomes our reality, and what we don't attend to fades out of reality.'[1]

In this chapter we explore the relationship between fear of death and suffering. We consider how, if unrecognized, this same fear in clinicians may be counterproductive, sabotaging our best intentions to alleviate the suffering of our patients; possibly even compounding the situation. While continuing our clinical efforts to lessen suffering by containing fear, we suggest that it may be helpful for us to move beyond models of care that focus exclusively on problem-solving and damage limitation to ones where, from the outset, care of the soul is prioritized. We propose that the most effective way for us as clinicians to do this is to cultivate and practice a 'therapeutic use of self' by attending to our own inner depths, and to that in us that is not afraid of death.

Map of the human psyche

What is it in us that is afraid of death? What is it in us that is not afraid of death? Why and how does this matter? We can approach a possible answer to the first two of these questions by considering a psycho-spiritual map of the psyche. This map is based on concepts from the work of depth psychologist Carl Gustav Jung and from Buddhist Philosophy. With this as a backdrop, we will consider the third question by examining some of the intra-psychic dynamics of fear.

A useful metaphor for the individual human psyche is that of a wave on the ocean (Figure 38.1). The tip of the wave is the conscious part of the psyche in which the ego, the executive aspect or 'control room' of the psyche, is most at home (Figure 38.2). Other than its very tip, the rest of the wave represents the unconscious aspects of the psyche. Of note, the wave does not end at its base. Rather, the base of any individual wave flows into the ocean currents and is in continuity with the other waves on the ocean's surface.

Within this model the unconscious has three dimensions—the personal unconscious, the collective unconscious, and what we refer to as 'the deeper stream' (Figure 38.3). The *personal unconscious,* also known as the subjective unconscious, contains, for example, memories, repressed instincts and emotions, and is specific to that particular wave. The *collective unconscious*, also known as the objective or universal unconscious, is comprised of content that is shared 'collectively' among all human beings. Depth psychologist Carl Gustav Jung calls this the 'two million wise person within.'[2] He hypothesizes that the collective unconscious contains 'archetypes', latent patterns of distilled human wisdom that are activated in specific life circumstances, for example, at times of crisis or major transition. Below these layers of the unconscious is the *deeper stream*; an energetic flux that connects the individual wave to other waves and to the ocean's infinite depths.

The three dimensions of the unconscious are taken here to comprise 'soul'—the *depths of psyche*. This connection between soul and depth was highlighted by Heraclitus of Ephesus, the pre-Socratic Greek philosopher who wrote, 'You could not discover the limits of soul even if you travelled every road to do so; such is the *depth* of its meaning.'[3] Archetypal psychologist James Hillman amplifies this as a defining aspect of soul when he says, 'The dimension of soul is depth (not breath or height) and the dimension of soul travel is downward.'[4] Throughout the rest of this chapter we use the terms 'soul' and 'depth' interchangeably.

Seeing the unconscious figuratively as multilayered or multidimensional gives us a metaphor that allows us to appreciate that there are qualitatively different energies within the unconscious. It is important to emphasize that depicting the unconscious in this way is not intended to imply a hierarchy of value or importance, nor that these are static, reified entities. Rather, it seems more likely that these energies are part of a dynamic weave that is constantly moving between the unconscious and the conscious, between being and matter and that these energies are not confined to an individual 'wave' (i.e. psyche).

The ego, therefore, is, within this model, that in us that is not afraid of death. For the ego, security and control are synonymous. The *raison d'être* of ego is *maintaining the status quo*. For the ego, death represents a loss of self and of control and is the ultimate dread.

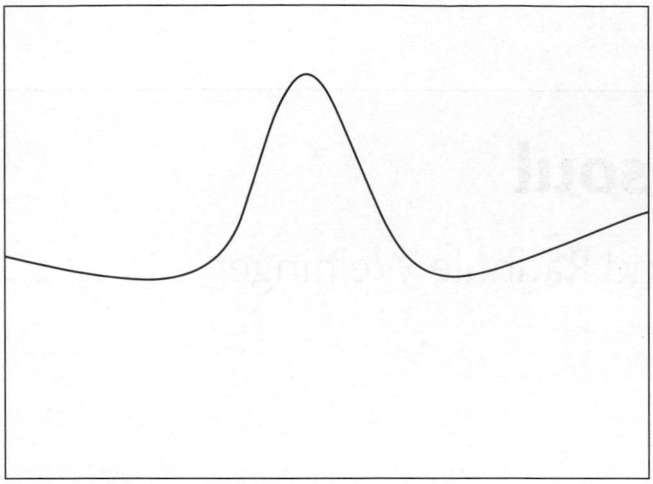

Figure 38.1 Metaphor for the individual human psyche.

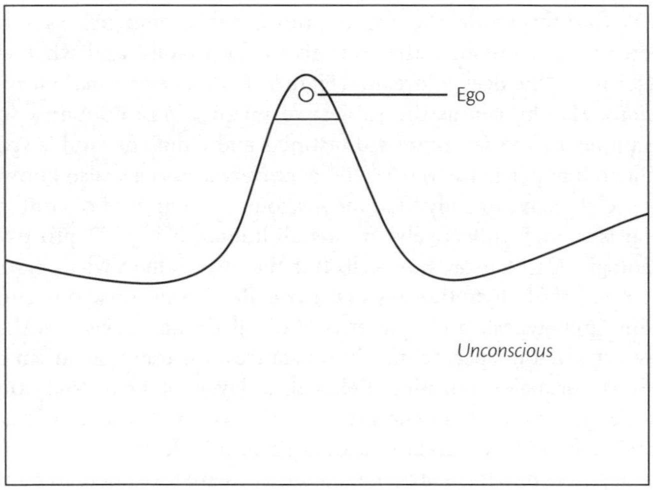

Figure 38.2 'Control room' of the psyche.

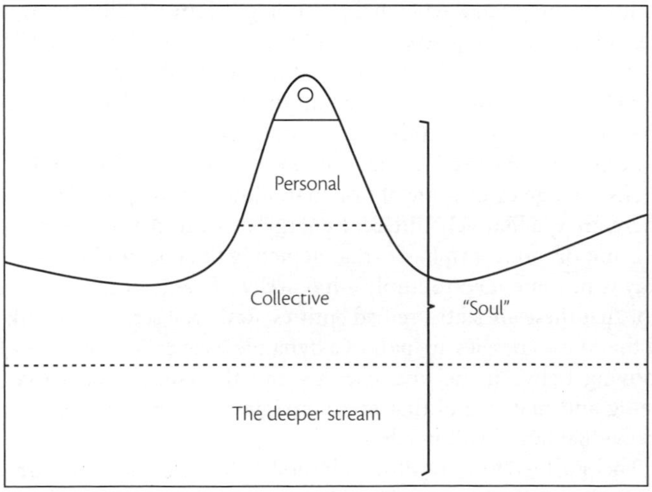

Figure 38.3 'The deeper stream.'

Understanding the dynamics of the frightened ego

In terms of the map of the psyche consider how might it be for the ego, perched on top of the wave, looking downwards (Figure 38.2):

> From the tip of the wave ego looks down into the ocean's depths and sees only darkness; a great unknown. Ego recoils to the tip of the tip of the wave. Ego feels safer there, closer to the light and in the driving seat. While this may bring some relief, this is, at best, temporary. What is more, there may be unforeseen and disturbing consequences ...

Understanding the dynamics of the frightened ego is clinically relevant. It enables us to more compassionately and effectively contain our patients' fear and facilitate the healing process. The dynamics are eloquently described by Ernst Becker in his book, 'The Denial of Death',[6] which inspired an approach called Terror Management Theory.[5] For over thirty years Solomon *et al.* have tested and validated these ideas. Their research is well summarized in the book, 'In the Wake of 911: The Psychology of Terror,'[7] and the award winning documentary film, 'Flight from Death'.[8] In essence, their findings confirm what we know from experience: that fear of death causes us to pull back from what is different or unfamiliar; to cling to what is familiar, and to distance, denigrate, and destroy what is perceived as a threat to the familiar.

In terms of the map of psyche we have outlined, 'the familiar' is the tip of the wave, with ego firmly in control. Threats to ego-control, such as reminders of mortality, terrify the ego, which retreats to the safety of the tip of the tip of the wave. The intra-psychic implications of Terror Management Theory are that we then act to support and maintain ego-control by over-valuing rational, materialistic, and literal forms of thinking, and distancing ourselves from perceived threats to ego control and reminders to our mortality; including the dark, alien, and unknown of the unconscious. While such strategies may have short-term benefits for the ego, as they reinforce its sense of control, they are, at best, short-lived. Furthermore, such distancing and disconnection from depth results in an anxious and rigid ego that is cut off from whatever healing potential there is in soul. This may manifest as intractable physical symptoms, as what hospice pioneer Cicely Saunders calls 'Total Pain,'[9] and/or as an experience of disassociation, alienation, isolation, and meaninglessness; 'soul pain.'[10]

The dynamics of the frightened ego are relevant throughout the illness trajectory. For example, with a new diagnosis the ego is given what is tantamount to a death sentence: 'Life as you knew it is over. Finished. However life will be from now on, it will never again be how it was'.

What is it in us that is not afraid of death?

Soul, as the unfathomable depths of psyche, includes that in us that is not afraid of death. Two authors, one writing from his lived experience of illness, the other from the perspective of years of meditation and spiritual practice, raise an intriguing possibility: could it be that that is us that is not afraid of death is that in us that does not die?

In his book, 'Body and Soul: The Other Side of Illness,'[11] Jungian analyst Albert Kreinheder chronicles his experience of living and dying with chronic illness. In the final pages of his book he writes:

> The more we are with soul, the less identified we are with the ego. We know our center to be a larger stream of life transcending ego and going on beyond our death. The soul is somehow in union with this larger being. And as I align myself more with soul and less with ego, the soul's story becomes my story. Then I cannot grieve unduly for the ego. It is like a candle that has had its hour and now must flicker and go out.[12]

Hindu scholar and teacher Sri Madhava Ashish, quoting from the *Kathopanishad* writes, 'Some wise man, seeking what does not die, with in-turned gaze beheld the Self'.[13] Commenting on this he says, 'That was neither mythology nor religious doctrine. It was a real man seeking a real answer to the emptiness of existential meaninglessness, seeking and finding at the very root of his being ... [It describes] the innate human capacity to experience the immaterial roots of self-awareness—call it the level of Self, soul, or what you will—and so receive the reassuring touch of what does not die, and with it the sense of a meaningful existence'.[14] He suggests that this process of self-discovery should not 'wait for the last days of terminal illness, when pain is the spur to try anything that promises relief, instead [it should be] seen as part of a life-long preparation for entry into a meaningful existence.'[15]

While Kreinheder writes from a Jungian and Sri Madhava Ashish from a Hindu perspective, there is a deep congruence in what they say. Common to both is a description of a transformational experiential encounter in realms beyond the ego. Both speak of a search, of a finding (or being found by), and of a letting go to and an aligning with 'soul' or 'Self'; portrayed here as a non-reified dynamic process. Then, 'the soul's story becomes my story.'[16] Then, I may find my 'self-identification with what does not die.'[17] Sri Madhava Ashish makes it clear that this inner quest is at least a lifetime's work. While it is evident that Kreinheder's final words are the fruit of years of analysis and introspection, there is also a sense that the illness experience has accelerated this process for him. The theme of illness as potentially catalytic to the spiritual journey is further explored by other authors: see 'Grace in Dying,'[18] 'The Alchemy of illness;'[19] 'Ego and Archetype;'[20] 'Learning to Fall.'[21]

How to care for the frightened ego?

We have considered what it is in us that is afraid of death: ego. We have considered what it is in us that is not afraid of death: soul. We have considered how the dynamics of the frightened ego can lead to a disconnection from soul and existential distress. How then might we go about caring for a fearful ego that can wreak such havoc?

The therapeutic approach we choose either increases or lessens the fear of the ego. A therapeutic approach that *only* attends to the biological aspects of disease can all too easily become an escalating spiral of fear. When the frightened ego of the patient meets the frightened ego of the clinician the dynamics of fight and flight are activated. While this may lead to a successful outcome, such as a cure or a helpful referral on to another clinician, if unsuccessful, which it is likely to be when the patient is experiencing existential suffering, it may instead compound the suffering as the patient experiences the excesses of over-treatment and/or abandonment.[22]

A more integrated therapeutic approach recognizes the importance of depth work and the need to attend to both body and soul.[23] Here, because we are aware and sensitive to the fundamental need to care for soul and appreciate the possible contribution that our colleagues from other disciplines can make in this, we include them in the care plan from the outset, in tandem with other clinical interventions. The plan of care then resembles a combination of disease and symptom modifying-treatments and approaches that also bring attention to soul, for example, by incorporating one or more of the approaches listed in Box 38.1.

However, here too there may be a problem. The prevailing norm in Western healthcare is, *first*—treat the disease and contain the suffering; then, if and when satisfactory results have been achieved and the necessary resources are available to do so, *then*—take care of the soul. In practice, within this linear schema, we rarely if ever get to care of the soul because the needs of the frightened ego are urgent and endless, and resources are limited. By comparison, care of the soul may seem an unnecessary luxury, of secondary importance; 'someone else's responsibility'.

There is a third possibility. To understand this, begin by calling to mind someone who you would consider to have 'died well'; someone, who, even if in some pain, was awake, alive, 'themselves'; someone in whose presence you too felt awake, alive, 'yourself'. What happened here? One possibility is that this individual encountered that in her/himself that is already well; that in her/himself that is not afraid of death. As we have already noted, this is not so much a reified thing or place as a process, a quality of awareness that arises from immersion in depth; from, in the deepest sense, 'going with the flow'.

How might we enable our patients to experience this way of seeing and of being? We suggest that the components of this response are similar to the prevailing approach outlined above, but with a different emphasis. Here, *we attend to and care for soul from the outset,* while simultaneously considering how best to treat the

Box 38.1 Approaches that bring attention to soul

- Art therapy
- Bodywork, e.g. massage, yoga, Qi Gong, Watsu
- Creative and artistic expression
- Dream work
- Gratitude journaling
- Humour, laughter, levity
- Meditation practice
- Music therapy
- Quality time with significant others
- Reflective writing
- Reminiscence therapy
- Spiritual and religious practice
- Time in nature

disease and contain the suffering. In other words, the therapeutic approach here, which we might call 'primary care of the soul', is one that positively biases towards depth; one that deliberately prioritizes care of soul. One reason why this is necessary is because Western healthcare is strongly, if unconsciously, 'psyche-phobic'. It is embedded in and wedded to a wider culture of materialism and empiricism that by default devalues, distances itself from, and denigrates soul.

So, what might primary care of the soul look like at the bedside? What this does *not* mean is offering a patient in pain 'meditation before medication'. That would be impractical, and cruel. First things first: pain needs to be taken care of before someone has the psychic space and energy to turn her/his attention inwards. What it means and what matters is that depth infuses our attitude and our work from the outset. And this is only possible if we ourselves are self-aware and grounded in depth. What matters is that we as persons, who happen to be clinicians, have embarked on our own, 'experiment in depth'.[24] For, as we do this we become familiar with those spaces and places and energies within that are not afraid of death; we are touched by the mysteries, and our quality of presence is transformed by immersion in the luminous dark. Then, even our simplest acts of care become depth work and care of the soul.

So, there is *a practice before the practice*; doing what we need to do as clinicians to become familiar enough with depth that it informs our quality of presence as we move towards another in crisis. If this has not happened, if we are not already familiar with depth through introspection, then approaches such as such as those outlined in Box 38.1 may be little more than a sham; ego-reinforcement techniques masquerading as complementary or integrative therapies. It's not about techniques or sophisticated skill-sets. It's about commitment to our own inner-journey. It's about immersion in depth. It's about allowing ourselves to be initiated into another way of seeing, another way of being, another way of behaving. It's not about what we do. It's about becoming the healers we already are.

'We are the medicine': An educational programme in the therapeutic use of self

Even if these ideas encourage us to set out on an inner journey, or to renew our commitment to the journey we are already on, we should not underestimate the challenges involved. We are embarking on what will most likely be a life-long process. We are choosing a path that is strongly countercultural and for which we may not get much if any support. We should be aware that we are in a culture that idealizes a version of the hero as one who conquers by over-powering others. What we are imagining here is another kind of heroism. Irish poet and philosopher John Moriarty describes this other kind of hero as, 'One who lays down her/his sword and lets nature happen to her/him.'[25] This kind of hero is one who can be passive as well as active; one who has the courage to make hard choices, but who is rarely, if ever, in control; one who heeds Jung's words, 'Don't drown—dive!'[26]

It may be helpful to consider what else we might expect as we begin this process. For example, in the early stages of introspection, while some will be lucky enough to sink into calm and quiet right away, this is not usually how it is. Much more commonly there will be a sense of agitation as we notice how many worries, plans, memories, day-dreams, fantasies, and feelings float to the surface, like a lake whose depths have been disturbed and whose surface is covered in debris. We may feel discouraged and troubled, and find ourselves agreeing with author Anne Lamott's comment: 'My mind is a neighborhood I try not to go into alone!'[27] At this point, we may be tempted to leave the 'neighborhood' and go outside and find whatever distractions will numb the pain. Either that or fall asleep. Agitation or somnolence.

These are some of the reasons why we should not attempt this journey alone. Having a guide is valuable—someone who knows the terrain from walking it; someone who is not overwhelmed by the process or the problems. We need encouragement. Someone alongside who says, 'Yeah! That's normal. You're not crazy or inept. Just human!' Having a teacher helps—someone to teach us how to avoid falling into distraction or drowsiness; how to be simultaneously relaxed and highly present. Being highly present in a relaxed way is something that most of us need to learn. It is possible to cultivate this as a way of attending to whatever arises and it helps to have good instruction in this rather than being left to our own devices.

There are four overlapping and complementary practices that can be helpful in developing a therapeutic use of self. These are self-knowledge, self-empathy, mindful-awareness, and contemplative awareness. We now briefly consider each of these:

1. *Self-knowledge* prepares the ground for the therapeutic use of self. This means becoming familiar with our family history, our cultural, racial and religious history, as well as our individual strengths and limitations. Having insight into our background allows us to work through emotional challenges so that these will not get repressed or projected onto others. This allows us to recognize *transference* (the unconscious redirection of feelings from one person to another, for example, from patient to clinician) and *counter-transference* (the clinician's unconscious projection onto the patient and/or his or her reaction to the patient),[28] enabling the clinician to engage in the therapeutic encounter with more awareness and less reactivity. Some possible ways for the clinician to increase self-knowledge include counseling or psychotherapy, peer-group or individual clinical supervision, and reflective writing.
2. *Self-empathy* is the essential complement to self-knowledge. As we become more familiar with ourselves through the practice of self-knowledge, we may not like what we see and become self-critical, judgmental, overwhelmed and/or discouraged. Self-empathy includes noticing how hard it is for us to accept our imperfections and mistakes with an attitude of warmth and self-acceptance, while simultaneously being committed to finding a way to become more forgiving and compassionate towards ourselves. Certain practices from the Buddhist tradition are especially helpful in developing self-empathy. Metta or Loving-Kindness Meditation is an explicit practice of opening the heart with empathy and compassion towards ourselves and others.[29]
3. *Mindful-awareness* refers to the cultivation of three particular awareness skills: focusing, noticing, and expanding. The development of mindful-awareness is helpful for introspection and in enabling us to relate to our patients in a sensitive and sustainable way.[30] Mindfulness meditation, another meditative practice from the Buddhist tradition that is now extensively

used within healthcare,[31] can be used to cultivate these three cognitive skills. Meditation teacher and author Jon Kabat-Zinn, describes Mindfulness meditation as a process of developing careful attention to minute shifts in body, mind, emotions, and environment, while holding a kind, non-judgmental attitude towards self and others.[32]

- *Focusing* is the foundational skill in mindful-awareness and refers to the steadying and direction of attention and, therefore, the mind. Tibetan Buddhist teacher and author Alan Wallace emphasizes the importance of deep relaxation, stabilization of the mind, and an attitude of vividness in his method of teaching mindfulness of breathing to focus the mind.[33]
- *Noticing* arises naturally from focused awareness. It means witnessing the stream of thoughts, physical sensations and feelings that arise from moment to moment, with gentleness and respect and without commentary, reaction, or comparison. A further aspect of noticing is becoming aware of the subtle stream of awareness itself, which runs concurrently yet on a finer frequency than other phenomena.
- *Expanding* is a cognitive stance that permits the clinician to enlarge her/his awareness so that it is possible to simultaneously monitor his or her own subjective experience and the needs of the patient and/or the work environment.

These three aspects of mindful-awareness work synergistically together. Expanding builds on the skills of focusing and noticing. Through focusing and noticing we stabilize our attention and witness our experience in a non-judgmental way. As we do so, we may be aware of moments of meta-awareness, when we are aware of the quality with which we attend to the object of our attention, or, possibly, that we have just been distracted by a thought. With practice we can deliberately chose this cognitive stance, use it to monitor the quality of our attention in meditation practice and introspection, and, with time, to self-monitor our interactions with our patients. This can help to prevent us from getting trapped in reactivity or self-preoccupation, allow us to respond to the patient with more flexibility and greater sensitivity, and to experience a form of empathic engagement called 'Exquisite Empathy', which may be mutually beneficial to patient and clinician.[34]

4. *Contemplative Awareness* is awareness that we as individuals are situated in a larger field of relationships. Psychologically this includes the recognition of the inter-subjective field in the therapeutic encounter, and of an archetypal or universally shared dimension to our experience. Spiritually, it can be understood as the experience of our relationship to 'the numinous' or the sacred. It includes becoming aware of how we find meaning through our values, our cosmology and our philosophy of life. Mount, Boston and Cohen describe this as a process of establishing 'healing connections', and observe how these healing connections can engender a sense of meaning.[35] Practices to develop contemplative awareness are unique to each individual. They may include some of the approaches outlined in Box 38.1.

The 'mystical' can be understood as the direct experience of the larger field of relationships in which we are embedded. A mystical process that may arise from practicing the three components of mindful-awareness, discussed above, is what is called 'awareness of awareness'. Here, we come to glimpse the deeper stream of awareness itself, which is always present as a backdrop to emerging phenomena with qualities of stillness, luminosity, and knowing. Alan Wallace describes this aspect of perception as follows:

> Discerning this fraction of a second as pure-perception, before concepts, classifications, and emotional responses overlay ... This brief instant is important because it is an opportunity for gaining a clearer perception of the nature of phenomena, including a subtle continuum of mental consciousness out of which all forms of sensory perception and conceptualization emerge.[36]

A metaphor for awareness of awareness is a grandmother standing quietly behind a playing grandchild. The child represents the breath or other focus of attention, and the grandmother the ever-present flow of awareness in the background. Sri Madhava Ashish reminds us of the radical potency of self-awareness for both the individual and others when he writes:

> The root of the mystery of being lies at the root of the awareness that perceives the universe. Every human being is human by virtue of that awareness. Every human being is or can be aware that he is aware. When that self-awareness is traced to its inner source, then only can the identity of the individual with the universal be found, then only can the mystery of being be solved. And only when there are enough such individuals can sanity return through them to our troubled world.[37]

The process begins with naked attention to bodily sensations. Next, as we attend to the breath and experience greater and greater stillness, we may become aware of awareness itself. Finally, even for moments, we may come to rest in that awareness. To rest in awareness, an awareness that is contiguous with the awareness that fills the universe, is deeply peaceful. We are now participating in the sacred interconnectedness of all things.

Conclusions

As we return to the bedside, to the ones who suffer, we now do so with a new mode of perception, one that affects how we see and what we see; one that affects the treatment choices we make; one that affects how we do what we do.

'Prayer is not something we say or do. Prayer is state of being. And once we are in that state of being, everything we do is prayer' (W. Wapepah, personal communication). So, too, soul-work is not something we say or do. Soul-work is a state of being. Once we are in that state of being, everything we do is soul-work. Then, each of our simple acts of attention and kindness become care of the soul. Offering a drink, bathing, giving medications, and suturing a wound, care of the soul.

While we may automatically assume that approaches such as those in Box 38.1 are soul-work, this may or may not be the case. They are soul-work when they are offered by a clinician who embodies soul, where they work synergistically with the quality of the clinician's presence to bring attention to depth; to what is not afraid of death; to what does not die; to what is already deeply well. As clinicians who offer these approaches we are not doing something to or even for our patients so much as joining with them in compassionate celebration of what is.

Facing fear through primary care of the soul is, ultimately, about who we are; our quality of presence. And the journey inwards, *our* journey inwards, is where we start. This is the journey to the heart. For a moment, imagine yourself rooted, like some great tree, in Grand Prismatic Spring in Yellowstone National Park.[38]

Here your roots descent into the depths of the universe, which flows through you like some great, breathing ocean. Here, through the rust-red chords of relationship, you are connected to your brothers and sisters; to all your relations. The poet TS Elliott describes how it begins: 'Quick now, here, now, always—, a condition of complete simplicity, (Costing not less than everything)'.[39] Novelist Henry Miller offers these words on how it ends: 'At Epidaurus, in the stillness, in the great peace that came over me, I heard the heart of the world beat. I know what the cure is: it is to give up, to relinquish, to surrender, so that our little hearts may beat in unison with the great heart of the world'.[40]

References

1 James, W. (1958). *The Principles of Psychology*. New York: Dover Publications.

2 Stevens, A. (1993). *The Two Million Year Old Self*, Carolyn and Ernest Fay Series in Analytical Psychology. College Station: A&M University Press.

3 Hillman, J. (1992). Heraclitus, cited in: *Re-visioning Psychology*, p. xvii. New York: Harper Perennial.

4 [3], p. xvii.

5 Solomon, S., Greenberg, J., Pyszczynski, T. (1991). Terror management theory. In: C.R. Snyder, D. Forsyth (eds) *Handbook of Clinical and Social Psychology: the Health Perspective*. New York: Pergamon.

6 Becker, E. (1974). *The Denial of Death*. New York: Free Press.

7 Solomon, S., Greenberg, J., Pyszczynski, T. (2003). *In the Wake of 9/11: the Psychology of Terror*. Washington DC: American Psychological Association.

8 Shen, P., Bennick, G. (2005). *Flight From Death: the Quest for Immortality*, DVD, Transcendental Media.

9 Saunders, C. (1978). *The Management of Terminal Malignant Disease*, p. 194. London: Edward Arnold. p.194.

10 Kearney, M. (2007). *Mortally Wounded: Stories of Soul Pain, Death and Healing*, pp. 45–50. New Orleans: Spring Journal Books.

11 Kreinheder, A. (1991). *Body and Soul: the Other Side of Illness*. Toronto: Inner City Books.

12 [11], p. 109

13 Ashish, S.M. (2007). Afterword. In: M. Kearney (ed.) *Mortally Wounded: Stories of Soul Pain, Death and Healing*, pp. 147–8. New Orleans: Spring Journal Books.

14 [13], p. 148

15 [13], p. 148

16 Kreinheder, A. (1991). *Body and Soul: the Other Side of Illness*, p. 110. Toronto: Inner City Books.

17 Ashish, S.M. (2007). Afterword. In: M. Kearney (ed.) *Mortally Wounded: Stories of Soul Pain, Death and Healing*, p. 148. New Orleans: Spring Journal Books.

18 Dowling Singh, K. (1998). *The Grace in Dying*. San Francisco: Harper Collins.

19 Duff, K. (1993). *The Alchemy of Illness*. New York: Bell Tower.

20 Edinger, E.F. (1992). *Ego and Archetype*. Boston & London: Shambala.

21 Simmons, P.E. (2003). *Learning to Fall: Blessings of an Imperfect Life*. New York: Bantam Books.

22 #[10], pp. 46–7.

23 Kearney, M. (2009). *A Place of Healing: Working With Nature and Soul at the End of Life*. New Orleans: Spring Journal Books.

24 Martin, P.W. (1955). *Experiment in Depth*. London: Routledge & Kegan Paul.

25 Moriarty, J. (2007). *Tridium Sacrum*, Vol. 2 (Audio CD). Dublin: Sli Na Firinne Publishing. Lilliput Press.

26 Jung, C.G., (1955). Cited in: Martin, P.W. (ed.) *Experiment in Depth*, p. 167. London: Routledge & Kegan Paul.

27 Lamott A. (2011). Quotes. Available at: http://www.goodreads.com/quotes/show/72582 (accessed 11 November 2011).

28 [23], pp. 118–30.

29 Salzburg, S. (2008). *The Kindness Handbook: a Practical Companion*. Boulder: Sounds True Inc.

30 Kearney, M.K., Weininger, R.B., Vachon, M.L.S., Harrison, R.L., Mount, B.M. (2009). Self-care of physicians caring for patients at the end of life. *J Am Med Ass* **301**(11): 1155–64.

31 Grossman, P., Niemann, L., Schmidt, S., Walach, H. (2004). Mindfulness-based stress reduction and health benefits: a meta-analysis. *J Psychosom Res* 57: 35–43.

32 Kabatt-Zinn, J. (2003). Mindfulness-based interventions in context: past, present, and future. *Clin Psychol Sci Proc* **10**(2): 144–55.

33 Wallace, B.A. (2006). *The Attention Revolution: Unlocking the Power of the Focused Mind*, pp. 16–55. Somerville: Wisdom Publications Inc.

34 Harrison, R.L., Westwood, M.J (2009). Preventing vicarious traumatization of mental health therapists: identifying protective practices. Psychother *Theory, Res Pract Training* **46**(2): 203–19.

35 Mount, B.M., Boston, P.H., Cohen, R.S. (2007). Healing connections: on moving from suffering to a sense of well-being. *J Pain Sympt Manag* **33**(4): 372–88.

36 [33], p. 67.

37 Ashish, S.M. (2010). *What is Man? Selected writings of Sri Madhava Ashish*, p. v. New Delhi: Penguin books.

38 Image at National Geographic Website (2011). *Grand prismatic spring*. Available at: http://www.nps.gov/features/yell/slidefile/thermalfeatures/hotspringsterraces/midwaylower/Images/17708.jpg (accessed 11 November 2011).

39 Eliot, T.S. (1971). *Little Gidding V; The Four Quartets*, p. 47. San Diego: Harvest.

40 Miller, H. (1958). *The Colossus of Maroussi*, p. 77. New York: New Directions.

CHAPTER 39

Counselling

William West

In this chapter I will briefly explore the origins of modern counselling and psychotherapy focusing on the role of religion as both a forebearer and a significant if minority contributor to current practice. I will then briefly consider how religion and spirituality can be defined within the counselling field. I will then examine some typical case examples to highlight some of the challenges faced when exploring religion and spirituality in counselling. Some reflections on working with spirituality in practice and on necessary skills are followed by a careful consideration of the ethical issues involved.

Introduction

Counselling and psychotherapy, like much of modern healthcare as a whole, are regarded as having their origins in religious forms of pastoral care.[1] However, the development of modern counselling and psychotherapy arguably began with Freud in the late Victorian era. Like the new discipline of psychology, therapy was keen to be seen as a science and to be scientific at that moment in time was to be secular. Freud himself was a critic of religion which he regarded as at best a 'crooked cure.' Speaking of religion he said, 'The whole thing is potentially so infantile, so foreign to reality ... it is painful to think that the great majority of mortals will never be able to rise above this view of life.'[2]

Not all counsellors and psychotherapists have followed Freud's view, for example Jung was an early supporter of the potentially healthy role of religion in people's lives and famously said, 'Among my patients in the second half of life—that is over 35 years of age—there has not been a single one whose problem has not been in the last resort that of finding a religious outlook on life.'[3] Jung also made clear that he was not necessarily speaking here of organized religion. Besides Jung there have been a number of therapists who have challenged this secular assumption underlying modern therapy including Assagioli,[4] Carl Rogers,[5] and more recently, Brian Thorne.[6,7]

In Britain the Christian and Jewish members of the Association for Pastoral Care and Counselling (formed in 1970, now called Association for Pastoral and Spiritual Care and Counselling) played a key role in the establishment of the Standing Conference for the Advancement of Counselling in 1971, renamed the British Association for Counselling in 1977 and renamed the British Association for Counselling and Psychotherapy in 2001.

Mainstream Western societies seem to define themselves largely in secular terms—as Tony Blair's spin doctor Alistair Campbell famously put it 'we don't do God' and in the USA Constitution there is a careful separation of church and state, despite their high levels of religious membership and practice. In this context the increasingly professionalization of counselling lends itself to problem solving and short-term approaches that are to all sense and purposes non- or even anti-religious. As John McLeod, probably the most authoritative figure writing on counselling today states 'It would be a mistake to imagine that all clients reporting religious, spiritual or mystical beliefs or experiences would be understood or well received by their counsellors.' He further gives us the background to this issue: 'few counselling training courses address religious or spiritual issues in any depth.'[8] This negative attitude to religion is not confined to some counsellors and therapists. Dein reports that 'many psychiatrists see religion as primitive, guilt-inducing, a form of dependency, irrational and having no empirical basis.'[9]

However, there is plenty of evidence that people still have religious faith, spiritual experiences and an interest in spirituality. For example, in the British 2001 census figure, we find that over 45 million people—76.8% of respondents claim to be religion and over 42 million of these to be Christian. This does not mean that all these people regularly attend churches, mosques, synagogues, and temples. Davie[10] coined the phrase 'believing not belonging' to cover this rather semi-detached relationship many have with organized religion in Britain. Research[11] into British reports of religious or spiritual experience suggests that over 76% of respondents in an opinion survey indicated at least one such experience. This compares with a similar survey reported in 1987 of 48%. The authors conclude, not that religious and spiritual experiences are happening to more people, but that there is a greater readiness to acknowledge them.

It also needs mentioning that, in a number of ways, religious groups have lagged behind this zeitgeist of a greater willingness to acknowledge and discuss spirituality in a spirit of equality. For example, the Church of England's struggles around accepting women as Bishops, the Catholic Church's refusal to ordain women at all, or accept the general use of condoms and the homophobic attitudes still found in many religious groups worldwide.

So, despite the continued contribution of religious people to the development of modern counselling, the secular framing of counselling theory and practice has proved to be a disservice to a significant number of its clients. This disservice has been a focus for research.[12–14] In the past decade spirituality has become more widely discussed within counselling and psychology.[15,16] However, this past decade has also seen a polarization around atheism and religion in a climate of Islamophobia within the Western world. This polarization is reflected in the writings of Dawkins[17] and Hitchens[18] who challenge religious beliefs from arguably a polemical and atheist position.

In terms of the varieties of counselling approaches available, the main approaches could be grouped into five categories namely: psychodynamic; cognitive behavioural, humanistic; transpersonal; multicultural and integrative.[19] Whilst any individual counsellor may have their own skills and understandings in relation to spirituality, these broader grouping do vary in their approaches to spirituality.[19] Many psychodynamic counsellors follow Freud in taking a negative view of spirituality and religion. Cognitive behavioural counsellors tend to be secularly minded, but are often convinced by the research evidence supporting the effectiveness of using of spiritual practices liked mindfulness and meditation. Humanistic counsellors vary, but tend to be pro-spiritual if sometimes anti-religious. Transpersonal counsellors have a positive view of spirituality, by and large, since their approach explicitly recognizes and values spirituality. The practice of multicultural counselling implies an acceptance of the possible role of religious and spirituality within counselling. Integrative counsellors vary in relation to spirituality depending on how they do and see their integration.

There is a range of views about what counselling is (for further details see the discussion in McLeod[20]). McLeod makes a strong that most definitions are written from the perspective of the professional counsellor and not the client, and offer the following 'user-centred' definition:

Counselling is a purposeful private conversation arising from the intention of one person to reflect on and resolve a problem in living, and the willingness of another person to assist in that endeavour.[20]

This 'resolving a problem in living' clearly involves meaning making on the client's behalf. For many clients meaning making involves spirituality and religion. Implicit in such a definition of counselling is a willingness by the counsellor to respectively accept and enter the client's world and world view. Thus, counsellors need a working understanding of the range of religious and spiritual experiences and frameworks together with how people use these to make sense of their lives. There is a discourse within the professional world of counselling about 'fitness to practice'. A deep understanding of spirituality and religion is, in my view, an essential part of such fitness to practice.

Definitions of religion and spirituality within the counselling field

There are a number of differing definitions particularly of spirituality, but also of religion that are particularly useful to counselling practice. There seems to be a developing Western consensus, reflected in most dictionary definitions, that spirituality relates to personal beliefs and religion to the organized group of believers including places of worships, rituals, and creeds. However, not everyone, especially those of a religious nature, accepts these distinctions and many people, whether religious believers or not, are dismissive of personal spirituality, especially if the word 'New Age' is added to the word 'spiritual'. From the viewpoint of the practitioner it is always best to explore what words mean for clients.

Elkins *et al.*[21] research into what people mean by 'spirituality' seems especially useful with its focus on experience, Rowan's[22] transpersonal approach reminds us that exploring what spirituality means can involves changes in our sense of self and Swinton[14] writing within a healthcare context draws our attention to spirituality being about making connections inside, between people, and with creation. Drawing on these ideas and clinical experience I came up with the following composite definition for spirituality within the counselling context:

- it is rooted in human experiencing rather than abstract theology, i.e. it helps to focus on spirituality as a human experience and what this means to people
- it is embodied, that spiritual experience often actively involves us as physical beings
- it involves feeling strongly connected to other people and the universe at large
- it involves non-ordinary consciousness, that is in altered states of consciousness or trance states
- active engagement with spirituality tends to make people more altruistic, less materialistic, and more environmentally aware
- it deals with the meaning that people make of their lives
- it faces suffering, its causes, and potentially its meaning to the individual
- it relates to God/Goddesses/divine/ultimate reality—these words are especially rich in meaning, not always unproblematic
- it often uses the word 'soul' or 'higher self:' these words often have powerful associations and meanings for people
- techniques such as prayer, meditation, contemplation, mindfulness, yoga, and Tai Chi are often used as spiritual practices.[16,23]

Many people continue to have experiences that they put the word 'spiritual' to. Other people having the same or similar experience may not use the word 'spiritual'. This use of the word 'spiritual' for a human experience—perhaps feeling of being at one with nature or a profound sense of togetherness with another human being—has many implications. For a start, such experiences may not be welcome or altogether pleasant, and even if they are, they may raise many issues. Such spiritual experiences are common among clients,[24] inevitably happen to therapists, and sometimes occur within the therapy room.[5,6]

Case studies

To highlight some of the challenges faced when counsellors aim to be respectful of their clients' spirituality I will here present and discuss some typical examples from counselling practice.

Case study I: Louise

Louise, a counsellor in training, described an unusual experience that occurred to her with a client. 'I was having a discussion with my client at the end of a counselling session when something happened. In that moment it was as if we were both suddenly 'held'. I had never felt anything like it before. Neither of us said anything, but we both knew that something had occurred ... like an imperceptible seismic shift. It was as if I had stepped out of normal time and space, and suddenly felt connected with everything that was, is, and would be. I had a feeling of joy and I remember thinking that if I died there and then, it would be OK, because I had experienced this and that was all that mattered! Bizarre. In that moment I felt Blessed and it was as if we had both received some 'healing' at the same time. When we discussed it the next week, my client described it as feeling some great need of wanting to get back into the room and be back with me immediately. However, I don't think it was 'me'. I think he needed to be back in the experience which, to me, felt like 'unconditional love' coming from someone or something other than me. It was difficult to discuss and describe, almost as if we didn't need to. To have experienced it was enough.

I then took [this experience] to [counselling] supervision, in great excitement and looking for some help on interpreting it. However, we did not discuss it as being a spiritual experience. As a group we described it, in psychodynamic terms, as the client becoming 'attached' to me, which he undoubtedly was, but I felt it was more than that. I felt that something else had happened, that wasn't created or facilitated by me or my client. So, without getting much further in being able to talk about it in spiritual terms, I put the experience to the back of my mind then, thinking that it wasn't valid and that it wasn't helping my psychodynamic training or supervision. During the session with my client that day, I truly felt that, for a few moments, the counselling room really did become a 'sacred space''.

This description of a 'spiritual' encounter between counsellor and client is not that unusual and there are a number of similar examples discussed in the writings of Brian Thorne[6] who talks in terms of 'tenderness' and Carl Rogers,[5] who uses the word 'presence'. This description also matches the work of the Jewish philosopher Martin Buber[25] who argues that people can treat one another as objects and thereby form I–It relationships or treat people as kin and from I–Thou relationships. This I–Thou relationship is a meeting of equals and has a definite spiritual quality to it.

It is interesting to note that Louise did not get a supportive response from her supervisor. Counsellors and psychotherapists in Britain in training, and beyond, usually have their work regularly supervised. Most training and accreditation bodies insist on lifelong supervision. It is not unusual for some supervisors to be negative about spiritual and religious experiences and beliefs.[26] For example, I have been told in research interviews of counsellors who hide their more spiritually informed work from their supervisors. In my research study into Quakers who were also counsellors, one respondent told me: 'I found that when I did have one client for whom the spiritual was very important, it was quite difficult to deal with, being supervised by someone who had no sense of the spiritual ... either I took what I'd done to supervision and got it rubbished, or I left it outside supervision, protected it increasingly by not getting it supervised, being quite sure that with this client that was the right way to go.'[27] Peter Gubi's[12,28] pioneering work into counsellors' use of prayer found that many counsellors in Britain did use prayer in counselling, but often did not share the matter with their supervisors.

Case study II: Chris

It is not just the counsellors who may struggle with talking about spirituality. Chris Jenkins did doctoral research into clients who felt that their spiritually was denied in counselling. Chris draws on one of his participant's story when he writes:

> Imagine being in a psychiatric unit, so ill and confused you aren't even sure of the year. Imagine, as the confusion begins to subside, having one source of clarity, an awareness of divine care and love. Imagine meeting your therapist and mentioning this and seeing her reaction, noticing your medication has been increased ... and is increased whenever you talk about your spiritual awareness. Then being in a therapy group when another patient names their sense of God, the group shutting them up and hearing, at the break, the patient being told: 'Don't talk about that stuff in here, you'll never get out ...' Slowly you are learning to play the game, to leave a vital spark of yourself outside the therapy room door.[29]

This theme from Chris's research of mental patients learning to 'play the game' in order to get out of psychiatric hospital is commonly heard and as John Swinton notes despite the rhetoric about spirituality and mental healthcare 'in practice, spirituality is frequently excluded, in terms of both research and practice.'[30] It is well worth reflecting on the truth that within some religious groups it is natural to seek and even hear the voice of God. In a mental health setting a patient claiming to hear the voice of God may well unwittingly invite a psychiatric diagnosis. The overlap between mystical experiences and psychosis is well known and there are problems in diagnosis not least bias on the part of the practitioner involved.[24] Lukoff[31,32] has usefully suggested that we think in terms of the possibility of mystical experiences with psychotic features or psychotic experiences with mystical features. The focus then is pragmatically on what support the patient needs.

Case study III: cults

Some years ago a man came to me for counselling who had recently left a residential Buddhist group that acted, in his words, as a 'cult'. He was struggling to adjust his new life outside of this community. There was a palpable sense of loss when he talked about the community and his friendships with people there, who he felt he could no longer see. These multiple losses needed exploring. There was also a challenge to his sense of religious faith: was he still a Buddhist or not, should he seek a new Buddhist group to become a member of? Leaving the group appeared to condemn him to a Buddhist equivalent of hell. These were big faith issues that needed careful addressing. I was challenged both to understand more about how religious groups can function as cults (INFORM[33] were a useful resource for this) and also to understand Buddhism more deeply. Thankfully, my client had embarked on a university degree, which at least gave his life a focus and gave him a whole series of new contacts with fellow students to explore. His experiences in the cult group challenged my limited and largely positive view of Buddhism causing me to realise that any human group can go off the rails and act in destructive ways.

Case study IV: loss of faith by a partner

A new client comes for counselling and says: 'I am a born-again Christian and so was my husband. In fact we were married in church and our children go to Sunday school at the church.

In recent weeks my husband has stopped going to church with me and the children, indeed he says he no longer believes. I find this very hard and (begins to sob) I don't think he will be saved ... we won't be in heaven together.'

Such a statement of faith may strike a secular counsellor as absurd and, indeed, a liberal-minded religious counsellor could struggle with accepting this client's religious viewpoint. However, this is the real world for some believers, and it needs and deserves a hearing and exploration. It is always worth considering why any particular person ends up seeking counselling and who they seek it from. This particular client would have been welcomed by their minister or religious pastoral team, but instead sought counselling for whatever reason. Maybe they want to understand their husband's viewpoint, maybe they want to voice some doubts of their own. Maybe there are some real relationships issue underneath the husband's apparent loss of faith. Whatever is going on for the client and her husband, she deserved good quality counselling from her counsellor who needed to be able to put aside their own personal viewpoint.

Counselling skill, spirituality, and healthcare

McLeod[1] has written eloquently about the embedded use of what he calls 'counselling skill' by professionals, including those working in healthcare, who do not define themselves as counsellors. Many healthcare professions face similar challenges and dilemmas to those highlighted in the case studies offered in this chapter. Indeed, when people are confronted by severe health issues, it is not surprising that challenges to their core beliefs arise and these often inevitably share a religious or spiritual dimension. It is for precisely this reason that chaplaincy is available in most hospitals.[34] However, spirituality is too big and widespread an issue to be left to chaplains alone. Indeed, the Royal College of Psychiatrists has a Spirituality and Psychiatry Special Interest Group (SPSIG) that was founded in 1999 to:

- help psychiatrists to share experiences and to explore spirituality in mental healthcare
- to increase knowledge of the research linking spirituality with better health
- to raise the profile of spirituality in patient care.[35]

They state: 'Spiritual practices can help us to develop the better parts of ourselves. They can help us to become more creative, patient, persistent, honest, kind, compassionate, wise, calm, hopeful and joyful. These are all part of the best healthcare.'

Reflections on counselling practice

There are at least three ways in which spirituality and/or religion can feature in the counselling session:

1. *As an issue for the client.* There are times when the client may be wrestling with issues to do with their spirituality. The client may have a troubled religious upbringing; tensions with their current religious group; spiritual experiences they find troubling; spiritual or faith questions arising from events in their life such as bereavement These issues can take as many forms as there are clients, but some common possibilities are issues of spiritual or religious beliefs in response to life crises (for example, why is this happening to me? Why does God allow these horrors to occur?) and spiritual experiences that clients find challenging ('I know since then that I need to lead a different life, but ...').
2. *As an issue for the counsellor.* The client's issue may raise important religious and spiritual issues for the counsellor, which may then take them by surprise or connect with current issues within the counsellor's own life. There are times when the counsellor is challenged either directly by the client or by her or his own processes in relationship to spirituality. These again are multiple. Many counsellors recognize that clients often work on issues of importance to them and, in supporting their clients, their own need for change and development is laid bare.
3. *As a shared experience within the counselling session.* Sometimes the counselling encounter itself can take on a spiritual feel much as described in the first case study above. There can be experienced as special moments which both therapist and client might well cause to label as 'spiritual' and be experienced as profoundly therapeutic. There is a rich literature and discourse around these moments, which Buber[25] called 'I/Thou,' Carl Rogers[5] called 'presence,' Brian Thorne[6] called 'tenderness,' etc. Such moments do not have to be discussed in spiritual terms. Indeed, Mearns and Cooper[36] discuss them in terms of relational depth. What is striking is how often clients (and therapists) spontaneously use the word 'spiritual' for such moments.

Having briefly summarized the part spirituality can play in healthy counselling practice it is another matter to spell out how this might be actually achieved. Briefly, I would recommend:[15,19,23]

- An inclusion of a substantial training around spiritual issues in basic counsellor training programmes, which would require support from the professional bodies involved for it to happen in practice
- The content of such a training package could include religion and spirituality in (post)modern multicultural society, maps of psychospiritual development, spiritual experiences, diagnostic issues, spiritual counter transference, religious pastoral care, and referrals and spiritual intervention in counselling
- Post-qualifying specialist training for counsellors around spirituality to equip and update existing and future trained counsellors
- Further development of theories, maps, and sensing making around spirituality and counselling
- Further research into the spirituality of counsellors and their attitude to spirituality; their use of spiritual interventions and outcomes of spiritual interventions
- Personal development work for counsellors around their own spiritual development.

Necessary skills

It is worth reviewing the guidance provided by the British Association for Counselling and Psychotherapy.[37] In their 'gold book,' which is their guide for BACP accredited training programmes there is little mention of religion and no mention of spirituality. Their mention of religion is in section 9.1 B 'Understanding the client' and states:

> 6. Demonstrate awareness of diversity and the rights and responsibilities of all clients, regardless of their gender, age, ethnicity, culture, class, ability, sexuality, religion and belief.

Whilst this commitment to awareness of religion is welcome it is located within a list that includes other hot topics demanding attention, for example, sexuality and ethnicity. Often exploration of diversity on counsellor training programmes will occur within a module in which religion and/or spirituality might well only attract brief coverage or possibly only feature as an optional item. Banks describes counsellor trainees' reactions to a case study of a woman with strong religious feelings who tolerated emotional neglect from her husband and teenage children because 'through suffering one will find the true meaning of God'. Subsequently, 'many angry feelings' were expressed by trainees some from a feminist viewpoint and from those who felt stunted by their own religious upbringings. Some stated that they had 'no time for religious [nutters]'. Banks comments 'A heated debate arose in which others attempted to get the dismissive individuals to reflect on whether their experience was unfortunate and distorted or whether this could be generalized to the experience of all ... in some cases this self-reflection was not possible.'[38]

Of course issues around religion and spirituality can feature within personal development groups, which are a common feature of counsellor training, but this is not always done in a positive light. Jenkins[29] was told by a counsellor reflecting on his experience of being trained 'The message there [on the PD group] was that a lot of counsellors had anti-religious feelings ... So I suppose there too there is a message being given that it is not okay to talk about your spirituality ... certainly never in my [counsellor] training have we talked about religion.'

Ethics

Counsellors are expected to have a high standard of ethical practice. This has particular relevance in relation to clients with religious or spiritual issues. The counsellor may be challenged by new scenarios that they are not familiar with, to work perhaps outside of their usual comfort zone. They may well encounter challenges that they are unprepared for. This will put a demand on their usual usage of supervision—a regular meeting between them and an experienced colleague in which they reflect on their practice. Such use of supervision is mandatory for counsellors in Britain and is an important part of counsellor training and beyond in the USA and elsewhere.

However, such supervision is not always without problems[26,39] and some of these are specific to religion and spirituality. For example, not all supervisors are supportive of counsellors working with clients' religious and spiritual issues and beliefs.[27] There may be specific problems in the counsellor is using prayer with a client.[28] Counsellors may find that their supervisors encourage them to refer such clients on to religious ministers, pastoral care teams or counsellors as their supervisor, especially those of a psychodynamic orientation, may view such work as being outside of the remit of counselling. If counsellors feel they are working beyond their own competence this might well be appropriate. However, there is no reason why a well-prepared and well-trained counsellor cannot be facilitative of such clients. As Wyatt reminds us: 'When I am clear about my faith and comfortable with it—whatever it looks like—then it is good. I know what I think. I know what I believe and I know what I do not believe. I know what my values are, or I know that I don't know. Then, when I am like that, I can listen to clients.'[40]

Conclusion

In these times of apparent polarization around religion in Britain and elsewhere it is not surprising that the challenges around working with clients religious and spiritual beliefs have become more marked and perhaps more apparent. The best counselling practices arises out of a good therapeutic alliance between counsellor and client.[1] To establish a good alliance the counsellor needs to demonstrate their acceptance of their client and the client's world. This might seem a tall order, but it is practiced every day by thousands of counsellors working with clients who will be significantly different to them in terms of gender, sexuality, ethnicity, class, age and religious and spiritual beliefs.

The tensions around counselling and spirituality reflect the tension in the wider society. Consequently, I do not expect these tensions to be easily resolved. However, one of the features of good counselling practice is its willingness to witness tensions in client's lives. Such tensions are not always resolvable; indeed, some seem part of the human condition. Nonetheless, the counsellor's willing to witness these tensions is an important part of the therapeutic encounter. Human problems do not always have easy solutions. Indeed, counselling and religion can both be seen as responses to human suffering.[16]

The careful training and supervision that causes counsellors to be as effective as they are with a wide range of clients and their problems needs improving in the light of themes explored in this chapter. Nonetheless, it is not beyond the reach of the best counsellors to work well with spirituality as it arises within the lives of their clients.

Acknowledgements

Whilst I accept full responsibility for the ideas and how they are expressed in this chapter, many people over the years have contributed to my understanding of issues in relation to spirituality religion and counselling. These include: Terry Biddington, Dee Brown, Fevronia Christodoulidi, Peter Gubi, the late Grace Jantzen, Chris Jenkins, John McLeod, Ann Scott, Brian Thorne and Dori Yusef.

References

1 McLeod, J. (2009). *An Introduction to Counselling*, 4th edn. Maidenhead: Open University Press.
2 Freud, S. (1963). *Civilization and its Discontents*, p. 11. New York: Basic Books.
3 Jung, C.G. (1933). *Modern Man in Search of a Soul*, p. 164. London: Routledge and Kegan Paul.
4 Assagioli, R. (1986). Self-realization and psychological disturbance. *Revision* **8**(2): 21–31.
5 Rogers, C.R. (1980). *A Way of Being*. Boston: Houghton Mifflin.
6 Thorne, B. (1998). *Person-centred Counselling and Christian Spirituality—the Secular and the Holy*. London: Whurr.
7 Thorne, B. (2002). *The Mystical Path of Person-centred Therapy: Hope Beyond Despair*. London: Whurr.
8 McLeod, J. (2009). *An Introduction to Counselling,* 4th edn, pp. 489–90. Maidenhead: Open University Press.
9 Dein, S. (2004). Working with patients with religious beliefs. *Adv Psychiat Treat* **10**: 287–95.
10 Davie, G. (1994). *Religion in Britain Since 1945*. Oxford: Blackwell.
11 Hay, D., Hunt, K. (2000). *Understanding the Spirituality of People Who Don't Go to Church,* Centre for the Study Of Human Relations. Notttingham: Nottingham University.

12 Gubi, P.M. (2008). *Prayer in Counselling and Psychotherapy: Exploring a Hidden Meaningful Dimension.* London: Jessica Kingsley Publishers.
13 Jenkins, C. (2011). When the clients' spirituality is denied in therapy. In: W. West (ed.) *Exploring Therapy, Spirituality and Healing.* Basingstoke: Palgrave.
14 Swinton, J. (2001). *Spirituality in Mental Healthcare.* London: Jessica Kingsley Publishers.
15 Richards, P.S., Bergin, A.E. (2005). *A Spiritual Strategy for Counseling and Psychotherapy.* 2nd edn. Washington DC: APA.
16 West, W. (ed.) (2011). *Exploring Therapy, Spirituality and Healing.* Basingstoke: Palgrave.
17 Dawkins, R. (2007). *The God Delusion.* London: Black Swan.
18 Hitchens, C. (2007). *God is not great: how religion poisons everything.* New York NY: Twelve, Hachette Book Group.
19 West, W. (2000) *Psychotherapy and Spirituality—Crossing the Line Between Therapy and Religion.* London: Sage.
20 McLeod, J. (2009). *An Introduction to Counselling,* 4th edn, pp. 4–9. Maidenhead: Open University Press.
21 Elkins, D.N., Hedstorm, J.L., Hughes, L.L., Leaf, J.A., Saunders, C. (1988). Toward a humanistic-phenomenological spirituality. *J Humanist Psychol* **28**(4): 5–18.
22 Rowan, J. (2005). *The Transpersonal: Spirituality in Psychotherapy and Counselling,* 2nd edn. London: Routledge.
23 West, W. (2004). *Spiritual Issues in Therapy: Relating Experience to Practice.* Basingstoke: Palgrave.
24 Allman, L.S., De Las Rocha, O., Elkins, D.N., Weathers, R.S. (1992). Psychotherapists' attitudes towards clients reporting mystical experiences. *Psychotherapy* **29**(4): 654–9.
25 Buber, M. (1970). *I–Thou.* Edinburgh: T and T Clark.
26 West, W.S. (2003). The culture of psychotherapy supervision. *Counsell Psychother Res* **3**(2): 123–7.
27 West, W. (2000). Supervision difficulties and dilemmas for counsellors and psychotherapists around healing and spirituality. In: B. Lawton, C. Feltham (eds) *Taking Supervision Forwards: Dilemmas, Insights and Trends,* pp. 113–25 London: Sage.
28 Gubi, P.M. (2011). Integrating prayer in counselling. In: W. West (ed.) *Exploring Therapy, Spirituality and Healing.* Basingstoke: Palgrave.
29 Jenkins, C. (2006). *Clients who feel their spirituality is denied by their counsellor,* p. 29, PhD thesis. Manchester: University of Manchester.
30 Swinton, J .(2001). *Spirituality in Mental Healthcare,* p. 8. London: Jessica Kingsley Publishers.
31 Lukoff, D. (1985). The diagnosis of mystical experience with psychotic features. *J Transpers Psychol* **17**(2): 155–81.
32 Lukoff, D. (1998). From spiritual emergency to spiritual problem: the transpersonal roots of the new DSM-IV category. *J Humanist Psychol* **38**(2): 21–50.
33 INFORM. Available at: www.inform.ac
34 Department of Health. (2003). *NHS Chaplaincy: Meeting the Religious and Spiritual Needs of Patients and Staff, Guidance for Managers and Those Involved in the Provision Of Chaplaincy-spiritual Care.* London: DHS.
35 SPSIG (2010). *Spirituality and Mental Health.* Available at: http://www.rcpsych.ac.uk/mentalhealthinfo/treatments/spirituality.aspx (accessed10 March 2011).
36 Mearns D, Cooper M (2005). *Working at Relational Depth in Counselling and Psychotherapy.* London: Sage Publications.
37 British Association for Counselling and Psychotherapy. (2010). *Accreditation of Training Courses.* Available at: www.bacp.co.uk/admin/structure/files/repos/416_course_accreditation_scheme_.pdf
38 Banks, N. (2003). Counselling and religion. In: C. Lago, B. Smith (eds) *Anti-discriminatory Counselling Practice,* p. 106. London: Sage.
39 Ladanby, N., Bradley, L.J. (eds) (2010). *Counselor Supervision,* 4th edn. New York: Routledge.
40 Wyatt, J. (2002). 'Confronting the Almighty God'? A study of how psychodynamic counsellors respond to clients' expressions of religious faith. *Counsell Psychother Res* **2**(3): 177–84.

CHAPTER 40

Dignity conserving care: research evidence

Shane Sinclair and Harvey M. Chochinov

Introduction

The concept of dignity and its implications for spiritual care was spelt out in Chapter 21. In this chapter we discuss the implications and effect of dignity-conserving care in clinical practice. While a growing body of empirical evidence related to dignity care will be reviewed, we also discuss how the intrinsic qualities of healthcare professionals serve as powerful modifiers of patient dignity.

The patient dignity inventory (PDI): evaluating the landscape of patient distress

The dignity model provided the basis for the development of the Patient Dignity Inventory (PDI), a 25-item measure of dignity related distress (Figure 40.1). Patients are provided the option of completing the PDI as a self-report or with the aid of a healthcare professional, with each item being rated on a five-point Likert scale (1 = not a problem; 2 = somewhat of a problem; 3 = a problem; 4 = a major problem; 5 = an overwhelming problem). The PDI was validated in a study of 253 palliative care patients, establishing its validity and reliability.[1] There was a significant correlation between the Functional Assessment of Chronic Illness Therapy—Spiritual Wellbeing (FACIT-sp) *Inner Peace Factor* and the PDI *Peace of Mind* factor. Unlike existential distress, the PDI *Peace of Mind Factor* consists of concerns that, even death itself, may not be seen as providing resolution (e.g. 'not having made a meaningful contribution in life,' 'concerns about spiritual life,' and 'feelings of unfinished business'). In a secondary study, PDI scores were further analysed utilizing descriptive statistics and demographic information in an attempt to describe a broad landscape of distress among terminally-ill patients. Patients who were younger, male, in-patients, more educated, and had a partner or were living with someone were more likely to experience certain kinds of distress. [2] Conversely, spirituality, particularly its meaning-making components, was shown to have a positive effect on the conservation of dignity. The significant correlations between many of the PDI items and the FACIT-Sp score, particularly the FACIT Meaning and Peace scale, suggests that spiritual wellbeing is more predictive of a personal and dynamic framework of meaning, than mere religious identification. While faith or religion can serve as a framework of meaning,[3,4] the experiential and relational nature of spirituality over time seems to have a marked and enduring influence. [5–7] While differentiating between specific PDI items and their relationship to overlapping constructs of wellbeing, quality of life and meaning is challenging, the utility of the PDI lies in its ability to provide a broad framework, wherein patients and their healthcare providers can identify and address issues that matter most at the end-of-life.

Dignity therapy: a meaning and purpose-enhancing intervention

Dignity therapy targets various aspects of distress amongst terminally ill patients, through a reflective process focusing on their lives, where meaning and purpose most strongly reside.[8] While much of Dignity Therapy's clinical utility seems to come from providing patients an opportunity to acknowledge dignity related issues, its individualized and semi-structured format allows patients to recognize the legacy they will leave, while identifying those unfinished matters which can still be addressed.[9] The Dignity Therapy question protocol, based on the Dignity Model, serves as a guide to illicit memories, offer wisdom and provide comfort to soon to be bereft loved ones[10] (Figure 40.2). The brief nature of the protocol (one or two sessions, one hour each in duration), unlike many other psychotherapeutic approaches, seems particularly well suited to palliative care populations, where issues of fatigue and alertness are prominent. Patient sessions are audio-recorded, transcribed, and edited, creating a generativity document that can be shared with family members and close friends, in accordance with the patient's wishes. A phase 1 trial of dignity therapy, involving 100 terminally-ill patients reported a 91% satisfaction rate, with 76% of patients reporting a heightened sense of dignity as a result of the therapeutic intervention.[11] In addition to these dignity-specific outcomes, 68% reported an increased sense of purpose, 67% reported a heightened sense of meaning, 47% reported an increased will to live and 81% reported that dignity therapy had been or would be of help to their family. McClement and colleagues investigated the benefits of Dignity Therapy from the perspective of 60 bereft family members, nine to twelve months after the patient had died. Ninety-five% of participants reported that Dignity Therapy had benefited the patient, while 78% reported that it heightened the patient's sense of dignity, 65% reported that it helped the patient

Patient Dignity Inventory

For each item, please indicate how much of a problem or concern these have been for you within the last few days.

1. Not being able to carry out tasks associated with daily living (e.g. washing myself, getting dressed).

1	2	3	4	5
Not a problem	A slight problem	A problem	A major problem	An overwhelming problem

2. Not being able to attend to my bodily functions independently (eg. needing assistance with toileting-related activities)

1	2	3	4	5
Not a problem	A slight problem	A problem	A major problem	An overwhelming problem

3. Experiencing physically distressing symptoms (such as pain, shortness of breath, nausea).

1	2	3	4	5
Not a problem	A slight problem	A problem	A major problem	An overwhelming problem

4. Feeling that how I look to others has changed significantly.

1	2	3	4	5
Not a problem	A slight problem	A problem	A major problem	An overwhelming problem

5. Feeling depressed.

1	2	3	4	5
Not a problem	A slight problem	A problem	A major problem	An overwhelming problem

6. Feeling anxious.

1	2	3	4	5
Not a problem	A slight problem	A problem	A major problem	An overwhelming problem

7. Feeling uncertain about my health and health care.

1	2	3	4	5
Not a problem	A slight problem	A problem	A major problem	An overwhelming problem

8. Worrying about my future.

1	2	3	4	5
Not a problem	A slight problem	A problem	A major problem	An overwhelming problem

9. Not being able to think clearly.

1	2	3	4	5
Not a problem	A slight problem	A problem	A major problem	An overwhelming problem

10. Not being able to continue with my usual routines.

1	2	3	4	5
Not a problem	A slight problem	A problem	A major problem	An overwhelming problem

11. Feeling like I am no longer who I was.

1	2	3	4	5
Not a problem	A slight problem	A problem	A major problem	An overwhelming problem

12. Not feeling worthwhile or valued.

1	2	3	4	5
Not a problem	A slight problem	A problem	A major problem	An overwhelming problem

Figure 40.1 The Dignity Model. Reprinted from (1) with permission from Elsevier.

13. Not being able to carry out important roles (e.g. spouse, parent).

1	2	3	4	5
Not a problem	A slight problem	A problem	A major problem	An overwhelming problem

14. Feeling that life no longer has meaning or purpose.

1	2	3	4	5
Not a problem	A slight problem	A problem	A major problem	An overwhelming problem

15. Feeling that I have not made a meaningful (and) OR lasting contribution in my life.

1	2	3	4	5
Not a problem	A slight problem	A problem	A major problem	An overwhelming problem

16. Feeling that I have 'unfinished business' (e.g. things that I have yet to say or do, or that feel incomplete)

1	2	3	4	5
Not a problem	A slight problem	A problem	A major problem	An overwhelming problem

17. Concern that my spiritual life is not meaningful.

1	2	3	4	5
Not a problem	A slight problem	A problem	A major problem	An overwhelming problem

18. Feeling that I am a burden to others.

1	2	3	4	5
Not a problem	A slight problem	A problem	A major problem	An overwhelming problem

19. Feeling that I don't have control over my life.

1	2	3	4	5
Not a problem	A slight problem	A problem	A major problem	An overwhelming problem

20. Feeling that my health and and care needs have reduced my privacy.

1	2	3	4	5
Not a problem	A slight problem	A problem	A major problem	An overwhelming problem

21. Not feeling supported by my community of friends and family.

1	2	3	4	5
Not a problem	A slight problem	A problem	A major problem	An overwhelming problem

22. Not feeling supported by my health care providers.

1	2	3	4	5
Not a problem	A slight problem	A problem	A major problem	An overwhelming problem

23. Feeling like I am no longer able to mentally cope with the challenges to my health.

1	2	3	4	5
Not a problem	A slight problem	A problem	A major problem	An overwhelming problem

24. Not being able to accept the way things are.

1	2	3	4	5
Not a problem	A slight problem	A problem	A major problem	An overwhelming problem

25. Not being treated with respect or understanding by others.

1	2	3	4	5
Not a problem	A slight problem	A problem	A major problem	An overwhelming problem

Figure 40.1 *(Continued).*

Dignity therapy question protocol
Tell me a little about your life history; particularly the parts that you either remember most or think are the most important? When did you feel most alive?
Are there specific things that you would want your family to know about you, and are there particular things you would want them to remember?
What are the most important roles you have played in life (family roles, vocational roles, community-service roles, etc)? Why were they so important to you and what do you think you accomplished in those roles?
What are your most important accomplishments, and what do you feel most proud of?
Are there particular things that you feel still need to be said to your loved ones or things that you would want to take the time to say once again?
What are your hopes and dreams for your loved ones?
What have you learned about life that you would want to pass along to others? What advice or words of guidance would you wish to pass along to your (son, daughter, husband, wife, parents, other[s])?
Are there words or perhaps even instructions that you would like to offer your family to help prepare them for the future?
In creating this permanent record, are there other things that you would like included?

Figure 40.2 The Dignity Therapy question protocol. Reprinted from with permission from [11] © 2008 American Society of Clinical Oncology. All rights reserved.

prepare for death and 65% reported that it was as important as any other aspect of care.[9] Dignity therapy was also beneficial to family members, with 78% reporting that the generativity document helped them during their time of grief, 77% indicating the document would serve as an ongoing source of comfort for both themselves and their families, while 95% reported that they would recommend dignity therapy to other patients and families. Dignity therapy addresses spiritual and existential distress, and can therefore be applied broadly, irrespective and independent of a specific religious or faith-based focus.

The role of caregivers in maintaining dignity: dignity-conserving care

The Dignity Model, the Patient Dignity Inventory and Dignity Therapy provide empirical tools to address dignity-related distress and patient spiritual needs. However, the intrinsic qualities of healthcare providers and the manner in which these qualities shape and inform the provision of care, also have a profound influence on patients' overall sense of dignity. With respect to promoting healing, wholeness, and wellness among patients facing serious illness, healthcare professional attributes such as compassion, caring, authenticity, and empathy have been identified as equally, or in some instances more, important than professional knowledge or technical competencies.[12–15] While overlapping significantly with terms, such as whole person care, humanistic medicine, and spiritual care, dignity-conserving care is both an aretic and deontic modality. The terms 'aretic' (based on virtue or character) and 'deontic' (based on duty or obligation) come from the field of virtue ethics, which emphasizes the characteristics of the moral agent, rather than ethical principles or consequences.[16] When applied to dignity-conserving care or spiritual care, aretic components of therapeutic efficacy involve aspects of the therapeutic relationship, the presence of the care provider and the care tenor. Deontic components, in comparison, are rooted in the language of treatment, skills, and tasks that are the predominant features of contemporary healthcare education.[17] The intrinsic qualities of healthcare providers, and their bearing on conserving patient dignity, are particularly applicable when dignity considerations are subsumed within the scope of spiritual care, which has long recognized the impact of the intrinsic qualities of the care provider in the delivery of care.[18] While the administration of Dignity Therapy and the Patient Dignity Inventory represent tangible, deontic approaches, investing them with the aretic qualities of compassion, authenticity, empathy, kindness, is more likely to preserve patient sense of dignity.[19–23] Recent research has identified these so called invisible ingredients of healing as being central components of spiritual care giving, with deontic approaches playing an important, but secondary role.[13,20,23–31]

The concept of the care tenor denotes the impact that 'healthcare provider presence' has on patient sense of dignity. While including a range of subtleties such as active listening, affirmation, body language and attitudes, care tenor broadly refers to the *tone of care* that healthcare professionals embody, which either enhances or undermines a patient's sense of dignity.[19] In fact, some authors have suggested that dignity be construed as an interactive process between patients and their healthcare providers, rather than a separate and prescriptive construct.[32] A study exploring patient and healthcare professional perspectives regarding essential components of spiritual care, identified a similar process termed 'co-creating', which involves a mutual and fluid interaction between patients, families and healthcare professionals.[20] The other key themes identified from the study were 'being present' and 'opening eyes,' a process whereby healthcare providers became aware of patients' humanity, further enunciating an aretic pathway of dignity conserving care. Similarly, a study of an interdisciplinary palliative care team identified spirituality as a relational process between team members and their patients, often embedded within acts of caring and routine patient interactions.[22] In a study investigating the delivery of spiritual care by twenty-two nurses in an Irish palliative care setting, participants identified 'being with' (77%) and intuitive knowing (68%) as significant components of spiritual care giving, both of which were contingent on a trusting nurse-patient relationship (55%).[21] The field of psychotherapy has also recognized the impact of a deep and trusting connection between therapist and patient in promoting healing [33–35]. As Christopher Perry summarizes, 'It is essential for therapists and health professionals to know more about the nature of wellbeing from within, as it lives inside of themselves, in order to better recognize and help awaken it in their clients and patients.[36] In summary, while dignity-related tools provide practitioners with the necessary knowledge and skills to address dignity-related distress, equally important to the healing process are the intrinsic qualities of the healthcare professional, as 'the more that healthcare providers are able to affirm the patient's value—that is, seeing the person they are or were, rather than just the illness they have—the more likely that the patient's sense of dignity will be upheld.'[37]

Recent research seems to suggest that the impact of aretic aspects of care extend beyond professionals self-interest in dignity-conserving or spiritual care, as the absence of such qualities have been shown to have a negative impact on patient's overall care experience. A large cohort study (n = 3424) of Canadian physicians reported that low scores in patient–physician communication and clinical decision making on a national accreditation exam significantly predicted retained complaints to provincial medical regulatory authorities over a twelve year period.[38] 17.1% of the sample had at least one retained complaint, with 81.9% of total registered complaints being communication or quality-of-care related, further fortifying the impact that the aretic qualities of healthcare professionals have in the patient experience. A number of studies have reported on the impact healthcare professionals have on patient sense of spirituality,[3,20,22,39] including adverse clinical experiences causing spiritual distress or iatrogenic suffering.[40] Addressing issues of dignity and spirituality, therefore consists of not only what is done to patients, but the manner in which one cares for patients across the various domains of care requiring healthcare providers to reflect on the deontic and aretic components of their care delivery.

Dignity conserving care: translating theory into practice

While empirical research related to dignity conserving care provides compelling evidence connecting dignity to spiritual care, the translation of this knowledge into practice is perhaps most challenging. While many patients have expressed a desire to have matters of 'spirit' or 'soul' addressed by the healthcare professionals,[41–50] healthcare professionals are reticent to do so,[51,52] even though most feel that spiritual issues fall within their scopes of practice [53–56]. While 41–94% of patients in various studies expressed a desire to have their spiritual needs addressed by their healthcare professionals,[13] a recent study reported that 75% of advanced cancer patients felt that their spiritual needs were not met during a recent hospital admission.[57] While issues of time, inadequate education and a lack of organizational support[20,22] have been cited as reasons for this phenomena, the nebulous quality of spirituality and the paucity of a codified operational framework for addressing concerns falling within this domain suggests more inherent and systemic challenges. A simple mnemonic framework—the A, B, C, and D of dignity conserving care—provides practitioners with pragmatic clinical guidance on how to maintain, and perhaps foster a sense of dignity, in patients across the spectrum of healthcare.[37]

'A'—attitude

'A'—attitude emphasizes the need for healthcare professionals to examine the attitudes and assumptions they bring to a patient encounter. *Attitude* can be defined as a learnt predisposition towards individuals or groups, treating them not as they are, but as they are perceived to be. Attitudes consist of conscious, sub-conscious and socially constructed assumptions, which often fall beyond the grasp of self-awareness. Michel Foucault, a post-structuralist philosopher, in *The Birth of the Clinic*[58] argues that underlying tenets of contemporary western medicine are built on epistemological assumptions, which directly affect the attitude or gaze of the physician towards their patients, in many cases reducing patients to objects or the location of their disease. Clinical examples of how attitude effects patient care range from value-laden terminology such as 'the difficult patient' or a 'good death';[59,60] to the way patients with a history of substance abuse or the socially disenfranchised are treated by healthcare providers. Studies have shown that attitudes impact: decisions related to the inclusion of new cancer drugs into provincial formularies;[61] and the provision of life-sustaining measures for patients with longstanding disabilities.[62]

Healthcare providers are implored to examine their own beliefs, values, and assumptions, and their impact on patients charged to their care. While numerous practices and questions could aid in this process, some examples might include: 'Who is the person behind this disease?'; 'Is this person the subject or object of my clinical attention?'; and, 'Am I aware of how my attitudes are affecting the way I care for this patient?' The spirituality of healthcare professionals has been identified as an essential factor in effective spiritual care delivery, which may in turn bestow healthcare providers with a framework for cultivating awareness and generating attitudes that affect the healing process in general.[3,18,22,39,63] Puchalski reminds healthcare professionals that a part of their patient's story will be carried in their heart.[64] The reverse is also true, as a part of healthcare professionals' story will be carried in patients' hearts, long after the clinical encounter has passed.

'B'—Behaviours

Attending to the attitudes that affect patient care can influence professional behaviours. The 'B' of dignity conserving care consists of actions or reactions to the patient, ranging from small acts of kindness to the coordination of their care in a personalized manner. Simple behaviours, even the healthcare providers' body language, have been shown to have a powerful effect on patients' perception of time and compassion. One study reported that patients overestimated time spent when providers were sitting and under-estimated time when they were standing.[65] Another study reported that physicians were perceived as more compassionate by patients when they sat down, rather than when they stood at the bedside.[66] Dignity conserving care and spiritual care can be achieved through simple, sincere gestures, such as offering a glass of water, acknowledging patients' personal space, inquiring about photographs adorning a patients' room and endless other behaviours that convey genuine regard, respect and honour for the whole person.[7,37] Over 40 years ago, Marshall McLuhan coined the phrase 'the medium is the message,'[67] a sentiment that was echoed clinically by Dame Cicley Saunders, the founder of the modern hospice movement who reminds clinicians that, 'Care, in how it is given can reach the most hidden places.'[68]

'C'—Compassion

Attitudes and behaviours influence the decorum of bedside care and communication. Compassion, however, is rooted in the feelings and virtues that healthcare providers carry within themselves. Compassion can be defined as a state of mind that is both calm and energetic, allowing one to feel connected through a deep desire to alleviate the suffering of another.[69] Patients, especially those at the end-of-life, continually identify healthcare provider's compassion as a vital component of quality palliative care.[18,40,70,71] While seemingly more ephemeral than either attitude or behaviour, compassion, and interrelated aspects of empathy have a beneficial effect on healthcare providers, including fostering an increased commitment by nurses to their jobs and protecting them against emotional burnout.[6,72] While compassion can be cultivated through various means, Wasner and colleagues reported improved and sustained levels of compassion among some healthcare providers who participated in spiritual care training.[73] A number of wisdom traditions attest to a 'compassion feedback loop', where personal compassion directly impacts individual's ability to bestow compassion on others. While the specific mechanism of achieving compassion may vary and possibly elude comprehension by even the individual it embodies, it is often manifested in a reassuring touch, a gentle look, a reassuring smile, and an acknowledgment of the meta narrative in which the story of suffering resides.[37,74]

'D'—Dialogue

While the A, B, C mnemonics seem particularly relevant to spiritual care, the 'D' of dignity conserving care—Dialogue—explicitly invites the patient's perspective and personhood into the provision of care. The Dignity Therapy Question Protocol, along with PDI, provide one way of entering this broader discourse of meaning and purpose. However, opportunities to acknowledge personhood through dialogue are present in virtually every clinical encounter. These range from statements such as 'I'm sorry to have to tell you this ...' to 'What do I need to know about you as a person to take the best care of you possible?' Words such as these provide consolation, and affirm an approach that intentionally seeks to care for the person and not just the patient. Other psychotherapeutic approaches including meaning centred therapy;[75] life review;[76,77] and other spirituality specific interventions [78–80] share the common goal of seeking to understand broader aspects of personhood, in order to inform the way that care is given.[37] The absence of the patients' perspective in dignity-conserving care is akin to trying to provide spiritual care without consideration of the spiritual background of the patient, or attempting to alleviate pain strictly through pharmaceutical means, without, for example, exploring the nature of a dying mother's suffering in knowing her newborn baby will not remember her. Daaleman and colleague identified 'co-creating' as one of the essential components of spiritual care, which in addition to the overarching interpersonal connection between the healthcare professional and their patient, also included more granular aspects of care, such as incorporating aspects of the patient's life experience into the care plan.[20] Various studies have enunciated patients' desires to have their voice heard in interactions with their healthcare providers, including having the opportunity to talk to someone about finding peace and having someone listen to their personal concerns.[31,81] While eliciting the story that extends beyond the location of disease and symptomatology may not cure illness, it may, nonetheless, provide the essential ingredients for healing.[82]

Conclusion

Dignity conserving care provides a framework and rhetoric for entering the realm of human spirituality. While this path traverses the patient's beliefs, values and experiences, it provides a means to explore an innately human quest for meaning and purpose. Clinicians working at the end-of-life are encouraged to address dignity related issues not only through the incorporation of tools and techniques, but also by examining the modifying effect that their intrinsic qualities have on their patient's sense of dignity. The role of healthcare providers in this journey cannot be underestimated. Dignity, while ultimately defined by the patient, is often distilled in the aretic qualities of those who provide care during the sacred season of life drawing to a close.

References

1 Chochinov, H., Hassard, T., McClement, S., Hack, T., Kristjanson, L., Harlos, M., *et al.* (2008). The patient dignity inventory: a novel way of measuring dignity-related distress in palliative care. *J Pain Sympt Manag* **36**(6): 559–71.

2 Chochinov, H., Hassard, T., McClement, S., Hack, T., Kristjanson, L., Harlos, M., *et al.* (2009). The landscape of distress in the terminally ill. *J Pain Sympt Manag* **38**(5): 641–9.

3 Cobb, M. (2003). Spiritual care. In: M. Lloyd-Williams (ed.) *Psychosocial Issues in Palliative Care*, pp. 135–47. London: Oxford.

4 Pesut, B., Fowler, M., Taylor, E., Reimer-Kirkham, S., Sawatzky, R. (2008). Conceptualizing spirituality and religion for healthcare. *J Clin Nurs* **17**: 2803–10.

5 Clark, L., Leedy, S., McDonald, L., Mueller, B., Lamb, C., Mendez, T., *et al.* (2007). Spirituality and job satisfaction among hospice interdisciplinary team members. *J Palliat Med* **10**(6): 1321–7.

6 Desbiens, J., Fillion, L. (2007). Coping strategies, emotional outcomes and spiritual quality of life in palliative care nurses. *Int J Palliat Nurs* **13**(6): 291–300.

7 Strang, S., Strang, P. (2009). Spiritual care. In: Bruera, E, Higginson, I., Ripamonti, C, VonGunten, C. (eds) *Textbook of Palliative Medicine*, pp. 1019–1028. London: Hodder Arnold.

8 Chochinov, H., Hack, T., Hassard, T., Kristjanson, L., McClement, S., Harlos, M. (2004). Dignity and psychotherapeutic considerations in end-of-life care. *J Palliat Care* **20**(3): 134–42.

9 McClement, S., Chochinov, H., Hack, T., Hassard, T., Kristjanson, L., Harlos, M. (2007). Dignity therapy: family member perspectives. *J Palliat Med* **10**(5): 1076–82.

10 Chochinov, H.M. (2004). Dignity and the eye of the beholder. *J Clin Oncol* **22**(7): 1336–40.

11 Chochinov, H., Hack, T., Hassard, T., Kristjanson, L., McClement, S., Harlos, M. (2005). Dignity therapy: a novel psychotherapeutic intervention for patients near the end of life. *J Clin Oncol* **23**(24): 5520–5.

12 Puchalski, C. (2002). Spirituality and end-of-life care: a time for listening and caring. *J Palliat Med* **5**(2): 289–94.

13 Sulmasy, D. (2006). Spiritual issues in the care of dying patients. *J Am Med Ass* **296**(11): 1385–92.

14 Bush, T., Bruni, N. (2008). Spiritual care as a dimension of holistic care: a relational interpretation. *Int J Palliat Nurs* **14**(11): 539–45.

15 Yedidia, M. (2007). Transforming doctor–patient relationships. *J Pain Sympt Manag* **33**(1): 40–56.

16 Pellegrino, E., Thomasma, D. (1993). *The Virtues in Medical Practice*. New York: Oxford University Press.

17 Campbell, A. (2003). The virtues (and vices) of the four principles. *J Med Eth* **29**(5): 292–6.

18 Puchalski, C. (2006). *A Time for Listening and Caring: Spirituality and the Care of the Chronically Ill and Dying*. New York: Oxford.

19 Chochinov, H. (2006). Dying, dignity, and new horizons in palliative end-of-life care. *CA* **56**(2): 84–103.

20 Daaleman, T., Usher, B., Williams, S., Rawlings, J., Hanson, L. (2008). An exploratory study of spiritual care at the end of life. *Ann Fam Med* **6**(5): 406–11.

21 Bailey, M., Moran, S., Graham, M. (2009). Creating a spiritual tapestry: nurses' experiences of delivering spiritual care to patients in an Irish hospice. *Int J Palliat Nurs* **15**(1): 42–8.

22 Sinclair, S., Raffin, S., Pereira, J., Guebert, N. (2006). Collective soul: the spirituality of an interdisciplinary team. *Palliat Support Care* **4**(1):13–24.

23 Puchalski, C. (2002). Spirituality. In: A. Berger, R. Portenay, D. Weissman (eds) *Principles and Practice of Palliative Care and Supportive Oncology*, pp. 799–812. Philadelphia: Lippincott Williams and Wilkins.

24 Chochinov, H. (2002). Dignity conserving care: a new model for palliative care. *J Am Med Ass* **287**(17): 2253–60.

25 Hinshaw, D. (2005). Spiritual issues in surgical palliative care. *Surg Clin N Am* **85:** 257–72.

26 Brock, C., Salmsky, J. (1993). Empathy: an essential skill for understanding the physician-patient relationship in clinical practice. *Fam Med* **25:** 245–8.

27 Kearney, M., Mount, B. (2000). Spiritual care of the dying patient. In: H. Chochinov, W. Breitbart (eds) *Handbook of Psychiatry in Palliative Medicine*, pp. 357–73. Oxford: Oxford University Press.

28 Larson, D., Swyers, J., McCullough, M. (1997). *Scientific Research on Spirituality and Health: a Consensus Report.* Rockville: National Institute for healthcare Research.

29 Larson, D., Tobin, D. (2000). End-of-life conversations: evolving practice and theory. *J Am Med Ass* **284**(12): 1573–8.

30 Weaver, M., OW, C., Walker, D., Degenhardt, E. (1993). A questionnaire for patients' evaluations of their physicians humanistic behaviours. *J Gen Intern Med* **8**(3): 1235–9.

31 Wright, M. (2001). Chaplaincy in hospice and hospital: findings from a survey in England and Wales. *Palliat Med* **15:** 229–42.

32 Johnson, P.R. (1998). An analysis of dignity. *Theoret Med Bioeth* **19:** 337–52.

33 Rogers, C., Kirschenbaum, H., Henderson, V. (1989). *The Carl Rogers Reader.* New York: Houghton Mifflin Harcourt.

34 Jung, C.G. (1962). *Memories, Dreams, Reflections.* New York: Vintage.

35 Satir, V., Banmen, J., Gerber, J., Gomori, M. (1991). *The Satir Model.* Palo Alto: Science and Behavioural Books.

36 Perry, C. (1997). Transference and countertransference. In: P. Young-Eisendrath, T. Dawson (eds) *The Cambridge Companion to Jung*, pp. 141–63. Cambridge: Cambridge University Press.

37 Chochinov, H.M. (2007). Dignity and the essence of medicine: the A, B, C, and D of dignity conserving care. *Br Med J* **335:** 184–7.

38 Tamblyn, R., Abrahamowicz, M., Dauphinee, D., Wenghofer, E., Jacques, A., Klass, D., *et al.* (2007). Physician scores on a national clinical skills examination as predictors of complaints to medical regulatory authorities. *J Am Med Ass* **298**(9): 993–1001.

39 Ross, L. (1994). Spiritual care: the nurses role. *Nurs Standard* **8**(39): 35–7.

40 Kuhl, D. (2002). *What Dying People Want.* Toronto: Anchor.

41 Astrow, A., Puchalski, C., Sulmasy, D. (2001). Religion, spirituality and heath care: social, ethical, and practical considerations. *Am J Med* **110:** 283–7.

42 Brown, A., Whitney, S., Duffy, J. (2006). The physician's role in the assessment and treatment of spiritual distress at the end of life. *Palliat Support Care* **4:** 81–6.

43 Emblen, J., Halstead, L. (1993). Spiritual needs and interventions: comparing the views of patients, nurses, and chaplains. *Clin Nurse Special* **7**(40): 175–82.

44 Gallup, G. (1997). *Spiritual beliefs and the dying process*: a report on a national survey. London: George H. Gallup International Institute.

45 McCord, G., Gilchrist, V., Grossman, S., King, B., McCormick, K., Oprandi, A., *et al.* (2004). Discussing spirituality with patients: A rational and ethical approach. *Ann Fam Med* **2:** 356–61.

46 Post, S., Puchalski, C., Larson, D. (2000). Physicians and patient spirituality: Professional boundaries, competency, and ethics. *Ann Intern Med* **132**(7): 578–83.

47 Pronk, K. (2005). Role of the doctor in relieving spiritual distress at the end of life. *Am J Hospice Palliat Med* **22**(6): 419–24.

48 Reed, P. (1991). Preferences for spiritually related nursing interventions Among terminally ill and nonterminally ill hospitalized adults and well adults. *Appl Nurs Res* **4**(3): 122–8.

49 Taylor, E. (2003). Nurses caring for the spirit: Patients with cancer and family caregiver expectations. *Oncol Nurs* **30**(4): 585–90.

50 Warr, T. (1999). The physician's role in maintaining hope and spirituality. *Bioethics Forum* **15**(1): 31–7.

51 Kuin, A., Deliens, L., van Zuylen, L., Courents, A., Vernooij-Dassen, M., van der Linden, B., *et al.* (2006). Spiritual issues in palliative care consultations in the Netherlands. *Palliat Med* **20:** 585–92.

52 Puchalski, C. (2008). Spiritual issues as an essential element of quality palliative care: a commentary. *J Clin Eth* **19**(2): 160–2.

53 Dane, B., Moore, R. (2005). Social workers' use of spiritual practices in palliative care. *J Soc Work End-of-life Palliat Care* **1**(4): 63–82.

54 Nagai-Jacobsen, M.G., Burkhardt, M.A. (1989). Spirituality: cornerstone of holistic nursing practice. *Holist Nurs Pract* **3**(3): 18–26.

55 Prochnau, C., Liu, L., Boman, J. (2003). Personal-professional connections in palliative care occupational therapy. *Am J Occupat Ther* **57**(2): 196–204.

56 Ross, L. (1997). The nurse's role in assessing and responding to patient's spiritual needs. *Int J Nurs Stud* **3**(1): 37–42.

57 Balboni, T., Vanderwerker, L., Block, S., Paulk, E., Lathan, C., Peteet, J., *et al.* (2007). Religiousness and spiritual support among advanced cancer patients and associations with end-of-life treatment preferences and quality of life. *J Clin Oncol* **25**(5): 555–60.

58 Foucault, M. (1973). *Birth of the Clinic.* New York: Pantheon.

59 Walters, G. (2004). Is there such a thing as a good death? *Palliat Med* **18:** 404–8.

60 Zimmermann, C., Rodin, G. (2004). The denial of death thesis: Sociological critique and implications for palliative care. *Palliat Med* **18:**121–8.

61 Sinclair, S., Hagen, N.A., Chambers, C., Manns, B., Simon, A., Browman, G.P. (2008). Accounting for reasonableness: exploring he personal internal framework affecting decisions about cancer drug funding. *Hlth Policy* **86:** 381–90.

62 Steinstra, D., Chochinov, H.M. (2006). Vulnerability, disability, and palliative end-of-life care. *J Palliat Care* **22:** 166–74.

63 Boston, P., Mount, B. (2006). The caregiver's perspective on existential and spiritual distress in palliative care. *J Pain Sympt Manag* **32**(1): 13–26.

64 Puchalski, C. (Speaker) (2006). *The Healing Encounter.* Boulder: Companion Arts.

65 Johnson, R.L., Sadosty, A.T., Weaver, A.L., Goyal, D.G. (2008). To sit or not sit? *Ann Emerg Med* **51**(2): 188–93.

66 Bruera, E., Palmer, J.L., Pace, E., Zhang, K., Willey, J., Strasser, F., *et al.* (2007). A randomized, controlled trial of physician postures when breaking bad news to cancer patients. *Palliat Med* **21**(6): 501–5.

67 McLuhan, M. (1964). *Understanding Media.* New York: Mentor.

68 Saunders C. (1988). Spiritual pain. *J Palliat Care* **4**(3): 29–32.

69 Ladner L. (2004). *The Lost Art of Compassion.* San Francisco: Harper Collins.

70 Cherlin, E., Schulman-Green, D., McCorkle, R., Johnson-Hurzeler, R., Bradley, E. (2004). Family perceptions of clinicians' outstanding practices in end-of-life care. *J Palliat Care* **20**(2): 113–16.

71 Lynn, J., Lynch-Schuster, J., Wilkinson, A., Simon, L. (2008). Supporting people in difficult times. In: J. Lynn, J. Lych-Schuster, A. Wilkinson, L. Simon (eds) *Improving Care for the End of Life*, pp. 133–61. New York: Oxford.

72 Holland, J., Neimeyer, R. (2005). Reducing the risk of burnout in end-of-life care settings: the role of daily spiritual experiences and training. *Palliat Support Care* **3:** 173–81.

73 Wasner, M., Longaker, C., Fegg, M., Borasio, G. (2005). Effects of spiritual care training for palliative care professionals. *Palliat Med* **19:** 99–104.

74 Frank, A.W. (1992). The pedagogy of suffering. *Theory Psychol* **2**(4): 467–85.

75 Breitbart, W. (2002). Spirituality and meaning in supportive care: Spirituality and meaning-centered group psychotherapy interventions in advanced cancer. *Support Care Cancer* **10:** 272–80.

76 Steinhauser, K.E., Alexander, S., Byock, I., George, L., Olsen, M., Tulsky, J. (2008). Do preparation and life completion discussions improve functioning and quality of life in seriously ill patients? Pilot randomized control trial. *J Palliat Med* **11**(9): 1234–40.

77 Ando, M., Tsuda, A., Morita, T. (2007). Life review interviews on the spiritual wellbeing of terminally ill cancer patients. *Support Care Cancer* **15**: 225–31.

78 Renz, M., Mao, M., Cerny, T. (2005). Spirituality, psychotherapy and music in palliative cancer care: research projects in psycho-oncology at an oncology center in Switzerland. *Support Care Cancer* **13**: 961–6.

79 Miller, D., Chibnall, J., Videen, S., Duckro, P. (2005). Supportive-affective group experience for persons with life-threatening illness: reducing spiritual, psychological, and death-related distress in dying patients. *J Palliat Med* **8**(2): 333–43.

80 Elias, A., Giglio, J., Pimenta, C., El-Dash, L. (2006). Therapeutical intervention, relaxation, mental images, and spirituality (RIME) for spiritual pain in terminal patients. *Scient World J* **6**: 2158–69.

81 Moadel, A., Morgan, C., Fatone, A., Grennan, J., Carter, J., Laruffa, G., *et al.* (1999). Seeking meaning and hope: Self-reported spiritual and existential needs among an ethnically-diverse cancer patient population. *Psycho-oncol* **8**: 378–85.

82 Waldfogel, S. (1997). Spirituality in medicine. *Prim Care* **24**(4): 963–76.

CHAPTER 41

Pastoral theology in healthcare settings: blessed irritant for holistic human care

Emmanuel Y. Lartey

Introduction

Pastoral theology may be understood as a critical reflection on the nature and caring activity of the divine, and of human persons in relation to the divine, within the personal, social, communal, and cultural contexts of the world. Pastoral theology is described as *pastoral* because of its focus on the care of persons and communities. It is *theological* because it reflects on the nature and activity of the divine, and of humanity in relation to the divine, as portrayed and understood through various practices and documents of faith. In line with the almost exclusive identification of 'theology' with the Christian faith, pastoral theology has been conceptualized as an activity related to Christian traditions. The term 'theology' itself has, in many circles and in the minds of many practitioners of different religious and cultural persuasions, become synonymous with Christian doctrine. However, with the growth of interest and concern for inter-religious dialogue, and the recognition of the riches that lie in different religious traditions, the term is increasingly being utilized in its etymologically more accurate sense as the study (*logos*) of the divine (*theos*). Pastoral theology is a constructive practical theology that seeks to make contributions to both disciplines of pastoral care and theology. As such the American Society for Pastoral Theology (SPT) comprising mostly of teachers and doctoral students in pastoral theology, pastoral care, and counselling, defines pastoral theology as 'a constructive practical theological enterprise focused on the religious care of persons, families and communities', emphasizing its constructive and practical nature.[1] By identifying 'religious care' as its focus, the Society expresses its interest and intention to pay attention to different religious traditions. Institutional chaplains in general and healthcare chaplains in particular, have long practiced in multi-religious settings, and with respect for the variety of religious and spiritual traditions in which we participate in today's world.

Pastoral theology

Pastoral theology includes interpretive, constructive, and expressive reflections on the caring activities of the divine and of human communities throughout history, as well as in the current contemporary world. Pastoral theologians engage 'the Divine' or 'God' and 'care' critically, raising questions, and exploring concepts and practices in order to examine their fidelity to particular understandings of faith and their effectiveness in caring for human persons, families, and communities in their respective contexts. Given that notions of 'God', 'the Divine', the 'Higher Self', 'Ultimate Reality', etc., abound in different religious traditions and beyond them, it is not necessary that pastoral theology be restricted to Christianity. Moreover, the existence of non-theistic religious traditions, such as Buddhism, calls for theological reflection that is neither singular nor theistic in its content. Pastoral theologians engage interpretively by examining the meanings—both manifest and unconscious—of statements and practices of faith as they impinge upon practices of care.[2]

Spirituality

Pastoral theology is constructive in that it seeks to assist in the refining and redefining of notions of the divine toward the end of more adequate ways of being present with and caring for human persons in the midst of the exigencies of life. Included in such examination, therefore, is an exploration of the term 'spirituality' as it has increasingly become used in the healthcare fields in particular. Recognizing the complexities of defining the term and the myriad ways in which 'spirituality' is employed and engaged, a consensus definition was arrived at in 2009 for usage in the healthcare disciplines. The consensus is that 'spirituality is the aspect of humanity that refers to the way individuals seek and express meaning and purpose, and the way they experience their connectedness to the moment, to self, to others, to nature and to the significant or sacred.'[3] Pastoral theologians may examine meanings and practices by which persons 'seek and express a sense of meaning and purpose,' as well as how they articulate or express their connections with the divine as a part of their necessary critical reflection. From a pastoral theological perspective spirituality emphasizes a 'human capacity for relationship with self, others, world, God and that which transcends sensory experience, which is often expressed in the particularities of given historical, spatial and social contexts and which often leads to specific forms of action in the world.'[4] Our spirituality has reference to our *characteristic manner of relating* and is manifest along at least five dimensions—relationship with transcendence, intra-personal (i.e. with self), interpersonal (i.e. with another), corporate (i.e. relationships among people, in groups, communities and institutions), and spatial (i.e. with places, spaces and objects). Pastoral theologians may be found expressing their work through practices of care that include creative, liturgical, and artistic activities, such as healthcare and healing, counselling, worship, preaching, teaching, group work, and community development.

A theology of pastoral care

Pastoral theology, then, is essentially a theology of pastoral care or a theological reflection upon practices and theories of care. The relationship between theology, on the one hand, and pastoral care, on the other, is largely conceived of in this discipline as *dialogical* and *mutual* in nature. Consequently, there is an expectation that theology will inform care and that care will also inform theology. The assumption is that both theory and practice are loci of learning and revelation. Pastoral theologians expect to encounter the divine and learn about this dimension of the human experience through the practices of care they engage in. As such, various practices are engaged in with the express purpose of discovering more about the divine dimension and learning more about the self that engages in acts of care. One such important practice is that of the writing and presentation of detailed accounts of encounters with patients and clients (called *verbatims*) to and in supervised groups. These accounts and the presentation and discussion of them become significant means of theological learning. Supervisors of clinical pastoral education groups are pastoral theologians who assist groups engage in pastoral theology at the coal face of practice in hospitals and other sites of human need and care.

Pastoral theology has a wide scope. It includes the study of the theological underpinnings, understandings and implications of the offices, roles, and functions of persons in religious ministry within, as well as outside communities of faith. Historically 'pastoral' theology was restricted to a study of the officially recognized rabbinical, clerical or religious leadership office. However, as the discipline has developed, especially during the twentieth century, there has been a deeper recognition of the multifarious and communal nature of the caring ministry within communities of faith. As such pastoral theology has focused increasingly on exploring the theological aspects of the care of persons, rather than exclusively upon caregivers, and their office and functions.

Paridigms of pastoral care

Traced historically, paradigms of pastoral care have morphed through *classical clerical*, *clinical pastoral*, *communal contextual* and *intercultural post-modern* phases. Elements of each of these distinguishable paradigms are still very much in evidence today in various parts of the world.

- *Classical clerical* pastoral care emphasized the office, role and functions of ordained clergy or officially sanctioned religious leaders as ministers and purveyors of the 'cure of souls' (cura *animarum*). Ordained religious leaders were theologically trained to offer ministrations that transmitted the grace of God to persons in need of healing, guiding, sustaining or reconciling. Pastoral theology in the classical clerical age, and in the practice of some communities of faith currently, is essentially a theology of ministry with a focus on the role and action of the ordained
- *Clinical pastoral* care is modelled upon medical practice with pastoral care givers occupying the role of trained clinicians. 'Pastoral care and counselling' here is conceived of as a mental health discipline with a spiritual component. Psychotherapy is the reigning paradigm and pastoral care is largely synonymous with counselling. Chaplains and pastoral counsellors acquire therapeutic skills to be utilized with patients or clients. Pastoral theology in the clinical-pastoral model consists of theological reflections upon clinical encounters, with explorations of how the presence of the divine is discernible in the therapeutic experience
- *Communal contextual* care raised questions about the individualistic tone and personal therapeutic nature of the practices of pastoral care. Pastoral theologians recognized the communitarian nature of the care of persons and emphasized the place of communities of faith and faith perspectives in the practice of care. The important influence of Liberation theology in the development of Feminist, Black, Womanist, Mujerista, Queer and various significant contextual theologies provided tools for the development of pastoral theology in different contexts. Pastoral theology in a communal contextual frame employs the methodologies of Liberation theologies in seeking social and communal justice, drawing attention as Feminist theologians in particular have, to the interconnectedness between personal distress and socio-political conditions.[5] Theology is examined for its liberative contributions to the human quest for wholeness and healing
- *Intercultural post-modern* pastoral care identifies gender, race, class, sexuality, and culture as significant elements in the practice and theorizing of care and seeks to incorporate socio-economic and cultural analysis into the theory and delivery of pastoral care exploring, as Womanist theologians have, the specific and cumulative influence of race, gender, class, sexuality, and other socially constructed realities upon the practices of care. Global cultures and differences in pastoral care in different world situations have began to play a more prominent role in pastoral care.

Pastoral theologians are beginning to pay closer attention to the way faith and religious tradition play a role in shaping the kind of care on offer and, indeed, upon the way in which meaning is made of human exigencies. Inter-religious dialogue and activity have begun to play a much more significant role in pastoral care and theology. Intercultural pastoral theology emphasizes theological anthropology arising from international contexts, is respectful of diversity, celebrates difference and seeks meaningful and honest dialogue across differences.[6]

Pastoral theology: methodology

The pastoral theology that has accompanied developments in pastoral care, growing out of classical and contemporary theological traditions has, in terms of methodology, taken the following forms: deductive, correlational, interdisciplinary, inductive, contextual, and constructive methodologies. *Deductive* pastoral theology arises where theological, experiential or documentary material is premised as the source out of which practices of care are derived. *Correlational* theological methods, made explicit in the work of Paul Tillich and later revised by David Tracy, lay the existential realities of human life alongside the symbols and teachings of Christian faith. Tillichian correlational approaches are unidirectional with questions arising from existence and answers from the symbols of faith. Revised correlational methods are more dialogical allowing for mutual questioning and answering. *Interdisciplinary* pastoral theology draws on a variety of disciplines in arriving at theologically recommended practices. Pastoral care has traditionally drawn on psychology as its scientific disciplinary partner. As such, pastoral theology has, under this paradigm, been a religion-and-science discussion with psychology being the science. More recently, sociology, and now brain and neuroscience are occupying that position. In *inductive* approaches to pastoral theology human experience is the main source out of which pastoral care practices are sought. *Contextual* approaches emphasize social location, cultural dynamics and anthropological considerations in the derivation of theologically appropriate practices of care. *Constructive* approaches largely in tune with process theology seek to advance theological notions that reflect creativity and development within the divine sphere.

Pastoral theology is practical theology that has a very clear praxis orientation. It emphasizes the necessary interaction between theory and practice in all practical theology. In pastoral theological terms the praxis orientation has often been expressed in at least four ways, namely theory–practice, practice–theory, theory–practice–theory or practice–theory–practice. These four are evident in the way pastoral theology is engaged in contemporaneously. Starting and ending points distinguish these approaches from each other. Nevertheless, each includes, as of necessity, both theory and practice in some form of interaction.

Core tasks

Pastoral theology fulfills the 'core tasks' of all practical theological endeavors. Rick Osmer[7] usefully articulates these four tasks as:

1. descriptive empirical
2. interpretive
3. normative
4. pragmatic.

1. The *descriptive empirical task* entails gathering information that helps in the discernment of patterns and dynamics in particular episodes, situations, or contexts. Pastoral theologians develop acute observational skills that enable them to carefully record what is going on. Listening is a core skill for the pastoral theologian, as is asking questions that elicit clearer expressions of what is being experienced. The usage of narrative therapy in pastoral care, for example, begins with the facilitation of the uninhibited articulation of one's story. Much of pastoral care, including pastoral counselling, begins with listening to and hearing descriptions of empirical experience. However, so does congregational or communal care engage social descriptive means to 'hear the story of the community.' Other important tools employed in pastoral care and pastoral theology include personal genograms, which are pictorial depictions of family relations and personal characteristics going back two or three generations, and community genograms, which identify significant social and cultural patterns in the historical development of communities.

2. *The interpretive task* draws on hermeneutical theories from the arts and sciences to unearth deeper understandings and explanations of the observed patterns and dynamics. In this activity, what is sought is to go beyond the superficial surface into deeper underlying forces and influences upon what is experienced or perceived. Meaning-seeking here employs an array of different possible theories in an attempt to account for experience. This task deliberately explores non-theological disciplines in the belief that they may also reflect the divine realm manifest through all of human experience. It also reflects the interdisciplinarity that is basic to pastoral theology.

3. *The normative task* is pursued in expressly theological language and forms of thought. Here, theological concepts are used to interpret particular episodes, situations, or contexts, constructing ethical norms to guide responses, and learning from 'good practice'. Pastoral theology *qua* theology engages critically in theological discourse with a deep sense of the value and importance of theological thinking in the quest for appropriate and effective means of care and healing. Theological interpretation, far from being an intrusive add-on to a therapeutic process, actually serves to offer fresh and needed perspectives for the task of providing adequate care. Theological concepts often critique social scientific ones in helpful ways when the two are engaged dialogically. Similarly, the human sciences can and do offer useful questions and critiques to theological interpretations.

4. *The pragmatic task* seeks to develop strategies of action that will influence situations in ways that are desirable. The goals of pastoral theology include the provision of appropriate and effective care of humans in our existential realities. 'God is love' is both a theological and a pastoral statement. Pastoral theologians seek to find ways in which this theological statement may be 'enfleshed' in the lives of living human persons within the networks of relationships in which we are embedded, in ways that will be beneficial for all. As such pastoral theologians tend not to end with the aesthetically satisfactory theological statement. Rather they push forward to find a pragmatically appropriate response that will be in keeping with theology, appropriate ethics, and effective care of persons.

Healthcare chaplains

Healthcare chaplains are the most obvious exemplars of pastoral theology within healthcare institutions and settings. Generally, healthcare chaplains view themselves as 'spiritual care professionals' whose tasks include attending to the religious needs of patients, staff, and families; attending to wider spiritual and existential needs expressed or implied in the conditions in which patients, staff, and families find themselves; providing general emotional support for all; acting as advocates, mediators, and agents of evaluation within hospitals and healthcare delivery systems.[8] Chaplains have often been seen as being in relatively advantageous positions to facilitate and empower debate concerning the critical role of values in healthcare. As such they are often to be found on the Ethics Boards or Committees of hospitals.

On the basis of an in-depth study of role of acute healthcare chaplains in Britain, Woodward suggested that:

> The chaplain's place in the organization gives him or her, a unique opportunity to engage in constructive and systematic evaluation of the systems and organizations within which he or she works. In other words, the chaplain can facilitate asking how comprehensiveness, quality of access to service, choice of user, and costs of these services relate to each other.[9]

Woodward argues, aware of the marginal space within healthcare institutions often occupied by chaplains, that 'chaplains might be described as liminal people. They are *in between;* and the freedom, or potential freedom, this position imparts gives them the possibility of relating to and interpreting reality in all kinds of creative ways.'[9]

Responsibilities

Healthcare chaplains as spiritual care professionals and pastoral theologians by no means see themselves as solely performing a service that is esoteric or not shareable with others. Rather than being solely responsible for the non-physical part of a person's experience, chaplains see themselves as partly (alongside others) responsible for the whole person's total health. It is a holistic vision of health that chaplains bring and they wish to work alongside other professionals and others in the coming into fruition of wholeness for all.[10] Health is about wholeness and its delivery is enhanced through partnerships. 'The patient, physician, nurse, and pastor, are the primary co-adventurers for health, assisted by family, friends, and associates ... All are agents of healing. God alone is the source of healing.'[11] Moreover, healthcare chaplains may help link hospitals with university or other institutions of learning where theologians and/or knowledgeable and reflective practitioners of different faith traditions may be engaged to assist in the quality assurance processes of hospitals. As pastoral theologians, then, healthcare chaplains together with others in the delivery of healthcare may engage in and stimulate the critical exploration of the very essence, meaning, and value of practices of healthcare, to the end of facilitating more holistic visions, and practices of health and healthcare, and facilitating the greater wellbeing of all persons.

Reflections and actions

Pastoral theological reflection and action within healthcare settings can be likened to the stimulating or indeed *irritating* role played by spices in a sumptuous dish of food. Imagery of this type is used in the Christian gospels where 'salt' (e.g. Matthew 5: 13) and 'yeast' (e.g. Matthew 13: 33) perform a necessary function of invigorating and stimulating to greater ends. Pastoral theology necessarily offers a supportive role to the enterprise of healthcare through being critical, constantly challenging and calling for holistic human care. The rallying cry of the theologian within care settings is for attention to the whole human person, the nature of human community and for care that not only leaves no aspect of humanity's wholeness unattended to, but also engages in practices of care that are ethically responsible and genuinely humane.

What then are some of the specific health issues to which a theological contribution might usefully be made? Let me mention five: (1) the very concept of health, (2) public or community health, (3) health inequities, (4) power issues and (5) compassionate care.

Notions of health

In contributing to the ongoing refining of practices of healthcare, notions of spirituality have increasingly been employed. As we have argued viewing spirituality in terms of characteristic styles of relating is one important way in which pastoral theologians may analyze the enterprise and undertakings of healthcare. The fundamental questions are 'What is health' and what is healthcare? In conceptualizing health theologians may raise questions that critically focus on the qualitative and relational aspects of health in complement to the physiological or quantitative. In settings in which notions of health appear to emphasize illness and its eradication, theologians may wish to draw attention to the promotion through relationship of more positive quality of life issues. Theologians are likely to raise questions of human worth, dignity and value and to require that these be on the table squarely in all understandings of health and practices of healthcare.

Health as a public good

Health as a public good requires the communal relational activities of interaction, education, and advocacy. Pastoral theologians as communicators and educators are skilled in hermeneutics and in the inter-subjective and corporate spheres. As such, they may be of great help in interpreting messages of health from the health disciplines to a wide public, whilst also being able to communicate to healthcare practitioners the felt needs and concerns of the public. This intermediary role is one that theologians by definition are perceived as playing in both secular and spiritual matters. In settings where financial considerations threaten to over ride the health needs of people, theologians will often want to draw attention to the ultimate significance of life over material wealth. In arriving at the best choices in the face of scarce financial resources, theologians will likely be in the forefront of calling for the usage of resources in the interest of wholesome living. Questions likely to be contributed by pastoral theologians in this kind of discussion include: what makes for the best utilization of resources in this particular human community in the service of their total wellbeing? How may the dignity and wellbeing of this community be enhanced by what is done in the name of healthcare? How could the solutions and treatments available be applied in ways that promote the wellbeing and wholeness of this particular community.

Health inequities

This leads naturally into discussions of health inequities—the great dilemmas of access, resource allocation, and distribution. Questions of social justice and compassion need to be taken together, but rarely are. The redistribution of resources in favour of the under-served and under-privileged would be a value that many in the theological fields would embrace. Very often what is needed in most communities is not the most sophisticated and technologically expensive equipment, but rather simple, appropriate interventions that are relational and that promote human dignity. A pastoral theological contribution in this arena would entail the promotion of education for self-care on both a personal and a communal dimension. The greater allocation of resources in the direction of increased specialization and crisis intervention tends to result in the lessening of awareness and sensitivity to the distribution of illness and need in populations. Localized areas of health assets need to be mapped out and encouraged for there will never be full resource possibility for all needs on the models of healthcare delivery that are current and favoured. The emphasis on pharmacological intervention, whilst increasing the wealth of producers of drugs, has not necessarily increased the health of populations. Pastoral theologians will not be silent on the issue of finance and its determinative power. Given an implicit commitment to holistic health for all, theologians are likely to raise the awareness of institutions to the deliberate or inadvertent development of communities of dependence, which are then exploited for the financial benefit of some.

As Michel Foucault pointed out repeatedly, all human relations involve power. Power is a relational given. All therapeutic relations, in fact all relations between professional helpers and their clients, are necessarily asymmetrical. Issues of power exist at all the dimensions of relationality we have defined as being constitutive of spirituality. Power issues exist not merely within professional groups and between them. Issues of power exist at the personal, collective, and cultural levels of healthcare delivery and practice. Theological analyses tend to point to the ambiguity and ambivalence of power. Pastoral theologians will tend therefore to encourage self-critical and institutional analyses of power relations among and between staff, patients, families, communities, and public. The theological call will entail an honest assessment of how power is being utilized, by whom and to what ends. It will include a desire that power be acknowledged as inevitable and that its exercise be examined to ensure that it serves the good of those most at risk or in need.

Compassionate care

Pastoral theologians' contribution to the chorus of voices calling for compassionate care will be in the direction of a greater awareness of the complexity of the physical-spiritual holism that lies at the heart of human nature. Human beings are complex composites of personal, physical, social, cultural, and spiritual components. Compassionate care requires attention to this mutli-dimensionality in totality. Reductionism is the thief of compassionate care. For care to be compassionate it needs to be attentive to all the dimensions of our human existence.[12]

Conclusion

As such, pastoral theologians, when they function in true integrity with their discipline and calling, will probably be a source of irritation to a healthcare enterprise that focuses narrowly on individualized bioethics. Pastoral theology will irritate those who would annex the language and practice of spirituality and spiritual care into the service of a healthcare delivery system that is more about illness than about health. Pastoral theologians might risk being charged with being out of touch with financial realities for calling for greater equity in the distribution of resources and social justice in seeking to uplift under-resourced groups. Pastoral theologians will be a source of irritation in healthcare systems that refuse to constantly review policies and practices to ensure that power is being utilized for the wellbeing of all. Pastoral theology when it functions best within healthcare settings serves as a 'blessed' irritation within corporate and institutional systems to nudge them in the direction of holistic human care.

References

1 The Society for Pastoral Theology.(2009). Available at: http://www.societyforpastoraltheology.com/ (accessed 14 November 2011).
2 Fabella, V., Sugirtharajah, R.S. (eds) (2000). *Dictionary of Third World Theologies*. Maryknoll: Orbis.
3 Puchalski, C.M., Ferrell, B. (2010). *Making Healthcare Whole: Integrating Spirituality into Patient Care*, p. 25. West Conshohocken: Templeton Press.
4 Lartey, E.Y. (2003). *In Living Color: an Intercultural Approach to Pastoral Care and Counseling*, pp. 140–1. London: Jessica Kingsley Publishers.
5 Ramsay, N.J. (ed.) (2004). *Pastoral Care and Counseling: Redefining the Paradigms*. Nashville: Abingdon.
6 Lartey, E.Y. (2006). *Pastoral Theology in an Intercultural World.* Cleveland: Pilgrim Press.
7 Osmer, R.R. (2008). *Practical Theology: an Introduction*, p. 4. Grand Rapids: William B. Eerdmans Publishing Company.
8 Orchard, H. (2000). *Hospital Chaplaincy: Modern, Dependable?* A research report of the Lincoln Theological Institute, University of Sheffield. Sheffield: Sheffield Academic Press.
9 Woodward, J.W. (1998). *A study of the role of the acute healthcare chaplain in England*, p. 268, Unpublished PhD thesis, School of Health and Social Welfare, The Open University, Milton Keynes.
10 Wilson, M. (1975). *Health is for People*. London: Darton, Longman and Todd.
11 Evans, A.R. (1999). *Redeeming Marketplace Medicine: a Theology of Healthcare*, p. 132. Cleveland: Pilgrim Press.
12 Willows, D., Swinton, J. (eds) (2000). *Spiritual Dimensions of Pastoral Care: Practical Theology in a Multidisciplinary Context.* London: Jessica Kingsley Publishers.

CHAPTER 42

Next steps for spiritual assessment in healthcare

George Fitchett

Introduction

The past 25 years have seen remarkable developments in the relationship between religion, spirituality, and health. There is a growing body of research investigating the relationship between religion and health[1] and there is growing acceptance of the role of religion and spirituality in health, especially in palliative care.[2,3] During this period numerous models for spiritual assessment have also been developed. In light of this, I believe we no longer need to develop new models for spiritual assessment. Rather, we need to focus attention on a critical review of the existing models and the dissemination of best practices in spiritual assessment. The chapter has three sections: it begins with a review of some existing models for spiritual assessment, then describes the research about spiritual assessment and concludes with a description of issues that will need to be considered in a critical review of models for spiritual assessment. Readers should be aware that the perspective I bring to this chapter is that of a liberal Quaker chaplain and chaplain-educator who has worked in a large, urban, academic medical centre in the USA for over 30 years.

Some models for spiritual assessment

There is a lot of diversity in the things that people call spiritual assessment. In an effort to make sense of all the existing models for spiritual assessment, my colleagues and I described three levels of inquiry about spiritual life: spiritual screening, spiritual history-taking, and spiritual assessment [4; see Table 42.1).

Spiritual screening

Like screening in other disciplines, spiritual screening is part of a two-tier approach to assessment.[12,13] It is designed to provide initial information about whether a patient is experiencing spiritual distress or a possible spiritual crisis and whether referral for a more in-depth spiritual assessment is indicated. A growing body of evidence describing the harmful effects of spiritual struggle, pain or distress points to the importance of being able to identify and refer patients who may be experiencing such pain.[14–16] Good models of spiritual screening employ a few, simple questions that can be asked by any health professional. Figure 42.1 describes one approach to spiritual screening.[5] This protocol was tested in a sample of 173 medical rehabilitation patients in which 12 (7%) were identified as possibly being in the midst of spiritual struggle.[5] The chaplain's spiritual assessment confirmed spiritual struggle in 11 (92%) of these patients.

Other approaches to screening for acute spiritual distress include the distress thermometer[17] and the nursing diagnosis of spiritual distress.[18] Steinhauser and colleagues[19] have reported evidence for the validity of the question, 'Are you at peace?' Chaplains have also developed other screening models.[20–22]

Spiritual history-taking

Spiritual history-taking is the process of interviewing a patient, asking them about their spiritual life, in order to develop a better understanding of their spiritual needs and resources. Compared to screening, spiritual history-taking employs a broader set of questions to capture salient information about spiritual needs and resources. These spiritual history questions are usually asked in the context of a comprehensive examination by a clinician such as a physician who is primarily responsible for providing direct care and referrals to specialists as indicated. The information obtained from the spiritual history permits the clinician to understand how spiritual concerns could either complement or complicate the patient's overall care. Box 42.1 shows the FICA model, a popular model for spiritual history-taking.[7] Other models for spiritual history-taking have been published.[8,23–25]

Spiritual assessment

I reserve the term spiritual assessment to refer to an in-depth, on-going process of evaluating the spiritual needs and resources of persons to whom we provide care. In this view, models for spiritual assessment do not consist of a set of interview questions. They are interpretive frameworks that are applied based on listening to the patient's story as it unfolds in the clinical relationship. An early and influential model for spiritual assessment was developed by the psychologist Paul Pruyser.[9] In it, he identified seven aspects of a person's religious life, including awareness of the holy, beliefs about providence, and connections with others or their absence. Pruyser did not intend to propose a definitive model for spiritual assessment, although the strengths of his work and the absence of other resources led others to develop models based on his work [26–28].

Another model for spiritual assessment is the 7 × 7 model, which my colleagues and I developed.[10] As can be seen in Table 42.2,

Table 42.1 Three levels of inquiry about spirituality and religion

Level of Inquiry	Context	Length	Mode	Examples
Spiritual screening	Initial contact	Very brief	Questions	Fitchett and Risk (5)
Spiritual history-taking	Initial contact and periodic reassessment	Brief	Questions	Stoll (6) FICA (7) HOPE (8)
Spiritual assessment	Initial contact and on-going reassessment	Extensive	Conceptual framework for interpretation	Pruyser (9) 7x7 (10) Brun (11)

the 7 × 7 model explicitly places spiritual assessment in the context of a holistic assessment. The model employs a multidimensional view of spirituality including spiritual beliefs, behaviour, emotions, relationships, and practices. My colleagues and I have published five case examples of spiritual assessment based on the 7 × 7 model.[4,10,29] Chaplain Arthur Lucas[30] described a model for spiritual assessment called the Discipline for Pastoral Care Giving. It focuses on the patient's concept of the holy, meaning, hope, and community. It places the work of spiritual assessment in the context of the clinical process and its cycle of assessment, care plan, intervention, and re-assessment. A case example of chaplain's care with a cancer patient that was informed by this model has been published.[31]

Research about spiritual assessment

There is limited research about spiritual assessment. This research includes validation studies of the nursing diagnosis spiritual distress. In one such study, 59 critical care nurses felt most of the defining characteristics for this diagnosis were major indicators of spiritual distress.[32] They also demonstrated an ability to distinguish the defining characteristics of spiritual distress from a diagnosis of ineffective individual coping. A similar study, using 26 board certified paediatric chaplains as raters, found the majority of the defining characteristics of the diagnosis of spiritual distress were not valid for use with children, especially those under age 13 years.[33] Other studies have found that many nurses report

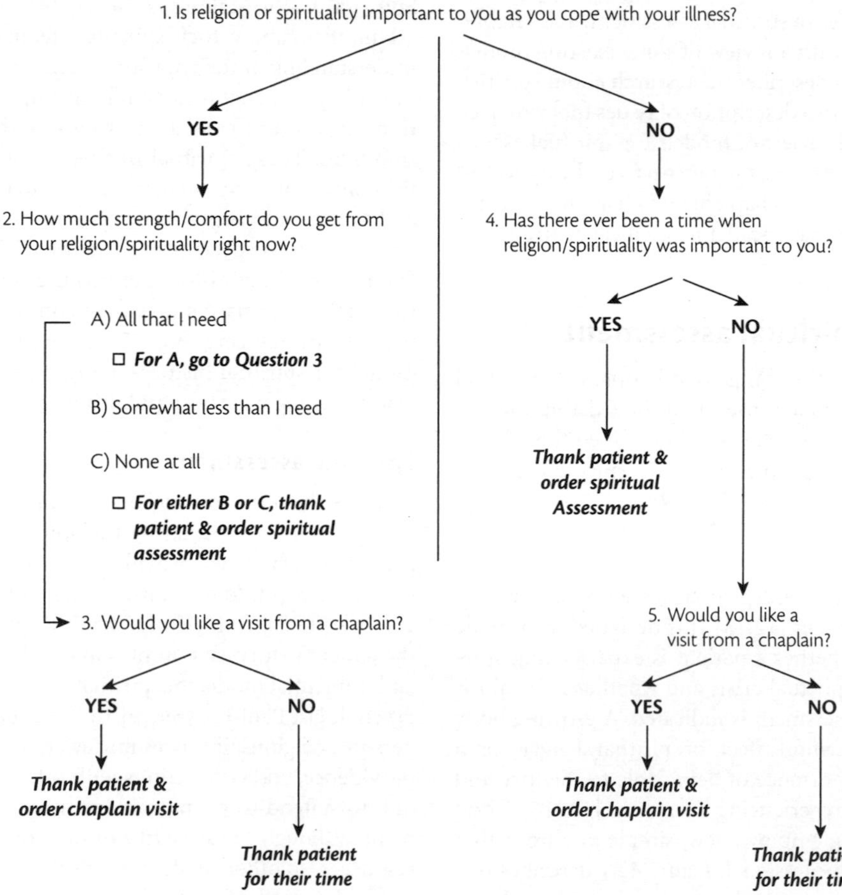

Figure 42.1 Religious Struggle Screening Protocol. Taken from [5].

Box 42.1 FICA Model for Religious/Spiritual History-taking

F—faith, belief, meaning

- What is your faith or belief?
- Do you consider yourself spiritual or religious?
- What things do you believe in give meaning to your life?

I—importance and influence

- Is it important in your life?
- What influences does it have on how you take care of yourself?
- How have your beliefs influenced your behaviour during this illness?
- What role do your beliefs play in regaining your health?

C—community

- Are you part of a spiritual or religious community?
- Is this of support to you and how?
- Is there a person or group of people you really love or who are really important to you?

A—address/action in care

How would you like me, your healthcare provider, to address these issues in your healthcare?

Taken from [7]. Reprinted with permission from Puchalski and Romer (2000). Copyright Christina M. Puchalski, MD, 1996.

problems in conducting spiritual assessments, including lack of time and inadequate training.[34] Several studies have found that educational programmes increase nursing students' awareness of the importance of spirituality and may increase their competence in providing spiritual assessment and spiritual care.[35]

Research nurses administered the FICA spiritual history-taking tool to 67 oncology clinic patients.[36] The investigators reported key themes in the patients' responses to the FICA questions, but did not evaluate the clinical impact of its use. Like nurses, physicians have described lack of training and time as barriers to conducting spiritual assessment. One study found that 38% of oncologists and 48% of oncology nurses felt they were primarily responsible for addressing their patients' spiritual distress, but significant majorities (97 and 90%, respectively) felt that chaplains were the ideal person for this work.[37] When they rated the most important three issues in a vignette of a patient with a poor prognosis very few of these doctors (12%) or nurses (9%) included spiritual distress.

Table 42.2 The 7 × 7 model for spiritual assessment

Holistic assessment	Spiritual assessment
Medical dimension	Belief and meaning
Psychological dimension	Vocation and obligations
Family systems dimension	Experience and emotions
Psychosocial dimension	Doubt (courage) and growth
Ethnic, racial, or cultural dimension	Ritual and practice
Social issues dimension	Community
Spiritual dimension	Authority and guidance

Taken from [10]. Used by permission from Academic Renewal Press, 5450 N. Dixie Highway, Lima, Ohio, 45807.

Courses about spirituality are now common in US medical schools. In one course, first-year students received training on taking a spiritual history using the HOPE model.[38] Faculty raters reported that 65% of these students were able to recognize spiritual issues in an interview with a standardized patient and 57% of those students asked at least one further question about those issues. Another study trained four haematologists/oncologists to conduct a brief inquiry about their patient's spiritual concerns.[39] The physicians reported they were comfortable making the inquiry in 85% of the cases. The majority of the patients who received the inquiry (76%) felt it was useful and three weeks later they reported a better quality of life and more sense of interpersonal caring from their physicians than those who had received usual care.

The research about spiritual assessment among chaplains gives a mixed picture. Gleason reported levels of agreement between 66 and 89%, when he asked 21 clinical pastoral education students to use his 'Four Worlds' model to assess patients described in their verbatim reports.[40] A survey of 159 board certified US chaplains found that 79% had received training in spiritual assessment and they often noted their spiritual assessment in patient's charts.[41] Another study found Canadian chaplains had positive and negative views about spiritual assessment.[42] Most did not use any published models for spiritual assessment, but about one in three had developed their own model or used one developed in their chaplaincy department. A Canadian palliative care chaplain reported that consistent use of the HOPE model for spiritual history-taking[8] increased staff colleagues' understanding and utilization of chaplaincy services.[43] According to a large survey of chaplains in England and Wales, 88% of hospices and 71% of hospitals had spiritual assessment protocols that recorded patients' religious preferences, requests for religious care (e.g. visit from clergy, sacraments), and religion-based preferences for specific services [e.g. diet; 44]. In 90% of the hospices and hospitals nurses conducted these interviews.

Next steps

In the past 25 years, many models, especially models for spiritual history-taking and spiritual assessment, have been published. (The George Washington Institute for Spirituality and Health (GWish) website, and especially its Spirituality and Health Online Education and Resource Center (SOERCE), is a good resource. www.gwumc.edu/gwish/soerce.) However, the current situation, where anyone can develop their own model for spiritual assessment,[42,45,46] has led to confusing variations in practice. In turn, this has inhibited the research needed to demonstrate the value of good spiritual assessment and spiritual care. In light of this, I would argue that the field does not need any new models at this time. Rather, what is needed is a critical review of the existing models. Some prior work has described criteria for evaluating models for spiritual assessment. For example, my colleagues and I developed criteria for evaluating models for spiritual assessment and used these criteria to examine a number of models.[10,47] These criteria included how spirituality was conceptualized in the model and whether the model included explicit attention to issues of norms and authority. Practical issues were also described such as amount of training required to understand and use the model, and the contexts in which the model would be useful. Others have also addressed the issue of criteria for evaluating and selecting the best approach for spiritual assessment for specific contexts.[46] Several critical reviews and overviews have also been published.[34,48,49]

Evaluations of spiritual assessment and spiritual care programs must reference norms or standards for these activities. An example of such a standard was developed by the Trent Hospice Audit Group in the UK. 'The spiritual needs of patients and caregivers are integrated into the assessment and delivery of palliative care.'[12] The Group also suggested structure, process, and outcome criteria that can be used to audit whether healthcare teams are meeting this standard. An example of one of the process criteria is that the multidisciplinary team 'uses consistent assessment processes to inform the planning of spiritual care interventions.'[12, p. 211]

The critical review I am proposing should examine the strengths and weaknesses of existing models, and identify gaps in the published work and areas for future research. Most importantly, this critical review should lead to identification of best practices in spiritual assessment. Based on the existing literature I see five issues that need to be addressed in this critical review.

Defining spirituality

Clear definitions of spirituality and religion form an essential basis for developing and evaluating models for spiritual assessment.[13,50] A lot is at stake in the debate about definitions since some definitions describe spirituality as beneficial and religion as restrictive or harmful.[51,52] Many authors argue that spirituality is a universal feature of human life.[13,53] Some clinicians and investigators see existential issues of meaning as the most important spiritual issues faced by patients with serious illness[54] and recommend meaning-focused treatment offered by mental health professionals.[55] Still others argue against the idea of a universal spirituality and focus on the important role of the distinct beliefs and teachings of specific religious groups.[56,57] Some who hold this view believe that spiritual assessment and spiritual care can only be offered by religious authorities who share the patient's religious traditions.[49]

Normative issues in spiritual assessment

It is difficult to engage in spiritual assessment without eventually identifying some of the patient's spiritual or religious beliefs or behaviours as unhelpful, if not limited or immature. Many health professionals feel unqualified to make judgments about such a complex and personal aspect of a patient's life. Some chaplains are also uncomfortable with diagnostic labels and prefer models of spiritual assessment with descriptive summaries.[58] Hodge[59] suggests models for spiritual assessment that focus on clients' strengths and resources.

However, there are models that are explicit about spiritual diagnoses. For example, the model developed by Denton, a pastoral counsellor, describes pathological struggles with guilt, betrayal, and defilement.[60] The model developed by Brun,[11] also a pastoral counsellor, describes ten issues in spiritual life (e.g. capacity for reverence, capacity for guilt/repentance/forgiveness, capacity to face death), each with healthy and pathological dimensions. In other models the focus is on spiritual distress,[18,61] spiritual pain,[62,63] or spiritual injury.[64] Several models conceptualize a continuum from spiritual suffering to spiritual wellness.[65–68]

A related issue is describing mature or immature features of a patient's spirituality. The language of 'growing in faith' is familiar, even central, in many religious traditions. Explicit models of faith development add a new perspective to this idea of growing in faith. The well-known model of James Fowler[69] describes stages of faith development that include increasing complexity in the treatment of symbols and moral decision-making. Several early models for understanding differences in patients' religious worldviews employed developmental perspectives that focused on patient's use of symbols.[40,70,71] Ivy described a model for spiritual assessment that focused on faith development.[72]

A few authors have addressed the issue of the authority that permits professionals to create normative models of spiritual life and to make assessments or diagnoses of whether another person's life conforms to those models.[9,10,49,73] Paul Pruyser believed the professionals' job was to be a consultant to the patient's own spiritual self-assessment.[9] A critical review of models for spiritual assessment should address practitioners' reluctance to evaluate another person's spiritual wellbeing or distress.

The quantification of spiritual assessment

While there are many published measures of religion and spirituality for use in research,[74,75] most models for spiritual assessment are descriptive or narrative. The psychologist Kenneth Pargament probably speaks for many clinicians when he writes that inviting clients to tell a story is the best way to learn about their spirituality and that fixed questions are 'more likely to interfere with the unfolding of the client's tale than to promote it' [76, p. 224]. Others would share Pargament's view.[58,59] One Canadian chaplain who participated in a survey about spiritual assessment commented, 'My image of sitting in front of somebody with a piece of paper and writing answers down ... is not a positive image.'[42]

A few models of spiritual assessment include quantification of the patient's spiritual needs and resources. An early example is the work of the US physician Elisabeth McSherry and her colleagues.[77] Building on McSherry's work, Gary Berg, a chaplain in the US Veterans Affairs health system developed the Computer Assessment Profile, which included a Spiritual Injury Scale.[64,78] With their numerical descriptions of a patient's spiritual needs and resources, the models developed by McSherry and Berg bring spiritual assessment closer to the quantitative language that is familiar to healthcare professionals. Despite the difficulty associated with developing quantitative descriptions of patient's spiritual needs and resources, such models make it possible to document on a routine basis, not just in limited investigations, whether spiritual care creates measurable improvement in spiritual needs or resources or other outcomes such as emotional wellbeing or quality of life.

The contexts for spiritual assessment

The great diversity in patients, for example, their age, illness, and religious background, makes spiritual assessment a challenge. In addition to models for general use that have been previously described, there are models for specific contexts including models for adults with psychiatric conditions[28,79] and for persons with intellectual disabilities.[80] Models for use in hospice and palliative care are available[2,12,81] as are models for spiritual assessment with older adults.[82,83] Several authors have described the spiritual needs of children,[84,85] and one model for screening for spiritual distress in children and adolescents has been published.[86] Faith-specific models have been proposed for Jewish patients.[87,88] Models have been developed by pastoral counsellors[11,60] and psychotherapists[76,89,90] to facilitate addressing the spiritual issues in their client's lives.

In the USA, the agency that sets standards for healthcare organizations, the Joint Commission, has a very modest requirement regarding spiritual assessment.[91] This leaves considerable room for tailoring the best approach to spiritual assessment for each context.[92] A critical review of the existing models for spiritual assessment will need to find the best mix of models for general and context-specific practice.

Spiritual assessment and professional authority

Many of those who write about spiritual assessment have approached the topic from within their professional discipline. For example, physicians have developed models for spiritual history-taking with acronyms such as HOPE,[8] SPIRIT,[25] and FICA.[7] Nurses write about the nursing process and the use of nursing diagnoses such as spiritual distress.[13] Social workers and chaplains have developed models for their colleagues.[58,65,93,94] This intradisciplinary focus should not be surprising since diagnostic models are 'touchstones of professional identity.'[9] However, it is unfortunate that many writers about the topic appear to have limited familiarity with work by authors from other disciplines. There has been a lack of disciplinary cross-fertilization in much writing about spiritual assessment.

A final issue that will need to be considered in a critical review of the literature on spiritual assessment is the role of different professions in spiritual assessment. Some nurses[13,63] and physicians[23,95] describe spiritual assessment as part of their professional responsibility. Chaplains see spiritual assessment as 'a fundamental process of chaplaincy practice.'[96] Others suggest that different members of the healthcare team should have different levels of involvement in spiritual assessment depending on their role in direct patient/family care and training in spiritual care. Using this perspective some professionals such as nurses and doctors may be seen as spiritual care generalists who can conduct spiritual screening and spiritual history-taking, while chaplains are seen as spiritual care specialists with the expertise for in-depth spiritual assessment.[2,12,97,98]

Conclusion

The past several decades have seen a growing acceptance of spirituality as a dimension of persons that is influenced by and influences their health. There is also growing recognition of the importance of spiritual care that focuses clinical attention on this dimension especially for patients with serious and life-limiting illness, or those with spiritual distress. The purpose of spiritual assessment is to help guide effective spiritual care. Clinicians can select from many models for spiritual assessment that have been published. A critical review of the existing models and further research about spiritual assessment are needed to help us identify and disseminate best practices.

Acknowledgments

I am grateful for the helpful comments of Mary Altenbaumer and Paul Derrickson on an earlier draft of this chapter.

References

1 Koenig, H.G., McCullough, M.E., Larson, D.B. (2001). *Handbook of Religion and Health*. Oxford: Oxford University Press.

2 Puchalski, C., Ferrell, B., Virani, R., Otis-Green, S., Baird, P., Bull, J., *et al.* (2009). Improving the quality of spiritual care as a dimension of palliative care: the report of the Consensus Conference. *J Palliat Med* **12**(10): 885–904.

3 Sulmasy, D.P. (2002). A biopsychosocial-spiritual model for the care of patients at the end of life. *Gerontologist* **42**(Special issue 3): 24–33.

4 Massey, K., Fitchett, G., Roberts, P.A. (2004). Assessment and diagnosis in spiritual care. In: K.L. Mauk, N.K. Schmidt (eds) *Spiritual Care in Nursing Practice*, pp. 209–42. Philadelphia: Lippincott, Williams and Wilkins.

5 Fitchett, G., Risk, J. (2009). Screening for spiritual struggle. *J Past Care Counsel* **63**: 1,2. [Available online.]

6 Stoll, R.I. (1979). Guidelines for spiritual assessment. *Am J Nurs* **79:** 1574–7.

7 Puchalski, C., Romer, A.L. (2000). Taking a spiritual history allows clinicians to understand patients more fully. *J Palliat Med* **3**(1): 129–37.

8 Anandarajah, G., Hight, E. (2001). Spirituality and medical practice: using the HOPE questions as a practical tool for spiritual assessment. *Am Fam Physic* **63**(1): 81–9.

9 Pruyser, P.W. (1976). *The Minister as Diagnostician*. Philadelphia: Westminster Press.

10 Fitchett, G. (2002). *Assessing Spiritual Needs: a Guide for Caregivers*. Lima: Academic Renewal Press. (This is a reprint of the 1993 volume published by Augsburg Fortress, Minneapolis.)

11 Brun, W.L. (2005). A proposed diagnostic schema for religious/spiritual concerns. *J Past Care Counsel* **59**(5 Suppl): 425–40.

12 Hunt, J., Cobb, M., Keeley, V.L., Ahmedzai, S.H. (2003).The quality of spiritual care—developing a standard. *Int J Palliat Nurs* **9**(5): 208–15.

13 Taylor, E.J. (2002). *Spiritual Care: Nursing Theory, Research, and Practice*. Upper Saddle River, New Jersey.

14 Pargament, K.I .(1997). *The Psychology of Religion and Coping*. New York: Guilford Press.

15 Pargament, K.I., Koenig, H.G., Tarakeshwar, N., Hahn, J. (2004). Religious coping methods as predictors of psychological, physical and spiritual outcomes among medically ill elderly patients: a two-year longitudinal study. *J Hlth Psychol* **9**(6): 713–30.

16 Fitchett, G., Murphy, P.E., Kim, J., Gibbons, J.L., Cameron, J.R., Davis, J.A. (2004). Religious struggle: prevalence, correlates and mental health risks in diabetic, congestive heart failure, and oncology patients. *Int J Psychiat Med* **34**(2): 179–96.

17 National Comprehensive Cancer Network. Distress Management V.1.2008. Available at: http://www.nccn.org (accessed 30 December 2010).

18 NANDA International. (2007). *NANDA-I Nursing Diagnoses: definitions and classification*, 2007–2008. Philadelphia: NANDA International.

19 Steinhauser, K.E., Voils, C.I., Clipp, E.C., Bosworth, H.B., Christakis, N.A., Tulsky, J.A. (2006). 'Are you at peace?': one item to probe spiritual concerns at the end of life. *Arch Intern Med* **166**(1): 101–5.

20 Derrickson, P.E (1994–1995). Screening patients for pastoral care: a preliminary report. *Caregiver J* **11**(2): 14–18.

21 Hodges, S. (1999). Spiritual screening: the starting place for intentional pastoral care. *Chaplaincy Today* **15**(1): 30–40.

22 Wakefield, J.L., Cox, D., Forrest, J.S. (2001). Seeds of change: the development of a spiritual assessment model. *Chaplaincy Today* **15**(1): 41–50.

23 Koenig, H.G (2007). *Spirituality in Patient Care: Why, How, When, and What*, rev 2nd edn. West Conshohocken: Templeton Foundation Press.

24 Kuhn, C.C. (1988). A spiritual inventory of the medically ill patient. *Psychiatr Med* **6**(2): 87–100.

25 Maugans, T.A. (1996). The spiritual history. *Arch Fam Med* **5**(1): 11–16.

26 Malony, H.N. (1988). The clinical assessment of optimal religious functioning. *Rev Religion Res* **30**(1): 3–17.

27 Stoddard, G., Burns-Haney, J. (1990). Developing an integrated approach to spiritual assessment: one department's experience. *Caregiver J* **7**(1): 63–86.

28 Weiss, F.S. (1991). Pastoral care planning: a process-oriented approach for mental health ministry. *J Past Care* **45**(3): 268–78.

29 Fitchett, G. (1995). Linda Krauss and the lap of God: a spiritual assessment case study. *2nd Opin* **20**(4): 41–9.

30 Lucas AM (2001). Introduction to the discipline for pastoral care giving. In: L. VandeCreek, A.M. Lucas (eds) *The Discipline for Pastoral Care Giving*, pp. 1–33. Binghamton: Haworth Pastoral Press.

31 Berger, J.A. (2001). A case study: Linda. In: L. VandeCreek, A.M. Lucas (eds) *The Discipline for Pastoral Care Giving*, pp. 35–43. Binghamton: Haworth Pastoral Press.

32 Twibell RS, Wieseke AW, Marine M, Schoger J (1996). Spiritual and coping needs of critically ill patients: validation of nursing diagnoses. *Dimens Crit Care Nurs* **15**(5): 245–53.

33 Pehler, S. (1997). Children's spiritual response: validation of the nursing diagnosis spiritual distress. *Nurs Diag* **8**(2): 55–66.

34 Taylor, E.J. (2006). Spiritual assessment. In: B.R. Ferrell, N. Coyle (eds) *Textbook of Palliative Nursing*, pp. 581–94. Oxford: Oxford University Press.

35 van Leeuwen, R., Tiesinga, L.J., Middel, B., Post, D., Jochemsen, H. (2008). The effectiveness of an educational programme for nursing students on developing competence in the provision of spiritual care. *J Clin Nurs* **17**(20): 2768–81.

36 Borneman, T., Ferrell, B., Puchalski, C.M. (2010). Evaluation of the FICA tool for spiritual assessment. *J Pain Sympt Manag* **40**(2): 163–73.

37 Kristeller, J.L., Zumbrun, C.S., Schilling, R.F. (1999). 'I would if I could': how oncologists and oncology nurses address spiritual distress in cancer patients. *Psycho-oncol* **8**(5): 451–8.

38 King, D.E., Blue, A., Mallin, R., Thiedke, C. (2004). Implementation and assessment of a spiritual history taking curriculum in the first year of medical school. *Teach Learn Med* **16**(1): 64–8.

39 Kristeller, J.L., Rhodes, M., Cripe, L.D., Sheets,V. (2005). Oncologist Assisted Spiritual Intervention Study (OASIS): patient acceptability and initial evidence of effects. *Int J Psychiat Med* **35**(4): 329–47.

40 Gleason, J.J. (1999). The four worlds of spiritual assessment and care. *J Religion Hlth* **38**(4): 305–17.

41 Spidell, S. (2005). A survey of beliefs and practices in professional chaplaincy. *Chaplaincy Today* **21**(1): 23–9.

42 O'Connor, T.S., O'Neill, K., Van Staalduinen, G., Meakes, E., Penner, C., Davis, K. (2005). Not well known, used little and needed: Canadian chaplains' experiences of published spiritual assessment tools. *J Past Care Counsel* **59**(1–2): 97–107.

43 Pierce, B. (2004). The introduction and evaluation of a spiritual assessment tool in a palliative care unit. *Scot J Hlthcare Chaplaincy* **7**(2): 39–43.

44 Wright, M.C. (2001). Chaplaincy in hospice and hospital: findings from a survey in England and Wales. *Palliat Med* **15**(3): 229–42.

45 Derrickson, P., Van Hise, A. (2009).Curriculum for a Spiritual Pathway Project: integrating research methodology into pastoral care training. *J Hlthcare Chaplain* **16**(1–2): 3–12.

46 Timmins, F., Kelly, J. (2008). Spiritual assessment in intensive and cardiac care nursing. *Nurs Crit Care* **13**(3): 124–31.

47 Fitchett, G. (1993). *Spiritual Assessment in Pastoral Care*. Decatur: Journal of Pastoral Care Publications.

48 Richards, P.S.(2010). *Discerning Patient Needs: Spiritual Assessment Perspectives for Healthcare Chaplains*. Available at: http://www.healthcarechaplaincy.org/userimages/pb-discerning-patient-needs-spiritual-assessment.pdf (accessed 26 November 2010).

49 VandeCreek, L. (2005). Spiritual assessment: six questions and an annotated bibliography of published interview and questionnaire formats. *Chaplaincy Today* **21**(1): 11–22.

50 Puchalski C, Ferrell B (2010). *Making Healthcare Whole: Integrating Spirituality in Patient Care*. West Conshohocken: Templeton Press.

51 Hill, P.C., Pargament, K.I., Hood, R.W., et al (2000). Conceptualizing religion and spirituality: points of commonality, points of departure. *Journal for the Theory of Social Behavior* **30**(1): 51–77.

52 Zinnbauer BJ, Pargament KI, Scott AB (1999). The emerging meanings of religiousness and spirituality: problems and prospects. *J Pers* **67**: 889–919.

53 Swinton, J., Narayanasamy, A. (2002). Response to: 'A critical view of spirituality and spiritual assessment' by P Draper and W. McSherry. *J Adv Nurs* **40**(2): 158–60.

54 Salsman, J.M., Yost, K.J., West, D.W., Cella, D. (2011). Spiritual well-being and health-related quality of life in colorectal cancer: a multi-site examination of the role of personal meaning. *Support Care Cancer* **19**(6): 757–64.

55 Breitbart, W. (2002). Spirituality and meaning in supportive care: spirituality- and meaning-centered group psychotherapy interventions in advanced cancer. *Support Care Cancer* **10**(4): 272–80.

56 Hall, D.E., Koenig, K.G., Meador, K.G. (2004). Conceptualizing 'Religion:' how language shapes and constrains knowledge in the study of religion and health. *Perspect Biol Med* **47**: 386–401.

57 Hall, D.E., Meador, K.G., Koenig, H.G. (2008). Measuring religiousness in health research: review and critique. *J Relig Hlth* **47**: 134–63.

58 Lewis, J.M. (2002). Pastoral assessment in hospital ministry: a conversational approach. *Chaplaincy Today* **18**(2): 5–13.

59 Hodge, D.R. (2001). Spiritual assessment: a review of major qualitative methods and a new framework for assessing spirituality. *Social Work* **46**(3): 203–14.

60 Denton, D. (2008). *Naming the Pain and Guiding the Care: the Central Tasks of Diagnosis*. Lanham: University Press of America Inc.

61 Stoddard, G.A. (1993). Chaplaincy by referral: an effective model for evaluating staffing needs. *Caregiver J* **10**(1): 37–52.

62 Millspaugh, C.D. (2005). Assessment and response to spiritual pain: part I. *J Palliat Med* **8**(5): 919–23.

63 O'Brien, M.E. (1999). *Spirituality in Nursing: Standing on Holy Ground*. Sudbury: Jones and Bartlett Publishers.

64 Berg, G.E. (1999). A statement on clinical assessment for pastoral care. *Chaplaincy Today*. **14**(2): 42–50.

65 Bartel, M. (2004). What is spiritual? What is spiritual suffering? *J Past Care Counsel* **58**(3): 187–201.

66 Kliewer, S.P., Saultz, J. (2006). *Healthcare and Spirituality*. Oxford: Radcliffe Publishing.

67 Nash, R. (1990). Life's major spiritual issues. *Caregiver J* **7**(1): 3–42.

68 Sanders, R. (2006). A comprehensive approach to pastoral care. *Chaplaincy Today* **22**(1): 3–12.

69 Fowler, J.W. (1981). *Stages of Faith: the Psychology of Human Development and the Quest for Meaning*. San Francisco: Harper & Row, Publishers.

70 Baldridge, W.E., Gleason, J.J. (1978). A theological framework for pastoral care. *J Past Care* **32**(4): 232–8.

71 Hemenway, J.E (1984). Four faith frameworks. *J Past Care* **38**(4): 317–23.

72 Ivy, S.S. (1987). A faith development/self-development model for pastoral assessment. *J Past Care* **41**(4): 329–40.

73 Browning, D.S. (1996). *The Moral Context of Pastoral Care*. Philadelphia: Westminster Press.

74 Hill, P.C., Hood, R.W .Jr. (eds) (1999). *Measures of Religiosity*. Birmingham: Religious Education Press.

75 Hill, P.C., Pargament, K.I. (2003). Advances in the conceptualization and measurement of religion and spirituality: implications for physical and mental health research. *Am Psychol* **58**(1): 64–74.

76 Pargament, K.I. (2007). *Spirituality Integrated Psychotherapy: Understanding and Addressing the Sacred*. New York: Guilford Press.

77 Salisbury, S., Ciulla, M., McSherry, E. (1989). Clinical management reporting and objective diagnostic instruments for spiritual assessment in spinal cord injury patients. *J Hlthcare Chaplaincy* **2**(2): 35–64.

78 Berg, G.E. (1994). The use of the computer as a tool for assessment and research in pastoral care. *J Hlthcare Chaplaincy* **6**(1): 11–25.

79 Eimer, K. (1989). The assessment and treatment of the religiously concerned psychiatric patient. *J Past Care* **43**(3): 231–41.

80 Gaventa, W.C. (2001). Defining and assessing spirituality and spiritual supports: a rationale for inclusion in theory and practice. In: W.C. Gaventa, D.L. Coulter (eds) *Spirituality and Intellectual Disability*, pp. 29–48. Binghamton: Haworth Press, Inc.

81 Hay, M.W. (1989). Principles in building spiritual assessment tools. *Am J Hospice Care* **6**(5): 25–31.

82 Monod, S.M., Rochat, E, Büla, C.J., Jobin, G., Martin, E., Spencer, B. (2010). The spiritual distress assessment tool: an instrument to assess spiritual distress in hospitalised elderly persons. *BMC Geriatr* **13**(10): 88.

83 Stranahan, S. (2008). A spiritual screening tool for older adults. *J Relig Hlth* **47**(4): 491–503.

84 Barnes, L.L., Plotnikoff, G.A., Fox, K., Pendleton, S. (2000). Spirituality, religion, pediatrics: intersecting worlds of healing. *Pediatrics* **104**(6): 899–908.

85 Mueller, C.R. (2010). Spirituality in children: understanding and developing interventions. *Pediat Nurs* **36**(4): 197–203, 208.

86 Grossoehme, D.H. (2008). Development of a spiritual screening tool for children and adolescents. *J Past Care Counsel* **62**(1–2): 71–85.

87 Shulevitz, S., Springer, M. (1994). Assessment of religious experience—a Jewish approach. *J Past Care* **48**(4): 399–406.

88 Davidowitz-Farkas, Z. (2001). Jewish spiritual assessment. In: D.A. Friedman (ed.) *Jewish Pastoral Care: a Practical Handbook from Traditional and Contemporary Sources*, pp. 104–24. Woodstock: Jewish Lights Publishing.

89 Chirban, J.T. (2001). Assessing religious and spiritual concerns in psychotherapy. In: T.G. Plante, A.C. Sherman (eds) *Faith and Health: Psychological Perspectives*, pp. 265–90. New York: Guilford Press.

90 Richards, P.S., Bergin, A.E. (2005). A *Spiritual Strategy for Counseling and Psychotherapy*, 2nd edn. Washington, DC: American Psychological Association.

91 Joint Commission. (2005). Evaluating your spiritual assessment program. *Source* **3**(2): 6–7. Available at: http://www.professionalchaplains.org/uploadedFiles/pdf/JCAHO-evaluating-your-spiritual-assessment-process.pdf (assessed 30 December 2010).

92 Hodge, D.R (2006). A template for spiritual assessment: a review of the JCAHO requirements and guidelines for implementation. *Soc Work* **51**(4): 317–26.

93 Hodge, D.R. (2003). *Spiritual Assessment: Handbook for Helping Professionals*. Bolsford: North American Association of Christians in Social Work.

94 Larocca-Pitts, M.A. (2008). FACT: taking a spiritual history in a clinical setting. *J Hlthcare Chaplain* **15**(1): 1–12.

95 King, D.E. (2000). *Faith, Spirituality, and Medicine: Toward the Making of the Healing Practitioner*. Binghamton: Haworth Pastoral Press.

96 Standards of Practice Acute Care Work Group. (2009). *Standards of Practice for Professional Chaplains in Acute Care*. Available at: http://www.professionalchaplains.org/index.aspx?id = 1210 (accessed 30 December 2010).

97 Gordon, T., Mitchell, D. (2004). A competency model for the assessment and delivery of spiritual care. *Palliat Med* **18**(7): 646–51.

98 Handzo, G.F. (2006). Best practices in professional pastoral care. *Sth Med J* **99**(6): 663–4.

SECTION IV

Research

CHAPTER 43

Methodology

David Hufford

Introduction

Definitions

Methodology comprises 'The system of principles, practices and procedures as applied to a specific branch of knowledge.'[1] That is, methodology is both the *methods*—the specific procedures of a field—and the assumptions, rationale and patterns of behaviour that underlie those procedures. Methodology is the framework of a field, and a new field such as spirituality and healthcare (SaH) needs time for methodology to develop and mature. In this chapter I will discuss the field's methodology in terms of definitions, common methods, problems of scope, and unexamined biases that hinder methodological development.

The definition of core terms is a basic aspect of methodology. However, SaH has had great difficulty defining and distinguishing between *spirituality* and *religion*. I will discuss the reasons for this below, in connection with the scope of the field. However, a brief statement is needed to start the discussion of methods. *Spirituality* is often defined as one's personal relationship to the transcendent. Although serviceable in many circumstances, this definition is ambiguous, because *transcendent* is itself ambiguous. Derived from the Latin, *transcendere*, 'climb over or beyond, surmount,' the word is used in different settings to refer to all kinds of 'rising above.' However, in ordinary English usage *spirituality* means that which is not material, having to do with the spirit, such as God (or gods) and the human soul.[2] This covers the relevant meaning of 'the transcendent' without ambiguity. When spirituality refers to something else it is by metaphorical extension to other intangible and invisible things, such as ideas, as in 'team spirit' or the 'spirit of democracy.' Religions are those institutions that that have developed around spirituality. Spirituality is the core aspect of religion, but is also found outside religious institutions.

In clinical practice the spirituality/religion distinction is crucial. No matter how powerful the scientific data showing positive health effects of a religious practice, clinical advice regarding a patient's religion would be ethically out of bounds. However, knowledge on the subject can be useful for medical education and institutional policy decisions; e.g. how best to deal with clinical obstacles arising from beliefs and practices of Jehovah's Witnesses. In areas of spirituality less bounded by specific religious doctrine, research may develop interventions based on the efficacy of particular practices, such as meditation. However, this research will not be valid or useful if it fails to understand the spirituality-religion distinction as that distinction operates in the society within which medicine finds itself.

The word research came into English from French in the late sixteenth century. Composed of the Old French *cerchier*, 'to search,' and the Latin *re-* meaning 'again,' the term refers to thorough investigation. Comparison is at the heart of systematic research. Meta-analyses compare reviewed publications in order to evaluate them and combine their implications. The concept of scientific control inherently involves comparison; experiments manipulate a variable in one set of observations and compare the results to those in a control set. Case series compare subjects with a known condition to 'control subjects.' Comparisons in research may be across groups of subjects or among subjects over time. Discovering variation and understanding its meaning, the central goal of research, requires comparison. This is as true in historical research or the study of literature as it is in medical research. One way of understanding the types of research design discussed below is as different ways of constructing systematic comparisons.

Constructing a research study

Guiding questions

Most systematic research arises from a guiding question. In SaH such questions may be clinically orientated, as in the question: 'Is spirituality good for people's health and wellbeing?' However, not all SaH questions must be clinical to be relevant to healthcare. For example, 'What is the prevalence of various religious groups, and how are they distributed in the United States?' is a question that would be very useful to administrators in developing appropriate religious accommodations and for medical educators in creating curriculum. Guiding questions are likely to be refined and narrowed as the researcher's thinking progresses.

Case study 1

In 2010 Fowler and Rountree published a study of 'the meaning and role of spirituality for women survivors of intimate partner abuse'.[3] This qualitative study used focus groups to explore the subject. There was no *a priori* hypothesis, rather the study was guided by the question of what spirituality means in the lives of subjects who have survived such trauma. The study concluded that 'spirituality provides strength, influences outcomes and assists in the regulation of behavioural responses in a positive manner in terms of participants' traumatic IPA victimization.' Practice implications are discussed in this Chapter, and it may also be used to develop hypotheses for further research.

Sampling and issues of measurement

Several methodological issues are important regardless of the research design selected. Validity is the most basic. There are many forms of validity with slightly different definitions. Validity is the soundness or accuracy of a study and its conclusions, e.g. a valid quantitative instrument measures what it is intended to measure. Lack of clarity is one obstacle to validity—if a survey question is hard to understand answers may not refer to the intended topic. Another common validity problem specific to SaH is the conflation of positive emotions such as hopefulness or optimism with spirituality.[4–6] If an instrument designed to 'measure' spirituality includes questions about these emotions, then positive 'spirituality' scores cannot validly show that they result from spirituality. Confounds are another validity problem. A confound is a variable that offers an alternative explanation for variation under study. For example, if a study of the association between church attendance and health does not control for the fact that church attendance requires a certain level of health and mobility to begin with (the confound), then for that study to conclude that something intrinsic to church produces health would not be valid. This has been a common criticism of SaH findings, and this confound is now usually taken into account. The subtypes of validity (face validity, convergent and discriminant, criterion validity, etc.) are various tests of an instrument's validity.

Good qualitative research must also be valid; its conclusions must follow logically from the information gathered. Errors such as conflation and confounds are pitfalls for qualitative research too. However, just as qualitative research addresses issues difficult to objectify numerically, the evaluation of qualitative studies is more difficult to reduce to a standard method. Nonetheless, all of the validity issues in quantitative research may be productively considered in planning and assessing qualitative research. The core issue is to watch for uncontrolled biases, usually unintended, that may account for some of what is reported.

Random variation might also account for some of what is found in a study. Reliability is the extent to which a research method is free from random error. The simplest assessment of reliability is repeating the procedure to see if the results are similar (test re-test reliability). This is best done during the pilot phase of a study. In qualitative research, reliability is harder to assess, but comparison of the results of similar studies approximates what is done in re-testing. For instance, if one qualitative study of Jehovah's Witnesses found intransigent resistance to blood transfusions for critically ill children and another found some willingness to accommodate, the inconsistency suggests a lack of reliability and calls for consideration of possible biases. In this case the problem may be that the sample in the first study did not include members of the Associated Jehovah's Witnesses for Reform on Blood, and the latter did.[7] This is the kind of variation that randomization is designed to avoid, but that qualitative research must usually take into account in other ways.

The appropriate selection of persons to study (the sample) is fundamental to validity and is a constraint on the generalizability of results. The gold standard is a true random sample of the population of interest, because randomization increases the likelihood that two resulting groups will be similar or that a randomly selected group is representative of the population from which it was selected. The more diverse the population the larger the sample required to achieve similarity. The larger the size of the anticipated effect being studied the smaller the sample required. The sample size required for significant results can be calculated from the effect size, or the necessary effect size can be determined for a given sample size. This statistical procedure is called power analysis, and it indicates the chance of false positive results. In randomized controlled trials randomization is used to sort a sample into experimental and control groups. In survey research randomization is used to select the sample of respondents to be surveyed.

Other forms of subject selection are less powerful, but true randomization can be difficult and expensive. Therefore, other systematic methods of selection are often used, such as consecutive patients entering a clinic. If these are alternately assigned to experimental and control groups the two are likely to be similar. However, simply selecting the most easily available individuals, a 'convenience sample,' introduces uncontrolled variability and reduces a study's validity.

Qualitative research must also select subjects, but qualitative sample selection is usually less formal. Members of focus groups may be selected in a process similar to that for quantitative studies, but such groups are usually too small for random selection to include members of all relevant sub-groups, so selection is likely to be purposive. When an anthropologist decides to do an ethnographic study of a Charismatic healing group all of the group's members become the study's potential sample. Selection of particular interview subjects is usually purposive, such as focusing on those who claim a healing or who exhibit ecstatic behaviour, such as being 'slain in the spirit,' depending on the investigator's guiding question. This selection process bears on the validity of qualitative research as much as in quantitative studies, and the problems of unintended bias require careful attention.

Hypotheses

Research showing causal connections between SaH variables is the most clinically useful, because it directly guides the development of effective interventions. Such research requires hypotheses stated in advance. Much SaH research has been conducted on the basis of guiding questions alone. For early exploratory work this can be useful, but the results cannot be conclusive.

Hypotheses developed after data collection can also be fruitful when the data are not fully explained or when a priori hypotheses appear questionable after data collection. Thoughtfully developed new hypotheses can inform and stimulate future research, and 'should be encouraged as a thinker's prime tool rather than be discouraged'.[8, p. 448]

Case study 2: a priori hypothesis

In 2010, Bonaguidi and colleagues published a study concerning the possible association of religiosity with prolonged survival in liver transplant patients. Their sample was comprised of 179 candidates for liver transplant. They report that 'We tested the hypothesis that religiosity (i.e. seeking God's help, having faith in God, trusting in

God, and trying to perceive God's will in the disease) is associated with improved survival in patients with end-stage liver disease who have undergone orthotopic liver transplantation'.[9, p. 1158] Note that they specify their measure of religiosity. For the hypothesis to be testable and the results to be interpretable it is crucial that a relatively broad concept, such as religiosity be defined in detail. Within the responses the researchers found that a single spiritual factor, which they called the 'searching for God factor,' was independently associated with prolonged survival in these patients. Their clearly stated *a priori* hypothesis, complete with specific measures, provided strong support for their conclusion.

Theory

Research grounded in existing theory and literature has the best chance of yielding interpretable results. In SaH much of the progress in the 1990s consisted of refuting theories that interpreted spirituality and religion (rarely distinguishing the two) in negative, even pathological ways. Sigmund Freud's view of religious thought as neurotic[10] was a major source of this idea, and by the mid-twentieth century it had become a largely unquestioned assumption. Research that undermined this viewpoint, especially the systematic reviews of David Larson and colleagues,[11–14] showed that although the psychiatric literature on spirituality was largely negative, most studies in psychiatry journals either gathered no religious data or used inadequate measures of religiosity.[11] Furthermore, the great majority of spirituality-health associations that were documented in the psychiatric literature were positive,[12] Now many empirical studies of spiritual practice have shown positive health effects of spiritual practice, contrary to the predictions of older theories. Situating a study in the context of the literature does not mean simply accepting current conclusions. However, to refute a position that is common in the scientific literature requires even more thorough grounding than simply supporting one.

Case study III

An excellent example of recent SaH research that is very well grounded in explicit theory is the work of Kevin Flannelly, linking positive spiritual beliefs to reduced stress as a mechanism leading to reduced morbidity and mortality.[15] Surveying a national sample of more than 1400 Americans regarding belief in life after death and six measures of psychiatric symptoms, this study found a statistically significant inverse relationship between these beliefs and the severity scores for all six symptom clusters after controlling for other factors known to affect mental health. The study also showed that there was no significant association between religious service attendance and any of the symptom measures, suggesting 'that it may be more valuable to focus on religious beliefs than on religious practices and behaviours' (p. 524). This study was designed to contrast with existing SaH literature that focuses on practice rather than belief.

The theoretical grounding of this study utilized the physiological literature on stress extending back through most of the twentieth century. The idea of *stress* as a reaction that can be either adaptive (eustress) or destructive (distress) emerged in the 1930s, especially from the work of Hans Selye building on Walter Cannon's concept of homeostasis. The process is captured in Selye's concept of the General Adaptation Syndrome (GAS: alarm, resistance, exhaustion), in which the exhaustion stage is characterized by a growing burden of dysfunction and morbidity.[16] Walter Cannon had pointed out in his classic article 'Voodoo Death' that overwhelming stress can be lethal, and that the level of stress is heavily dependent on perception (hence, the use of 'Voodoo' as a metaphor for an overwhelming—but imaginary—stressor).[17] In the 1960s psychologist Richard Lazarus argued that psychological stress is a product of cognitive appraisal, comprised of an assessment of the balance between threats and resources.[18,19] These two points—that stress can produce morbidity and death, and that cognitive appraisal (i.e. beliefs) modulates stress; provide the background for the idea that beliefs in spiritual resources (and/or threats) can be potent mediators of the stress response and, therefore, health (emotional and physical). While stress has been a consistent focus in SaH research, the second point, the importance of belief, has received little attention,[4, p. 22; 5, p. 101; 15, p. 524; 20] the focus being instead on practices and overt behaviours. This development of a specific theory linking the cognitive domain (belief) to physiology could dramatically enhance future studies of spirituality and stress.

Pilot studies

While published studies are helpful, many study design questions require new empirical data. Preliminary pilot studies are used for this. Pilot studies are relatively small and are not expected to produce statistically significant results. Their purposes include showing feasibility, providing estimates of likely effect sizes, and assessing the reliability of a new questionnaire or a questionnaire planned for use in a new kind of population.

Feasibility is important because many unforeseen obstacles arise in human subjects research. A common obstacle is approval by the relevant human subjects protection review committee (IRB—institutional review board). IRBs provide a convenient opportunity to acquire critical input on study design. IRBs are not only watchful for direct risks of harm to subjects (from physical injury to embarrassment or other psychological issues). They are also mandated to ensure that a proposed study is well designed and focused on an important topic; that is, that the research is not trivial. It is assumed that trivial research is a waste of the subjects' time and therefore not justifiable. Response burden, another common obstacle, refers to the time and effort required to complete a survey form (self-report) or to be interviewed. Questionnaires that may seem 'easy,' 'quick,' or interesting to the researcher may be difficult, time-consuming, and boring to most respondents. That will reduce compliance and respondent accuracy, and may ruin a study. The pilot study is also a good opportunity to make certain that subjects understand questions as intended by the researcher. Focus groups are helpful for this purpose.

Case study IV

Along with assessing feasibility and estimating effect size for power analysis, the reliability of instruments that are new or that will be used in a novel setting should be evaluated during pilot testing. For example, Beardsley *et al.* wished to study patient satisfaction with chaplaincy care in the United Kingdom. They intended to use an existing instrument that has been reliable in the United States. When the instrument was piloted in the UK it proved reliable only in part.[21] Enough difficulty was found related to 'patient acuity, ethical concerns about standard follow-up protocols, and the Western Christian origins of the instrument' to suggest either revision or even the construction of a new instrument because of the religious diversity in the UK population.

The evidence pyramid

In the health sciences information is generally ranked hierarchically, often displayed within an 'Evidence Pyramid'[22] organized by design type. Those at the lowest levels are usually supported by the most published literature, while those at the higher levels yield greater clinical relevance. For practical purposes the pyramid image mixes the characteristics of rigor and clinical relevance in its ranking.

Typical hierarchy of medical information sources

- Systematic reviews (including meta-analyses)
- Experimental studies: randomized controlled trials (RCTs)
- Observational studies (some control)
- Cohort
- Case control
- Observational studies (no controls)
- Case series
- Case reports
- Editorials
- Animal research
- *In vitro* laboratory research

Randomized, controlled trials (RCTs) are far more rigorous than editorials and expert opinion; animal and laboratory studies are often the most rigorous research, but their results must be subjected to methods 'further up the pyramid' to demonstrate clinical effectiveness. Each method is important, and studies utilizing methods in the lower tiers contribute to the development and understanding of those 'further up.' Many RCTs would never have been undertaken without the evidence from *in vitro* and animal studies. Differences in definition across these design types in the literature can be confusing. I have used the most common meanings.

Reviews

Systematic (literature) reviews

Systematic reviews use formal criteria to select publications focused on a particular research question. For example, a review to analyse the field of 'spirituality and health' described its search parameters as follows:

> In February 2005 several searches of Ovid MEDLINE were carried out to identify health outcome studies involving spirituality and/or religion for the year's 2000 to the present. These searches combined the search terms 'health outcome' OR 'pregnancy outcome' OR 'exp treatment outcome' OR 'Outcome Assessment (Healthcare)', with either 'spirituality OR Spiritual Therapies' or 'religion.' The spirituality and the religion searches were carried out separately. The 'spirituality and health' search yielded a total of 323 references. The 'religion and health' search yielded 219. Of the total of 542 references, 103 were duplicates, leaving a set of 439 references on spirituality and/or religion and health outcomes, indexed on MEDLINE for the years 2000 through February 2005.[4, p. 2; 5, p. 76]

Such reviews then apply explicit criteria to evaluate the literature reviewed.

Systematic reviews, including meta-analyses, are scholarship utilizing documentary sources, not empirical studies. They obtain their clinical relevance by organizing numerous empirical studies orientated toward a particular clinical purpose.

Case study V

In 1986 David Larson and colleagues published a systematic review of research published in four major psychiatry journals, from 1978 to 1982.[11] Their guiding questions concerned the metrics for religion used in psychiatric studies and the associations found. During the period examined there were 3777 articles and the authors considered them all. They excluded 17 that were specifically devoted to 'sects' and 'cults,' because they deemed these outside the mainstream Western religious tradition. In the remaining articles they found 2348 quantitative studies. Of these, only 59 included at least one religious variable; of these, only 3 were focused on religion. As the authors put it, 'Thus in the 5 years reviewed, these four journals included 17 articles on cults or sects and only three on traditional religious phenomena' (p. 331). They then assessed the 59 articles on the following 5 issues: '1) the frequency of inclusion of religious variables ..., 2) the robustness of statistical analysis; 3) the type of measure of religion used; 4) the conceptual basis for measurement of religion; and 5) awareness of the scientific data base on religious research' (p. 332). They found that religious variables were rarely included and less robust statistical analysis was typically used when they were. Regarding metrics, 'the majority of articles used a single, weak denotative measurement (denomination), while a small proportion used appropriate multiple measures of religiosity' (p. 332). The conceptual basis of measurement was weak, which was not surprising because of the 59 articles with at least one religious variable only eight included at least one reference to scientific research on religion! (p. 332). This systematic review began a serious reconsideration of the scholarship regarding religion in the scientific medical literature, and helped to stimulate the rapid growth of SaH research.

Meta-analysis

A meta-analysis is 'any systematic method that uses statistical analyses for combining data from independent studies to obtain a numerical estimate of a particular ... variable on a defined outcome'.[23] The purpose of a meta-analysis is to aggregate data, yielding substantially more power than each individual study could provide.

Case study VI

In 2006, Masters *et al.* conducted a meta-analysis of studies of distant intercessory prayer (IP) 'to assess the impact of potential moderator variables'.[24, p. 337] 'Distant IP' is prayer offered outside the presence of the one being prayed for. Most IP studies are blinded to prevent recipients from knowing whether they are being prayed for. Thus, IP studies assess an effect for which there is no known causal mechanism. Moderator variables are variables that change the strength of a causal relationship between independent and dependent variables.

The Masters et al. meta-analysis selected studies as follows:

> PsycINFO and Medline databases were searched using the term intercessory prayer, and articles published prior to August 2005 were eligible for inclusion. References in relevant review articles (6–9) were also searched as were reference lists from articles included in the meta-analysis. To meet inclusion criteria, studies must have (a) used IP as an intervention to treat any type of medical or mental health problem, (b) provided data that allowed for calculation of an effect size, (c) compared IP to a control group, and (d) blinded participants as to their experimental condition.' (p. 22, with kind permission from Springer Science+Business Media: Annals Behavioral Medicine, Are there demonstrable effects of distant intercessory prayer? A meta-analytic, Volume 32, 2006.)

Fourteen studies met the inclusion criteria. When the data from these studies were statistically aggregated the overall effect was not significant, although some individual studies had achieved statistical significance. However, the reviewers recognized the possibilities of an important confound: the highly likely administration of intercessory prayer to members of the control group. Given the widespread use of prayer for health reasons in the USA,[25] one must assume that non-experimental prayer was as substantial in the control group as in the experimental group, perhaps even exceeding that of the IP intervention. This would reduce any effect size (difference between experimental and control group outcomes) and, therefore, power, in the IP studies. Also, we have no basis for estimating (or even assuming) a dose–response relationship between prayer and the medical conditions of the experimental subjects, so the crucial factor might be 'prayer/no prayer.' As the authors note, 'it could be argued that virtually all participants receive prayer or at least believe they do'.[24, p. 25] Therefore the reviewers state that they could find 'no scientifically discernable effect that differentiates the status of individuals who are the recipients of IP initiated by a research team from those who do not receive research team initiated IP'.[24, p. 25] This caution, limiting conclusions to the specific conditions of the study, is admirable.

Experimental studies

Randomized controlled trials

RCTs are experimental studies in which independent variables such as treatments are manipulated under controlled conditions in order to observe the effects on outcomes (dependent variables). An initial sample of subjects, all of whom would be appropriate recipients of the experimental condition (e.g. all having the same diagnosis), is randomly divided between the experimental condition (receiving the actual intervention) and the control condition (not receiving the intervention). Depending on the homogeneity of the initial sample (e.g. age, sex, severity of condition, etc.) randomization applied to the proper size sample will yield two groups that do not differ in ways relevant to the study. Therefore, an effect in the experimental group larger than expected random variation may be inferred to have been caused by the intervention.

'Blinding' refers to hiding the difference between the experimental and control conditions to prevent bias. It is assumed that there will be a certain amount of effect from *any* intervention, based on the subject's hope and expectation, the 'placebo effect.' This bias can be avoided by providing the control group with a 'mock intervention,' giving them a similar expectation and, therefore, bias. Double-blind studies, the ideal, are those in which both subjects and investigators are blinded to the distinction. This adds the strength of avoiding any 'experimenter effect,'[26] a collection of unintentional biases introduced by the experimenter's hope to achieve positive results.

Blinding is relatively easy in drug therapy where an inert pill, shot, etc. (a placebo) can be administered to controls. It is much harder in surgery or psychotherapy. It is also much harder for most spiritual interventions. Prayer, for example, has been studied for its effect on both physical and mental health. Two kinds of prayer have been studied. One form is 'distant intercessory prayer,' in which someone prays for the health of another who is not physically present. This common kind of prayer is relatively easy to control for, because the intervention occurs beyond the view of subjects, their families and the investigators. If randomization is adequate, significant effects should be attributable to the prayers offered. The results of such studies have been equivocal.[24]

Other studies have examined the effect of prayer offered directly with the subject. This is also a common kind of prayer for healing. Unlike distant intercessory prayer, blinding is not practical for this kind of prayer because there is no plausible 'placebo prayer.' Still such studies can be controlled, for example by randomizing the sample between the experimental group and a 'no treatment group,' such as subjects on a waiting list. This control is less powerful than use of a mock treatment because of the placebo effect.

Case study VII

In 2009, Boelens *et al.* published a study of 'direct contact person-to-person prayer on depression, anxiety, positive emotions and salivary cortisol levels.'[27, p. 377] (Salivary cortisol is a biomarker indicative of stress level.) There were 63 participants, all of them adult and suffering from depression, randomized either to the experimental or the 'no treatment' control group. The experimental subjects received one hour of direct person to person prayer per week for six weeks; the controls received no intervention (randomized and controlled, but not blinded). After six weeks the controls 'crossed over' to the experimental arm of the study and commenced six weeks of person-to-person prayer. Using the controls as experimental subjects through the crossover design reduced the total number of subjects needed for the trial, and it also allowed the crossover group to be examined as 'their own controls.' In this case the investigators were able to conclude that 'Direct contact person-to-person prayer may be useful as an adjunct to standard medical care for patients with depression.'[27, p. 377]

Observational studies

Observational studies are those in which the researcher cannot assign subjects to investigational and control groups. Controls are standards for comparison that help to assess the validity of observations. Although observational studies cannot randomly assign subjects, there are some other forms of comparison.

Cohort studies

A cohort study compares subjects with a particular characteristic to either the general population or a subset thereof that does not share that characteristic; the comparison is usually made over time (these are longitudinal) to look at the occurrence of some medical condition; e.g. comparing church members (the defining cohort characteristic) to the general population for the development of alcoholism (the medical condition). The comparison provides a measure of control, but lacking random assignment there may be confounds, relevant differences between the cohort and the comparison group in addition to the characteristic being studied. (The difference from *case control* studies: In cohort studies the study population does not have the medical condition at the beginning of the study. Both are epidemiological.)

Case study VIII

In 2010, Schnall *et al.* published a study of the relationship between religion and both cardiovascular outcomes and all cause mortality.[28] The study was based on the Women's Health Initiative Observational Study, a longitudinal collection of data involving 92,395 women begun by the National Institutes of Health in 1991. The Schnall study 'examined the prospective association of religious affiliation, religious service attendance, and strength and comfort from religion with subsequent cardiovascular outcomes and death'[28, p. 249] over a period of 7.7 years. Religious data had been collected at enrolment in the study. After controlling for various demographic, socio-economic, and prior health variables, measures of religion were found significantly associated with reduced overall mortality risk, but not with any reduction in coronary heart disease morbidity and mortality.

Case control studies

Case control studies compare a group of subjects who have a particular health condition (the 'case' group) with another group that does not have that condition, typically during a single period of time (then they are a kind of cross-sectional study), looking for factors that may have contributed to development of the condition under study. These studies may also add a retrospective or prospective dimension (then they are not cross-sectional). Control may be sought by matching subjects across the two groups for personal characteristics (sex, age, etc.). (The difference from cohort studies: in case control studies the study population *does* have the medical condition.)

Case study IX

In 2010, Sisask *et al.* published 'Is religiosity a protective factor against attempted suicide: a cross-cultural case-control study.'[29] This study compared suicide attempters (the 'case' group] with community controls on measures of 'subjective religiosity' in four different societies (Estonia, Iran, Sri Lanka, and South Africa). They found major variations in this association, concluding that 'subjective religiosity (considering him/herself as religious person] may serve as a protective factor against non-fatal suicidal behaviour in some cultures'.[29, p. 44]

Case study, case series (or clinical series)

A case study examines a patient with a known condition, risk, or treatment, and describes the outcome of the case. A case series does the same for a group of cases. These reports may be either retrospective (using charts) or prospective. Although obviously weaker than case control or cohort studies, or RCT's, the case studies and series are useful to generate hypotheses for further study and to bring rare or previously unknown issues to light.

Case study X

In 2009 Glueckauf *et al.* published two case reports describing the use of 'cognitive-behavioural and spiritual counseling (CBSC) for rural dementia caregivers (CGs) ... for treating depression in this population,'[30] using a pre–post-evaluation design. The authors reported that 'Case study findings provided evidence of substantial improvement in caregiving problems and reductions in depression.' This is a useful starting point for this intervention, but as the authors note in their conclusion, 'replication across the sample is required to evaluate the overall effectiveness of CBSC for reducing CG depression'.[30, p. 449]

Cross-sectional studies

Cross-sectional studies seek to describe the relationship of a health state (disease or wellness) and some other factor in a particular population at a single point in time. Although most cross-sectional studies lack controls (cross-sectional case control studies are an important exception), such studies are inexpensive and can be useful in generating hypotheses.

Case study XI

In 2009, Beckelman *et al.* published a cross-sectional study of the relationship of 'symptom burden, psychological wellbeing, and spiritual wellbeing in heart failure and cancer patients,' finding 'that heart failure patients, particularly those with more severe heart failure, need the option of palliative care just as cancer patients do.'[31, p. 592]

Editorials

Editorials, commentaries and other essays that do not present original empirical data carry less weight than formal studies. Nonetheless they have value as background and may be influential in a field.

Case study XII

In 2008, the *Journals of Gerontology Series A—Biological Sciences & Medical Sciences* published a guest editorial by Terence D. Hill, PhD, then Assistant Professor of Sociology at the University of Miami, entitled 'Religious involvement and healthy cognitive aging: patterns, explanations, and future directions.'[32] Dr Hill presented an overview of research published in the *Journals of Gerontology*, suggesting that religious involvement favours healthy cognitive ageing, and the author outlines promising avenues for future research. The editorial included 19 bibliographic references. This editorial would be very helpful for one formulating a research project on the subject of religion and ageing.

Animal research and in vitro studies

Note: *in vitro*, from Latin meaning 'within glass,' referring to test tubes, petri dishes, etc.

Laboratory studies are usually tightly controlled experiments. So they are often more rigorous than the human study designs described above in the 'pyramid,' because they can employ more rigorous controls than would be practical (or ethical) in human subjects. For example, much of our knowledge of the health effects of stress have come from animal studies, and stress is generally considered to be an important pathway through which spirituality affects human health. However, the initial human relevance of such findings was uncertain until human trials provided evidence.

Case study XIII

Herbert Benson, the discoverer of the 'Relaxation Response' has said that his initial decision to study possible health effects of Transcendental Meditation, a spiritual practice brought to the USA from India, came from what he had seen of animal studies showing the effect of stress on hypertension.[33]

The scope of the field: beyond the evidence pyramid

Modern medicine emerged during the late nineteenth century, as the 'German model' led medical schools to organize their curricula around science. A strong connection between spirituality and health had been assumed throughout history, but the new scientific medicine disentangled itself from spirituality explicitly and intentionally. By the 1920s, many intellectuals considered traditional spirituality 'primitive,' certain to die out in the modern world.[34] Not until the late twentieth century did this view give way as new data about spirituality and religion emerged.

During the 1960s the nexus of spirituality, religion, and health was undergoing a renaissance in the United States, as Neo-Pentecostalism and the Charismatic Movement grew in influence.[35] By the mid-1970s, spiritual healing had a firm place within virtually every Christian denomination. Now survey data consistently shows the important role of spirituality in health for most Americans. For example, a national survey published in *Archives of Internal Medicine* found that in 1998 '35% of respondents used prayer for health concerns; 75% of these prayed for wellness, and 22% prayed for specific medical conditions. Of those praying for specific medical conditions, 69% found prayer very helpful.'[25, p. 858] Illness elicits prayer from a majority of Americans, as it has for people around the world throughout history. Even in Europe, generally considered less spiritual than the USA, the 2005 Eurobarometer Poll[36] found that only an average 14% of respondents in Europe did not 'believe there is any sort of spirit, God or life force.' Modern spirituality has been rediscovered and the field of SaH has developed rapidly, primarily arising within medicine itself.

As SaH emerged within medicine the modern paradigm of medical research, illustrated by 'the evidence pyramid,' provided the basic template for the field. However, that paradigm developed to test the efficacy of medical treatments, especially drugs. Spiritual practices are very different. Like eating, exercise, and marriage, spirituality is a behaviour with health relevance (either positive or negative in a given situation), but that is utilized for many other reasons. Such complex behaviours cannot be reduced to single independent variables. Cultural, social, and psychological factors must be included. As Wayne Jonas has shown in detail, healthcare research requires more than an 'evidence pyramid,' it needs an 'evidence house' with a variety of rooms for different kinds of information.[37,38] Unfortunately, the disciplines that traditionally study religion, such as religious studies, anthropology, and the sociology and history of religion have not focused on health relevance, and have been largely ignored in SaH. (Nonetheless, those scholars and scholar/scientists who have studied and written on SaH topics should receive more attention than they have; for example, physicians Larry Dossey[39–41] and Rex Gardner,[42] religion scholar Robert Fuller[43,44] and political scientist Fred Frohock.[45])

Lacking interdisciplinary scope, SaH methodology has a narrow scholarly base, and omits many important topics and methods. To illustrate this problem I will describe several major gaps in SaH research:

- insufficient use of qualitative (and mixed) methods
- problems of definition (linguistics)
- implicit biases against the 'spiritual, but not religious' (linguistics and history), minority religions (anthropology and sociology), complementary and alternative medicine (sociology), and extraordinary spiritual experiences (phenomenology).

Qualitative research

Many relevant disciplines currently under-utilized in SaH emphasize qualitative, rather than quantitative methods. Whereas quantitative methods (as in the 'Evidence Pyramid') study numerically measureable properties, qualitative research gathers information better expressed in words than numbers. For example, in open-ended interviews subjects are encouraged to give accounts in their own words as opposed to the closed-ended questions typical in questionnaires. Participant observation immerses the observer in the setting being studied, providing a first-person, experiential view. Documents such as letters, diaries, court records, etc., are studied and analysed. Qualitative research may be quite formal, as when focus groups composed of representative individuals are engaged in semi-structured conversations with researchers; or it can much less formal, as when an observer participates in a healing service. Qualitative research requires the investigator to engage in complex, reflexive analysis and interpretation, quite different from the statistical analysis characteristic of quantitative methodology. In quantitative research questionnaires and scales are often called 'instruments.' In qualitative research it is the investigator who serves as 'the instrument.'

For example, in 2010 Grossoehme and colleagues published a qualitative study entitled 'We can handle this: Parents' use of religion in the first year following their child's diagnosis with cystic fibrosis.'[46] The study was intended to develop a theory of the way parents of children newly diagnosed with CF use religion and their understanding of how this religious coping affects their adherence to medical regimens for their child. Based on 15 interviews, the study found that 'Parents imagined God as active, benevolent, and interventionist; found hope in their beliefs; felt supported by God; and related religion to their motivation to adhere to their child's treatment plan.'[46, p. 95] Linking this study to the same team's study of positive and negative coping styles,[47] the investigators made clinical recommendations to improve adherence by including spiritual issues. In this study, the qualitative approach allowed the investigators to understand aspects of the parents' lived experience with their child's illness, a subjective dimension of coping that cannot be fully captured by quantitative studies.

A study such as this provides a sound basis for new hypotheses that can then be examined in larger, representative samples using quantitative methods to allow broader generalization. However, this study was not merely preliminary. It set out to learn about the way these parents experience their children's devastating diagnosis in the context of their spiritual beliefs. It succeeded and was able to use the findings, coupled with another study that employed some quantitative measures, to offer clinical advice. This is comparable to the case series design, but with a richer description of the experiential dimension.

Quality of life (QOL) is a topic that is especially open to SaH effects and that requires a combination of quantitative and qualitative approaches by definition. QOL studies in SaH are becoming more common, especially among cancer patients,[48–51] but QOL has not yet received the attention that it deserves (see, however, Chapter 46).

Mixed methods

The results of qualitative and quantitative research are different, but complementary, so researchers have increasingly combined the two, the 'mixed methods' approach. Sometimes this is done for very specific, limited purposes, such as improving the validity of a quantitative instrument.

For example, King *et al.* created a questionnaire intended to measure spirituality as a characteristic distinct from religion.[52] They began with a cross-sectional qualitative study using a purposive sample of 39 people, some with advanced cancer and some without cancer, to discuss spirituality. They employed a combination of focus groups and individual interviews with a semistructured format, 'using prompts such as 'What does your life mean to you?' 'What are your beliefs?' 'What makes your life worthwhile?' 'Do you have any spiritual understanding of your life?' 'How do you express your spiritual beliefs?'[52, p. 418] They also recruited palliative care nurses into focus groups to discuss their perception of the role of spirituality in the dying process. The sessions were audiotaped, transcribed and independently analysed by theme by the four senior members of the research team. The themes were discussed jointly to develop a set of statements, which were then discussed with a group of patients and care givers who rated the statements on a 5-point Likert scale (from strongly agree to strongly disagree). From this they created a scale with 47 statements which was evaluated for clarity and reliability in 4 diverse groups (patients and non-patients, total 372). This led to creation of a 24-item scale that was evaluated by another group of 284 subjects. 'The final 20-item questionnaire performed with high test–retest and internal reliability and measures spirituality across a broad religious and non-religious perspective.[52, p. 417]

In this example we see the extensive use of qualitative methods in the development of a quantitative instrument, the Beliefs and Values Scale. In other cases quantitative and qualitative methods are combined to serve the broader overall research goal. [e.g. 53]

Definitions and linguistic methods

SaH's difficulty in defining *spirituality* illustrates the problem of the field's narrow scope. In the 1997 *Scientific Research on Spirituality and Health: A Consensus Report*,[54] 'Definitions of religion and spirituality' begins with the following statement: 'An immediate consensus among Panel members was the need to ground definitions of religion and spirituality in scientific and historical scholarship.'[54, p. 15]

However, of 21 panel members, only one had a humanities appointment (an endowed chair of Liberal Arts), one was a sociologist and the rest held medical or psychology appointments. They may be excellent researchers, but that does not make them historians, linguists, or philosophers. The panel's resulting definitions of spirituality are ambiguous and excessively complex, centering on 'a search for the sacred ... The term 'sacred' refers to a divine being or Ultimate Reality or Ultimate Truth as perceived by the individual;'[54, p. 21] religion may involve 'non-sacred goals,' such as 'meaning' in a primarily sacred seeking context *plus* 'The means and methods of the search' validated and supported by a group. As George *et al.* say, these are 'highly abstract definitions that do not lead to straightforward operationalization.'[55, p. 105]

In the authoritative *Handbook of Religion and Health*[56] Koenig *et al.* further developed the concepts from the *Consensus Report*, giving the following definition: 'Spirituality is the personal quest for understanding answers to ultimate questions about life, about meaning and about relationship to the sacred or transcendent, which may (*or may not) lead to or arise from the development of religious rituals and the formation of community.'[56, p. 18]

The meaning of the word spiritual in the SaH literature is inconsistent, 'fuzzy'[57] and 'vague and contradictory.'[58, p. 8] There have been complaints that the meanings of each has changed over time.[59, p. 60]

Spirituality is a natural language term and, therefore, inherently ambiguous. Meanings shift, expand, and contract as words travel in different speech communities. Research on human behaviour requires language-based methods (surveys, interviews, etc.), and natural language words appropriated as technical terms create a problem. Operationalized to meet the conceptual criteria of investigators, the words lose their ordinary speech meanings and questionnaire responses lose validity. For naturally occurring language the only correct meanings are those found in customary usage. Correct meaning, as Emblen concisely points out 'depends on how the ambient community commonly uses the terms.'[60, p. 41] Community usages are discovered through lexicology, a branch of linguistics based on substantial numbers of naturally occurring usages within a representative sample of speakers. This is not asking respondents for definitions, something most people find difficult, but rather analysing the natural utterances of words in context. The closest to this generally found in SaH is surveys of usages in the literature.[e.g. 61] Less frequently, there have been surveys with small convenience samples of ordinary speakers.[57] These studies are useful, but they do not provide the basis for a definition that matches the meaning of most ordinary speakers, and that is what is required for solid research and interpretation. Ironically, a wealth of data on the meaning of spirituality and religion in English is easily available in the lexicology literature, and the meanings are concise and clear. Spirituality means the quality relating to spirit, that which is not material, having to do with spirits, such as God (or gods) and the human soul. This has been the meaning in English for more than five centuries.[62] Religion has more complex meanings within particular settings. For example, in Catholicism the state of clergy who live within a specific religious order, often a monastic setting, is called religion. Such narrow meanings are of little use in SaH generally, but traditionally *religion* also means a system of spiritual belief, a spiritual institution or organization.[2, p. 2538] This distinguishes spirituality from religion without dichotomizing. Beliefs are spiritual on the basis of their content; they are religious on the basis of their location. Belief in God is a spiritual belief, and in many religions it is a religious belief, 'a spiritual belief found in a religious setting.'

Spirituality is defined by a kind of belief, but using the term properly does not require holding such beliefs. The beliefs that fall within this definition vary sufficiently to be cross-culturally applicable: spiritual beliefs may be more about forces (e.g. *qi*) or processes (e.g. reincarnation) than about deities or other entities, as in some forms of Buddhism, or they may be very theo-centric, like Judaism, Christianity and Islam. Being religious, that is, having commitment to a particular spiritual institution, varies by degrees. These definitions make clear why some Americans say they are 'spiritual, but not religious:' they hold spiritual beliefs, but do not accept the authority of a given religious institution. This also explains why so few say they are 'religious, but not spiritual,' since religions are basically spiritual.

'Spiritual, but not religious' and historical methods

Surveys estimate that between 20[63] and 30%[64] of Americans identify as 'spiritual, but not religious.' With Catholics being the largest American religious group at about 24%, the 'spiritual, but not religious' are one of the most numerous groups of spiritual believers in the country. It has been suggested that their beliefs are a mere hodgepodge of uninformed opinions, defying analysis. It has also been assumed that this group represents a recent development in American spirituality.[59] George *et al.*, for example, say that 'it is only recently that spirituality began to acquire meanings separate from religion.'[55] However, in fact this phenomenon is older than the Republic. In the late 1600s less than 1/3 of colonist adults were church members, and by the time of the Revolutionary War this had dropped to about 15%.[44, p. 13]. Nonetheless, the colonists were avidly spiritual in their orientation, engaging in astrology, divination, and folk healing practices that were fundamentally spiritual, decried by colonial clergy as wicked and heretical, and influenced by the Freemasons (most of the men who signed the Declaration of Independence were Masons) and Rosicrucianism. During the nineteenth century movements from Transcendentalism to Mesmerism, New thought and spiritualism flowered in the United States.[44, pp. 13–44; 65–67] Spiritual language was widely used in all of these discourses. This strand of unchurched American spirituality is what Sydney Ahlstrom has called 'harmonial piety,'[67, p. 1019] and its message, summarized by Fuller as being that 'spiritual composure, physical health, and even economic wellbeing are understood to flow from a person's rapport with the cosmos.'[44, p. 51], is readily recognizable in today's 'spiritual, but not religious.' The history of 'unchurched spirituality' is important to understanding contemporary American spirituality, especially regarding health. This kind of issue requires SaH researchers to be conversant with historical methods and the relevant research published by professional historians.

Despite the salience of the spiritual-but-not-religious group in America, the SaH literature tends to disparage this viewpoint. *The Handbook of Religion and Health* refers to it as 'unmoored spirituality.'[56, p. 18] The authors subdivide spirituality categories in a way that results in a low estimate of this group's size, and illustrates it with references to crystals, astrology and Shirley MacLaine.[56, p. 19] George *et al.* in 2000 stated that:

> So long as most individuals do not distinguish between religion and spirituality, separating these concepts operationally will be impossible. Of course, we can study individuals who report that they are spiritual, but not religious—there are a few studies of this kind (e.g. Legere, 1984; Roof, 1993). However, such studies will not generate distinct, broadly applicable measures of religiousness and spirituality. (In theory we could also study individuals who describe themselves as religious, but not spiritual, but research suggests that the numbers of such persons are too small for meaningful analysis.) [55, p. 104]

This kind of misunderstanding illustrates the problems caused by lack of familiarity with linguistic and historical research within SaH. In fact, most English speakers do distinguish the terms, and spiritual beliefs can be studied in all kinds of settings, within various religions and among those with no particular religion. The effects of religion and spirituality have varied through history, and may be distinct or synergistic depending on context.

Minority religions (anthropology and sociology)

SaH attention has been deflected not only from the spiritual, but not religious, but also from many other spiritual traditions, such as the diverse spirituality of Native Americans, new immigrant groups, the regional 'folk healing' traditions of other ethnic minorities, and other religions outside the Protestant Christian mainstream, such as Judaism, Islam, Buddhism, Hinduism, Mormons and Catholics. This may simply reflect greater familiarity with mainstream Protestantism among SaH researchers. However, in the modern world all spiritual traditions, ancient and new, are present and influential. The fields of anthropology and the sociology of religion have produced a vast literature on this subject and have the potential to reduce the ethnocentrism characteristic of SaH. As the largest religious denomination, Catholicism provides a good example.

Catholicism has the longest continued tradition of spiritual healing and commentary on medical practice of any branch of Christianity in the world. And since the Charismatic movement in Catholicism began in the late 1950s, Catholicism also includes most of the healing practices found in Protestant denominations. Catholicism also exerts major influence in medical policy areas such as reproductive health and end-of-life care. Catholics are often included in epidemiological studies, but studies of distinctively Catholic healing practices, such as pilgrimage and 'the cult of the saints,' are largely absent from the SaH literature. The MEDLINE searches reported in my 2005 analysis of the SaH field[4] yielded only four references citing Catholicism,[68–71] and none of these referred to distinctive Catholic spiritual practices. *The Handbook*[56] mentions pilgrimage, a major aspect of Catholic healing practice, only five times, and three of these are disparaging. Millions of Americans and others visit healing shrines in the Americas and Europe every year, and there is a large literature on pilgrimage in the social scientific study of religion. My own ethnographic work on pilgrimage suggests that the majority of pilgrims find support in coping with illness and many explicitly deny that they are primarily concerned with the possibility of a miraculous physical healing.[72] Yet even Pargament's excellent book on religious coping[73] has only a single reference to Catholicism and coping, and that involves Catholic Charismatic practice. The rich and varied healing practices of Catholics offer a major opportunity for SaH research, but have as yet received very little attention.

Research on these topics requires what anthropologists call 'thick description,'[74, p. 6.] and SaH is relatively weak in descriptive methods. The specific beliefs of spiritual groups and their particular effects on health have received cursory treatment.[4, p. 22; 5, p. 101; 15, p. 524; 20] They tend to be described globally (e.g. 'belief in God'), and though often included in survey instruments such as King *et al.*'s Beliefs and Values Scale,[52] belief has not received much attention as a specific variable. For example, George *et al.* note that the Fetzer/NIA conference group that developed the Fetzer/NIA multi-dimensional measurement 'did not recommend' religious/spiritual belief 'as particularly important for understanding the links between religion/spirituality and health.'[55 p. 106] Although the relationship of prayer to various health measures has frequently been investigated, the SaH literature devotes little attention to the specifics of prayer belief and practice, although there is solid social science research that suggests the scope, variety, and importance of the distinct forms.[25,75] Clearly, beliefs about the efficacy of prayer comprise a major perceived resource among American patients, and the impact of that belief influences both decision-making and coping. These beliefs are associated both with positive coping and with religiously motivated non-compliance. However, the specific beliefs themselves and the ways that patients arrive at and maintain those beliefs have received very little attention in the SaH literature. The Fetzer/NIA instrument section on 'Beliefs' has seven questions, and all, but one ('Do you believe there is life after death?') are general, largely metaphysical beliefs (e.g. 'God's goodness and love are greater than we can possibly imagine').[76, p. 32] Although several studies have supported the connection of specific beliefs to mental health,[e.g. 15,77–80] the description and utilization of specific beliefs is an understudied area in SaH.

The lack of belief description is related to the lack of ethnographic, qualitative and historical work within SaH, because these forms of scholarship are heavily committed to description. In the contemporary SaH literature such methodologies are typically assumed to be primarily useful for the generation of hypotheses,[e.g. 56, p. 482] but they are also very helpful in extending and clarifying the findings of quantitative studies and as studies in their own right.

Complementary and alternative medicine

Both SaH and Complementary and Alternative Medicine (CAM) research have recently emerged among health researchers from a history of neglect, marginalization and stigma, and both currently strive with considerable success for legitimacy. Basically all SaH health interventions fit the conventional definition of CAM.[81] The best quantitative studies of CAM utilization show strong associations between CAM use and use of prayer.[25,75] Studies of why patients use CAM indicate that a spiritual point of view is among the strongest reasons and that CAM use is associated with the use of prayer.[25,75,82] Most CAM practices show a variety of affinities to both spirituality and religion. Both SaH and CAM researchers are engaged in studies of the prevalence, distribution and health impact of the practices that they are investigating. And both groups are working toward the appropriate integration of the practices they study into clinical medicine. Yet there is a clear and apparently intentional divide between the two research domains. For example, the *Handbook of Religion and Health*[56] cites Eisenberg's seminal survey research published in *Journal of the American Medical Association* in 1998 showing that CAM use was very high among Americans and was directly related to better education[83] as support for the statement that lack of 'psychosocial-spiritual care ... has opened the door to a whole host of charlatans and alternative medicine practitioners.'[83, p. 5] In the *Handbook*'s index there are only two entries for CAM, 'alternative medicine' leads to the 'charlatans' quote, and 'unconventional therapies (UT)' leads to Eisenberg's 1993 study, which is only used to document Americans' frequent use of prayer.[84] Neither the affinities nor the antipathies between these areas is new in America. They are readily traced back to colonial days.[43]

Extraordinary spiritual experiences (ESEs) and phenomenology

During the past thirty years research on dramatic spiritual experiences, such as the 'near-death experience' (NDE), has grown rapidly, much of it carried out by psychologists and physicians.[85,86] The experiences of bereaved people being 'visited by a deceased loved one,' a very powerful spiritual experience, has been shown to be common, normal and psychologically helpful; it is now incorporated into the conventional psychiatric literature.[78,87,88] The terrifying experience of sleep paralysis with a spiritual presence has great impact on the experiencer's beliefs, and it has been misdiagnosed consistently as various disorders over the years; it is now known to be common in all cultures.[78,89,90] Historically medicine consistently assimilated experiences such as these to psychiatric symptomatology.[78,91] Contemporary research shows those assumptions of pathology to be false and has documented new associations with health: (1) some of these experiences are triggered by serious health events, often in medical settings (e.g. NDEs), and (2) they often have positive effects on emotional health.[78,87,88,92] Yet SaH research consistently ignores all such experiences in favour of more ordinary, daily spiritual experiences.

The study of subjective experience requires phenomenological methods. Phenomenology began within philosophy as a method for studying consciousness *per se*. However, its methods and applications have been adopted in a variety of fields where experience is important, from architecture to psychology and anthropology. Phenomenological methods are essentially qualitative. For example, those who report NDEs are usually asked to give descriptions in their own words, followed by probing questions, in open ended interviews. This is often combined with the use of quantitative metrics[e.g. 93] in a mixed method approach. Recently, some instruments with good psychometric properties have been developed, allowing the broad range of ESEs and ordinary spiritual experiences to be studied together in relation to health.[94,95] Phenomenological inquiry has brought discovered robust, complex patterns across subjects in different cultures in several ESEs.[78] The study of NDEs and of spiritual experiences in sleep paralysis has particularly emphasized phenomenological description and analysis.[89]

The SaH aversion to extraordinary spiritual experiences parallels the lack of interest in the topic shown in the theological and pastoral care literature.[85] This leaves another gap in the field that parallels the preference for religion over non-institutional spirituality and the avoidance of unconventional topics, even when those topics are receiving serious investigation with studies published in peer reviewed journals.

Conclusion

The greatest methodological challenge to SaH is the need to broaden its scope. A very simple place to start would be understudied populations with unique health concerns, such as the military.[96] More challenging is the need to include the full range of relevant disciplines and their methods, and to break through the field's current ethnocentric focus on a particular segment of mainstream Christianity. This challenge results from unrecognized biases with historical and social roots.

Intellectuals have frequently asserted that modern science and traditional spirituality are incompatible. It is the core spiritual beliefs of religion that are at issue: 'Man's knowledge and mastery of the world have advanced to such an extent through science and technology. . . . Now that the forces and the laws of nature have been discovered, we can no longer believe in *spirits, whether good or evil*' (theologian Rudolf Bultmann, 1953);[97 p.5] 'Religion and science seem to be mutually exclusive perspectives' (sociologist Rodney Stark, 1963);[98] 'Religion and science are mutually exclusive realms of thought whose presentation in the same context leads to misunderstanding of BOTH scientific theory and religious belief' (from a resolution of the Council of the National Academy of Sciences in 1981).[99] The recent rapid growth of SaH is a direct contradiction to such assertions.

We now know that most modern people simultaneously hold spiritual beliefs and scientific knowledge with ease. This includes a majority of scientists[100] and other academics,[101] showing that this is not scientific ignorance at work. Even among Europeans, generally considered one of the world's most secular populations, a large majority in all countries hold explicitly spiritual beliefs.[36] Yet the idea that scientific knowledge and traditional spiritual beliefs are incompatible persists.[102,103] For SaH this creates a major challenge that is at once social and epistemological.

Through most of the twentieth century medicine ignored spirituality or considered it an unhealthy impediment to healthcare. However, in the 1980s and 1990s SaH emerged through research showing that these negative assumptions lacked evidence and that spirituality and religion can actually have positive health effects. However, the core of both spirituality and religion is belief in a non-material reality: God or gods, human souls, prayer, the afterlife. And these are the beliefs that were thought to have lost viability in the modern world. Freud and others insisted such beliefs are neurotic and irrational.[104] Yet the majority of American physicians are quite spiritual and/or religious by a variety of measures; a large majority of them believe spirituality has a positive effect on health (less than 5% take the opposite view),[105,106] and a majority believe that God intervenes in patients' lives, at least occasionally.[106,107]

The tension between the conventional 'science vs. spirituality' view and sympathetic (or at least respectful) scientific research on spirituality as a health resource is obvious. This tension has produced a variety of effects, some obvious and some subtle.

Spirituality is an emotionally charged subject, and religious differences provoke strong reactions. So avoiding bias in SaH research is difficult since all investigators have their own spiritual position. Not only the devout have spiritual commitments; atheists and agnostics also have 'an axe to grind.' Bias is a problem in all research domains, but SaH is particularly fraught with sources of bias. Even though most of the public favors medical attention to spiritual issues,[108,109] the topic remains controversial in scientific terms.[110–115] This reflects a kind of 'split personality' among scientists, the majority of whom hold spiritual beliefs, but tend to avoid public disclosure because of peer pressure.[100] This pressure is not only personal, but can also affect careers.[116] Partly in response to this situation SaH has developed an orientation much like what is generally called 'liberal theology,' descended from spiritual ideas developed during the Enlightenment and influential in mainstream Protestantism. This position is illustrated by the Christian Existentialism of Protestant theologian Paul Tillich.[117,118]

Tillich's idea of faith, and therefore religion, as 'ultimate concern'[117, p. 5] and spirituality simply meaning all human capacities,[119] lie behind many of the SaH definitions of spirituality that have been criticized as 'fuzzy' and ambiguous. Tillich's theology rejects what he calls the God of 'theological theism'[117, p. 184], saying that God is not a being, but rather 'the ground of all being.' This approach emphasizes the symbolic meaning of all spiritual language, embraces doubt, and seeks to accommodate spirituality to the modern world. The ambiguity of Tillich's symbolic framework and his 'ultimate concern' definition leave ample room for all sorts of believers and disbelievers. This has some advantages for SaH. It creates a spiritual/religious language that is broadly inclusive: all humans are equally spiritual (regardless of their beliefs), all spiritual beliefs are symbolically meaningful (regardless of their ontological status), and contradiction of any scientifically founded belief is virtually impossible. True to its Enlightenment roots, liberal theology is strongly accommodative regarding conventional science.

However, despite the apparent inclusiveness of this framework it has led SaH to omit from study a great swath of spiritual beliefs and practices that make unambiguous reference to non-material spiritual causes, effects and realities. Complementary and alternative medicine (CAM) incorporates many ideas regarding spiritual forces and 'subtle energies;' and it has received scant attention in the main stream of SaH literature, despite its strong spiritual associations.[25,75,82,83,84] To those who have them extraordinary 'mystical' spiritual experiences (ESEs) appear to reveal a non-material reality, and they are rarely included within the scope of SaH, even though they have numerous well documented health effects.[78] ESEs and spiritual healing forces obviously relate to ancient beliefs in folk and shamanic healing, as well as in several major spiritual traditions (e.g. Judaism, Islam, Buddhism, Hinduism, and several branches of Christianity, such as Catholicism and Mormonism); all of these beliefs and traditions are conspicuously absent from most of the SaH literature. The 'spiritual, but not religious' tradition is focused on wellness and healing, but it is ignored and disparaged in SaH, often referred to with the popular term 'New Age' for the same reasons, although ironically Tillich has been as influential to this tradition as to mainstream Protestantism—a testament to Tillich's ambiguity!

The challenge is for SaH is to recognize that the framework for the scientific study of spirituality need not and should not embody a particular theological stance. Furthermore, investigators must not allow their own personal spiritual commitments to influence their research. In the study of beliefs and practices it is prevalence and effects that are central, not a belief's 'truth' or how it conforms to current theory. Even if one accepted the common call for 'methodological atheism' or agnosticism,[120,121] based on the assumption that spiritual/religious beliefs are not testable, one could still investigate theistic and other 'supernatural' beliefs in useful ways. However, for the practically oriented domain of spirituality in healthcare the accuracy of beliefs sometimes has great importance, and some spiritual beliefs make empirical claims that can be studied. The very controversial topic of distant intercessory prayer studies illustrates this. Although the studies to date have problems, it is not obvious that the topic cannot be investigated productively. SaH might better follow Ninian Smart's advice that studies of spiritual matters need not be 'neutral, but simply open and pluralist'.[122, p. 23] The 'open and pluralist' stance might also encourage investigators to attend more to the negative potential of some spiritual factors.[73,123,124]

If the scope of field were broadened, a wide variety of disciplines and their methods would enter SaH. For example, the *Handbook of Religion and Health*[56] is presented as a comprehensive overview of research on the relationship of religion and health, but its index includes no references to the disciplines of anthropology or history, fields with extensive literatures on spirituality and health. The 'Research Methods' chapter notes qualitative methods and grants they can be helpful for generating hypotheses, but there is no discussion of ethnography or historical methods. Medical anthropology and medical history are absent along with many other relevant disciplines. The inclusion of the omitted topics noted above would immediately bring these fields, their methods and their extensive literatures into view in SaH. With the exception of medical anthropology and medical sociology these other fields have not concentrated on yielding clinically useful results, but their inclusion would be salutary in both directions. Just as medical interest created the enormously productive field of medical ethics, so might we expect inclusion to encourage anthropologists, linguists, historians and other scholars to develop applied approaches in SaH.

Acknowledgement

The research on which this manuscript was based was supported in part by Award Number W81XWH-08–1-0615 (United States Army Medical Research Acquisition Activity) to the Samueli Institute in Alexandria, Virginia, and the writing of this manuscript was supported by the Center for Brain, Mind and Healing of the Samueli Institute.

References

1 DeVinne, P.B, (ed.) (1991). *The American Heritage Dictionary of the English Language*, 2nd College edn. Boston: Houghton Mifflin Co. Methodology, p. 791.

2 Brown, L, editor. (1993). *The New Shorter Oxford English Dictionary on Historical Principles*, p. 1178. Oxford: Clarendon Press.

3 Fowler, D.N., Rountree, M.A. (2010). Exploring the meaning and role of spirituality for women survivors of intimate partner abuse. *J Past Care Counsel* **64**(2): 3.1–13. Available at: http://www.researchgate.net (accessed 7 July 2011).

4 Hufford, D. (2011). *An Analysis of the Field of Spirituality, Religion and Health* (S/RH). Available at: http://www.templetonadvancedresearchprogram.com/field.analyses.htm (accessed 5 May 2011).

5 Hufford, D. (2010). Strengths and weaknesses in the field of spirituality and health. In: W. Grassie (ed.) *Advanced Methodologies in the Scientific Study of Religion and Spirituality*, pp. 73–116. Philadelphia: Metanexus Institute.

6 King, M.B., Koenig, H.G. (2009). Conceptualising spirituality for medical research and health service provision. *BMC Hlth Serv Res* **9**: 116. Available at: http://www.biomedcentral.com/1472–6963/9/116 (accessed 4 May 2011).

7 Elder, L. (2000). Why some Jehovah's Witnesses accept blood and conscientiously reject official Watchtower Society blood policy. *J Med Eth* **26**: 375–80.

8 Erren, T.C. (2007). The case for *a posteriori* hypotheses to fuel scientific progress. *Med Hypoth* **69**(2): 448–53.

9 Bonaguidi, F., Michelassi, C., Filipponi, F., Rovai, D. (2010). Religiosity associated with prolonged survival in liver transplant recipients. *Liver Transpl* **16**(10): 1158–63.

10 Freud, S. (1928). *The Future of an Illusion*. London: Hogarth Press.

11 Larson, D.B., Pattison, E.M., Blazer, D.G., Omran, A.R., Kaplan, B.H. (1986). Systematic analysis of research on religious variables in four major psychiatric journals, 1978–1982. *Am J Psychiat* **143**: 329–4.

12 Larson, D.B., Sherrill, K.A., Lyons, J.S., Craigie, F.C., *et al.* (1992). Dimensions and valences of measures of religious commitment found in the *American Journal of Psychiatry and the Archives of General Psychiatry*, 1978–1989. *Am J Psychiat* **149**: 557–9.

13 Townsend, M., Kladder, V., Ayele, H., Mulligan, T. (2002). Systematic review of clinical trials examining the effects of religion on health. *Sthn Med J* **95**(12): 1429–34.

14 Weaver, A.J., Samford, J.A., Larson, D.B., Lucas, L.A., Koenig, H.G., Patrick, V. (1998). A systematic review of research on religion in four major psychiatric journals: 1991–1995. *J Nerv Ment Dis* **186**(3): 187–90.

15 Flannelly, K.J., Koenig, H.G., Ellison, C.G., Galek, K., Krause, N. (2006). Belief in life after death and mental health: findings from a national survey. *J Nerv Ment Dis* **194**(7): 524–9.

16 Selye, H. (1950). Stress and the general adaptation syndrome. *Br Med J* **1**(4667): 1383–92.

17 Cannon, W. (1942). 'Voodoo' death. Am Anthropolog **44** (new series): 169–81.

18 Lazarus, R. (1966). *Psychological Stress and the Coping Process*. New York: McGraw-Hill.

19 Lazarus, Richard, S. (1991). Progress on a cognitive-motivational-relational theory of emotion. *Am Psycholog* **46**(8): 819–34.

20 Exline, J.J (2002). The picture is getting clearer, but is the scope too limited? Three overlooked questions in the psychology of religion. *Psychol Inquiry* **13**: 245–7.

21 Beardsley, C., (2009). 'In need of further tuning': using a US patient satisfaction with chaplaincy instrument in a UK multi-faith setting, including the bereaved. *Clin Med* **9**(1): 53–8.

22 SUNY Downstate Medical Center. *Guide to Research Methods: The Evidence Pyramid*. Available at http://library.downstate.edu/EBM2/2100.htm (accessed 12 June 2011).

23 Levinton, L.C., Cook, T.D. (1981). What differentiates meta-analysis from other forms of review? *J Personal* **49**: 231–6.

24 Masters, K.S., Spielmans, G.I., Goodson, J.T. (2006). Are there demonstrable effects of distant intercessory prayer? A meta-analytic review. *Ann Behav Med* **32**: 21–6.

25 McCaffrey, A.M., Eisenberg, D.M., Legedza, A.T.R, Davis, R.B., Phillips, R.S. (2004). Prayer for health concerns: results of a national survey of prevalence and patterns of use. *Arch Intern Med* **164**L 858–62.

26 Rosenthal, R. (1976). *Experimenter Effects in Behavioral Research*. New York: Irvington.

27 Boelens, P.A., Reeves, R.R., Replogle, W.H., Koenig, H.G. (2009). A randomized trial of the effect of prayer on depression and anxiety. *Int J Psychiat Med* **39**(4): 377–92.

28 Schnall, E, Wassertheil-Smoller, S., Swencionic, C., *et al.* (2010). The relationship between religion and cardiovascular outcomes and all-cause mortality in the Women's Health Initiative Observational Study. **25**(2), 249–63.

29 Sisask, M., Varnik, A., Kolves, K, Zemon, V., Tinker, L., O'Sullivan, M.J., *et al.* (2010). Is religiosity a protective factor against attempted suicide: A cross-cultural case-control study. *Arch Suicide Res* **14**(1): 44–55.

30 Glueckauf, R.L., Davis, W.S., Allen, K., Chipi, P., Schettini, G., Tegen, L., *et al.* (2009). Integrative cognitive-behavioral and spiritual counseling for rural dementia caregivers with depression. *Rehab Psychol* **54**(4): 449–61.

31 Bekelman, D.B., Rumsfeld, J.S., Havranek, E.P., (2009). Symptom burden, depression, and spiritual wellbeing: a comparison of heart failure and advanced cancer patients. *J Gen Intern Med* **24**(5): 592–8.

32 Hill, T.D. (2008). Religious involvement and healthy cognitive aging: Patterns, explanations, and future directions. *J Gerontol Series A—Biolog Sci Med Sci* **63**(5): 478–9.

33 The faith factor: mind/body pioneer Herbert Benson on the health benefits of spirituality. Shambala Sun, July 1998. Available at: http://www.shambhalasun.com/index.php?option = com_content&task=view&id=1987&Itemid=0 (accessed 20 July 2011).

34 Leuba, J.H. (1912). *The Psychological Study of Religion: Its Origin, Function, and Future.* New York: Macmillan.

35 Harrell, D.E., Jr. (1975). *All Things are Possible: The Healing and Charismatic Revivals in Modern America.* Bloomington: Indiana University Press.

36 Eurobarometer Poll (2005). Social values, science, and technology. Available at: http://ec.europa.eu/public_opinion/archives/ebs/ebs_225_report_en.pdf (accessed 15 July 2011).

37 Jonas, W.B. (2001). The evidence house: how to build an inclusive base for complementary medicine. *West J Med* **175**(2): 79–80.

38 Jonas, W.B. (2005). Building an evidence house: challenges and solutions to research in complementary and alternative medicine. *Forsch Komplement Klass Naturh* **12**(3): 159–67.

39 Dossey, L. (1993). *Healing Words: The Power of Prayer and the Practice of Medicine.* San Francisco: Harper Collins.

40 Dossey, L. (1999). *Reinventing Medicine.* San Francisco: Harper.

41 Dossey, L. (2000). Prayer and medical science. *Arch Intern Med* **160**: 1735–8.

42 Gardner, R. (1983). Miracles of healing in Anglo-Celtic Northumbria as recorded by the Venerable Bede and his contemporaries: a reappraisal in the light of twentieth century experience. *Br Med J (Clin Res Ed)* **287**(6409): 1927–33.

43 Fuller, R.C. (1989). *Alternative Medicine and American Religious Life.* New York: Oxford University Press.

44 Fuller, R.C. (2001). *Spiritual, but not Religious: Understanding Unchurched America.* New York: Oxford University Press.

45 Frohock, F.M. (1992). *Healing Powers: Alternative Medicine, Spiritual Communities, and the State.* Chicago: University of Chicago Press.

46 Grossoehme, D.H., Ragsdale, J., Wooldridge, J.L., Cotton, S., Seid, M. (2010). We can handle this: parents' use of religion in the first year following their child's diagnosis with cystic fibrosis. *J Hlthcare Chaplaincy* **16**(3–4): 95–108.

47 Grossoehme, D.H., Ragsdale, J., Cotton, S., Wooldridge, J.L., Grimes, Seid, M. (2010) Parents' religious coping styles in the first year after their child's cystic fibrosis diagnosis. *J Hlthcare Chaplaincy* **16**(3–4): 109–22.

48 Brady, M.J., Peterman, A.H., Fitchet, G., Mo, M., Cella, D. (1999). A case for including spirituality in quality of life measurement in oncology. *Psycho-Oncol* **8**(5): 417–28.

49 Carlson, L.E., Speca, M., Patel, K.D., Goodey, E. (2003). Mindfulness-based stress reduction in relation to quality of life, mood, symptoms of stress, and immune parameters in breast and prostate cancer outpatients. *Psychosom Med* **65**(4): 571–81.

50 Demierre, M.F., Kim, Y.H., Zackheim, H.S. (2003). Prognosis, clinical outcomes and quality of life issues in cutaneous T-cell lymphoma. *Hematol-Oncol Clin N Am* **17**(6): 1485–507.

51 Tate, D.G., Forchheimer, M. (2002). Quality of life, life satisfaction, and spirituality: comparing outcomes between rehabilitation and cancer patients. *Am J Phys Med Rehab* **81**(6): 400–10.

52 King, M., Jones, L., Barnes, K., Low, J., Walker, C., Wilkinson, S., *et al.* (2006). Measuring spiritual belief: development and standardization of a Beliefs and Values Scale. *Psychol Med* **36**(3): 417–25.

53 Bormann, J., Warren, K.A., Regalbuto, L., Glaser, D., Kelly, A., Schnack, J., *et al.* (2009). A spiritually based caregiver intervention with telephone delivery for family caregivers of veterans with dementia. *Fam Comm Hlth* **32**(4): 345–53.

54 Larson, D.B., Swyers, J.P., McCullough, M.E., editors. (1998). *Scientific Research on Spirituality and Health: A Consensus Report.* Rockville: National Institute for Healthcare Research.

55 George, L.K., Larson, D.B., Koeing, H.G., McCullough, M.E. (2000). Spirituality and health: what we know, what we need to know. *J Soc Clin Psychol* **19**(1): 102–16.

56 Koenig, H.G., McCullough, M.E., Larson, D.B. (2001). *Handbook of Religion and Health.* Oxford: Oxford University Press.

57 Zinnbauer, E.J., Pargament, K.I., Cole, B., *et al.* (1998). Religion and spirituality: unfuzzying the fuzzy. *J Scient Study Relig* **36**: 459–64.

58 Egbert, N., Mickley, J., Coeling, H. (2004). A review and application of social scientific measures of religiosity and spirituality: assessing a missing component in health communication research. *Hlth Commun.* **16**(1): 7–27.

59 Pargament, K.I. (1996). *What is the Difference Between Religiousness and Spirituality?* Toronto: Symposium conducted at the annual meeting of the American Psychological Association.

60 Emblen, J.D. (1992). *Religion* and *spirituality* defined according to current use in the nursing literature. *J Profess Nurs* **8**(1): 41–7.

61 Unruh, A.M. (2002). Spirituality unplugged: a review of commonalities and contentions, and a resolution. *Canad J Occupat Ther* **69**(1): 5–19.

62 Skeat, W.W. (1909). *An Etymological Dictionary of the English Language.* Oxford: Clarendon Press.

63 Blum and Weprin Associates (2001). A national survey. Spiritual Hlth, (Spring):28.

64 Gallup Organization. (1999). Americans remain very religious, but not necessarily in conventional ways. Available at: http://www.gallup.com/poll/3385/Americans-Remain-Very-Religious-Necessarily-Conventional-Ways.aspx (accessed 1 August 2011).

65 Butler, J. (1990). *Awash in a Sea of Faith.* Cambridge: Harvard University Press.

66 Schmidt, L.E. (2005). *Restless Souls: The Making of American Spirituality.* New York: Harper Collins.

67 Ahlstrom, S. (1972). *A Religious History of the American People.* New Haven: Yale University Press.

68 Kemkes-Grottenthaler, A. (2003). God, faith, and death: The impact of biological and religious correlates on mortality. *Hum Biol* **75**(6): 897–915.

69 Latkovic, M.S., Nelson, T.A. (2001). Conjoined twins of Malta: a survey of Catholic opinion. *Nat Cathol Bioeth Q* **1**(4): 585–614.

70 Panicola, M.R. (2001). Withdrawing nutrition and hydration. The Catholic tradition offers guidance for the treatment of patients in a persistent vegetative state. *Hlth Progr* **82**(6): 28–33.

71 White, S.V., Savitsky, M.J. (2003). Interview with a quality leader. Sister Mary Jean Ryan on the first Baldrige Award in healthcare. *J Hlthcare Qual* **25**(3): 24–5.

72 Hufford, D.J. (1985). Ste. Anne de Beaupre: Roman Catholic pilgrimage and healing. *West Folklore* **44**: 194–207.

73 Pargament, K.L. (1997). *The Psychology of Religion and Coping: Theory, Research and Practice.* New York: Guilford Press.

74 Geertz, C. (1973). *The Interpretation of Cultures.* New York: Basic Books.

75 Barnes, P.M., Powell-Griner, E., McFann, K., Nahin, R.L. (2004). *Complementary and alternative medicine use among adults: United States, 2002. Advance Data from Vital and Health Statistics (343).* Available from http://www.cdc.gov/nchs/data/ad/ad343.pdf (accessed 1 August 2011).

76 Fetzer Institute. (1999). *Multidimensional Measurement of Religiousness/Spirituality for Use in Health Research.* Kalamazoo: John E. Fetzer Institute.

77 Flannelly, K.J., Galek, K., Ellison, C.G., Koenig, H.G. (2010). Beliefs about God, psychiatric symptoms, and evolutionary psychiatry. *J Relig Hlth* **49**: 246–61.

78 Hufford, D. (2010). Visionary spiritual experiences in an enchanted world. *Anthropol Hum* **35**(2): 142–58.

79 Alvarado, K.A., Templer, D.I., Bresler, C., Thomas-Dobson, S. (1995). The relationship of religious variables to death depression and death anxiety. *J Clin Psychol* **51**: 202–4.

80 Schafer, W.E. (1997). Religiosity, spirituality, and personal distress among college students. *J Coll Student Devel* **38**: 633–44.

81 O'Connor, B. (1997). Defining and describing complementary and alternative medicine. *Altern Therap Hlth Med* **3**(2): 49–57.

82 Astin, J. (1998). Why patients use alternative medicine: results of a national survey. *J Am Med Ass* **19**: 1548–53.

83 Eisenberg, D.M., Davis, R.B., Ettner, S.L., Appel, S., Wilkey, S., Van Rompay, M., *et al.* (1998). Trends in alternative medicine use in the United States 1990–1997. *J Am Med Ass* **280**: 1569–75.

84 Eisenberg, D.M., Kessler, R.C., Foster, C., Norlock, F.E., Calkins, D.R., Delbanco, T.L. (1993). Unconventional medicine in the United States. *N Engl J Med* **328**(4): 246–79.

85 Fox, M. (2002). *Religion, Spirituality and the Near-death Experience.* New York: Routledge.

86 Holden, J.M., Greyson, B., James, D., Editors (2009). *The Handbook of Near-death Experiences.* Santa Barbara: Praeger Publishers.

87 Rees, D. (1971). The hallucinations of widowhood. *Br Med J* **4**(5778): 37–41.

88 Rees, D. (2001). *Death and Bereavement: The Psychological, Religious and Cultural Interfaces*, 2nd edn. London: Whur Publishers.

89 Hufford, D. (1982). *The Terror That Comes in the Night: An Experience-centered Study of Supernatural Assault Traditions.* Philadelphia: University of Pennsylvania Press.

90 Hufford, D. (2005). Sleep paralysis as spiritual experience. *Transcult Psychiat* **42**(1): 11–45.

91 Hufford, D. (1985). Commentary: mystical experience in the modern world. In: The World Was Flooded with Light: A Mystical Experience Remembered, pp. 87–183. Pittsburgh: University of Pittsburgh Press.

92 van Lommel, P., van Wees, R., Meyers, V., Elfferich, I. (2001). Near-death experience in survivors of cardiac arrest: a prospective study in the Netherlands. *Lancet* **358**(9298): 2039–45.

93 Greyson, B. (1983). The near-death experience scale: construction, reliability, and validity. *J Nerv Ment Dis* **171**(6): 369–75.

94 Kohls, N., Walach, H. (2008). Validating four standard scales in spiritually practising and non-practising samples using propensity score matching. *Eur J Psycholog Assess* **24**(3): 165–73.

95 Kohls, N., Walach, H., Wirtz, M. (2009). The relationship between spiritual experiences, transpersonal trust, social support, and sense of coherence and mental distress—a comparison of spiritually practising and non-practising samples. *Ment Hlth, Relig Cult* **12**(1): 1–23.

96 Hufford, D.J., Fritts, M.J., Rhodes, J.E. (2010). Spiritual fitness. In: W.B. Jonas, G. O'Connor, P. Deuster, C. Macedonia (eds) Military Medicine, pp. 175, 733–87. Supplement: *Total Force Fitness.*

97 Bultmann, R. (1953). The New Testament and mythology. In: H. W. Bartsch (ed.) *Kerygma and Myth*, pp. 1–44. Transl. by R.H. Fuller. London: SPCK.

98 Stark, R. (1963). On the incompatibility of religion and science: a survey of American graduate students. *J Scient Study Relig* **3**: 3–20.

99 Steering Committee on Science and Creationism, National Academy of Science. (1984). *Science and Creationism: A View from the National Academy of Science.* Atlanta: National Academies Press.

100 Ecklund, E.H. (2010). *Science vs. Religion: What Scientists Really Think.* Oxford: Oxford University Press.

101 Gross, N., Solon, S. (2009). The religiosity of American college and university professors. *Sociol Relig* **70**(2): 101–29.

102 Barbour, I.G. (2000). *When Science Meets Religion.* New York: HarperCollins.

103 Farah, M.J., Murphy, N. (2009) Neuroscience and the Soul (Letter). *Science* **323**: 1168.

104 Freud, S. (1959). Obsessive actions and religious practices (1907). In: J. Strachey (ed. and transl.) *The Standard Edition of the Complete Psychological Works of Sigmund Freud*, Vol. IX, pp. 126–7. London: Hogarth.

105 Daaleman, T.P., Frey, B. (1999). Spiritual and religious beliefs and practices of family physicians: a national survey. *J Fam Pract* **48**(2): 98–104.

106 Curlin, F.A., Sellergren, S.A., Lantos, J.D., Chin, M.H. (2007). Physicians' observations and interpretations of the influence of religion and spirituality on health. *Arch Intern Med* **167**(7): 649–54.

107 Louis Finkelstein Institute for Religious and Social Studies at the Louis Stein Center. Survey of physicians' views on miracles. Available at: http://www.jtsa.edu/research/finkelstein/surveys/physicians.html (accessed 21 April 2005).

108 Ehman, J.W., Ott, B.B., Short, T.H., Ciampa, R.C., Hansen-Flaschen, J. (1999). Do patients want physicians to inquire about their spiritual or religious beliefs if they become gravely ill? *Arch Intern Med* **159**: 1803–6.

109 MacLean, C.D., Susi, B., Phifer, N., Schultz, L., Bynum, D., Franco, M., *et al.* (2003). Patient preference for physician discussion and practice of spirituality. *J Gen Intern Med* **8**(1): 38–43.

110 Sloan, R.P., Bagiella, E. (2001). Religion and health [comment]. *Hlth Psychol* **20**(3): 228–9.

111 Sloan, R.P., Bagiella, E. (2001). Spirituality and medical practice: a look at the evidence. *Am Fam Physic* **63**(1): 33–4.

112 Sloan, R.P., Bagiella, E. (2002). Claims about religious involvement and health outcomes. *Ann Behav Med* **24**(1): 14–21.

113 Sloan, R.P., Bagiella, E. (2004). The literature on religion and health: caveat emptor [comment]. *J Past Care Counsel* **58**(3): 271–6.

114 Sloan, R.P., Bagiella, E., Powell, T. (1999). Religion, spirituality and medicine. *Lancet* **353**: 664–7.

115 Sloan, R.P., Bagiella, E., VandeCreek, L., Hover, M., Casalone, C., Jinpu Hirsch, T., *et al.* (2000). Should physicians prescribe religious activities? *N Engl J Med* **342**(25): 1913–16.

116 Sherrill, K.A., Larson, D.B. (1994). The anti-tenure factor in religious research in clinical epidemiology and aging. In: J. S. Levin (ed.), Religion in Aging and Health, pp. 149–77. Thousand Oaks: Sage Publications.

117 Tillich, P. (1952). *The Courage to Be.* New Haven: Yale University Press.

118 Tillich, P. (1957). *Dynamics of Faith.* New York: Harper and Row.

119 Thomas, O.C. (2000). Some problems in contemporary Christian spirituality. *Anglic Theolog Rev* **82**: 267–81.

120 Berger, P.L. (1967). *The Sacred Canopy: Elements of a Sociological Theory of Religion.* Garden City: Doubleday.

121 Kunin, S.D. (2003). *Religion; the Modern Theories.* Edinburgh: University of Edinburgh Press.

122 Smart, N. (2009). *Ninian Smart on World Religions*, Vol. 1: Religious Experience and Philosophical Analysis, J.J. Shepherd (ed.). London: Ashgate.

123 Pargament, K.I., Kennell, J., Hathaway, W., Grevengoed, N., Newman, J., Jones, W. (1988). Religion and the problem-solving process: Three styles of coping. *J Sci Study Relig* **27**: 90–104.

124 Pargament, K.I., Ensing, D.S., Falgout, K., *et al.* (1990). God help me (I): religious coping efforts as predictors of the outcomes to significant negative life events. *Am J Comm Psychol***18**: 798–824.

CHAPTER 44

Measures

Arndt Büssing

Introduction

There are various instruments which were developed to measure spirituality/religiosity (SpR) in their unique context, either on religious studies, theology, psychology, sociology, medicine, nursing, etc. These instruments differ not only with respect to their underlying concepts of SpR.

For research, it is useful to distinguish between spirituality and religiosity. Spirituality is a complex and multi-dimensional construct, and can be defined as an open and individual experiential approach in the search for meaning and purpose in life (content). In contrast, religion is an institutional and culturally determined approach, which organizes the collective experiences of people (faith) into a closed system of beliefs and practices (form). Spirituality can be found through religious engagement, through an individual experience of the divine, and/or through a connection to others, environment, and the sacred. One could differentiate between spirituality *in* religion (which connotes a more open, individual and pluralistic faith) and spirituality as opposed to religion (which rejects organized religiosity).

Conceptualizations

Spirituality can be globally defined as humans' search for meaning in life, while religion involves an organized entity with rituals and practices about a higher power or God.[1] Spirituality can also be described as an 'individual and open approach in the search for meaning and purpose in life, as a search for "transcendental truth", which may include a sense of connectedness with others, nature, and/or the divine.'[2] Also Pargament argued that spirituality is the search for significance in ways related to the sacred.[3] Koenig stated that spirituality can then be found through religious engagement, through an individual experience of the divine, and/or through a connection to nature.[4]

We defined recently:[5] Spirituality refers to an attitude of search for meaning in life. The searching individual is aware of its divine origin (either transcendent or immanent, i.e. God, Allah, JHWH, Tao, Brahman, Prajna, Unity, etc.), and feels a connection with others, nature and the Divine, etc. Because of this awareness one strives towards the realization (either formal or informal) of the respective teachings, experiences or insight, which have a direct impact on conduct of life and ethical commitments.' A similar attempt was presented by Engebretson:[6] 'Spirituality is the experience of the sacred other, which is accompanied by feelings of wonder, joy, love, trust and hope. Spirituality enhances connectedness within the self, with others and with the world. Spirituality illuminates lived experience. Spirituality may be expressed in relationships, prayer, personal and communal rituals, values, service, action for justice, connection with the earth. Spirituality may be named in new and redefined ways or through the beliefs, rituals, symbols, values, stories of religious traditions'.

A recent empirical attempt to analyse which aspects of spirituality are of relevance also in secular societies identified 7 main dimensions:[7]

- prayer, trust in God and shelter
- insight, awareness and wisdom
- transcendence conviction
- compassion, generosity and patience
- conscious interactions
- gratitude, reverence and respect
- equanimity.

Thus, spirituality is not only the 'experiential core' (content) of ritualized religiosity (form), but in fact a complex construct which shares relevant topics with secular aspects of spirituality. Therefore, the required broader conceptualizations of spirituality/religiosity may be less specific and the underlying constructs may overlap. Nevertheless, because of the trend to individualization and secularization, and thus often rejection of ecclesiastic approaches with subsequent development of new forms of 'secular spirituality' or even 'religious patchwork', there is a need for adequate measures of the 'un-measurable' which are suited also for secular societies.

The traditional view assumes spirituality as the core of any religion, and both contrast with secular attitudes (Figure 44.1A). In fact, a profound spiritual experience (content) is highly individual and not easily communicated and shared by a group of individuals who lack this unique experience. Nevertheless, they may share similar rituals and forms of practice within a referential system of interpretation (form). Today spirituality is often viewed as an individual, non-formal approach which contrasts with formal institutional religiosity (Figure 44.1B). In a more secular context,

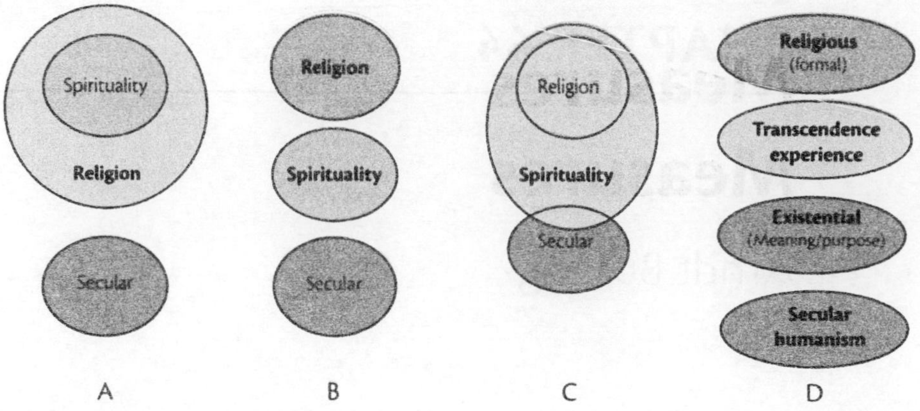

Figure 44.1 Different concepts to address spirituality and religiosity.

spirituality can be viewed as a general concept which includes religiosity and may share defined aspects with secular forms of spirituality (Figure 44.1C); however, this 'all inclusive' conceptualization is difficult to measure.

If it is true that spirituality/religiosity can have an impact on mortality,[8] one has to ask which aspect of spirituality/religiosity. The systematic review of Chida *et al.*[8] indicated that organizational activities (i.e. involvement in religious community and attendance at services) were associated with better survival, while neither non-organizational activities such prayer, meditation, study of sacred books, nor intrinsic aspects were effective. On the other hand, it is unclear whether secular forms of spirituality may have an impact too, particular in secular societies with reduced engagement in organizational religious activities. Thus, it is important for future studies to differentiate actional aspects of spirituality (i.e. frequency of engagement in specific forms of spirituality) and cognitive/emotional aspects (i.e. specific attitudes and convictions). These aspects could be measured as independent dimensions, i.e. formal religiosity, experiential aspect of spirituality, existential aspects (meaning and purpose), and secular humanism (Figure 44.1D)—with respect to cognition, emotion, and behaviour. While this differentiation (spirituality versus religiosity) is important in countries with a more secular and liberal background (i.e. Europe), this distinction is meaningless in countries with conservative, but vital theistic beliefs.

The aim of this chapter is to pay attention to established instruments which measure aspects of spirituality/religiosity in the context of health care, but also to describe unique features and intentions of newly developed instruments which may have potential to be used in larger studies to develop knowledge relevant for spiritual care and practice.

Categorization of questionnaires

There are different ways to categorize the available instruments (Table 44.1). One a first glance one may differentiate generic instruments which measure SpR in general populations, or contextual questionnaires addressing spirituality/religiosity as a strategy to cope with illness.

With respect to the underlying aspects, one may differentiate:

- Intensity of attitudes/convictions and experiences
- Frequency of distinct practices/activities
- Spiritual wellbeing and meaning/purpose
- Coping strategies and resources
- Psychosocial and spiritual needs.

Before one chooses an instrument, one has to consider the purpose and context of the intended assessment:

1. Is it used in healthy populations or in patients with distinct (chronic) diseases?
2. Is the focus of the intended assessment spiritual wellbeing, spiritual coping, intensity of distinct attitudes, or the differentiation of practices (forms and frequency)?
3. Is the intention of the study to make a diagnosis (spiritual distress, spiritual needs), or is it to evaluate the effects of distinct spiritual interventions in a unique health care setting?
4. What are the modalities of the assessment, i.e. self-administered standardized questionnaires for research purpose (Table 44.1), or semi-structured interview tools to assess patients' spiritual history in the clinic (i.e. FICA)?[59]

One has to be aware that spirituality is a highly subjective and multidimensional construct which shares several aspects of psycho-social wellbeing,[60,61] i.e. self-awareness, stress adjustment, relationships/connectedness, sense of faith, meaning and hope, etc. Thus, particularly spiritual wellbeing may overlap with mental health associated dimensions. Another pitfall for research is the fact that the conceptual background of several instruments refer to an exclusive Judeo-Christian perspective or a specific belief in God, while there are just a few assessment tools that refer to a broader concept of spirituality. Particularly in more secular or diverse societies the former instruments may not accurately map patients' spirituality. It is thus an option to use assessment tools which cover a larger spectrum of specific aspects of the complex whole.

Short description of validated instruments

For this description, the questionnaires suited for health care research were identified as generic or contextual instruments, and categorized according to five major categories, i.e. (1) intensity, (2) wellbeing, (3) resource, (4) coping strategy, and (5) needs (Table 44.1).

Table 44.1 Selected instruments to measure aspects of spirituality/religiosity

Author	Instrument	Scales	Comments
Allport and Ross[9]	Religious Orientation Scale (ROS)	20 items, 2(-3) factors: Intrinsic; Extrinsic; (Indiscriminately Pro-religious)	Generic; Intensity
Hoge et al. [10]	Intrinsic Religious Motivation Scale	10 items, 1 scale	Generic; intensity
Paloutzian and Ellison [11]	Spiritual Wellbeing Scale (SWBS)	20 items, 2 scales: Religious; Existential	Generic; wellbeing
Idler [12]	Idler Index of Religiosity (IIR)	4 items, 2 scales: public religiousness; private religiousness	Generic; intensity
Gomez and Fisher[13,14]	Spiritual Wellbeing Questionnaire (SWBQ)	20 items, 4 scales: personal, transcendental, environmental, communal wellbeing	Generic; wellbeing
Holland *et al.* [15]	Systems of Belief Inventory (SBI-15R)	5 items, 2 scales: spiritual beliefs and practices; support from a religious/spiritual community	Generic; intensity
Reed *et al.* [16,17]	Spiritual Perspective Scale (SPS)	10 items: frequency of SpR activities; role of SpR in daily life	Generic; intensity
Batson and Schoenrade[18]	Quest scale	12 items, 3 subscales: readiness to face existential questions, self-criticism and perception of religious doubts as positive, Openness to change	Generic; intensity
Genia[19] Genia and Cooke [20]	Spiritual Experience Index (SEI)	23/38 items, 2 scales: spiritual support, spiritual openness	Generic; intensity
Veach and Chappel[21]	Spiritual Health Inventory (SHI)	18 item scale: personal spiritual experience, spiritual well-being, sense of harmony, and personal helplessness	Generic; intensity and wellbeing
Kass *et al.* [22,23]	Index of Core Spiritual Experiences (INSPIRIT)	6 items, 1 checklist of 12 spiritual experiences: experiential and relational aspects	Generic; intensity
Plante *et al.* [24–26]	Santa Clara Strength of Religious Faith Questionnaire (SCSORF)	10 items, 1 scale	Generic; intensity
Pargament *et al.* [27,28]	Brief RCOPE	10 items, 2 scales: positive/negative religious coping	Generic; coping
Koenig *et al.* [29]	Duke Religious Index (DRI)	5 item Index: organizational, non-organizational, and intrinsic religiosity	Generic; intensity
Belschner;[30] Albani *et al.* [31]	Transpersonal Trust (TPV)	11 items, 1 scale	Generic; intensity
Daalemann *et al.*[32] Daalemann and Frey[33]	Spirituality Index of Wellbeing (SIWB)	12 items, 2 scales: self-efficacy, life schema (i.e. meaning and purpose); psychological focus	Generic; wellbeing
Underwood and Teresi;[2] Underwood[34]	Daily Spiritual Experience Scale (DSES)	6 or 16 items, 1–2 scales	Generic; intensity
Peterman *et al.*;[35] Bredle *et al.*[36]	Functional Assessment of Chronic Illness Therapy—Spiritual Well-Being (FACIT-Sp)	12 items, 2 scales: faith, meaning/peace	Contextual; wellbeing
Ryan and Fiorito[37]	Means-ends Spirituality Questionnaire (M-E SQ)	MEANS scale: 17 items, 2 scales (devotional and transformational means); ENDS scale: 25 items, 5 scales (relationship with devine; protection against social loss; seeking a better self; protection against metaphysical punishment; avoiding life's ordinary challenges)	Generic; intensity
Huber[38,39]	Centrality of Religiosity (C-10; C-7)	10/7 items: 5 core dimensions (ideology, experience, private practice, public practice, intellect) and 2 indicators	Generic; intensity
Ostermann *et al.*,[40] Büssing *et al.*[41,42]	Spiritual/religious attitudes in dealing with illness (SpREUK)	15 items, 3 scales: search (for support/access to spirituality/ religiosity); trust (in higher guidance/source); reflection (positive interpretation of disease)	Contextual; resource
Büssing *et al.* [43–45]	Spiritual/religious practices (SpREUK-P)	17/25 items, 5 scales to measure forms and frequency of engagement: religious; (spiritual) mind/body; existentialistic; humanistic; gratitude/reverence	Generic; intensity
Galek *et al.*;[46] Flanelly *et al.* [47]	Spiritual Needs Assessment Scale	24 items, 6 factors: divine, appreciation of beauty; meaning/ purpose; love/belonging; death/resolution; positivity/ gratitude/hope/peace	Contextual; needs
Herrmann[48]	Spiritual Needs Inventory (SNI)	27/17 items, 5 factors: outlook; inspiration; spiritual activities; religion; community	Contextual; needs
Zwingmann et al.[49]	Scales of Religious Coping	16 items, 2 factors: positive religious coping; negative religious coping	Contextual; coping

Table 44.1 (*Cont'd*) Selected instruments to measure aspects of spirituality/religiosity

Author	Instrument	Scales	Comments
Büssing and Koenig[50]	BENEFIT Scale	6 items, 1 scale: support of patients' life concerns through SpR	Contextual; resource
Büssing *et al.*,[44,51]	Trust in God's Help (TGH) scale	5 items, 1 scale: coping strategy in the context of external locus of health control part (part of the AKU questionnaire)	Contextual; resource
Büssing *et al.* [52,53]	Aspects of Spirituality (ASP 2.0) Questionnaire	25 items, 4 scales: religious orientation (prayer/trust in God); search for insight/wisdom; conscious interactions; transcendence conviction	Generic; intensity
Yong *et al.*[54]	Spiritual needs	26 items, 5 factors: love/connection; hope/peace; meaning/purpose; relationship with God; acceptance of dying	Contextual; needs
Cole *et al.*[55]	Spiritual Transformation Scale (STS)	40 items, 2 scales: spiritual growth; spiritual decline	Contextual; intensity
Bowman *et al.* [56]	Cancer and Deity Questionnaire (CDQ)	12 items, 2 scales: benevolence; abandonment	Contextual; intensity
Büssing *et al.*,[57] Büssing and Koenig[58]	Spiritual Needs Questionnaire (SpNQ)	19 items, 4 factors: religious; existential (reflection/meaning); inner peace; actively giving (solace/forgiving)	Contextual; needs

Intensity of spiritual/religious attitudes, convictions and practices

Duke Religious Index (DRI)

The instrument assesses organized and non-organized religious activities, and intrinsic religiosity.[29,62]

Generic: 5 items with a 3-item intrinsic religiosity subscale (alpha = 0.75): i.e. experience presence of good, religious beliefs are what lies behind whole approach in life, carry religion over into all other dealings in life, and two items assessing the frequency of religious attendance (church/religious meetings) or private religious activities (praying, meditation, Bible reading).

The advantage of the index, its brevity, can be regarded as its limitation too, because particularly the measurement of organized and non-organized religious activities by a single item each reduces its reliability.

Daily Spiritual Experience Scale (DSES)

The instrument was developed for use in health studies as a measure a person's perception of the transcendent in daily life, and thus the items measure experience rather than particular beliefs or behaviours.[2,34]

Generic: 16 items, 2 factors (Cronbach's alpha = 0.94 and 0.95):[2] Relation to God (i.e. feel God's presence, guided by God, feel God's love, joy when connecting with God, etc.). Peace and Harmony (i.e. feel inner peace and harmony; touched by beauty of creation; connecting to all life, etc.); and 2 items (factor 2): Selfless caring, accept others.

Generic: 6 items, 1 factor (alpha = 0.91),[2] i.e. feel God's presence, God's love, desire to be closer to God (union), find strength / comfort in SpR, touched by beauty of creation.

The scale can be regarded as a measure of daily spiritual experiences for surveys (response categories: many times a day, every day, most days, some days, once in a while and never/almost never).

Santa Clara Strength of Religious Faith Questionnaire (SCSRFQ)

The instrument was designed to measure strength of religious faith, without assuming that the person is religious, or assuming that the person is of a specific religious denomination.[24,26]

Generic: 10 items (alpha = 0.95), 1 factor:[24,25,63], i.e. religious faith is important, daily praying, faith as a source of inspiration, faith as providing meaning and purpose, active in faith/church, faith is an important part of who I am as a person, relationship with God is extremely important, enjoy being around with others who share my faith, faith as a source of comfort, faith impacts decisions

Strength of the instrument is its exclusive focus on religious faith; it does not significantly correlate with depression or anxiety, or character traits.

Aspects of Spirituality (ASP)

To measure a wide variety of vital aspects of spirituality beyond conventional conceptual boundaries in more secular societies, expert representatives of various spiritual orientations (and also atheists) were asked which aspects of spirituality are relevant to them.[64] Identified motifs we condensed to 40 items of the Aspects of Spirituality (ASP) questionnaire (7 factors; Cronbach's alpha = 0.94),[52] which differentiates and quantifies cognitive, emotional, intentional and action-oriented matters of theism/belief, (esoteric) transcendence, existentialism, humanism etc. The shortened 25-item ASP 2.1 was re-validated in a sample of 1,191 healthy individuals.

Generic: 25 items, 4 factors.[53]

1. *Religious orientation* (alpha = 0.93), i.e. praying, guided and sheltered, trust in and turn to God, spiritual orientation in life, distinct rituals, reading SpR books, etc.
2. *Search for Insight/Wisdom* (alpha = 0.88), i.e. insight and truth, develop wisdom, beauty/goodness, frankness/wideness of the spirit, broad awareness, etc.
3. *Conscious interactions* (alpha = 0.83), i.e. conscious interactions with others, environment, self, compassion, generosity
4. *Transcendence conviction* (alpha = 0.85), i.e. existence of higher beings, rebirth of man/soul, soul origins in higher dimensions, man is a spiritual being

Strength of the instrument is the operationalization of non-formal aspects of spirituality in terms of relational consciousness, particularly secular humanism and existential awareness.

Forms and frequency of spiritual practices (SpREUK-P)

The instrument was designed to measure the engagement frequencies of a large spectrum of spiritual, religious, existential and philosophical practices.[43,44,65]

Generic: 17 items, 5 factors (SpREUK-P SF17):

1. *Religious* (alpha = 0.82), i.e. praying, church/mosque/synagogue attendance, religious events, religious symbols
2. *Humanistic* (alpha = 0.79), i.e. help others, consider their needs, do good, etc.
3. *Existential* (alpha = 0.77), i.e. self-realization, insight, meaning in life
4. *(Spiritual) mind/body* (alpha = 0.72), i.e. meditation, rituals, etc.
5. *Gratitude/reverence* (alpha = 0.77), i.e. feeling of gratitude, awe, experience beauty.

Strength of the instrument is the differentiation of both religious and secular forms of spirituality also in secular societies.

Spiritual Transformation Scale (STS)

The instrument was developed to measure changes in spiritual engagement in cancer patients.

Contextual: 40 items, 2 scales:[55]

1. *Spiritual growth* (alpha = 0.98), i.e. experience life around as spiritual, act more compassionately towards other people since my diagnosis, changed priorities, see own life as sacred, stronger sense of the Sacred, stronger connection to nature, pray for others, etc.
2. *Spiritual decline* (alpha = 0.86), i.e. spiritually lost, failed in faith, spirituality less important to me, etc.

The Spiritual Growth scale correlates strong with the Positive RCOPE, the Daily Spiritual Experiences Scale and the Posttraumatic Growth Inventory, while the Spiritual Decline scale correlated with the Negative RCOPE and depression.

Item wording is appropriate for individuals who identify themselves as spiritual rather than religious; the Growth scale contains also existential and humanistic issues.

Spiritual/religious wellbeing

Spiritual Well-Being Scale (SWBS)

The instrument was designed to assess people's perception of their own sense of spiritual wellbeing, either religious or nonreligious, in the context of quality of life respectively subjective wellbeing (Paloutzian and Ellision, 1982; Ellision 1983).[112,66]

Generic: 10 items, 2 subscales:[66]

1. *Religious wellbeing* (alpha = 0.87): self-assessment of one's relationship with God (i.e. private prayer, God loves and cares, meaningful relationship with God; God is concerned about my problems, satisfying relationship with God, etc.)
2. *Existential wellbeing* (alpha = 0.78): self-assessment of one's sense of life purpose and life satisfaction (i.e. life is a positive experience, unsettled about future, satisfied with life, enjoy much about life, life has meaning, purpose for life, etc.)

About half of the items are worded in a reversed direction. Ten items specifically rely on a personal God and thus at least the Religious scale is not appropriate in atheistic/agnostic individuals, while the Existential is suited also for secular societies.

Spiritual Well-Being Questionnaire (SWBQ)

The instrument was developed as a multidimensional instrument which is based on a broader conceptualization of spiritual wellbeing.[13,14]

Generic: 20 items, 4 subscales.[13,14]

1. *Personal* (alpha = 0.89), i.e. identity, self-awareness, joy in life, inner peace, meaning in life
2. *Transcendental* (alpha = 0.86), i.e. relation with God, worship of creator, oneness/peace with God, prayer
3. *Environmental* (alpha = 0.76), i.e. connect to nature, awe at view, oneness with nature, harmony with environment, see magic in environment
4. *Communal wellbeing* (alpha = 0.79), i.e. love towards people, forgive, trust, respect others, kindness to others.

Compared with Ellison's Spiritual Wellbeing Scale (SWBS), the Spiritual Wellbeing Questionnaire (SWBQ) more clearly differentiates existential wellbeing, and thus is of relevance also in secular societies. Although the scale was tested so far exclusively in healthy (younger) individuals, the instrument is worth to be used in health care research.

Functional Assessment of Chronic Illness Therapy-Spiritual (FACIT-Sp)

The instrument was developed to measure spiritual wellbeing,[35] and uses a careful language avoiding traditional religious terminology, without implying a very particular religious perspective.[36]

Contextual: 12 items, 2 subscales (alpha = 0.87):[35]

1. *Meaning/Peace* (alpha = 0.81), i.e. feel peaceful, peace of mind, have reason for living, life has been productive, purpose in life, meaning and purpose, comfort, harmony with myself)
2. *Faith* (alpha = 0.88), i.e. find comfort/strength in spiritual beliefs, illness has strengthened spiritual beliefs, whatever happens with illness, things will be alright.

The existential scale Meaning/Peace correlated strongly with mental health and weakly with physical health, while the Faith scale was just marginally associated with mental health, and not with the physical.[35,67,68]

Canada *et al.* [67] suggested a more appropriate 3-factor model, because Meaning addresses cognitive aspect of spirituality, while Peace is an affective component:

1. *Meaning*: i.e. have reason for living, life has been productive, purpose in life, life lacks meaning and purpose
2. *Peace*: i.e. feel peaceful, trouble feeling peaceful, feel comfort, harmony with myself
3. *Faith*: i.e. find comfort/strength in faith; difficult times has strengthened spiritual beliefs; whatever happens with illness, things will be alright.

Peace was strongly related only to mental health, while Meaning was weakly related to physical and mental health; in contrast, Faith was weakly (negatively) associated with mental health.

Particularly the Faith scale refers to experience of illness and thus is a contextual scale, while Meaning and Peace have to be regarded as generic scales. The FACIT-Sp lacks specific religious terminology and is appropriate for a diverse population.

Spirituality/religiosity as a resource

SpREUK: Spiritual/religious attitudes in dealing with illness

The instrument was developed to examine how patients with chronic diseases view the impact of spirituality/religiosity on their health and how they cope with illness, in terms of reactive coping.[11,40,41,44,53] It relies on essential motifs found in counselling interviews with chronic disease patients (i.e. having trust/faith; search for a transcendent source to rely on; hint to change life).[69]

Contextual: 15 items, 3 factors:[40]

1. *Search (for Support/Access to Spirituality/Religiosity)* (alpha = 0.91), deals with patients' search for a spiritual source to cope with illness (i.e. searching for an access to spirituality/religiosity; renewed interest; finding access to a spiritual source can have a positive influence on illness; urged to spiritual/religious insight whether disease may improve or not, etc.)
2. *Trust (in Higher Guidance/Source)* (alpha = 0.91) is a measure of intrinsic religiosity dealing with patients' view to be sheltered and guided by a transcendental source (i.e. whatever may happen, trust in a higher power which carries through; trust in spiritual guidance in life; feel connected with higher source, etc.)
3. *Reflection (Positive Interpretation of Disease)* (alpha = 0.86) deals with cognitive reappraisal because of illness and subsequent attempts to change (i.e. reflect on what is essential in life; hint to change life; chance for development; illness has meaning, etc.)

The instrument avoids exclusive religious terminology and appears to be a good choice for assessing patients' interest in spiritual/religious concerns which is not biased for or against a particular religious commitment. Particularly in Arabic Muslims and Orthodox Jews, the factors *Search* and *Trust* were interconnected, while differentiated in German patients with a Christian background.

The cognitive appraisal scale operationalizes the unique point of view that disease can be viewed as an opportunity, a hint to change life, or to reflect upon what is essential in life. Because of this reflection, patients may change aspects of their life or behaviour (transformation). Nevertheless, it is strongly inter-correlated with *Search* and *Trust* and thus has a spiritual connotation.

Benefit through spirituality/religiosity

The intention was to design a brief and compact scale which measures the beneficial effects of spirituality/religiosity on several dimensions of patients' life.[50]

Contextual: 6 items, 1 factor (alpha = 0.92): i.e. spirituality/religiosity helps to manage life more consciously, cope better with illness, deeper connection with others and the world around, spirituality/religiosity promotes inner strength, engaged in spirituality/religiosity restores mental and physical health; feeling of inner peace

The resource scale correlates strongly with SpREUK's *Trust* and *Search* scales, with frequency of *Religious Practices* and *Spiritual (Mind Body) Practices*, and just weakly with internal adaptive coping strategies such as *Conscious Living/Positive Attitudes*.[50] It correlates moderately with positive disease interpretations, and with patients' satisfaction with future perspectives and satisfaction with themselves.[70]

Spirituality/religiosity as a coping strategy

Religious coping (Brief RCOPE)

The instrument was developed to operationalize religious coping strategies to deal with religious struggles and life stressors.[71] The instrument needs three major strategies, collaborative (cooperation with God to deal with stressful events), deferring (everything is left to God), and self-directed (solve problems by own efforts).

Generic: 14 items, 2 scales:[71]

1. *Positive religious coping:* i.e. stronger connection with God; sought God's love and care; sought help from God in letting go of anger; put plans into action together with God; focused on religion to stop worrying about problems; forgiveness of sins, etc.
2. *Negative religious coping:* i.e. God had abandoned me; punished by God for lack of devotion; wondered what I did for God to punish me; questioned the power of God; questioned God's love; devil made this happen; wondered whether my church had abandoned me, etc.).

The instrument in its original version is appropriate for populations with a theistic background. There are attempts to operationalize the topic for individuals with a Buddhist background (Phillips *et al.*, 2009).[72] This BCOPE contains 66 items across 14 subscales (i.e. Morality, Sangha support, Loving kindness, Meditation, Mindfulness, Right understanding, Dharma, Impermanence, Interbeing, Not-self, Active karma, Passive karma, Bad Buddhist, Its not easy being Buddhist), and is also a measure of reactive coping. Preliminary findings with the BCOPE indicate that the addressed ways of dealing with stress predicted outcomes, better than demographic and general religious variables.

In a recent attempt to adapt Pargament's concept,[49] developed 16 items for the use in cancer patients avoiding strong religious phrases such as 'devil' or 'sin'. The instrument differentiates positive religious coping (alpha = 0.97; i.e. a confident and constructive turning to religion), and negative religious coping (alpha = 0.89; i.e. religious struggle and doubt).

Spiritual needs

Spiritual Needs Inventory (SNI)

The instrument was developed from a qualitative study of spiritual needs of dying patients.[48]

Contextual: 17 items, 5 factors (alpha = 0.85):

1. *Outlook* (alpha = 0.78), i.e. see the smiles of others, think happy thoughts, talk about day-to-day things, be around children, laugh
2. *Inspiration* (alpha = 0.76), i.e. talk with someone about spiritual issues, sing/listen to inspirational music, be with people who share spiritual beliefs, read a religious text
3. *Spiritual activities* (alpha = 0.68), i.e. use/inspirational material, phrases from religious text
4. *Religion* (alpha = 0.74), i.e. pray, religious services
5. *Community* (alpha = 0.62), i.e. be with friend/family, have information about family and friends.

An important feature of this instrument is the rating of needs (Never, Rarely, Sometimes, Frequently, Always), the assessment

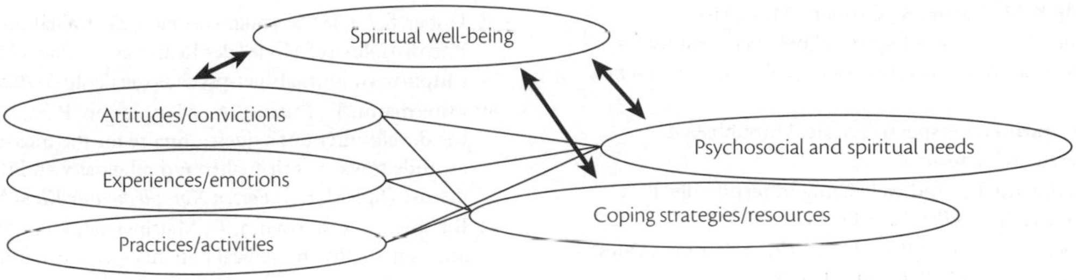

Figure 44.2 Spiritual issues to be addressed in research and clinic.

whether the respective activities are really a spiritual need to the patients, and whether these needs are met in the patients' life or not.

Spiritual Needs Questionnaire (SpNQ)

The intention was to develop an instrument addressing the spiritual needs of patients with chronic diseases in secular societies). [45,57,58]

Contextual: 19 items, 4 factors:

1. *Religious* (alpha = 0.90), i.e. praying for and with others, and by themselves, participate at a religious ceremony, reading religious/spiritual books, turning to a higher presence
2. *Inner peace* (alpha = 0.83), i.e. wish to dwell at places of quietness and pace, plunge into the beauty of nature, finding inner peace, talking with other about fears and worries, devotion by others
3. *Existential* (reflection/meaning) (alpha = 0.84) i.e. reflect previous life, talk with someone about meaning in life/suffering, dissolve open aspects in life, talk about the possibility of a life after death, etc.
4. *Actively giving* (alpha = 0.82) addresses the active and autonomous intention to solace someone, to give away something from yourself, and turning to others.

The patients rate whether they currently have the respective needs, and how strong they were to them. Spiritual needs are conceptually different from life satisfaction, and can be interpreted as the patients' longing for spiritual wellbeing.

Conclusion

Addressing patients' spirituality in health care can be done by semi-structured interviews, which have the benefit to provide more in-depth insights and engaging the patient in dialogue, or with standardized questionnaires, which have the benefit to compare the respective scores with those of other cohorts and studies. Each approach has advantages and limitations. When addressing spirituality in health care, one has to be aware that some instruments may share overlapping constructs.

Thus, one has to clearly define the intention of the assessment and to specify primary and secondary end points (to avoid weak design and statistical problems such as multiple testing, and false positive inter-correlations), and subsequent selection of appropriate instruments. Short and circumscribed measures can be easily integrated in larger studies, but may represent just a limited facet of a complex spectrum of spirituality/religiosity. In contrast, broader conceptualizations of spirituality/religiosity may require more differentiated measures, and thus a higher number of items and scales which are often difficult to integrate. Depending on your intention, one may choose either circumscribed uni-/bi-dimensional scales (diagnostic), or a wide spectrum of different aspects of spirituality (differentiating analyses) which have to fit to the spiritual context of culture and country.

Because spirituality/religiosity is a complex construct involving cognitive, emotional and behavioural aspects, one may address the following interconnected layers of spirituality (which all may have an impact on an individual's wellbeing and quality of life) with specific instruments as described above (Figure 44.2).

References

1 Tanyi, R.A. (2002). Nursing theory and concept development or analysis. Towards clarification of the meaning of spirituality. *J Adv Nurs* **39:** 500–9.

2 Underwood, L.G., Teresi, J.A. (2002). The Daily Spiritual Experience Scale: development, theoretical description, reliability, exploratory factor analysis, and preliminary construct validity using health-related data. *Ann Behav Med* **24:** 22–33.

3 Pargament, K.I. (1997). *The Psychology of Religion and Coping: Theory, Research, Practice.* New York: Guilford.

4 Koenig, H.G. (2008). Concerns about measuring 'spirituality' in research. *J Nerv Ment Dis* **196:** 349–55.

5 Büssing, A., Ostermann, T. (2004). Caritas und ihre neuen Dimensionen: Spiritualität und Krankheit. In: M. Patzek M (ed.) *Caritas plus. Qualität hat einen Namen*, pp.110–33. Kevelaer: Butzon & Bercker.

6 Engebretson, K. (2004). Teenage boys, spirituality and religion. *Int J Child Spiritual* **9:** 263–78.

7 Büssing, A., Ostermann, T. Matthiessen, P.F. (2007). Distinct expressions of vital spirituality. The ASP questionnaire as an explorative research tool. *J Relig Hlth* **46:** 267–86.

8 Chida, Y., Steptoe, A., Powell, L.H. (2009). Religiosity/spirituality and mortality. A systematic quantitative review. *Psychother Psychosom* **78:** 81–90.

9 Allport, G.W., Ross, J.M. (1967). Personal religious orientation and prejudice. *J Personal Soc Psychol* **5:** 432–43.

10 Hoge, D. (1972). A validated intrinsic religious motivation scale. *J Sci Study Relig* **11:** 369–76.

11 Paloutzian, R.F., Ellison, C.W. (1982). Loneliness, spiritual well-being and the quality of life. In: L.A. Peplau, D. Perlman, D. (eds) *Loneliness: A Sourcebook of Current Theory, Research and Therapy*, pp. 224–37. Harlow: Wiley-Interscience.

12 Idler, E. (1987). Religious involvement and the health of the elderly: some hypotheses and an initial test. *Soc Forces* **66:** 226–38.

13 Gomez, R., Fisher, J.W. (2003). Domains of spiritual well-being and development and validation of the Spiritual Well-Being Questionnaire. *Personal Individ Diff* **35:** 1975–91.

14 Gomez, R., Fisher, J.W. (2005). The Spiritual Well-Being Questionnaire: testing for model applicability, measurement and structural equivalencies and latent mean differences across gender. *Personal Individ Diff* **39:** 1383–93.

15 Holland, J.C., Kash, K.M., Passik, S., Gronert, M.K., Sison, A., Lederberg, M., *et al.* (1998). A brief spiritual beliefs inventory for use in quality of life research in life-threatening illness. *Psycho-oncol* **7:** 460–9.

16 Reed, P.G. (1986). Spiritual Perspective Scale. Unpublished instrument, University of Arizona.

17 Reed, P.G. (1987). Spirituality and well-being in terminally ill hospitalized adults. *Res Nurs Hlth* **10:** 335–44.

18 Batson, C.D., Schoenrade, P.A. (1991). Measuring religion as Quest: validity concerns. *J Scient Study Relig* **30:** 416–29.

19 Genia, V. (1991). The spiritual experience index: a measure of spiritual maturity. *J Relig Hlth* **30:** 337–47.

20 Genia, V., Cooke, B.A. (1998). Women at midlife: Spiritual maturity and life satisfaction. *J Relig Hlth* **37:** 115–23.

21 Veach, T.L., Chappel, J.N. (1992). Measuring spiritual health: a preliminary study. *Subst Abuse* **13:** 139–47.

22 Kass, J., Friedman, R., Leserman, J., Caudill, M., Zuttereister, P., Benson, H. (1991). An inventory of positive psychological attitudes with potential relevance to health outcomes. *Behav Med* **17:** 121–9.

23 Kass, J., Friedman, R., Leserman, J., Zuttermeister, P., Benson, H. (1991). Health outcomes and a new measure of spiritual experience. *J Scient Study Relig* **30:** 203–11.

24 Plante, T.G., Boccaccini, M.T. (1997). The Santa Clara Strength of Religious faith Questionnaire. *Past Psychol* **45:** 375–87.

25 Plante, T.G., Vallaeys, C., Sherman, A.C., Wallston, K.A. (2002). The development of a brief version of the Santa Clara Strength of Religious Faith Questionnaire. *Past Psychol* **50:** 359–68.

26 Plante, T.G. (2011). The Santa Clara Strength of Religious Faith Questionnaire: assessing faith engagement in a brief and nondenominational manner. *Religions* **1:** 3–8.

27 Pargament, K.I. (1997). *The psychology of religion and coping: Theory, research, practice.* New York: Guilford.

28 Pargament, K., Feuille, M., Burdzy, D. (2011). The Brief RCOPE: current psychometric status of a short measure of religious coping. *Religions* **2:** 51–76.

29 Koenig, H.G., Meador, K., Parkerson, G. (1997). Religion Index for Psychiatric Research: a 5-item measure for use in health outcome studies. *Am J Psychiat* **154:** 885–6.

30 Belschner, W. (2001). Tun und Lassen—Ein komplementäres Konzept der Lebenskunst. *Transpers Psychol Psychother* **7:** 85–102.

31 Albani, C., Bailer, H., Blaser, G., Geyer, M., Brähler, E., Grulke, N. (2002). Psychometrische Überprüfung der Skala 'Transpersonales Vertrauen' (TPV) in einer repräsentativen Bevölkerungsstichprobe. *Transpers Psychol Psychother* **2:** 86–98.

32 Daaleman, T.P., Frey, B.B., Wallace, D., Studenski, S.A. (2002). Spirituality Index of Well-Being Scale: development and testing of a new measure. *J Fam Pract* **51:** 952.

33 Daalemann, T.P., Frey, B.B. (2004). The Spirituality Index of Well-Being: A new instrument for health related quality of life research. *Ann Fam Med* **2:** 499–503.

34 Underwood, L.G. (2011). The Daily Spiritual Experience Scale: overview and results. *Religions* **2:** 29–50.

35 Peterman, A.H., Fitchett, G., Brady, M.J., Hernandez, L., Cella, D. (2002). Measuring spiritual well-being in people with cancer: the functional assessment of chronic illness therap—Spiritual Well-being Scale (FACIT-Sp). *Ann Behav Med* **24:** 49–58.

36 Bredle, J.M., Salsman, J.M., Debb, S.M., Arnold, B.J., Cella, D. (2011). Spiritual well-being as a component of health-related quality of life: the Functional Assessment of Chronic Illness Therapy—Spiritual Well-Being Scale (FACIT-Sp). *Religions* **2:**77–94.

37 Ryan, K., Fiorito, B. (2003). Means-ends spirituality questionnaire: Reliability, validity, and relationship to psychological well-being. *Rev Relig Res* **45:** 130–54.

38 Huber, S. (2003). *Zentralität und Inhalt: Ein neues multidimensionales Messmodell der Religiosität.* Opladen: Leske & Budrich.

39 Huber, S. (2008). Kerndimensionen, Zentralität und Inhalt. Ein interdisziplinäres Modell der Religiosität. *J Psychol* **16**(3): Article 05 (http://www.journal-fuer-psychologie.de/jfp-3-2008-05.html) 2008-5.

40 Ostermann, T., Büssing, A., Matthiessen, P.F. (2004). [Pilot study for the development of a questionnaire for the measuring of the patients' attitude towards spirituality and religiosity and their coping with disease (SpREUK)]. *Forsch Komplementär Klass Naturheilk* **11:** 346–53.

41 Büssing, A., Ostermann, T., Matthiessen, P.F. (2005). Role of religion and spirituality in medical patients—confirmatory results with the SpREUK questionnaire. *Hlth Qual Life Outcomes* **3:** 1–10.

42 Büssing, A. (2010). Spirituality as a resource to rely on in chronic illness: The SpREUK Questionnaire. *Religions* **1:** 9–17.

43 Büssing, A., Matthiessen, P.F., Ostermann, T. (2005). Engagement of patients in religious and spiritual practices: Confirmatory results with the SpREUK-P 1.1 questionnaire as a tool of quality of life research. *Hlth Qual Life Outcomes* **3:** 1–11.

44 Büssing, A., Keller, N., Michalsen, A., Moebus, S., Dobos, G., Ostermann, T., *et al.* (2006). Spirituality and adaptive coping styles in German patients with chronic diseases in a CAM health care setting. *J Complement Integrat Med* **3**(1): 1–24.

45 Büssing, A., Lux, E.A., Janko, A., Kopf, A. (2011). Psychosoziale und spirituelle Bedürfnisse bei Patienten mit chronischen Schmerz- und Krebserkrankungen. *Deut Zeitsch Onkol* **41:** 39–73.

46 Galek, K., Flannelly, K.J., Vane, A., Galek, R.M. (2005). Assessing a patient's spiritual needs: a comprehensive instrument. *Holist Nurs Pract***19:** 62–9.

47 Flanelly, K.J., Galek, K., Flannelly, L.T. (2006). A test of the factor structure of the patient spiritual needs assessment scale. *Holist Nurs Pract* **20:** 187–90.

48 Hermann, C. (2006). Development and testing of the spiritual needs inventory for patients near the end of life. *Oncol Nurs Forum* **33:** 737–44.

49 Zwingmann, Ch, Wirtz, M., Müller, C., Körper, J., Murken, S. (2006). Positive and negative religious coping in German breast cancer patients. *J Behav Med* **29:** 533–47.

50 Büssing, A., Koenig, H.G. (2008). The Benefit through spirituality/religiosity scale—a 6-item measure for use in health outcome studies. *Int J Psychiat Med* **38:** 493–506.

51 Büssing, A., Fischer, J., Ostermann, T., Matthiessen, P.F. (2008). Reliance on God's help, depression and fatigue in female cancer patients. *Int J Psychiat Med* **38:** 357–72.

52 Büssing, A., Ostermann, T., Matthiessen, P.F. (2007). Distinct expressions of vital spirituality. The ASP questionnaire as an explorative research tool. *Journal of Religion and Health* **46:** 267–86.

53 Büssing, A., Föller-Mancini, A., Gidley, J., Heusser, P. (2010). Aspects of spirituality in adolescents. *Int J Child Spiritual* **15:** 25–44.

54 Yong, J., Kim, J., Han, S.S., Puchalski, C.M. (2008). Development and validation of a scale assessing spiritual needs for Korean patients with cancer. *J Palliat Care* **24:** 240–6.

55 Cole, B.S., Hopkins, C.M., Tisak, J., Steel, J.L., Carr, B.I. (2008). Assessing spiritual growth and spiritual decline following a diagnosis of cancer: reliability and validity of the spiritual transformation scale. *Psycho-oncol* **17:** 112–21.

56 Bowman, E.S., Beitman, J.A., Palesh, O., Perez, J.E., Koopman, C. (2009). The Cancer and Deity Questionnaire: a new religion and cancer measure. *J Psychosoc Oncol* **27:** 435–53.

57 Büssing, A., Balzat, H.J., Heusser, P. (2010). Spiritual needs of patients with chronic pain diseases and cancer—validation of the Spiritual Needs Questionnaire. *Eur J Med Res* **15**(6): 266–73.

58 Büssing ,A., Koenig, H.G. (2010). Spiritual needs of patients with chronic diseases. *Religions* **1:** 18–27.

59 Puchalski, C., Romer, A.L. (2000). Taking a spiritual history allows clinicians to understand patients more fully. *J Palliat Med* **3:** 129–37.

60 Sawatzky, R., Ratner, P.A., Chiu, L. (2005). A meta-analysis of the relationship between spirituality and quality of life. *Soc Indicat Res* **72:** 153–88.

61 Stefanek, M., McDonald, P.G., Hess, S.A. (2005). Religion, spirituality and cancer: current status and methodological challenges. *Psycho-oncol* **14:** 450–63.

62 Koenig, H.G., Büssing, A. (2010). The Duke University Religion Index (DUREL): a five-item measure for use in epidemiological studies. *Religions* **1:** 78–85.

63 Lewis, C.A., Shevlin, M., McGuckin, C., Navr'atil, M. (2001). The Santa Clara Strength of Religious Faith Questionnaire: confirmatory factor analysis. *Past Psychol* **49:** 379–84.

64 Büssing, A., Ostermann, T., Glöckler, M., Matthiessen, P.F (2006). Spiritualität, Krankheit und Heilung – Bedeutung und Ausdrucksformen der Spiritualität in der Medizin. Frankfurt: VAS - Verlag für Akademische Schriften; 2006.

65 Büssing, A., Reiser, F., Michalsen, A., Uahn Zahn, A., Baumann, K. (2012). Engagement of patients with chronic diseases in spiritual and secular forms of practice: Results with the shortened SpREUK-P SF17 Questionnaire.

66 Ellison, C. (1983). Spiritual well-being: conceptualization and measurement. *J Psychol Theol* **11:** 330–8.

67 Canada, A.L., Murphy, P.E., Fitchett, G., Peterman, A.H., Schover, L.R. (2008). A 3-factor model for the FACIT-Sp. *Psycho-oncol* **17:** 908–16.

68 Levine, E.G., Aviv, C., Yoo, G., Ewing, C., Au, A. (2009). The benefits of prayer on mood and well-being of breast cancer survivors. *Support Care Cancer* **17:** 295–306.

69 Büssing, A., Ostermann, T., Glöckler, M., Matthiessen, P.F. (2006). *Spiritualität, Krankheit und Heilung—Bedeutung und Ausdrucksformen der Spiritualität in der Medizin.* Frankfurt: VAS—Verlag für Akademische Schriften.

70 Büssing, A., Michalsen, A., Balzat, H.J., Grünther, R.A., Ostermann, T., Neugebauer, E.A.M., *et al.* (2009). Are spirituality and religiosity resources for patients with chronic pain conditions? *Pain Med* **10:** 327–39.

71 Pargament, K.I., Koenig, H.G., Perez, L.M. (2000). The many methods of religious coping: Development and initial validation of the RCOPE. *J Clin Psychol* **56:** 519–43.

72 Phillips, R.E. III, Cheng, C., Pargament, K., Oemig, C., Colvin, S., Abarr, A., Dunn, M., Reed, A. (2009). An exploratory study of Buddhist methods of coping in the United States. *International Journal for the Psychology of Religion* **19**: 231–43.

CHAPTER 45

On the links between religion and health: what has empirical research taught us?

Hisham Abu-Raiya and Kenneth I. Pargament

Introduction

Religion is a significant human phenomenon. Religious beliefs and practices are widespread, and play a central role in the lives of many people in almost all societies and cultures around the globe.[1–2] Consider the following examples: 96% of persons living in the United States believe in God, over 90% pray and 69% are church members;[3] 78% of Canadians surveyed in 1993 affirmed belief in God, with 67% ascribing to the basic tenets of Christianity;[4] 60% of Lebanese Muslims surveyed considered themselves either religious or very religious, 49% reported praying daily, 53% indicated fasting regularly during the month of Ramadan, and 61% reported reading the Holy Qur'an weekly or more;[5] and about 60% of Israeli Jews identify themselves as either traditional or religious.[6]

Yet, although religion continues to be an important component of life, mainstream psychology has paid little attention to this phenomenon.[7] The relationship between religion and psychiatry or clinical psychology has been also controversial. Historically, psychologists have taken both sides in the debate on the value of religious experience (for a thorough review, see[8]). For example, Freud[9] associated religious beliefs and practices with the repression of instincts, intrapsychic conflicts and helplessness. On the other hand, Jung[10] suggested that religion is a source of meaning and stability in an uncertain world.

Before the 1990s, the relationship between religion and health was for the most part a neglected area of research: researchers often buried religious variables in the methods and results sections of their studies.[11] In the last two decades, this picture has changed dramatically—a considerable body of research has emerged regarding the relationship between religion and health.[12–15] These studies have led to some important insights into the links between religious beliefs and practices, and the wellbeing of the individual. These ties between religion and health outcomes are the focus of this chapter.

In what follows, we start by referring to issues of definition and measurement of religion. Then, we summarize the important findings on the relationship between religion, health and wellbeing that has emerged from research in four main areas: religious involvement, religious motivation, religion and prejudice, and religious coping. We conclude by pointing to some of the limitations of this body of research and suggesting directions for research that might further advance the empirically-based psychology of religion and spirituality

Religion: definition and measurement issues

What is religion? According to Wulff,[8] the word 'religion' originated from the Latin *religio,* which some scholars say was initially used to designate a greater-than human power that requires a person to respond in a certain way to avoid some dreadful consequences. Smith postulates that the word *religio* referred to 'something that one does, or that one feels deeply about, or that impinges one's will, exacting obedience or threatening disaster or offering reward or binding one into one's community.'[16, p. 20] Social scientists and theologians have suggested a variety of definitions of religion, but have failed to reach a consensus which led sociologist J. Milton Yinger to conclude, 'any definition of religion is likely to be satisfactory only to its author.'[17, p. 108]

Pargament[18] asserts that because religion is so complex and personal, no single definition is likely to be completely adequate. Therefore, our task is to construct a definition of religion that is relevant to the phenomena of interest. Because our focus here is on health and wellbeing, an operational definition of religion is needed that is appropriate for psychological research. Pargament offers such a definition. According to Pargament, religion is a 'search for significance in ways related to the sacred.' [18, p. 32]. This perspective is tailored to the psychological venture, and it excludes concerns about the nature of the sacred that have little to do with significant human issues.[19]

This definition includes two important elements: *search for significance,* and the *sacred.* The search refers to the process of discovery of the sacred, conservation of the sacred once it has been found, and transformation of the sacred when internal or external pressures require a change.[18,20) The search can also be understood in terms of the multiple pathways people take to reach their goals and the goals themselves. Religious pathways can be manifested through multiple dimensions in which the sacred is involved, such as ideology, ethical conduct, emotional experience, social intercourse, and study. The goals to be reached are just as diverse. They include achieving personal ends, such as meaning in life and self-regulation, social ends, such as intimacy with others and justice in the world, and spiritual ends, such as closeness to God and living a moral and ethical life.[21]

According to the Oxford Dictionary, the sacred refers to the holy, those things that are 'set apart' from the ordinary and deserve veneration and respect. Pargament and Mahoney[20] define the sacred as divine beings, higher powers, or God and other aspects of life that take on spiritual character by virtue of their association with the divine. According to this definition, any aspect of life can be imbued with extraordinary character through its association with, or representation of, divinity. What makes religion distinctive is the involvement of the sacred in the pathways and destinations that define the individual's search for significance.

One of the pivotal characteristics of religion as reflected by the definition of Pargament is its multi-dimensionality. Theorists and researchers have generally viewed religion as a multi-dimensional phenomena though they do not necessarily agree on the content of these dimensions (for a thorough review, see[18]). Psychologist Gordon Allport, in a classic work, distinguished between two religious orientations: the *extrinsic* and *intrinsic*. These two orientations, in spite of conceptual and psychometric difficulties, have received a great deal of attention. According to Allport and Russ,[22] the extrinsic orientation is characteristic of those who:

> are disposed to use religion for their ends. The term is borrowed from axiology, to designate an interest that is held because it serves other, more ultimate interests. Extrinsic values are always instrumental and utilitarian. Persons with this orientation may find religion useful in variety of ways- to provide security and solace, sociability and distraction, status and self-justification. The embraced creed is lightly held or else selectively shaped to fit more primary goals. In theological terms, the extrinsic type turns to God, but without turning away from self. (p. 441)

On the other hand, the intrinsic orientation characterizes those who:

> find their master motive in religion. Other needs, strong as they may be, are regarded as of less of ultimate significance, and they are, so far as possible, brought into harmony with the religious beliefs and prescriptions. Having embraced a creed, the individual endeavors to internalize and follow it fully. It is in this sense that he lives his religion. (p. 441)

Allport and Ross measured extrinsic and intrinsic religion by the Religious Orientation Scale.[22] Actually, this scale consists of two subscales, one designed to measure extrinsic religion (items such as 'the primary purpose of prayer is to gain relief and protection,' and 'occasionally I find necessary to compromise my religious beliefs in order to protect my social and economic wellbeing'), and one to measure intrinsic religion (items such as 'it is important for me to spend periods of time in private religious thought and meditation,' and 'quite often I have been keenly aware of the presence of God or the divine being').

Allen and Spilka[23] suggested a slightly different distinction. They differentiated between *committed* and *consensual religion*. They defined committed religion as a discerning, highly differentiated, candid, open, self-critical, abstract, and relational approach to religious questions. Moreover, for the committed individual, religion is a central value. They defined consensual religion as the opposite of each of these characteristics.

Daniel Batson and his colleagues[24] introduced a third orientation to religion. This orientation grew out of some dissatisfaction with Allport's work. While they did not argue with Allport's conceptualization of the extrinsic orientation, they claimed that his conceptualization of the intrinsic orientation is rigid and dogmatic, and does not leave room for other factors central to the religious experience. As a result, Batson *et al.*[24] suggested a third orientation:

> religion as a *quest*, an 'approach that involves honestly facing existential questions in all their complexity, while at the same time resisting clear-cut, Pat answers. An individual who approaches religion in this way recognizes that he or she does not know, and probably never will know, the final truth about such matters. Still, the questions are deemed important, and however tentative and subject to change, answers are sought. There may or may not be a clear belief in a transcendent reality, but there is a transcendent, religious aspect to the individual's life. (p. 166)

Based on a factor analysis, Batson *et al.*[24] developed a measure of religion that includes three scales: means (extrinsic), ends (intrinsic) and quest. While the means and the ends scales are quite similar to those of Allport's scales, the quest was a new scale. This scale was designed to measure the basic component of the quest dimension- the degree to which an individual's religion involves an open-ended, responsive dialogue with existential questions raised by the contradictions and tragedies of life. This scale includes items, such as 'as I grow and change, I expect my religion to grow and change,' and 'questions are far more central to my religious experience than are answers.'

Empirical evidence is consistent with the theoretical view of religion as multi-dimensional. Glock and Stark[25] developed a comprehensive way of measuring religiousness. Their work is considered a key step in the evolution of sociologically oriented attempts to measure religion. Using factor analysis with a sample of 1,976 participants who took part in the National Opinion Research Center (NORC) survey in 1964, they identified five dimensions of religiousness. These dimensions are the *experiential* (subjective and emotional religious experience as an expression of personal religiousness), the *ideological* (acceptance of the belief system), the *ritualistic* (participation in religious activities and practices), the *intellectual* (knowledge of the belief system), and the *consequential* (ethical consequences of these dimensions and the prescriptions derived from them).

Based on factor analysis, they developed the Dimensions of Religious Commitment Scale. The consequential dimension was omitted from this scale because it was not strictly a measure of religiousness itself. The remaining four dimensions are assessed by 48 different items, many with multiple subsections.

Working with four independent Christian samples, Ryan *et al.*[26] concluded that two types of internalization (the process through which an individual transforms a formerly externally prescribed regulation or value into internal one) characterize the interplay between the individual and religion. The first is *introjection* and represents a partial internalization of religiousness based on self and other-approval-based pressures. The second is *identification* which represents adoption of beliefs as personal values. They found differential relations between these two constructs and measures of mental health and self-related outcomes. For example, introjection was associated with higher levels of anxiety and depression; in contrast, identification was linked with greater identity integration. They also found that evangelical teenagers scored higher on both introjection and identification measures than controls.

Idler *et al.*[27] developed an instrument to measure religiousness and spirituality, intended explicitly for studies of health. They tested the instrument in a nationally representative sample of Americans from the 1998 General Social Survey ($n = 1445$). Drawing on existing theory and research, they identified nine dimensions of religiousness and spirituality that were correlated with variables of physical and mental health: *public religious activities*, *private religious activities*, *positive religious coping*, *negative religious coping*, *religious intensity*, *forgiveness*, *daily spiritual experience*, *beliefs and values*, and *giving-to-income ratio*.

It should be noted that these dimensions of religiousness and their associated instruments are the outcome of empirical research that has focused almost exclusively on Christian populations, mainly in the United Sates, and largely neglected people from other traditional faiths. Recently, this picture has begun to change as empirical studies on religious dimensions among non-Christian groups have grown in number. Consider the following examples.

Tarakeshwar, Pargament, and Mahoney[21] developed measures of the religious pathways of a convenience sample of Hindus in the United States. Consistent with Hindu theology, they identified four religious pathways through factor analysis: *path of devotion* (in which the devotee submits himself or herself to the will of God, and through devotional practices, such as prayer, aims to become one with God and attain spiritual liberation), *path of ethical action* (in which the individual chooses to perform work without attachment to its effects; this attitude purifies his or her mind so that he or she can attain a sense of God-vision), *path of knowledge* (in which the individual dedicates himself or herself to acquiring knowledge that reveals the impermanence and ineffectuality of things in the world, and thereby frees the self from the bondage of ignorance, leading to spiritual liberation), and *path of mental concentration* (in which the devotee practices disciplinary measures that involve physiological and psychological restrains to free the self from all impurities so that the divine self of the person can then manifest itself, leading to spiritual liberation).

Lazar, Kravetz and Fredrich-Kedem[6] examined the content and structure of self-reported motivation for Jewish behaviour. Through factor analysis in a sample of 323 Jewish participants from different religious orientations, they identified five reliable factors: *belief in divine order*, *ethnic identity*, *social activity*, *family activity*, and *upbringing*.

Working with a sample of 340 Muslims from all over the world, Abu-Raiya *et al.*[28] developed a valid and reliable Psychological Measure of Islamic Religiousness (PMIR). The PMIR yielded seven distinct and reliable factors: Islamic Beliefs ('I believe in the Day of Judgment'); Islamic Ethical Principles and Universality ('I consider every Muslim in the world as my brother or sister'); Islamic Religious Struggle ('I find myself doubting the existence of afterlife'); Islamic Religious Duty, Obligation, and Exclusivism ('How often do you pray?'); Islamic Positive Religious Coping and Identification ('When I face a problem in life, I read the Holy Qur'an to find consolation'); Punishing Allah Reappraisal ('When I face a problem in life, I wonder what I did for Allah to punish me'); and Islamic Religious Conversion ('All at once, I felt that my life has no meaning without Islam').

To summarize, theoretical and empirical evidence indicate that people practice religion in different ways, connected to their thoughts, emotions, actions and relationships. Religion can be individualistic as well as collectivistic, and provides various pathways to various destinations.

The psychology of religion and spirituality: four main areas of research

The field of psychology of religion and spirituality has tested the links between various facets of religiousness and health and wellbeing. Among these, four areas of inquiry seem more developed: religious involvement, religious motivation, religion and prejudice, and religious coping. In what follows, we refer in detail to the empirical literature pertaining to each of these areas.

Religious involvement

A large body of empirical research has demonstrated links between religious involvement and physical health, drug/alcohol abuse, and mental health. By religious involvement we mean self-rated religiousness, endorsement of religious beliefs and participation in religious rituals. Cross-sectional and longitudinal studies have consistently found significant associations between religious attendance and health status indicators, including specific conditions such as hypertension, general measures of functional disability, and overall mortality.[13] For example, McCullough *et al.*[29] conducted a meta-analysis of data from 42 independent samples examining the association of a measure of religious involvement and all causes of mortality. They found that, even after controlling for a variety of potential confounding variables, religious involvement was significantly associated with lower mortality, indicating that people with higher religious involvement were more likely to be alive at a follow-up than people lower in religious involvement.

There is consistent evidence that religiousness and substance use are negatively related to each other. For example, of 38 studies covered in a review by Benson,[30] 29 indicated a negative relationship between religiousness and alcohol use, and 26 with marijuana use. Working with high school students, Corwyn and Benda[31] found that a measure of personal religiousness (e.g. private prayer, evangelism) was a significant predictor of lower levels of drug use. Investigations of tobacco use and illicit drug use also show a negative relationship with religion. Using a sample of 1092 twins, Kendler *et al.*[32] found that religious devotion was significantly and negatively linked to current levels of drinking and smoking as well as lifetime risk for alcoholism and nicotine dependence.

In a meta-analysis of 100 studies examining the relationship between religiousness and mental health conducted by Koenig and Larson,[2] religious beliefs and practices were related to greater life satisfaction, happiness, positive affect and higher morale in 79 (nearly 80%) of the studies. Of 12 prospective cohort studies identified in their meta-analysis, 10 reported a significant relationship between greater religiousness and greater wellbeing. Similar levels of positive association were found between religiousness and hope, optimism, purpose and meaning; of 14 studies examining these relationships, 12 reported significant positive associations among these variables and two found no association with religion.

Salutary effects of religion have also been demonstrated with other dimensions of mental health and illness, such as self-esteem and mastery,[33] depressive symptoms and anxiety.[34,35] Overall, this literature indicates that there is a positive relationship between religious and spiritual involvement and wellbeing.

Religious motivation

As mentioned earlier, the psychology of religion literature distinguishes between two basic types of religiousness: intrinsic and extrinsic. Overall, research conducted mostly among Christian samples has shown a positive correlation between an intrinsic orientation to religion and wellbeing, and a negative correlation between extrinsic religiousness and wellbeing (see [36–7] for review). For example, in a study of religious college students, Bergin *et al.* [36-37] found a positive correlation between intrinsic religiousness and sociability, sense of wellbeing, and tolerance, and a negative correlation between extrinsic religiousness and the same criteria. Similarly, Ryan *et al.*[26] found that higher levels of identification were associated with higher self-esteem, less depression, anxiety, and social functioning, while higher levels of introjection were negatively associated with these variables.

In the last few years, researchers have been testing the intrinsic-extrinsic religiousness framework with non-Christian samples. For example, in a recent comprehensive review of the empirically based psychology of Islam, Abu-Raiya and Pargament[38] identified multiple studies conducted among Muslim populations, which tested the applicability of Allport and Ross's[22] religious orientation framework to the Muslim context.[39–42] By and large, this group of studies has yielded support for the usefulness of Allport and Ross's[22] framework and identified three religious orientations relevant to Muslims: intrinsic, extrinsic-personal, and extrinsic-social. The pattern of relationship between these orientations and outcomes has been quite consistent: intrinsic religiousness and extrinsic-personal were related to positive outcomes while extrinsic-social religiousness was related to negative or no outcomes.

Religion and prejudice

Does religion encourage tolerance or intolerance? This question has concerned social scientists for a number of years. Gordon Allport, one of the influential researchers on the subject of prejudice in the twentieth century and one of the first psychologists to focus on this question, summarized his findings in a classic statement 'it (religion) makes prejudice and it unmakes prejudice.'[43, p. 494] To explain this seemingly paradoxical statement, Allport referred to the religious orientation of the individual; extrinsic religiousness, he claimed, 'makes' the prejudice, while intrinsic religiousness 'unmakes' it. Since Allport's classic work, abundant studies have studied the relationship between religion and prejudice. (see [8,24] for a review). Although several researchers in the field of psychology of religion have pointed to serious methodological and conceptual problems in Allport's work (e.g.[44–5]), the original question still elicits controversy and research.

Numerous studies have found a link between religion and prejudice. Reviewing the literature on this topic, Wulff[8] concluded, 'Using a variety of measures of piety-religious affiliation, church attendance, doctrinal orthodoxy, rated importance of religion, and so on-researchers have consistently found positive correlations with ethnocentrism, authoritarianism, social distance, rigidity, intolerance of ambiguity, and specific forms of prejudice, especially against Jews and blacks' (p. 223). Reviewing the literature, Batson[24] found that 37 out of 47 studies included in the review showed a positive relationship between religion and prejudice, while only two showed a negative relationship.

However, the results of these studies should be interpreted in the light of two major limitations. First, they have referred to religion as a whole without specifying particular types of religiousness. Second, they are based mostly on Christian samples.[12] To overcome the first shortcoming, researchers in the field have tried recently to identify religious variables other than intrinsic-extrinsic orientations that might have the potential to predict prejudice and tolerance. One of the variables that has been identified is religious fundamentalism. In a seminal study, Altemeyer and Hunsberger[46] defined religious fundamentalism as follows:

> the belief that there is one set of religious teachings that clearly contains the fundamental, basic, intrinsic, essential, inerrant, truth about humanity and deity; that this essential truth is fundamentally opposed by forces of evil which must be vigorously fought; that this truth must be followed today according to the fundamental, unchangeable practices of the past; and that those who believe and follow these fundamental teachings have a special relationship with the deity. (p. 118)

Based on this conceptualization, the authors developed a 20-item Religious Fundamentalism Scale. This scale includes items such as 'Of all the people on this earth, one group has a special relationship with God because it believes the most in his revealed truths and tries the hardest to follow His laws' and 'God will punish severely those who abandon His true religion.' Altemeyer and Hunsberger[46] established the reliability and validity of their scale by administering it to 491 Canadian parents of university students in five different studies. They found that individuals who scored higher on the Religious Fundamentalism Scale also scored higher on measures of prejudice and lower on measures of tolerance.

Since this seminal work, studies, in general, have found a positive relationship between fundamental or exclusivist orientations to religion and prejudice, and a negative relationship between a pluralistic orientation to religion (i.e. one that espouses multiple pathways to religious ends) and prejudice (see [12] for review). It should be stressed, though, that some recent studies conducted by Altemeyer and Hunsberger have raised questions about the direct effects of fundamentalism on prejudice. Their research suggests that the relationship between fundamentalism and prejudice is at least partially mediated by authoritarian personality traits (see [46] for a detailed review of these studies).

Desecration (i.e. the perceptions that sacred aspects of members of the in-group have been violated by members of religious out-group) has been proposed more recently as another religiously based variable that has a potential to predict prejudice and tolerance.[47] A few empirical studies have supported this proposition. For example, Pargament *et al.*[47] found that prejudice toward Jews among Christians was associated with the perception that this group threatened Christian values and teachings. Similarly, using a sample of 192 Christian participants, Abu-Raiya *et al.*[49] examined the links between the appraisal that Muslims desecrate Christian values and teachings, religious coping methods, and anti-Muslim attitudes. They found that Christians who reported greater perceptions of Muslims as desecrators of Christianity were more likely to report anti-Muslim prejudice and perceived conflict with Muslims.

Religious coping

The relationship between religion and coping is the subject of a growing body of psychological research. For many people, religion appears to be an important resource in coping. Numerous studies have revealed the extensive use of religious coping methods in stressful situations (see [15,18,48] for review). For example, Conway,[50] Kesseling *et al.*[51] Gilbert,[52] Greil *et al.*,[53] Segall and Wykle,[54] and Schuster *et al.*[55] found that religion is used in coping by the large majority of their participants, with prevalence figures reaching as high as 92%.

Pargament[18] asserts that, faced with life stressors, many people apply religious and non-religious coping methods to deal with these stressors. According to Pargament and Abu- Raiya,[15] religious coping methods can be defined as ways of understanding and dealing with negative life events that involve the sacred. Pargament *et al.*[56] identified two higher-order patterns of religious coping: one pattern made up of positive religious coping methods and the other made up of negative religious coping methods. The positive religious coping methods reflect the perception of a secure relationship with God, a belief that there is a greater meaning to be found, and a sense of spiritual connectedness with others. In contrast, the negative religious coping pattern involves expressions of a less secure relationship with God, a tenuous and ominous view of the world, and a religious struggle to find and conserve significance in life.

Ample studies have examined the relationship between religious coping and wellbeing. Overall, positive religious coping has been positively associated with desirable wellbeing indicators,[57–60] while negative religious coping has been linked to undesirable physical and mental health indicators.[61–3]

Recently, researchers have begun to examine religious coping methods and their associations with health and wellbeing in samples of Muslims,[64–8] Jews[58] and Hindus.[69] The findings of these studies are similar to those obtained from non-Christian samples. For example, working with an international sample of 340 Muslims, Abu-Raiya *et al.*[28] identified three subscales of the Psychological Measure of Islamic Religiousness (PMIR) that tapped into religious coping: one assesses positive religious coping (Islamic Positive Religious Coping and Identification) and two measure assess negative religious coping (Islamic Religious Struggle, Punishing Allah Reappraisal). Their findings indicated that greater levels of Islamic Positive Religious Coping were consistently and strongly tied to greater levels of positive wellbeing (general Islamic wellbeing, purpose in life, satisfaction with life) and lower levels of negative wellbeing (physical health, alcohol use). On the other hand, greater levels of Islamic Religious Struggle were linked consistently and strongly with more negative outcomes (angry feelings, alcohol use, depressed mood) and less positive outcomes (positive relations with others, purpose in life). Punishing Allah reappraisals were also related to negative outcomes (e.g. depressed mood, angry feelings), though less strongly.

Conclusion

Clearly, the existing scientific research on psychology of religion has offered numerous insights on the relationship between religion and physical and psychological wellbeing. Specifically, this research has shown that: (1) religion is a multidimensional phenomenon; (2) there is an overall positive relationship between religious involvement and wellbeing; (3) there is a positive correlation between an intrinsic orientation to religion and wellbeing, and a negative correlation between extrinsic religiousness and wellbeing; (4) some religiously based variables (e.g. fundamentalism, desecration) are strong predictors of prejudice; (5) overall, positive religious coping is positively associated with desirable wellbeing indicators while negative religious coping is negatively linked to undesirable wellbeing indicators.

However, this research is not free of limitations. There are four major weaknesses in this body of research. First, much of the research is either atheoretical or lacks an overarching theoretical perspective. Secondly, current scientific findings are overwhelmingly based on a few items as indices of the multi-faceted complex domain of religion. For example, Mahoney *et al.*[71] found that 83% of the studies published in journals in the past 20 years on religion, marriage and parenting relied on one or two items to assess family members' general religiousness (e.g. denominational affiliation, church attendance) or conservative Christian beliefs. Thirdly, possible harmful aspects of religion are generally not considered, with the exception of studies of religious struggles (i.e. negative religious coping). Finally, the studies that have been conducted and the measures that have been developed have focused almost exclusively on Christian samples,[72] and have been geared largely to members of Judeo-Christian traditions.[73] Other traditional faiths have been neglected for the most part.

Let us conclude our discussion by pointing to some of the exciting new directions on the links between religion and health and wellbeing. First, we should look further into the links between religion and health among different cultures and religious traditions. Researchers are beginning to examine these connections among members of different religious traditions including Jews[58,73], Hindus,[21,69] and Muslims.[28,63] However, though this accumulating body of research is beginning to yield important insights into religious diversity, it is still in its 'infancy.' Further empirical studies are needed to reveal a clearer picture of the relationship between religion and health among different religious groups, especially non-Western religious traditions.

Secondly, the vast majority of studies on the relationship between religion and health have used psychological and physical outcome measures. One type of outcome, the spiritual, has been particularly neglected. Because religion is designed primarily to serve spiritual functions, the effects of religious beliefs and practices on spiritual outcomes (e.g. spiritual maturity, commitment to faith, religious stewardship, and spiritual security) seem crucial to consider.

Thirdly, much of the research in the psychology of religion has focused on the conservational functions of religion (i.e. the role religion plays in helping people preserve, protect, and sustain whatever they hold sacred). The role religion plays in personal transformation, what has been called 'quantum change,'[74] has been largely neglected. Given that religion, at times, serves as a catalyst for profound changes in underlying goals, values and lifestyles, researchers should take a serious look at religion's capacity for promoting life transformations.

Fourthly, we should investigate the links between religion and health among some relatively neglected groups. Though religious ideas have their roots in childhood and extends throughout the lifespan, most of the research on religion has been conducted with adult populations. It is time to learn more about the developmental aspects of religious beliefs and practices and how they evolve over the course of the individual's lifetime. For instance, it would be interesting to examine whether religious coping methods change at different phases of life, or whether certain forms of religiousness are especially helpful to certain groups, such as the elderly.

Finally, many individuals rely on religious resources to cope with difficulties and crises. Thus, it is important to study the impact of such resources in psychotherapy. Moreover, because studies have linked signs of religious struggle to poorer mental health and even psychopathology, it seems natural to assume that interventions targeting religious struggles may help improve the mental health status of the individual and prevent distress and psychopathology.[61] This assumption has received some empirical support,[76–7] but further evidence is needed to verify the effectiveness of efforts to address religious struggles in psychotherapy. Promising steps in this direction have already been taken (e.g.[75–8]

We hope that researchers will find these new directions for research in the psychology of religion as intriguing as we do. We believe that answers to the questions we outlined will help us better understand how religion impacts the health and wellbeing of people. Because religion is perhaps the most distinctively human dimension of life, any psychological approach that neglects the religious dimension is necessarily incomplete. However, by expanding our understanding of religious life, we can enhance our more general understanding of what it means to be human and, in turn, apply this knowledge to our efforts to enhance the lives of people in their communities.

References

1 Haque, A. (1998). Psychology and religion: their relationship and integration from an Islamic perspective. *Am J Islamic Soc Sci* **15**(4): 97–116.

2 Koenig, H.G., Larson, D.B. (2001). Religion and mental health: Evidence of association. *Int Rev Psychiat* **13**: 67–78.

3 Princeton Religion Research Centre Religion in America (1996). *Gallup Poll*. Princeton: Princeton Religion Research Center.

4 Baetz, M., Larson, D.B., Marcoux, G., Bowen, R., Griffin, R. (2002). Canadian psychiatric inpatient religious commitment: An association with mental health. *Can J Psychiat* **47**: 159–66.

5 Khashan, H., Kreidie, L. (2001). *The Social and Economic Correlates of Islamic Religiosity- Statistical Data Included*. World Affairs.

6 Lazar, A., Kravetz, S., Frederich-Kedem, P. (2003). The multidimensionality of motivation for Jewish religious behaviour: Content, structure, and relationship to religious identity. *J Sci Study Relig* **41**: 509–19.

7 Al-Issa, I. (2000). Does the Muslim religion make a difference in psychopathology? In: I. al-Issa (ed.) *Al- junun: Mental Illness in the Islamic World*, pp. 315–53. International Universities Press, Connecticut.

8 Wulff, D.M. (1997). *Psychology of Religion: Classic and Contemporary*, 2nd edn. New York: Wiley.

9 Freud, S. (1927). *The Future of an Illusion*, pp. 1–56. London: Hogarth Press.

10 Jung, C.G. (1938). *Psychology and Religion*. New Haven: Yale University Press.

11 Miller, W.R., Thoresen, C.E. (2003). Spirituality, religion, and health. *Am Psychol* **58**: 24–35.

12 Hood, R.W. Jr, Hill, P.C., Spilka, B. (2009). *The Psychology of Religion: An Empirical Approach*, 5th edn. New York: Guilford Press.

13 Koenig, H.G., McCullough, M.E., Larson, D.B. (2001). *Handbook of Religion and Health*. New York: Oxford University Press.

14 Paloutzian, R.F., Park, C.L. (2005). Integrative themes in the current science of the psychology of religion. In: R.F. Paloutzian, C.L. Park (eds) *Handbook of the Psychology of Religion and Spirituality*, pp. 3–20. New York: Guilford Press.

15 Pargament, K.I., Abu-Raiya, H. (2007). A decade of research on the psychology of religion and coping: Things we assumed and lessons we learned. *Psyke Logos* **28**: 742–66.

16 Smith, W.C. (1963). *The Meaning of Religion: A New Approach to the Religious Traditions of Mankind*. New York: Macmillan.

17 Yinger, J.M.. (1967). Pluralism, religion and secularism. *J Sci Study Relig* **7**: 104–18.

18 Pargament KI (1997). *The Psychology of Religion and Coping: Theory, Practice, Research*. New York: Guilford Press.

19 Pargament KI (2002). The bitter and the sweet: An evaluation of the costs and benefits of religiousness. *Psychol Inq* **13**: 168–81.

20 Pargament KI, Mahoney A (2002). Spirituality: discovering and conserving the sacred. In: C.R. Snyder, S.J. Lopez (eds) *Handbook of Positive Psychology*, pp. 646–59. New York: Oxford University Press.

21 Tarakeshwar, N., Pargament, K.I., Mahoney, A. (2003). Measures of Hindu pathways: Development and preliminary evidence of reliability and validity. *Cult Divers Ethn Minor Psychol* **9**: 316–32.

22 Allport, G.W., Ross, J.M. (1967). Personal religious orientation and prejudice. *J Pers Soc Psychol* **5**: 432–43.

23 Allen, R.O., Spilka, B. (1967). Committed and consensual religion: A specification of religion-prejudice relationships. *J Sci Study Relig* **6**: 191–206.

24 Batson, C.D., Schoenrade, P., Ventis, W.L. (1993). *Religion and the individual: A social-psychological perspective*. New York: Oxford University Press.

25 Glock, C.Y., Stark, R. (1966). *Christian Beliefs and Anti-Semitism*. New York: Harper & Row.

26 Ryan, R.M., Rigby, S., King, K. (1993). Two types of religious internalization and their relations to religious orientations and mental health. J *Pers Soc Psychol* **65**: 586–96.

27 Idler, E.L., Musick, M.A., Ellison, C.G., George, L.K., Krause, N., Ory, M.G., *et al.* (2003). Measuring multiple dimensions of religion for health research: Conceptual background and findings from the 1998 General Social Survey. *Res Aging* **25**: 327–65.

28 Abu-Raiya, H., Pargament, K..I., Mahoney, A., Stein, C. (2008). A psychological measure of Islamic Religiousness: Development and evidence of reliability and validity. *Int J Psychol Relig* **18**(4): 291–315.

29 McCullough, M.E., Hoyt, W.T., Larson, D.B., Koenig, H.G., Thoresen, C. (2000). Religious involvement and mortality: a meta-analytic review. *Hlth Psychol* **19**: 211–22.

30 Benson, P.L. (1992). Religion and substance use. In: J.F. Schumaker (ed.) *Religion and Mental Health*, pp. 211–20. New York: Oxford University Press.

31 Corwyn, R.F., Benda, B.B. (2000). Religiosity and church attendance: The effects on use of 'hard drugs' controlling for sociodemographic and theoretical factors. *Int J Psychol Relig* **10**: 241–58.

32 Kendler, K.S., Gardner, C.O., Prescott, C.A. (1997). Religion, psychopathology, and substance use and abuse; a multimeasure, genetic-epidemiologic study. *Am J Psychiat* **154**: 322–9.

33 Koenig, H.G. (1998). *Handbook of Religion and Mental Health*. Academic Press, California.

34 Smith, T.B., McCullough, M.E., Poll, J. (2003). Religiousness and depression: Evidence for a main effect and the moderating influence of stressful life events. *Psychol Bull* **129**: 614–36.

35 Shreve-Neiger, A.K., Edelstein, B.A. (2004). Religion and anxiety: a critical review of the literature. *Clin Psychol Rev* **24**(4): 379–97.

36 Donahue, M.J. (1985). Intrinsic and extrinsic religiousness: review and meta-analysis. *J Pers Soc Psychol* **48**: 400–19.

37 Bergin, A.E., Master, K.S., Richards, P.S. (1987). Religiousness and mental health reconsidered: A study of an intrinsically religious sample. *J Counsel Psychol* **34**: 197–204.

38 Abu-Raiya, H., Pargament, K.I. (2011). Empirically based psychology of Islam: Summary and critique of the literature. *Ment Health Relig Cult* **14**(2): 93–115.

39 Khan, Z.H., Watson, P.J. (2004). Religious orientations and the experience of Eid-ul-Azha among Pakistani Muslims. *J Sci Study Relig* **43**(4): 537–45.

40 Ghorbani, N., Watson, P.J., Ghramaleki, A.F., Morris, R.J., Hood, R.W. (2002). Muslim-Christian Religious Orientations Scale: Distinction, correlations, and cross-cultural analysis in Iran and the United States. *Int J Psychol Relig* **12**(2): 69–91.

41 Ghorbani, N., Watson, P.J., Mirhasani, V.S. (2007). Religious commitment in Iran: Correlates and factors of quest and extrinsic religious orientations. *Arch Psychol Relig* **29**(1): 245–57.

42 Khan, Z.H., Watson, P.J., Habib, F. (2005). Muslim attitudes toward religion, religious orientation and empathy among Pakistanis. *Ment Health Relig Cult* **8**(1): 49–61.

43 Allport, G.W. (1954). *The Nature of Prejudice*. Cambridge: Addison-Wesley.

44 Hunsberger, B. (1995). Religion and prejudice: the role of religious fundamentalism, quest and right wing authoritarianism. *J Soc Issues* **51**: 112–29.

45 Altemeyer, B., Hunsberger, B. (1992). Authoritarianism, religious fundamentalism, quest, and prejudice. *Int J Psychol Relig* **2**: 113–33.

46 Altemeyer, B., Hunsberger, B. (2005). Fundamentalism and authoritarianism. In: R.F. Paloutzian, C.L. Park (eds) *Handbook of the Psychology of Religion and Spirituality*, pp. 378–93. New York: Guilford Press.

47 Pargament, K.I., Trevino, K., Mahoney, A., Silberman, I. (2007). They killed our Lord: The perception of Jews as desecrators of Christianity as a predictor of anti-Semitism. *J Sci Study Relig* **46**: 143–58.

48 Pargament, K.I. (2010). Religion and coping: the current state of knowledge. In: S. Folkman (ed.) *Handbook of Stress, Health and Coping*, pp. 269–88. New York: Oxford University Press.

49 Abu-Raiya, H., Pargament, K.I., Mahoney, A., Trevino, K. (2008). When Muslims are perceived as a religious threat: Examining the connection between desecration, religious coping and anti-Muslim attitudes. *Basic Appl Soc Psychol* **30**(4): 311–25.

50 Conway, K. (1985–6). Coping with the stress of medical problems among black and white elderly. *Int J Aging Hum Devel* **21**: 39–48.

51 Kesseling, A., Dodd, M.J., Lindsey, A.M., Strauss, A.L. (1986). Attitudes of patients living in Switzerland about cancer and its treatment. *Cancer Nurs* **9**: 77–85.

52 Gilbert, K.R. (1989). *Religion as a Resource for Bereaved Parents as They Cope With the Death of Their Child*. New Orleans: Proceedings of the National Council on Family Relations.

53 Greil, A.L., Porter, K.L., Leitko, T.A., Riscilli, C. (1989). Why me? Theodicies of infertile women and men. *Sociol Hlth Illn* **11**: 213–29.

54 Segall, M., Wykkle, M. (1988–89). The black family's experience with dementia. *J Appl Soc Sci* **13**: 170–91.

55 Schuster, M.A., Stein, B.D., Jaycox, L.H., Collins, R.L., Marshall, G.N., Elliott, M.N. *et al.* (2001). A national survey of stress reactions after the September 11, 2001, terrorist attacks. *N Engl J Med* **345**: 1507–12.

56 Pargament, K.I., Koenig, H.G., Perez, L. (2000). The many methods of religious coping: initial and validation of the RCOPE. *J Clin Psychol* **56**: 519–43.

57 Narin, R., Merluzzi, T. (2003). The role of religious coping in adjustment to cancer. *Psycho-oncol* **12**: 428–41.

58 Rosmarin, D.H., Pargament, K.I., Krumrei, E.J., Flannelly, K.J. (2009). Religious coping among Jews: development and initial validation of the JCOPE. *J Clin Psychol* **65**(7): 670–83.

59 Smith, B.W., Pargament, K.I., Oliver, J.M. (2000). Noah revisited: religious coping by church members and the impact of the 1993 Midwest flood. *J Commun Psychol* **28**: 169–86.

60 Fitchett, G., Rybarczyk, B.D., DeMarco, G.A., Nicholas, J.J. (1999). The role of religion in medical rehabilitation outcomes: a longitudinal study. *Rehabil Psychol* **44**: 1–22.

61 McConnell, K.M., Pargament, K.I., Ellison, C.G., Flannelly, K.J. (2006). Examining the links between spiritual struggles and symptoms of psychopathology in a national sample. *J Clin Psychol* 62, 1469–84.

62 Sherman AC, Simonton S, Latif U, Spohn R, Tricot G (2005). Religious struggle and religious comfort in response to illness: Health outcomes among stem cell transplant patients. *J Behav Med* **26**: 359–67.

63 Abu-Raiya, H., Pargament, K.I., Mahoney, A. (2011). Examining coping methods with stressful interpersonal events experienced by Muslims living the U.S. following the 9/11 attacks. *Psychol Relig Spirit* **3**(1): 1–14.

64 Ghorbani, N., Watson, P.J. (2006). Religious orientation types in Iranian Muslims: Differences in alexithymia, emotional intelligence, self-consciousness and psychological adjustment. *Rev Relig Res* **47**(3): 303–10.

65 Aflakseir, A., Coleman, P.G. (2009). The influence of religious coping on mental health of disabled Iranian war veterans. *Ment Hlth Relig Cult* **12**(2): 175–90.

66 Aguilar-Vafaie, M.E., Moghanloo, M. (2008). Domain and facet personality correlates of religiosity among Iranian college students. *Ment Hlth Relig Cult* **11**(5): 461–83.

67 Ai, A.L., Peterson, C., Huang, B. (2003). The effects of religious-spiritual coping on positive attitudes of adult Muslim refugees from Kosovo and Bosnia. *Int J Psychol Relig* **13**: 29–47.

68 Khan, Z.H., Watson, P.J. (2006). Construction of the Pakistani Religious Coping Practices Scale: Correlations with religious coping, religious orientation, and reactions to stress among Muslim university students. *Int J Psychol Relig* **16**: 101–12.

69 Tarakeshwar, N., Pargament, K.I., Mahoney, A (2003). *Initial development of a measure of religious coping among Hindus. J Commun Psychol* **31**(6): 607–28.

70 Mahoney, A., Pargament, K.I., Murray-Swank, A., Murray-Swank, N. (2003). Religion and the sanctification of family relationship. *Rev Relig Res* **44**: 220–36.

71 Mahoney, A., Pargament, K.I., Tarakeshwar, N., Swank, A.B. (2001). Religion in the home in the 1980s and 1990s: A meta-analytic review and conceptual analysis of links between religion, marriage, and parenting. *J Fam Psychol* **15**(4): 559–96.

72 Gorsuch, R.L. (1988). Psychology of religion. *Annu Rev Psychol* **39**, 201–21.

73 Dubow, E.F., Pargament, K.I., Boxer, P., Tarakeshwar, N. (2000). Initial investigation of Jewish early adolescents' ethnic identity, stress, and coping. *J Early Adolesc* **20**: 418–41.

74 Miller, W.R., C'de Baca, J. (2001). *Quantum Change: When Epiphanies and Sudden Insights Transform Ordinary Lives*. New York: Guilford Press..

75 Pargament, K.I. (2007). *Spirituality Integrated Psychotherapy: Understanding and Addressing the Sacred*. New York: Guilford Press.

76 Murray-Swank, N.A., Pargament, K.I. (2005). God, where are you? Evaluating a spiritually-integrated intervention for sexual abuse. *Ment Hlth Relig Cult* **8**: 191–203.

77 Richards, P.S, Bergin, A.E. (2005). *A Spiritual Strategy for Counseling and Psychotherapy*, 2nd edn. Washington, DC: American Psychological Association.

78 Abu-Raiya, H., Pargament, K.I. (2010). Religiously integrated psychotherapy with Muslim clients: from research to practice. *Prof Psychol Res Pr* **41**(2): 181–88.

CHAPTER 46

Quality of life

Bella Vivat

Spirituality and quality of life ('QOL') are both highly debated and frequently contested concepts. If they are juxtaposed, therefore, this results in even more debate, not least because, since some definitions of QOL include a spiritual dimension, the two concepts are already interwoven and overlapping. This interweaving of spirituality and quality of life is particularly evident in the field of palliative care, with some definitions of palliative care including both QOL and spiritual issues. This chapter explores some of the ongoing debates around these concepts, and related issues and consequences for the provision of spiritual care, with a particular focus on care for people with cancer who are approaching the ends of their lives.

Debates and definitions

Quality of life

Many quality of life (QOL) measures have been developed in the last few decades, most particularly for people with cancer, and the term 'quality of life' has become less problematic in recent years than when it first began to be used on a wide scale in the early 1980s. The term is now commonly used and often simply referred to by the abbreviation 'QOL.' However, the term was regularly challenged when first used, and the concept is still contested by some.[1] One key issue has always been whether it is possible to have standardized measures of QOL, or whether QOL is always, unavoidably, subjective and specific to each individual.[2,3] Other, ongoing debates concerning QOL generally revolve around how the concept is defined, including arguments over whether it is a single construct or multi-dimensional,[4] and also whether it is appropriate to explore those dimensions collectively, or whether they should be examined separately. If agreement is reached that the concept is multi-dimensional, and should be investigated as such, further debates occur, concerning which specific domains or dimensions are relevant.

In the 1980s both the Quality of Life Group of the European Organization for Research and Treatment of Cancer (EORTC) and the Functional Assessment of Cancer Therapy (FACT) [later Functional Assessment of Chronic Illness Therapy (FACIT)] organization in the USA began developing tools to measure the quality of life of people with cancer. The EORTC QLQ-C30 has 30 items, which mostly comprise six functional scales (physical functioning, role functioning, emotional functioning, cognitive functioning, and social functioning, and a global QOL item), plus a fewer shorter scales, mostly for physical symptoms such as nausea, but also including financial issues.[5] FACT-G, the general questionnaire of FACIT.org, has 27 items in four domains (physical wellbeing, social/family wellbeing, emotional wellbeing, and functional wellbeing).[6] Thus, neither of these widely used general QOL measures includes a spiritual dimension.

However, at more or less the same time in the USA, Ferrell *et al.* [7] were developing a definition of QOL, which included a spiritual dimension. They defined QOL as having four domains: physical wellbeing, psychological wellbeing, social wellbeing, and spiritual wellbeing. In Canada, the McGill Quality of Life Questionnaire was developed to include an existential domain.[8] The 1996 definition of QOL by the World Health Organization (WHO) also includes a domain relating to spirituality; this definition states that QOL has six domains: physical health, psychological state, levels of independence, social relationships, environmental features, and spiritual concerns.[9] The WHOQOL measure was developed to include all six of these domains.[9] However, the 100-item WHOQOL was later reduced to a 26-item instrument, the WHOQOL-BREF, with four domains: physical health, psychological health, social relationships, and environment,[10] thus removing the spiritual dimension. Later, a WHO measure of spirituality, religion and personal beliefs (SRPB)[11] was developed to address this dimension separately.

Thus, those definitions of QOL that include a dimension relating to spirituality all clearly distinguish these dimensions from the psychological or emotional. Interestingly, however, despite this, some key debates concerning spirituality revolve around whether spiritual issues are distinct from psychological issues.

Spirituality/spiritual wellbeing

It is repeatedly stated[12–15] that there seems to have been a rapid growth of interest in spirituality in the last few decades, and it is certainly the case that there is an ever-increasing number of published research studies relating to spiritual issues. Unfortunately, however, some of these publications revisit issues that have been exhaustively addressed in previous years, often linked to the attempt to find definitions that are universally acceptable, by conducting small-scale qualitative interview studies.

Current debates regarding spirituality strongly parallel those which previously concerned QOL. Similar questions to those regarding definitions of QOL, which were prevalent in the 1990s are now encountered for the concepts of spirituality or spiritual wellbeing, and similar debates occur regarding the specific dimensions that comprise spirituality/spiritual wellbeing.

Parallelling the arguments that QOL is individual and standardized measures cannot therefore capture an individual's understanding of their QOL,[2,3] similar arguments are made regarding spiritual issues. Some critics argue that the concept of 'spirituality' is amorphous, and only has the meaning that an individual ascribes to it. People who take this position ask how it is possible to make any general statements, when respondents to measures of spirituality or related concepts understand these concepts in a personal, idiosyncratic way.[16] David Moberg[17] highlights the variations of interpretations of spirituality, and argues that any attempt to be universal in defining spirituality therefore inevitably excludes some groups.

For those who accept that it is possible to produce a measure of spiritual issues, other debates are dominant. One of these debates centres on whether QOL subsumes spirituality or vice versa, which links to related debates concerning whether spiritual wellbeing subsumes psychological wellbeing or vice versa.[12,17–19] Linked to this, a rather reductionist perspective identifies spiritual beliefs and practices as one coping process amongst others.[20] From this perspective, finding a positive meaning in one's experiences is simply a way of coping psychologically, rather than one outcome of a connection with someone or something beyond or greater than oneself. Relatedly, some authors use terms such as 'negative religious coping' for religious struggle, such as questioning God's love.[21,22] However, spiritual or religious doubt or uncertainty is surely a much wider issue than an indicator that someone is not coping; rather than spiritual wellbeing being a way of coping, therefore, perhaps it is rather the opposite, i.e. that coping may be one consequence of spiritual wellbeing. In contrast, Mako *et al.*[23] argue that spiritual struggles are connected with psychological distress, but do not equate the two. Some authors categorize feelings of meaning and purpose in life, positive relations with others, and personal growth as psychological wellbeing, and distinguish these from spiritual perceptions.[24] Others[25] respond to the problem of definitions/domains by collapsing spiritual and psychological wellbeing into a single concept, such as 'psycho-spiritual wellbeing,' which Lin and Bauer-Wu[26] define as including both emotional health and meaning-in-life concerns. A further, linked field of study explores meaning-in-life;[27] again, identifying this as distinct from spirituality or spiritual wellbeing. Fegg *et al.*[27] cite Merviglia's claim that meaning-in-life is not a dimension of, but an outcome of spirituality,[28] and argue that meaning-in-life is related to spirituality and self-trancendence, whereas quality-of-life reflects current, subjective wellbeing.[29]

Another, similar, debate concerns whether existential issues are part of spirituality or a separate category.[30,31] Mount *et al.*[30] distinguish the two concepts, discussing the 'existential and spiritual domains to suffering, healing and quality of life (QOL)'. They point out that suffering does not solely equate with lack of physical wellbeing, and state that suffering and subjective wellbeing are at the two extremes of QOL. However, it is not clear how they consider that the existential and spiritual domains are distinct, nor how they contribute differently to suffering. The distinction between the spiritual and the existential has also been made by the Last Acts Task Force[32] in the US, who state: 'Palliative care refers to the comprehensive management of the physical, psychological, social, spiritual and existential needs of patients [...] The goal of palliative care is to achieve the best possible quality of life.' Yet, similarly, although spiritual and existential needs are presented as separate, how they differ from one another is not clear in this document. Likewise, Boston *et al.*[31] review the palliative care literature on existential suffering, arguing that the concepts of spiritual and existential issues are sometimes used interchangeably and conflated with one another.[33] Boston *et al.* argue that the meanings of these two terms are not always clearly defined, and that spiritual measures are unsuitable for addressing existential needs. However, they do not clearly define their own understanding of either concept, or how they distinguish the two concepts from one another. Other authors argue that existential concerns include loss of personal meaning, and distinguish this from spirituality, which they identify as general beliefs about the meaning of life.[34]

Koenig[35] argues that measures of spiritual wellbeing which include positive psychological traits are flawed, since they are tautological, so positive data from such measures will of course correlate with positive mental health, and de Jager Meezenbroek *et al.*[12] echo this. Monod *et al.*[13] argue that spiritual distress is not the absence of spiritual wellbeing, and that therefore measures of spiritual wellbeing do not capture spiritual distress. They claim that no current instrument measures poor spiritual wellbeing, and argue that an instrument that measures a person's spiritual wellbeing cannot provide information on the respondent's need for spiritual intervention. Yet, it seems clear that the absence of physical wellbeing indicates physical need, and it is difficult to see why the equivalent should not also hold for spiritual wellbeing.

There seems to be a tendency amongst some authors to perceive psychological concepts as subsuming all others, even when citing other authors who do make a clear distinction between psychological and other issues. Thus, in a systematic review of psychological distress,[36] the authors state that the term 'distress' was first introduced as a working concept, based on expert consensus, to refer to emotional or psychological problems in people with cancer. However, they frame their study by referring to the US National Comprehensive Cancer Network's definition of distress as: '... a multifactorial unpleasant emotional experience of a psychological (cognitive, behavioural, emotional), social, and/or spiritual nature ... Distress extends along a continuum ... from common normal feelings of vulnerability, sadness ... to problems that can become disabling, such as depression, anxiety, panic, social isolation, and existential and spiritual crisis.'[37] This definition clearly distinguishes between psychological/emotional and spiritual or existential issues, yet Thekkumpurath *et al.*'s paper itself collapses all these issues into a psychological dimension.[36]

Similarly, in a study by Morasso *et al.*[38] of the 'psychological and symptom distress' of terminal care patients in Italy, patients' needs were identified using a semi-structured interview, which sought to explore five areas: physiological needs, safety needs, love and belonging needs, self-esteem needs, self-fulfilment needs, and identify which of these needs were most frequently not met. Over 50% of the respondents spoke of unmet needs for emotional support, and Morasso *et al.* classify these needs, and related needs for emotional closeness and self-fulfilment, as psychological,[39] despite their reference[40] to a study with terminally ill people[41] in which Greisinger *et al.* distinguish between existential, spiritual and emotional issues, stating that respondents commented that it was rare for the care they received to address the existential, spiritual, familiar, and emotional aspects of their illness. Nevertheless, Morasso *et al.* do not make the same distinction in their own study.

Fisher *et al*[42] point out that the concept of 'spiritual health' is not straightforward because not only has the term 'spiritual' been developed and revised so that it now pertains to a much broader concept than matters relating to the soul, but also the understanding of 'health' has similarly widened to include the whole person, not only treatment of disease, but a sense or state of wellbeing. Yet, interestingly, at the same time as general understandings of 'spiritual' and 'health' are becoming broader, theoretical conceptualizations of spirituality and related issues seem to be becoming narrower.

Bekelman *et al.*[43] compare the FACIT-Sp[44] with another measure, the Ironson–Woods Spirituality/Religiousness Index.[45] They point out that instruments that claim to be measuring the same spiritual domains may in fact be measuring different concepts,[46] and one goal of their study was to identify whether these two instruments obtained the same or different information from respondents[47] and also to address the criticism [e.g. 35] that the FACIT-Sp measures psychological, rather than spiritual wellbeing. They argue that their data demonstrate that, while there is some overlap between psychological and spiritual wellbeing, they are distinct phenomena.[48]

Thus, there is considerable debate over the definition of spirituality/spiritual wellbeing and the related issue of the content of measures of these and related concepts. A particularly prevalent strand of this debate is that of how psychological and spiritual issues relate to one another, and whether they are distinct, or whether one subsumes the other. As yet, there is no sign of these debates being resolved, rather an increasing fragmentation between different concepts, which nevertheless seem fundamentally rather closely related.

Palliative care/palliative medicine

In the UK palliative medicine was established as a subspecialty of general medicine in 1987, and in 1994 became a specialty in its own right.[49] The origins of palliative medicine are usually considered to be rooted in the work of Cicely Saunders, generally understood to be the founder of the modern hospice movement[49,50] (although the term 'palliative care' was itself introduced in 1973 by Balfour Mount in Canada[51]). Cicely Saunders was always explicit that the needs of people who were coming to the ends of their lives were not only physical, but also emotional, social, and spiritual, as she made clear in her concept of 'total pain.'[49,52–54] 'Total care' in modern hospices has therefore always been assumed to include spiritual care, although studies in hospices or other palliative care settings increasingly explore what total or holistic care actually means in practice.[55]

The National Hospice Organization in the US identifies a goal of palliative care as improving or enhancing patients' quality of life.[56] The definition of palliative care of the World Health Organization (WHO) in 1990 includes both quality of life and spiritual issues,[57] stating that, in palliative care: 'Control of pain, of other symptoms and of psychological, social, and spiritual problems, is paramount. The goal of palliative care is achievement of the best quality of life for patients and their families'. This definition was revised in 2002,[58,59] to state: 'Palliative care is an approach that improves the quality of life of patients and their families facing the problems associated with life-threatening illness, through the prevention and relief of suffering by means of early identification and impeccable assessment and treatment of pain and other problems, physical, psychosocial and spiritual. Palliative care provides relief from pain and other distressing symptoms; affirms life and regards dying as a normal process; intends neither to hasten or postpone death; integrates the psychological and spiritual aspects of patient care.'[59]

Thus, from the outset palliative medicine/palliative care have been explicitly associated with both QOL and spirituality, and this, together with its origins in Cicely Saunders' work, might therefore lead to the expectation that palliative care would be the area of healthcare where the identifying and addressing of spiritual issues would be the most advanced. However, there is no clear consensus around this, and debates are ongoing in this field also, beginning in the early 1990s (i.e. not long after palliative medicine was first established as a subspecialty in the UK) with Derek Doyle[60] in the UK and Michael Kearney[61] in the US almost simultaneously expressing the concern that palliative medicine could become merely 'symptomatology' (i.e. that the expertise offered by palliative medicine would amount merely to effective management of physical symptoms).

The issue of whether psychological and spiritual dimensions are distinct is also pertinent to palliative care. The Liverpool Care Pathway for the Dying Patient (LCP)[62] identifies four key domains of care: physical, psychological, social, spiritual. Yet the National Care of the Dying Audit conducted using the LCP in 2008–9 groups psychosocial and spiritual aspects of care together as a single domain of care.[63]

Problems similar to those concerning the definitions of QOL and of spirituality also arise when seeking to define palliative care/palliative medicine/end-of-life care, and, as Pastrana *et al.*[64] point out, the definition of palliative care continues to be contested. Pastrana *et al.* argue that this is not due to a lack of conceptual clarity, but rather the opposite, that is, because of attempts to achieve precision in meaning. They point out that the multiplicity of terms for related and overlapping fields such as palliative care, terminal care, end-of-life care, hospice care, 'do not simply reflect a jumble of terms, but point to the diversity of meanings.'[65]

Tools and tribulations

It is frequently argued that there is a need for suitable, high quality measures of spirituality or spiritual issues for people receiving end-of-life or palliative care.[14,66,67] Associated with this, another frequent activity in research related to spirituality, often conducted in tandem with the attempt to construct the definitive definition of the term, is reviewing the literature for measures of spirituality or related issues, such as spiritual wellbeing. Part of the ever-increasing published literature in spirituality research, therefore, includes reviews (systematic and otherwise) of existing measures, and papers reporting on the development of new measures.

As noted, neither the QLG in Europe nor FACT/FACIT in the US included a spiritual dimension in their original general measures of QOL for people with cancer, and it took some time for either organization to begin developing measures which took account of spiritual issues. The Functional Asssessment of Chronic

Illness Therapy—Spiritual Wellbeing Scale (FACIT-Sp)[44] began development in the late 1990s, at the same time as several other standalone measures were also being developed in the US, and in Europe the EORTC QLG had also begun developing a measure of palliative care, which would include a spiritual dimension.[14] This later evolved into a project to develop a single stand-alone measure of spiritual wellbeing for people receiving palliative care for cancer.[14,68]

There is, however, what could be considered a strange reticence within palliative medicine to engage with spiritual issues, and the concern that palliative medicine could become 'just another specialty'[60,61] is still not entirely resolved.[50] In 1992, Derek Doyle[60] argued that palliative care providers should not be 'merely symptomatologists,' but 'have no choice, but to be alert to and responsive to human spiritual needs.' Yet, although the European Association of Palliative Care (EAPC) was founded in 1988, an EAPC 'Task Force' to focus on spiritual care in palliative care was only established in April 2010.[69,70] There continues to be a lack or even a complete absence of spiritual care in some end-of-life/palliative care contexts.[54,55,71–74] This is perhaps due to anxiety and uncertainty by some staff concerning how to address patients' spiritual needs, and a felt lack of expertise on their part.[54,55,72] Saguil *et al.*[75] argue that the lack of spiritual care may be partly due to 'the potential reticence of patients to broach the subject in the clinical encounter.'[76] However, Saguil *et al.*'s study investigated whether a random sample of US family physicians said that they would explore spiritual issues with hypothetical patients; they did not explore those physicians' actual practices.

The gap between policy, clinicians' stated goals, and actual practice is evident in a recent publication, 'Route to success: the contribution of nursing to end of life care,' produced by the Royal College of Nurses jointly with the NHS,[73] as part of the End of Life Care Strategy of the UK Department of Health. This document states that one of the core principles for end of life care is to 'Recognize and respect an individual's spiritual and religious needs' (p. 7), and later states that nurses are to 'Ensure that access to spiritual care is available' (p. 22), and 'Ensure that spiritual and religious needs are addressed and appropriate referrals made' (p. 23). The relative document says nothing about how nurses should recognize spiritual and religious needs, nor how they should address these needs once recognized, other than brief notes in a case study included as a single page appendix on p. 41. This case study indicates that a local audit of the Liverpool Care Pathway in the West of Sussex Community NHS Trust demonstrated a significant gap in the provision of spiritual care, and that nursing teams in this Trust expressed a lack of confidence in discussing spiritual issues and a lack of clarity as to their role, and its limits, in this area.

However, the lack of spiritual care may also perhaps be associated with the pursuit of definitions, and, in the absence of any single accepted definition, a particular uncertainty regarding what comprises spiritual care. However, although it does seem difficult to find a single definition of spirituality with which everyone can agree, and although some say that this is impossible,[77] there does seem to be some shared understanding. Threads of this are evident throughout much of the literature, and have been for some time. In 1997 Hall said that the link between religion and spirit is the search for meaning, which can culminate in an understanding of self, others, God, and the meaning of one's life.[78] Sawatzky *et al.*[79] argue that, while definitions of spirituality are diverse, it is possible to extract some common characteristics: having a relationship to something that lies beyond the physical, psychological, or social; an existential search for meaning and purpose; that spirituality is defined by subjective experiences; and that spirituality and religion are distinct.

Similarly, the Scottish Government's recent document 'Spiritual care and chaplaincy'[80] argues (p. 1, points 5 and 6) 'that the spiritual dimension is a natural dimension of what it means to be human' and that this dimension includes an awareness of self, and of relationships with others and with creation. This document distinguishes between spiritual and religious care, stating that religious care might be said to be a part of the umbrella term spiritual care, so spiritual care is not necessarily religious, but religious care should always be spiritual, seeking to meet spiritual need. The document continues to state (p 2, point 7) that among the basic spiritual needs that might be addressed within the normal, daily activity of healthcare are: giving and receiving love; being understood; being valued; finding forgiveness, hope and trust; exploring beliefs and values; honestly expressing feelings; finding meaning and purpose in life.

Lemmer[81] argues that since a clear definition of spirituality is lacking, nurses might think more usefully of caring for the spiritual dimension of a person, rather than for their spirituality, and focus their assessments on key elements of the spiritual dimension: sense of meaning; hope; forgiveness; self-transcendence; and relatedness/connectedness with other people, and, for many people, also with a higher power.

Conclusion

There seems to be an intimate, perhaps inextricable, interweaving between spirituality, QOL, and palliative care, which is made explicit in some definitions of palliative care. This interweaving is also evident in struggles to find generally agreed definitions for all three concepts.

The pursuit of a single agreed definition seems currently a major stumbling block for moving forward with research connected to spirituality, and, more importantly, with the provision of spiritual care. Perhaps it is necessary, as in the early days with QOL, to grasp the imperfection and, while recognizing that any understanding is incomplete and imperfect, act nevertheless. Although there is still not a generally accepted single definition of QOL, the concept seems to now be in general use, and the way in which debates over definitions seem to have been at least partially resolved was not that general agreement on definition was reached. Rather, the point was reached where sufficient numbers of people were using the term 'quality of life' (albeit with slightly different, individual interpretations of its meaning) for it to become generally accepted—as Ludwik Fleck[82] argues, changes in understandings of valid knowledge occur not so much because members of existing thought collectives are convinced that new ideas are valid, but rather because those thought collectives become transformed and/or replaced by new thought collectives. Perhaps a similar thing will happen with spirituality, but there is as yet no sign of that occurring. Instead, the fragmentation which Pastrana *et al.*[64] point to with various terms for fields related to palliative care seems also to be happening for spirituality and related issues, resulting in ever narrower and smaller categories being produced.

Possibly measures of spirituality are not needed, and some argue that measuring spirituality or spiritual concerns is *per se* a contradictory activity.[80] However, there does seem to be uncertainty amongst some healthcare providers concerning how to identify and address spiritual issues for people receiving care, including in palliative care settings, despite claims that holistic or total care is practiced in such settings. Given the emphasis on evidence-based healthcare, associated with the rise in the use of measurement tools to justify and assess healthcare, perhaps it is better to have an imperfect measure than no measure at all. Rather than (or while) waiting for the 'perfect' measure to be developed, a possible strategy would be to select a measure from those currently available which seems to address the key elements of relevance to a particular healthcare setting, while bearing in mind the inevitable limitations of all such measures.

References

1 Grant, M., Sun, V. (2010). Advances in quality of life at the end of life. *Sem Oncol Nurs* **26**(1): 26–35.

2 Joyce, C.R.B., McGee, H.M., O'Boyle, C.A. (1999). *Individual Quality of Life: Approaches to Conceptualization and Assessment*. Amsterdam: Harwood Academic Publishers.

3 Waldron, D., O'Boyle, C.A., Kearney, M., Moriarty, M., Carney, D. (1999). Quality-of-life measurement in advanced cancer: assessing the individual. *J Clin Oncol* **17**(11): 3603–11.

4 Bush, S.H., Parsons, H.A., Palmer, J.L., Li, Z., Chacko, R., Bruera, E. (2010). Single- vs. multiple-item instruments in the assessment of quality of life in patients with advanced cancer. *Journal of Pain and Symptom Management* **39**(3): 564–71.

5 Aaronson, N.K., Ahmedzai, S., Bergman, B., Bullinger, M., Cull, A., Duez, N.J., *et al.*(1993) For the European Organization for Research and Treatment of Cancer. The QLQ-C30: a quality-of-life instrument for use in international clinical trials in oncology. *J Nat Cancer Inst* **85**: 365–76.

6 Cella, D.F., Tulsky, D.S., Gray, G., Sarafian, B., Linn, E., Bonomi, A., *et al.* (1993). The Functional Assessment of Cancer Therapy (FACT) scale: development and validation of the general measure. *J Clin Oncol* **11**(3): 570–9.

7 Ferrell, B.R., Dow, K.J., Leigh, S. Ly, J., Gulasekaram, P. (1995). Quality of life in long-term cancer survivors. *Oncol Nurs Forum* **22**: 915–22.

8 Cohen, S.R., Mount, B.M., Bruera, E., Provost, M., Rowe, J., Tong, K. (1997). Validity of the McGill Quality of Life Questionnaire in the palliative care setting: a multi-centre Canadian study demonstrating the importance of the existential domain. *Palliat Med* **11**: 3–20.

9 WHOQOL Group (1996). What is quality of life? The World Health Organization Quality of Life Assessment. *Wld Hlth Forum* **17**: 354–6.

10 World Health Organization Division of Mental Health. (1998). *WHOQOL user manual.* Available at: www.who.int/entity/mental_health/evidence/who_qol_user_manual_98.pdf (accessed 17 July 2011).

11 WHOQOL SRPB Group. (2006). A cross-cultural study of spirituality, religion, and personal beliefs as components of quality of life. *Soc Sci Med* **62**: 1486–97.

12 de Jager Meezenbroek, E., Garssen, B., van den Berg, M., van Dierendonck, D., Visser, A., Schaufeli, W.B. (2010). Measuring spirituality as a universal human experience: a review of spirituality questionnaires. *J Relig Health*. Available at: Springerlink.com (accessed 20 July 2010).

13 Monod, S., Brennan, M., Rochat, E., Martin, E., Rochat, S., Büla, C.J.(2011). Instruments measuring spirituality in clinical research: a systematic review. *J Gen Intern Med* **26**(11): 1345–57.

14 Vivat, B. on behalf of the EORTC Quality of Life Group (2008). Measures of spiritual issues for palliative care patients: a literature review. *Palliat Med* **22**: 859–68.

15 Weaver, A.J., Pargament, K.I., Flannelly, K.J., Oppenheimer, J.E. (2006). Trends in the scientific study of religion, spirituality and health: 1965–2000. *J Relig Hlth* **45**: 208–14.

16 Sawatzky, R., Pesut, B. (2005). Attributes of spiritual care in nursing practice. *J Holist Nurs* **23**(1): 19–33.

17 Moberg, D.O. (2002). Assessing and measuring spirituality: confronting dilemmas of universal and particular evaluative criteria. *J Adult Devel* **9**(1): 47–60.

18 Monod, S., Rochat, E., Büla, C., Jobin, G., Martin, E., Spencer, B. (2010). The spiritual distress assessment tool: an instrument to assess spiritual distress in hospitalized elderly persons. *BMC Geriat* **10**: 88.

19 Moreira-Almeida, A., Koenig, H.G. (2006). Retaining the meaning of the words religiousness and spirituality: a commentary on the WHOQOL SRPB group's 'a cross-cultural study of spirituality, religion, and personal beliefs as components of quality of life.' *Soc Sci Med* **63**: 843–5.

20 Folkman, S. (1997). Positive psychological states and coping with severe stress. *Soc Sci Med* **45**(8): 1207–21.

21 Hills, J., Paice, J.A., Cameron, J.R., Shott, S. (2005). Spirituality and distress in palliative care consultation. *J Pall Med* **8**(4): 782–8.

22 Pargament, K.I., Koenig, H.G., Perez, L.M. (2000). The many methods of religious coping: development and initial validation of the RCOPE. *J Clin Psychol* **56**: 519–43.

23 Mako, C., Galek, K., Poppito, S.R. (2006). Spiritual pain among patients with advanced cancer in palliative care. *J Pall Med* **9**(5): 1106–13.

24 Greenfield, E.A., Vaillant, G.E., Marks, N.F. (2009). Do formal religious participation and spiritual perceptions have independent linkages with diverse dimensions of psychological wellbeing? *J Hlth Sci Behav* **50**(2): 196–212.

25 Lin, H.R., Bauer-Wu, S.M. (2003). Psycho-spiritual wellbeing in patients with advanced cancer: an integrative review of the literature. *J Adv Nurs* **44**(1): 69–80.

26 Lin, H.R., Bauer-Wu, S.M. (2003). Psycho-spiritual wellbeing in patients with advanced cancer: an integrative review of the literature. *J Adv Nurs* **44**(1): 70.

27 Fegg, M.J., Brandstätter, M., Kramer, M., Kögler, M., Haarmann-Doetkotte, S., Borasio, G.D. (2010). Meaning in life in palliative care patients. *J Pain Sympt Manage* **40**(4): 502–9.

28 Meraviglia, M. (1999). Critical analysis of spirituality and its empirical indicators. Prayer and meaning in live. *J Holist Nurs* **17**: 18–33.

29 Fegg, M.J., Brandstätter, M., Kramer, M., Kögler, M., Haarmann-Doetkotte, S., Borasio, G.D. (2010). Meaning in life in palliative care patients. *J Pain Sympt Manage* **40**(4): 503.

30 Mount, B.M., Boston, P.H., Cohen, S.R. (2007). Healing connections: on moving from suffering to a sense of wellbeing. *J Pain Sympt Manage* **33**(4): 372–88.

31 Boston, P., Bruce, A., Schreiber, R. (2011). Existential suffering in the palliative care setting: an integrated literature review. *J Pain Sympt Manage* (published online ahead of press)

32 Last Acts Task Force. (1997). *Precepts of palliative care*. Princeton, NJ: Robert Wood Johnson Foundation.

33 Boston, P., Bruce, A., Schreiber, R. (2011). Existential suffering in the palliative care setting: an integrated literature review. *J Pain Sympt Manage* **41**(3): 608–18.

34 Henoch, I., Danielson, E. (2009). Existential concerns among patients with cancer and interventions to meet them: an integrative literature review. *Psycho-oncol* **18**: 225–36.

35 Koenig, H.G. (2008). Concerns about measuring 'spirituality' in research. *J Nerv Ment Dis* **196**(5): 349–55.

36 Thekkumpurath, P., Venkateswaran, C., Kumar, M., Bennett, M.I. (2008). Screening for psychological distress in palliative care: a systematic review. *J Pain Sympt Manage* **36**(5): 520–8.

37 National Comprehensive Cancer Network. (2007). Clinical Practice Guidelines in Oncology. Available at: http://www.nccn.org/professionals/physician_gls/PDF/distress.pdf (accessed 17 July 2011).

38 Morasso, G., Capelli, B., Viterbori, P., Di Leo, S., Alberisio, A., Costantini, M., *et al.* (1999). Psychological and symptom distress in terminal cancer patients with met and unmet needs. *J Pain Sympt Manage* **17**(6): 402–9.

39 Morasso, G., Capelli, B., Viterbori, P., Di Leo, S., Alberisio, A., Costantini, M., *et al.* (1999). Psychological and symptom distress in terminal cancer patients with met and unmet needs. *J Pain Sympt Manage*, **17**(6): 405.

40 Morasso, G., Capelli, B., Viterbori, P., Di Leo, S., Alberisio, A., Costantini, M., *et al.* (1999). Psychological and symptom distress in terminal cancer patients with met and unmet needs. *J Pain Sympt Manage* **17**(6): 408.

41 Greisinger, A.J., Lorimor, R.J., Aday, L.A., Winn, R.J., Baile, W.F. (1997). Terminally ill cancer patients: their most important concerns. *Cancer Pract* **5**: 147–54.

42 Fisher, J.W., Francis, L.J., Johnson, P. (2000). Assessing spiritual health via four domains of spiritual wellbeing: the SH4DI. *Past Psychol* **49**(2): 133–45.

43 Bekelman, D.B., Parry, C., Curlin, F.A., Yamashita, T.E., Fairclough, D.L., Wamboldt, F.S. (2010). A comparison of two spirituality instruments and their relationship with depression and quality of life in chronic heart failure. *J Pain Sympt Manage* **39**(3): 515–26.

44 Peterman, A.H., Fitchett, G., Brady, M.J., Hernandez, L., Cella, D. (2002). Measuring spiritual wellbeing in people with cancer: the Functional Assessment of Chronic Illness Therapy-Spiritual Wellbeing Scale (FACIT-Sp). *Ann Behav Med* **24**(1): 49–58.

45 Ironson, G., Solomon, G.F., Balbin, E.G., O'Cleirigh, C., George, A., Kumar, M., *et al.* (2002). The Ironson–Woods Spirituality/ Religiousness Index is associated with long survival, health behaviours, less distress, and low cortisol in people with HIV/AIDS. *Ann Behav Med* **24**(1): 34–48.

46 Bekelman, D.B., Parry, C., Curlin, F.A., Yamashita, T.E., Fairclough, D.L., Wamboldt, F.S. (2010). A comparison of two spirituality instruments and their relationship with depression and quality of life in chronic heart failure. *J Pain Sympt Manage* **39**(3): 515–26, p. 523.

47 Bekelman, D.B., Parry, .C, Curlin, F.A., Yamashita, T.E., Fairclough, D.L., Wamboldt, F.S. (2010). A comparison of two spirituality instruments and their relationship with depression and quality of life in chronic heart failure. *J Pain Sympt Manage* **39**(3): 515–26, p. 517.

48 Bekelman, D.B., Parry, C., Curlin, F.A., Yamashita, T.E., Fairclough, D.L., Wamboldt, F.S. (2010). A comparison of two spirituality instruments and their relationship with depression and quality of life in chronic heart failure. *J Pain Sympt Manage* **39**(3): 515–26, p. 524.

49 Clark, D. (2007). From margins to centre: a review of the history of palliative care in cancer. *Lancet Oncol* **8**: 430–8.

50 Byock, I. (1998). Hospice and palliative care: a parting of the ways or a path to the future? *J Palliat Med* **1**(2): 165–76.

51 Billings, J.A. (1998). What is palliative care? *J Palliat Med* **1**: 73–81.

52 Clark, D. (1999). 'Total pain', disciplinary power, and the body in the work of Cicely Saunders 1958–67. *Soc Sci Med* **49**: 727–36.

53 Saunders, C.M. (1981). The founding philosophy. In: C. Saunders, D.H. Summers, N. Teller (eds) *Hospice: the Living Idea*, p. 4. London: Edward Arnold.

54 Vivat, B. (2004). *The Whole and the Parts: Spiritual Aspects of Care in a West of Scotland Hospice*. Unpublished PhD, University of Edinburgh.

55 Vivat, B. (2008). 'Going down' and 'getting deeper': physical and metaphorical location and movement in relation to death and spiritual care in a Scottish hospice. *Mortality* **13**(1): 42–64.

56 National Hospice Organization. (1993). *Standards of a Hospice Program of Care*. Arlington: National Hospice Organization.

57 World Health Organization. (1990). *Cancer Pain Relief and Palliative Care*, WHO Technical Report Series 804. Geneva: World Health Organization.

58 Sepúlveda, C., Marlin, A., Yoshida, T., Ullrich, A. (2002). Palliative care: the World Health Organization's global perspective. *J Pain Sympt Manage*, **24**: 91–6.

59 World Health Organization. (2002). *WHO Definition of Palliative Care*. Available at: http://www.who.int/cancer/palliative/definition/en/(accessed 17 July 2011).

60 Doyle, D. (1992). Have we looked beyond the physical and psychosocial? *J Pain Sympt Manage* **7**: 302–11.

61 Kearney, M. (1992). Palliative medicine: just another specialty? *Palliat Med* **6**(1): 39–46.

62 Marie Curie Palliative Care Institute Liverpool. (2009a). Liverpool Care Pathway for the Dying Patient (LCP): Core Documentation. Available at: http://www.mcpcil.org.uk/liverpool-care-pathway/documentation-lcp.htm (accessed 17 July 2011).

63 Marie Curie Palliative Care Institute Liverpool. (2009b). *National Care of the Dying Audit—Hospitals (NCDAH): Round 2 Generic Report 2008/2009*, p. 4. Available at: http://www.liv.ac.uk/mcpcil/liverpool-care-pathway/national-care-of-dying-audit.htm (accessed 17 July 2011).

64 Pastrana, T., Jünger, S., Ostgathe, C., Elsner, F., Radbruch, L. (2008). A matter of definition—key elements identified in a discourse analysis of definitions of palliative care. *Palliat Med* **22**: 222–32.

65 Pastrana, T., Jünger, S., Ostgathe, C., Elsner, F., Radbruch, L. (2008). A matter of definition—key elements identified in a discourse analysis of definitions of palliative care. *Palliat Med* **22**: 222–32, p. 222.

66 Chochinov, H.M., Hassard, T., McClement, S., Hack, T., Kristjanson, L.J., Harlos, M., *et al.* (2008). The Patient Dignity Inventory: a novel way of measuring dignity-related distress in palliative care. *J Pain Sympt Manage* **36**(6): 559–71.

67 Mularski, R.A., Dy, S.M., Shugarman, L.R., Wilkinson, A.M., Lynn, J., Shekelle, P.G., *et al.* (2007). A systematic review of measures of end-of-life care and its outcomes. *Hlth Serv Res* **42**(5): 1848–70.

68 Vivat, B., Young, T., Efficace, F. *et al.* on behalf of the EORTC Quality of Life Group (forthcoming). Developing the EORTC QLQ-SWB36: a measure of spiritual wellbeing for palliative care patients with cancer. *Eur J Cancer.*

69 European Association of Palliative Care (EAPC). (2011). *EAPC Task Force on Spiritual Care in Palliative Care*. Available at: http://www.eapcnet.eu/Themes/Clinicalcare/Spiritualcareinpalliativecare/tabid/1520/Default.aspx (accessed 17 July 2011).

70 Nolan, S., Saltmarsh, P., Leget, C. (2011). Spiritual care in palliative care: working towards an EAPC Task Force. *Eur J Palliat Care* **18**(2): 86–9.

71 Carr, T. (2008). Mapping the processes and qualities of spiritual nursing care. *Qual Hlth Res* **18**(5): 686–700.

72 Lemmer, C.A. (2005). Recognizing and caring for spiritual needs of clients. *J Holist Nurs* **23**(3): 310–22.

73 National End of Life Care Programme (NEoLCP). (2011). Route to Success: the Key Contribution of Nursing to End of Life Care. London: Royal College of Nursing/NHS. Available at: http://www.endoflifecareforadults.nhs.uk/publications/rts-nursing (accessed 17 July 2011).

74 Williams, J.A., Meltzer, D., Arora, V., Chung, G., Curlin, F.A. (2011). Attention to inpatients' religious and spiritual concerns: predictors and association with patient satisfaction. *J Gen Intern Med* **26**(11): 1265–71.

75 Saguil, A., Fitzpatrick, A.L., Clark, G. (2011). Are residents willing to discuss spirituality with patients? *J Relig Hlth* **50**: 279–88.

76 Saguil, A., Fitzpatrick, A.L., Clark, G. (2011). Are residents willing to discuss spirituality with patients? *J Relig Hlth* **50**: 279–88.

77 McSherry, W., Cash, K. (2004). The language of spirituality: an emerging taxonomy. *Int J Nurs Stud* **41**: 151–61.

78 Hall, B.A. (1997). Spirituality in terminal illness. *J Holist Nurs* **15**(1): 82–96.

79 Sawatzky, R., Ratner, P.A., Chiu, L. (2005). A meta-analysis of the relationship between spirituality and quality of life. *Soc Indicat Res* **72**: 153–88.

80 NHS Scotland. (2009). *Spiritual Care and Chaplaincy*. Edinburgh: Scottish Government.

81 Lemmer, C.A. (2005). Recognizing and caring for spiritual needs of clients. *J Holist Nurs* **23**(3): 310–22.

82 Fleck, L. (1935/79). *Genesis and Development of a Scientific Fact*, eds T.J. Trenn, R.K. Merton; transl F. Bradley, T.J. Trenn. Chicago: University of Chicago Press.

CHAPTER 47

Cognitive sciences: a perspective on spirituality and religious experience

Kevin S. Seybold

Psychology is typically defined as the scientific study of human behaviour and mental processes, and for the psychologists of the late nineteenth and early twentieth centuries, religious experience was an important subject of investigation. Leading psychologists took care to present this new discipline as a practical tool for the understanding of religion. Perhaps the best example of this approach is the work of William James whose book *The Varieties of Religious Experience* brought the new psychology to the analysis of the 'religious propensities of man,' which must, according to James, 'be at least as interesting as any other of the facts pertaining to his mental constitution.'[1] Influenced by the work of Freud and Skinner, however, who both took decidedly negative views of religion, psychology for most of the twentieth century considered the study of religion and religious behaviour taboo. Few psychologist interested in developing a publication resume investigated this seemingly universal human concern. The last two decades of the century saw a dramatic change with more and more researchers from a variety of disciplines (psychology, sociology, anthropology, medicine, etc.) investigating religion and religious experiences. Much of this renewed interest was motivated by studies suggesting that religion and spirituality have a positive effect on both physical and mental health.[2]

The cognitive sciences consist of a group of disciplines interested in studying the mind. Psychology, linguistics, computer science, artificial intelligence, philosophy, and neuroscience are just a few of the fields that contribute to this approach to mind, and religious and spiritual experiences are now included as subject matter in this method. The current chapter will review how spirituality and religious experience are understood from the perspective of the cognitive sciences. Included in this review will be a discussion of current thinking in the field regarding the origin of religion. A leading approach to this issue comes from evolutionary psychology, which argues that behaviour (including religious behaviour) can be understood as evolving through natural selection, often involving the social emotions, altruism, and cooperation. An important controversy within this approach is the extent to which religion (and its associated behaviours and experiences) is an evolutionary adaptation. In addition, the question of why a person believes in God or gods will be considered, particularly the view that humans use 'mental tools' that bias how we develop all of our mental concepts, including religious/spiritual ones. The chapter will also review evidence from the neurosciences dealing with what religion/spirituality and the associated experiences look like in the brain. Is there a consistent set of brain areas or brain circuitry associated with religious and spiritual experiences? If so, what might that tell us about the function of religion? Finally, the chapter will consider what the evidence from the cognitive sciences and the neurosciences suggest regarding the relationship between spirituality and health, and what the putative mechanisms involved in this interface might entail for healthcare.

Before beginning an overview of the literature, however, a question to consider in this discussion is whether religious/spiritual experiences are different from other experiences. Are religious experiences unique or similar to all the other experiences we have? One approach argues that religious/spiritual experiences are *sui generis*. According to this model, religiousness in inherent in the experience itself and is, therefore, a unique kind of experience tapping into a common core of experiences that refer to the numinous and mystical. Certain experiences are, by definition, religious and are always understood as such. A different approach suggests that experiences are not inherently religious or spiritual; instead, the person having the experience ascribes it as being religious. There is no common core for religious experiences. Different kinds of experiences can be deemed religious by the person having the experience. This ascription model[3] is similar to the view taken by James in *Varieties* where, talking about the role of emotion in religious experience, he argued that there is no elementary religious emotion, 'but only a common storehouse of emotions upon which religious objects may draw.'[4] For the cognitive or neural scientist, one is either investigating the cognitive and brain mechanisms involved in these inherently spiritual experiences or studying how these mental and neural mechanisms are involved in making a given experience special or religious. Either way it is the mental modules that are investigated in the cognitive sciences and the corresponding neural mechanisms that the neuroscientist is attempting to identify. In this respect, considerable advances were made in the last 10–15 years, and these developments will be reviewed in this chapter.

In this chapter the terms religion and spirituality are used more or less interchangeably. While society today often distinguishes between religion and spirituality, from the perspective of cognitive science/neuroscience, the cognitive and neural structures that underlie these beliefs are thought to be essentially the same. Individuals' decisions to identify with religious institutions or spiritual movements, or to dissociate from them, has a social and cultural, not a neurological, basis.

Spirituality from a cognitive science perspective

The cognitive science of religion (CSR) uses theories in the cognitive sciences to understand the basic structure of those human thoughts and actions that can be deemed religious. It typically does not concern itself with trying to define religion, but to understand why thoughts and behaviours considered religious take the form they do, and why these forms of thought and behaviour are so common and recurrent across cultures.[5] These cognitive structures of the mind shape and bias the kinds of concepts we form and influence how we experience the world, including those aspects of the world considered to be religious. Religious beliefs, like all beliefs, reflect the underlying structures of the mind.[6,7] CSR also does not necessarily assume that its understanding of religious thoughts and actions is exhaustive. While some (for example, Boyer) seek a complete and reductionistic account of religion and believe that current findings in CSR present a problem for theism, others do not see evidence from CSR (or evolutionary biology or neuroscience for that matter) as providing a threat for theological versions of religious beliefs.[8] Seen through this lens, reality is multi-levelled and stratified, and so can be studied from a variety of perspectives and on a number of levels. Religion, therefore, can be approached from different levels, each with its own methods of investigation. While one could, theoretically, exhaustively know about some aspect of reality using methods appropriate for a given level of analysis, other types of analyses can always be applied to further understand that particular phenomenon. It is appropriate, therefore, to study religion or spirituality from a cognitive science perspective (or from a neuroscience perspective) without doing so in a reductionistic manner. Religion and spirituality can always be known more completely by applying methods appropriate from other levels of reality. (Of course, CSR and the neurosciences, or theology for that matter, cannot tell us the truth or falsity of any belief. Identifying, for example, what area of the brain is activated when we express the belief that 2 × 2 equals 4, tells us nothing about the truth of that belief.)

A central issue in CSR is why people have religious beliefs in the first place. According to evolutionary psychology, the mind's structures or tools exist because they, like physical characteristics, confer a survival advantage. Are the specific mental constructs that are deemed religious adaptations that provide survival advantage? One view is to say yes, religious and spiritual concepts are the products of natural selection and serve to benefit the religious individual. Those individuals with mental concepts that bias them to see reality in religious or spiritual terms will have a reproductive advantage over those individuals who lack these mental tools.[9] The adaptationist argument is supported, some suggest, by evidence of a salubrious effect of religion on physical (and mental) health. Among other findings, people who score high on measures of spirituality and religion tend to live longer, have lower rates of disease, and have a higher satisfaction with life. If a spiritual/religious person lives longer, so the argument goes, then spirituality/religion is adaptive. A version of this adaptation approach is to argue that selection occurs at the level of the group, and that it is the group, not the individual, that benefits from religious and spiritual mental constructs. Those groups showing greater degrees of cohesion, trust, and cooperation (fostered by religion/spiritual beliefs and practices) would also be more likely to survive, and the individual members of those groups would pass these traits to their offspring.

Another perspective suggests that religion/spirituality is not adaptive, *per se*, but is a by-product of adaptations that serve non-spiritual/non-religious practices. For example, a cognitive structure that promotes group solidarity and cooperation would be selected because it serves to make the group stronger (perhaps aiding in hunting for food and defence of the group). This cognitive tool could also, as a secondary benefit, foster religious beliefs, but it is not the religious beliefs that are selected, it is the tendency toward cooperation with members of one's group that is selected. Religion is, therefore, a by-product, not directly adaptive.

Sosis and Alcorta argue that selective pressures did, in fact, shape the human capacity for religion and that physical, psychological, and reproductive benefits result. They see these benefits developing because religious beliefs and practices promote group solidarity. Groups form in order to obtain resources, and this group activity requires coordinated action among many individuals. Moral systems (part of a group's religious practices) help to regulate behaviour which is needed for coordinated and effective group behaviour. To the extent that religion enhances cooperation among individuals and fosters coordinated group behaviour, it provides a selective advantage over a competing group that is less coordinated and efficient.[10] A potential danger in groups, however, is the problem of free-riders, those who take advantage of the success of the group without providing any behavioural support for the group's action. Consider, for example, the individual who repeatedly eats the group's food, but does not participate, in an active way, in the hunt itself. The potential for a free-ride on the backs of others in the group must be reduced for any large-scale cooperative endeavours. Sosis and Alcorta suggest that religious rituals can be seen as hard to fake, costly signals that demonstrate an individual's commitment to the group and engender trust in that individual. Taboos can also serve this function in a group. Giving up something desired to belong to the group can be seen as a show of commitment, a desire to be a part of that group. These religious practices are adaptations, not by-products, and a religion's ability to promote cooperation is its evolutionary function.[11] The cognitive mechanisms that support such religious beliefs and rituals evolved to ensure this cooperation. Religious rituals also activate the autonomic nervous system and limbic system structures eliciting emotions. Because they have a neurological foundation and are largely outside of conscious control, emotions are difficult to fake and are, therefore, good communication signals. Rituals, in non-humans, increase communication of social information and coordinate social behaviours.[12] While potentially costly, rituals are useful in that they provide signals of a person's intent vis-à-vis the group, readying the participants for social interaction.

The moral sense, an important part of human nature, also evolved to encourage cooperation, altruism, and virtue.[13] Prosocial behaviour was encouraged in groups through these moral judgments. According to this view, early humans inherited social instincts which induced pleasure in the presence of others of the group and to feel sympathy for them. With the development of higher mental processes such as language, the proper way to treat others in the group could be effectively communicated which developed into a sense of morality. These evolved mechanisms lead individuals to behave in prosocial ways that produce psychological states experienced as awe, righteousness, gratitude, love, forgiveness, empathy, loyalty, etc. (the so-called social emotions).[14] Some behaviours are deemed acceptable to the group, others not acceptable. The primatologist Frans de Waal sees the social emotions, especially empathy, as important in promoting group cohesion. Empathy evolved as the primary mechanism for altruism that is directed toward those with whom one has a positive or close relationship. Altruism is withheld from strangers or defectors from the group.[15]

To what extent are religious belief and experience the same among cultures, and to what extent are they the same from one society to another? From a CSR perspective, the similarities among religious beliefs suggest a framework for understanding why a person would believe in gods or in God. Justin Barrett is a cognitive psychologist who, representing the position of many researchers in the cognitive science of religion, argues that religious beliefs are common in humans because they are supported by intuitive mental tools that all humans possess. In his analysis of these religious beliefs, Barrett[16] distinguishes between reflective and non-reflective beliefs. Non-reflective beliefs are arrived at automatically and instantaneously without conscious activity. Reflective beliefs, however, are arrived at using conscious and deliberate thought processes. While religious beliefs typically have reflective components, they are, nevertheless, supported by non-reflective elements. The question then becomes, 'What is the origin of these non-reflective beliefs that serve as the basis for strongly held reflective, religious beliefs?' According to a CSR approach, these non-reflective beliefs emerge out of the mental tools that bias the way we understand and explain events in our environment.

Some of these mental tools act as categorizers in that they utilize information from the senses to determine what sort of thing is being perceived. An example of such a categorizer is the Agency Detection Device (ADD), which looks for agents or beings that might be the cause of some action perceived in the environment. Another kind of mental tool is a describer that attributes properties to an identified agent. For example, a Living Thing Describer ascribes nutritional, growth, and reproductive needs to a thing categorized as an animal. Another describer is Theory of Mind (ToM), which ascribes a host of mental abilities to an agent identified by the ADD. All humans have the same mental tools, which evolved in our species through the process of natural selection. According to a CSR approach, which is strongly influenced by evolutionary psychology, these mental tools provide survival advantage to those individuals who possess them and give rise to non-reflective beliefs. Consider the situation where a person is walking in the woods and hears a 'rustling' noise from behind. According to CSR, the human mind is biased to non-reflectively come to believe (or assume) that the ambiguous noise is generated by some kind of agent (the activity of the, now, hypersensitive ADD or HADD) that might be a threat or, perhaps, a possible source of food for a hunter-gatherer. While this ascription might later prove to be false (it was, after all, just the wind blowing through the trees), better to be 'biased' to make a false positive than to miss a real threat or potential meal.

How do these evolved mental tools lead to religious beliefs? While reflective beliefs certainly vary from person to person, non-reflective beliefs are similar among individuals because they are tied to mental tools that function similarly among individuals. Religious beliefs, emerging as they do from non-reflective beliefs, are common (universal?) because they are supported by the human mind's intuitive mental tools. Religious beliefs are also common because they represent a class of concepts termed Minimally Counterintuitive (MCI)[17] which are concepts that meet most of the assumptions that categorizers and describers create, but violate just a few. By violating a few of these assumptions (being minimally counterintuitive), the concept becomes interesting and memorable.[18] Because the categorizers and describers set the parameters for what is intuitive and counterintuitive, what is MCI in one culture (or in one person) will be MCI in another culture (or in another person). Being counterintuitive can activate other mental tools (e.g. ToM), which increase the non-reflective evidence for the belief. (The wind storm that destroyed my neighbour's house, but spared mine was caused by an agent that has certain purposes and goals for me, and so it was by the agent's will that my home and family were spared.) The more such evidence, the greater the likelihood of developing a reflective belief. To become a religious belief, however, the belief must spread to or be shared with others. Beliefs about gods, for example, spread to others because these MCI concepts meet most of the requirements for categorizers and describers, but violate just enough to make them memorable and interesting. A concept that is memorable and interesting is more likely to be talked about to others. In addition, MCI concepts are used to explain, predict and make sense of experiences, activating a number of mental tools and enhancing the concept's credibility.[19]

Regularity across cultures as to what constitutes moral behaviour suggests that morality is neither arbitrary nor relative. A third type of mental tool (in addition to categorizers and describers), known as facilitators, organize social behaviours in order to help predict and understand human behavior, where beliefs or desires provided by ToM are not adequate. According to CSR, an example of such a facilitator is intuitive morality, a product of our biological heritage that enables necessary instincts regarding what behaviour and expectations are proper for a given community and situation. As a general rule, these behaviours and expectations refer to survival and reproductive issues within a community and also play a role in the development of non-reflective beliefs.

Specific religious beliefs for which a CSR approach might account include belief in life after death. According to CSR, humans have an ability to imagine, via ToM, psychological states in the absence of a physical body. For example, it is easy to imagine what one's partner is feeling or thinking, even if the partner is not physically present (away at work, visiting the in-laws, etc.). The same ToM processes can readily imagine psychological processes occurring after physical death of a person; thoughts, feelings, etc., can still be ascribed to that individual. The same mental tools are used for a person who is deceased as are used every day for a person we know who is still living, but not physically with us.

One issue in the CSR literature is the extent to which belief in gods or in God is a natural thing. That is to say, is a belief in an agent with superhuman powers (omnipotence, omniscience, etc.) a belief that comes naturally to a child (it is intuitive) or is it unnatural in that it is difficult for the child to accept and hold such views. While there is disagreement on this subject, CSR generally suggests that such beliefs are natural and that a child's cognitive mechanisms assume that many superhuman properties are the norm.

[20] To develop this further, a brief discussion of the timing of the development of a child's ToM is necessary. A child develops a ToM around the age of 5 years and is illustrated in what is known in the developmental psychology literature as the surprising-contents false-belief task. A child is shown a cracker box that is filled, not with crackers, but with stones. When asked what her mother, who has not looked in the box, will think is in the box, a child under 5 years of age will typically indicate a belief that her mother will think that there are stones in the cracker box because that is what the child knows to be true. At the age of 5 years and above, however, the child will report that her mother will believe that there are crackers in the box. At this point, the child has developed a ToM, which allows her to understand that the mother will have a false belief; the mother does not know what the child knows, and the child can make this distinction. So, the default position for the child is to accept this superhuman power for the mother, and God concepts play upon this default assumption rather than violate it. Children develop a ToM by the age of 5 and no longer believe that their mothers think there are stones in the box instead of crackers. A 5-year-old child, however, still believes that God would correctly know what is actually in the box. So, the mother is fooled, but God is not suggesting that children are using a prepared (or natural) mental concept when thinking about God's powers and abilities.[21] Additionally, children easily distinguish between the natural world and the artificial. They understand that there are some things that humans just cannot make and so naturally see the world as created by a non-human super-being. Belief in a concept of God as creator is an easy (perhaps natural) step for the child to take. Comparable results are found in studies of children from different cultures using various culture-appropriate tasks, leading many CSR researchers to propose that belief in a super-knowing, -perceiving, -powerful being is non-reflective and is, therefore, a natural product of the human mind.

Children are also biased in favour of teleological explanations when trying to understand both living and non-living natural objects. They tend to reason about these objects in terms of purpose making children, according to psychologist Deborah Kelemen, intuitive theists.[22] Kelemen reports that this bias diminishes around 10 years of age, but is seen in children in a variety of countries suggesting that the preference is not due to cultural religiosity, but is a natural human tendency to use intentional explanations for the world.

Paul Bloom, professor of psychology at Yale University, also argues that belief in divine agents comes naturally to children. While culture certainly plays a role in the development of religious beliefs, Bloom suggests that some religious concepts (such as dualism and divine agents) are unlearned and emerge out of the cognitive biases that characterize a child's mind.[23]

From this CSR perspective, belief in gods emerges from the same mental processes as do the majority of all beliefs: the operation of mental tools that give rise to non-reflective beliefs used to make sense of the world. Because these beliefs are natural or intuitive, they are widespread among people of various cultures.[24] We use these non-reflective beliefs to make inferences and to provide explanations, and they provide best guesses for our reflective beliefs unless there are compelling reasons to believe otherwise. We believe in gods (or in God, specifically) because such beliefs are an inevitable consequence of the kind of minds we have and the kind of world in which we live.[25]

What does spirituality look like in the brain?

The brain is involved in all that we think, feel, do, and believe. Neuroscientists use the term neural representation to refer to how a particular experience is registered in the nervous system. We should not be surprised, therefore, to discover brain activity correlated with experiences deemed to be religious or spiritual. Biologically orientated psychologists and neuroscientists use various kinds of imaging technology to see what the brain looks like when a particular experience occurs. For example, using imaging technologies such as PET and fMRI, a brain scientist can get a picture of which brain areas are active when a person reports having a particular kind of spiritual experience. If there is a consistent set of brain sites or circuits that turn on during a spiritual experience, then knowing the function of those brain regions can provide information about the possible function of the spiritual experience.[26] This section will discuss the role of three general brain regions in religious and spiritual experience: the temporal lobe and associated limbic system structures, areas of the parietal lobe, and structures of the frontal lobe. In addition, the role of neurotransmitter systems in spiritual experiences will be reviewed followed by a discussion of the implications of this literature for understanding the function of spirituality/religion and its relevance to the cognitive science of religion.

Much of the early work in what has come to be called neurotheology (the study of the brain's involvement in religious experience) focused on the role of the temporal lobe and limbic system structures. Evidence from a variety of sources suggests a correlation between seizures in the temporal lobe and reported religious experience.[27] Some researchers (e.g. Persinger) suggest that religious/spiritual experience can be reduced to short-term electrical activity localized within the temporal lobe. We are able to have a God experience because the temporal lobe developed the way it did. Had it developed differently, the 'God experience would not have occurred.'[28] Joseph also points to the limbic system (especially the amygdala and hippocampus) as providing a foundation for spiritual experience speculating that, if a spiritual reality exists, these structures would, just like other evolved structures and networks in the brain, increase the likelihood of survival by helping the individual make contact with this aspect of reality.[29]

Other researchers note activity not only in temporal lobe structures during religious experiences, but in a variety of areas found throughout the brain. For example, Newberg reports increased activity in the frontal lobe and decreased activity in neural areas found in the parietal lobe. The inhibition of parietal activity is, Newberg suggests, in the area responsible for orientating us in space by creating a distinction between the self and the rest of the world. When this parietal region is inhibited, as Newberg found in his study of both Franciscan nuns in prayer and Buddhist monks during meditation, the reported experience is one of 'timelessness' or 'infinity' in the Buddhist meditators and of being 'close to God' in the Franciscan nuns.[30] The increased activity in the frontal lobes was interpreted to represent a heightened level of attention during the religious activities. Other studies have also noted decreases in parietal lobe activity, particularly in the right hemisphere, during reported religious experiences. Johnstone and Glass[31] observed a decrease in right parietal lobe, which they, like Newberg, associated with a reduction in awareness of the self (or an elevated sense of the transcendent). The authors also reported an increase in activity in the left temporal lobe, which they suggest is associated with the experience of particular religious figures or symbols. The authors use these data to develop a model of spirituality that includes specific and universal neurophysiological and neuropsychological processes that reflect the multifaceted nature of the religious/spiritual experience. These natural processes, however, can be interpreted differently depending on how religious symbols and figures are culturally defined.

Selective damage to parietal regions induces increases in self-transcendence, operationalized to mean a tendency to see the self as an integral part of the universe as a whole.[32] Self-transcendence measures were taken prior to and after patients experienced surgical removal of brain glioma involving the parietal region. Damage to right and left posterior parietal cortex was associated with higher self-transcendence; this increase was especially noted following right hemisphere damage.

Evidence from temporal lobe epilepsy and obsessive-compulsive disorder suggests that not only the limbic system and temporal lobe structures are involved in these disorders, but also frontal and prefrontal regions as well. These disorders are associated with hyperreligiosity, and McNamara postulates, based on clinical data, that structures in each of these regions are involved in brain circuits that mediate religiosity including the amygdala, basal ganglia, medial and superior temporal lobe, and dorsomedial, orbitofrontal, and right dorsolateral prefrontal cortex.[33] Overall, imaging studies support the involvement of these structures in religious experiences, with increases in activity seen in prefrontal and temporal lobes, as well as the limbic system, most notably on the right side. This circuit is regulated by dopamine and serotonin neurotransmitter systems, and increases in dopaminergic activity are observed during religious practices.[34] This circuit partially overlaps that of the neural system involved in reinforcement and addiction, activation of which is rewarding.

McNamara notes that the frontal and temporal lobes mediate capacities and functions that are considered to be involved in defining us as free human beings, and that successful religious practices are, at least partially, those that foster activity in and development of the frontal (especially prefrontal) and temporal circuits.[35] These practices also serve to foster long-term social co-operation, which supports McNamara's position that religion serves an adaptive function. According to McNamara, an adaptive trait would have a genetic component (i.e. gene behaviour correlations), a brain component, as well as have a chemical component, and religion tends to have each of these features.[36]

Azari and colleagues also report involvement of prefrontal areas in mediating religious experiences. Their imaging data show activation of right prefrontal cortex during religious experience (e.g. the reading of Psalm 23), which they suggest supports the notion that religious experience is primarily a cognitive, rather than an emotional, experience because the prefrontal cortex is involved in the conscious monitoring of thought.[37] They also distinguished neural patterns that mediate religious experience from those mediating emotional states. Specifically, religious experiences were reported during activation of prefrontal regions involved in cognition, while, in their studies, limbic system structures that mediate emotion remained inactivated. Wide-spread neural areas were involved, but a clear distinction was seen between the circuits involved in religious experience and those involved in emotional experiences. The regions activated during the religious experiences overlapped those used in establishing and maintaining social relationships which the authors saw as support for the importance of relationships in many religions (e.g. Christianity's emphasis on a relationship with Christ). The authors suggest that an experience is deemed religious, in part, because of the perception of a relationship that emerges from the experience.[38] Additional support for the suggestion that religious experiences are associated in some manner with relationships comes from Schjoedt *et al.* who found that religious subjects who believe they are praying to a real, personal God used neural circuits involved in social cognition. The authors interpreted these results to mean that praying to God, for these subjects, was similar to any other interpersonal interaction and utilized circuits involved in ToM, specifically the anterior medial prefrontal cortex and the temporal-parietal junction.[39]

How is the cognitive science and neuroscience of religion/spirituality related to health?

The question of a relationship between spirituality/religion and health is considered controversial by some. As reported in this volume, however, there is abundant evidence of a positive association between spirituality/religion and health (both physical and mental) including positive correlations with healthy habits and longevity, and negative correlations with heart disease, stroke, depression, suicide, and mortality.[40] If a true relationship between spirituality/religion and health does exist, what might be the mechanism to account for this association? Various mediators have been proposed for religion's and spirituality's effect on health, including better health habits (regarding the use of tobacco, alcohol, etc.), psychosocial resources such as self-esteem and the attribution of purpose and meaning to events, social support coming from membership and participation in a community, and biological/physiological mechanisms. In regard to these biological and physiological pathways, evidence suggests an involvement of the endocrine, immune, and autonomic systems as well as participation of the central nervous system in mediating a spirituality/religion effect on health.[41] The activity in brain areas involved in spirituality and religious behaviour (described above) provides potential mechanisms whereby changes in neurotransmitter levels, immune system responses, hormonal levels, etc. can influence the body's response to infections, cardiovascular reactivity, and stress.

Activity in the frontal lobes, for example, is associated with certain forms of prosocial actions (e.g. forgiveness, empathy, etc.) and also mediates approach-withdrawal behaviour. As discussed above, one understanding of the development of religion is to consider it a product of behavioural mechanisms that evolved to encourage social behaviour. The neural circuitry that mediates approach–withdrawal overlaps with the circuitry that influences social affiliation. These neural areas include sections of the prefrontal cortex and the amygdala. According to this model, affiliation with or approach to others (mediated through these neural systems) activates hormones such as oxytocin as well as the dopaminergic reward system serving to reduce the stress response of the body and producing the salutary benefits of spirituality/religion on health.[42]

Understanding spirituality and religion from the perspective of the cognitive sciences and elucidating the cognitive and neural mechanisms involved in belief, ritual, and religious experience can provide insight into the possible functions of spirituality/religion. Knowledge of these functions and mechanisms can also help in the planning of approaches to the care and treatment of individuals who are seen by healthcare professionals. Knowing that social affiliation, for example, activates hormones and neurotransmitters that help to reduce the body's stress response could lead healthcare professionals to encourage their patients to seek out and engage in social interactions with others, even in religious settings. There are also individuals who suggest that a patient's religious/spiritual history, along with the standard medical history, be taken by a physician or nurse in order to develop an effective treatment plan. This is a controversial idea, resisted by many, but as cognitive science and neuroscience proceed in their study of religion and spirituality, these proposals and more will no doubt continue to be made to healthcare professionals.

References

1 James, W. (1902/1999). *The Varieties of Religious Experience*, p. 4. New York: Modern Library.
2 Koenig, H.G., McCullough, M.E., Larson, D.B. (2001). *Handbook of Religion and Health*. Oxford: Oxford University Press.
3 Taves, A. (2009). *Religious Experience Reconsidered*. Princeton: Princeton University Press.
4 James, W. (1902/1999). *The Varieties of Religious Experience*, p. 33. New York: Modern Library.
5 Barrett, J.L. (2007). Cognitive science of religion: what is it and why is it? *Relig Compass* **1**: 1–19.
6 Barrett, J.L. (2007). Is the spell really broken? Bio-psychological explanations of religion and theistic belief. *Theol Sci* **5**(1): 57–72.
7 Boyer, P. (2001). *Religion Explained: the Evolutionary Origin of Religious Thought*. New York: Basic Books.
8 Peterson, G.R. (2010). Are evolutionary/cognitive theories of religion relevant for philosophy of religion? *Zygon* **45**(3): 545–57.
9 Sosis, R., Alcorta, C. (2003). Signaling, solidarity, and the sacred: the evolution of religious behaviour. *Evolut Anthropol* **12**: 264–74.
10 Ibid
11 Alcorta,C., Sosis, R. (2005). Ritual, emotion, and sacred symbols: the evolution of religion as an adaptive complex. *Hum Nature* **16**(4): 323–59.
12 Ibid
13 Krebs, D.L. (2008). Morality: an evolutionary account. *Perspect Psycholog Sci* **3**(3): 149–68.
14 Ibid
15 de Waal, F.B.M. (2008). Putting the altruism back into altruism: the evolution of empathy. *Ann Rev Psychol* **59**: 279–300.
16 Barrett, J.L. (2004). *Why Would Anyone Believe in God?* New York: AltaMira Press.
17 Boyer, P. (2001). *Religion Explained: the Evolutionary Origin of Religious Thought*. New York: Basic Books.
18 Barrett, J.L. (2004). *Why Would Anyone Believe in God?* New York: AltaMira Press.
19 Ibid p. 44.
20 Barrett, J.L., Richert, R.A. (2003). Anthropomorphism or preparedness: exploring children's God concepts. *Rev Relig Res* **44**(3): 300–12.
21 Ibid
22 Kelemen, D. (2004). Are children 'intuitive theists'? Reasoning about purpose and design in nature. *Psycholog Sci* **15**(5): 295–301.
23 Bloom, P. (2007). Religion is natural. *Develop Sci* **10**(1): 147–51.
24 Barrett, J.L., Richert, R.A., Driesenga, A. (2001). God's beliefs versus mother's: the development of nonhuman agent concepts. *Child Develop* **72**(1): 50–65.
25 Barrett, J.L. (2004). *Why Would Anyone Believe in God?* New York: AltaMira Press.
26 McNamara, P. (2009). *The Neuroscience of Religious Experience*. New York: Cambridge University Press.
27 Ramachandran, V.S., Blakeslee, S. (1998). *Phantoms in the Brain: Probing the Mysteries of the Human Mind*. New York: HarperCollins.
28 Persinger, M. (1987). *Neuropsychological Bases of God Beliefs*, p. 14. New York: Praeger.
29 Joseph, R. (2001). The limbic system and the soul: evolution and the neuroanatomy of religious experience. *Zygon* **36**: 105–36.
30 Newberg, A., d'Aquili, E. (2001). *Why God Won't Go Away*. New York: Ballantine Books.
31 Johnstone, B., Glass, B.A. (2008). Support for a neuropsychological model of spirituality in persons with traumatic brain injury. *Zygon* **43**(4): 861–74.
32 Urgesi, C., Aglioti, S.M., Skrap, M., Fabbro, F. (2010). The spiritual brain: selective cortical lesions modulate human self-transcendence. *Neuron* **65**: 309–19.
33 McNamara, P. (2009). *The Neuroscience of Religious Experience*, p. 105. New York: Cambridge University Press.
34 Ibid, p. 127.
35 Ibid, p. 163.
36 Ibid, p. 249.
37 Azari, N.P., Nickel, J.P., Wunderlich, G., Niedeggen, M., Hefter, H., Tellmann, L. *et al.* (2001). Neural correlates of religious experience. *Eur J Neurosci* **13**: 1649–52.
38 Azari, N.P., Missimer, J., Seitz, R.J. (2005). Religious experience and emotion: evidence for distinctive cognitive neural patterns. *Int J Psychol Relig* **15**(4): 263–81.
39 Schjoedt, U., Stødkilde-Jørgensen, H., Geertz, A.W., Roepstorff, A. (2009). Highly religious participants recruit areas of social cognition in personal prayer. *Soc Cogn Affect Neurosci* **4**: 199–207.
40 Koenig, H.G., McCullough, M.E., Larson, D.B. (2001). *Handbook of Religion and Health*. Oxford: Oxford University Press.
41 Seybold, K.S. (2007). Physiological mechanisms involved in religiosity/spirituality and health. *J Behav Med* **30**: 303–9.
42 Taylor, S.E. (2006). Tend and befriend: biobehavioural bases of affiliation under stress. *Curr Direct Psycholog Sci* **15**: 273–7.

CHAPTER 48

Spiritual Well-Being Scale: mental and physical health relationships

Raymond F. Paloutzian, Rodger K. Bufford, and Ashley J. Wildman

Introduction

The existence of this handbook documents the recent increase in research on and practical attention to the role of spirituality in healthcare. One essential companion to the concept of spirituality is spiritual well-being (SWB).[1] That is, although the degree and type of spirituality *per se* can no doubt play an important role in how well a person faces the dilemmas related to health issues,[2,3] the degree to which a person perceives or derives a sense of well-being from that spirituality may be equally or more important. In this connection, SWB is an outcome indicator, or barometer, of how well a person is doing in the face of whatever the person is confronting.[4] Therefore, although SWB is not synonymous with spirituality, it is closely related to it. Similarly, SWB is not synonymous with mental health or physical health, but is likely to be related to both of them. SWB connotes one's subjective perception of well-being in both the religious and/or existential dimensions in accord with whatever is implicitly or explicitly conceived of as a spiritual umbrella for the individual. The Spiritual Well-Being Scale (SWBS)* was developed in order to be a tool for self-assessment of these aspects of general perceived well-being.[4,5]

Since its first publication in 1982, a large body of research has been done with the SWBS. In preparation for writing this chapter, a literature search documented the scale's use in over 300 published articles and chapters, 190 doctoral dissertations and Masters theses, 35 posters and presentations, and 50 unpublished papers. It has also been reprinted in no less than 4 books on palliative care and counseling.[6–9] An exhaustive review of all of this research is beyond the scope of this chapter; the interested reader is referred to a companion review article.[10] Here, we focus specifically and selectively on research related to healthcare. We highlight those studies using the SWBS that are related to mental health variables or to the mental and well-being issues that are consequences or correlates of physical health conditions.

In order to maximize the usefulness of this chapter, it is necessary to (1) summarize the intellectual roots of the concept of SWB and what the SWBS does and does not measure, (2) explain the meaning and utility of its religious well-being (RWB) and existential well-being (EWB) subscales, (3) summarize the literature with the SWBS as related to mental and physical health variables, (4) note any strengths and weaknesses, research directions, and applications of the SWBS, and (5) summarize implications of SWB research for healthy healthcare practice.

Brief Roots of the Spiritual Well-Being Scale

The SWBS was created a generation ago to be a social indicator of the quality of life,[4,5] but one that would be different from the common social indicators of that era. At the time, social indicators were developed to assess many aspects of life quality. Some of them were measures that reflected access to or the number of tangible or countable goods, services, or things. Countering this trend, however, Campbell[11] proposed that 'the quality of life lies in the experience of life' (p. 118), rather than merely or only in the tangible aspects of it. Many years later, research on happiness, which is not identical to SWB, but is related to it and is part of the burgeoning research on general subjective well-being, would make the same point. For example, Diener and colleagues[12,13] document that increased income predicts increased happiness only until most ordinary needs are met. After that, having more money, which is directly associated with having more tangible goods and services, does not predict more happiness, subjective well-being, or a feeling of being OK. Overall, such results are strong evidence that once basic needs are met, one does not become happier or experience greater well-being, tranquility, or internal peace by having more wealth or the things obtained by it. The findings are instead consistent with notions rooted in the existential psychiatry of Frankl[14] and with the building-block model of personality proposed by Maslow[15] that after basic needs are satisfied, higher-order 'spiritual' values and motives take priority as human strivings. Such values, motives, and strivings are sometimes couched in

Note: We dedicate this chapter to Craig W. Ellison.

'spiritual' terms, but as established by Emmons,[16] are nevertheless basic functional aspects of human personality. Research with the SWBS was a manifestation of these trends.

Implicit in the idea behind SWB is the notion that people need transcendence. However, this does not mean that people have a subjective 'need for transcendence,' as if they should be in a certain state of consciousness for its own sake or because it is an interesting state of mind. Rather, it means that they need to focus on whatever transcends them because it is psychologically functional to do so. That is, by transcending immediate concerns, people's minds go beyond themselves and make attributions about the meaning of events in their environment—past, present, and future. Such processes have increased the probability of survival of those whose minds adapted this skill. There are psychological and evolutionarily functional benefits to attending to and making meaning out of the stimuli that surround us;[17–19] thus meaning-making processes including those operative under the label 'spirituality,' and their correlates, such as SWB, could be seen as one kind of healthy psychological manifestation of the tendency to put one's attention on things that lie outside of oneself.

The Spiritual Well-Being Scale

The scale, subscales, and properties

In ordinary language people refer to whatever is connotes 'spirituality' to them in religious and/or in nonreligious, existential terms. Because of this, and based on interviews and literature on what was meant by 'spiritual,' the SWBS is comprised of two subscales, one as an assessment of one's perception of well-being in ordinary religious language, called religious well-being (RWB), and the other as an assessment of one's perception of well-being in existential terms, called existential well-being (EWB). There are a total of 20 items on the SWBS, with 10 items on the RWB subscale and 10 items on the EWB subscale. The RWB items contain the word 'God.', and some researchers have found it useful to indicate that 'God' can be taken to mean 'god or higher power' in whatever sense is meaningful to the subject or in his or her religious or cultural context. The EWB items contain no specifically religious language, but are instead worded in terms of meaning, connection, and general satisfaction. Thus, RWB can be thought of as a 'vertical' dimension and EWB can be thought of as a 'horizontal' dimension. About half of the items are reverse worded (and therefore reverse scored) as a guard against response set bias. Each item is scored from 1–6 with a higher number reflecting more well-being. The scale yields three scores: (1) a total score for overall SWB, (2) an RWB subscale score, and (3) an EWB subscale score.

The face validity of the SWBS is evident by an examination of its items, especially in light of the procedures used to develop them. Standard statistical tests have been run in order to assess the statistical properties of the scale and its subscales with various datasets. Alpha reliability coefficients typically are in the 0.8 and 0.9 range, test-retest reliabilities show that the scale score remains stable, and, as expected, RWB and EWB subscale scores do not necessarily behave the same way.[20,10] Conceptually, EWB and RWB would seem to overlap, but not be synonymous. The correlation coefficients between RWB and EWB subscale scores have ranged from about 0.20 to 0.71 with various samples,[20] which suggests that these two subscales, as operational representations of their constructs, are statistically distinct while they also share common variance in some datasets. This would be expected on theoretical grounds, since it is possible for someone to perceive well-being both religiously and existentially at the same time, even though they are not identical.

Factor analyses of the datasets through which the SWBS was developed yielded 2 factors consistent with the above conceptualization and operationalization of the constructs.[4,5] All of the 'God' items loaded on the RWB factor and all of the a-religious items loaded on the EWB factor. The EWB subscale also yielded two small subfactors, one connoting life satisfaction and one connoting life purpose. Subsequent examinations of the factor structure of the SWBS with datasets similar to those in the original studies report a similar structure.[21,22] However, examination of the factor structure with data from different samples shows more diverse results. For example, Scott et al.[23] reported that SWBS data from a sample of hospitalized mental patients yielded 3 factors, but these clustered into different factors than those in the college student datasets of Genia,[21] and Paloutzian and Ellison.[4,5] Ledbetter et al.[24,25] also showed that the factor structure of the SWBS can vary in complexity depending on the dataset under examination. Such variations are valuable, as may be revealed by an examination of the difference in the factor structure as well as the descriptive statistics [e.g. 26] obtained by in-hospital subjects compared with other outpatient clinical and counselling, convict, caregiver, or other normal samples. For example, the factors obtained in the data of Paloutzian and Ellison is what one would expect based upon item content (God and non-God items loading on two relatively independent factors), but those obtained for the hospitalized subjects by Scott et al.[23] do not fit this to-be-expected grouping. Such differences may be clinically revealing, and useful.

The predictive and discriminate validity of the SWBS is supported by the large number of research findings that have consistently shown that the scale scores are associated with other variables in ways that they ought to be on theoretical grounds. For example, low scores on the SWBS and its subscales have been repeatedly found to predict higher scores on measures of depression and anxiety, lower marital satisfaction, lower hardiness in coping with terminal disease, greater alcohol and other substance abuse, higher loneliness, higher PTSD, and so forth.[10] These and similar subsequent findings are consistent with the initial normative data for various samples published by Bufford et al.[26]

Translations

Reliable and tested translations of the SWBS have been made in Spanish,[27] Portuguese,[22] Chinese,[28,29] Malay,[30] and Arabic.[31] Translations at various stages of development are underway in Korean, Hebrew, Dutch, German, Urdu, Farsi, Latvian, and others. Especially important for a translated version of a psychological scale is that the meaning of the items, not merely the words in each item, be translated so that its psychological content and implications are represented in the translated scale to mean the same thing that they mean in the original English scale, to the maximum degree possible for a different population, culture, and language. In addition, the meaning of the answer format must be accurately transferred from one language and culture to the other, so that the mathematical weight of each item is the same and a total score obtained on the translated tool can be meaningfully compared to the same score on the original English scale. Factor structures and validity predictions in the datasets obtained with translated versions of the SWBS have been partly similar to those obtained in the original English-speaking work on the scale, and the alpha and test-retest reliabilities typically show the same strength. At the same time, the factor structures also show characteristics perhaps unique to the local culture. Therefore, there may be room for cross-cultural research on clinical and non-clinical populations, since relatively comparable versions of the scale are emerging in different languages.

Applied use of Spiritual Well-Being Scale

Depending on the specific sample from which data are obtained, scores on the SWBS can show a ceiling effect[26] or not.[20] A ceiling effect may occur especially in religiously conservative samples. When it is observed, it is probably due to a high grouping of scores on the RWB subscale; such a pattern of scores is considerably less evident for the EWB subscale. Data from various samples shows distributions ranging from normality to different degrees of skewness; however, if the data are skewed, they are virtually always skewed in the negative direction.[26] This means that SWBS total scores, and especially RWB subscale scores, are not likely to be useful if the researcher's goal is to test differences in SWB, EWB, or RWB on the high end. However, it also means that the scale can be especially useful for clinical, counselling, or other helping relationships in which a scale sensitive at the low end is needed. That is, the scale property that makes the SWBS not particularly useful for testing differences in high degrees of SWB, is the very property that makes it more sensitive, and therefore more useful, at the low end. Thus, the scale is applicable for helping work for which an easy-to-use tool can be applied that will help point to and identify problems to solve or dilemmas to raise and deal with.

Research on the Spiritual Well-Being Scale, and mental and physical health

Space constraints allow only a brief sketch of recent research in which the SWBS has been used to explore psychological well-being dimensions in association with mental and physical health. They include studies of stress response, blood pressure, heart rate, domestic violence, health-risk and health-promotion behaviour and status, HIV-AIDS and immune health, poor vision or blindness, diabetes, irritable bowel syndrome (IBS), kidney failure, depression, anxiety, coping, intimate partner violence, sleep quality, juvenile delinquency, 12-step programmes, schizophrenia, and suicidal ideation. Some have examined differences among intact groups, many have been correlational, and several studies have examined SWB changes as a result of psychotherapy. In the vast array of studies the variables overlap a great deal; thus, digesting the findings into meaningfully separate chunks is difficult. Nevertheless, we try to present the information in units that highlight the most prominent aspects of the study as related to SWB.

Physical health

Stress

In a laboratory study, Edmonson et al.[32] examined the effects of an induced stress experience on perceived stress, subjective well-being, heart rate, and systolic blood pressure. EWB was inversely related to perceived stress and physical health symptoms; RWB was also inversely related to perceived stress. SWB was inversely related with self-reported use of medications. SWB, EWB, and RWB were all positively related to self-reported mental health. EWB was associated with both lower heart rate and lower heart rate reactivity to the stressful interview, while RWB was inversely related to increases in systolic blood pressure during the stressful interview.

Family predictors

Paranjape and Kaslow[33] explored the relationship between spirituality and coping with exposure to family violence among older African American women. They found that with family violence and demographic factors controlled, SWB predicted both better physical and mental health status. They proposed efforts to promote spiritual well-being as a way to cope with and buffer the exposure to family violence. In a twin study, in an effort to examine the relationship of SWB to health status among Vietnam era twins, Tsuang et al.[34] found that EWB predicted health outcomes in this sample.

Youth risk and education

In a sample of mostly white high school students, Cotton et al.[35] found that after controlling for demographics and religiosity, EWB and RWB contributed an additional 17% of variance in predicting health-risk behaviours. However, EWB was the only predictor that contributed significantly to the final model. Similarly, Douchand Brown[36] found that along with education and number of children, EWB made a statistically significant unique contribution to health promotion behaviours among African American women.

HIV/AIDS

Studies among African-American HIV or AIDS patients by Coleman and Holzemer[37] found that EWB was significantly related to psychosocial well-being. Similarly, Dalmida et al.[38] reported a strong relationship between SWB scores and health functioning in a predominantly African American sample of HIV-positive women; both EWB and RWB were positively related to CD4 cell count, an index of healthy immune functioning; they accounted for a significant amount of the variance beyond that explained by demographic variables, HIV medication adherence, and HIV viral load. Finally, Philips et al.[39] examined the role of RWB and EWB in ameliorating the adverse effects of HIV infection in a mixed sample of male and female patients. EWB predicted better sleep quality, and both better mental and physical health status, while RWB predicted only better physical health status.

Other physical conditions

In an examination of well-being among a sample of individuals with vision impairment, Yampolosky et al.[40] found that RWB was a predictor of more effective coping with this challenge, but EWB was not. An exploration of the contribution of SWB as an added predictor of psychosocial well-being in patients with diabetes mellitus, Landis[41] showed that both RWB and EWB were inversely related to self-reported uncertainty. Uncertainty accounted for 43% of the variance in psychosocial well-being; EWB explained an additional 10%. In a predominantly White sample, Cotton et al. [42] compared individuals with and without IBS on RWB and EWB; scores were similar. However, the relationships of RWB and EWB with depression were significantly increased when IBS was present—more so for EWB. Finally, among patients with end-stage renal disease, Tanyi and Werner[43] found that RWB was related to lower psychological and total distress scores on the Psychosocial Adjustment to Illness Scale. EWB was significantly related to these scores as well as to lower distress about extended family relationships.

Mental health

Correlational studies

Several studies show inverse relationships between RWB or EWB and depression. Fehring et al.[44] reported two studies that showed EWB had a strong inverse relationships with negative moods. Cotton et al.,[35] in a sample of mostly white high school students, found that after controlling for demographics and religiosity, EWB and RWB contributed an additional 29% of variance in predicting depression. EWB was the only predictor that contributed significantly in their final model. Coleman[45] found that RWB and EWB accounted for 32% of the variance in depression in a sample of African American heterosexuals with HIV infection. Dalmida et al.[38] reported a strong relationship between SWB scores and psychological functioning in a predominantly African American sample of HIV-positive women; both EWB ($r = -0.62$) and RWB ($r = -0.36$) were negatively related to depressive symptoms. Phillips et al.[39] found that spiritual well-being was a significant predictor of sleep quality and mental and physical health status among a sample of HIV infected individuals. As related to a very serious mental disorder, Compton and Furman[46] studied the relationship between general psychopathology symptoms on the SCID-IV and well-being in a small sample of African Americans hospitalized for a first-episode schizophrenia-spectrum disorder at a public urban hospital. Results showed negative symptoms were inversely related with RWB (rho = –0.614; $p = 0.007$) and general psychopathology symptoms were inversely related with EWB (rho = –0.539; $p = 0.021$).

Anxiety, depression, and suicide

In a complex study, Mela et al.[47] investigated a sample of Canadians that was predominantly male and about half aboriginal. EWB correlated negatively with anxiety and depression, and positively with life satisfaction. RWB correlated positively with life satisfaction. Dunn et al.[48] found that SWB was inversely related and accounted for 22, 32, and 64% of the variance for anxiety, depression, and combined anxiety and depression respectively. Consistent with these findings, Kocot and Goodman[49] found that low SWB was associated with higher psychological distress and parenting stress. Similarly, Mitchell et al.[50] found SWB to be inversely related to depression, anxiety, and parenting stress. Further, they found that SWB played a mediating role between intimate partner violence and both depression and parenting stress, but not anxiety. Extending these findings to concerns about suicide, Anglin et al.[51] found that RWB was negatively related to suicide attempts among a low-income African American group (ES = –1.0). Taliaferro et al.[52] studied suicidal ideation among college students and found that EWB, but not RWB, added significant unique variance in addition to that from several other predictors.

Group differences

Bufford et al.[26] reported significantly different means for mental health patients and normal samples on both RWB and EWB. Kaslow et al.[53] and Meadows et al.[54] reported that abused women have lower levels of SWB than non-abused peers and use more mental health services. Ganje-Fling et al.[55] found that outpatient mental health clients who reported childhood sexual abuse did not differ from other clients in their sample, but both groups scored significantly lower on EWB, RWB and SWB than hospice workers and medical outpatients; they also scored significantly lower than Bufford et al.'s[26] adult and sexually abused mental health outpatients on RWB.

In an investigation of well-being among three groups of antepartum women, Dunn et al.[48] found that women who had been on enforced bed rest for at least seven days scored significantly lower on SWB than those without known high-risk pregnancies. In a study of African American women who either had or had not been the victim of intimate partner violence, Mitchell et al.[50] found a significant difference on SWB between those who had experienced such violence and a control group who had not.

Outcome Studies

A few studies explored the effects of counseling and psychotherapy on SWB. First, Richards et al. explored the effectiveness of a religiously-oriented group treatment on self-defeating perfectionism in a group of 15 religiously-devout university students, most of whom were probably Mormon.[56] Interventions included religious imagery, relaxation exercises, religious bibliotherapy, and discussion of religious perfectionism. Improvements were found in perfectionism, depression, self-esteem, and EWB. Because a single group pre- and post-test design was used, causal conclusions were not established.

Second, in studies of Christian lay counseling conducted through a local church, Toh et al.[57] investigated SWB gains following both 10 and 20 sessions of Christian counseling. In an uncontrolled study, they demonstrated reduced emotional distress and significant gains on EWB and RWB. In a controlled follow-up study, Toh and Tan[58] again found significant gains in SWB and the treatment group showed significantly greater gains than a no-treatment control group, thus providing evidence that gains were the result of counseling rather than other factors. In related studies, Bufford and Renfroe[59] studied outpatients at two clinics, one associated with a Baptist seminary that had a reputation for Christian counseling and one with no religious affiliation or identity. They found significant reductions in depression and significant gains in RWB and EWB for both samples. There were no differences between groups, and no interactions.

Third, Howard and others[60,61] examined changes in SWB in two groups of adolescents. The first was a group of adolescents hospitalized in a private psychiatric hospital for substance abuse, severe misconduct, or severe affective disorders. The second group was comprised of adolescents incarcerated in a juvenile detention facility; this group was considered a non-equivalent control group since treatment was not a normal feature of their setting. Religious or spiritual interventions were not an explicit aspect of treatment in either facility, except that substance abuse treatment incorporated 12-step elements including appeals to a 'higher power.' About half of the inpatient group, and over 80% of the detention group professed no traditional religious affiliation. Results showed that the two groups did not differ on RWB, EWB, or SWB at the pretest. The psychiatric groups showed significant gains in both EWB and RWB, and scored significantly higher than the detention group at post-test when pre-test scores were controlled.

Fourth, two studies have explored the relationship between SWB and substance abuse outcomes. Borman and Dixon[62] found that SWB increased significantly among participants in both a 12-step programmes and an alternative programme; no differences were found between the two groups. Brooks and Matthews[63] also found an increase in SWB scores for participants in substance abuse counselling. In their study, increases in SWB were found to be positively correlated with the SWB scores of participants' counsellors: as the counsellor's score increased, gains in counselee SWB also increased.

Spiritual well-being and healthy healthcare practice

The above summary of research with the SWBS suggests that people's sense of well-being, as they perceive it in terms that they deem to be spiritual, is related to a number of mental and physical health conditions. It seems, therefore, that SWB ought to be taken into account in healthcare policy side-by-side with other factors. In their assessment, Hill and Killian[64] concluded that 'there is evidence of a moderately positive relationship between Ellison's ... measure of spiritual well-being ... and physical as well as mental health (see Ellison & Smith, 1991)' (p. 155). This does not mean that particular forms of spirituality should be promoted or that patients should be encouraged or manipulated into 'being spiritual.' It means, instead, that patients' sense of well-being, as they perceive it in terms meaningful to them, ought to be properly taken into account in a comprehensive program of patient care,[3] with the particular form that this might take being chosen by the patient. Simply put, when it comes to patient comfort, it is the patient that calls the shots. We would argue, too, that the priority that is given to this should increase as the severity of the disease or disorder that the patient is suffering increases, and that this is maximally so when a patient is terminally ill.

Summary and conclusions

The research on relationships between SWB and mental and physical health suggests that the larger perceptual umbrella under which a person sees, interprets, and faces life's difficulties may play an important role in his or her health, and coping with the issues that come with deficiency or illness. In addition to what happens to a person being important in determining his or her well-being, the larger meaning umbrellas under which such things occur also play a part. They seem to be important in helping a person cope and suffer less, and feel less dread, and greater peacefulness and comfort, in the face of harsh realities. There is no evidence that higher SWB has any causally curative effect on a purely organic disease, but there seems to be ample evidence that high SWBS scores predict greater comfort and peace in the face of them. Finally, the research seems clear that SWB is not one thing; it is multidimensional. Each dimension must be understood independently as well as in combination with the whole, for what it is and is not, and can and cannot do, for people who are suffering.

References

1 Moberg, D.O. (1979). The development of social indicators of spiritual well-being for quality of life research. In: Moberg, D.O. (ed.), *Spiritual Well-Being: Sociological Perspectives*. Washington, DC: University Press of America.

2 Piedmont, R.L. (2001). Spiritual transcendence and the scientific study of spirituality. *J Rehabil* **67**: 4–14.

3 Masters, K.S., Hooker, S.A. (in press). Religion, spirituality, and health. In: R.F. Paloutzian, C.L. Park (eds), *Handbook of the Psychology of Religion and Spirituality*, 2nd edn. New York: Guilford Press.

4 Ellison, C.W. (1983). Spiritual well-being: conceptualization and measurement. *J Psychol Theol* **11**: 330–40.

5 Paloutzian, R.F., Ellison, C.W. (1982). Loneliness, spiritual well-being and the quality of life. In: L.A. Peplau, D. Perlman (eds) *Loneliness: a Sourcebook of Current Theory, Research and Therapy*, pp. 224–37. New York: Wiley-Interscience.

6 Dow, K.H. (2006). *Nursing Care of Women With Cancer*. St Louis: Mosby Elsevier.

7 Kuebler, K.K., Heidrich, D.D., Esper, P. (2007). *Palliative and End-of-life Care: Clinical Practice Guidelines*, 2nd edn. St Louis: Saunders Elsevier.

8 Kelly, E.W. Jr. (1995). *Spirituality and Religion in Counseling and Psychotherapy: Diversity in Theory and Practice*. Alexandria: American Counseling Association.

9 Topper, C. (2003). *Spirituality in Pastoral Counseling and the Community Helping Professions*. New York: Haworth.

10 Bufford, R.K., Paloutzian, R.F., Wildman, A.J. (in press). Spiritual Well-Being Scale: research and assessment. *Religions*.

11 Campbell, A. (1976). Subjective measures of well-being. *Am Psychol*, **31**: 117–24.

12 Diener, E., Biswas-Diener, R. (2008). *Happiness: Unlocking the Mysteries of Psychological Wealth*. Oxford: Blackwell.

13 Myers, D., Diener, E. (1995). Who is happy? *Psychol Sci* **6**: 10–19.

14 Frankl, V. (1963). *Man's Search for Meaning*. New York: Washington Square Press.

15 Maslow, A. (1954). *Motivation and Personality*. New York: Harper.

16 Emmons, R.A. (1999). *The Psychology of Ultimate Concerns: Motivation and Spirituality in Personality*. New York: Guilford Press.

17 Park, C.L. (in press). Religion and meaning. In: R.F. Paloutzian, C.L. Park (eds) Handbook of the Psychology of Religion and Spirituality, 2nd edn. New York: Guilford Press.

18 Park, C.L. (2010). Making sense of the meaning literature: an integrative review of meaning making and its effects on adjustment to stressful life events. *Psychol Bull* **136**(2): 257–301.

19 Kirkpatrick, L.A. (2005). *Attachment, Evolution, and the Psychology of Religion*. New York: Guilford.

20 Brinkman, D.D. (1989). *An Evaluation of the Spiritual Well-Being Scale: Reliability and Measurement*. Portland: Western Conservative Baptist Seminary.

21 Genia, V. (2001). Evaluation of the Spiritual Well-Being Scale in a sample of college students. *Int J Psychol Relig* **11**(1): 25–33.

22 Marques, L.F., Sarriera, C., Dell'Aglio, D.D. (2009). Adaptacao e validacao da Escala de Bem-Estar Espiritual (EBE) [Adaptation and validation of Spiritual Well-Being Scale]. *Aval Psicol* **8**(2): Porto Alegre ago. [In Portuguese].

23 Scott, E.L., Agresti, A.A., Fitchett, G. (1998). Factor analysis of the Spiritual Well-Being Scale and its clinical utility with psychiatric inpatients. *J Scient Study Relig* **37**: 314–21.x

24 Ledbetter, M.F., Smith, L.A., Fischer, J.D., Vosler-Hunter, W.L. (1991). An evaluation of the research and clinical usefulness of the Spiritual Well-Being Scale. *J Psychol Theol* **19**(1): 49–55.

25 Ledbetter, M.F., Smith, L.A., Fischer, J.D., Vosler-Hunter, W.L., Chew, G.P. (1991). An evaluation of the construct validity of the Spiritual Well-Being Scale: a confirmatory factor analytic approach. *J Psychol Theol* **19**(1): 94–102.

26 Bufford, R.K., Paloutzian, R.F., Ellison, C.W. (1991). Norms for the spiritual well-being scale. *J Psychol Theol* **19**: 56–70.

27 Bruce, K.C. (1997). *A Spanish translation of the Spiritual Well-Being Scale: preliminary validation* [dissertation]. Newberg: George Fox University, 1995.

28 Tang, W.R. (2008). *Spiritual Assessment and Care of Cancer Patients*. Taiwan: School of Nursing, Chang Gung University.

29 Liu, Y.H. (2010). *Spiritual Well-Being and Acculturative Stress Among Older Chinese Immigrants in the United States*. Long Beach: Gerontology Program, California State University.

30 Imam, S.S., Karim, N.H., Jusoh, N.R., Mamad, N.E. (2009). Maylay version of the Spiritual Well-Being Scale: is the Malay Spiritual Well-Being Scale a psychometrically sound instrument? *J Behav Sci* **4**(1): 59–69.

31 Musa, A.S., Pevalin, D.J. (2012). An Arabic version of the Spiritual Well-Being Scale. *Int J Psychol Relig*, **22**(2): 119–34.

32 Edmondson, K.A, Lawler, K.A, Jobe, R.L, Younger, J.W, Piferi, R.L, Jones, W.H. (2005). Spirituality predicts health and cardiovascular responses to stress in young adult women. *J Relig Hlth* **44**(2): 161–71.

33 Paranjape, A., Kaslow, N. (2010). Family violence exposure and health outcomes among older African American women: does spirituality and social support play a protective role? *J Womens Hlth* **19**: 1899–904.

34 Tsuang, M.T., Williams, W.M., Simpson, J.C., Lyons, M.J. (2002). Pilot study of spirituality and mental health in twins. *Am J Psychiat* **159**(3): 486–8.

35 Cotton, S., Larkin, E., Hoopes, A., Cromer, B.A., Rosenthal, S.L. (2005). The impact of adolescent spirituality on depressive symptoms and health risk behaviours. *J Adolesc Hlth* **36**(6): 529.

36 Douchand Brown, S.E. (2009). *Health promotion behaviours among African American women* [dissertation]. Coral Gables: University of Miami.

37 Coleman, C.L., Holzemer. (1999). Spirituality, psychological well-being, and HIV symptoms for African-Americans living with HIV disease. *J Ass Nurses AIDS Care* **10**(1): 42–50.

38 Dalmida, S.G., Holstad, M.M., Diiorio, C., Laderman, G. (2009). Spiritual well-being, depressive symptoms, and immune status among women living with HIV/AIDS. *Women Hlth* **49**(2–3): 119–43.

39 Phillips, K.D., Mock, K.S., Bopp, C.M., Dudgeon, W.A., Hand, G.A. (2006). Spiritual well-being, sleep disturbance, and mental and physical health status in HIV-infected individuals. *Iss Ment Hlth Nurs* **27**(2): 125–39.

40 Yampolosky, M.A.,Wittich, W., Webb, G., Overbury, O. (2008). The role of spirituality in coping with visual impairment. *J Vis Impairment Blindness* **102**(1): 28–39.

41 Landis, B.J. (1996). Uncertainty, spiritual well-being, and psychosocial adjustment to chronic illness. *Iss Ment Hlth Nurs* **17**(3): 217–31.

42 Cotton, S., Kudel, I., Roberts, Y.H., Palleria, H., Tsevat, J., Succop, P., et al. (2009). Spiritual well-being and mental health outcomes in adolescents with or without inflammatory bowel disease. *J Adolesc Hlth* **44**(5): 485–92.

43 Tanyi, R.A., Werner, J.S. (2007). Spirituality in African American and Caucasian women with end-stage renal disease on hemodialysis treatment. *Hlth Care Women Int* **28**(2): 141–54.

44 Fehring, R.J., Brennan, P.F., Keller, M.L. (1987). Psychological and spiritual well-being in college students. *Res Nurs Hlth* **10**(6): 391–8.

45 Coleman, C.L. (2004). The contribution of religious and existential well-being to depression among African American heterosexuals with HIV infection. *Iss Ment Health Nurs* **25**(1): 103–10.

46 Compton, M.T., Furman, A.C. (2005). Inverse correlations between symptom scores and spiritual well-being among African American patients with first-episode schizophrenia spectrum disorders. *J Nerv Ment Dis* **193**(5): 346–9.

47 Mela, M.A., Marcoux, E., Baetz, M., Griffin, R., Angelski, C., Deqiang, G. (2008). The effect of religiosity and spirituality on psychological well-being among forensic psychiatric patients in Canada. *Ment Hlth Relig Cult* **11**(5): 517–32.

48 Dunn, L.L., Handley, M.C., Shelton, M.M. (2007). Spiritual well-being, anxiety, and depression in antepartal women on bedrest. *Iss Ment Health Nurs* **28**(11): 1235–46.

49 Kocot, T., Goodman, L.A. (2003). The roles of coping and social support in battered women's mental health. *Violence Against Women* **9**: 1–24.

50 Mitchell, M.D., Hargrove, G.L., Collins, M.H., Thomson, M.P., Reddick, T.L., Kaslow, N.J. (2006). Coping variables that mediate the relation between intimate partner violence and mental health outcomes among low-income, African American women. *J Clin Psychol* **62**(12): 1503–20.

51 Anglin, D.M., Gariel, K.O.S., Kaslow, N.J. (2005). Suicide acceptability and religious well-being: a comparative analysis in African American suicide attempters and non-attempters. *J Psychol Theol* **33**: 140–50.

52 Taliaferro, L.A., Rienzo, B.A., Pigg, R.M. Jr., Miller, M.D., Dodd, V.J. (2009). Spiritual well-being and suicidal ideation among college students. *J Am Coll Hlth* **58**(1): 83–90.

53 Kaslow, N.J., Thompson, M.P., Okun, A., et al. (2002). Risk and protective factors for suicidal behaviour in abused African American women. *J Consult Clin Psychol* **70**: 311–19.

54 Meadows, L.A., Kaslow, N.J., Thompson, M.P., Jurkovic, G.J. (2005). Protective factors against suicide attempt risk among African American women experiencing intimate partner violence. *Am J Commun Psychol* **36**: 109–21.

55 Ganje-Fling, M., Veach, P.M., Kuang, H., Houg, B. (2000). Effects of childhood sexual abuse on client spiritual well-being. *Couns Values* **44**: 84–91.

56 Richards, P.S., Owen, L., Stein, S. (1993). A religiously-oriented group counseling intervention for self-defeating perfectionism: a pilot study. *Couns Val* **37**: 96–105.

57 Toh, Y.M., Tan, S.Y., Osburn, C.D., Faber, D.E. (1994). The evaluation of a church-based lay counseling program: some preliminary data. *J Psychol Christian* **13**: 270–5.

58 Toh, Y.M., Tan, S.Y., Osburn, C.D., Faber, D.E. (1994). The evaluation of a church-based lay counseling program: some preliminary data. *J Psychol Christianity* **13**: 270–5.

59 Bufford, R.K., Renfroe, T.W. (1994). Spiritual well-being and depression in psychotherapy outpatients. Paper presented at The Annual Meeting of the Christian Association for Psychological Studies/Western Region, June 1994, Del Mar (CA).

60 Howard, G.T. (1995). *The effect of short-term hospitalizations on the spiritual well-being of psychiatric, adolescent inpatients* [dissertation]. Newberg: George Fox University.

61 Bufford, R.K., Renfroe, T.W., Howard, G. (1995). Spiritual changes as psychotherapy outcomes. Paper presented at the Annual Meeting of the American Psychological Association; August 1995, New York.

62 Borman, P.D., Dixon, D.N. (1998). Spirituality and the 12 steps of substance abuse recovery. *J Psychol Theol* **26**(3): 287–91.

63 Brooks, C.W., Matthews, C.O. (2000). The relationship among substance abuse counselor's spiritual well-being, values, and self-actualizing characteristics and the impact of clients' well-being. *J Addict Offender Couns* **21**: 23–33.

64 Hill, P.C., Kilian, M.K. (2004) Assessing clinically significant religious impairment in clients: applications from measures in the psychology of religion and spirituality. *Ment Hlth Relig Cult* **6**(2): 149–60.

CHAPTER 49

Prayer and meditation

Marek Jantos

Introduction

Prayer and meditation are spiritual practices central to the world's oldest faith traditions and cultures, as Section I indicates. From earliest human history to the present day these practices have found expression in varied forms, rituals, and arenas of life. Prayer for some conjures images of a bowed head and bended knees, or of arms raised to heaven, but it can also take the form of singing, chanting, ecstatic whirling, or the spinning of a prayer wheel. Prayers may have set times of the day, or be spontaneous expressions of petition and praise. Likewise meditation, with its predominantly Biblical and Eastern origins, can conjure images of thoughtful reflection, meditative postures and contemplative practices focussed on attention regulation, breathing, chanting and movement. Each of these practices, whether in the context of personal growth or as a response to a health crisis, reflects an innate human yearning for the sacred and a relationship with a higher power.

Recognizing the continued centrality of prayer and meditation in modern life, peak bodies such as the United States National Centre for Complementary and Alternative Medicine (NCCAM) at the National Institutes of Health (NIH), and individual researchers continue to examine the efficacy of prayer and meditation in relation to health and wellbeing. The results have generated considerable discussion and controversy, particularly in relation to the metaphysical assumptions underpinning empirical investigation and potential mechanisms by which they impact health.

Prayer

Prayer is an important part of the religious and spiritual life of a large proportion of the world's population. Whether in the form of Christian prayer, the Moslem Salah or the Jewish Tefilah, prayer forms a 'thread in the fabric of beliefs about a meaningful world.'[1] The practice of prayer varies from culture to culture. In the United States, for example, 95 out every 100 people profess belief in God and nine out of ten pray weekly, one out of two pray daily, and one out of four pray several times a day.[2] In more secularized cultures the prevalence of the practice of prayer may be different, but evidence nevertheless shows that praying continues to be a core practice in the spiritual life of people throughout the world.[3]

The perceived relationship of prayer with health has been highlighted in several recent population surveys. The National Center for Complementary and Alternative Medicine (NCCAM) found that 62% of a sample of 31,000 adults had used complementary and alternative medicine in relation to health.[4] They included prayer as a CAM strategy, and found that a total of 45% had used prayer for health reasons, with 43% praying for their own health and 25% asking others to pray for them. Among all the complementary and alternative medicine therapies, including meditation, yoga, tai chi, qi gong, and reiki, prayer was most frequently used.[5] A Harvard Medical School survey[6] of 2055 participants found 35% used prayer for health concerns, and among these 75% prayed for wellness and 22% for specific medical conditions. Other studies confirm the importance of private prayer to coping with illness.[7–12]

Two fundamental questions arise in relation to prayer; *why do we pray*? And, *what is prayer?* In considering the first, William James, a nineteenth century philosopher and psychologist spoke of a human 'impulse to pray,' of an inner desire which cannot be quantified through empirical studies of human nature. It is through the act of prayer, according to James, that a person finds his or her true identity 'the intimate, the ultimate, the permanent me which I seek.' In his view, this identity can only be established by relating to the one who is the 'The Great Companion,' 'the Absolute Mind,' God himself.[13] From James' perspective, prayer is the process through which an individual, and in a broader sense humankind, finds purpose and meaning.

Not all contemporary researchers of prayer would concur with this viewpoint. Neurotheologians Andrew Newberg and Eugene d'Aquili suggest that to search for the divine is a human form of comfort seeking to pacify brain-generated existential fears linked to living in a baffling and dangerous world.[14] The same brain that gives rise to fear invents ideas and myths to pacify them. Myths of God, of heroes, of heaven and hell, of sin and suffering, are simply cognitive pairings of incompatible opposites that seek to alleviate anxiety. It is however evident that people are drawn to prayer because of their belief in, or at least hope for, the existence of an infinite and supernatural being. Levin in his review of epidemiological studies on the role of prayer states,

> Indeed, the possibility that there is a creator-God who volitionally chooses to answer or not answer petitionary prayers by means which entirely transcend any naturalistic mechanism may be the most commonly held belief of people who use prayer interventions for friends or loved ones who are ill.[15]

In considering what prayer is, James, in *The Varieties of Religious Experience,* defines prayer as a communion with God, an act that goes well beyond the exercise of 'vain words and repetitions of sacred formulae,' it is 'the very movement itself of the soul, putting itself in the personal relation of contact with the mysterious power of which it feels the presence.'[16] Similarly Friedrich Heiler, in *Prayer: A Study in the History and Psychology of Religion,* defined prayer as a living communion with God, an act which enables a 'spontaneous emotional discharge, a free outpouring of the heart.'[17]

It is evident that prayer is both an action and a state of mind. As an action it is said to lead to communion between the human and divine realms, but when people are engaged in prayer they are said to be 'in prayer,' in a unique state of being.[18] As a state, it is not defined by body language, words or posture. Some have sought to define prayer through exclusions of things not considered to be a part of prayer. Prayer is not centred on self, nor is it the repetition of sounds and syllables, it is not dependent on breathing techniques and visualizations, but consists of a conversation with God, a dialogue, which enables 'the loftiest experience within our reach—the ability to connect with the creator and ruler of the universe on a personal level.'[19] As human beings enter into the state of prayer and commune with God, prayer becomes an expression of a relationship with God.

Efficacy of prayer in relation to health

The first published empirical data on the efficacy of prayer were provided by Sir Francis Galton, a cousin of Charles Darwin.[20] Galton, a sceptic, proposed that if prayer bestowed any benefits upon those praying or being prayed for, then it would be a 'perfectly appropriate and legitimate subject for scientific inquiry.'[20] The question of efficacy, from Galton's perspective, can be reduced to a simple statistical comparison—are prayers answered, or are they not? Adopting this transactional view, Galton assumed that those who pray should attain their objects more frequently than those who do not. In relation to health those who pray and are prayed for should recover on average more rapidly than others. This question could be resolved without endeavouring to understand channels by which prayer reached its fulfilment. Galton's review of the research conducted by others, together with his own findings, found no evidence for the efficacy of prayer. He pointed out that those who were most prayed for—royalty and missionaries serving in foreign lands—were not supernaturally endowed with better health, but rather experienced shorter life spans than other groups. Likewise, those who were a part of the praying class, the clergy, showed no health benefit from their practice of prayer, their life spans being shorter than those of other professionals like lawyers and medical practitioners. Galton concluded that the praying classes did not appear to be specially favoured; if anything, they were likely to be disadvantaged by the practice. He also expressed appreciation for the 'eloquence of the silence' among medical professionals of repute, who refrained from such spiritual practices. To Galton, God does not intervene in human affairs by suspending natural laws. Some have suggested that all subsequent research on prayer has been in some respects a reaction to Galton's devastating conclusions of 140 years ago.[18, p.340]

A number of reviews of prayer research have been published to date. Some have explored the efficacy of prayer in relation to biological entities, enzymes, plants and animals, while others have focused on prayer in relation to human health.[21] This has generated much discussion, but the focus of this chapter is on prayer research in relation to human health.

A recent systematic review of prayer research identified 17 clinical studies utilizing standardized measures and double-blind randomized control trial methodology to examine the effects of prayer on physical and psychological outcomes.[22] Eleven studies found that intercessory prayer exhibited little or no effect. The no-effect studies examined the effect of prayer on clients receiving treatment for alcohol dependence;[23] on physical and psychological outcomes among patients receiving kidney dialysis;[24] on children coping with psychiatric disorders;[25] on heart surgery outcomes;[26] on patients with deteriorating rheumatic disease;[27] and children with leukaemia.[28] In six studies there were statistical trends in the direction of effectiveness; three explored outcomes for patients in coronary care;[29–31] one examined patients with AIDS utilizing various prayer traditions and secular forms of bioenergy healing;[32] one considered retroactive prayer for past events;[33] and one examined pregnancy rates in patients undergoing *in vitro* fertilization-embryo transfer.[34] Meta-analysis suggested evidence of a small, but significant effect of intercessory prayer, concluding that even though intercessory prayer does not meet the American Psychology Association's criteria for empirically supported treatment, it should be classified as an experimental intervention until additional research confirms its therapeutic efficacy.[22]

Three of the landmark studies will be reviewed in more detail. Each utilized a randomized, controlled, double-blind study design with large patient samples. The first was carried out in the late 1980s by Randolph Byrd, a cardiologist at the San Francisco General Hospital, who studied the impact of prayer on coronary patients post myocardial infarction.[29] Byrd sought answers to two research questions: does intercessory prayer to the Judeo-Christian God have any effect on the patient's medical condition and recovery while in hospital? and: how are these effects characterized, if present? Three-hundred-and-ninety-three patients, admitted over a 10-month period to the coronary care unit of San Francisco General Hospital, were randomly assigned to either an intercessory prayer group (IP) or a no prayer group (NP). Patients and medical staff were unaware of which patients were being prayed for. The 192 patients in the IP group were prayed for daily by off campus Christian intercessors. The NP group of 201 patients received no prayer from the study's intercessors. After 10 months, analysis showed no significant difference on 26 of the study's indicators, but further analysis found that the prayed-for patients were five times less likely to need antibiotics, required fewer artificial breathing aids (intubation), suffered less pulmonary oedema and that fewer had died. Byrd concluded that 'intercessory prayer to the Judeo-Christian God had a beneficial therapeutic effect in patients admitted to the CCU [coronary care unit].'[29] Byrd's study is considered a benchmark study in prayer research. The double-blinding has been criticized because clerical staff making computer entries knew to which group each patient belonged. A more substantial reservation about study design is that there was no way of eliminating prayer on behalf of the NP group from, for example, family members or the patients themselves.

In 1999 William Harris and associates[30] sought to replicate Byrd's findings in a randomized, controlled, double-blind study of

990 consecutive patients newly admitted to a coronary care unit. Patients were assigned to either an intercessory prayer group or a regular care group. The first names of patients in the prayer group were given to an external team of intercessors who prayed for them daily for 4 weeks. The patients were not aware that they were prayed for and the intercessors did not know and had never met the patients. Analysis found that the prayed-for group had lower coronary care unit scores, indicating better medical outcomes, when compared with the control group. Harris *et al.* suggested that prayer may be an effective adjunct to standard medical care. They justified the lack of informed consent by participants on the grounds that there was no known risk associated with receiving remote intercessory prayer.

In 2006 Herbert Benson and associates reported on a large controlled study on the therapeutic effects of prayer,[26] seeking to establish whether intercessory prayer itself, or knowledge that prayer is provided, may affect recovery following coronary artery bypass grafts. Patients were randomly assigned to one of three groups; the first received intercessory prayer after being informed that they may or may not receive prayer ($n = 604$); the second did not receive intercessory prayer after being informed that they may or may not receive prayer ($n = 597$); and the third group received intercessory prayer after being informed that they would receive prayer. Intercessory prayer was provided for 14 days starting one day prior to the surgery. Primary measures were based on complications within 30 days of surgery, and relevant secondary outcomes, major events and mortality, were noted. In the two groups uncertain of receiving intercessory prayer complications occurred in 52% of patients who received intercessory prayer as compared with 51% of patients who did not. In the group of patients certain of receiving prayer, complications occurred in 59% of cases. Individuals certain to be receiving prayer were thus more likely to experience complications than individuals who were uncertain of receiving prayer, but in fact did receive it. Major events and mortality were similar across all three groups for the 30 days post-surgery. The results indicate that intercessory prayer had no effect on those who did not know they were being prayed for, while those who were certain of receiving prayer fared somewhat worse.

A critique of research on intercessory prayer

While there is evidence that links prayer, spirituality and religion positively with general health and wellbeing,[35] and that private prayer is an important source of personal support,[36] there is little evidence that prayer is an effective treatment intervention. Conversely there is little evidence of harm,[37] although Benson's findings raise this possibility. Current research on the efficacy of prayer has however come under considerable criticism from both scientific and theological sectors.

To facilitate empirical research scientists make assumptions about prayer that may be vastly different to those of scholars of religion and of the lay people engaged as petitioners in research studies.[38] As just one example, prayer is characteristically relational, yet the primary focus of empirical studies is on the transactional, not the relational aspects, of prayer.

In the studies reviewed, most of the individuals recruited to offer prayer had a Christian background, although their views of God and of the process of prayer varied.[30,38] Operationalizing prayer as a clinical intervention imposes requirements never seen in religious practice. Praying only for individuals unknown to the intercessor and specifying the number and duration of prayers that could be offered each day has no religious rationale and only a tenuous relationship with traditional prayer practices. With the exception of the Harris study,[30] where patients were asked about their religious preference, most of the studies failed to take into consideration the prayer practices and beliefs of the patients in the experimental and control group. Harris and associates found that half of their patients had religious preferences and it was probable that they were studying the effects of intercessory prayer supplementing the prayers offered by the patients, their families and friends.

Gaudia[39] in his critique of intercessory prayer research makes two pertinent observations. He highlights the lack of any theoretical and theological framework for research into the efficacy of prayer, and acknowledges that attempting to validate religious rituals, such as prayer, on clinical grounds trivializes both the ritual and its religious context. As Masters and Spielman point out,[40] the study of prayer requires methodologies that focus on the meaning and personal experience of prayer, rather than framing prayer as a therapeutic technique to be evaluated in terms of clinical outcomes.

Meditation

Meditation has a long and rich history embedded in the Hebrew Bible and the Vedic beliefs of the Indus civilization. The term meditation can refer to many different practices rooted in various traditions. The word 'meditation' is derived from the Latin *meditari*, 'to engage in contemplation or reflection'. Historically, religious and spiritual goals of growth, enlightenment and personal transformation were intrinsic to all forms of meditation. The discussion of meditation in this section will focus predominantly on practices of eastern origin. Since the 1950s eastern meditation has become increasingly popular in western countries both as a spiritual practice and a complementary therapy. However, the role of spirituality and belief in the modern day practice of meditation has diminished.[41] Current research rarely attends to the spiritual, religious, and belief components of meditation, investigating for the most part western versions that are secular adaptations of eastern traditional meditative practices.

As with prayer, definitions of meditation vary and recent literature reviews have proposed parameters to describe and identify its practice. In general, meditation is defined as a form of mental training that requires either stilling or emptying the mind, with the goal of achieving a state of 'detached observation' in which practitioners are aware of the environment, but do not become involved in thinking about it. Meditation practices differ in terms of their primary goal (therapeutic or spiritual), the direction of attention (whether mindfulness or concentrative), the anchor employed (a word, breath, sound, object or sensation), the posture used (motionless sitting or active movement), and whether the practices occur in conjunction with other therapies or as stand-alone therapy.[41]

The ultimate aim of meditation is to assist in the development of a deeper knowledge of the intricate connections between mind and body and of how the mental and spiritual states of individuals affect their psychological and physical health and well-being. As the modern day Buddhist spiritual leader the Dalai Lama explains, every kind of happiness and suffering can be classified as mental and physical. Of the two 'it is the mind that exerts the greatest influence on most of us. Unless we are either gravely ill or deprived of basic necessities, our physical condition plays a secondary role ... The mind however, registers every event, no matter how small. Hence we should devote our most serious efforts to bringing about mental peace.' The purpose of meditation is to 'wage a struggle between the negative and positive forces in your mind. The meditator seeks to undermine the negative and increase the positive.' The Dalai Lama further explains that by listening to the teachings and practicing them each individual can progressively learn to recognize and eliminate personal delusions that lead to suffering and enter 'a path that eventually leads to freedom from suffering and to the bliss of enlightenment.'[42]

The earliest eastern spiritual traditions focused on the primordial human need to find meaning in life and purpose in existence. The meditation practices of the major eastern traditions recognized the spiritual significance of these existential questions and the contribution of a healthy body to spiritual development and personal enlightenment.[43]

Common meditation practices

The recent NCCAM meta-analysis of research on meditation practices proposed five categories: Yoga, Mantra meditation, Mindfulness meditation including Zen Buddhist meditation, Tai Chi, and Qi Gong.[41] Each category is distinctive in its use of postures, breathing, focus of attention, use of a mantra, or accompanying belief system.

Yoga

Classical Yoga forms the basis of the meditative practices of Hinduism, Buddhism and Jainism.[43] According to the writings of Yogi Ramacharaka, those who dissociate the spiritual aspects from the practice of yoga constitute 'the masses being satisfied with the crumbs which fall from the tables of the educated classes.'[44] The modern day practice of yoga is, however, predominantly secular.

Hindu Yoga teaches how to control the body through the breath. Deep rhythmic breathing, facilitated by correct posture, is believed not only to oxygenate the blood, but also improve management of the energy that revitalizes body organs and the mind. A Yogi thus develops the ability to send to any organ or body part 'an increased flow of vital force or 'prana' thereby strengthening and invigorating the part or organ' and becoming able to 'cure disease in himself and others, [and] also practically do away with fear and worry and the base emotions.'[44] Yoga teaches that intelligent control of breathing power has the potential to lengthen life through increased vitality and enhanced powers of resistance, while unintelligent and careless breathing will shorten life, decreasing vitality and laying open the path to disease. While in ordinary breathing the body inhales atmospheric air that is charged with *prana*, through controlled breathing (Yogi breathing) it is possible to extract a greater supply which can be stored away in the brain and other centres of the body. Thus,

> One who has mastered the science of storing away prana, either consciously or unconsciously, often radiates vitality and strength which is felt by those coming in contact with him, and such a person may impart this strength to others, and give them increased vitality and health.[44]

Mantra Meditation

A mantra is a sound, syllable, word or group of words believed to be capable of having a transformative effect. The type of mantra and its use varies according to the school and philosophy with which it is associated. Transcendental meditation [TM] practitioners, for example, utilize 'mental sounds' such as 'Om' or 'Mu' to which no meaning is attached, enabling the mind to settle to its simplest non-active state in pursuit of greater happiness.[41] Practitioners sit in a comfortable posture, with eyes closed repeating the mantra, using a passive breathing technique. 'Relaxation response' (RR) developed by Harvard Cardiologist Herbert Benson in the early 1970s[45] is one secular technique using mantras. As Benson states, the relaxation response is more than a state of relaxation and requires adherence to a specific set of instructions. Practitioners sit in a comfortable position, progressively relaxing body muscles from the feet upwards while focusing on a natural rhythm of breathing and silently repeating a neutral one-syllable word like the word 'one.' The mantra is linked to the breath and helps avoid distracting thoughts. Practitioners are encouraged to elicit the relaxation response twice daily, for 15–20 min.

Mindfulness meditation

Using bodily sensory inputs (breath, smell, taste or hearing) the mind is kept in touch with the present as opposed to focusing on the past or future. Practitioners discipline themselves to avoid 'default' mental activities like worrying, ruminating or catastrophizing. The technique assists in establishing a natural state of awareness that is claimed to lead to greater happiness and simplicity.

Zen Buddhist Meditation

Zen Buddhist meditation, or Zazen, originated in India and in time was introduced to Japan from China. Zazen attends to all aspects of life, including good nutrition and adequate rest. A quiet sitting posture enables a shift in focus from external things to the inner self.[41]. The preferred posture is either the full-lotus or the half-lotus positions, which create the most stable foundation for both body and mind. Hands are held in prescribed ways, eyes are open and attention is directed at a point 1 or 2 m in front of the meditator. Various breathing patterns maintain an energetic and attentive focus. With tanden breathing (effortless diaphragmatic breath focusing on the body's centre of gravity) the body, the breathing, and the mind come into a state of harmony. Attention then focuses on counting breaths, maintaining, with practice, a frequency of three to six breaths per minute.

Other meditation practices

These include popular practices such as Tai Chi, a martial art practice that focuses on exercises that promote relaxation, flexibility, mental concentration and movement coordination, and Qi Gong, an 'energy healing' discipline. Qi Gong has two forms: internal (nei qi) or individual practice and external (wai qi), where a Qi Gong practitioner 'emits' qi for the purpose of healing another person.[41]

Efficacy of meditation

Advocates of meditation have in general been open to 'establishing the truth or falsity of claims' independent of 'wishful thinking and metaphysical assumptions.'[46] However, as with some prayer researchers, the same zeal to obtain empirical evidence of efficacy has influenced research efforts, leading to claims that:

> … meditation can produce such highly practical results as enhanced intelligence, happiness, creativity, self-actualization, physical health, improved interpersonal relationships… remarkable experiences of pure consciousness, pure positive affect and various 'higher' states of consciousness gained through meditation … extreme sorts of claims about supernormal abilities, immortality, divine beings, etc.[46]

Positive outcomes range from self-actualization and 'pure happiness,' to growth of a fulfilled society of healthy, happy, energetic people moving in the direction of peace and harmony.[46]

The report *Meditation Practices for Health: State of the Research* by the University of Alberta Evidenced-Based Practice Center, provides the most comprehensive review of literature on the efficacy of meditation.[41] From an initial 11,030 citations, the review panel selected 2285 potentially relevant articles, of which only 813 ultimately met their criteria of providing relevant measurable health-related outcomes. Even these 813 research studies the EPC deemed to be 'predominantly poor-quality', commenting:

> Overall, we found the methodological quality of meditation research to be poor, with significant threats to validity in every major category of quality measured, regardless of study design.[41]

As with prayer studies, the main criticisms were directed at the quality of randomization, blinding, attrition, and loss to follow-up. Other concerns raised were bias in selecting target populations, lack of criteria for what constitutes successful meditation practice, and lack of clarity in relation to the role that spiritual and beliefs systems play in the successful practice of meditation. Less than 5% of the studies explicitly identified the mediation practice being used. The majority of the studies (61%) were conducted in North America.

Of the 813 studies, 65 intervention studies examined the therapeutic efficacy of meditation on hypertension (27 trials), other cardiovascular diseases (21 trials), and substance abuse disorders (17 trials). Meta-analyses based on poor quality studies with small numbers of hypertensive participants showed that TM, Qi Gong, and Zen Buddhist meditation significantly reduced blood pressure and Yoga helped reduce stress, with most significant changes noted in healthy participants. A few studies reported non-significant results. The report noted that:

> TM had no advantage over health education to improve measures of systolic blood pressure and diastolic blood pressure, body weight, heart rate, stress, anger, self-efficacy, cholesterol, dietary intake, and level of physical activity in hypertensive patients … Yoga did not produce clinical or statistically significant effects in blood pressure when compared to non-treatment; Zen Buddhist meditation was no better than blood pressure checks to reduce systolic blood pressure in hypertensive patients. Yoga was no better than physical exercise to reduce body weight in patients with cardiovascular disorders.[41]

Meta-analysis was difficult to carry out because of the diversity of practices, comparison groups and outcome measures used. Results of the highest quality trials showed inconclusive outcomes for Mindfulness meditation, Relaxation response, and Yoga in substance abuse. The study comparing Mindfulness meditation with usual care for alcohol and cocaine abuse found little indication that Mindfulness meditation enhances treatment outcomes for substance abuse patients. One positive finding came from comparing Yoga with exercise in alcohol abuse where a significantly greater recovery was reported for the Yoga group.

The report concludes that 'the therapeutic effects of meditation practices cannot be established based on the current literature' and states in its executive summary that 'firm conclusions on the effects of meditation practices in healthcare cannot be drawn based on the available evidence.'[41] It recommends that research establish a definition of meditation so that it can be clearly separated from other relaxation techniques such as visualization and self-hypnosis, and that subsequent studies be rigorous in their design, execution, analysis and reporting of results. Similar conclusions were reached by the only Cochrane review currently available,[47] which also notes the absence of reporting of adverse findings.

Recent reviews, focused on the use of meditation in highly specialized applications with well-defined groups reveal promising trends. These include mind-body therapies in relation to metabolic syndrome,[48], neurological disorder,[49] and attention-deficit/hyperactivity disorder,[47] mindfulness mediation in relation to chronic pain,[50] and psychiatric disorders.[51,52] Results have been particularly promising for stress reduction and treating mood problems,[53,54] although less so for treating substance abuse.[55] The reviews recommend further study in adequately powered controlled trials.

A critique of research on meditation

Considerably more research has been carried out on meditation than on prayer. Given the NCCAM finding that of all the complementary therapies prayer is most commonly used, the quantity of research reported is disproportionate. While there may be cultural, socio-religious and scientific reasons for such a trend, quantity has not resulted in quality. Research on meditation has been conducted primarily in North America, where its application to health has become increasingly secularized and commercialized, as exemplified by TM and Yoga. Divorced from their religious and spiritual origins, TM and Yoga are no longer seen as spiritual practices by the majority of their practitioners. Similarly Mantra or Mindfulness meditation and Tai Chi have been developed as 'secular, clinical interventions' in which there is no need to adopt 'any specific spiritual orientation or belief system.'[41]. It could be argued that 'in extracting the technique from its theoretical and belief context, the meaning and effect of meditation is deprived of its essence.'[55]

Definitional issues are a significant problem for research. Meditation is an umbrella term for a range of practices with a spiritual, philosophical or psychophysiological focus. Since relaxation is one of the defining characteristics of meditation, and meditation itself is often considered to be a relaxation response, it is difficult to differentiate within current research the benefits derived from relaxation alone, from relaxation combined with meditation, or meditation itself. Secular meditation practices, such as the Relaxation response, illustrate this dilemma. There is little doubt about the value of relaxation in stress management, chronic pain and other illnesses, but further work is required to identify any distinctive contribution of meditation itself.

Amid the claims of benefits associated with practicing meditation there is virtually no mention of earlier findings of the negative effects of meditation.[56–58] These studies found that more than half of long-term meditators experienced some adverse effects, including relaxation induced anxiety and panic, paradoxical increases in tension, less motivation in life, boredom, anger, pain, impaired reality testing, confusion, disorientation, feeling 'spaced out', depression, and increased negativity.[57] Other studies have identified psychosis-like symptoms, mild dissociation, grandiosity, elation, destructive behaviour and suicidal feelings.[58] The adverse effects of meditation were stronger the longer the practice was maintained. Clinicians and health care professionals should be mindful of these possible adverse effects.

Conclusion and recommendations

Prayer and meditation have a long history of involvement in healthcare and treatment of the sick. In both illness and health, spiritual practices bring comfort, meaning, and reassurance. Through prayer and meditation individuals seek to commune, and enter into a closer relationship with God or a higher power. However, the attempt to measure the efficacy of spiritual practices as healthcare interventions has had marginal success at best.

The studies of prayer and meditation reviewed in this chapter are not directly comparable. Participants in prayer studies have been generally recipients of interventions, while in meditation studies participants have been agents of their own care. Even the studies of private prayer are not directly comparable, as it has been assumed that North American patients know how to pray, but meditation techniques have been taught, thus introducing the therapeutic alliance as a possible confounding factor.[59] In both cases, however, the underlying assumption is that these activities might be the active ingredients associated with better health status and longer lifespan.

Clearly, the assumption that prayer or meditation is the primary active component of belief cannot be sustained. The improved health status associated with religious or spiritual lifestyles is not attributable to a single activity, nor is the activity simply an intervention to be administered in isolation. No major religion claims that one active belief or practice will necessarily confer benefits as some religious and spiritual practices have positive effects, while some have harmful effects.[60] The idea that a deity might be persuaded to intervene on the terms of researchers is theologically controversial. It is also clear that RCT methodologies will fail to identify any 'supernatural' or singular events that occur within a study group.[61] All they can show is that such events, if they occur, are rare and unpredictable, and are not related to spiritual practices in any sustained and causal way.

Considering that a majority of people use prayer, and a significant minority use meditation, in relation to health concerns[4–6] it is necessary to acknowledge that these practices assist in coping with both symptoms and treatment. Accordingly, the beliefs, values and requests of individuals should be considered by healthcare practitioners in delivering healthcare services.[22,62] Rather than investigate prayer as a clinical intervention, prayer research should attend to people's experience of prayer, both private and public, and the ways in which prayer might facilitate a sense of self-efficacy and of social participation that promote health.[63–66] Unlike the reductionist RCT studies, such investigations would open up possibilities of constructive dialogue with religious and spiritual traditions.

References

1 Bishop, J.P. (2003). Prayer, science, and the moral life of medicine. *Arch Intern Med* **163**: 1408.

2 Greeley, A. (1991). Keeping the Faith: Americans hold fast to the Rock of Ages. *Omni* 6–13.

3 Zeiders, C.L., Pekala, R. (1995). A Review of the Evidence Regarding the Behavioural Medical and Psychological Efficacy of Christian Prayer. *J Christian Heal* **17**(3): 17–28.

4 National Institutes of Health; National Centre for Complementary and Alternative Medicine. (2005). Prayer and spirituality in health: ancient practices, modern science. *CAM at the NIH* **12**, 1–5. Available at: http://nccam.nih.gov/news/newsletter/2005_winter/prayer.htm (accessed Mar 2007).

5 Bell, R., Suerken, C., Quandt, S., Gryzywacz, Lang, W., Arcury, T. (2002). Prayer for health among US adults: the 2002 National Health Interview Survey. *Complement Hlth Pract Rev* **10**(3): 175–88.

6 McCaffrey, A.M., Eisenberg, D.M., Legedza, A.T., Davis, R.B., Phillips, R.S. (2004). Prayer for health concerns: results of a National Survey on Prevalence and Patterns of Use. *Arch Intern Med* **164**(8): 858–62.

7 McNeill, J.A., Sherwood, G.D., Starck, P.L., Thompson, C.J. (1998). Assessing clinical outcomes: patient satisfaction with pain management. *J Pain Sympt Manage* **16**(1): 29–40.

8 Barnes, P., Powell-Grinter, E., McFann, K., Nahin, R. (2002). *Complementary and alternative medicine use among adults: United States*, CDC Advance Data Report 343. Available at: http://www.cdc.gov/nchs/data/ad/ad343.pdf (accessed 4 July, 2011)

9 Zaza, C., Sellick, S.M., Hillier, L.M. (2005). Coping with cancer: what do patients do? *J Psychosoc Oncol* **23**(1): 55–73.

10 Ai, A.L., Peterson, C., Tice, T., Huang, B., Rodgers, W., Bolling, S. (2007). The influence of prayer coping on mental health among cardiac surgery patients. *J Hlth Psychol* **12**(4), 580–96.

11 Ai, A.L., Corley, C.S., Peterson, C., Huang, B., Tice, T.N. (2009). Private prayer and quality of life in cardiac patients: pathways of cognitive coping and social support. *Soc Work Hlth Care* **48**: 471–94.

12 Ai, A.L., Ladd, K.L., Peterson, C., Cook, C.A., Shearer, M., Koenig, H. (2010). Long-term adjustment after surviving open heart surgery: the effect of using prayer for coping replicated in a prospective design. *Gerontologist* **30**(6): 798–809.

13 James, W. (2001). *Psychology: the Briefer Course*, p. 59. Mineola: Dover .

14 Newberg, A., D'Aquila, E., Rause, V. (2002). *Why God Won't go Away*. New York: Ballantine.

15 Levin, J.S. (2001). *God, Faith and Health: Exploring the Spirituality-Healing Connection*. New York: John Wiley and Sons.

16 James, W. (1978). *The Varieties of Religious Experience*. New York: Image Books.

17 Heiler, F. (1932). *Prayer: a Study in the History and Psychology of Religion*. Oxford: Oxford University Press.

18 Zaleski, P., Zaleski, C. (2005). *Prayer: A History*. New York: Houghton Mifflin.

19 Tolson, C.L., Koenig, H.G.(2003). *The Healing Power of Prayer*. Grand Rapids: Baker Books.

20 Galton, F. (1872). Statistical Inquiries into the Efficacy of Prayer. *Fortnightly Rev* **1**: 123–35.

21 Benor, D. (1992). Lessons from spiritual healing research and practice. *Subtle Energ* **3**: 73–88.

22 Hodge, D.R. (2007). A systematic review of the empirical literature on intercessory prayer, research on social work practice. *Res Soc Work Pract* **17**(2): 174–87.

23 Walker, S.R., Tonigan, J.S., Miller, W.R., Comer, S., Kahlich, L. (1997). Intercesorry prayer in the treatment of alcohol abuse and dependence: a pilot investigation. *Altern Therap* **3**(6): 79–86.

24 Matthews, D.A., Conti, J.M., Sireci, S.G. (2001). The effects of intercessory prayer, positive visualization, and expectancy on the wellbeing of kidney dialysis patients. *Altern Therap* **7**(5): 42–52.

25 Mathai, J., Bourne, A. (2004). Pilot study investigating the effect of intercessory prayer in the treatment of child psychiatric disorders. *Austral Psychiat* **12**(4): 386–8.

26 Benson, H., Dusek, J.A., Sherwood, J.B., Lam, P., Bethea, C.F., Carpenter, W. (2006). Study of the Therapeutic Effects of Intercessory Prayer (STEP) in cardiac bypass patients: a multi-center randomized trial of uncertainty and certainty of receiving intercessory prayer. *Am Hrt J* **151**: 934–42.

27 Joyce, C.R.B., Welldon, R.M.C. (1965).The objective efficacy of prayer: a double-blind clinical trial. *J Chron Dis* **18**: 367–77.

28 Collipp, P.J. (1969). The efficacy of prayer: a triple blind study. *Med Times* **97**: 201–4.

29 Byrd, R.C., (1988). Positive Therapeutic Effects of Intercessory Prayer in a Coronary Care Unit Population. *Sthn Med J* **81**: 826–9.

30 Harris, A., Thoresen, C.E., McCullough, M.E., Larson, D.B. (1999). Spiritually and religiously oriented health interventions. *J Hlth Psychol* **4**: 413–33.

31 Furlow, L., O'Quinn, J.L. (2002). Does prayer really help? *J Christian Nurs* **19**(2): 31–4.

32 Sicher, F., Targ, E., Moore, D., Smith, H.S. (1998). A randomized double blind study of the effects of distant healing in a population with advanced AIDS: report from a small scale study. *West J Med* **169**: 356–63.

33 Leibovic, L. (2001). Effects of remote, retroactive intercessory prayer on outcomes in patients with blood stream infection: randomized controlled trial. *Br Med J* **323**: 1450–1.

34 Cha, K.Y., Wirth, D.P. (2001). Does prayer influence the success of *in vitro* fertilization-embryo transfer? report of a masked randomized trial. *J Reprod Med* **46**: 781–7.

35 Koening, H.G., McCullough, M.E., Larson, D.B. (2001). *Handbook of Religion and Health*. New York: Oxford University Press.

36 Hollywell, C., Walker, J. (2008). Private prayer as a suitable intervention for hospitalised patients: a critical review of the literature. *J Clin Nurs* **18**: 637–51.

37 Roberts, L., Ahmed, I., Hall, S., Davison, A. (2011). Intercessory prayer for the alleviation of ill health. *Cochr Datab Systemat Rev 2009.* Issue 2 Art No CD 000368. DOI: 10.1002/14651858.CD000368.pub3.

38 Cage, W. (2009). Saying your prayers, constructing your religions: medical studies of intercessory prayer. *J Religion* **89**(3): 299–327.

39 Gaudia, G. (2007). About intercessory prayer: the scientific study of miracles. *Med Gen Med* **9**(1): 56.

40 Masters, K.S., Spielmans, G.I. (2007). Prayer and health: review, meta-analysis, and research agenda. *J Behav Med* **30**: 329–38.

41 Ospina, M.B., Bond, T.K., Karhaneh, M., Tjosvold, L., Vandermeer, B., Liang, Y. (2007). *Meditation Practices for Health: State of Research*, Evidence Report/Technology Assessment No 155. (Prepared by the University of Alberta Evidence-Based Practice Center under Contract No. 290–02-0023.). Rockville, MD: AHRQ Publication No 07-E010 Agency for Healthcare Research and Quality.

42 Shou-Yu, L., Wen-Ching, W. Taoist Qigong. (2006) In: J. Shear (ed.) *The Experience of Meditation: Experts Introduce the Major Traditions*. St Paul: Paragon House.

43 Feuerstein, G (2006). Yogic meditation. In: J. Shear (ed.) *The Experience of Meditation: Experts Introduce the Major Traditions*. St Paul: Paragon House.

44 Ramacharaka, Y. (1903). *The Hindu-Yogi Science of Breath: A Complete Manual of the Oriental Breathing Philosophy of Physical, Mental, Psychic and Spiritual Development*. Chicago: Yogi Publication Society.

45 Benson, H. (1975). *The Relaxation Response*. New York: Avon Books.

46 Shear, J. (2006). Conclusion. In: J. Shear (ed.) *The Experience of Meditation: Experts Introduce the Major Traditions*, p. 259. St Paul: Paragon House.

47 Krisanaprakornkit, T., Sriraj, W., Piyavhatkul, N., Laopaiboon, M. (2009). Meditation therapy for anxiety disorders. *Cochr Datab Systemat Rev* Issue 1 Art No CD004998. DOI: 10.1002/14651858.CD004998.pub2.

48 Anderson, J.G., Taylor, A.G. (2011). The metabolic syndrome and mind-body therapies: a systemic review. *J Nutr Metab* **2011:** 276419.

49 Erwin, Wells, R., Phillips, R.S., McCarthy, E.P. (2011). Patterns of mind-body therapies in adults with common neurological conditions. *Neuroepidemiol* **36**(1): 46–51.

50 Chiesa, A., Serretti, A. (2011). Mindfulness-based interventions for chronic pain: a systematic review of evidence. *J Altern Compl Med* **17**(1): 83–93.

51 Chiesa, A., Serratti, A. (2011). Mindfulness based cognitive therapy for psychiatric disorders: a systematic review and meta-analysis. *Psychiat Res* **187**(3): 441–453.

52 Freeman, M.P., Fava, M., Lake, J., Trivedi, M.H., Wisner, K.L., Mischoulon, D. (2010). Complimentary and alternative medicine in major depressive disorder: the American Psychiatric Association Task Force report. *J Clin Psychiat* **71**(6): 669–81.

53 Greeson, J.M. (2009). Mindfulness research update: 2008. *Compl Hlth Pract Rev* **14**(1): 10–18.

54 Hofman, S.G., Sawyer, A.T., Witt, A.A., Oh, D. (2010). The effect of mindfulness-based therapy on anxiety and depression: a meta-analytic review. *J Consult Clin Psychol* **78**(2): 169–83.

55 Zgierska, A., Rabago, D., Chawla, N., Kushner, K., Koehler, R., Marlatt, A. (2009). Mindfulness meditation for substance abuse disorders: a systematic review. *Subst Abuse* **30**(4): 266–94.

56 Perez-de Albeniz, A., Holmes, J. (2000). Meditation: concepts, effects, and uses in therapy. *Int J Psychother* **5**(1): 49–58.

57 Shapiro, D.H. (1992). Adverse effects of meditation: a preliminary investigation of long term mediators. *Int J Psychosom* **39**: 62–7.

58 Otis, L.S. (1984). Adverse effects of transcendental meditation. In: D.H. Shapiro, R.N. Walsh (eds) *Meditation: Classic and Contemporary Perspectives*, pp. 201–8. New York: Aldine.

59 Schnur, J., Montgomery, G. (2010). A systematic review of therapeutic alliance, group cohesion, empathy, and goal consensus/collaboration in psychotherapeutic interventions in cancer: uncommon factors. *Clin Psychol Rev* **30**(2): 238–47.

60 Griffith, J.L. (2010). *Religion that Heals, Religion that Harms: a Guide for Clinical Practice*. New York: Guilford Press.

61 Chibnall, J.T., Jeral, J.M., Cerullo, M.A. (2001). Experiments on distant intercessory prayer: God, science, and the lesson of Massah. *Arch Intern Med* **161**: 2529–35.

62 Seybold, K.S., Hill, P.C. (2001). The role of religion and spirituality in mental and physical health. *Curr Direct Psycholog Sci* **10**(1): 21–4.

63 Breslin, M., Lewis, A.L. (2008). Theoretical models of the nature of prayer and health: a review. *Ment Hlth, Relig Cult* **11**(1): 9–21.

64 Dein, S., Littlewood, R. (2008). The psychology of prayer and the development of the Prayer Experience Questionnaire. *Ment Hlth, Relig Cult* **11**(1): 39–52.

65 Maselko, J., Kubzansky, L.D. (2006). Gender differences in religious practices, spiritual experiences and health: results from the US General Social Survey. *Soc Sci Med* **62**: 2848–60.

66 Baker, J.O. (2008). An investigation of the sociological patterns of prayer frequency and content. *Sociol Relig* **69**(2): 169–85.

CHAPTER 50

Resiliency and coping

Gregory Fricchione and Shamim Nejad

Introduction

Resiliency is a term used in structural engineering. and refers to the ability to rebound or bounce back from a stressor or adversity. Resiliency, as it pertains to psychiatry, reflects good adjustment across different domains in the face of significant adversity. It consists of 5 major capacities: the capacity to:

- experience reward and motivation nested in dispositional optimism and high positive emotionality
- circumscribe fear responsiveness so that one can continue to be effective through active coping strategies despite fear
- use adaptive social behaviours to secure support through bonding and teamwork and to provide support through altruism
- the ability to use cognitive skills to reinterpret the meaning of negative stimuli in a more positive light
- the integration of a sense of purpose in life along with a moral compass, meaning and spiritual connectedness.[1]

Only recently have scientific advances made it possible to begin to elucidate the underlying biological processes associated with resilient phenotypes.[1–3] A variety of hormones, neurotransmitters, and neuropeptides are involved in the acute biological response to stress, and the different interactions and function of these underlie the individual variability that is observed in stress-resistance among individuals.

Stress physiology

Being alive involves *stress* as a stimulus; stress requires biological, psychological, and social adaptations. *Eustress* can be thought of as the normal physiological workings of the living organism. It consists of homeostatic mechanisms called 'eustasis'. *Pathogenic stress* or *distress* occurs when homeostasis is threatened or perceived to be so in the setting of overwhelming or sustained external and internal stressors. Distress is accompanied by over-activity of the stress response systems mediated primarily by hypothalamic corticotrophin-releasing hormone (CRH) and locus coeruleus A1–A2 derived norepinephrine (NE). Focusing on the sympathetic nervous system and its production of *'the flight–fight response,'* Walter Cannon in the early 1900s did groundbreaking work on one axis of the stress response system, the autonomic nervous system and first described the term *homeostasis*.[4] Hans Selye, another twentieth century stress researcher, focused on the hypothalamus-pituitary-adrenal (HPA) axis.[5]

Stress as *distress* refers to a disruption of the dynamic equilibrium among the person's physiological, psychological and social dimensions, as a result of the perceived presence of an external or internal threat.[6] Alterations in the environment may provoke a physiological response mediated by several interconnected physiological systems constituting the so-called stress response system. Stressors, the stress system, and the stress response are the three key elements in this process.

The stress response system is composed of elements of the central nervous system (CNS), the HPA axis, and the immune system. The CNS and the peripheral nervous system (PNS) have sympathetic and parasympathetic components. All these systems constitute a complex matrix with overlapping boundaries under the ultimate top-down control of the brain. This interconnected system maintains homeostasis by modulating different bodily functions and controlling the administration, distribution, and use of energy. In this way, the brain adapts the level of functioning of different organs to global corporeal demands under each specific circumstance. It is constantly functioning, at varying levels of intensity, autoregulated by negative feedback and feed-forward mechanisms. Despite the ability to auto-regulate, the system can become over-activated by persistent or overwhelming stressors that make adaptation difficult. It is at this point where there is development of *distress*, which can either be acute, in the face of an enormous insult, or chronic, in the setting of persistent unrelenting stressors.

When the stress response is activated, some functions can be stimulated, such as metabolism, cardiac output, vascular tone, respiration, and muscle contraction. Other functions can be suppressed, such as the excretory system, and gastrointestinal and reproductive activity.[7] The stress response is characterized by an increased heart rate, increased breathing rate, increased metabolism, increased oxygen consumption, and increased brain wave activity.

Hypothalamus-pituitary-adrenal axis

Activation of the HPA axis results in secretion of glucocorticoids, hormones that act at many levels to modulate the body's energy resources and restore the body to homeostasis after acute disruption.[8] The medial parvocellular division of the paraventricular hypothalamic nucleus (PVN) houses CRH neurons that release the CRH required for adrenocorticotrophin (ACTH) secretion from the pituitary along with arginine vasopressin (AVP). CRH is also expressed outside of the hypothalamus in the hippocampus, amygdala, nucleus accumbens, bed nucleus of the stria terminalis (BNST), thalamus, hypothalamus, cerebral cortex cerebellum, and hindbrain.[9] There are at least two G-protein-coupled receptors (CRF1 and CRF2) that mediate CRH functioning. CRH binds to CRF1 receptors in the pituitary where signal transduction involving protein kinase A (PKA) and protein kinase C (PKC) leads to ACTH synthesis and secretion. ACTH moves through the systemic circulation arriving at the adrenal cortex where it promotes synthesis and secretion of corticosteroids like cortisol in the human. The CRH neurons are regulated by direct somatic, visceral and humoral sensory afferents relayed from nuclei like the nucleus of the solitary tract (NTS), the raphe, the subfornical organ, and lamina terminalis, other parts of the hypothalamus, the BNST and the thalamus. These 'reactive' stimuli are generally excitatory. At the same time, limbic forebrain structures, such as the paralimbic medial prefrontal cortex, hippocampus, amygdala, and lateral septum along with parts of the hypothalamus and thalamus are thought to provide indirect 'anticipatory' signals through projected connections to select brainstem, hypothalamic and BNST regions that, in turn, enervate the PVN. It is thought that limbic areas that service 'anticipatory' voluntary stress responses, when integrated with 'reactive' reflexive stress responses, can modulate the HPA axis through tuning of the PVN CRH output.

Glucocorticoids can stimulate energy mobilization (glycogenolysis) in the liver, sympathetic nervous system mediated vasoconstriction, proteolysis, and lipolysis, and suppress innate immunity, reproductive function, and bone and muscle growth, as well as mood leading to behavioural depression. This profile can become pathogenic if prolonged. Thus, a premium is placed on multiple feedback control mechanisms to shut this response down.

Central nervous system

The CNS plays an essential role in the regulation of the stress response. The autonomic nervous system (ANS) controls a wide array of functions—cardiovascular, respiratory, gastrointestinal, renal, endocrine, immune and others—that are affected under conditions of stress.[10] While the sympathetic nervous system (SNS) activates the stress response, the parasympathetic nervous system (PNS) can dampen this effect, and restore balance in the autonomic response.

The SNS efferent output flows down the intermediolateral cell column in preganglionic fibres to synapse in a bilateral chain of sympathetic ganglia from where postganglionic mostly NE fibres proceed to innervate vascular smooth muscle, the heart, the gut, the kidney and other organs. The SNS through its innervation of the adrenal medulla has a humoral component resulting in the secretion of circulating epinephrine. The great vagus nerve is the major PNS cholinergic outflow tract. The ANS also contains SNS and PNS subdivisions with neuronal subpopulations that collocate special peptide transmitters. These peptide hormones CRH, Neuropeptide Y (NPY), somatostatin, and galanin are co-localized in NE neurons of this type. Vasoactive intestinal peptide (VIP), substance P and calcitonin gene-related peptide co-localize within cholinergic neurons.[10]

A stressor is 'stressful' only when it is perceived as such. Cognitive appraisal is personalized, and thus each individual determines what is stressful. Certain events or experiences are universally threatening, but there is a lot of room for personification of particular threats. Depending on the appraisal, the mediators of the stress response may or may not emerge.[11] In fact, it has recently been shown that anticipatory cognitive appraisal is an important determinant of the cortisol stress response.[12] On the other hand, the brain also determines the physiological and behavioural responses to stress. The limbic system is a set of structures related to the control of emotional responses, behaviour, and long-term memory. The main structures involved are the hippocampus and the amygdala. The amygdala, which is responsible for fear conditioning, serves as a trip wire for the stress response. It has connections with the prefrontal cortex (PFC), which is related to attention and motivation and can inhibit amygdalar tone, and with the hypothalamus, which regulates endocrine and autonomic system functioning. The hippocampus is a target of stress hormones, and chronically increased levels of cortisol induce a structural remodelling, associated with selective atrophy and altered behavioural and physiological responses.[13]

The PFC regions (dorsolateral—DLPFC, dorsomedial—DMPFC, ventromedial—vmPFC and inferior—iPFC) co-operate to help us plan for the future and manage higher order decision making in concert with the anterior cingulate cortex (ACC). During times of low stress, the PFC, and its extensive connections to cortices and subcortices orchestrate behaviour, thought, and emotion in a reasonable, goal-directed, and regulated way. Direct and indirect connections to the aminergic cell bodies in the brainstem allow the PFC to modulate NE flow from the locus coeruleus, DA from the ventral tegmentum and serotonin from the nucleus raphe. When unstressed there is the potential for optimal levels of amine releases in the PFC creating what is called a 'delicious cycle.'[14] This situation potentiates a top down guidance of attention and thought (DLPFC), error monitoring and reality testing (DMPFC), inhibition of inappropriate actions (iPFC) and regulation of emotions (vmPFC).[14]

During times of distress, on the other hand, the amygdala stimulates the stress response pathways in the HPA axis and the brainstem with outpourings of cortisol, NE and DA. Interaction of the basolateral nucleus (BLA) and central nucleus (CeA) of the amygdala with modulatory regions such as the medial prefrontal cortex (mPFC) is significant during these episodes.[15,16]

Central nervous system and neurocircuitry of fear

The basolateral nucleus of the amygdala is thought to compare conditioned stimulus (CS) inputs and unconditioned stimulus (US) inputs regulating central nucleus activation of the hardwired fear and stress circuitry, leading to inhibition or activation of the fear response. Recent research has begun to determine the role of inhibitory neural circuitry in modulating the fear response at the cellular level.[17–19] Sensory inputs, as well as associative inputs from the hippocampus and cortex project directly and indirectly to the central amygdalar nucleus. 'On' and 'off' inhibitory circuits within the central nucleus are thought to differentially modulate fear output and extinction of fear. Additionally, direct projections from the infralimbic region of the mPFC activate inhibitory neurons in the intercalated region between the basolateral and central nuclei, serving to inhibit, in a top-down manner, the stress enhancing fear output of the central nucleus.

The neurochemical environment of elevated cortisol and NE impairs PFC top-down regulation and strengthens amygdala driven bottom-up dynamics. Stress induced catecholamine excess impairs PFC higher order functioning while activating amygdala fear conditioning accompanied by bottom up sensory hypervigilance and habituated motor responses as opposed to thoughtful pliant approaches characteristic of top down PFC control. Stress can thus set up an amygdala-centred 'vicious cycle'.[14]

Immune system

The immune system also plays an important role in the stress response, and it is well integrated in the psychoneuroendocrinology system. Psychosocial stress stimulates the stress response system resulting in the output of CRH and catecholamines. It is of interest that postganglionic sympathetic nerve fibres secrete CRH, and that norepinephrine and epinephrine stimulate IL-6 release by immune cells and other peripheral cells through effects on beta-adrenergic receptors.[20] Stress activates transcription factor NF-kB, which then produces pro-inflammatory cytokines.[21] This signalling molecule is an essential mediator at the blood brain barrier that translates peripheral immune signals to the CNS. Catecholamines from SNS fibres increase NF-kB DNA binding in immune cells including the macrophage resulting in inflammatory response syndrome.[22] Pro-inflammatory cytokines can access the brain directly through fenestrated endothelium zones (area postrema, subfornical organ, median eminence, pineal gland) and indirectly through cellular active transport, endothelial cell, and perivascular macrophage activation and peripheral vagal paraganglia activation, which is transmitted through the NTS and hypothalamus into the brain, and proceeds to interact with neurotransmitter metabolism, neuroendocrine action, and neuroplasticity.[23] This interaction may result in excitotoxicity, oxidative stress, aminergic changes, and trophic factor reductions.

Microglial cells are the primary central targets of pro-inflammatory signals originating in the periphery. Once activated, they release cytokines, chemokines, and reactive oxygen species (ROS), which then initiate a sequence of effects including activation of astroglial cells. The CNS inflammatory response syndrome is amplified as a result. Eventually IL-1, IL-6, and TNF-alpha and interferons stimulate the enzyme indoleamine 2,3-dioxygenase (IDO), which breaks down tryptophan into kynurenine, reducing brain serotonin stores, and increasing quinolinic acid, a potent NMDA agonist that can produce excitotoxicity and severe oxidative stress. At the same time, oligodendrocytes are also sensitive to this cascade, and particularly to TNF-alpha, which may have a toxic effect, leading to apoptosis and demyelination. Cytokines also stimulate the CRH and HPA axis. In acute stress situations, cortisol elevation will, along with PNS vagal stimulation, tend to reduce NF-kB activation, with the potential goal of dampening the inflammatory response.

These aspects of the immune response's physiology hypothetically have relevance in the genesis or progression of multiple diseases. Distress has been related to proneness to viral infections, progression from HIV to AIDS, flares of multiple sclerosis, lupus, arthritis and risk of developing coronary heart disease and Alzheimer's disease.[24–29]

Both catecholamines and glucocorticoids control the amplitude of immune response by negative feedback mechanisms. In physically threatening situations, inflammatory cytokines, mainly IL-6, stimulate the HPA axis, and the elevation of cortisol levels induce the suppression of the immune/inflammatory reaction. Simultaneously, the SNS causes systemic secretion of cytokines, which will eventually suppress the immune system.[30] Thus, acute activation of the HPA axis helps to regulate the activity of the immune response, and in the case of psychological distress, the immune system can be suppressed. However, under conditions of chronic stress such as extensive caregiving, marital strife or even perceived stress, there are increases in acute phase proteins (C-reactive protein- CRP), IL-6 and other inflammatory mediators.[31] Maltreatment in early childhood is associated with elevated CRP 20 years later.[32]

Resiliency and neurobiology

Molecular adaptations within the dopamine (DA) reward and motivation circuitries are associated with vulnerability and resiliency.[33] For example, a naturally occurring single nucleotide polymorphism (SNP) (G196A Met/Met) promotes insusceptibility to stress by virtue of deficits in activity dependent BDNF release in the nucleus accumbens. In another study, the ratio of CRH to neuropeptide Y (NPY) also seems to reflect a relationship between vulnerability and resiliency. High CRH increase (increase stress response + negative affect) with low NPY (decrease anxiolysis) correlates with high allostatic loading and low resilience and increased propensity to alcohol abuse.[34] When there is lower haplotype driven NPY expression (SNPrs 16147 in NPY promoter region) in limbic areas associated with amygdala arousal and emotional valencing, there is higher amygdala activation and diminished resiliency.[35] Dihydroepiandrosterone–S (DHEA) over cortisol and NPY over norepinephrine ratios reflect resiliency in Navy Seal commandos exposed to a stressful capture exercise.[36] In a human depression study, the serotonin transporter allele 5-HTTLPR with 2 short arms SS, thought to be a risk for depression in and of itself, when combined with maltreatment in childhood plus low social support will be twice as likely to cause depression as those with 5-HTT SS, and no maltreatment and low social supports. Further, this latter profile is more likely than the 5-HTT SS group with maltreatment and good social supports to cause depression, which in turn is more likely to cause depression than the group with 5-HTT SS plus no maltreatment and good social supports.[37] It should be noted however that a recent meta-analysis found no evidence that the 5-HTTLPR conveyed extra risk for depression beyond the stressful life events.[38] There are HPA axis-related genes that may interact with resiliency to stress. For example, single nucleotide polymorphisms (*SNPs*) of the *CRH type 1* receptor gene may moderate the effects of child maltreatment on susceptibility to depression in adulthood[39] and four *SNPs* of the gene (*FKBP5*) that codes for a protein chaperone that regulates glucocorticoid receptor (GR) sensitivity modulate the association of child abuse with the risk of PTSD in adulthood.[40] In addition, there is a catechol-O-methyltransferase (COMT) polymorphism (Val158Met) that has relevance to resiliency. Those with low activity Met158 develop higher levels of catecholamines in response to stress resulting in lower resilience to anxiety and negative mood states.[41]

There are also epigenetic mechanisms of resiliency in which the environment can change chromatin structure through methylation or acetylation of histones or direct methylation of DNA. In the rat model, maternal nurturance has been shown to increase levels of the transcription factor nerve growth factor-inducible protein A (NGFI-A) known as EGR1 in the hippocampus of the nurtured pup. This allows for hypomethylation and stimulation of the hippocampal GR gene. Higher levels of hippocampal GR translates into certain neurobehavioural phenotypes in the adult including lower baseline and post-stress glucocorticoid secretion levels, lower anxiety-like behaviours, and in females improved nurturance of their own offspring.[42] In resilient mice, chronic stress activates several potassium channel subunits in VTA DA neurons and this blocks a stress induced increase in VTA excitability and downstream release of BDNF in the nucleus accumbens.[33]

If evolution made us a species that relies on social support for our survival and health, then it had to create a species that had the capacity to give social support, to be pro-social, to be altruistic. Indeed, altruistic behaviour has been associated with good health outcomes as long as stress does not overwhelm the individual's ability to cope.[43]

Placebo

In medicine, most of the available treatment for underlying illnesses, until only recently in history, has been the placebo effect. Calling some responses 'the placebo effect' is not an epithet, even though in medicine it has developed that connotation. Integral to the effect of placebo is the belief that a patient has in the ability of either the clinician or the treatment itself to heal him or her. This positive conscious expectation of a return to wellness has the power to stimulate the brain reward and motivation circuitries in a way that results in the reduction of the stress and allostatic loading brought about by either real or perceived stress. Thus, top-down control of the stress response becomes engaged dampening underlying anxiety or fear, particularly when belief and positive expectation diminish the underlying 'dis-ease.'

There has been focus on three main disorders—pain, depression, and Parkinson's disease that establish the importance of the placebo response. The main reason why the placebo is so active in these three disease processes is probably because placebo is actually working on the brain mesolimbic/mesocortical reward and motivation circuitries.[44] There are now neuroimaging studies that support this. One experiment shows that if a standard heat pain paradigm is applied to subjects, the ACC becomes activated while the DLPFC is relatively deactivated. That is a signature of human pain. The ACC is the place that modulates all forms of human pain. If the same experiment is conducted, but a placebo cream is applied prior to the heat stimulus, you will see the exact opposite—ACC activation goes down, DLPFC activation goes up and pain is reduced.[45] The endogenous opioid mu receptor system is of importance in placebo pain response, and this receptor can be blocked by the administration of naloxone, which then eliminates the placebo's effectiveness.

In elegant studies with Parkinson's disease (PD) patients, researchers using positron emission tomography (PET) with the DA ligand raclopride, have been able to show that a placebo of subcutaneous saline can improve PD symptoms coinciding with the displacement of the raclopride presumably by DA from the substantia nigra and the ventral tegmentum DA cell bodies.[46]

In depression, it has been known that a considerable number of depressed patients will improve with antidepressant medication or placebo medication, with estimates ranging from 25 to 60% of depressed patients responding to placebo treatment.[44,47,48] Mayberg and colleagues utilized PET to study regional brain metabolism associated with the placebo response in patients with major depression.[49] In their double blind controlled study, symptom remission at 6 weeks was seen in 8 of 15 study completers, 4 of whom received fluoxetine and 4 placebo. Placebo response at 6 weeks was associated with metabolic decreases in the subgenual cingulate, hypothalamus, thalamus, parahippocampus, and supplementary sensory insula.

With this background understanding of the power of belief to enhance brain reward and motivation while reducing the stress response, it is reasonable to place belief in the category of human resiliency responses.

Building resiliency and coping capacity

Whether one is disease free or has risk factors for disease, or has the disease already, there are ways to reduce stress and allostatic loading (the metabolic wear and tear sustained in an effort to maintain physiological stability in the face of change) and to enhance resiliency thus improving one's health profile. In other words lifestyle modification and individual and group therapies designed to reduce stress and strengthen resiliency will provide primary, secondary, and tertiary prevention.

Building on the earlier work of medical sociologist George Albee,[50] if one thinks about the numerator as being stress or allostatic loading and about the denominator as being resiliency, a pretty good picture of one's vulnerability to illness in the future will emerge. This might be called an heuristic Illness Index or the propensity to illness (see Figure 50.1).[51,52]

Conversely, if one switches the numerator to resiliency and the denominator to stress, you get the quotient changed to propensity to health—a Health Index. For example, if one studies women with systemic lupus erythematosis, when you populate the variables in the equation and you stratify the groups into low social support leading to a decrease in the denominator, the propensity to a lupus flare will increase. There are many examples of this relationship in the literature.[53–60]

Because of this relationship, it is advisable that doctors and nurses take heed of this equation when they evaluate patients and create treatment plans. There should be some ability in the clinical encounter to get an objective feel for the level of patient stress and the level of the patient's resiliency. The problem is compounded once illness takes hold because illness itself is an enormous stress because it ignites the threat of separation.

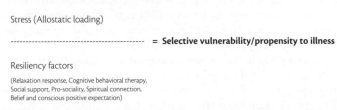

Stress (Allostatic loading)

-- = **Selective vulnerability/propensity to illness**

Resiliency factors

(Relaxation response, Cognitive behavioral therapy, Social support, Pro-sociality, Spiritual connection, Belief and conscious positive expectation)

Figure 50.1 Mind Body Medicine Equation.

Here is where spirituality can be health promoting by supporting secure attachment, a key component in human resiliency (see Figure 50.2). The recent 'Improving the Quality of Spiritual Care as a Dimension of Palliative Care Consensus Conference' recommended the following definition for spirituality: 'Spirituality is the aspect of humanity that refers to the way individuals seek and express meaning and purpose and the way they experience their *connectedness* to the moment, to self, to others, to nature, and to the significant or sacred.'[61] This definition includes the critical elements of connectedness, meaning, and the search for the significant and the sacred in life.

Examples of resiliency building approaches include individual- and group-based relaxation response and meditation training, including elements such as:

- mindfulness-based stress reduction, yoga, tai chi and qi gong
- cognitive skills training
- positive psychology and positive expectation
- spiritual connectedness
- exercise
- nutrition
- sleep hygiene.

The somatic symptoms, pain complaints and depression that often accompany chronic diseases can be reduced by these strategies.[62] At the same time the resiliency that emerges after these trainings will help the coping of patients who are facing the physical and emotional challenges of acute and chronic illnesses (see Figure 50.3).

- Decrease in perceived stress/threat
- Increase in benign appraisal
- Increase in positive expectations and optimism
- Increase in social support
- Increase in pro-social behavior and altruistic love
- Increase in support from a Source greater than oneself
- Downstream benefits for coping and healing

Figure 50.2 Spirituality, resiliency and health.

Conclusion

Resilience to stress is multi-determined. In the face of extreme stress or trauma, an individual may develop psychopathology with significant functional decline or may recover quickly, with minimal psychological sequelae. When response emerges depends upon an interconnected and dynamic mix of factors, including the individual's neurobiological and psychological profile, personal trauma history, and peri-traumatic circumstances, such as availability of social support networks.[2,63,64]

The growing body of knowledge regarding the many factors that affect an individual's response to stress will likely lead to the development of new therapies, both pharmacological and psychotherapeutic, for enhancing resilience to stress. Stress inoculation training, via exposure to manageable stressors, may be useful in building resistance to adversity in both children and adults. It may also be possible to enhance resilience with pharmacological means. The likelihood and/or severity of stress-induced psychopathology in the future may be reduced with the use of NPY, DHEA, CRH-1 antagonists, and GAL-1 agonists. Further research will be

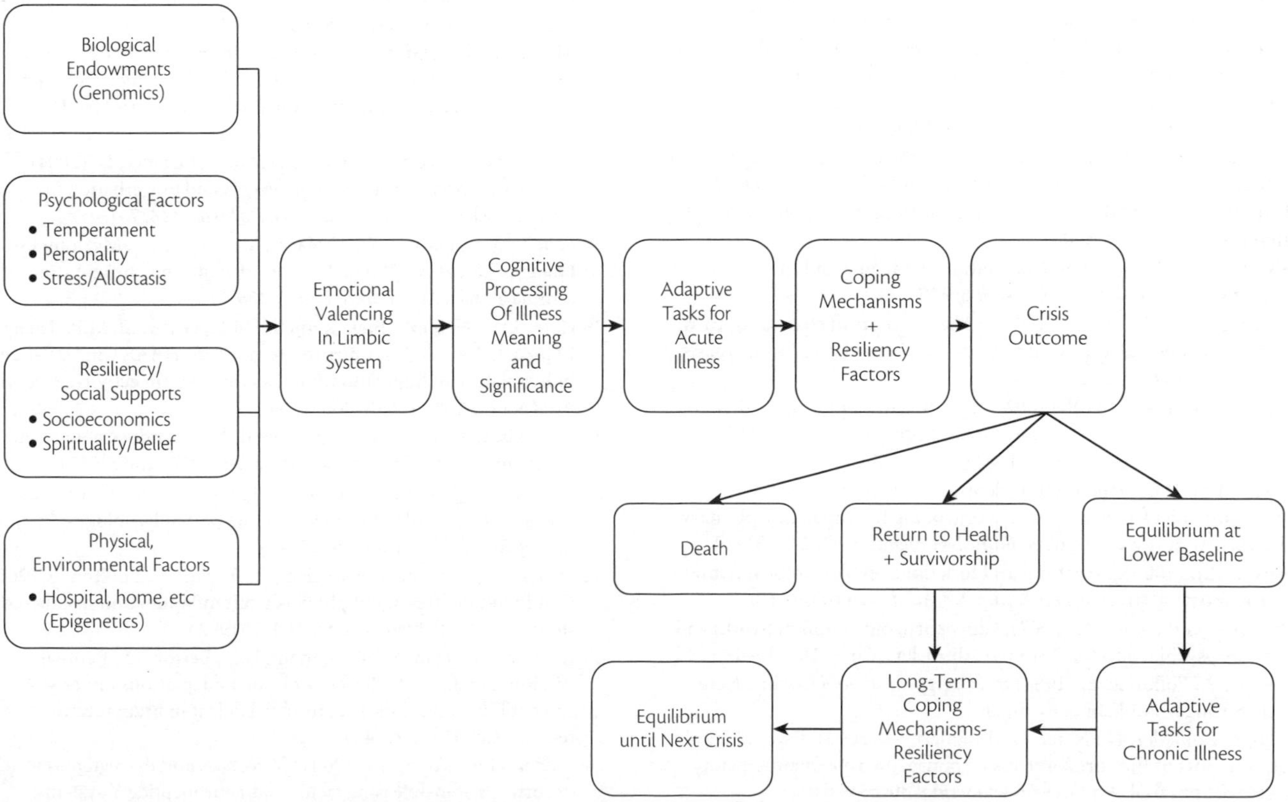

Figure 50.3 An approach to the patient with the medical illness experience.
[Adapted from Fricchione & Marcantonio (1998) & Moos and Tsu, (1977)] 51, 63

necessary to investigate the potential of these and other molecules and compounds to dampen the stress response in humans.

In addition, it will be necessary to evaluate the efficacy of agents that target receptors involved in fear conditioning and fear extinction, that is, voltage-gated calcium channels, beta adrenergic receptors, tyrosine kinase b receptors, and NMDA receptors. By weakening fear-conditioning mechanisms and enhancing fear-extinction pathways, it may be possible to attenuate the progress and encoding of traumatic memories that often occurs upon exposure to trauma.

All of the potential new pharmacotherapies for preventing and/or treating stress related disorders can be coupled with psychotherapy. Cognitive behavioural therapies can assist patients in learning how to reframe adverse events and cognitive distortions, how to adopt active coping techniques when faced with problems, and how to achieve greater cortical control over negative emotions. Prolonged exposure therapy is particularly useful in helping patients to extinguish learned fear associations. Individual and group mind body approaches designed to enhance the core components of human resiliency as discussed above can have benefits for primary, secondary, and tertiary prevention.

Continued progress in understanding the genetic, developmental, biological, and psychological underpinnings of resilience and vulnerability to stress, as well as the interactions between these factors, will aid in moving the field toward the identification, prevention and treatment of those at risk of developing stress-related psychopathology.

References

1 Feder, A., Nestler, E.J., Charney, D.S. (2009). Psychobiology and molecular genetics of resilience. *Nat Rev Neurosci* **10**: 446–57.

2 Charney, D.S. (2004). Psychobiological mechanisms of resilience and vulnerability: implications for successful adaptation to extreme stress. *Am J Psychiat* **161**: 195–216.

3 Cicchetti, D., Blender, J.A. (2006). A multiple-levels-of-analysis perspective on resilience: implications for the developing brain, neural plasticity, and preventive interventions. *Ann NY Acad Sci* **1094**: 248–58.

4 Cannon, W.B. (1929). Pharmacological injections and physiological inferences. *Science* **70**: 500–1.

5 Selye,H. (1946). The general adaptation syndrome and the diseases of adaptation. *J Clin Endocrinol Metab* **6**: 117–230.

6 Chrousos, G.P., Gold, P.W. (1992). The concepts of stress and stress system disorders. Overview of physical and behavioural homeostasis. *J Am Med Ass* **267**: 1244–52.

7 Tsigos, C., Chrousos, G.P. (2002). Hypothalamic-pituitary-adrenal axis, neuroendocrine factors and stress. *J Psychosom Res* **53**: 865–71.

8 Herman, J.P., Figueiredo, H., Mueller, N.K., Ulrich-Lai, Y., Ostrander, M.M., Choi, D.C., *et al.* (2003). Central mechanisms of stress integration: hierarchical circuitry controlling hypothalamo-pituitary-adrenocortical responsiveness. *Front Neuroendocrinol* **24**: 151–80.

9 Denver, R.J. (2009). Structural and functional evolution of vertebrate neuroendocrine stress systems. *Ann NY Acad Sci* **1163**: 1–16.

10 Chrousos, G.P., Kino, T. (2007). Glucocorticoid action networks and complex psychiatric and/or somatic disorders. *Stress* **10**: 213–19.

11 Lazarus, R., Folkman, S. (1984) *Stress, Appraisal, and Coping*. New York: Springer Publishing Company.

12 Gaab, J., Rohleder, N., Nater, U.M., Ehlert, U. (2005). Psychological determinants of the cortisol stress response: the role of anticipatory cognitive appraisal. *Psychoneuroendocrinol* **30**: 599–610.

13 McEwen, B.S. (1999). Stress and hippocampal plasticity. *Ann Rev Neurosci* **22**: 105–22.

14 Arnsten, A.F. (2009). Stress signalling pathways that impair prefrontal cortex structure and function. *Nat Rev Neurosci* **10**: 410–22.

15 Jovanovic, T., Ressler, K.J. (2010). How the neurocircuitry and genetics of fear inhibition may inform our understanding of PTSD. *Am J Psychiat* **167**: 648–62.

16 Lanius, R.A., Vermetten, E., Loewenstein, R.J., Brand, B., Schmahl, C., Bremner, J.D., *et al.* (2010). Emotion modulation in PTSD: Clinical and neurobiological evidence for a dissociative subtype. *Am J Psychiat* **167**: 640–7.

17 Herry, C., Ciocchi, S., Senn, V., Demmou, L., Müller, C., Lüthi A. (2008). Switching on and off fear by distinct neuronal circuits. *Nature* **454**: 600–6.

18 Likhtik, E., Popa, D., Apergis-Schoute, J., Fidacaro, G.A., Paré, D. (2008). Amygdala intercalated neurons are required for expression of fear extinction. *Nature* **454**: 642–5.

19 LeDoux, J.E., Gorman, J.M. (2001). A call to action: overcoming anxiety through active coping. *Am J Psychiat* **158**: 1953–5.

20 Chrousos, G.P., Kino, T. (2009). Glucocorticoid signaling in the cell. Expanding clinical implications to complex human behavioural and somatic disorders. *Ann NY Acad Sci* **1179**: 153–66.

21 Bierhaus, A., Humpert, P.M., Nawroth, P.P. (2004). NF-kappaB as a molecular link between psychosocial stress and organ dysfunction. Pediat Nephrol **19**: 1189–91.

22 Miller,G.E., Chen, E., Sze, J., Marin, T., Arevalo, J.M., Doll, R., *et al.* (2008). A functional genomic fingerprint of chronic stress in humans: blunted glucocorticoid and increased NF-kappaB signaling. *Biol Psychiat* **64**: 266–72.

23 Saper, C.B., Breder,C.D. (1994). The neurologic basis of fever. *N Engl J Med* **330**: 1880–6.

24 Cohen, S., Williamson, G.M. (1991). Stress and infectious disease in humans. *Psychol Bull* **109**: 5–24.

25 Dong, H., Goico, B., Martin, M., Csernansky, C.A., Bertchume, A., Csernansky, J.G. (2004). Modulation of hippocampal cell proliferation, memory, and amyloid plaque deposition in APPsw (Tg2576) mutant mice by isolation stress. *Neuroscience* **127**: 601–9.

26 Matthews, K.A., Gump, B.B. (2002). Chronic work stress and marital dissolution increase risk of posttrial mortality in men from the Multiple Risk Factor Intervention Trial. *Arch Intern Med* **162**: 309–15.

27 Mohr, D.C., Hart, S.L., Julian, L., Cox, D., Pelletier, D. (2004). Association between stressful life events and exacerbation in multiple sclerosis: a meta-analysis. *Br Med J* **328**: 731.

28 Sandberg, S., Paton, J.Y., Ahola, S., McCann, D.C., McGuinness, D., Hillary, C.R., *et al.* (2000). The role of acute and chronic stress in asthma attacks in children. *Lancet* **356**: 982–7.

29 Cole, S.W., Naliboff, B.D., Kemeny, M.E., Griswold, M.P., Fahey, J.L., Zack, J.A. (2001). Impaired response to HAART in HIV-infected individuals with high autonomic nervous system activity. *Proc Natl Acad Sci USA* **98**: 12695–700.

30 Stratakis, C.A., Chrousos, G.P. (1995). Neuroendocrinology and pathophysiology of the stress system. *Ann NY Acad Sci* **771**: 1–18.

31 Miller, A.H., Maletic, V., Raison, C.L. (2009). Inflammation and its discontents: the role of cytokines in the pathophysiology of major depression. *Biol Psychiat* **65**: 732–41.

32 Danese, A., Pariante, C.M., Caspi, A., Taylor, A., Poulton, R. (2007). Childhood maltreatment predicts adult inflammation in a life-course study. *Proc Natl Acad Sci USA* **104**: 1319–24.

33 Krishnan, V., Han, M.H., Graham, D.L., Berton, O., Renthal, W., Russo, S.J., *et al.* (2007). Molecular adaptations underlying susceptibility and resistance to social defeat in brain reward regions. *Cell* **131**: 391–404.

34 Valdez, G.R., Koob, G.F. (2004). Allostasis and dysregulation of corticotropin-releasing factor and neuropeptide Y systems: implications for the development of alcoholism. *Pharmacol Biochem Behav* **79**: 671–89.

35 Zhou, Z., Zhu, G., Hariri, A.R., Enoch, M.A., Scott, D., Sinha, R., *et al.* (2008). Genetic variation in human NPY expression affects stress response and emotion. *Nature* **452:** 997–1001.

36 Southwick, S.M., Vythilingam, M., Charney, D.S. (2005). The psychobiology of depression and resilience to stress: implications for prevention and treatment. *Ann Rev Clin Psychol* **1**: 255–91.

37 Kaufman, J., Yang, B.Z., Douglas-Palumberi, H., Houshyar, S., Lipschitz, D., Krystal, J.H., *et al.* (2004). Social supports and serotonin transporter gene moderate depression in maltreated children. *Proc Natl Acad Sci USA* **101**: 17316–21.

38 Risch, N., Herrell, R., Lehner, T., Liang, K.Y., Eaves, L., Hoh, J., *et al.* (2009). Interaction between the serotonin transporter gene (5-HTTLPR), stressful life events, and risk of depression: a meta-analysis. *J Am Med Ass* **301**: 2462–71.

39 Bradley, R.G., Binder,E.B., Epstein, M.P., Tang, Y., Nair, H.P., Liu, W., *et al.* (2008). Influence of child abuse on adult depression: moderation by the corticotropin-releasing hormone receptor gene. *Arch Gen Psychiat* **65**: 190–200.

40 Binder, E.B., Bradley, R.G., Liu, W., Epstein, M.P., Deveau, T.C., Mercer, K.B., *et al.* (2008). Association of FKBP5 polymorphisms and childhood abuse with risk of posttraumatic stress disorder symptoms in adults. *J Am Med Ass* **299**: 1291–305.

41 Heinz, A., Smolka, M.N. (2006). The effects of catechol O-methyltransferase genotype on brain activation elicited by affective stimuli and cognitive tasks. *Rev Neurosci* **17**: 359–67.

42 Meaney, M.J., Szyf, M. (2005). Environmental programming of stress responses through DNA methylation: life at the interface between a dynamic environment and a fixed genome. *Dialog Clin Neurosci* **7**: 103–23.

43 Post, S.G. (2009). It's good to be good: science says it's so. Research demonstrates that people who help others usually have healthier, happier lives. *Hlth Prog* **90**: 18–25.

44 Fricchione, G., Stefano, G.B. (2005). Placebo neural systems: nitric oxide, morphine and the dopamine brain reward and motivation circuitries. *Med Sci Monit* **11**: MS54–65.

45 Zubieta, J.K., Bueller, J.A., Jackson, L.R., Scott, D.J., Xu, Y., Koeppe, R.A., *et al.* (2005). Placebo effects mediated by endogenous opioid activity on mu-opioid receptors. *J Neurosci* **25**: 7754–62.

46 de la Fuente-Fernandez, R., Stoessl, A.J. (2004). The biochemical bases of the placebo effect. *Sci Eng Eth* **10**: 143–50.

47 Quitkin, F.M. (1999). Placebos, drug effects, and study design: a clinician's guide. *Am J Psychiat* **156**: 829–36.

48 Shapiro, A., Shapiro, E. (1997). *The Powerful Placebo: From Ancient Priest to Modern Physician*. Baltimore: Johns Hopkins University Press.

49 Mayberg, H.S., Silva, J.A., Brannan, S.K., et al. (2002). The functional neuroanatomy of the placebo effect. *Am J Psychiat* **159**: 728–37.

50 Albee, G.W. (1982). The politics of nature and nurture. *Am J Commun Psychol* **10**: 4–30.

51 Fricchione, G., Marcantonio, E (1998). Approach to the patient with chronic illness. In: T.A. Stern, J.P. Herman, P. Slavin (eds) *Massachusetts General Hospital Practical Guide to Psychiatry for Primary Care Clinicians*, pp. 199–206. New York: McGraw Hill Publ.

52 Fricchione, G.L. (2010). The new science of mind body medicine. In: Yano E, Kawachi I, Nakao M (eds) *The Healthy Hospital. Maximizing the Satisfactions of Patients, Health Workers and Community*, pp. Tokyo, Japan.

53 Ward, M.M. (1999). Health-related quality of life in ankylosing spondylitis: a survey of 175 patients. *Arthrit Care Res* **12:** 247–55.

54 Sutcliffe, N., Clarke, A.E., Levinton, C., Frost, C., Gordon, C., Isenberg, D.A. (1999). Associates of health status in patients with systemic lupus erythematosus. *J Rheumatol* **26**: 2352–6.

55 Sewitch,M.J., Abrahamowicz, M., Bitton, A., Daly, D., Wild, G.E., Cohen, A., *et al.* (2001). Psychological distress, social support, and disease activity in patients with inflammatory bowel disease. *Am J Gastroenterol* **96**: 1470–9.

56 Seeman, T.E. (2000). Health promoting effects of friends and family on health outcomes in older adults. *Am J Hlth Promot* **14**: 362–70.

57 Case, R.B., Moss, A.J., Case, N., McDermott, M., Eberly, S. (1992). Living alone after myocardial infarction. Impact on prognosis. *J Am Med Ass* **267**: 515–19.

58 Horsten, M., Mittleman, M.A., Wamala, S.P., Schenck-Gustafsson, K., Orth-Gomér, K. (2000). Depressive symptoms and lack of social integration in relation to prognosis of CHD in middle-aged women. The Stockholm Female Coronary Risk Study. *Eur Heart J* **21**: 1072–80.

59 Ruberman, W., Weinblatt, E., Goldberg, J.D., Chaudhary, B.S. (1984). Psychosocial influences on mortality after myocardial infarction. *N Engl J Med* **311**: 552–9.

60 Albee, G.W. (1982). Preventing psychopathology and promoting human potential. *Am Psychol* **37**: 1043–50.

61 Puchalski, C., Ferrell, B., Virani, R., Otis-Green, S., Baird, P., Bull, J., *et al.* (2009). Improving the quality of spiritual care as a dimension of palliative care: the report of the Consensus Conference. *J Palliat Med* **12**: 885–904.

62 Astin, J.A., Shapiro, S.L., Eisenberg, D.M., Forys, K.L. (2003). Mind-body medicine: state of the science, implications for practice. *J Am Bd Fam Pract* **16**: 131–47.

63 Moos, R., Tsu, V. (1977). The crisis of physical illness. In: R. Moos (ed.) *Coping with Physical Illness*. New York: Plenum Press.

64 Yehuda, R. (2004). Risk and resilience in posttraumatic stress disorder. *J Clin Psychiat* **65**(Suppl 1): 29–36.

CHAPTER 51

Spiritual experience, practice, and community

Fiona Gardner

It is clear that in Western cultures religious participation is declining, whilst interest in exploring spirituality is increasing.[1,2] Links between these trends remain under-investigated, but research into their communal context is beginning to provide some answers. This chapter draws upon a range of research findings that explore the changing place of community in expressions of religion and spirituality.

Community in relation to spiritual practice

We are accustomed to thinking about community as it relates to religion in a geographical or place-based way. This is the conventional understanding of community as grounded in a sense of local identity and belonging, and mutual support or obligation on a human scale.[3] Local religious communities, congregations, are typically situated in a neighbourhood, or town or rural area, so that membership draws upon those living in a particular district. This reinforces the congregational connections in other ways: people also meet during other activities such as shopping, taking children to school or offering each other support. Engaging the plumber or lawyer who is also in your congregation reinforces community bonds. Increasingly, however, communities are becoming thought of more widely as including networks of association, people coming together because of a shared interest or purpose. People now meet in regional or online communities for religious and spiritual reasons creating a sense of belonging and mutual support and interest with little or no geographical connection.[4–6]

Heelas' and Woodhead's pioneering study, reported in their book The Spiritual Revolution,[7] is a useful place to begin considering community in relation to spiritual experience and practice. They chose a case study approach focusing on a specific geographic community, the small rural town of Kendal, in northwest England. Kendal, in 1999, when the research commenced, had a population of 27,610. While it was chosen partly for convenience, it also mirrored English society in its gender and age distributions, though not in cultural diversity, having no significant ethnic communities. 'By taking a single relatively small locality', the researchers considered 'we could be fairly confident of systematically exploring what was going on by way of face-to-face, *associational* religious and spiritual activity'(p. 8). A combination of quantitative and qualitative methods was used to map the nature and extent of religious and spiritual activity. Researchers visited all 25 (Christian) congregations to observe activity before, during and after Sunday morning services. They also investigated what they called the 'holistic milieu' or others might call 'New Age' activities. They listed all groups, organizations and services that identified as being spiritual in some way; yoga, tai chi, Buddhist mediation groups and nearly one hundred practitioners of complementary medicine. Seven 'communities' or associations' were chosen for in-depth study: three in the holistic milieu and four in the congregational domain. Research on these was carried out through participant observation and 200 interviews. Quantitative data collected included attendance at church services and other group activities.

Heelas and Woodhead's findings illuminate the relationship between individuals and communities in their religious or spiritual journeys. Central to their research is the idea of the 'subjective'—'life lived in deep connection with the unique experience of my self-in-relation as opposed to life lived as particular roles'.[7, p. 3] An example of this would be expressing individual beliefs through the role of being a parent or spouse rather than living according to a role dictated by others, such as a religious community. From a subjective perspective, the 'goal is not to defer to higher authority, but to have the courage to become one's own inner authority'. [7, p. 4] This idea of subjectivity, they suggest is embedded in the cultural expectation of 'being yourself' rather than living according to other people's expectations. This informs their distinction between religion and spirituality. Those who are religious, sacralize 'life-as' their 'subjectivity subordinate to the 'higher' authority of transcendent meaning, goodness and truth' generally expressed in a collective way which they call 'congregational life' [7, p. 5]. In comparison, those in the holistic milieu who consider themselves as 'spiritual' see the 'sacred in the cultivation of unique subjective life' [7, p. 5] with emphasis on personal growth and development, movement towards wholeness, making their own decisions without apparent reference to a community.

In the religious congregations, Heelas and Woodhead found more consistent identification with the community of the church, often expressed as a belief that individuals should conform with the church's view of 'truth and goodness'. However, they also found significant differences between congregations and named four categories:

1. *Congregations of difference:* typically evangelical congregations, emphasizing their separation from the world around them,

and with a high expectation of conformity to congregational life[7, p. 17]

2. *Congregations of humanity:* typically liberal Catholic and Anglican congregations that emphasize that humanity is something that God and humans have in common, and that people worship God by serving humanity
3. *Congregations of experiential difference:* typically charismatic evangelicals who believed that God could enter directly into subjective experience with them through the holy spirit, be with people in their suffering, for example
4. *Congregations of experiential humanity:* more often Universalists or Quakers who thought the 'divine more likely to be found in inner experience than in externals of religion.'[7, p. 18]

There are, of course, more connections and complexities within and between categories. The congregations of difference and experiential difference both attend more to individual hopes and fears than do congregations of humanity. However, in these congregations there was often a difference between the older and younger members of the congregation. Older members were more comfortable with the community's structure and expectations, and possessed a strong sense of duty of humanitarian care. Younger members emphasized subjective-life and often formed small spiritual groups that provided a more immediate sense of community outside the main worship service.

In comparison, the emphasis in the holistic milieu was on three themes: being holistic (encouraging growth and connection to the 'true self'), personal development within relationships, and the value or quality of personal experience. Overall, the aim was 'to work with their participants to enable them to be true to their deepest experiences of themselves, to know themselves.... Spirituality as integral to the 'wholeness' of their being...is thereby experienced as flowing through subjectivities, without violating or harming the unique'(p. 30). It wasn't clear whether people were generating a sense of community from their holistic activities, but there were certainly many group activities undertaken in addition to consultations with individual practitioners. Smerdon's study of the New Age in popular culture similarly found that in at least some New Age activities 'we can see these sites as a ritual space for the rehearsal of norms and values for our mutual wellbeing, spaces in which we see and experience our interdependence as we strive for personal wholeness.'[8, p. 8] This suggests that a sense of community or association was also important in the holistic milieu.

Heelas and Woodhead set the Kendal findings in the context of an overall decline of congregational life and rise in holistic activity shown in other data from the UK and US. Their comparison of the number of people who reported their attendance at church services and the number actually attending—15% saying they attended weekly to 8% actually present was matched with US data, where about 40% said they attend church weekly, but actual attendance was more like 22–24%. While this may suggest a decline in community activity related to religious practice, it is interesting to note also the rise in small groups in the United States, many of them connected to a church or synagogue, with a spiritual focus. This suggests that people may be finding their own ways to generate a sense of community that are complementary, or alternative, to traditional church attendance.

This latter suggestion is supported by other investigations carried out around the time of the Kendal study. Two categories of findings are particularly relevant; studies of emerging spiritual practices; and research into online communities and associations.

Emerging spiritual practice

Forman[9] explored what he called grass roots spirituality in the United States during the period 1997 to 2002, and Kavanagh[10] wrote what she calls 'a guide to modern religious life'. Both based their conclusions on interviews with people from a range of religious and spiritual backgrounds, using purposive sampling. Both studies suggested an increase in the number of people seeking to develop their spirituality in their own unique ways—as Heelas and Woodhead found—but by blending what they find useful from existing traditions as well as from the 'holistic milieu' or new age spirituality. Forman and Kavanagh both suggest that there is a significant change for people who would see themselves as religious as well as those who would call themselves spiritual in how these connections are expressed.

Forman interviewed 92 people in the United States 'strategically chosen' to sample a variety of religious and spiritual traditions. They included Catholics and Protestants of various kinds, Jews, Buddhists, Hindus, Native American, African Americans, Muslims, Sufis, etc. He sought people who 'had made sense of what they were doing and could talk about it.'[9, p. 22] From these interviews he concluded that there were three categories of people interested in spirituality: first was the one-third of Americans who 'understand God in the traditional way: a personal God;'[9, p. 7] second was between one-fifth and one-third for whom 'ultimate reality is not personal, but more like a universal energy or spirit'[9, p. 10] and the third was about one quarter who do 'identify with a religious tradition, but remain open-minded, exploring a range of traditions, tools and paths. The attitudes of this third group include an open-minded interest in the spiritual, but they retain their church- or synagogue-going patterns and much of their language.'[9, p. 14] Forman's focus was upon people in the second category, particularly whether they formed a coherent group, what caused their development, and whether they could develop better relationships with those in the other two categories.

This second category he named as 'grassroots spirituality'. While expressed varied, he suggested it 'generally involves a vaguely panentheistic ultimate that is indwelling, sometimes bodily, as the deepest self and accessed through not-strictly rational means of self-transformation and group process that becomes the holistic organization for all of life.'[9, p. 51]

Panentheism is believing that everything is made up of one principle that is both transcendent and immanent—having a sense of being that is greater than the world, but also in the world. Forman's view of spirituality then is that it is a form of holistic organization: 'spirituality becomes a guiding value orientation for our whole lives'. Community is also important. 'Many people told us ... that they longed for long term and deep dialogue between committed spiritual people from a variety of paths. Given the surprisingly deep level of agreement we discovered, no matter which tradition they hail from, folks in this movement should be able to communicate relatively easily with each other.'[9, p. 68] This implies the formation of other kinds of communities that provide some of the support and nurture usually associated with religious traditions, but these communities are organized around a shared quest (orthopraxis) more than shared beliefs (orthodoxy).

Kavanagh, working in the UK, also interviewed 'dozens' of people from a variety of traditions including 'Quakers, Christians of many denominations, Hindus, yogis, Buddhists, a Jain, a Sufi, Kabbalists, a devotee of Hare Kirshna, as well as many without labels, both the unchurched and those who consider they have gone beyond the confines of one religion.'[10, p. 3] All of them, Kavanagh says, would consider that they are on a spiritual path and that they are committed to living their lives according to that path. Her book explores 'what is means to be a contemplative in the world; it attempts to examine how people face the difficulties of being in the world, but not of it—and what that means.' [10, p. 107] While she affirms the essence of the holistic milieu saying: 'The objective is to help people grow into the precious individuals they have it in themselves to become,' she also suggests that many individuals see their spirituality as combining faiths or moving beyond religion. For example, one of her interviews is with a primary school learning mentor, who visited a Hindu temple in London and felt transformed by an experience there. She then explored many spiritual paths and was finally confirmed in a high Anglican church, but remained 'interested in the Quakers, Christian meditation and gnosticism, Sufism, Kabbalah and paganism/earth religions'. Kavanagh suggests this is the case for many of those she interviewed, as well as for many others. These people find their own ways into supportive communities or networks. Gilmour[11] names this as 'polyreligious practice,' where people have to navigate 'uncharted territory' with varying degrees of support from traditional congregations.

Forman's and Kavanagh's findings provide further nuances to Heelas' and Woodhead's concluding reflection 'that the future of associational forms of the sacred in Britain depends on the future of 'the massive subjective turn of modern culture', and the ways in which religion and spirituality relate to it.'[7, p. 129] Heelas and Woodhead further suggest that contemporary culture reinforces the subjective through increased pluralization and wider choices related to greater affluence. Overall, their sense is that the holistic milieu may continue to grow to some extent, and that congregational life overall is likely to decline, unless there is a change in the approach of at least some congregations. Rightly, they conclude that they have demonstrated 'that we are living through a period of unique change'.

Modern spiritual communities

Forman's and Kavanagh's work, however, suggests that there are other, more varied ways in which people may associate. Some may continue to be involved in their local church community and in selected activities offered there, whilst also developing or continuing broader interfaith interests and/or connections to the holistic milieu. If this is the case, Heelas' and Woodhead's finding that people say they go to church more often than they actually do might be seen differently. People might perceive their attendance at church as greater than it is because they still see this as part of how religion/spirituality is expressed in their lives; though they may be more likely to attend small group activities related to church life. The new interest in spirituality is also driving change in the traditional or established churches. Appointments to teach spirituality and spiritual direction have been made in many theological schools that hitherto had no tradition of such appointments. Spirituality centres are emerging to link local congregations with their neighbourhoods and other similar centres nationally and internationally. Spiritual direction, formerly a specialized ecclesial task, is now being taught and provided through the burgeoning spirituality centres. All these activities provide further forms of community or at least opportunities for longer-term connectedness and a sense of belonging. In popular culture other less-recognized expressions of spiritual community abound including the 'conscious partying movement' where music and dance with implicit spiritual messages encourages a sense of oneness 'a merging between the self and its auditory/sensory environment and in terms of a sense of profound connection with other dancers'.[12]

The concept of association is further broadened by the relatively recent formation of online 'communities'–interest groups or mutual support groups. The importance of including such groups in research is only now being recognized.[13] Kozinets[6] suggests that online communities are typically between 20 and 200 people, tend to be open rather than closed, have a 'subjective sense of authentic contact ... emotional matters as disclosure, honesty, reciprocal support' and 'the creation of a sense of the group as a discrete collection of these relationships,' which may extend beyond the online community into people's lives. He identifies four categories of online community, each built around different kinds of connection. His fourth category of 'building communities' is particularly used for spiritual and religious connections and has a 'strong sense of community as well as detailed information and intelligence about a central, unifying interest and activity.'[6, p. 36] These kinds of associational communities would not have been detected in Heelas' and Woodhead's geographically based study, which in turn raises a general issue for contemporary social research. In general, most of our survey methods continue to be neighbourhood based, but an increasing proportion of the population is engaged in networks as well as, or instead of, their neighbourhood. Using standard research survey strategies, such as fixed-line 'phone polling, to obtain data about particular neighbourhoods, will fail to capture data from the increasing proportion of residents who use only mobile and online technologies.

While a research literature concerning online religious and spiritual communities is still small, there is clearly an increased interest in them as 'places' where people seek spiritual and religious connection.[4] O'Leary,[14] in order to explore this, joined a Religious Forum on line and writes:

> What intrigued me about this type of connection to the network was that it allowed for group interaction of a sort not possible through basic email, people were not merely exchanging letters with each other, but actually engaged in collective devotion, much as they would at church or in a Bible study group. For some regular participants this activity was a significant part of their spiritual life.[14, p. 794]

This sense of surprise is echoed by Muller and colleagues[5] who offered a special interest group at an information technology conference asking 'can we have spiritual experiences on line?'. All 50 participants affirmed that they had had a significant emotional and/or spiritual experience on line. Other writers affirm the vast range of ways in which people experience communities of spirituality online, while suggesting that these practices are likely to complement rather than replace 'offline' spiritual and religious expression.[15]

Online communities reflect the same diversity of spiritual and religious expression identified by the research outlined earlier in this chapter. This in turn identifies a need for continuing work that maps the emerging forms of social connectedness, including spiritual communities, emerging within online social media. The 'mobile lives'[16] of the early twenty-first century appear to be creating new forms of social connection, including blends of physical and electronic communities. How this will shape spiritual expression and spiritual understanding, and how these expressions and understanding will relate with the traditional place-based religious traditions, is yet to be seen.

Nor is it clear how this new social connectedness might impact upon health. The data we have that positively correlate social connection with health status overwhelmingly come from geographical neighbourhood contexts.[17,18] The role of religious community in enhancing neighbourhood social connectedness and therefore health also seems reasonably clear. Whether similar health benefits will stem from connectedness that extends, or even replaces, physical connection, remains to be investigated, as does the role of spirituality in facilitating such connections.

Implications for healthcare professionals

There are at least two principal questions for healthcare practice emerging from the research findings reviewed above. The first is whether spiritual care assessment—in so far as it exists—is capable of identifying the new patterns of spiritual expression outlined above. The second is the extent to which communal aspects of spiritual expression are recognized.

Clearly, it is important in spiritual assessment to discover what individuals mean by spirituality. Some, of course, will respond to the religious categories on health service admission forms, but for others these will not be relevant. Their spirituality may be expressed in their alignment with complementary therapeutic practices, or through music[19] or gardening.[20] Haynes and colleagues[21] based at a large Australian metropolitan hospital, point out that '(T)he phraseology of the admission form fails to identify patients who see themselves as spiritual, but not religious—nearly a quarter of those surveyed.'[21, p. 6] In response to healthcare providers feeling ill equipped to care spiritually for patients, two hospitals in the United States initiated training for healthcare professionals with the aim of integrating spiritual care into their roles. 'This led to a cultural shift for patients and staff, a capacity to be to be present to spiritual issues for ourselves and each other.'[22, p. 32]

As well as demonstrating the diversity of religious and spiritual commitments, the research findings reviewed above affirm the desire of most that spirituality be connected to an experience of community, whether this is geographically defined, or a virtual community or a mixture of ways of being connected to others. These communities may not have the sense of stability or continuity of a community linked with a traditional religious body and its related organizational structure. However, even people still affiliated with these traditional communities may not see them as their only or even their central association; their online community or links with a centre for spirituality may offer the connectedness they seek. This corporate or associational aspect of belief is downplayed or neglected in much of the research carried out into individuals' spiritual/religious beliefs and attitudes.

These findings have major implications for the training of health and social care professionals who wish to develop what Canda[23] calls 'spiritually sensitive practice'. Tacey[24] says 'The fields of public health, social work and psychology are now facing a crisis situation, where secular-trained therapists are no longer sure how to respond to this new and urgent cry for spiritual meaning.' Despite increased interest in spirituality and religion, professional courses have been slow to incorporate teaching about practice in this area.[25,26] Current practitioners acknowledge the challenges this presents, and express a desire to work more holistically despite the recent trend towards managerialism in health organizations.[27] White says 'I believe that a better understanding of spirituality is the key to attempting to re-establish health service that is both holistic and effective...Both patients and staff want to work in a more holistic way; discussions about the nature of spirituality and spiritual care could help make this a reality.'[28, p. 40] Such training needs to include awareness of the complexity of this field, and recognition that there is now a more subjective and post-modern sense of spirituality and a multitude of ways of expressing the spiritual. This means exploring with each individual person what spirituality means to them, rather than making assumptions about individuals or about what it means to be associated with a particular religious or spiritual group.

Healthcare practitioners should be trained to recognize and work effectively with the fundamental connection between spirituality and community. This means asking individuals where their sense of community comes from so that they can be helped to maintain connections that support their resilience and their decision-making. These supportive communities may be diverse. Much of the literature on social inclusion stresses links with neighbourhoods or other geographical communities,[29,30] but increasingly virtual communities matter. Carroll and Landry,[31] for example, point out that people who are grieving can find mutual support through websites such as MySpace, where memorial networks can be centred upon or tethered to the page of someone who has died.

Recognizing people's desire to be connected to spiritual communities can challenge current professional practice. Most health practitioners tend to focus on working with individuals, rather than seeing that person in the context of significant relationships, including associations with communities. Ideally, the emphasis could shift from enquiries focused solely around individual beliefs to asking about connectedness, which is after all often the aspect most disrupted by healthcare treatment.

The current literature on spiritual assessment tools is beginning to facilitate this by including questions, or inviting observations, about people's relationships with their community. Rumbold[32] describes an Australian project using a 'web of relationships' approach in three health settings, which identified what were seen as five significant areas: relationship to the transcendent, to self, to other people, to social networks and to 'space' (places and things). Puchalski's 'FICA' tool—Faith, Importance, Community and Action, asks: 'are you part of a spiritual or religious community? Do you find this community supportive? in what way? Is there a group of people you really love or who are important to you?'[33,34] Similarly, Bryson[35] asks questions about both the social self—what relationships are important–and the environmental self—about connections to neighbourhood. In an analogous way Hearle *et al.*'s[36] research reinforces the value of place, demonstrating significantly more positive attitudes to life in older adults living in their community compared with those in residential care. Resilience or recovery may be aided as much by enabling people to remain connected to community, perhaps particularly their spiritual community, as by any other forms of treatment.

Another issue that needs to be addressed in training concerns limits to spiritual expression. Professional practice generally emphasizes inclusivity and acceptance of diversity, but individual expression needs to be sensitive to the shared life of a family, a ward, or an institution. Subjectivity exists in dynamic tension with community. This tension, while not unfamiliar to healthcare, might be experienced more frequently with the growing acceptance of the validity of personal experience. Critical social theory, or liberation theology, however suggest the need for professionals to work toward achieving socially-just practice, which might mean not only defending rights of expression, but also questioning some religious and cultural practices. The clearest examples would be when one person's expression is experienced as violence by another or disrupts someone else's expression of the spiritual. While Tacey writes about a spirituality revolution as 'a democratization of the spirit ... individuals taking authority into their own hands, and refusing to be told what to think or believe,'[24, p. 4] he also points out that 'spiritual energy can set society alight with enthusiasm, but such energy needs to be directed towards the good and history has shown that this is by no means automatic.'[24, p. 28). Clearly, there are forms of religion and spirituality that exploit individuals, and professionals will be appropriately reluctant to support clients in these.

Healthcare professionals will have their own combination of spiritual or religious practices.[37] They will also need processes that help them reflect on their 'subjective life-as', so that they do not impose this on their clients. A reflective approach encourages professionals to identify their own assumptions and values and how these might influence their practice. Critically reflective processes can also remind professionals of the importance of history and context in considering spiritual expression in individuals and communities as well as enabling them to articulate their own values and beliefs.[38–40] Furthermore, professionals need supervisors able to explore both how to work with the client's spirituality and the implications for their own.

Conclusion

The research findings explored in this chapter demonstrate the diversity of spiritual expression in at least some Western countries. Looking for evidence of spiritual and religious practice requires clarity about the breadth of what is meant by spirituality and an ability to ask about this in a variety of ways. Increasingly people are finding their own ways to explore and nurture their spirituality, and last century's questions may not capture this century's practice.

It is clear that the many contemporary expressions of spirituality include the desire to experience spirituality in community. Not surprisingly, the diversity of spiritual and religious expressions that exist in 'real' communities is also found in virtual or online communities. A person can, online, be part of a bible study group offering shared discussion and mutual support, take part in a pagan ritual or be part of a group exploring what spirituality means. While some would argue that there is an obvious difference between being physically present at a spiritual event and participating on line,[15] others would affirm that they still experience being part of this spiritual expression on line and that this sense of shared experience and of belonging and/or of mutual support is important to them.[5]

For healthcare professionals, these findings affirm the necessity of including the spiritual: recognizing how spirituality influences their own practice, and how their own and their clients' spirituality influences health and wellbeing. From the Kendal research, it appears that most people experience a more internal and subjective sense of the spiritual or holistic—their own sense of how the spiritual would be expressed—while others continue to value to varying degrees the external guidance of a religious tradition. Overall, those interested in the spiritual seek a sense of something greater or beyond the self as well as valuing their own inner authority.

For most people connections to community are a vital part of their sense of who they are and what makes life meaningful for them. Healthcare professionals and agencies need ways to embed recognition of this in practices and structures that affirm and actively engage with such community connections. A key question becomes: how do we structure care so that professional interventions minimize disruption to the settings that hold people and support their spiritual lives? To practice in this way will mean, for many, a shift from focusing solely on individuals to seeing each person in the context of his or her relationships and community, whatever that community may be. This, in turn, raises questions about training and supporting professionals to work with complex issues: respecting diversity and the individual's own subjective experience of the spiritual, while at the same time affirming broader values of working for the greater good or for a non-violent and socially just society. Critical reflection can help here as a process for articulating assumptions and values and encouraging the connection between the spirituality of individuals and their interactions with their immediate and their broader communities.

Finally, the questions raised by these preliminary findings extend to questions about research priorities and methodologies. How can the social dimensions of spiritual expression and belief be represented in spirituality research, so that we see spirituality as more than an individual's preference? How can communal or associational dimensions be theorized appropriately given the 'methodological secularism'[41] of sociology?[42] These are questions that need to be explored further if we are to approach spiritual care through multi-disciplinary research and practice[43].

References

1 Bouma, G. (2006). *Australian Soul.* Port Melbourne: Cambridge University Press.

2 Tacey, D. (2011). *Gods and Diseases: Making Sense of Our Physical and Mental Wellbeing.* Sydney: Harper Collins.

3 Ife, J., Tesoriero, F. (2006). *Community Development Community Based Alternatives in an Age of Globalization*, 3rd edn. French's Forest: Pearson.

4 Zaleski, J. (1997). *The Soul of Cyberspace: How New Technology is Changing Our Spiritual Lives.* New York: HarperCollins.

5 Muller, M., Uller, E.J., Christiansen, B.N., Dray, S. (2001). Spiritual Life and Information Technology. *Comm Ass Comput Machinery* **44**(3): 82–3.

6 Kozinets, R.V. (2010). *Netnography: Doing Ethnographic Research Online.* London: Sage.

7 Heelas, P., Woodhead, L. (2005). *The Spiritual Revolution Why Religion is Giving Way to Spirituality.* Oxford: Blackwell Publishing.

8 Smerdon, G. (2007). *New age in popular culture and everyday life: mapping and critical appraisal,* PhD Thesis. Bundoora: La Trobe University.

9 Forman, R. (2004). *Grassroots Spirituality.* Exeter: Imprint Academic.

10 Kavanagh, J. (2007). *The World is Our Cloister: A Guide to the Modern Religious Life*. Winchester: John Hunt Publishing.
11 Gilmour, P. (2000). Spiritual Borderlands: Practicing More Than A Single Religious Tradition. Listening. *J Relig Cult* **35**(1): 17–24.
12 Beck, G.A., Lynch, G. (2009). 'We Are All One, We Are All Gods': Negotiating Spirituality in the Conscious Partying Movement. *J Contemp Relig* **24**(3): 339–55.
13 Liamputtong, P. (ed.) (2006). *Health Research in Cyberspace: Methodological, Practical and Personal Issues*. New York: Nova Science.
14 O'Leary, S.D. (1996). Cyberspace as Sacred Space: Communicating Religion on Computer Networks. *J Am Acad Relig* **LX1V**(4): 781–808.
15 Cowan, D.E. (2005). Online Utopia: cyberspace and the mythology of placelessness. *J Scient Study Relig* **44**(3): 257–63.
16 Elliott, A., Urry, J. (2010). *Mobile Lives*. London: Routledge.
17 Pickett, K., Wilkinson, R. (eds) (2009). *Health and Human Inequality: Major Themes in Health and Social Welfare*, Vols 1–4. London: Routledge.
18 World Health Organization Commission on the Social Determinants of Health. (2008). *Closing the gap in a generation: health equity through action on the social determinants of health*, final report of the Commission on Social Determinants of Health. Geneva: World Health Organization.
19 Lynch, G. (2006). The role of popular music in the construction of alternative spiritual identities and ideologies. *J Scient Study Relig* **45**(4): 481–8.
20 Unruh, A., Hutchinson, S. (2011). Embedded spirituality: gardening in daily life and stressful life experiences. *Scand J Caring Sci* **25**(3): 567–74.
21 Haynes, A., Hilbers, J., Kivikko, J., Ratnavyuha, D. (2007). *Spirituality and Religion in Healthcare Practice: a Person-centred Resource for Staff at the Prince of Wales Hospital Sydney*. Sydney: South Eastern Sydney Illawarra Area Health Service.
22 Puchalski, C.M.A., McSkimming, S. (2006). Creating healing environments. *Hlth Progr* **87**(3): 30–3.
23 Canda, E.R. (2005). Transpersonal theory. In: S.P. Robbins, P. Chatterjee, E.R. Canda (eds) *Contemporary Human Behavior Theory: A Critical Perspective for Social Work*. Boston: Pearson.
24 Tacey, D. (2003). *The Spirituality Revolution*. Sydney: HarperCollins.
25 Lindsay, R. (2002). *Recognizing Spirituality: The Interface Between Faith and Social Work*. Crawley: University of Western Australia Press.
26 Crisp, B.R. (2010). *Spirituality and Social Work*. Ashgate, Farnham.
27 Gardner, F. (2006). *Working with Human Service Organizations: Creating Connections for Practice*. Melbourne: Oxford University Press.
28 White, G. (2006). *Talking about Spirituality in Healthcare Practice*. London: Jessica Kingsley.
29 Smale, G., Tuson, G.A., Statham, D., Statham, G. (2000). *Social Work and Social Problems: Working Towards Social Inclusion and Social Change*. Basingstoke: Palgrave.
30 Pierson, J. (2002). *Tackling Social Exclusion*. London: Routledge.
31 Carroll, B.A., Landry, K. (2010). Logging On and Letting Out: Using Online Social Networks to Grieve and to Mourn. *Bull Sci Technol Soc* **30**(5): 341–9.
32 Rumbold, B. (2007). A review of spiritual assessment in healthcare practice. *Med J Aust* **186**(10): S60–2.
33 Puchalski, C., Romer, A.L. (2000). Taking a spiritual history allows clinicians to understand patients more fully. *J Palliat Med* **3**: 129–37.
34 Borneman, T., Ferrell, B., Puchalski, C.M. (2010). Evaluation of the FICA tool for spiritual assessment. *J Pain Sympt Manage* **40**(2): 163–74.
35 Bryson, K.A. (2004). Spirituality, meaning and transcendence. *Palliat Support Care* **2**: 321–8.
36 Hearle, D., Prince, J., Rees, V. (2005). An exploration of the relationship between the place of residence, balance of occupation and self-concept in older adults as reflected in life narratives. *Qual Ageing Policy Pract Res* **6**(4): 24–33.
37 Gale, F., Bohan, N., McRae-McMahon, D. (eds) (2007). *Spirited Practices: Spirituality and the Helping Professions*. Crows Nest: Allen & Unwin.
38 Fook, J., Gardner, F. (2007). *Practising Critical Reflection: A Resource Handbook*. Maidenhead: Open University Press.
39 Gardner, F. (2011). *Critical Spirituality A Holistic Approach To Contemporary Practice*. Farnham: Ashgate.
40 Rolfe, G., Jasper, M., Freshwater, D. (2011). *Critical Reflection in Practice: Generating Knowledge for Care*. Basingstoke: Palgrave Macmillan.
41 Beck, U. (2010). *A God of One's Own*. Cambridge: Polity Press.
42 Gray, M. (2008). Viewing spirituality in social work through the lens of contemporary social theory. *Br J Soc Work* **38**(1): 175–96.
43 Meier, A., James, O.C.T.S., Vankatwyk, P.L. (2005). *Spirituality & Health: Multidisciplinary Exploration*. Waterloo: Wilfred Laurier University Press.

SECTION V

Policy and Education

CHAPTER 52

Policy

Bruce Rumbold, Mark Cobb, and Christina Puchalski

Introduction

This chapter outlines the development of spiritual care policy within the wider healthcare policy environments of the editors' home countries. All three nations—UK, USA, and Australia—face similar challenges in delivering healthcare. These include an increasing proportion of aged citizens, increasing prevalence of chronic disease, the impact of new medical technologies, higher public expectations coupled with eroding public confidence, and increasing access to diverse health information through digital technologies. All three also share similar concerns about improving safety and quality in healthcare.

The three nations however approach these challenges in markedly different ways.[1] The UK has a nationalized, centrally-driven healthcare system (albeit devolved into four national networks). US healthcare, in contrast to this monolithic structure, uses a pluralistic, private-sector-driven, market-based approach that is implemented through a variety of healthcare systems, funded by varied insurance arrangements, and subject to differing regulation at state and federal levels. Australia's healthcare stands between these approaches, combining an established universal access system with a market-driven private sector that accounts for one-third of health expenditure. Responsibilities for funding, regulating, and delivering healthcare overlap between federal and state governments.

The place of spirituality in existing healthcare policy

The UK, Australia, and USA thus span a continuum of approaches to healthcare delivery and policy development. For each, the question of how spiritual care engages healthcare has taken shape over many years. Formative influences include an emerging public discourse around spirituality, growing consumer input into healthcare policy and practice, a research literature that connects religious belief or spiritual practices positively (for the most part) with health status, and increasing attention to cultural perspectives upon health and illness, in many of which religious or spiritual viewpoints are embedded. These influences, most of which are reviewed in this book, have brought public consciousness to the point that conversation around spirituality in healthcare has moved from 'why should it be included' to discussion of 'how should it be included'. Recognition is reflected in references to 'spiritual care' and 'spiritual need' in much contemporary healthcare policy. Further influences are the differing relationships between religion and the state in each nation. This is most obvious with regard to chaplaincy practice, but these differences also shape public policy in general.[2]

These allusions to spirituality in current policy, however, acknowledge professional and community interest, rather than express a strong desire at the national level to develop and implement policy that will drive changes in society's perceptions of health and illness. In this respect, at a health system level, spiritual care policy is in its infancy. It is on the policy agenda, but detailed and comprehensive policy has yet to be developed.

United Kingdom

The United Kingdom has a National Health Service founded over 60 years ago that provides a comprehensive public health service funded through national taxation administered by government. In 1998, a legislative framework was introduced to devolve central government powers to the countries of Scotland, Wales, and Northern Ireland. Each has its own settlement and therefore each has developed its own particular structures. Devolution is not a form of federalism that is found in other parts of Europe as the United Kingdom Parliament at Westminster retains legislative supremacy, and the devolved countries are constitutionally subordinate. Health is one area that has been transferred to the control of the Scottish Parliament, the National Assembly for Wales and the Northern Ireland Assembly. This means in effect that there are four NHS systems within the UK (including England's), each with its own administration and approach, but all founded on the principles of a welfare state to provide a health service to all that is generally free of charge.

The NHS in Scotland has the most developed and integrated policy context with government sponsored national guidelines that regional health boards are required to comply with through the development and implementation of their own spiritual care policy.[3] Health service providers are in turn required to develop and implement a local plan for a spiritual care service that complies with the overarching Board policy.

Spiritual care in the NHS is further influenced by two national policy-drivers in healthcare. The first driver is the quality agenda and the requirement for health services to attain specific quality standards. The National Institute for Health and Clinical Excellence (NICE) provides clinical guidelines and sets quality standards that apply to England, Wales, and Northern Ireland. These are generally condition-specific and when they refer to spiritual needs this is within the principles of person-centred care. A notable exception is the NICE Guidance on cancer services that contains a chapter on Spiritual Care.[4] Healthcare Improvement Scotland provides a similar quality standards function to the NHS in Scotland.

The second driver that relates to spiritual care is UK legislation that enshrines the European Convention on Human Rights and includes the provision that, 'Everyone has the right to freedom of thought, conscience and religion; this right includes freedom to change his religion or belief and freedom, either alone or in community with others and in public or private, to manifest his religion or belief, in worship, teaching, practice and observance.' (Human Rights Act 1998). Further legislation places a duty of equality on public services that means it is unlawful for health services to discriminate on the grounds of religion and belief. A guidance document 'Religion or belief: a practical guide for the NHS' was issued by the Department of Health in 2009 to help health services comply with the legislation,[5] but this rights-based approach has little to say about the practice of spiritual care and renders complex and nuanced issues into simplistic and functional points.

Spiritual care policies

At the level of service provider, healthcare organizations such as hospitals and hospices have a spiritual care policy (see for example Harrogate Healthcare Spiritual Care Policy).[6] This policy, and others like it, typically links the provision of spiritual care with NHS guidance concerning privacy, dignity, patient-centred care, and a commitment to holistic care. While named as a policy, it is in effect a guidance document, containing statements about spiritual care, some clarification of concepts, and check lists for assessing implementation. These are supported, at least in Harrogate's case, by an eclectic collection of references from which evidence reviews are notably absent.

Chaplaincy practice guidelines

When the NHS was founded, the then Archbishop of Canterbury ensured that the Ministry of Health included chaplaincy as a core service and hospitals were advised to make appropriate appointments. Since then, the Department of Health has issued guidance on chaplaincy from time to time, the most recent being a best-practice guide for '... the provision of chaplaincy–spiritual services for patients and staff.'[7] The Scottish Healthcare Chaplaincy Training and Development Unit is responsible for the provision of chaplaincy training, chaplaincy service standards, and a capability and competence framework.[8,9] The Scottish guidance on capabilities and competences has been adopted by the UK Board of Healthcare Chaplaincy and subsequently endorsed by NHS Wales,[10] while NHS Northern Ireland has endorsed the Code of Conduct for Healthcare Chaplains developed by the UK Board.[11]

Professional groups

There are four professional associations of healthcare chaplains in the UK: the Association of Hospice and Palliative Care Chaplains (AHPCC), the College of Healthcare Chaplains (CHCC), the Northern Ireland Healthcare Chaplains Association (NIHCA), and the Scottish Association of Chaplains in Healthcare (SACH). At a UK level the UK Board of Healthcare Chaplaincy (UKBHC) works on behalf of these professional associations to maintain a register of practitioners, develop standards and guidelines, and advance and disseminate the knowledge and practice of healthcare chaplaincy. A number of healthcare professions also have spiritual care interest groups, such as the Spirituality and Psychiatry Special Interest Group.

Faith communities and belief groups

There are many bodies representing a wide variety of faiths and beliefs with an interest in healthcare that lobby government, and the departments of health, undertake research, and promote their own concerns and issues. The most notable representation is that of the established Church of England in the House of Lords, the second chamber of the UK parliament that scrutinises proposed legislation. By merit of their ecclesiastical office the two Archbishops of the Church along with 24 other senior bishops are members of this chamber as 'Lords Spiritual' and in addition to their legislative role take it in turns to read prayers each legislative day. In Scotland, the churches have a parliamentary office that supports them in engaging with both Scottish and UK parliaments and governments. The representation and consultation of other religious communities' groups in the UK is less consistent, particularly for religions that do not have clear representative bodies. Regional faith forums and an Inter Faith Network foster dialogue, and co-operation between religious groups and provide a forum to address local and national issues.

Summary

In the UK, national legislation and healthcare policy enunciate principles and values that are congruent with spiritual care and give protection to the observance of religion. England, Wales and Northern Ireland appear to rely on established conventions and assumptions about spiritual care at a national level maintaining mostly a low-key involvement, all of which is in stark contrast to the progressive stance taken in Scotland where is there is a clear aim and resources to address the contemporary dynamics of religion and spirituality and promote positive approaches that can contribute to effective healthcare.

In the clinical context there is some evidence of the inclusion of spirituality in guidelines and standards, but often without any clear statement as to how these might be addressed. Palliative and end-of-life care along with mental health stand out as exemplars in this field where some attempt has been made to develop systematic reviews of evidence, establish policy and service standards, and promote practical guidelines.[4,12,13] There are many other areas of health and social care where spiritual care is poorly addressed or unacknowledged in clinical guidelines despite evident interest in health research and professional publication. This disconnection will remain without some combination of informed champions, evidence, external lobbying and government will.

United States of America

The Department of Health and Human Services is the United States government's principal agency for protecting the health of Americans and providing essential human services, especially for those least able to help themselves. Spiritual care is a component of the Department's interest, most evidently, albeit indirectly, through the Center for Faith-based and Neighbourhood Partnerships,[14] an initiative of President George W. Bush that has continued under the Obama administration. Links to spiritual care research findings and resources are also provided on the Department's web sites, particularly through the Department's principal research division, the National Institutes of Health.[15] It is however notable that, in the Strategic Plan 2010–2015[16] the only reference to 'religion' is in a section on Faith-Based Partnerships, while the sole mention of 'spiritual' is made in reference to native American healthcare.

The National Institutes of Health provide guidance on spirituality principally in cancer care,[17] although spiritual care is also a component of research funding in HIV/AIDS, substance abuse, and adolescent development. A spiritual care programme is included in the National Cancer Institute's Community Cancer Centers Program Palliative Care Matrix. More generally, the *NIH Clinical Center Patient Handbook*[18] has a section devoted to spiritual care, outlining spiritual services available to patients/families. Apart from this, references to 'spiritual care' or 'spiritual health' appear in conference proceedings or speeches, commonly as a 'complementary' or 'alternative' form of care.

References to spiritual care on national health web sites are largely concerned with informing the health systems that take direction from these resource networks. In addition, access to spiritual services is a criterion for accreditation of healthcare organizations.[19] Further weight for the inclusion of spiritual care as an integral aspect of healthcare is added by an emerging focus upon whole person and patient-centred care,[20] and a recent development has been to mandate spiritual assessment as an accreditation requirement.[21] These various mentions of spirituality and spiritual care for the most part indicate that a spiritual domain should be taken into account. How this might be done, and according to which standards, is left to the healthcare organizations implementing the requirements and the professional bodies to which responsibility is devolved[19] (see Chapter 29). Most health systems accordingly provide on their web sites information about spiritual care and links to resources for spiritual care, often an eclectic mix of local agencies and providers.

The need to provide bridges between the requirements of national agencies and the range of initiatives undertaken at the local level is being addressed, in particular, by collaborative activities and forums established with the support of major philanthropic foundations and trusts (Templeton Foundation, Pew Trust, Fetzer Institute, Archstone Foundation, Arthur Vining Davis Foundations). These include consensus-building strategies utilizing guidelines established by the NIH.[22] A particular example of this is the Spiritual Care Consensus Conference[23,24] referred to in many places in this volume. The conference, sponsored by the Archstone Foundation, was held early in 2009 to develop the spiritual care component of the 2004 National Consensus Project (NCP) for Quality Palliative Care.[25] The guidelines developed by the NCP had in 2006 formed the basis of National Quality Framework (NQF) preferred practices for palliative care.[26] The NQF, the nation's major private-public partnership responsible for identifying evidence-based quality measures linked with reimbursement in all part of the health system, identified 38 preferred practices. These included, in the domain of spiritual, religious and existential aspects of care, spiritual assessment (preferred practice 20), spiritual services (preferred practice 21), spiritual training and certification (preferred practice 22) and community partnerships (preferred practice 23). These practices were linked in the NQF report with NHPCO (National Hospice and Palliative Care Organization) standards (somewhat ironically, accessible only by members) or existing accreditation schemes (such as CPE-trained chaplains for practice 22).[27]

The Consensus Conference aimed to develop recommendations consistent with the earlier NCP and NQF frameworks, and thereby contribute to revision of these frameworks to include recommendations of the Conference. In the meantime, because the NCP guidelines and subsequent NQF preferred practices for spiritual care were very general, the more detailed standards of the National Consensus Conference are being used for palliative care and hospice quality. Thus, the Consensus Conference recommendations stand as a description of best practice in end-of-life spiritual care.

Plans are also being developed by the George Washington Institute for Spirituality and Health to conduct a consensus process more generally within healthcare. One goal is to establish spiritual history taking as a required part of total patient assessment. An argument to this effect has already been submitted to The Centers for Medicare and Medicaid Services regarding the Medicare Program: Medicare Shared Savings Program: Accountable Care Organizations. To practise truly patient-centred care, based on transparency, individualization, recognition, respect, dignity, and choice in all matters important to each person, and his/her circumstances and relationships, the patient's spirituality must be given equal weight with all other factors when conducting the patient assessment to identify health strengths and risks.

Chaplaincy practice

North America has a strong tradition of professional healthcare chaplaincy represented in a number of professional associations that train and accredit their members. In late 2000 five of the largest of these—The Association for Clinical Pastoral Education, The Association of Professional Chaplains, The Canadian Association for Pastoral Practice and Education, The National Association of Catholic Chaplains, and The National Association of Jewish Chaplains—issued a joint White Paper in which they presented a consensus statement on the spiritual care they provide for the benefit of individuals, healthcare organizations, and communities.[28] The paper, while evidence-informed, was however more about promoting chaplaincy than about contributing to the emerging spiritual care conversation. Since then collaboration between the associations has been extended more widely within the spiritual care movement. Recent standards of practice for professional chaplains [29] thus incorporate understandings that were part of the Consensus Conference and the Conference Report, in turn integrating board-certified chaplains in a systematic institution-wide approach to spiritual care.

Summary

As with the UK, the US demonstrates both a groundswell of interest and activity in spiritual care at the grassroots and formal acknowledgement of, but little or no strategic direction for, spiritual care at the level of national policy. The different structure of the US health system, however, allows more opportunity to advocate for the inclusion of spiritual care in healthcare practice through consensus processes. These processes involve a complex network of private–public partnerships mediated through philanthropic organizations, universities, healthcare organizations, and professional associations.

While this advocacy is focused on spiritual care, the goal is to include spiritual care in mainstream healthcare practice and make more effective use of existing resources, chaplains in particular. A key strategy for achieving this is to have spiritual care guidelines and practices included in national regulatory programs.

Consensus processes thus seek to influence the healthcare system through professional persuasion and by influencing financial regulation. Persuasion depends upon the reputation and status of the practitioners involved in the consensus process. Financial regulation depends upon the capacity of the process to mobilize evidence that convinces the NQF to incorporate it in guidelines. NQF involvement is in turn an essential step in attracting the attention of policy-makers in the diverse networks that comprise the US health system.

Australia

In Australia, the federal government is by far the most significant funder of health services, in 2007–8 providing 43.2% of costs. States and territories in this same year provided 25.5%, while the non-government sector funded the remaining 31.3%. The latter included individuals' out-of-pocket expenses at 16.8% and health insurance funds at 7.6%, with the remainder coming from other non-government sources such as injury-compensation agencies.[30]

These figures illustrate clearly the mixed character of the Australian health system. In addition, shares are distributed unevenly across programmes. The federal government has primary responsibility for primary and specialist medical services through the Medicare programme. In- and out-patient services in public hospitals are the responsibility of the states, which also provide a range of public health, community health, and primary health services. Medical services in private hospitals receive a federal subsidy. Residential aged care is a federal responsibility, as is a large portion of pharmaceutical expenditure. Joint responsibilities are negotiated between the federal government and state and territory governments through health services agreements, and regulation similarly is jointly negotiated.[31] It is easy to infer even from this incomplete overview the possibilities for both service redundancies and service gaps within the system overall, and for different policy interests and emphases at federal and state levels due to their different responsibilities.

Despite the different context, spiritual care in Australia shows similarities to both UK and USA in that federal policy and programmes tend to identify spiritual care as a requirement for, or a desirable component of, at least some areas of healthcare provision, while leaving actual issues of implementation to organizational providers and accreditation to professional bodies. Furthermore, as with the UK and USA, the majority of spiritual service development has been in relation to palliative care and, to a lesser extent, cancer care. Spiritual care protocols for aged care and dementia care, however, appear at federal level reflecting commonwealth responsibility for residential aged care.[32] Recently published guidelines for a palliative approach in community-based aged care also contain a substantial section on spiritual care.[33] Spiritual need is similarly an aspect of assessment in palliative care[34] and supportive cancer care.[35]

The states and territories have differing patterns of policy and fiscal support for spiritual care. Spiritual care is identified as a desired aspect of care for a range of conditions on most government sites, and links made to resources available from both government and private providers. There are, however, no stand-alone spiritual care policies. Rather, spiritual care is included in integrated care guidelines.

Guidelines that incorporate spiritual care have been developed at various levels of the health system, often using consultative or consensus processes. Thus, a consultative process that includes consumer input is built into the development of clinical practice guidelines in general.[36] Most palliative care guidelines are the product of extensive consultation with palliative care practitioners and provider organizations, usually facilitated through a government-funded tender or project brief. As a consequence, formal consensus processes like those in the USA are less used, although conversations are currently proceeding about developing a spiritual care enquiry process within states (palliative care in Victoria) and nationally (Spiritual Care Australia). A further difference as compared with the US is that government funding is likely to be available to support such initiatives.

Chaplaincy

Accreditation of healthcare practitioners has, until very recently, been a matter for the states, albeit subject in most cases to explicit national standards. Chaplaincy and pastoral care requirements have however varied from state to state, with the national body Australian Health and Welfare Chaplains Association (AHWCA) being simply an association, not an accrediting body. AHWCA has recently re-formed itself as Spiritual Care Australia (SCA),[37] adopting a constitution that provides for levels of certified membership, recognized according to a capabilities framework. SCA has thus positioned itself to participate in a new national accreditation scheme as this is rolled out by the federal government.[38]

Victoria is one state where government funding has been provided to enable benchmarking of pastoral care/spiritual care practice and to develop cooperative spiritual care projects within the health system in general, not just in the niche areas of palliative care and aged care.[39]

Summary

Australia thus has elements of both the UK and US systems, being a largely-nationalized health system, which still retains significant flexibility through consultative pathways linking local activity with state and federal policy and guidelines. This is essential given the geographical extent and small population of some health regions: solutions that might work for the densely-populated and well-resourced coastal cities are not feasible or sustainable for most of regional or rural Australia. In the latter in particular, community and volunteer contributions are needed to supplement professional care. Provision of spiritual care will require a multi-skilled professional workforce and trained volunteers. Considerable work remains to be done in this respect, although as Chapter 59 illustrates, a start has been made.

Discussion

In all three nations spiritual care interest has arisen initially within palliative care. Thus, we see the earliest collections of evidence, the most detailed presence of spiritual care in policy, in this specialism. We also see that spiritual care policy comes from the grassroots: it emerges on the levels at which spiritual care is practised. Spiritual need and spiritual care are recognized at national or federal levels, but such policy that exists appears at state, regional, or local levels. While spiritual care clearly is emerging beyond the confines of end of life care, its spread remains somewhat uneven, at least in terms of its presence in policy and guidelines. The interest in spirituality being expressed by healthcare practitioners from a wide range of professions and practice contexts, however, suggests that spiritual care perspectives are being brought to bear far more widely than this.

In all three nations there is a groundswell of interest in spirituality and spiritual care that supports the organized activities of those hoping to develop an intentional practice of spiritual care within the health services. In all three countries there are networks of practitioners and academics involved in this work, and there is an increasing degree of collaboration across these national networks (of which this book is one example). The presence of medical practitioner champions is most evident in the USA. In the UK and Australia, nursing is the profession with the greatest involvement in promoting spiritual care. Nevertheless, in all three contexts knowledge translation appears to an issue. Expert research-based knowledge is available, but does not inevitably inform either grassroots practice or health service policy. Knowledge-translation is a skill that merits further attention.[40]

Most references to spiritual care at the health system level identify it as a component of care. Spiritual care is recognized as an expansion of other aspects of care. It is embedded within care of the person. The implication—and the practice of most policies—is to see spiritual care as something that can be incorporated within or added to the caring responsibilities of the existing workforce, nurses in particular. Health bureaucrats are not likely to approve new specialities or provide new funding for spiritual care specializations without major community demand and political endorsement.

In taking this route, no new policy is required, just the insertion of further clauses or the expansion of existing clauses in the old. One practical implication of this is that the practitioners responsible for the domains that have been expanded tend to be given the responsibility for the addition. Thus, the expanded domain of 'emotional and spiritual care' means that nurses and counsellors become the new spiritual carers—and the spiritual care they offer can look very much like psychological care.

The specialist spiritual care providers, chaplains, pastoral counsellors, and pastoral care workers, occupy a curious place in these developments. On the one hand, government policy tends to look to the accredited professional bodies that have traditionally been the providers of religious care; but on the other hand these bodies are no longer the sole providers of spiritual care, but are asked to be the leaders of, or consultants to, an interdisciplinary spiritual care team. In some cases professional standards and training programmes struggle to keep pace with the changing workplace.

Public policy formation

This overview of spiritual care policies and guidelines shows a field in flux. John Kingdon's[41] multiple-stream model of public policy formation provides one way of setting this in context. There is, he notes, a range of influences on how problems come to be on the policy agenda. He identifies three largely-unrelated streams:

1. A problem stream consisting of information about contemporary 'issues' and effects of past government responses
2. A policy stream made up of a community of experts—researchers, advocates, policy specialists—who analyse problems and consider alternative approaches
3. A political stream comprising elected decision-makers.

Major policy initiatives or reforms occur when a window of opportunity joins these three streams: a problem is recognized, the policy community develops a proposal that is both financially and technically feasible, and politicians find it advantageous to approve it.[42]

The term 'problem' is of course no longer popular—search any government website and you'll be hard-pressed to find the word. Today we have 'issues,' not problems. By problem, however, Kingdon means the recognition that 'something should be done to change [a condition],'[43] or as the *Oxford English Dictionary* defines it, a problem is 'a doubtful or difficult matter requiring a solution'. The current debates around spiritual care fit well within this definition.

Clearly in the spiritual care field there is significant action taking place in streams (1) and (2). Continuing development of expertise and evidence over the past decade is notable in all three countries, although this has not added markedly to the policy presence of spiritual care—it was part of policy well before substantial evidence was available, underlining the fact that evidence may be desirable, but it is not entirely necessary or sufficient to form policy. Impetus from the political stream (3) is less evident both due to other pressing contemporary fiscal pressures and continuing debates around church-state issues in all three constituencies.[2]

A critical transition for spiritual care policy development is the point where expert- and practice-based knowledge engages the policy structures of the health system, which comes within stream (2) in Kingdon's model. This occurs at a different place for each of the three systems—early for the UK, late for the USA, early, middle, or late for Australia. One implication might be that one nation's relative ease in dealing with a particular phase of development that is difficult for another nation could inform and support the others through their transition.

While spiritual care is increasingly expressed through guidelines and beginning to be included in policy, it is unlikely to be enshrined in legislation. Failing to carry out a spiritual needs assessment, for example, is unlikely to be defined as a breach of the duty of care. Actively discriminating against a person on the basis of religious or spiritual belief however is already actionable.

The most compelling argument available to the proponents of spiritual care is that it provides a means by which government might achieve quality goals already articulated in health policy, namely person-centred or whole-person care.

Governance

Political scientist Carolyn Tuohy argues that accountability in the healthcare arena demonstrates an evolution of ideas from agency-based approaches through contracting approaches toward indirect or third-party governance.[44] The agency-based approaches located regulation and distribution of health services in trusted healthcare practitioners, principally physicians, to whom the state delegated authority. This approach began to be replaced under the new managerialism of the 1980s, where contracting took its place, partly because of abuse of trust by some practitioners, but mainly because the state saw the need to constrain healthcare costs. Contracting made the state a purchaser of services and introduced the possibility of competition between providers. It also shifted trust from healthcare practitioners to the managers of services. According to Tuohy, this model too is changing and governance is increasingly located in collaborative arrangements that involve multiple stakeholders, across a range of barriers. The skills of management have become 'enablement skills' whereby a common goal is sought through negotiation and persuasion, not command and control.

Looking at the processes outlined above, this shift from agency and contracting toward network governance seems clear. No longer is spiritual care identified with a specific profession or even contracted as a specific service. Increasingly, it seems that spiritual care is part of an integrated approach to care promoted throughout a network that is not only interdisciplinary, but also cross-institutional and cross-contextual. The role of policy is less to dictate responsibilities and strategies to parts of the network, more to give permissions and encourage constructive responses.

Implementing policy

Ferlie and Shortell argue that efforts to improve clinical performance through traditional continuing medical education or through dissemination of practice guidelines and protocols—that is, agency and contracting approaches—have not had a marked effect.[45] Congruent with Tuohy's perspective, they argue that a multi-level change strategy is required, involving individuals, group/teams, organizations, and larger systems/environments. Implementing such a strategy involves, for each country reviewed here, choices between very different trade-offs. The UK needs to balance its centralized approach to financing and change initiatives with a more bottom-up approach that encourages innovation and implementation at the local level. The USA needs to balance its decentralized pluralistic approaches with national standards, measures, and accountability. Australia needs to make good choices amongst the flexible options available, adapting the best, rather than reproducing the worst in a mixed system of care. From what has been reviewed here, all three systems are taking these choices into account.

Clearly, in seeking an appropriate balance each system can learn from the others. The UK's insistence on sharing responsibility and accountability can translate into appropriate liaison with the community and in workforce development. However, unless there are good links with community resources, bureaucratic resistance to anticipated increases in healthcare expenditure may marginalize spiritual care. US strategies for improving quality through consensus processes would seem to be a helpful resource here. The US, however, risks over-professionalizing spiritual care if consensus processes draw primarily upon experts and embed these expert contributions into regulation of the system. This can easily marginalize community resources for spiritual care—or at least make access to those resources dependent upon the quality of professional, usually chaplaincy, liaison. This may be questionable—professional chaplains tend to link more with the healthcare system and their profession than with local congregations and community spiritual care resources. Australia's involvement in community capacity building and developing a flexible healthcare workforce that can offer spiritual care provides insights and strategies relevant beyond its own shores, but flexibility and community involvement can also be used to avoid intentional policy and skills development. The UK and US systems stand as reminders here.

Conclusion

Spiritual care, as an interdisciplinary and cross-contextual activity and approach, is inherently suited to network approaches to care. It provides specific strategies for grounding the aspirational values expressed in current health policy (person-centred care etc) that as yet lack consistent implementation. It compensates for the contracting approaches that translated the scientific discourse of the health professions into actions that marginalized or neglected the art of care. It re-establishes values at the centre of care. In all these respects it can be seen to make a constructive contribution to contemporary health policy.

References

1 McLoughlin, V., Leatherman, S., Fletcher, M., Owen, J.W. (2001). Improving performance using indicators. Recent experiences in the United States, the United Kingdom, and Australia. *Int J Qual Hlthcare* **13**(6): 55–462.

2 Hjelm, T. (ed.) (2010). *Religion and Social Problems*. London: Routledge.

3 Scottish Executive Health Department. (2002). *Spiritual Care in NHS Scotland*. Edinburgh: Scottish Executive Health Department.

4 National Institute for Clinical Excellence. (2004). *Improving Supportive and Palliative Care for Adults with Cancer*. London: National Institute for Clinical Excellence.

5 Department of Health. (2009). *Religion or Belief: A Practical Guide for the NHS*. London: Department of Health.

6 Harrogate Healthcare. (2004). *Spiritual Care Policy*. Available at: http://www.mfghc.com/resources/resources_24.pdf (accessed 14 January 2011).

7 Department of Health. (2003). *NHS Chaplaincy: Meeting the Religious and Spiritual Needs of Patients and Staff—Guidance for Managers and Those Involved in the Provision of Chaplaincy Spiritual Care*. London: Department of Health.

8 NHS Education for Scotland. (2008). *Spiritual Care and Chaplaincy in NHS Scotland 2008—Revised Guidance—Report and Recommendations*. Edinburgh: NHS Education for Scotland.

9 NHS Education for Scotland. (2008). *Spiritual and Religious Care Capabilities and Competences for Healthcare Chaplains*. Edinburgh: NHS Education for Scotland.

10 NHS Wales. (2010). *Guidance on Capabilities and Competences for Healthcare Chaplains/Spiritual Care Givers in Wales 2010*. Cardiff: NHS Wales.

11 UK Board of Healthcare Chaplaincy (2010). *Code of Conduct for Healthcare Chaplains*. Cambridge: UKBHC.

12 Universities of Staffordshire, Hull, and Aberdeen. (2010). *Systematic Review of Spiritual Care in End of Life Care*. London: Department of Health. Available at: http://www.dh.gov.uk/publications (accessed 14 February 2011).

13 NHS Wales. (2003). *Mental Health Policy Wales Implementation Guidance*. Cardiff: NHS Wales.

14 US Department of Health and Human Services. *The Center for Faith-based and Neighborhood Partnerships*. Available at: http://www.hhs.gov/partnerships/index.html (Accessed 28 July 2011).

15 National Institutes of Health (2011). *NIH—Turning Discovery into Health*. Available at: http://nih.gov/about/discovery/ (accessed 21 November 2011).

16 US Department of Health and Human Services. (2010). *Strategic Plan: Fiscal Years 2010–2015*. Washington DC: DHHS.

17 National Cancer Institute. *Spirituality in Cancer Care*. Available at: http://www.cancer.gov/cancertopics/pdq/supportivecare/spirituality/patient (Accessed 14 January 2011).

18 NIH Clinical Center. (2011). *Patient Handbook*. Available at: http://www.cc.nih.gov/participate/_pdf/pthandbook.pdf (accessed 1 August 2011).

19 Joint Commission on Accreditation of Healthcare Organizations (1996). *Implementation Section of the 1996 Standards for Hospitals*. Terrace: Oakbrook.

20 Committee on Quality Healthcare in America (2001). *Crossing the Quality Chasm: a New Health System for the 21st Century*. Washington DC: National Academy Press. Available at http://www.nap.edu/catalog/10027.html (accessed 30 July 2011).

21 Joint Commission on Accreditation of Healthcare Organizations. (2008) *Provision of Care, Treatment and Services (CAMH/Hospitals): Spiritual Assessment*. Available at: http://www.jointcommission.org/standards_information/edition/aspx (accessed 31 July 2011).

22 NIH. NIH Consensus Development Program (2001). Available at: http://consensus.nih.gov/edition/aspx (accessed 30 April 2011).

23 Puchalski, C., Ferrell, B., Otis-Green, S., Baird, P., Bull, J., *et al.* (2009). Improving the quality of spiritual care as a dimension of palliative care: the report of the consensus conference. *J Palliat Med* **12**(10): 885–904.

24 Puchalski, C., Ferrell, B. (2010). *Making Healthcare Whole: Integrating Spirituality into Patient Care*. West Conshohocken: Templeton Press.

25 National Consensus Project for Quality Palliative Care. (2004). *Clinical Practice Guidelines for Quality Palliative Care; 2004*. Available at: http://www.nationalconsensusproject.org (accessed 1 August 2011).

26 National Quality Forum. (2006). *A National Framework and Preferred Practices for Palliative and Hospice Care Quality*. NQF, Washington DC. Available at: http://www.qualityforum.org/Topics/Palliative_and_End-of-Life_Care.aspx (accessed 29 July 2011).

27 National Quality Forum. (2006). *A National Framework and Preferred Practices for Palliative and Hospice Care Quality*, pp. 36–7. Washington DC: NQF. Available at: http://www.qualityforum.org/Topics/Palliative_and_End-of-Life_Care.aspx (accessed 29 July 2011).

28 VandeCreek, L., Burton, L. (eds) (2001). *Professional chaplaincy: its role and importance in healthcare. Journal of Pastoral Care*, **55**(1), 81–97.

29 Association of Professional Chaplains. *Standards of Practice*. Available at: http://www.professionalchaplains.org/index.aspx?id = 1210 (accessed 2 August 2011).

30 Australian Institute of Health & Welfare. (2010). *Australia's Health 2010*, pp. 413–14. Cat no AUS 122. Canberra: AIHW.

31 Swerissen, H., Duckett, S. (2008). Federalism and health. In: S. Barraclough, H. Gardner (eds) *Analysing Health Policy: a Problem-oriented Approach*, pp. 69–82. Sydney: Churchill Livingstone.

32 Australian Government Department of Health and Ageing. *Palliative Care*. http://www.health.gov.au/internet/main/publishing.nsf/Content/Palliative+Care-1 (accessed 15 January 2011).

33 Australian Government Department of Health and Ageing. (2011). *Guidelines for a Palliative Approach for Aged Care in the Community Setting—Best practice guidelines for the Australian context*. Canberra: Australian Government Department of Health and Ageing.

34 Girgis, A., Johnson, C., Currow, D., Waller, A., Kristjanson, L., Mitchell, G., *et al.* (2006). *Palliative Care Needs Assessment Guidelines*. Newcastle: Centre for Health Research & Psycho-oncology.

35 Supportive Cancer Care Victoria (2011). *Framework for Professional Competency in the Provision of Supportive Care*. Melbourne: Department of Health Victoria.

36 National Institute of Clinical Studies. *Clinical Practice Guidelines Portal*. http://www.clinicalguidelines.gov.au/(accessed 30 July 2011).

37 Spiritual Care Australia (2011). Available at: http://www.spiritualcareaustralia.org.au/website/home.html (accessed 6 July 2011).

38 Australia Health Practitioner Regulation Agency (2011). http://www.ahpra.gov.au/ (accessed 18 July 2011).

39 Healthcare Chaplains Council of Victoria Inc (2011). Available at: http://www.hccvi.org.au/ (accessed 15 July 2011).

40 Chambers, D., Wilson, P.M., Thompson, C.A., Hanbury, A., Farley, K., Light, K. (2011). Maximizing the impact of systematic reviews in healthcare decision making: a systematic scoping review of knowledge-translation resources. *Milbank Q* **89**(1): 131–56.

41 Kingdon, J.W. (1984). *Agendas, Alternatives, and Public Policies*. Boston: Little, Brown & Co.

42 Sabatier, P.A. (1991). Toward better theories of the policy process. *Polit Sci Politics* **24**: 147–56.

43 Kingdon, J.W. (1984). *Agendas, Alternatives, and Public Policies*. Boston: Little, Brown & Co. p. 118.

44 Tuohy, C.H. (2003). Agency, contract, and governance: shifting shapes of accountability in the healthcare arena. *J Hlth Polit Policy Law* **28**(2–3): 195–215.

45 Ferlie, E.B., Shortell, S.M. (2001). Improving the quality of healthcare in the United Kingdom and the United States: a framework for change. *Milbank Q* **79**(2): 281–315.

CHAPTER 53

Healthcare organizations: corporate spirituality

Neil Pembroke

Introduction

There are now dozens of books and hundreds of articles available on the topic of organizational spirituality (OS). When one engages with this literature, it very quickly becomes obvious that there is no consensus either on what 'spirituality' means or on what the term 'organizational spirituality' means. Some have become quite sceptical. Reva Berman Brown states that '[t]he more I read on the topic of Organizational Spirituality (OS), the more apparent it became that the concept is not unclear—it is opaque.'[1] Aside from the definitional problem, there is the question of whether the components that are commonly identified as core elements in OS can legitimately be labelled 'spiritual'. Writers include experiences such as meaning-making, being part of a good team, having fun at work, and realizing individual potential. It could be argued that to call positive experiences such as these 'spiritual' is to trivialize the term.[2]

When it comes to OS in a healthcare context, there are added challenges. While a great deal has been written on the topic of spiritual care by clinicians, there is relatively little literature available on corporate spirituality. There is also the fact that there are differences between a healthcare organization and other organized entities. The most prominent is that something is required beyond the care of staff—namely, the care of patients and their families. Finally, the fact that many healthcare organizations are not-for-profit must be taken into account. It is therefore not possible to simply transpose the central principles and practices from OS onto a healthcare setting.

The aim of this chapter is to present an adequate model of corporate spirituality in a healthcare setting. This will involve developing working definitions of spirituality, organizational spirituality, and corporate spirituality in a healthcare institution. The key definition is this: corporate spirituality in a healthcare setting indicates a spiritualized organizational culture characterized by a shared commitment to a set of personal virtues, relational practices, and social ethics orientated both to the care of staff and the care of patients/families, and grounded in life-enhancing ideals, such as service, empathy, compassion, and justice. The second and final step in developing the model that will be undertaken is a discussion of the core elements in the definition—viz., personal virtues, relational practices, and social ethics. It is recognized that a further task is required to complete the model: identifying strategies for developing corporate spirituality in healthcare organizations. However, due to the limitations of space this task cannot be undertaken.

Defining our terms: spirituality, organizational spirituality, and corporate spirituality in a healthcare setting

Some writers on OS launch into their discussion without any attempt to define what they mean by 'spirituality'. Given that it is widely acknowledged that this is an elusive term, one that is assigned a variety of meanings, this is clearly not helpful. Although there is no consensus amongst OS scholars on what 'spirituality' means, there are common elements in the various definitions.

What is spirituality?

Dehler and Welsh[3] view spirituality as simply an energized feeling. While it is true that spirituality is (often, at least) associated with a positive mental state and personal vitality, much more needs to be said to capture the full meaning of the term. It is an inner reality: '[T]hat which is spiritual comes from within … beyond our programmed beliefs and values.'[4] Spirituality is 'something very personal and yet very communal.'[5]

Meaning-making, self-transcendence, and a sense of connectedness are included in definitions.[5–10] The authors of a report from a consensus conference on spiritual care capture all the main elements: 'Spirituality ... refers to the way individuals seek and express meaning and purpose and the way they experience their connectedness to the moment, to self, to others, to nature, and to the significant or sacred.'[11]

While there is quite a bit of variation in the way spirituality is defined by scholars, it is possible to identify some common themes. Spirituality is both personal and communal; it gives meaning and purpose to life; it both energizes, and induces calm and serenity; and, finally, it involves self-transcendence and a sense of the interconnectedness of all things.

It is common in the literature for authors to make a distinction between spirituality and religion.[10,12,13] Writers commonly frame the discussion this way: spirituality is personal, involves an inner search for meaning or fulfillment, and is open to anyone, whereas religion is institutional, hierarchical, doctrinal, and restricted to adherents.

It is obvious why authors feel a need to make this distinction. If OS involved the support of particular religious beliefs, values, and practices, many in the organization would be alienated. It is clearly improper to promote religiosity in a secular setting. Spirituality, on the other hand, is viewed as something that virtually everyone can embrace. Meaning-making, community-building, and self-actualization are valued by most individuals.

That being said, the way in which the distinction is made is not particularly helpful. The impression that is created is that religion and spirituality are separate realities. That is, the message that comes across is that one can choose either to be religious or spiritual. It is important to recognize that there are both secular and religious forms of spirituality; moreover, there is usually a significant degree of overlap between the two. Gibbons'[14] three-fold typology—religious spirituality, secular spirituality, and mystical spirituality—is more helpful than the dualism that is often presented.

As was indicated above, the main reason that a number of authors writing on OS make such a stark contrast between religion and spirituality is that it is not legitimate to promote religious values and beliefs in a secular, pluralistic organization. The simple fact is, that in any given organization, there will be a variety of positions on religion and spirituality. If the culture of that organization is to be spiritualized, the values and practices that are promoted need to be ones that can be universally—or at least very widely—accepted. With this in mind, it is common for scholars contributing to the OS literature to make a statement along the lines of: 'My focus is on spirituality, not religion.' There seems to be no good reason, however, to make this over-simplified and misleading distinction. It is contended here that a more helpful way to go about things is to state that attention will be given to both secular spirituality and to those forms of religious spirituality that are likely to have wide appeal and application. Secular and religious spiritualities are not completely separate practices; there is often a good deal of overlap between the two (it needs to be noted that religious spiritualities vary considerably and not all of them embrace all of the central values in secular spirituality). There is an overlap in that both commonly involve a search for meaning, a valuing of self-transcendence, and a desire for communion with others. Furthermore, both are usually grounded in the values of love, peace, compassion, justice, and care of the natural environment.

It is neither necessary nor helpful to make a sharp distinction between religion and spirituality, the end-result of which is the exclusion of religious discourse in discussions of OS. Over the millennia, the religious traditions have developed spiritual wisdom that can be profitably applied. There are a number of useful studies in OS that appropriately draw on various religious traditions.[2,15–22] In building a model of corporate spirituality in a healthcare setting, insights from both secular and religious spiritualities will be utilized. When drawing on the latter, only principles and values that can be embraced by believers and non-believers alike will be employed. To be sure, there are some spiritual values that make no sense when lifted out of a matrix of either a commitment to love and serve God or to tread the path to Enlightenment. However, there are other values that can be appropriated by secular persons without compromise or distortion.

What is organizational spirituality?

Having developed a working understanding of spirituality, we now turn our attention to the task of defining workplace or organizational spirituality. As with the term 'spirituality', there is no consensus amongst scholars as to how to define OS. The first thing to note is that 'organizational spirituality' can only be legitimately used as shorthand for spirituality in organizational life. If it is taken literally, the term implies that an organization is an entity that has its own reality and its own spirituality.[1] An organization is not a thing—it is a collection of people who work together to achieve particular ends or goals. In any case, OS is defined in a variety of ways:

> ... a framework of organizational values evidenced in the culture that promote employees' experience of transcendence through the work process, facilitating their sense of being connected to others in a way that provides feelings of completeness and joy.[23]

> ... the recognition that employees have an inner life that nourishes and is nourished by meaningful work that takes place in the context of community.[24]

> ... [the] need to find meaning and purpose and develop our potential.[25]

> ... achieving personal fulfillment or spiritual growth in the workplace.[26]

In reviewing these frequently cited definitions, it is evident that there are some features that are taken to be essential in an adequate description of OS. These components are as follows: meaning and purpose, positive feelings (joy, wholeness, fun), self-actualization (developing personal potential), and an experience of community. As helpful as it is to identify these core elements, it does not take us very far in our quest to construct a model of corporate spirituality. What is described in most of these definitions is an *individual* employee's quest for enjoyment at work, meaning, personal fulfillment, and the experience of fellowship. The approach taken by Jurkiewicz and Giacalone is an exception. In their definition, they situate self-transcendence, the experience of community, and a positive emotional state in the context of organizational culture and the values that shape it. The culture of an organization is certainly built up by and expressed in individual actions, but it also transcends the personal. Culture is, by definition, a shared or corporate phenomenon.

Towards a definition of corporate spirituality in a healthcare setting

The first step in the process is to recognize that culture needs to feature prominently in our definition. The second step is to acknowledge that a healthcare organization is both similar to and different from other organizations. Like all other organized entities, it is made up of executives, managers, and workers who seek to express themselves on a spiritual level. Corporate spirituality in this setting should therefore be taken to mean a working environment in which all agents are encouraged in their quest for self-realization, self-transcendence, care, service, meaning and purpose, and community. A healthcare organization is different from other organizations in that its primary concern is not care of staff, but care of the patients and their families. This does not mean, of course, that a concern for the wellbeing of staff is deemed unimportant. It is simply recognition of the fact that the mission of a healthcare organization is care of the sick and their loved ones. Their suffering and distress is much more profound than that of the staff members who provide them with cure and care.[27]

These considerations lead to the following definition of corporate spirituality in a healthcare setting. It refers to a spiritualized organizational culture characterized by a shared commitment to a set of personal virtues, relational practices, and social ethics orientated both to care of staff and to care of patients/families and grounded in life-enhancing ideals such as service, empathy, compassion, and justice. Before moving to a discussion of the core elements in this definition—personal virtues, relational practices, and social ethics—it is necessary to offer some comment on what are obvious omissions. Nowhere in this definition are meaning-making, self-fulfillment, and self-actualization mentioned. The reason for this has to do with the way in which some strands in the humanistic and religious traditions construct the relationship between meaning-making and self-actualization on the one hand, and compassionate and loving service on the other. The position that is taken by the thinkers who represent these approaches is in the view of this author a compelling one. They contend that, for a person with a humanistic or spiritual approach to life, service to individuals and communities constitutes a higher ideal than either finding meaning or realizing one's potential. Some contend that meaning-making and self-actualization are best viewed as by-products of a life of compassion, care, self-giving, and justice. With this in mind, the decision was made to place compassionate and just care and life-enhancing relationality at the forefront of the definition. We need now to engage with the elements in the humanistic and religious traditions that put service above self-actualization.

Abraham Maslow is perhaps the best known of the self-actualization theorists. Late in his career, he decided it was necessary to produce a critique of his theory. The reason for this is that he had identified a construct—self-transcendence—that he thought should be placed at a higher level in his motivational hierarchy.[28] In a public lecture, entitled 'The farther reaches of human nature', he avers that '[t]he fully developed human being working under the best conditions tends to be motivated by values which transcend his *self*', and that 'living outside one's own skin' is essential in the attaining of full humanness.[29] In another place, Maslow states that in order to reach maturity as an individual, 'the good of other people must be invoked.'[30, p. 31]

Another prominent humanist and self-actualization theorist, Rollo May, shows how the three loves—*eros*, *philia*, and *agape*—are all inextricably bound together.[31] *Eros* is desire for the beloved. *Philia* is friendship love; it is based on mutuality, on give and take. *Agape*, lastly, is disinterested, selfless love. It is grounded in a concern for the wellbeing of others that is (largely) free of calculations of personal gain. May contends that an experience of fulfillment and wholeness is not possible if a person expresses love only as *eros* and *philia*. *Agape* makes our love for others complete, and it therefore makes us complete.

The view that *agape* needs to be the central priority in the spiritual life is a core principle in Christian moral theology. Some theologians see self-fulfillment and self-actualization as side-effects of loving service of others.[32–4] These theologians all tie in serving others with vocation. Vocation is defined as working in partnership with God through making available one's personal virtues and learned skills to advance God's project of liberation, reconciliation, peace, and justice. What is required, according to these theologians, is the dedication of body, mind, and soul to cooperation with God in God's redemptive work in the world. All the other states that human beings desire—a sense of meaning and purpose, personal fulfillment, and self-actualization—are by-products of living one's vocation faithfully.

In Mahāyāna Buddhism, the Bodhisattva ideal bears eloquent testimony to compassionate service as the highest human ideal. Bodhisattvas are 'Buddhas-to-be'. Out of compassion for all the sentient beings locked into the cycle of suffering (*samsara*), they commit themselves to helping others attain liberation through enlightenment. In an act of profound selflessness, they postpone complete attainment of *nirvana* in order to make themselves available for this service.

In the humanistic and religious traditions that we have (very briefly) surveyed, there is an affirmation of this general principle: Seek first not personal fulfillment and the realization of one's potential; seek first the wellbeing and flourishing of others. Service is higher than self-fulfillment; self-transcendence is above self-actualization.

Essential elements in corporate spirituality in a healthcare setting

It was necessary to take this excursion into the relationship between service and self-fulfillment because the definition of OS developed here differs significantly from the commonly adopted ones. In these alternative definitions, meaning-making and self-actualization are considered to be central components. It was therefore necessary to justify the decision to omit an explicit reference to these elements. They are certainly included on an implicit level. On the view adopted here, in developing the personal/social ethics and relational practices described below, the basic human needs and desires that others highlight will automatically follow.

Core personal virtues: availability and compassion

There are a number of personal virtues that play an important role in a spiritualized form of relating to others. Love, compassion, humility, and patience come quickly to mind. Given the limitations of space, our discussion will be limited to two fundamental ones—namely, availability and compassion. A further consideration is that while these virtues are crucial in any form of relationship, including relationships in the workplace, they are especially important in the context of care—something that we have identified as a central element in corporate spirituality in a healthcare setting. Availability is giving of oneself for the sake of others. It is therefore really another name for love. It has been described with great insight and eloquence by the French personalist philosopher, Gabriel Marcel. Marcel[35–7] uses the word *disponibilité* to capture the notion of disposing of oneself for others. The word has a financial connotation and is linked to the notion of disposable assets. The available person is the one who is prepared to put her assets at the disposal of the other.

Marcel[36] also interprets *disponibilité* in terms of receptivity. Receptivity involves a readiness to make one's personal centre available to others. I receive others in a room, in a house, or in a garden, but not on unknown ground or in the woods. Receptivity means that I invite the other *chez soi*.[35] That is, I invite her to 'be at home' with me.

The meaning of hospitality can also be broadened to include receiving into oneself the appeal of another for understanding. When I open myself to the call of the other to be with her in her pain and confusion, I am able to spontaneously feel with her.

Availability as receptivity has close links with *compassion*. The deep meaning of compassion is brought out in the rich descriptions provided in both biblical and Buddhist teaching. Bergant[38] observes that in the cluster of Hebrew words for compassion found in the Old Testament, *rhm* is the most prominent. It has the primary meaning of 'cherishing', 'soothing', or 'a gentle attitude of mind'. It refers to a tender parental love. The word *rehem*, meaning womb, is also derived from this root. Hence, Bergant concludes that this Hebrew word-group indicates a bond like that between a mother and the child of her womb.

The New Testament writer, Paul, uses the Greek word *splánchnon* for compassion. It is 'a very forceful term to signify an expression of the total personality at the deepest level.'[39]

We have just seen that in both the Hebrew Scriptures and the New Testament compassion is viewed essentially as taking the pain and distress of the other 'to heart'. Buddhists have a similar notion.[40,41] The Pali and Sanskrit word *karuṇā*, 'compassion', literally means 'experiencing a trembling or quivering of the heart in response to a being's pain.'[42]

It is held by Buddhists that compassion and loving-kindness are (potentially at least) fundamental characteristics of all human beings.[43–5] However, the compassion that exists naturally in human beings is not particularly strong and neither is it universal; it needs to be developed. While persons naturally feel compassion towards those that they like, the situation may be quite different in relation to strangers. Certainly, it is not often the case that a person responds with compassion to the suffering of an enemy. In contrast, the Buddha held up the very challenging and noble ideal of compassion for all sentient beings.

Core relational practices: inclusion, empathy, and confirmation

There is a close link between personal virtues and relational practices. The depth of one's relational presence depends on the quality of one's personal spirituality. The personalist philosopher, Martin Buber, has produced a highly influential approach to interpersonal dialogue. Two of his central concepts are inclusion and confirmation. Buber is best known for his work, *I and Thou*.[46] Buber uses the terms 'I' and 'thou' to identify a relationship involving two subjects. This relationship is contrasted with the I–It relation. In this way of relating, the other is treated as an object, a thing. Inclusion is essential if an I–Thou relation is to be established. In essence, it means including oneself in the personal reality of the other. This requires an imaginative projection into her inner world of experience.

Buber uses terms such as 'personal making present' and 'imagining the real' to describe this process in which one imaginatively enters the inner domain of the other. In order to enter into a relation with a person it is necessary to become aware of the other as 'a whole, as a unity, and as unique.'[47]

'Imagining the real' is essential if there is to be a genuine meeting between two persons. It has an important application in relation to care of patients and family members—something that we have identified as a central aspect of corporate spirituality in a healthcare context. In order to connect in a meaningful way with those she cares for, a clinician needs to reach out and into their inner universe of experience. That is, she needs to be empathic.

Clinical empathy involves an emotional as well as a cognitive connection with the other. Emotional attunement, however, is considered by some to be a liability in medical practice. They contend that it militates against clear thinking and composed action.[48,49] While recognizing that passion in a clinical context needs to be controlled, this author contends that emotional resonance has an important part to play in clinical empathy. It is not possible for clinicians to gain a comprehensive understanding of the subjective experience of the patient without feeling some of the emotion that she feels.[50–54] It is only when the patient senses that her healthcare provider has received her personal suffering as a real presence that she experiences genuine care.

'Confirmation' is the second of Buber's important dialogical notions selected for attention. It is grounded in an acknowledgement of otherness.[55] As I enter into dialogue with the other, I accept her uniqueness and particularity, and struggle with her in the realizing of her potential as a person. It depends on the capacity for inclusion that we have just discussed. Through 'imaging the real' in a relationship one is able to catch hold of otherness. This grasp of the particularity of the other is the first step in confirmation.

Confirmation is also closely related to responsibility.[55] Responsibility refers to a readiness to listen for the moral claim of others and to follow through on it. The responsible person is the one who, first of all, tunes in to the claim the other is making, and then, aware of what is being asked, applies her resources to the task of responding. Confirmation refers to a particular kind of claim, namely, a call for help in the realization of inner potential.[56]

On becoming a more caring clinician

The information provided above on the essential nature of compassion, availability, empathy, and confirmation can be profitably used in helping clinicians become more caring. However, it is recognized that a transformational element needs to be included along with a didactic one.[10,57] In the major religious traditions, transformation is associated with prayer and meditation. In the Western traditions, God is viewed as the ground of all love and compassion. The person who wants to become more compassionate and kind, is advised to pray for greater openness to divine power in her life. The Spirit of God is viewed as the transforming agent. In Buddhism, followers are counselled to use the meditation on compassion. In this meditation, a phrase such as 'May you be free of your pain and sorrow' is used. The one meditating first directs the blessing toward a person who is experiencing great physical or mental suffering. He or she then directs the benevolent wish toward a series of other select individuals. Included in the list is him- or herself, a benefactor, a friend, a neutral person (someone about whom the mediating person has neither positive nor negative feelings) and a difficult person. Finally, the blessing is radiated out to all sentient beings.

Story-telling is recognized as a powerful tool in the transformative process.[10,58] Reflecting on one's own story of caring (and failures in caring) and hearing the stories other tell are important pathways to becoming a more compassionate and empathic clinician. Leaders in healthcare organizations are using retreats to provide space for these reflective, experiential opportunities.

A commitment to social justice

It is commonly recognized that spirituality needs to have both a personal and a social dimension. The spiritual life is expressed through personal virtues and practices on the one hand, and social engagement on the other. Those who adopt a social justice ethic contend that in every society—to a greater or lesser extent—there are entrenched and fiercely defended systems of power and privilege that result in social and economic inequalities. That is, the prevailing socio-economic and political systems result in advantages for some and disadvantages for others. What is required, according to advocates of social justice, is, first, a critical analysis of social systems aimed at identifying injustice, and, secondly, action for change that goes to the root of the inequality and oppression.

A spirituality of social justice is very well-developed in Judaism[59–61] and Christianity,[62–4] and is emerging in Islam.[65–7] The social ethic in these traditions in grounded in a conviction that God exercises a preferential option for the poor. This view correlates well with that of healthcare advocates for social justice who argue that the healthcare system needs to privilege the disadvantaged.[68–71]

Justice advocates within the healthcare system express a deep concern for the wellbeing of people in marginalized groups. Included here are groups such as refugees, people suffering from serious mental illness, and substance abusers. What is required is an inclusive approach on the part of healthcare staff to those who are different from them. A person belonging to a disadvantaged social group looks different, speaks differently, (may) smell differently, and holds different attitudes and values. As a result, s/he may pose a threat to staff members, as s/he triggers certain fears and brings to mind their own vulnerabilities.[70]

A commitment to just healthcare is expressed at both the macrocosmic and the microcosmic level.[68] It involves working towards a healthcare system that offers equal access to all, regardless of ability to pay. At the clinical service delivery level, a just distribution of resources is required. This is a complex issue[72–5]—one that cannot be adequately handled here. However, it should be noted that there is evidence that scarce resources are often distributed according to considerations and principles other than those of social justice.[76,77] Just healthcare requires self-awareness, the practice of inclusivity, a critical focus on social inequality and power imbalances, and a commitment to work for change.

It is not possible in a short essay to discuss all of the personal virtues, relational practices, and social ethics that contribute to spiritualizing a healthcare organization. It is contended that what has been offered covers at least the really essential elements.

Conclusion

The aim in this essay has been the development of an adequate model of corporate spirituality in a healthcare context. In building our model, we have drawn from theories of organizational spirituality and influential thinking in secular and religious spirituality. We sought to describe what a spiritualized organizational culture looks like in a healthcare setting. The importance of care of patients and family members was highlighted. It was also argued that self-transcendence and service are higher spiritual ideals than meaning-making and self-actualization. With these considerations in mind, the model that was presented consists of the personal virtues of availability and compassion, a commitment to social justice, and the relational practices of inclusion, empathy, and confirmation. When these ethics and practices are generally embraced and enacted across a healthcare organization, it can rightly be called a spiritual place.

References

1 Brown, R.B. (2003). Organizational spirituality: the sceptic's version. *Org* **10**(2): 393–400.

2 Benefiel, M. (2003). Irreconcilable foes? The discourse of spirituality and the discourse of organizational science. *Org* **10**(2): 383–91.

3 Dehler, G.E., Welsh, M.A. (1994). Spirituality and organization transformation: Implications for the new management paradigm. *J Manager Psychol* **9**(6): 17–26.

4 Guillory, W.A. (2000). *The Living Organism: Spirituality in the Workplace.* Salt Lake City: Innovations International.

5 Gull, G.A., Doh, J. (2004). The 'transmutation' of the organization: toward a more spiritual workplace. *J Manage Inq* **13**(2): 128–39.

6 Mitroff, I.I., Denton, E.A. (1999a). *A Spiritual Audit of Corporate America: A Hard Look at Spirituality, Religion, and Values in the Workplace.* San Francisco: Jossey-Bass.

7 Mitroff, I.I., Denton, E.A. (1999b). A study of spirituality in the workplace. *Sloan Manage Rev* **40**: 83–92.

8 Ashmos, D.R., Duchon, D. (2000). Spirituality at work: a conceptualization and a measure. *J Manage Inq* **9**(2): 134–45.

9 Gozdz, K. (2000). Toward transpersonal learning communities in business. *Am Behav Sci* **43**(8): 1262–85.

10 Burkhart, L., Solari-Twadell, P.A., Hass, S. (2008). Addressing spiritual leadership: an organizational model. *J Nur Admin* **38**(1): 33–9.

11 Puchalski, C., Ferrell, B., Virani, R., Otis-Green, S., Baird, P., Bull, J., *et al.* (2009). Improving the quality of spiritual care as a dimension of palliative care: the report of a consensus conference, *J Palliat Care* **12**(10): 885–904.

12 Graber, D.R., Johnson, J.A., Hornberger, K.D. (2001). Spirituality and healthcare organizations. *J Hlth Manage* **46**(1): 39–50.

13 Duchon, D., Plowman, D.A. (2005). Nurturing the spirit at work: impact on work unit performance. *Lead Q* **16**: 807–33.

14 Gibbons, P. (2000). Spirituality at work: definitions, measures, assumptions, and validity claims. In: J. Biberman, M. Whitty (eds), *Work and Spirit: A Reader of New Spiritual Paradigms for Organizations*, pp. 111–31. Suanton: University of Saunton Press.

15 Fox, M. (1994). *The Reinvention of Work: A New Vision of Livelihood in our Time.* San Francisco: Harper Collins.

16 Louis, M.R. (1994). In the manner of friends: learnings from the Quaker practice for organizational renewal. *J Org Ch Manage* **7**(1) 42–60.

17 McCormick, D.W. (1994). Spirituality and management. *J Manage Psychol* **9**(6): 5–9.

18 Craigie, F.C. (1999). The spirit and work: observations about spirituality and organizational life. *J Psychol Christ* **28**: 43–53.

19 Kriger, M.P., Hanson, B.J. (1999). A value-based paradigm for creating truly healthy organizations. *J Org Ch Manage* **12**(4): 302–17.

20 Sass, J.S. (2000). Characterizing organizational spirituality: an organizational communication culture approach. *Com St*, **51**(3): 195–217.

21 Krisnakumar, S., Neck, C.P. (2002). The 'what', 'why', and 'how' of spirituality in the workplace. *J Manage Psychol* **17**(3): 153–64.

22 Pembroke, N. (2004). *Working Relationships: Spirituality in Human Services and Organisational Life.* London: Jessica Kingsley.

23 Jurkiewicz, C.L., Giacalone, R.A. (2004). A values framework for measuring the impact of workplace spirituality on organizational performance. *J Bus Eth* **49**, 129–42.

24 Ashmos, D.R., Duchon, D. (2000). Spirituality at work: a conceptualization and a measure. *J Manage Inq* **9**(2): 134–45.

25 Howard, S.A. (2002). A spiritual perspective on learning in the workplace. *J Manage Psychol* **17**(3): 230–42.

26 Graber, D.R., Johnson, J.A., Hornberger, K.D. (2001). Spirituality and healthcare organizations. *J Hlth* Manage **46**(1): 39–50.

27 Kilpatrick, A.O. (2009). The healthcare leader as humanist. *J Hum Ser Admin* **31**: 451–65.

28 Koltko-Rivera, M.E. (2006). Rediscovering the later version of Maslow's hierarchy of needs: Self-transcendence and opportunities for theory, research, and unification. *Rev Gen Psychol* **10**(4): 302–17.

29 Maslow, A.H. (1969). The farther reaches of human nature. *J Trans* Psychol **1**(1): 1–9.

30 Maslow, A.H. (1996). Critique of self-actualization theory. In: E. Hoffman (ed.), *The Unpublished Papers of Abraham Maslow*, pp. 26–32. Thousand Oaks: Sage.

31 May, R. (1969). *Love and Will*. New York: Norton.
32 Badcock, G. (1998). *The Way of Life: A Theology of Christian Vocation*. Grand Rapids: Eerdmans.
33 Fowler, J.W. (1999). *Becoming Adult, Becoming Christian*. San Francisco: Jossey-Bass.
34 Pembroke, N. (2007). *Moving Toward Spiritual Maturity: Psychological, Contemplative, and Moral Challenges in Christian Living*. Binghamton: Haworth Pastoral Press.
35 Marcel, G. (1950). *The Mystery of Being*, vol. I. London: Harvill Press.
36 Marcel, G. (1964). Phenomenological notes on being in a situation. In his *Creative Fidelity*. New York: Noonday Press.
37 Marcel, G. (1964). Belonging and Disposability. In his *Creative Fidelity*. New York: Noonday Press.
38 Bergant, D. (1996). Compassion. In: C. Stuhlmueller (ed.) *The Collegeville Pastoral Dictionary of Biblical Theology*, pp. 154–7. Collegeville: Liturgical Press.
39 Köster, H. (1985). Splánchnon. In: G. Kittel, G. Friedrich (eds) *Theological Dictionary of the New Testament*, 1 vol., pp. 1067–9, transl. G. Bromiley. Grand Rapids: Eerdmans.
40 Dalai Lama (1999). *Ethics for the New Millennium*. New York: Riverhead Books.
41 Salzberg, S. (1995). *The Revolutionary Art of Happiness*. Boston: Shambala.
42 [41], p.104.
43 Dalai Lama (2002). Understanding our fundamental nature. In: R.J. Davidson, A. Harrington (eds) *Visions of Compassion: Western Scientists and Tibetan Buddhists Examine Human Nature*, pp. 66–80. Oxford: Oxford University Press.
44 Dreyfus, G. (2002). Is compassion an emotion? A cross-cultural exploration of mental typologies. In: R.J. Davidson, A. Harrington (eds) *Visions of Compassion: Western Scientists and Tibetan Buddhists Examine Human Nature*, pp. 31–45. Oxford: Oxford University Press.
45 Master Sheng-yen. (1999). *Subtle Wisdom: Understanding Suffering, Cultivating Compassion Through Ch'an Buddhism*. New York: Doubleday.
46 Buber, M. (1937). *I and Thou*, transl. Gregor Smith R. New York: Scribner.
47 Buber, M. (1957). Elements of the interhuman. *Psychol*, **20**: 105–13.
48 Landau, R.L. (1993) … And the least of these is empathy. In: H.M. Spiro (eds), *Empathy and the Practice of Medicine: Beyond Pills and the Scalpel*, pp. 103–9. New Haven: Yale University Press.
49 Hojat, M., Gonnella, J., Nasca, T., Mangione, S., Vergare, M., Magee, M. (2002). Physician empathy: definitions, components, measurement, and relationships to gender and speciality. *Am J* Psychol, **159**(9): 1563–9.
50 Spiro, H.M. (1993). What is empathy and can it be taught? In: H.M. Spiro, (eds) *Empathy and the Practice of Medicine: Beyond Pills and the Scalpel*, pp. 7–14. New Haven: Yale University Press.
51 Halpern, J. (1993). Empathy: using resonance emotions in the service of curiosity. In: H.M. Spiro (eds), *Empathy and the Practice of Medicine: Beyond Pills and the Scalpel*, pp. 160–73. New Haven: Yale University Press.
52 Halpern, J. (2003). What is clinical empathy? *J Gen Int Med*, **18**: 670–4.
53 Coulehan, J.L. (1995). Tenderness and steadiness: emotions in medical practice. *Lit Med* **14**(2): 222–36.
54 Pembroke, N. (2007). Empathy, emotion, and ekstasis in the patient-physician relationship. *J Rel Hlth* **46**(2): 287–98.
55 Buber, M. (1947). *Between Man and Man*, transl. R. Gregor Smith. London: Routledge & Kegan Paul.
56 Buber, M., Rogers, C. (1965). Dialogue between Martin Buber and Carl R. Rogers. In: M. Buber (ed.) *The Knowledge of Man*, pp. 166–84, transl. M. Friedman, R. Gregor Smith R. London: George Allen & Unwin.
57 Watson, J. (2009). Caring science and human caring theory: Transforming personal and professional practices of nursing and health care. *J H Hum Serv Admin*, **31**(4), 466–482.
58 Smeltzer, C.H., Vlasses, F. (2004). Storytelling: A tool for leadership to shape quality. . .Listen to nurses' stories, *J Nurs Care Qual* **19**, 74–75.
59 Mackler, A.L. (1991). Judaism, justice, and access to health care. *Kennedy Inst Eth J* **1**(2): 143–61.
60 Schwarz, S. (2008). *Judaism and Justice: the Jewish Passion to Repair the World*. Woodstock: Jewish Lights.
61 Jacobs, J. (2009). *There Shall Be No Needy: Pursuing Social Justice Through Jewish Law and Tradition*. Woodstock: Jewish Lights.
62 Wallis, J. (2005). *God's Politics: Why the Right Gets It Wrong and the Left Doesn't Get It*. San Francisco: HarperCollins.
63 Brondos, D.A. (2007). *Fortress Introduction to Salvation and the Cross*. Minneapolis: Fortress.
64 Nangle, J. (2008). *Engaged Spirituality: Faith and Life in the Heart of the Empire*. Maryknoll: Orbis.
65 Munir, L.Z. (2003). *Islam, modernity, and justice for women*, unpublished paper presented as the Islam and Human Rights Fellow Lecture, Emory University, October 2003.
66 Muqtedar Khan, M.A. (2005). Islamic democracy and moderate Muslims: the straight path runs through the middle. *Am J Islamic Soc Sci* **22**(3): 39–50.
67 Moll, Y. (2009). 'People like us' in pursuit of God and rights: Islamic feminist discourse and Sisters in Islam in Malaysia. *J Int Wom Stud* **11**(1): 40–55.
68 Wear, D., Kuczewski, M.G. (2004). The professionalism movement: can we pause? *Am J Bioeth* **4**(2): 1–10.
69 Murphy, N., Canales, M.K., Norton, S.A., DeFilippis, J. (2005). Striving for congruence: the interconnection between values, practice, and political action. *Policy Polit Nurs Pract* **6**(1): 20–9.
70 Myhrvold, T. (2006). The different other—towards an including ethics of care. *Nurs Philos* **7**: 125–36.
71 Kagan, P.N., Smith, M.C., Cowling, W.R., Chinn, P.L. (2009). A nursing manifesto: An emancipatory call for knowledge development, conscience, and praxis. *Nurs Philos* **11**: 67–84.
72 Nord, E. (1999). *Cost-value Analysis in Health Care: Making Sense Out of QALYs*. Cambridge: Cambridge University Press.
73 Daniels, N. (2008). *Just Health: Meeting Health Needs Fairly*. Cambridge: Cambridge University Press.
74 Persad, G., Wertheimer, A., Emanuel, E.J. (2009). Principles for the allocation of scarce medical interventions. *Lancet* **373**: 423–31.
75 Kerstein, S.J., Bognar, G. (2010). Complete lives in the balance. *Am J Bioeth* **10**(4): 27–45.
76 Pedersen, R., Nortvedt, P., Nordhaug, M., Slettebø, Å., Grøthe, K.H., Kirkevold, M., *et al.* (2008). In quest of justice? Clinical prioritization in healthcare for the aged. *J Med Eth* **34**: 230–5.
77 Halvorsen, K., Førde, R., Nortvedt, P. (2009). The principle of justice in patient priorities in the intensive care unit: the role of significant others. *J Med Eth* **35**, 483–7.

CHAPTER 54

Utility and commissioning of spiritual carers

Lindsay B. Carey

Introduction

For centuries spiritual care, in its various forms, has been formally undertaken by designated individuals trained and commissioned by religious organizations or spiritual communities to be their priests, imams, rabbis, ministers, pastors, chaplains, monks, nuns, or other such bestowed practitioners. Irrespective of the particular religious/spiritual faith, the commissioning and subsequent professional engagement of such individuals was to ensure that the objectification of a deity or deities, and/or the philosophy of transcendental ordering, was systematically taught and reinforced, plus their legendary narratives and myths were reiterated along with their developed rituals that were enacted and re-enacted—all of which helped to 'sacralize the identity' and thus the commitment of individuals and communities to a particular faith and belief system.[1]

Concurrently with this formal process, there has always been an 'informal' spiritual care undertaken by those who have voluntarily given their time and energy to nurture others in their particular beliefs and faith. Today it is possible to discern three levels of 'spiritual care volunteerism'; namely:

- voluntary-idiosyncratic based on existing personal and/or familial relationships
- voluntary-organizational by an institution (secular or religious) that co-ordinates volunteers to undertake spiritual care
- voluntary-professional by those professionally qualified healthcare practitioners (e.g. physicians, nurses, occupational therapists, social workers, speech pathologists, psychologists, etc) who voluntarily (i.e. not as a core task or remunerated duty) provide spiritual care given their person-centred philosophy being inclusive of the religious and spiritual needs of their clients/patients.

It is important to note of course (as will be mentioned later), that for some professionally qualified healthcare practitioners, the provision of spiritual/religious care may be expected to be more than simply a voluntary response. Depending on the training and employment context of some healthcare practitioners, spiritual care could be considered to be an expected holistic 'duty of care' so as to aid the wellbeing of their patients.

Around the turn of the twenty-first century, however, there has been increasing debate about 'who should actually provide spiritual care?'[2,3] Should spiritual care be left to the traditional and formal practitioners (e.g. clerics and chaplains)? Should it be left to the devices of family, friends and/or volunteers? Should occupations that are predominantly secular occupations, such as medicine, nursing, and allied health, take responsibility for the various mechanisms that help to sacralize an individual's spiritual and/or religious identity?

To resolve such issues, particularly whom should be commissioned to provide spiritual care, it is first important to define exactly who these 'spiritual carers' are, and then to consider their actual and potential 'utility'. For the purposes of this chapter, 'spiritual carer' within the healthcare context, will refer (unless otherwise indicated) to those individuals who have been commissioned and appointed by a religious, spiritual and/or other organizations either as:

- *a professionally employed spiritual carer* (e.g. designated as a 'chaplain', 'pastoral care practitioner', 'pastoral carer', 'spiritual care therapist' or other such bestowed title)
- *volunteer spiritual carer* (e.g. 'chaplain assistant', 'pastoral care worker', 'pastoral care visitor', 'spiritual care assistant' or other such lay-person title)—but all having the primary purpose to help provide for and facilitate the spirituality of patients, their families and staff (refer Figure 54.1).

Following the consensus definition, 'spirituality' herein shall mean:

> '... the aspect of humanity that refers to the way individuals seek and express meaning and purpose and the way they experience their connectedness to the moment, to self, to others, to nature, and to the significant or sacred.'[4]

While spirituality is increasingly being understood more broadly (as reflected in the escalating material about spirituality within healthcare journals),[5] and while there is some momentum for traditionally bestowed titles to shift from 'chaplain' to more holistic designations such as 'spiritual care provider' (particularly given increasing spiritual/religious pluralism),[6] nevertheless in practice, the data about spiritual carers within most Western countries, derives predominantly from research into the specific role of 'chaplains' and associated 'pastoral care' volunteers. Such research, for now at least, provides the most reliable source of information about the utility and commissioning of spiritual carers within healthcare and will be used extensively through-out this chapter.

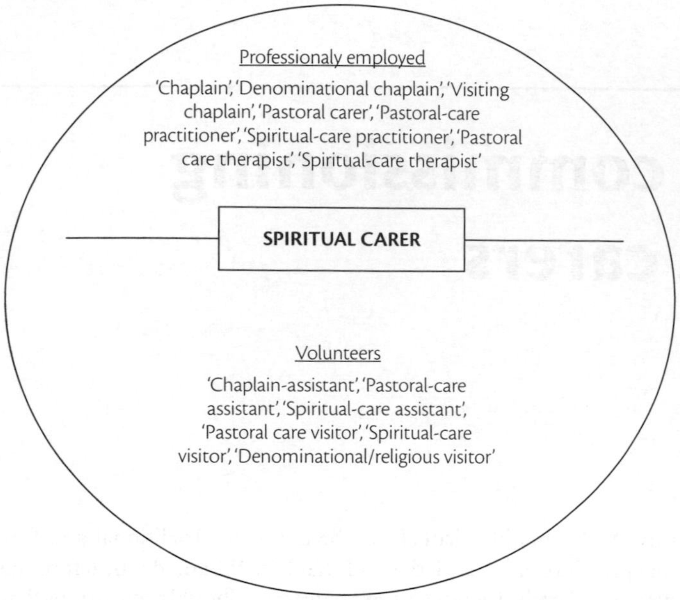

Figure 54.1 Spiritual carers: examples of professional and voluntary bestowed titles.

Utility of spiritual care providers

The term utility derives from the word 'utile' meaning useful or being of use or service—its antonym would be 'futile'—that is useless, ineffective and pointless. Pragmatically the term utility is extensively used within a number of fields when referring to such things as a public utility or 'public service' (i.e. providing a structured service to the public), 'communication' (e.g. a utility for receiving/sending information), providing 'protection and advocacy' (i.e. personal rights), being 'multipurpose' (i.e. a utility vehicle) and being 'multi-competent' (i.e. someone able to negotiate multiple roles) and finally with regard to 'economics' (i.e. being a measure of cardinal or ordinal economic value).[7] Interestingly, it can be argued, that each of these understandings of 'utility' is also relevant to spiritual cares and particularly those working within the healthcare context.

Public service

Within post-modern societies, spirituality and religious belief have predominantly been considered a private affair, so the concept of spiritual care being a 'public service' may seem somewhat incongruous. Yet formally recognized providers of spiritual care, traditionally categorized as, 'priests ', 'ministers of religion' or collectively 'clergy', have offered their services not only within the private sphere, but also the public domain for over three millennia (i.e. since the beginning of the Judaic priesthood 'Kohanim,' 1000 BC). Through various contemporary religious and spiritual traditions, the 'clergy' have continued to provide a public service within a variety of institutions today (e.g. hospitals, prisons, schools, universities, and military forces). Indeed, historically the clergy and thus spiritual carers should be considered one of the longest continuing formal public service 'professions'.

Within Western healthcare contexts numerous literature has indicated that spiritual carers (in various ways and relevant to their time) performed a number of public service roles. Traditionally, these roles have largely been perceived to be purely religious functions (e.g. administering the sacraments, conducting weddings, church and chapel services, plus religious counselling and education). Since the middle of the twentieth century much of the literature reflected a recognition that the role of spiritual carers within the healthcare context (particularly undertaken by chaplains and volunteer pastoral workers), had increased considerably. Not only had their contribution involved traditional services to patients and their families, but also non-traditional ministrations such as 'team-working' with clinical staff, providing pastoral counselling to clinical staff, providing pastoral care to the wider institution, including ethics committees, undertaking pastoral and spiritual assessments and education, plus assisting clinical staff and their employing institution with bioethical decisions. To put it simply, the role categories of spiritual carers (more specifically 'chaplains') have been, and continue to be, considerably broad (Table 54.1).

Communication

An important utility with regard to healthcare is communication. Within all healthcare contexts, poor communication quickly leads to a breakdown in the provision of appropriate care and subsequently a lack of trust by patients and families towards medical and other clinical staff, potentially leading to frustration, conflict and a costly impasse. It has been argued, however, that healthcare communication can be expansively facilitated by those involved in religious and spiritual care.[8]

Within the Western healthcare context for example, chaplains have been noted to act as communication facilitators, consulting with clinical staff on behalf of patients and families,[9] which may involve assisting bioethical discussions and healthcare treatment decisions.[10–12] Chaplains have also served as members of hospital ethics committees (requiring dialogue with medical scientists, researchers, and lawyers) and other communicative roles, such as being a community link between hospitals and faith community groups (i.e. churches, mosques, temples), plus communicating with government health services, universities, schools and community health professionals.[13] In overall terms, what is distinctly noticeable, is the increasing communication-reciprocity that will be demanded of all spiritual carers, whereby the traditional 'dialogue' between patient and their spiritual carer, will increasingly become a 'multilogue', requiring spiritual carers to communicate with a diverse range of professionals and groups (see Figure 54.2).

An interesting point of contention, however, is the difference in communication patterns by professionally employed spiritual carers compared with that of volunteers. For example, evidence suggests, that for a variety of reasons, staff appointed chaplains undertake physician consultancy and engage significantly more frequently with other clinical staff than do volunteer chaplains.[14–16] While some note that volunteer spiritual and pastoral carers/chaplaincy assistants are considered valuable, even indispensable[17,18] (particularly given the limited number of stipended positions for professional spiritual carers and the comparatively miniscule funds offered to spiritual/pastoral care departments), nevertheless, it is important to recognize that volunteer spiritual carers may *not* be able to enter into dialogue with professional healthcare staff to the same extent as professionally employed spiritual carers, thus potentially reducing direct communication opportunities with clinical staff that would otherwise ensure maximum care for patients and families. Professional communication

Table 54.1 Classification of professional role categories of spiritual carers—chaplains

Chaplaincy roles categories	Literature (Chronological order)
(1) Healing, (2) guiding, (3) sustaining, (4) reconciling	Clebsch & Jackle (1964)[66]
(1–4 above) + (5) nurturing, (6) ecologist	Clinebell (1966; 1992)[67,68]
(1) Traditional functions, (2) non-traditional functions	Knights & Kramer (1964)[69]
(1) Clinical non-religious functions, (2) evangelistic functions, (3) standard activities	Morrow & Matthews (1966)[70]
(1) Witness, (2) thanatonic, (3) sacramental, (4) prayer, (5) teacher, (6) counselor, (7) team-worker	Carey (1972)[71]
(1) Pastoral care to patients, (2) pastoral care staff, (3) pastoral care to wider institution	Dagenais (1985)[72]
(1) Friend, (2) surrogate parent, (3) godly representative, (4) religious link to church community.	Hesche (1987)[73]
(1) Ministry to patients and families, (2) ministry to staff, (3) ministry to physicians, (4) ministry to ethics committees	Wagner & Higdon (1996)[74]
(1) Healing, (2) guiding, (3) sustaining, (4) reconciling (5) nurturing (6) liberating, (7) empowering.	Lartey (1997)[75]
(1) Pastoral assessment and identification, (2) manage and develop a chaplaincy service, (3) provide worship and religious expression, (4) provide pastoral care, counselling and spiritual direction/guidance, (5) provision of ethical, theological, and pastoral resources.	Healthcare Chaplaincy Standards (UK) (1998)[76]/ Healthcare Chaplaincy Guidelines (AU) (2000)[77]
(1) Pastoral assessment, (2) pastoral ministry, (3) pastoral counselling and education, (4) pastoral ritual and worship	WHO (2002);[78] Carey *et al.* 2005 [79] Carey *et al.* (2006);[80] Carey (2010)[81]

is an important component when considering the utility and commissioning of spiritual carers.

Multi-purpose and multi-competent

Another utility, that needs to be considered, concerns whether spiritual carers are multipurpose and multi-competent. This is an important aspect as spiritual cares may be required at short notice to provide a service to the public within any number of departments or specialist units of a healthcare facility. Much of the literature to date highlights the broad ranges of areas in which spiritual carers (such as chaplains—both employed and volunteers) have ministered. These areas have not just been in general ward contexts, but within a diverse range of specialist facilities (e.g. paediatrics, organ transplant units, etc.) (refer Table 54.2).

Despite the serious concerns within some Western countries about post-modern healthcare reforms challenging spiritual care and (more particularly) the utility of chaplains,[19] nevertheless it is often overlooked that at an international level, the value

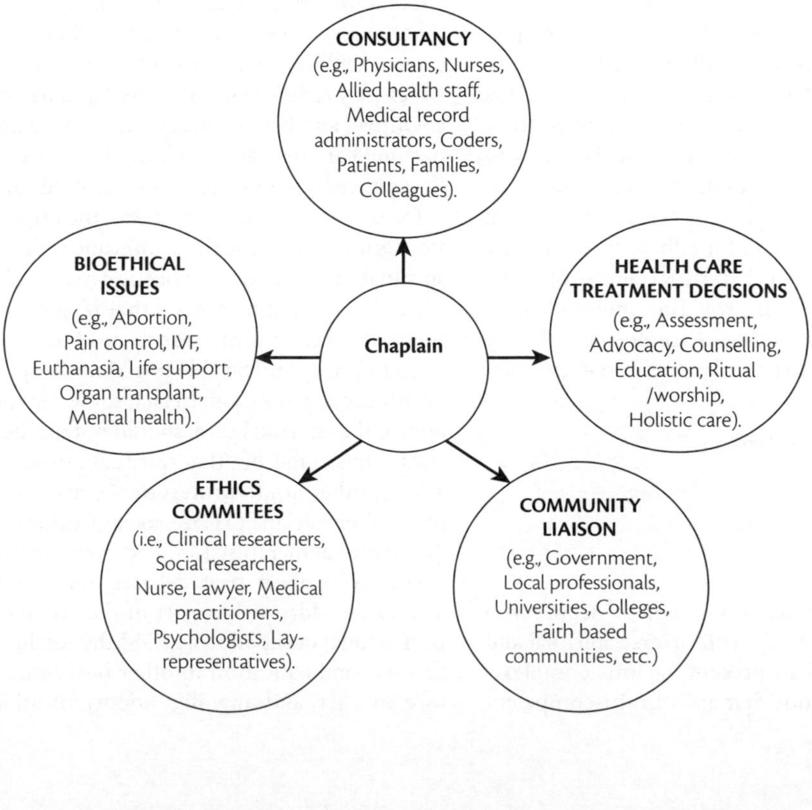

Figure 54.2 Examples of 'multilogue' healthcare communication [65]. Reproduced from Carey LB (2011). Chaplains and health care communication, in Miller AN, Rubin DL (eds) Health Communication and Faith Based Communities, (pp.263-278) Hampton Press, Cresskill, New Jersey.

Table 54.2 Examples of specialist healthcare areas utilizing spiritual carers—chaplains

Specialist Service	Literature
Physical rehabilitation and permanent disabilities	Ritter, 1994;[82] Stainton, 1994[83] Blair & Blair, 1994;[84] McCarthy, 1989;[85] Samson & McColgan, 2000[86]
Terminal illnesses: AIDS, cancer, palliative care	Bohne 1986;[87] Dugan, 1987;[88] Milne, 1988;[89] Rumbold, 1989;[90] Hodder & Turley, 1990;[91] Goodell, 1992;[92] Handzo, 1992;[93] Fraser, 2004;[94] Carey *et al.*, 2006;[95] Nolan, 2011[96]
Transplants/organ donation: kidney, liver, heart	Browning, 1988;[97] Copeland, 1993;[98] Delong, 1993 [99], 1990;[100] Elliot & Carey, 1996;[101] Carey *et al.*, 2009;[102] Carey *et al.* 2011[103].
Surgery/intensive care	Bryce, 1988;[104]; Sharp, 1991;[105] Wagner & Higdon, 1996;[106] Robinson *et al.*, 2006;[107], Carey & Newell, 2007[108,109]
Out-patients/ Aged care/gerontology	McSherry, 1994;[110]; Mandziuk, 1996;[111] Mowat, 2004;[112] MacKinlay (2002);[113]
Paediatrics and women	Hesch, 1987;[114] Stoter, 1987;[115] Donnelly, 1993;[116] Carey *et al.*, 1997;[117] Ryan, 1991;[118] Gilchrist, 2001;[119] Meese & Carey, 2006;[120] Cadge *et al.*, 2011[121]
Mental health	Knights & Kramer 1964;[122] Morrow & Matthews 1966;[123] Stephens 1994;[124] Macritchie 2004;[125] Ratray 2002;[126] Swinton 2006[127]

of religion and spirituality and the role of spiritual carers, is regaining some traction. For example, the multipurpose and multi-competent utility of spiritual carers is both explicitly and implicitly reflected in the World Health Organization's 'International Classification of Diseases' (ICD-10-a.m)[20] and within the World Health Organization's 'International Classification of Functioning, Disability and Health' (ICF)[21] (Table 54.3). The benefits of these codings, if they are utilized, is that such systems not only identify the multi-purpose and multi-competent roles of spiritual carers across the world, but such systems also provide a unified and comparable method for recording religious and spiritual activities plus the actual role of spiritual carers which in-turn assists with evidence-based evaluations and appropriate decision-making that is particularly important given rapidly changing societies.

Rapidly changing and increasingly pluralistic communities world-wide, highlights another particular area of multi-competency that is becoming increasingly important—interfaith spiritual care. There can be no question that the face of healthcare within most capital cities across the Western world has changed substantially, particularly in terms of meeting the various needs of people from other cultures with different spiritual beliefs who have migrated from distant shores as a result of poverty, persecution and war. While there has been some concern about spiritual carers from one spiritual tradition caring for adherents of another tradition,[22] nevertheless, it is clear that spiritual carers (of whatever tradition) have and are capable of providing interfaith spiritual care,[23] particularly if they are trained to understand the key mechanisms of 'sacralization' that are fundamental to every spiritual/religious faith, namely their:

- objectification or transcendental ordering
- myths/legends
- rituals
- acts of commitment.[24]

Providing spiritual care to an increasing number of people who are from different cultural backgrounds with diverse spiritual and religious beliefs has the potential to present various complexities within clinical contexts and thus demands multi-competent personnel to deal with the various religious and spiritual issues that inevitably arise—spiritual carers are the ideal personnel to address such issues.[25]

It has been suggested, however, that spiritual carers can only be as multi-purpose and multi-competent as what other clinical staff will allow. Galek *et al.*'s[26] research, for example, indicated that clinical staff often overlooked the inclusion of spiritual carers when it came to healthcare. Their research involving 1207 US hospital departmental directors (i.e. 278 medical, 230 nursing, 229 social workers, and 470 pastoral care directors), sought to 'gauge the impression of the importance' that departmental directors placed on referring patients to chaplains. Galek *et al.* found that while nurses, physicians, and social work directors indicated it was important to refer patients to chaplains for end-of-life issues, they thought it much less important to make referrals to chaplains for issues unrelated to death, dying, and bereavement. It can be argued that the results suggest a diminished value for the role of spiritual carers (held by the majority of clinical and allied health directors), which may reflect a lack of understanding not only about the social, cognitive, and behavioural benefits of religiosity, spirituality, and pastoral care intervention, but also a lack of appreciation for the fundamentals of holistic person-centred care.[27]

Despite such short-sightedness, the importance of health professionals understanding the significance of spirituality and the role of spiritual carers as part of holistic care, should not be underestimated. Indeed, it can be argued that if spiritual care is so important, then other health professionals need to be educated to understand its significance and be able to add to the spiritual care utility of any healthcare organization. In fact, some healthcare professionals have argued that spiritual care, should not just be left to traditional spiritual carers alone, but that spiritual care also lies within the boundaries of other health professional occupations (e.g. nurses,[28–30] medical physicians,[31,32] social workers,[33] psychologists,[34] occupational therapists[35] and even speech pathologists[36]).

However, given past debates about whether spiritual issues should be addressed as part of the scope of practice within such professional occupations[37,38] the teaching of spiritual, religious and pastoral education to other healthcare professionals is therefore another, and ongoing, important utility that spiritual carers

Table 54.3 WHO 'Pastoral Intervention Codings' and 'Religion and Spirituality Categories'

International Classification of Diseases and Health Related Illnesses (ICD-10- AM) [World Health Organization] 'Pastoral Interventions'	International Classification of Functioning, Disability and Health (ICF), [World Health Organization] Religion and Spirituality'
Pastoral assessment (ICD code 96186–00) [Major Heading : 1824] *Description*: an appraisal of the spiritual wellbeing, needs, issues, and resources of a person within the context of a pastoral encounter. (Elements of this intervention may include initial introductory or exploratory pastoral conversations that are 'informal assessments' or structured 'formal assessments' utilizing a religious/spiritual wellbeing scale)	*Religion and spirituality* (ICF Section D: Activities and Participation, Chapter 9 Community, Social and Civic Life; d930 Religion and Spirituality) *Description:* engaging in religious or spiritual activities, organizations and practices for self-fulfillment, finding meaning, religious, or spiritual value and establishing connection with a divine power, such as is involved in attending a church, temple, mosque, or synagogue, praying or chanting for a religious purpose, and spiritual contemplation. (*Subcategories:* d9300 Organized religion—Engaging in organized religious ceremonies, activities and events; d9301 Spirituality—engaging in spiritual activities or events, outside an organized religion)
Pastoral ministry/support (ICD code 96187–00; Major Heading: 1915) *Description*: the provision of the primary expression of the service, which may include: establishment of relationship, engagement with another, hearing their narrative, and the enabling of pastoral conversation in which spiritual wellbeing and healing may be nurtured and the companioning of persons confronted with profound human issues of death and dying, loss, meaning and aloneness. (Predominantly a 'ministry of presence and support' that may include advocacy or other supportive facilitation)	*Products And Technology—Religion & Spirituality* (ICF Section E: Environmental Factors; Chapter 1 Products and Technology; e145—products and technology for the practice of religion and spirituality) *Description:* products and technology, unique, or mass-produced that are given or take on a symbolic meaning in the context of the practice of religion or spirituality, including those adapted or specially designed. *Inclusion:* general and assistive products and technology for the practice of religion and spirituality. (*Subcategories:* e1450—general products and technology for the practice of religion or spirituality; e1451—assistive products and technology for the practice of religion or spirituality)
Pastoral counselling or education (ICD code 96087–00; Major Heading: 1869) *Description*: an expression of pastoral care that includes personal or familial counsel, ethical consultation, a facilitative review of one's spiritual journey and support in matters of religious belief or practice. The intervention expresses a level of service that may, for example, include counselling and catechesis, and the following elements may be identified: 'emotional/spiritual counsel', 'ethical consultation', 'religious counsel/catechesis', 'spiritual review', 'death and dying', 'Bereavement care/counsel', and 'Crisis care/debriefing'	*Social norms, practices and ideology* (ICF Section E: Environmental Factors) (Chapter 4 Attitudes; e465—Social norms, practices and ideologies) *Description:* customs, practices, rules, and abstract systems of values and normative beliefs (e.g. ideologies, normative world views, and moral philosophies) that arise within social contexts and that affect or create societal and individual practices and behaviours, such as social norms of moral and religious behaviour or etiquette; religious doctrine and resulting norms and practices; norms governing rituals or social gatherings
Pastoral ritual/worship (ICD code 96109–01; Major Heading 1873) *Description*: this intervention contains the pastoral expressions of informal prayer and ritual for individuals or small groups, and the public and more formal expressions of worship, including Eucharist and other services, for faith communities and others. Elements of this intervention may include: 'private prayer and devotion', bedside 'Communion' and 'Anointing' services, 'Blessing and Naming' services for the stillborn and miscarried, and other 'sacrament' and ritual expressions; 'public ministry'—'Eucharist/Ministry of the Word', funerals, memorials, seasonal and occasional services.	Association *and organizational services* (ICF Section E: Environmental Factors; Chapter 5 Services, Systems and Policies; e555—Associations, Services, Systems and Policies) *Description:* associations and organizational services, systems and policies relating to groups of people who have joined together in the pursuit of common, non-commercial interests, often with an associated membership structure—such as associations and organizations providing recreation and leisure, sporting, cultural, religious and mutual aid services *Subcategories*: e5550—Services and programmes; e5551—Administrative control and monitoring mechanisms; e5552—Policies, legislation, regulations

WHO (2001). *International Classification of Functioning, Disability and Health (ICF)*. Geneva: World Health Organization.
WHO (2002). *International Classification of Diseases: Australian Modification of Health Interventions of the International Classifications of Diseases and Related Health Problems*, Vol. 3, 10th edn. Geneva: World Health Organization.

can provide.[39] One particularly important role in which most healthcare practitioners could be trained by spiritual carers, is the ability to undertake patient spiritual screenings and spiritual histories.[40–43] Healthcare practitioners trained in spiritual screenings would then be supporting the appointed spiritual carers who can undertake further assessments and if required additional spiritual and/or pastoral interventions,[44] which in turn would assist teamwork and holistic practice.

Protection and advocacy

An important utility fulfilled by most spiritual cares within the healthcare context is that of providing support to patients and their families in terms of helping to advocate and ensure that fundamental bioethical principles are protected within the healthcare context; namely autonomy, beneficence, non-maleficence, and justice.[45]

For example, healthcare chaplains have been noted to provide spiritual and ethical safeguards at the ward level by supporting patient and family rights concerning issues such as not for resuscitation orders,[46] withdrawal of life support[47] and organ transplantation.[48,49] Furthermore, while there has been some criticism about 'ministers of religion' or other spiritual carers fulfilling advocacy roles on hospital or institutional ethics committees,[50] nevertheless most spiritual carers tend to affirm their role on ethics committees; not only in terms of being an advocate and providing an alternative specialist and holistic perspective, but also by helping to provide a continuum of spiritual care through encouraging bioethical moral discourse between healthcare institutions and the community.[51,52] While it is not a requirement for chaplains to be on human research ethics committees in most countries, nevertheless some countries mandatorily endorse the role of spiritual carers on such committees believing spiritual carers to be an important utility to ensure the protection and advocacy of patients, their families and the community.[53]

In particular, the role of spiritual carers as advocates for the community should not be underrated. Spiritual carers are inherently connected to a community base beyond the healthcare context and thus help to reinforce a community link—a reminder to patients and staff of the 'social self' beyond the hospital bedside—and thus the importance of 'community involvement' and the relevance of 'community care' being ultimately fundamental to all forms of healthcare.[54]

Economics

Another important utility to consider is the provision of spiritual care from an economic perspective. One can argue that a 'cardinal' economic benefit of having the utility of spiritual carers is actually due to an ethical and behavioural outcome that avoids additional costs. That is to say, spiritual carers who help to facilitate communication between patients and clinical staff, plus provide protection and advocacy for patients and their families, assist in reducing costs simply by developing and improving patient–staff rapport, which minimizes frustration, alleviates conflict, helps to avoid ethical mistakes and avoids offensive errors that could otherwise lead to expensive litigation. It has also been argued that, for example, the various pastoral interventions undertaken by chaplains, assist staff to maintain a level of personal congruence and wellbeing within the working environment that can reduce work place stress, absenteeism and accidents—thus caring for staff and further reducing costs.[55]

Another economic utility gained from having spiritual carers is simply an 'ordinal' benefit. That is, in addition to any ethical or behavioural advantage produced by the intervention of spiritual carers, spiritual care is relatively inexpensive (in terms of ranked health-care costs). For example, when considering healthcare chaplaincy, four key economic benefits have been identified, namely:

- spiritual care is a professional service at a reduced cost (i.e. compared with other professional services such as social work and psychological services, the cost for spiritual care is usually much less)
- patient and staff therapeutic benefits are achieved (e.g. chaplains assist in pro-actively supporting patients, families and staff which aids their wellbeing during crises and facilitates their decision-making reducing costs)
- the administration of a free support service is orchestrated (i.e. the coordination and use of volunteer spiritual carers)
- the use of additional services at no cost are procured (e.g. coordination and links to community and spiritual care services paid by external sources).[56]

When one considers the considerable multi-purpose and multi-competent roles undertaken by spiritual carers, it can be argued that the utility and commissioning of spiritual cares is an economically efficient decision for any healthcare service.

Commissioning of spiritual care providers

The term commissioning has numerous meanings.[57] Interestingly many of these meanings are pertinent to the appointment of spiritual care providers. Perhaps most commonly, 'commissioning' refers to

- a formal ceremonial process to officially install or induct someone or some-thing into active service given appropriate accreditation and recognition of training, skills and competencies
- commissioning may also be defined as a specific formal deed and/or official document implemented by a recognized institution granting certain powers or authority to an individual, group, organization, or vessel, to ensure certain utilities, roles, tasks, and duties are fulfilled
- commissioning can also refer to the remuneration entitlements of an individual, group or organization to undertake the agreed roles, tasks and duties to which they have been contracted or covenanted to complete.

These definitions raise several questions when one considers the commissioning of spiritual carers within the healthcare context. Questions such as, 'Who or what authority, should officially commission and appoint spiritual carers within the healthcare context?', 'Who should be commissioned to offer spiritual care?', 'How should they be accredited and, more fundamentally, based on what training, qualifications and competencies?' and finally, 'How should they by renumerated?'

Appointment

Currently, within most Western countries, spiritual carers within both public and private healthcare institutions are appointed by a combination of two key authorities; namely a religious or spiritual organization that has some form of statutory recognition either under national or state legislation and, secondly, by the authority of the public or private institution that is appointing the spiritual carer to provide a service within its organization (e.g. hospital, hospice, palliative care facility). Within some countries/states, it is also expected that spiritual carers will be approved by certification, or recognized by membership with a spiritual care, pastoral care or chaplains association. The combination of these authorities, serve as gatekeepers to help ensure that the most appropriate individuals are endorsed and, usually through a dedication service or other ceremony, are commissioned.

Of course, given certain circumstances, some institutions (e.g. a hospital) may decide to appoint a spiritual carer without the accompanying authority of a religious organization, and vice versa; a religious authority may appoint a spiritual carer to an institution, without regard to normal institutional protocols. Irrespective of whether it is a unilateral decision or the preferred bilateral decision, the key criteria for appointing a spiritual carer by a religious and/or other institutional authorities, should always be based on the level of training and accreditation of the individual commissioned to ensure a high level of professional utility—something that should be a critical priority for both religious/spiritual authorities and the institution concerned.

Accreditation

The training and accreditation of spiritual carers, of whatever title (e.g. chaplain, pastoral-care worker, pastoral-care practitioner, minister of religion, pastors, rabbi, imam, etc.), was traditionally and exclusively undertaken by various religious authorities for centuries. This 'in-breeding' style of education was predominantly to ensure that the appropriate 'sacralization' of each spiritual carer was in accordance with the theological or philosophical teachings of the particular sponsoring religious/spiritual authority. This, in turn, ensured the continuing sacralization of an adherent's identity to a specific religious or spiritual belief.

Since the middle of the twentieth century, it has been commonly accepted (though not mandatory) that spiritual carers would complete tertiary level training, either through their own denominational colleges or through a secular university or, increasingly and preferably, a combination of both. In addition, however, for those entering the healthcare field, it has usually been expected, particularly within the United States, Canada, Australia and New Zealand, that training in clinical pastoral education (CPE) would also be required for spiritual carers to work within healthcare contexts.[58] Similar to the increasing educational standards required of all healthcare practitioners and their assistants, most Western healthcare institutions and spiritual care/chaplaincy organizations have required minimal standards in order for spiritual carers to be appointed (Box 54.1).

However, while minimum standards might be true for most professionally employed spiritual carers, this has not always been the case for most volunteers. A review of both Australian and New Zealand healthcare chaplaincy personnel at the commencement of the twenty-first century, indicated that while the majority of professionally employed spiritual carers had completed both tertiary level education and a recognized clinical pastoral education training program (CPE), this was not so among voluntary spiritual carers. Approximately half of Australian chaplaincy volunteers (47.7%) and nearly 70% of New Zealand volunteer chaplain assistants (69.9%) had *not* undertaken CPE training.[59] This, of course, raises issues regarding the appropriate training and recognition of spiritual carers (particularly volunteers) and whether some form of statutory commission or government authority needs to formalize or even legislate the minimum requirements of training and accreditation required for all spiritual carers, the same way it does for other allied health occupations.

Measures have been taken by some healthcare authorities to establish capability frameworks for professional spiritual care and chaplaincy accreditation. Capability describes the extent to which a person can apply, adjust and synthesize new knowledge from experience and continue to improve his/her performance.[60,61] Assessing such capabilities and performance will probably vary from place to place; nevertheless, such capabilities seek to assess standard professional qualities such as:

- personal competencies
- general workplace abilities
- pastoral/spiritual care practice
- spiritual/theological reflection
- teamwork and accountability capabilities each of which can be further assessed according to different levels of experience (Table 54.4).[62,63]

Such capability qualities and levels of experience not only help to assess spiritual carer competency, but also provide a means for determining remuneration.

Remuneration

The last, but not least issue regarding commissioning, is that of remuneration. Remuneration for spiritual carers has varied enormously, from country to country, state to state and even between healthcare facilities within the same state. While there are some health authorities that have recommended payment levels for spiritual carers or 'pastoral carers,' nevertheless, generally speaking, the salaries for professional spiritual carers (within both public and private sectors) have usually not been commensurate with the income of other allied health occupations.

The lack of comparative remuneration for spiritual carers, has largely been due to factors such as

- historical precedence (e.g. clergy compensation has traditionally been minimally proportional in comparison to other professional occupations)
- increasing secularization leading to the devaluing of the metaphysical benefits of spiritual care
- tokenistic attitudes about holistic care held by governments and healthcare institutions thus failing to facilitate and resource adequate religious and spiritual care
- lack of recognition by governments, healthcare institutions and other healthcare occupations concerning the professional training, multi-competency and multi-utility of spiritual carers

Box 54.1 Common international professional minimal standards for appointing/commissioning of professional spiritual carers

- Member of a national/state recognized religious/spiritual organization or community
- Recognized formal tertiary level qualification or tertiary level training in theology, ministry, religious studies, pastoral care or spiritual education
- Specialist training in Clinical Pastoral Education (CPE) [minimum hours) or evidence of graduate/postgraduate tertiary level pastoral care or spiritual education and experience
- Member of, or eligibility to join, a registered spiritual, pastoral care or chaplains association with an established code of ethics
- Endorsement to practice by a recognized/authorized religious institution or spiritual entity
- Institutional Approval and Commissioning by recipient organization

Table 54.4 Professional spiritual carer levels of capability

Level	Professional Capabilities[128,129]
Level 1	Entry level—first professional appointment as pastoral/spiritual care practitioner
Level 2	Indicates capabilities of an autonomous spiritual care/pastoral care practitioner with minimum of 2 years experience, able to seek out, and respond to the spiritual and religious needs of individuals, their families, and staff
Level 3	Capable of providing both general and specialist care in dedicated units (such as intensive care units, paediatrics, oncology, palliative care, etc.) plus team responsibilities and mentoring roles of other practitioners
Level 4	Capable of advanced skills/and or specialization and ability to contribute to the education and training of others in the profession of chaplaincy and pastoral/spiritual care. Level 4 practitioner could hold a section leadership role or Departmental Head in a non-tertiary hospital or other facility (e.g. Aged Care)
Level 5	Highly experienced and credentialled practitioner, capable of leading and managing a spiritual/pastoral care department in a tertiary facility, and overseeing an entire programme of service delivery and education/training programme

Healthcare Chaplaincy Council of Victoria Inc. (2009). Capabilities Framework for Pastoral Care and Chaplaincy. Melbourne: Healthcare Chaplaincy Council of Victoria Inc. and National Health Service (2005). Spiritual and Religious Care Capabilities and Competencies for Healthcare Chaplains. Edinburgh: National Health Service Education for Scotland.

- a reluctance of healthcare facilities to employ or increase the employment and remuneration of spiritual carers, particularly given financial constraints and the available supply of volunteers.

A further and possibly contentious issue that will challenge the remuneration and employment of spiritual carers is the 'competition' from a number of other professions[64] (e.g. social workers, psychologists) who would either voluntarily or, as a part of their professional duty of care, deliberately seek to independently administer spiritual care. It can be argued, of course, that encroaching upon the traditional vocational and professional boundaries of spiritual carers, however, would add another task to workloads of other professional occupations already under stress—and although willing, may not be able to properly fulfill such duties given other professional and personal philosophies and priorities.

Nevertheless, taking over spiritual care tasks, would provide other professional groups (and their respective departments) with the political and strategic leverage to lobby for additional staff and resources in order for them to attempt to provide spiritual care—a shifting of resources that would fundamentally (and somewhat unethically) undermine spiritual and pastoral care departments and penultimately limit the remuneration and professional employment of spiritual carers. However given the cardinal and ordinal benefits of spiritual care and related departments, such strategies of simply relocating resources are of no real economic advantage to an employing institution (indeed, it could prove disadvantageous *not* to employ spiritual carers who have direct influential communication links to external organizations within the community). Furthermore, such strategies would undervalue the role and remuneration of spiritual carers within the healthcare context and eventually thwart the very aims of holistic care, and undermine the efficiency and effectiveness of a heath care facility. Rather what is required is for spiritual carers, who are duly trained, accredited and commissioned, to be treated equally with their allied health counterparts.

Conclusion

Spiritual care and spiritual carers have formed part of the history of health and wellbeing within most Western healthcare contexts for centuries—particularly through the traditional cleric and chaplaincy professions. It can be argued that the utility of spiritual carers (e.g. as a public service, communication facilitators, being multi-competent, multi-purpose, assisting with patient and family advocacy, plus being of economic worth) brings considerable benefit to healthcare institutions, governments, and the wider community. Given the beneficial utility that spiritual carers can bring to multiple areas within the healthcare context, the commissioning of spiritual carers and the practice of spiritual care, should be taken seriously, affirmed within health policy, plus fully endorsed, and supported by governments and healthcare institutions.

The appointment of spiritual carers, and/or those wanting to provide spiritual care (in whatever capacity), should be based upon appropriate tertiary level training and accreditation recognized by both spiritual/religious organizations, plus related professional associations, healthcare institutions and state authorities. Mandatory requirements should be endorsed necessitating tertiary education in spiritual/pastoral care, plus clinical pastoral education (or perhaps 'clinical spiritual education') for those wanting to engage in spiritual care—whether professionally or voluntarily. Similar to other healthcare occupations, legislation is also necessary to require professional registration of spiritual carers working within healthcare contexts, to ensure that expert practice and ethical standards are supported and maintained. Subsequently the remuneration of spiritual carers should also be of equal compensation to their allied health peers to help make certain the ongoing utility and holistic provision of professional spiritual care within healthcare facilities.

References

1 Mol, H. (1976). *The Sacred and Identity: A Sketch for a New Social-scientific Theory of Religion*. Oxford: Basil Blackwell.

2 Kellahear, A. (2002). Spiritual care in palliative care, In: B. Rumbold (ed.) *Spirituality and Palliative Care: Social and Pastoral Perspectives*, pp. 166–77. Melbourne: Oxford University Press.

3 Handzo, G., Koenig, H.G. (2004) Spiritual care: whose job is it anyway? *Sthn Med J* **97**(12): 1242–4.

4 Puchalski, C., Ferrell, B., Virani, R., Otis-Green, S., Baird, P., Bull, J., *et al.* (2009) Improving the quality of spiritual care as a dimension of palliative care: the report of the Consensus Conference. *J Palliat Med* **12**(10): 885–904.

5 Harding, S.R., Flannelly, K., Galek, K., Tannenbaum, H.P. (2008) Spiritual care, pastoral care and chaplains: trends in the healthcare literature. *J Hlthcare Chaplaincy* **14**: 99–117.

6 Pesut, B., Reimer-Kirkham, S., Sawatzky, R., Woodland, G., Perverall, P. (2010) Hospitable hospitals in a diverse society: from chaplains to spiritual care providers. *J Relig Hlth* 14 Sep, Online DOI 10.1007/s10943-010-9392-1

7 Stevenson, A. (ed) (2010). *Oxford Dictionary of English*, 3rd edn. Oxford: Oxford University Press.
8 Miller, A.N., Rubin, D.L. (eds) (2011). *Health Communities and Faith Communities*. Cresskill: Hampton Press.
9 Carey, L.B., Cohen, J. (2009). Chaplain–physician consultancy: when chaplains and doctors meet in the clinical context. *J Relig Hlth* **48** (3): 353–67.
10 Wagner, J.T., Higdon, T.L. (1996). Spiritual issues and bioethics in the intensive care unit: The role of the chaplain. *Crit Care Clin* **12**(1): 15–27.
11 Carey, L.B., Cohen, J. (2008). Religion, spirituality and healthcare treatment decisions: the role of chaplains in the Australian clinical context. *J Hlthcare Chaplaincy* **15**: 25–39.
12 Simmonds, A.L. (1994). The chaplain's role in bioethical decision-making. *Hlthcare Manage Forum* **7**(4): 5–17.
13 Carey, L.B. (2011). Chaplains and healthcare communication. In: A.N. Miller, D.L. Rubin (eds) *Health Communication and Faith Communities*, pp. 263–78. Cresskill: Hampton Press.
14 Carey, L.B., Rumbold, B., Newell, C., Aroni, R. (2006). Bioethical issues and healthcare chaplaincy in Australia. *Scot J Hlthcare Chaplaincy* **9**(1): 23–30.
15 Carey, L.B. (2010) Bioethical issues and healthcare chaplaincy in Aotearoa New Zealand. *J Relig Hlth* August. Online DOI 10.1007/s10943-010-9368-1
16 Carey, L.B., Cohen, J. (2009). Chaplaincy physician consultancy: When chaplains and doctors meet in the clinical context. *J Relig Hlth* **48**(3): 357–67.
17 Hochstetler, C. (2006). Pastoral ministers and volunteers: qualifications, training and functions. In: L.D. Bueckert, D. Schipani (eds) *Spiritual Caregiving in the Hospital: Windows to Chaplaincy Ministry*, pp. 55–72. Ontario: Pandora Press.
18 Munro, G. (2001). A chaplaincy volunteer service. *Scot J Hlthcare Chaplaincy* **4**(2): 29–31.
19 Orton, M.J. (2008). Transforming chaplaincy; The emergence of healthcare pastoral care for a post-modern world. *J Hlthcare Chaplaincy* **15**: 114–31.
20 WHO (2002). *International Classification of Diseases: Australian Modification of Health Interventions of* the International Statistical Classification of Diseases and Related Health Problems, Vol. 3, 10th edn. Geneva: World Health Organization.
21 WHO (2001). *International Classification of Functioning of Disability and Health (ICF)*. Geneva: World Health Organization.
22 Abu-Ras, W., Laird, L. (2010). How Muslim and non-Muslim chaplains serve Muslim patients? Does the interfaith chaplaincy model have room for Muslims' experiences? *J Relig Hlth* May. Online DOI 10.1007/s10943-010-9357-4
23 Davoren, R., Carey, L.B. (2008). Interfaith pastoral care and the role the healthcare chaplain. *Scot J Hlthcare Chaplaincy* **11**(1): 21–32.
24 Mol, H. (1976). *The Sacred and Identity: A Sketch for a New Social-scientific Theory of Religion*. Oxford: Basil Blackwell.
25 Carey, L.B., Davoren, R., Cohen, J. (2009). The sacralisation of identity: An interfaith spiritual care paradigm for chaplaincy in a multi-faith context. In: D. Schippani, L. Beuckert (eds) *Interfaith Spiritual Care: Understandings and Practices*, Chapter 13. Ontario: Hampton Press.
26 Galek, K., Flannelly, K. J., Koenig, G. H., Fogg, S. L. (2007). Referrals to chaplains: the role of religions and spirituality in healthcare settings. *Ment Hlth, Relig Cult* **10**(4): 367–77.
27 Tudor, L. E., Keemar, K., Tudor, K., Valentine, J., Worrall, M. (2004). *The Person-centred Approach: A Contemporary Introduction*. New York: Palgrave Macmillan.
28 Hussey, T. (2009). Nursing and spirituality. *Nurs Philos* **10**(2): 71–80.
29 McSherry, W. (2012). Nursing. In: M. Cobb, C. Puchalski, B. Rumbold (eds) *Oxford Textbook of Spirituality in Healthcare*, Chapter 30. Oxford: Oxford University Press.
30 VanLoon, A. (2011). Faith community (parish) nursing. In: M. Cobb, C. Puchalski, B. Rumbold (eds) *Oxford Textbook of Spirituality in Healthcare*, Chapter 31. Oxford: Oxford University Press.
31 Hamilton, D.G. (1998). Believing in patient's beliefs. Physicians attunement to the spiritual dimension as a positive factor in patient health and health. *Am J Hospice Palliat Care* September/October, **15**(5): 276–9.
32 Washam, C. (2009). Helping patients by including spirituality in discussions. *Oncol Times* **31** (13): 14–19.
33 Canda, E.R., Furman, L.D., (2009). *Spiritual Diversity in Social Work Practice: the Heart of Helping*. New York: Oxford University Press.
34 Schafer, R.M., Handal, P.J., Brawar, P.A., Ubinger, M. (2011) Training and education in religion/spirituality within APA-Accredited clinical psychology programs: 8 years later. *J Relig Hlth* **50**(2): 232–9.
35 Smith, S. (2008). Toward a flexible framework for understanding spirituality. *Occup Ther Hlthcare* **22**(1): 39–54.
36 Mathisen, B., Yates, P., Crofts, P. (2010). Palliative care curriculum for speech-language pathology students. *Int J Lang Commun Disord* **46** (3): 273–85.
37 Collins, J.S., Paul, S., West-Frasier, J. (2002). The utilization of spirituality in occupational therapy: Beliefs, practices and perceived barriers. *Occup Ther Hlthcare* **14**(3/4): 73–92.
38 Curlin, F., Hall, D. (2005). Strangers or friends? A proposal for a new spirituality-in-medicine ethic. *J Gen Intern Med* **20**: 370–4.
39 Grosvenor-Lovell, D. (2000). Teaching spiritual care to nurses. *Scot J Hlthcare Chaplaincy* **3**(2): 29–33.
40 Puchulski, C., Ferrell, B., Virani, R., Otis-Green, S., Baird, P., Bull, J., *et al.* (2009). Improving the quality of spiritual care as a dimension of palliative care: the report of the consensus conference, *J Palliat Med* **12**(10): 885–904.
41 Fitchett, G., Risk, J.L. (2009). Screening for spiritual struggle. *J Past Care Counsel*, Spring-Summer;**63**(1-2): 4–1–12.
42 Fitchett, G. (2012). Spiritual assessment in health care: an assessment. In: M. Cobb, C. Puchalski, B. Rumbold (eds) *Oxford Textbook of Spirituality in Healthcare*, Chapter 42. Oxford: Oxford University Press.
43 Pulchalski, C. (2012). Restorative Medicine. In: M. Cobb, C. Puchalski, B. Rumbold (eds) *Oxford Textbook of Spirituality in Healthcare*, Chapter 29. Oxford: Oxford University Press.
44 WHO-ICD-10-AM—Pastoral Intervention Codings (2002). *World Health Organization International Classification of Diseases and Hlth Interventions*, Vol. **10**(3) Pastoral Intervention Codings. Geneva: World Health Organization.
45 Beachamp, T.L., Childress, J.F. (2009). *Principles of Biomedical Ethics*, 6th edn. New York: Oxford University Press.
46 Carey, L.B., Newell, C. (2007). Chaplaincy and resuscitation. *Resuscitation* **75**: 12–22.
47 Carey, L.B., Newell, C. (2007). Withdrawal of life support and chaplaincy in Australia. *Crit Care Resus* **9**(1): 34–9.
48 Carey, L.B., Robinson, P., Cohen, J. (2009). Organ procurement and healthcare chaplaincy in Australia. *J Relig Hlth*.
49 Carey, L.B., Robinson, P., Cohen, J. (2012). Organ procurement and healthcare chaplaincy in Aotearoa New Zealand. *J Relig Hlth* (In press).
50 McNeil, P.M., Bergland, C.A., Webster, I.W. (1996). Ethics at the borders of medical research: How much influence do various members have within research ethics committees? *Camb Q Hlthcare Eth* **3**: 522–32.
51 Carey, L.B., Cohen, J. (2010). Healthcare chaplains and their role on institutional ethics committees: An Australian study. *J Relig Hlth* **49**(2): 221–32.
52 Van Loon, A.M., Carey, L.B. (2002). Faith community nursing and healthcare chaplaincy in Australia: a new collaboration. In: L. VandeCreek, S. Moon (eds) *Parish Nurses, Healthcare Chaplains and Community Clergy: Navigating the Maze of Professional Relationships*, pp. 143–57. New York: Haworth Press.

53 National Health and Medical Research Council. (2007) *Statement on Ethical Conduct in Research*. Canberra: Australia Commonwealth Government.
54 Kellahear, A. (2002). Spiritual care in palliative care. In: B. Rumbold (ed.) *Spirituality and Palliative Care: Social and Pastoral Perspectives*, p. 166–77. Melbourne: Oxford University Press.
55 Carey, L.B. (2010). Bioethical issues and healthcare chaplaincy in Aotearoa New Zealand. *J Relig Hlth* Online DOI 10.1007/s10943-010-9368-1.
56 Newell, C.J., Carey, L.B. (2000). Economic rationalism and the cost efficiency of hospital chaplaincy: An Australian study. *J Hlthcare Chaplaincy* **10**(1): 37–52.
57 Stevenson, A. (ed.) (2010). *Oxford Dictionary of English*, 3rd edn. Oxford: Oxford University Press.
58 Lartey, E.Y. (2012). Pastoral theology in healthcare settings: blessed irritant for holistic human care. In: M. Cobb, C. Puchalski, B. Rumbold (eds) *Textbook of Spirituality in Healthcare*, Chapter 41. Oxford: Oxford University Press.
59 Carey, L.B., Newell, C.J. (2002). Clinical pastoral education and the value of empirical research: Examples from Australian and New Zealand Datum. *J Hlthcare Chaplaincy* **12**(1): 53–65.
60 Healthcare Chaplaincy Council of Victoria Inc. (2009). *Capabilities Framework for Pastoral Care and Chaplaincy*. Melbourne: Healthcare Chaplaincy Council of Victoria Inc.
61 National Health Service. (2005). *Spiritual and Religious Care Capabilities and Competencies for Healthcare Chaplains*. Edinburgh: National Health Service Education for Scotland.
62 Healthcare Chaplaincy Council of Victoria Inc. (2009). *Capabilities Framework for Pastoral Care and Chaplaincy*. Melbourne: Healthcare Chaplaincy Council of Victoria Inc.
63 National Health Service. (2005). *Spiritual and Religious Care Capabilities and Competencies for Healthcare Chaplains*. Edinburgh: National Health Service Education for Scotland.
64 Gardner, H. (1997). *Health Policy in Australia*, p. 8. Melbourne: Oxford University Press.
65 Clebsch, W., Jaeckle, C. (1964). *Pastoral Care in Historical Perspective: An Essay with Exhibits*. Nashville: Abingdon Press.
66 Clinebell, H. (1984). *Basic Types of Pastoral Care and Counselling: Resources for the Ministry of Healing and Growth*. London: SCM Press.
67 Clinebell, H. (1990). Pastoral care movement. In: R. Hunter (ed.) *Dictionary of pastoral care and counseling*. Nashville: Abingdon Press, pp. 857–8.
68 Knights, W., Kramer, D. (1964). Chaplaincy role functions as seen by mental patients and staff. *J Past Care* **18**: 154–60.
69 Morrow, W., Matthews, A.T.J. (1966). Role definitions of hospital chaplains in mental health, *J Scient Study Relig* **5**: 421–34.
70 Carey, R. (1972). *Hospital Chaplains: Who Needs Them?* St Louis: Catholic Chaplains Association.
71 Dagenais, R. (1985). Pastoral care in modern hospitals. *CHAC Rev* **13**(2): 20–3.
72 Hesch, J. (1987). *Clinical Pastoral Care for Hospitalized Children and Their Families*. New Jersey: Paulist Press.
73 Wagner, J.T., Higdon, T.L. (1996). Spiritual issues and bioethics in the intensive care unit: the role of the chaplain. *Crit Care Clin* **12**(1): 15–27.
74 Lartey, E. (1997). *In Living Colour: An Intercultural Approach to Pastoral Care and Counseling*. London: Cassell.
75 National Health Service (1993) Healthcare Chaplaincy Standards, Bristol, National Health Service Training Directorate.
76 Cross, R., Carey, L., Allen, N. (eds) (2002). *Healthcare Chaplaincy Guidelines*. Melbourne: Australian Healthcare Chaplaincy Inc.
77 WHO-ICD-10-AM—Pastoral Intervention Codings. (2002). *World Health Organization International Classification of Diseases and Health Interventions*, Vol. **10** (3) Pastoral Intervention Codings. Geneva: World Health Organization.
78 Carey, L.B., Cobb, M., Equeall, D. (2005). From pastoral contacts to pastoral interventions, *Scot J Hlthcare Chaplaincy* **8**(2): 14–20.
79 Carey, L.B., Rumbold, B., Newell, C., Aroni, R. (2006). Bioethical issues and healthcare chaplaincy in Australia. *Scot J Hlthcare Chaplaincy* **9**(1): 23–30.
80 Carey, L.B. (2010). Bioethical issues and healthcare chaplaincy in Aotearoa New Zealand. *J Relig Hlth* Online DOI 10.1007/s10943-010-9368-1.
81 Carey, L.B. (2011). Chaplains and healthcare communication, in Miller, A.N., Rubin, D.L. (eds) *Hlth Communication and Faith Based Communities*, (pp.263–78) Cresskill, New Jersey: Hampton Press.
82 Ritter, H. (1994). Desperation and abandonment as themes for disability in rehabilitation. *J Religion in Disability and Rehabilitation*. **1** (4), 71–8.
83 Stainton, M. (1994). Healing stories: critiquing old and creating new, *J Relig Disabil Rehab* **1**(4): 71–8.
84 Blair, W.A., Blair, D.D. (1994). Ministry to persons with disabilities: can we do better, *J Relig Disabil Rehab* **1**(1): 1–9.
85 McCarthy-Power, M. (1989). How can I help? Healthcare chaplaincy with developmentally disabled persons. *J Hlthcare Chaplaincy* **2**(2): 27–34.
86 Samson, M., McColgan, S. (2000). Chaplaincy in action … and inaction. *J Relig Disabil Hlth* **3**(3): 41–9.
87 Bohne, J. (1986). AIDS: ministry issues for chaplains. *J Past Psychol* **34**(3): 173–91.
88 Dugan, D.O. (1987). Death and dying: emotional, spiritual and ethical support for patients and families. *J Psycholog Nurs Ment Hlth Serv* **25**(7): 21–9.
89 Milne, J. (1988). Patients and their families reflection on pastoral care in their cancer experience—report of a survey. *Cancer Forum* **12**(3): 115–23.
90 Rumbold, B. (1989). Spiritual dimensions in palliative care. In: P. Hodder, A. Turley (eds) *The Creative Option of Palliative Care*. Melbourne: Melbourne City Mission.
91 Turley, B. (1982). *Being There for Others: A Pastoral Resource for Lay People*. Melbourne: Joint Board of Christian Education.
92 Goodell, E. (1992). Cancer and family members. *J Hlthcare Chaplaincy* **4**(1): 2.
93 Handzo, G.M. (1992). Where do chaplains fit in the world of cancer. *J Hlthcare Chaplaincy* **4**(1): 29–44.
94 Fraser, D. (2004). Integrating chaplaincy and spiritual care within palliative care. *Scot J Hlthcare Chaplaincy* **4**(2): 8–11.
95 Carey, L.B., Newell, C.J., Rumbold, B. (2006). Pain control and chaplaincy in Australia. *J Pain Sympt Manage* **32**(6): 589–601.
96 Nolan, S. (2011). Hope beyond (redundant) hope: how chaplains work with dying patients. *Palliat Med* **35**(1): 21–5.
97 Browning, D. (1988). Hospital chaplaincy as public ministry. *J Hlthcare Chaplaincy* **2**(1): 3–16.
98 Copeland, J. (1993). The chaplain's role: a cardiac surgeon's view. *J Hlthcare Chaplaincy* **5**(1/2): 5–10.
99 DeLong, W. (1993). Waiting: pastoral care to the cardiac bridge to transplant patient. *J Hlthcare Chaplaincy* **5**(1/2): 63–71.
100 DeLong, W. (1990). Organ donations and hospital chaplains: attitudes, beliefs and concerns. *Transplantation* **50**(1): 25–9.
101 Elliot, H., Carey, L.B. (1996). Organ transplantation and the role of hospital chaplains, *Minist Soc Theol* **10**(1): 66–77.
102 Carey, L.B., Robinson, P., Cohen, J. (2011). Organ procurement and healthcare chaplaincy in Australia. *J Relig Hlth* **50**: 743–59.
103 Carey, L.B., Robinson, P., Cohen, J. (2012). Organ procurement and healthcare chaplaincy in Aotearoa New Zealand. *J Relig Hlth* (in press).
104 Bryce, B.E. (1988). Using chaplain in the OR. *AORN J* **48**(6): 5.
105 Sharp. (1991). Use of chaplaincy within the neo-natal intensive care unit. *Sthn Med J* **84**(12): 1482–6.
106 Wagner, J.T., Higdon, T.L. (1996). Spiritual issues and bioethics in the intensive care unit: The role of the chaplain. *Crit Care Clin* **12**(1): 15–27.

107 Robinson, M., Thiel, M., Meghan, M, Backus, M.M., Meyer, E.C. (2006). Matters of spirituality at the end of life in the pediatric intensive care unit. *Pediatrics* **118**: 719–29.

108 Carey, L.B., Newell, C.J. (2007). Chaplaincy and resuscitation. *Resuscitation* **75**: 12–22.

109 Carey, L.B., Newell, C.J. (2007) Withdrawal of life support. *Crit Care Resus* **9**(1): 34–9.

110 McSherry, E. (1994). Outpatient care: the modern chaplains new impact in healthcare reform. *J Hlthcare Chaplaincy* **6**(1): 83–108.

111 Mandziuk. (1996). Is there a chaplain in your clinic? *J Relig Hlth* **35**(1): 5–9.

112 Mowat, H. (2007). Gerontological chaplaincy. *Scot J Hlthcare Chaplaincy* **10**(1): 27–31.

113 MacKinlay, E. (2002). Health, healing and wholeness in frail elderly people. *J Relig Gerontol* **13**(2): 25–34.

114 Hesch, J. (1987). *Clinical Pastoral Care for Hospitalized Children and Their Families.* New Jersey: Paulist Press.

115 Stotter,D.J. (1987). Childhood illness: the chaplain's role. *Nursing* **24**: 910–11.

116 Donnelley, N.H. (1983). When children suffer. *Leadership* **4**(2): 45–51.

117 Carey, L.B., Aroni, R., Edwards, A. (1997). Health and wellbeing: hospital chaplaincy. In: H. Gardner (ed.) *Health Policy in Australia*, pp. 190–210. Melbourne: Oxford University Press.

118 Ryan, V. (1991). The spiritual needs of children in hospital. *Minist Soc Theol* **5**(2): 54–9.

119 Gilchrist, K. (2004). Chaplaincy and spiritual care in a children's hospital. *Scot J Hlthcare Chaplaincy* **4**(1): 26–8.

120 Carey, L., Meese, C. (2005). Do pastoral care and spirituality services make a positive difference: An evaluation at the Royal Women's Hospital. *Melb Minist Soc Theol* **19**(1): 114–27.

121 Cadge, W., Calle, K., Dillinger, J. (2011) What do chaplains contribute to large academic hospitals? The perspectives of pediatric physicians and chaplains. *J Relig Hlth* **50**(2): 300–12.

122 Knights, W., Kramer, D. (1964). Chaplaincy role functions as seen by mental patients and staff. *J Past Care* **18**: 154–60.

123 Morrow, W., Matthews, A. (1966). Role definitions of hospital chaplains in mental health. *J Scient Study Relig* **5**: 421–34.

124 Stephens, J. (1994). A personal view of the role of the chaplain at the Reaside Clinic. *Psychiat Bull* **18**: 677–9.

125 Macritchie, I. (2004). Worlds apart? A comparison of mental health and acute chaplaincy. *Scot J Hlthcare Chaplaincy* **7**(2): 23–7.

126 Ratray, L.H. (2002). Significance of the chaplain within the mental healthcare team, *Psychiat Bull* **26**: 190–1.

127 Swinton, J. (2001). *Spirituality and Mental Healthcare: Rediscovering a 'Forgotten' Dimension.* London: Jessica Kingsley Publishers.

128 Healthcare Chaplaincy Council of Victoria Inc. (2009). *Capabilities Framework for Pastoral Care and Chaplaincy.* Melbourne: Healthcare Chaplaincy Council of Victoria Inc.

129 National Health Service (2005). *Spiritual and Religious Care Capabilities and Competencies for Healthcare Chaplains.* Edinburgh: National Health Service Education for Scotland.

CHAPTER 55

Social care

Holly Nelson-Becker and Mary Pat Sullivan

Introduction

Spirituality is drawing increasing attention as an important aspect of social discourse. This chapter discusses the role of spirituality in social care from a professional practice perspective. We address the scope of spirituality in social care, spiritual care policy, educational and training models, spiritual leadership in organizations, ethical dimensions of practice, and evaluation and outcomes of spirituality in social care. Finally, we provide recommendations for best practices. We have integrated policies and education models of care principally from the UK and the USA. This is not because spiritual social care is not being addressed in Europe and third world countries, but rather that some of this is not yet accessible and a multinational comparison would be beyond the reach of this chapter.

Vignette

Claire Stewart was a 48-year-old-woman who had not considered herself to be very religious when she left home at age 22 to begin a career, although she had always professed belief in a Transcendent Power. She had been living for the past two months in a nursing care rehabilitation facility due to a car accident that resulted in a severe spinal cord injury leaving her paraplegic. At the time the social worker visited, she was expected to remain there for at least six months more. Claire had a vibrant personality, was physically attractive, and created an active social life with many friends. Although she had nurtured friendships, few friends now visited, as they felt uncomfortable seeing her unable to walk. Never married and independent with her own successful marketing business, she had no family support, other than a brother who lived about three hours away with his family. Under stress due to his recent unexpected termination from work due to company downsizing, he was not able to visit often.

For the first time in her life, Claire experienced unrelenting depression. Included in her depressive thoughts were questions about why this unfortunate event had happened to her at this point in her life when everything seemed to be going so well. Many of her feelings centred on her anger toward God who she had mostly considered a benevolent, if passive, force. She had been raised in an Anglican faith tradition, but had never taken time to explore the meaning of her faith. She had warm memories of the congregation she attended as a youth, but wondered if there was anything there relevant to the struggles she faced. Now she felt lost and sad, as if she were drifting alone in a vast and violent storm-lashed ocean. Only her own initiative could change anything, but the one thing she most wanted to change, to learn to walk again, was not likely to occur. Her anger and sadness caused her to see her life as over. The social worker had expected to work with her initially on reframing her cognitions and depressive thoughts and then move towards planning for the future, but what Claire most wanted to discuss were her questions about the meaning of life and the existence of God. These were questions to which the social worker did not perceive she could respond well because of limited professional training in this area. She herself was neither religious nor particularly spiritual. Furthermore, the worker wondered if policies at her organization permitted discussion of these service user-initiated questions.

As this vignette illustrates, spiritual distress, religious disconnection, and concerns about greater existential questions of life's purpose and meaning form part of the background of our being and may be especially prevalent at health status change points. Spiritual pain, anxiety, alienation, loss, anger, and guilt may appear alongside positive spiritual coping and personal spiritual strengths that achieve benefits of peace, joy, comfort, and hope. Thus, spirituality should be assessed whenever service users seek social care. Although spiritual and religious issues are not relevant to everyone, they do matter to significant numbers of individuals and may form part of an overall plan of intervention in the community. In the USA, 78% of all adults are affiliated with a Christian faith and 4.7% are affiliated with other faiths including Judaism, Buddhist, Muslim, and Hindu religions.[1] Sixteen per cent are unaffiliated, but the numbers who consider themselves spiritual and not religious are unknown. In the UK, 72–81% of the population is Christian followed by Muslims at 2.6%,[2] although both surveys have a margin of error. Australia is noted as 75.6% Christian, followed by Buddhist and Muslim combined at about 4%.[2] Other nations vary considerably in types and degrees of religious affiliation. India, for example, has approximately 73% of citizens who endorse Hinduism and 14% who endorse Islam.[2] Clearly, religion does hold value and gives meaning to many individuals worldwide.

The scope of spirituality in social care

Social care is the process of providing assistance to individuals and families at their point of deep need to change behaviour, obtain resources, prevail over discouragement, build strengths, and achieve their full capacity. Innate coping resources may be overwhelmed by unexpected events such as disability, an illness or other health challenge, or environmental factors such as poverty, oppression, and other global turmoil that may have upset life balance.[3] Social care includes the efforts of many mental health disciplines, particularly social work, counselling, and psychology, but also nursing and ancillary health professions, to provide various types of service, whether founded in material need, mental or physical health need, social or spiritual need.[4,5] Social care is often used to reference international contexts of care outside of the US, but is not limited to social needs. In the biopsychosocial spiritual model of personhood dimensions largely adopted now in social work,[6–8] social care includes attention to creation of healing contexts and modalities. The biological, psychological, and social dimensions of life are integrated with the spiritual dimension. All of these dimensions affect each other and thus should be assessed with the service user.

The healing and helping relationship includes two key individuals, the service user and social worker/health professional, who interact in a context of social care (Figure 55.1). Although each meets each other as a whole and integrated being, aspects of each dimension may be more salient at different points. The psychological skills of the worker will be used to intervene with a specific aspect of the service user, such as the biological or spiritual dimension, for example. The inside spheres on the diagram rotate so the same or different aspects may touch. At times, the spiritual sensitivity of the worker is called forth to meet other dimensions of the service user. The helping relationship unfolds against an organizational environment with its standards and tasks that brought both together. Other important environments include the family environment of each, the religious background or environment, the community and cultural environment, and the social justice principle of subsidiarity, explained later in the text. The dotted line separating the organizational and other environments signifies interactive effects between them. While the religious background may be active or individually dormant in the larger context for any service user, there is also an implicit spiritual background that forms the larger backdrop of the outer circlet.

Spirituality has been increasingly recognized and validated by the helping professions as a life dimension that should be included in initial assessment.[9,10] Dialogue in this area has expanded as professionals have begun to understand the importance and value of spirituality and religion in providing comfort, care, and/or guidance to some service users. Many schools of social work, nursing, and counsellor education are including the topic in their curricula along with physician education,[11–14] yet professionals still typically consider themselves less prepared to address this area than they would prefer.

There is a distinction between curing spaces where care is provided to a service user and healing spaces, where care is in 'being with' a service user.[15] Cure, or return to pre-illness functioning level, is sometimes an unrealizable goal. Healing spaces can empower service user coping by helping him/her process and understand the illness or life difficulty from an alternative vantage point. Creating room for both avenues can lead to healing on several levels, to enhanced meaning-making, and to phronesis, or practical wisdom about how to meet life aspirations. In community work accomplished with service users, lasting benefit often comes from attention to the healing space when curing is no longer possible.

Pursuit of spiritual goals

Spiritual goals often become salient during times of health or social crisis. Occupational therapists and non-professional workers

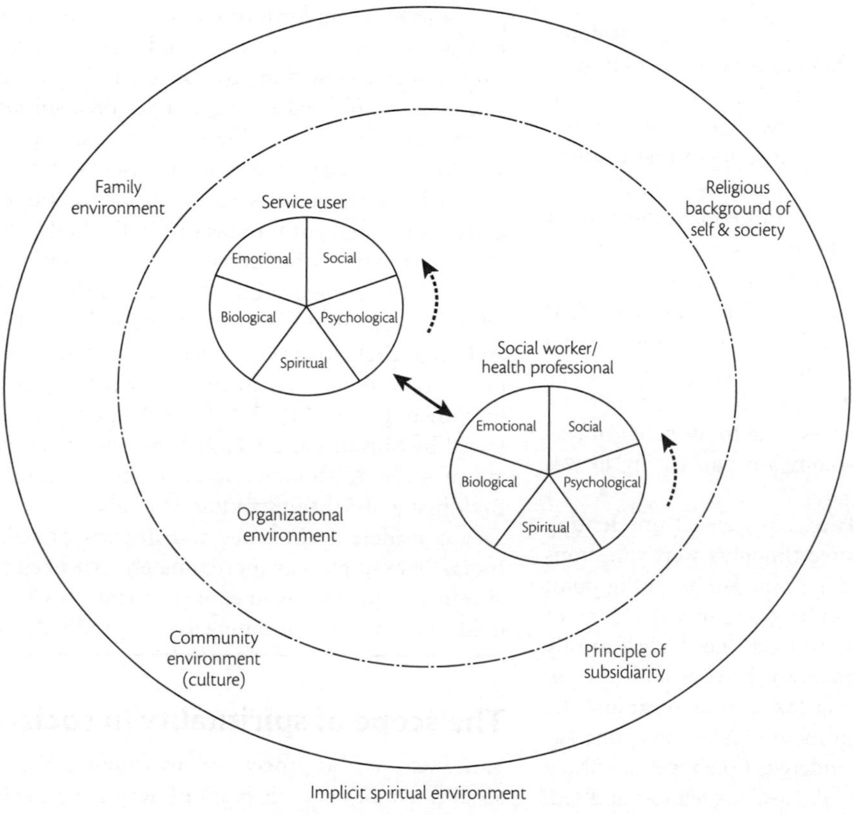

Figure 55.1 Healing and helping relationship.

in social care (e.g. care assistants, home care workers, residential care workers) are also involved in care provision and may support or obstruct spiritual goals of the service user. Spirituality shapes human development through the search for personal meaning and purpose, the desire to achieve harmony and wholeness in relationships, and acknowledgment of the presence of sacred space that sometimes leads to transformational change. It is often defined through the language of connections to self, to others, to nature, to a sacred source of meaning or transcendent power, and sometimes at the end of life, to deceased loved ones.[16] Seeking or offering forgiveness, dealing with guilt, shame, or other maladies of the soul may be part of this work.

Rumpold[17] called for attention to inclusion of spirituality particularly in the settings where older adults resided. In these places the bureaucratic style of many residential care organizations historically edited out attention to spirituality because it did not lend itself to being measured nor managed. In the USA, the Joint Commission that accredits healthcare organizations has recognized that access to spiritual supports can have a positive effect on service user wellbeing.[18] Spirituality also may include attention to social justice, particularly where the most vulnerable individuals find their right to self–determination or other human rights truncated or denied.

Subsidiarity supports the view of the individual as the center of life and defends social justice.[19,20] This perspective aligns with principles of the social work ethical code and assumes that every individual holds inherent worth and dignity. Thus, the role of the community, social organizations, and institutions is to serve the individual and help that person flourish by creating conditions to achieve fulfillment. Fulfillment is accomplished through the social interaction that fosters full authenticity. The individual may reciprocally be motivated to give back to society through civic engagement. The best decisions are made at the lowest hierarchical levels of society by those closest to the experience. Where an organization employs a physician, social worker, or nurse, the highest quality decisions will be made in the interlocution or nexus between the service user and the practitioner, where the practitioner holds trust from the organization to carry out tasks to his/her best ability and in turn develops trust outward with service users. Individual service users always retain their freedom to choose how to respond, but also do well when they adapt their actions to their shifting understanding of their own needs.

In the vignette above, Claire was at a beginning stage of voicing despair and confusion, and hopefully would be able to shift her view of the world that had so completely changed for her to one that still recognized her capacity and skills. All communities and organizations are ideally interconnected to help individuals achieve their finest goals. Spiritual care keeps this social justice component in mind as it addresses the needs of service users where they are.

Spirituality defined

Spirituality has been defined in a number of ways across the disciplines. It is the essence of what it is to be human,[21,22] the ground of existence,[23] connection with a purpose, power, idea, or the self in a way considered sacred,[16] the unfolding and opening of the heart.[24] It may also be known through connection with angels, supernatural guides, or deceased loved ones; it is often experienced through connection with nature and all of life. Spiritual awareness develops across time through relationships with one's inner self, others, and the universe however one understands this.[25] Paradoxically, it may be both the totality of the person that is holistic and integrative or one dimension of many (biological, psychological, social, emotional, and spiritual). Spirituality may be related to religion or expressed apart from it. It is usually viewed as personal and individual, although it may have corporate or social elements. Any definition of spirituality should be expansive and inclusive enough so that the subtlety and complexity of how it is perceived is not diminished. Not only should the professional views of spirituality be discussed, but client views should also be solicited where these domains appear to be valued.[26]

Religion is often regarded as a subset of spirituality in the mental health professions and is defined as the beliefs, values, rituals, and practices shared in community and associated with a particular faith tradition.[6] In the realm of social care, spirituality may be life-affirming where new avenues are explored, or life-denying where such exploration is shut down or individuals feel oppressed or excluded by dogma or religious leaders, for example. Social engagement and social relationships fostered by faith communities are valuable functions of religion.[27] Existentialism is a related spiritual concept that denotes a fundamental task to find what determines one's own level of meaning in life.[28] Meaning is as personal and unique as is the spatial location of every molecule in an ocean, or one's image outlined against the backdrop of a deep blue sky.

Cultural environmental context

Culture consists of one's unique location on age, gender, ethnicity, race, and socioeconomic status among other traditional factors such as language, traditions, customs, rituals, expectations and goals shared by a group and transmitted across time. Culture is both a basis for spiritual beliefs and values and also defines the spiritual expression of these aspects. Individuals often carry both individual and collective spiritual identity.[7,29] Seeking information from a cultural framework helps differentiate both universal and specific worldviews—identifying where a service user matches or deviates from normative behaviour of their groups—and assists in creating trans- or cross-cultural connections in spirituality and religion between service user and practitioner.

Furthermore, spiritual beliefs and values usually do not remain stable and static, but evolve as a person encounters spiritual challenges and grows in spiritual ways. Physiological distress may also contain elements of psycho-spiritual distress, so engaging in spiritual discourse or dialogue helps clarify the nature of the need. In the Qur'an, Hindu, and Buddhist texts, suffering creates resolve 'sabr' and thus illness awakens one to the faculties of the heart,[26] leading to greater compassion.

Indigenous peoples, such as American Indians and Maori may believe that there is an integrating force in the universe that unites all living things, whether they are human or non-human.[30,5] Included in this are environmental elements such as lakes, hills, forests, and stones. Indeed, people who are sensitive to these integrating factors often feel a call to connect with nature, even though they lie in a hospital room. Spiritual symbols and rituals can be incorporated into any care plan, and can lead to greater self-understanding, forgiveness for self and others, hope, peace, joy, and compassion. The latter four attributes have the potential to lift one over immediate difficulty to see larger purpose and pattern. Often individuals facing serious health and social care issues cannot leap this hollow and empty place alone. Wellness involves encouraging and supporting self-determination, and honouring the values of the client that are not necessarily the same values held by a system of care.

Policies related to social care

In the UK, the *Equality Act (2006)* and the new *Equality Act (2010)* refer to the right to hold, or not hold, religious or other philosophical beliefs (e.g. humanism), and requires equal access to all public services regardless of sex, race, disability, gender, sexual orientation, and religion or belief. Local authorities, who deliver various forms of social care, must therefore ensure no one is disadvantaged by reason of religion or belief. Under the auspices of the Department of Health in England, various other policy documents require social care practitioners to assess the religious or spiritual needs of service users. Most notably, the personalization agenda[31] marks a major transformation in adult social care. Here, the prominence of holistic person-centred care recognizes the uniqueness of each individual in the assessment and care process, and an emphasis on self-directed support permits more user control and choice to identify what is personally important to them and how they would like to see support delivered. Similarly, the *Common Assessment Framework*[32] requires practitioners to assess religious and spiritual needs within the family of concern.

In England, the Primary Care Trusts oversee the delivery of healthcare, but work in close partnership with social care providers. Policy guidance within this sector is more explicit in its response to meeting the religious or spiritual needs of patients. For example, the *National Service Frameworks* provide national standards 'for respect for privacy and dignity, religious beliefs and people's spirituality.'[33, p. 5]. More specifically, the Department of Health[33] published *NHS Chaplaincy: Meeting the Religious and Spiritual Needs of Patients and Staff: Guidance for Managers and those Involved in the Provision of Chaplaincy-Spiritual Care* to set out a framework for best practice. While the focus is on in-patient healthcare, it would be expected that chaplaincy-spiritual care managers would link with community and social care providers as appropriate. Although there is support for consideration of spirituality in healthcare, some suggest that spirituality undermines society's secular principles and departs from evidence-based care.[34] However, a functional perspective understands that 'four fifths of those who use it [the NHS] and work for it are not secular' (p. 26) and lack of faith (or belief including secularism), fellowship, fulfilling work, and free giving (volunteerism) may be root causes of unhealthy behaviour.[34]

Increasingly, the role of spirituality in social care is entering into health policies in the USA. The Joint Commission accredits healthcare organizations and references attention to spiritual values, service user rights to pastoral and other spiritual services, and a psychosocial assessment that includes spirituality.[35] The content and format of the spiritual assessment adopted is left to the choice of the agency, but at a minimum it does need to ask about religious affiliation and beliefs or practices important to the service user. Spiritual assessment should be multidisciplinary and professional staff should receive training on conducting such assessment.[36]

A guide titled *Native American Spirituality* has been developed as an informational tool for healthcare providers.[37] This guide suggests that native healers should be considered 'an adjunct to treatment, not a barrier,' and should be appreciated for religious, spiritual, and psychological support. Religious ceremonies are a right protected by law and American Indians may integrate Native American rites with other mainstream religious practices, including requesting services from both a shaman or medicine man and a priest, for example. It is 'the policy of the United States to protect and preserve for American Indians their inherent right of freedom to believe, express, and exercise [their] traditional religions ... including, but not limited to ... use and possession of sacred objects, and the freedom to worship through ceremonials and traditional rites according to the American Indian Religious Freedom Act (US Code, Title 42, Chapter 21, Subchapter I, 1996 cited in[37]). Furthermore, since the government does not certify religious faith and some historically recognized Indian tribes have even been decertified, healthcare professionals should accept the validity of a person's faith declaration. These principles also could apply as guidance in providing care to any minority groups.

Education and training models

Developing spiritual competency, or the ability to gain knowledge, skills, and learn actions to facilitate work with service users on a transcultural basis, is a relatively new area for social care workers. This might include conducting assessments, listening for spiritual themes, and providing spiritual care or referral to those who are trained to provide it in deeper ways such as chaplains. For example, a qualitative study of 20 hospice patients found that they expected *any* healthcare professional to be able to meet spiritual needs, and to be able to elicit the priority of spirituality alongside other concerns in a sensitive manner, although they understood professionals with specialized training might be better able to meet needs of service users.[14] While this study was done in a palliative care in-patient setting, in many countries hospice is often just as likely to be provided in community settings. One model suggests that audits can provide evidence of competency through such mechanisms as multidisciplinary team discussions, case reviews, and even employee performance appraisals.[38] It is important to recognize that specific service workers will have different training needs depending on their professional roles. If provision of spiritual care remains a specialization of a few professions, there is a risk that spiritual needs will not be wholly met due to restricted reach and lack of availability at critical times.

Despite a growing interest in spiritual need and spiritual care,[39] explicit models for educating and training social care practitioners in the UK are not well documented. This gap is particularly noteworthy in social work.[40–43] More specifically, the General Social Care Council, which currently regulates training and practice in social work in England established a *Code of Practice for Social Care Workers* (2002) and makes no reference to either religion or spirituality.

A small body of existing research literature has also documented that social work practitioners and students report little to no content on religion and spirituality in their training. For example, a national survey of social workers in the UK found that 47% of respondents believed that religion and spirituality were important in social work practice, 76% indicated that they had received no content on religion and spirituality in their social work education, and 57% felt that social workers did not have the skills to assist service users with these matters.[43] Interestingly, even in

Northern Ireland, where religion is intimately bound within the lives of all citizens, religious content in social work education was reported to be absent.[43]

In the UK, Furness and Gilligan[44] and in the US Furman *et al.* [43] among others, suggest that training curricula in health and social care and social work models are essential given current practice complexities as a result of recent social trends (e.g. immigration). A more recent initiative is *Spirited Scotland*, an independent development that has attempted to foster greater awareness of spiritual issues in health and social care.[45] Using a variety of approaches, including funded research exploring spiritual need and spiritual care, *Spirited Scotland* emphasizes education and training in health and social care. Examples include multidisciplinary courses for practitioners to build confidence in dealing with spiritual issues and cultural competence, and local conferences on person-centred and spiritual care aimed at fostering networking between the statutory, private, and voluntary sectors and the acute and community sectors.

Another example is a general guide that targets healthcare staff training on religious issues, *Religion or Belief: A Practical Guide for the NHS* available online.[46] This guide provides a legal context on protections against discrimination and offers a view of the changing dynamics of religious adherence in the UK over a ten-year time span. It also suggests specific consideration of employee religious issues in the work environment, stressing the need for flexibility and respect. Along with practice content directed to patients and service users such as consideration given to patient dietary and clothing/modesty desires, this guide also includes a framework for action planning around religious content that intersects with the workplace and community. This type of training resource is helpful in providing both micro (individual level) and macro (policy and organizational level) information in managing religion and religious belief at work. Spirituality is addressed here in a more minor way, but overall this initiative does help fill a gap in British society.

In the USA a survey conducted in 2004 found that of 171 master's programmes in social work that were accredited or in candidacy status for accreditation, 57 offered a course with a spiritual or religious content with at least seven others planning to initiate such a course.[47] That number likely continues to expand. The inclusion of discussion and teaching about spirituality and religion related to clinical practice with clients in social work is supported by the social work profession in the US, including mandates from the National Association of Social Workers (NASW) and the Council on Social Work Education (CSWE).[48] Content on spiritual and religious diversity is considered important in understanding human behaviour. This approach is also supported by the Canadian Society for Spirituality in Social Work.[30]

The number of medical schools in the USA that offered courses on spirituality increased from three in 1992 to 84 in 2004.[49,50] Other chapters in this text will provide information on the increasing interest and need for spiritual training in medical education. Nursing literature, too, suggests that more attention needs to be given to developing spiritual competency in nursing care within institutional settings and the community.[51,52] Van Leeuwen *et al.*[53] review studies of nursing education related to building spiritual competence and suggest that nursing students who are exposed to specialized training in this area develop greater spiritual self-awareness, greater knowledge about spirituality, and a more holistic and client-centred approach to spiritual care. Nursing can also contribute to social care in the community through interdisciplinary collaboration with professionals working in schools and other community settings.[54]

Spiritual leadership in organizations

Spiritual leadership within organizations attends to the potential of the environment to promote spiritual growth for both service workers and users. Even as service workers attend to multidimensional needs of clients, they also benefit when the organizations in which they work allow them opportunities to reflect on experiences in the workplace and their meaning.[55] While chaplains are often considered spiritual care experts within health facilities, not all health facilities or places where health and social care are delivered have access to chaplains. Social workers, occupational therapists, and nurses especially interact with service users in the community. It is thus particularly valuable when the organizations that sponsor them are able to offer ongoing training in such areas as spiritual assessment and offer time and space for collective reflection on their work.[56] This ongoing reflection may arise at points of daily need, as part of weekly team meetings, monthly meetings, or accomplished in retreat forms. It is important that the reflection period be non-denominational in tone, and open to many forms of spiritual and/or religious expression, inclusive rather than exclusive. In this context, even people who report being non-spiritual, non-religious may be able to remain connected and feel their experiences are accepted and appreciated.

Controversies in spiritual care provision

A concern has been raised in the literature about government sponsorship of programs that include holistic care.[57] In pre-World War II Germany, some social welfare programmes, such as preventive care for 'overwhelmed mothers' were connected to ideological purposes. While government initiatives can ensure standards of care are met, there still must be room for local programmes to integrate social and spiritual care. In this current tighter economic climate, for local programmes to survive, higher costs of providing service need to be justified by their effectiveness, effectiveness that includes measuring the effect of spiritual care. Thus, according to Hofman, 'spiritual care becomes a question of visible effects and measurable quantities.'[58, p. 144]

Another critique about provision of spiritual care comes from the hospice literature. A concern has arisen that spirituality has become 'politicized.'[58] Focus on religious supports has been marginalized in favour of a spiritual discourse that is thought to have broad appeal, but in fact may be disrespectful to those who are atheist, as well as those who identify as strongly religious. In the USA particularly, people of colour who may tend to be more religious are less likely to utilize hospice services.[59,60] There is a question about whether spirituality has become a cultural alternative to religion, rather than an adjunct to it. These criticisms remind us that provision of spiritual care in the community needs to find balance, as well as meet prevailing standards of effectiveness.

Ethical dimensions of practice

Social care in the community needs to abide by ethical standards, most especially in addressing spiritual concerns. Value clarity is important for social care professionals to seek through self-reflection prior to assessing spiritual care needs and as spiritual needs arise *in situ*.[16] While chaplains, priests, ministers, imams, shamans, and other religious leaders would typically be sought for singular religious problems, in health and community care, spiritual distress may arise in the context of other needs. Thus, community religious leaders may be brought in as part of a treatment team or involved as referral resources. However, social care professionals should be adequately trained to direct the work of the team in a holistic manner, including collaboration on addressing spiritual need. Some helping professionals may feel more adequately prepared both through specialized study and personal interest to discuss aspects of spiritual care. Chaplains are particularly trained for this, however, in the event they are not available, spiritual care should still be provided if desired. Other trained professionals may experience a certain comfort level in this domain, but some may be highly uncomfortable, finding such conversations difficult and awkward. Personal comfort levels in working with spiritual concerns are important to take into consideration, and professionals should not be forced to move beyond their zone of comfort or level of expertise.

There are several provisions of the ethical code of practice for social work that indirectly or directly address religion in care. Other professional codes such as nursing and psychology also address standards that seek to protect clients from inadequate or harmful practice in this area. Competency is one important provision. Practicing at a level consistent with one's level of competency is in accord with professional codes of conduct including the National Association of Social Workers (US) code *1.04 Competence* that asks social workers to work within the bounds of their education, training, and professional experience.[61] However, social workers also are asked to demonstrate competence in social care that recognizes culture difference and to understand the nature of social diversity concerning religion. The language of faith varies greatly, especially across religious traditions. Social workers should refer service users when additional expertise is needed to fully serve clients, particularly in understanding and responding to religious nuances.

Awareness of potential conflicts of interest is also crucial. Service user preferences need to be honoured by professionals. Professionals must never take advantage of the vulnerability of others and the natural power imbalance between professional and service user to proselytize or press their own religious, non-religious, or spiritual viewpoints. This kind of practice is always exploitive and disrespects service user choice. Some religious and spiritual beliefs may be so private or sacred (such as in aboriginal, American Indian, or other indigenous tribes) that service users may not wish to discuss them publicly. These beliefs should also not be included in records to respect patient preferences. Furthermore, some spiritual or religious beliefs may diverge from the interests of the service worker in providing efficient or what the professional deems to be most effective or 'best practice' care. However, opening up dialogue in spiritual areas and asking questions that can help service users such as Claire Stewart (in the chapter vignette) come to terms with their illness or assist them in coping are always well-advised. When one follows a service user's lead rather than proposing a certain direction in spiritual care, a professional will typically be protected from ethical violations and concomitantly promote the service user's dignity and wellbeing in the community.

Evaluation and outcomes of spiritual care

Evaluation of spiritual care is a different form of measurement than many typical healthcare measures which detail the types of care provided and the amount of time allotted to care provision. In fact some evaluation possibilities lie outside of standard measures. Quantitative and qualitative measures offer complementary tools to determine quality of spiritual care as one facet of social care in health settings. Quantitative tools may consist simply of documentation of whether any type of spiritual assessment was completed and whether a community referral, or spiritual type of helping activity, was provided. Rapid assessment tools to measure bereavement or spiritual practices, repeated over time, can assist professional service workers in determining positive coping. Spirituality, too, has multidimensional components which make measurement perplexing. There are many tools to assess different dimensions of spirituality and religion such as belief, attitudes, commitment, organizational religiousness and orientation, coping, use of spiritual practices, etc.,[62–64] but not all would meet the needs for use in a social care setting. Further research is needed to study instrument use in different settings and with multireligious and multispiritual populations.

Qualitative spiritual tools allow a richer base for understanding of unique aspects of the interactive components of care as well as a service user's perception of positive change. Global measures such as a spiritual assessment or spiritual history (longer in-depth form) may be completed. Interview guides may elicit information about life meaning and purpose, guilt, shame, forgiveness, and other areas of spiritual distress as well as spiritual strengths.[16] Life review work often may touch on spiritual development over the lifespan. Spiritual care in the community understands that in many situations professional responses must be open-ended, understanding that sometimes there is no answer, except to share one's presence with an individual and to listen.

In a quality improvement framework, the structure and process of care can each be considered. One well-developed protocol for assessing spiritual care standards is provided in a document titled *Standards for Spiritual Care Services in the NHS in Wales 2010*.[65] This document addresses seven standards including: spiritual and religious care; access to spiritual care services; working with faith communities and belief groups; staff support; education, training, and research; resources, and spiritual care to the hospital or unit. An opportunity for a self-audit in this same document asks such questions as. 'How do you ensure that patients have had the opportunity for their spiritual and religious needs to be assessed and addressed? (Describe the process and how audited).'[65, p. 15] Outcomes sought include not only patient satisfaction with the service provided, but also a positive change in quality of life, where possible.

Conclusion

Spirituality in social care is a relatively new area of interest. Until now, much of the interest centred on attention to spiritual care was directed to in-patient facilities rather than community care. The spiritual discourse has often been a hidden discourse. Service users were not comfortable disclosing intimate spiritual beliefs with care workers and care workers were less than enthusiastic about creating space for this. Sometimes this was due to their own discomfort with clients who were more spiritual than they were and sometimes because of perceived questions about agency and other organizational support for its inclusion.

Spiritually-sensitive practice suggests that the goals of social care are to include a place for a conversation about spirituality and its potential to enhance quality of life. If it is of interest to the service user, it can be included in the work. If it is not of interest, it can be dropped from further engagement. As the opening chapter vignette with Claire suggested, at times of health crisis, spiritual concerns may be elevated. Professional service users should prepare in advance to assess this area, and increasingly there is both information available in the community and support to do this.

From an organizational standpoint, we recommend the following as best practices in supporting the interaction of social care with spirituality:

1. Just as they would with any important life domain that has potential to affect health trajectories, professional service workers should routinely include some form of preliminary assessment of *first,* the role of spirituality and/or religion in the service user's life, and *secondly*, whether the client wishes these to be directly included in care or does not
2. Organizations should identify spiritual assessment and spiritual history tools that have particular relevance to their mission statement, and can capture movement towards change that provides information for quality improvement. These tools should be specific enough to provide unique service user information, but have some components that are general enough for comparability
3. Employees with direct service user contact, whether they themselves are spiritual or religious or not, should be required to participate in training about use of these tools that includes discussions about ethical parameters
4. Spiritual care is a skilled task. It is best to include service workers who have particular training in pastoral or spiritual care and to collaborate with spiritual leaders in the community with whom service user views are aligned. Organizational protocol for guidance in collaboration and to protect service user rights should be developed
5. Direction for spiritual care through and by service workers should be included in organizational policy
6. An organizational director should delegate monitoring of important published research findings in this area and ongoing development of best practice standards, particularly in provision of multi-faith, interdenominational religious and spiritual care
7. Within the organization, a culture of respect for team member spiritual and religious views should be fostered, as well as attention given to such spiritual concerns as compassion fatigue of staff. Employees should be considered as invaluable resources and encouraged to become all they can be in environments that promote resilience and appreciate diversity
8. All employees should take responsibility for the co-creation of organizational environments that include balance and heart to support staff in their difficult work with service users.

Inclusion of spirituality in social care involves attention to a complex interplay of individual service user perceptions, service worker perceptions, organizational supports or lack of supports, and background characteristics of the larger ebb and flow of spiritual and religious interests in society. This is a dynamic environment, but one that cannot be ignored. Preparing our organizations to better understand what spirituality is and how it should be addressed in the workplace will help create learning and healing environments for both professional staff and service users.

References

1 Pew Forum on Religion & Public Life. Pew Forum on Religion & Public Life. (2010). *US religious landscape survey: report*. Available at: http://religions.pewforum.org/reports (accessed 19 October 2010).

2 Association for Religious Data Archives (2010). *National Profiles*. Available at: http://www.thearda.com/internationalData/intmap.asp (accessed 16 January 2012).

3 D'Zurilla, T.J., Nezu, A. (2007). *Problem-solving Therapy: A Positive Approach to Clinical Intervention.* New York: Springer.

4 Greenstreet, W. (ed.) (2006). *Integrating Spirituality in Health and Social Care: Perspectives and Practical Approaches.* Oxford: Radcliffe Publishing.

5 Nash, M., Stewart, B. (2002).*Spirituality and Social Care: Contributing to Personal and Community Well-being.* London: Jessica Kingsley Publishers.

6 Canda, E.R., Furman, L.D. (1999). *Spiritual Diversity in Social Work Practice: The Heart of Helping.* NewYork: Free Press.

7 Canda, E.R., Furman, L.D. (2010). *Spiritual Diversity in Social Work Practice: the Heart of Helping*, 2nd edn. New York: Oxford Press.

8 Sulmasy, D.P. (2002). A biopsychosocial-spiritual model for the care of service users at the end of life. *Gerontologist* **42**(Spec 3): 24–33.

9 Marty, M.E. (1980). Social service: Godly and godless. *Soc Serv Rev* **54**: 463–81.

10 Nelson-Becker, H. (2005). Religion and coping in older adults: a social work perspective. *J. Gerontolog Soc Work* **45**(1/2): 51–68.

11 Association for Spiritual Ethical Religious Values in Counseling, ASERVIC. (2009). *Competencies for Addressing Spiritual and Religious Issues in Counseling.* Available at: http://aservic.org/?page_id = 133 (accessed 18 August 2010).

12 Council on Social Work Education (2008). *Educational policy and accreditation standards.* Available at: http://www.cswe.org/File.aspx?id=13780 (accessed 8 July 2010).

13 Miner-Williams, D. (2006). Putting a puzzle together: making spirituality meaningful for nursing using an evolving theoretical framework. *J Clin Nurs* **15**(7): 811–21.

14 Yardley, S., Walshe, C., Parr, A. (2009). Improving training in spiritual care: A qualitative study exploring patient perceptions of professional educational requirements. *Palliat Med* **23**(7): 601–7.

15 Milstein, J.M. (2008). Introducing spirituality in medical care: transition from hopelessness to wholeness. *J Am Med Ass* **299**(20): 2440–1.

16 Nelson-Becker, H., Nakashima, M., Canda, E. (2006). Spirituality in professional helping interventions. In: B. Berkman, S. D'Ambruoso (eds) *Handbook of Social Work in Health and Aging*, pp. 797–807. New York: Oxford University Press.

17 Rumbold, B. (2006). The spirituality of compassion: a public health response to ageing and end-of-life care. *J Relig Spirit Aging* **18**(2/3): 31–44.

18 The Joint Commission (2010). *Spiritual Assessment.* Available at: http://www.jointcommission.org/accreditationprograms/longtermcare/standards/09_faqs/pc/spiritual-assessment.htm(accessed 16 January 2012)

19 Carozza, P.G. (2003). Subsidiarity as a structural principle of international human rights law. *Am J Int Law* **97**(1): 38–79.

20 Consedine, J. (2003). Spirituality and social justice. In: M. Nash, B. Stewart, (eds) *Spirituality and Social Care*, pp. 49–68. London: Jessica Kingsley Publishers.

21 Teilhard de Chardin, P. (1959). *The Phenomenon of Man*. New York: Harper.
22 Carroll, M. (1998). Social work's conceptualization of spirituality. *Soc Thought: J Relig Soc Sci* **18**(2): 1–14.
23 Tillich, P. (1963). *The Eternal Now*. New York: Scribner.
24 Hanh, T.N. (2001). *Anger: Wisdom for Cooling the Flames*. New York: Penguin/Putnam.
25 James, W. (1982). *The Varieties of Religious Experience*. New York: Penguin Books.
26 Khan, F. (2008). An Islamic appraisal of minding the gap: Psycho-spiritual dynamics in the doctor-patient relationship. *J Relig Eth* **36**(1): 77–96.
27 Wulff, D.M. (1997). *Psychology of Religion: Classic and Contemporary Views*. New York: John Wiley & Sons.
28 Nelson-Becker, H. (2006). Voices of resilience: older adults in hospice care. *J Soc Work End-of-life Palliat Care* **2**(3): 87–106.
29 Lee, M.Y., Ng, S., Leung, P.P., Chan, C.L. (2009). *Integrative Body-mind-spirit Social Work*. New York: Oxford Press.
30 Graham, J.R., Coholic, D., Coates, J. (2007). Spirituality as a guiding construct in the development of Canadian social work: Past and present considerations. In: Canadian Scholars' Press (eds) *Spirituality and social work: Selected Canadian readings*,. pp. 23–46. Toronto: Canadian Scholars' Press.
31 Department of Health. (2007). *Putting People First: A Shared Vision and Commitment to the Transformation of Adult Social Care*. London: Stationary Office.
32 Children's Workforce Development Council. (2009). *The Common Assessment Framework for Children and Young People: Practitioner's Guide*. Leeds: CWDC.
33 Department of Health. (2003). *NHS Chaplaincy: Meeting the Religious and Spiritual Needs of Patients and Staff: Guidance for Managers and Those Involved in the Provision of Chaplaincy-spiritual Care*. Available at: http://www.dh.gov.uk/en/Publicationsandstatistics/Publications/PublicationsPolicyAndGuidance/DH_4062016. (accessed 11 January 2012).
34 Wright, S. (2009). Believe it or not—religion has a place in NHS care. *Nurs Standard* **23**(47): 26.
35 Joint Commission. (2008). *Comprehensive Accreditation Manual for Hospitals*. Oak Brook; JCAHO,
36 Joint Commission. (2005). *The Source*. **3**(2): 6–7.
37 Manataka American Indian Council (2006). *Native American spirituality*. Available at: http://www.blueskywaters.com/page_82.pdf (accessed 23 October 2010).
38 Marie Curie Cancer Care (2003). *Spiritual and Religious Care Competencies for Specialist Palliative Care*. Available at: http://www.mariecurie.org.uk/forhealthcareprofessionals/spiritualandreligiouscare (accessed 23 September 2010).
39 Holloway M. (2007). Spiritual need and the core business of social work. *Br J Soc Work* **37**: 265–80.
40 Gilligan, P. (2003). 'It isn't discussed': religion, belief and practice teaching—missing components of cultural competence is social work education. *J Pract Teach Hlth Soc Care* **15**(1): 75–95.
41 Furness, S. (2003). Religion, belief and culturally competent practice. *J Pract Teach Hlth Soc Care* **15**(1): 61–74.
42 Gilligan, P., Furness, S. (2006). The role of religion and spirituality in social work practice: Views and experiences of social workers and students. *Br J Soc Work* **36**: 617–37.
43 Furman, L.D., Benson, P.W., Grimwood, C., Canda, E. (2004). Religion and spirituality in social work education and direct practice at the millennium: a survey of UK social workers. *Br J Soc Work* **34**: 67–792.
44 Furness S., Gilligan P. (2010). Social work, religion and belief: Developing a framework for practice. *Br J Soc Work* **40**(7): 2185–202.
45 Mowat, H., Ryan, D. (2003). Spiritual issues in health and social care: practice into policy? *J Relig Gerontol* **14**(1): 51–67.
46 Department of Health (2009). *Religion or Belief: A Practical Guide for the NHS*. [updated 2009 Jan 5; cited 2010 Sept 19]. Available at: http://www.dh.gov.uk/en/Publicationsandstatistics/Publications/PublicationsPolicyAndGuidance/DH_093133 (accessed 11 January 2012).
47 Russel, R., Ferraro, G., Russo, A. (2005). *The development of MSW courses with a spiritual or religious focus*. Paper presented at the meeting of the Council on Social Work Education, New York, Feb 26th–March 4th, 2005.
48 Barker, S. (2007). The integration of spirituality and religion content in social work education: where we've been, where we're going. *Soc Work Christ* **34**(2): 146–66.
49 Nash, D.B., Yuen, E. (c2009) The role of spirituality in healthcare. *Medpage Today*, June 16. Available at: http://www.medpagetoday.com/columns/FocusonPolicy/14725 (accessed 16 January 2012).
50 Puchalski, C.M. (2006). Spirituality and medicine: curricula in medical education. *J Cancer Educ* **21**(1): 14–18.
51 McSherry, W. (2006). *Making Sense of Spirituality in Nursing and Healthcare Practice: An Interactive Approach*. London: Jessica Kingsley Publishers.
52 Ross, L. (2006). Spiritual care in nursing: an overview of the research to date. *J Clin Nurs* **15**(7): 852–62.
53 Van Leeuwen, R., Tiesinga, L.J., Middel, B., Post, D., Jochemsen, H. (2008). The effectiveness of an educational programme for nursing students on developing competence in the provision of spiritual care. *J Clin Nurs* **17**(20): 2768–81.
54 Stern, J., James, S. (2006). Every person matters: enabling spirituality education for nurses. *J Clin Nurs* **15**(7): 897–904.
55 Burkhart, L., Solari-Twadell, P.A., Haas, S. (2008). Addressing spiritual leadership: an organizational model. *J Nurs Adm* **38**(1): 33–9.
56 Puchalski, C., Ferrell, B. (2010). *Making Healthcare Whole: Integrating Spirituality into Patient Care*. West Conshohocken: Templeton Press.
57 Hofmann, B. (2009). Health and nurturing for body, mind, and soul: The German Muttergenesungswerk between family politics and healthcare. *Christ Bioeth* **15**(2): 136–46.
58 Garces-Foley, K. (2006). Hospice and the politics of spirituality. *Omega* **53**(1/2): 117–36.
59 Reese, D.J., Ahern, R.E., Nair, S., O'Faire, J.D., Warren, C. (1999). Hospice access and use by African Americans: Addressing cultural and institutional barriers through participatory action research. *Soc Work* **44**(6): 549–59.
60 US Census Bureau (2000). *State and County Quick Facts. Data derived from Population Estimates, 2000 Census of Population and Housing*. Washington DC: US Census Bureau. Available at: http://quickfacts.census.gov/qfd/states/00000.html (accessed 23 July 2010).
61 National Association of Social Workers (2008). *Code of Ethics*. Available at: http://www.socialworkers.org/pubs/code/code.asp (accessed 16 January 2012).
62 Fetzer Institute. (1999). *Multidimensional Measurement of Religiousness/Spirituality for Use in Health Research*. Kalamazoo: Fetzer Institute.
63 Hill, P.C., Hood, R.W. (1999). *Measures of Religiosity*. Birmingham: Religious Education Press.
64 Nelson-Becker, H. (2005). Development of a spiritual support scale for use with older adults. *J Hum Behav Soc Environ* **11**(3/4): 195–212.
65 NHS Wales (2010). *Standards for Spiritual Care Services in the NHS in Wales 2010*. Available at: http://wales.gov.uk/docs/dhss/publications/100525spiritualcarestandardsen.pdf (accessed 23 November 2010).

CHAPTER 56A

Curriculum development, courses, and CPE

Part I: Curriculum development in spirituality and health in the health professions

Christina M. Puchalski, Mark Cobb, and Bruce Rumbold

Introduction

Curriculum development in Spirituality and Health, which focuses on formal teaching of this topic, is a relatively new field within medicine, nursing and other health professions, in terms of formal courses in this subject area. Inspired by the advances of scientific technology, medical, and nursing schools focuses their training primarily on the scientific and technical aspects of their disciplines. It is important to note that, historically, some aspects of spirituality, which included religion, ethics, and caring presence, were part of medicine and nursing academic settings. However, spirituality was gradually omitted in favour of the technical and biomedical aspects, with the humanities and other non-technical subject matter deemed less important. In this chapter we are focusing primarily on major efforts in the USA, UK, and Australia. We also cover pastoral counselling, spiritual direction, and chaplaincy as these professionals work closely within the health system to provide spiritual care for patients and families.

United States perspectives

Medical schools

In the mid-1980s in United States, a few medical schools, particularly schools associated with a particular religious denomination, developed courses in religious traditions and healthcare, or included religious values as part of ethics courses. In 1993 only three US medical schools provided teaching on religious and spiritual issues as applied to medicine;[1,2] this figure has since risen to over 80% of medical school schools.[3] Now, more than 100 US medical schools have such training. This increase is in part due to a John Templeton Foundation funded programme entitled the GWish Spirituality and Medical Education Program directed by the George Washington Institute for Spirituality and Health at the George Washington University.[3] This was a competitive award programme in which medical schools proposed a curriculum in spirituality and health, and the curricula were rigorously judged by leading academic deans and curriculum faculty. Schools with the highest score were given a small amount of funding to develop their curricula. Interestingly, even schools that were not awarded funding, but who applied to the award programme developed courses in spirituality and health. Anecdotal evidence supports the idea that this was driven by schools' interest in developing courses that humanized the curriculum.

The first required medical school course in Spirituality and Health, with spirituality broadly defined, was developed at the George Washington University School of Medicine and Health Sciences in Washington, DC.[2,3] A committee of faculty and community clinicians helped develop it as an elective in 1992; four years later, the course was integrated into the four-year medical school curriculum. The strengths of the curriculum and perhaps one reason it was accepted was that the course built on existing goals of the medical school to enhance more holistic, person-centred care through curricular changes. The curriculum in spirituality and health also met the goals of the Medical School Objectives Project, an Association of American Medical Colleges (AAMC) ten-year project to change medical school education with increased focus on humanities, communication skills, and compassion.[4] Thus, when the Awards for Curriculum Development Program was started other medical schools could also build upon other programmatic curricular goals which courses in spiritual could support.

Awards for Curriculum Development for Medical Schools have recognized the best curriculum proposals and brought oversight to the integration process at award recipients' schools, medical schools have implemented such courses in their own fashion, resulting in a wide variety of topics, pedagogies, and timelines—and different definitions of the knowledge, attitudes, and specific patient-care competencies medical students should attain from these courses. Since the inception of this programme, now known as the GWish Curricular Awards in Spirituality and Health, there has been significant success integrating spiritual care in the healthcare practices taught by US medical schools and building consensus among national organizations regarding the significant role spirituality plays in patient-focused, quality healthcare. Currently 80% of US medical and osteopathic schools offer courses in spirituality and health—a marked increase from the few schools that taught courses about twenty years ago.[3]

A significant factor in the development of curricula in spirituality and health has been the partnership with the Association of American Medical Colleges (AAMC). In response to empirical, ethical and philosophical principles, the Association of American Medical Colleges (AAMC), the World Health Organization (WHO), and the Joint Commission on Accreditation of Healthcare Organizations (JCAHO) recommended including spirituality in clinical care and education.[5] In collaboration with the Association of American Medical Colleges (AAMC), the work of GWish has had impact on medical education in this subject area. Learning objectives and criteria for teaching were developed in 1998 with the AAMC, but with the development of courses, the field has developed substantially and has increased the sophistication of teaching as well as content of learning objectives.[4]

The support of the AAMC occurred because the objectives of the course in Spirituality and Health that were beginning to be developed in the early 1990s were aligned with a larger national curricular initiative led by the AAMC. In 1998, the Association of American Medical Colleges (AAMC), responding to concerns by the medical professional community that young doctors lacked humanitarian skills related to patient-centred care, undertook the Medical School Objectives Project (MSOP). The final project report notes, 'Physicians must be compassionate and empathetic in caring for patients ... they must act with integrity, honesty, respect for patients' privacy, and respect for the dignity of patients as persons. In all of their interactions with patients they must seek to understand the meaning of the patients' stories in the context of the patients' and family, and cultural beliefs and values.'[4]

In the follow-up MSOP III report, published in 1999, the AAMC further supported the development of courses in spirituality and health in medical schools by identifying seven spirituality-related learning objectives medical students should demonstrate to the satisfaction of faculty prior to graduation. The objectives include the ability to elicit a spiritual history and a cultural history, an understanding that the spiritual dimension of people's lives is an avenue for compassionate care-giving and the ability to apply that understanding to a patient's spirituality, knowledge of research data on the impact of spirituality on health and healthcare outcomes, an understanding of and respect for the role of clergy and other spiritual leaders, and an understanding of their own spirituality and how it can be nurtured as part of professional growth.[6]

One of the recommendations of this report was to encourage schools to develop spirituality content in a vertically integrated required curriculum. Thus, spiritual history was integrated into the part of the curriculum that taught history-taking; spirituality and chronic illness into the problem-based learning case that dealt with chronic illness, and spirituality as a way people understand illness was integrated into a humanities course. Thus, spirituality is a theme that is woven into a curriculum and integrated in such a way as it is part of the whole patient care. It is not just a course that students learn in one year, but not integrate more fully in the understanding of the whole patient. It is also a theme that recurs throughout the four year curriculum and is thus reinforced in the student's learning. A sample curriculum is included in Table 56.1. For other examples see www.gwish.org.

Chaplains play a role as faculty in the United States medical schools, particularly in sessions that involve communication skills, ethics, and compassion. In some primary care residency programmes, and palliative care fellowship programmes, residents and fellows shadow chaplains to get a better understanding of the role of spirituality in the care of the patient, what chaplains do and

Table 56.1 Spirituality and medicine course at George Washington University School of Medicine and Health Sciences

Year 1 *Required*	POM* 1: Taking a spiritual history (integrated with history taking course) Compassionate presence, attentive listening integrated throughout POM 1 & 2 communication skills Reflections on gross anatomy Service of Remembrance for body donors Humanities courses include spirituality, art and humanities themes integrated Problem-based learning where spiritual issues are integrated into cases
Year 2 *Required*	POM 2: Spirituality and chronic illness: breaking bad news PBL: problem-based learning cases where spiritual issues are integrated into cases
Year 3 *Required*	POM 3: Spirituality and end-of-life care Self-care Professionalism Medicine clerkship: GWish-Templeton reflective rounds
Year 4 *Elective*	POM 4: Palliative care Spirituality integrated as required domain of palliative care Additional lectures to physical therapy, physician assistant students, as well as residents

*Practice of Medicine (POM) is a four-year integrated required curriculum in which spirituality is integrated as part of larger courses.

how the resident or fellow can address spiritual issues with patients and families.

In addition to medical schools the John Templeton Foundation with the National Institutes for Health Research (NIHR), and later GWish also funded primary care and psychiatry residency programs in spirituality and health curricular development. In psychiatry, specific learning objectives were developed which formed the basis of what is now a requirement within the American Psychiatric Association to teach spirituality, religion and mental health.[7]

Canadian medical schools and residency programs also competed for the awards in spirituality and health; several of those programs developed some course material particularly in psychiatry.[8] One of the awardees built her course on data she gathered from clinicians and patients that demonstrated a patient desire to have their clinicians address patient spirituality.[8] A needs assessment survey was done in 2005, which demonstrated an interest by the Deans of several of the medical colleges in exploring spirituality in the context of cultural competency courses or palliative care.[9]

Spirituality-based medical school national competencies

While the number of medical schools addressing the role of spirituality in medicine is impressive, the growing variances in content and approach are of significant concern, as well as a major impediment to gathering outcome data. Medical schools continue to implement spirituality courses in their own fashion, resulting in a wide variety of topics, pedagogies, and timelines—and differing skills, knowledge, and attitudes medical students are to attain from these courses. These variances have contributed to the absence of large-scale, long-term research on the impact of spirituality courses on medical students' spiritual competency and consequent clinical outcomes.

In addition, most curricula in spirituality and health assess student satisfaction or self-reported changes in attitudes or knowledge using institution-based evaluation methodologies. Competency-focused outcome assessments are lacking primarily because no national spirituality-related competencies or widely accepted evaluation model exist. Most curricula in spirituality and health do not assess competency outcomes, focusing instead on assessing student satisfaction or self-reported changes in attitudes or knowledge.[10,1]

Evaluation methodologies and analysis also are institution-based, lacking an outcomes orientation primarily because no national or widely accepted model exists. Recent reviews of resident research, as well as evidence-based health curricula reveal that few programmes utilize sophisticated evaluation methodologies that address competency or patient outcomes.[11,12]

The AAMC summarized the lack of outcomes research and the impact medical education has on patient care, 'There is a lack of empirical evidence of the relationship between medical preparation (education and training) and the quality of care. While it is presumed that more comprehensive education and training better prepares a physician to provide high quality of care, there have not been studies to confirm this. It is also possible that certain types or elements of education and training may have a greater impact on some physician activities than other activities. Given the national concern with quality and outcomes, additional resources should be invested in research in this area.'[13]

To address these challenges, GWish led a F.I.S.H. Foundation-sponsored 2009 National Initiative to Develop Competencies in Spirituality for Medical Education (NIDCSME) that was based on the courses developed in Spirituality and Health over the past 15 years. The NIDCSME developed competency behaviours in healthcare systems, knowledge, compassionate presence, patient care, personal and professional development, and communications through a consensus process. These competences provide standards for learning objectives, teaching methods and evaluation that can be used to address these challenges. (See Figure 56.1) These competencies are based in the already accepted The Accreditation Council for Graduate Medical Education (ACGME) competencies for residency training and add compassionate presence as its own category given the importance of presence in clinical care.[14]

Twenty-seven representatives from eight medical schools, which were competitively chosen, participated in the National Initiative to Develop Competencies in Spirituality for Medical Education. Using the framework of the ACGME competencies, participants formulated spirituality-related competencies for medical students and the behaviours, teaching methods, and assessment tools required to demonstrate student attainment of those competencies.

GWish-Templeton reflective rounds for medical students

Building upon a clinical interprofessional spiritual care consensus conference (National Consensus Conference, further described in Chapter 29) where spirituality was linked to personal and professional development of clinicians, the GWISH developed a clinical course titled GWish-Templeton Reflective Rounds funded by the John Templeton Foundation. The G-TRR focus on students' personal and professional formation through the exploration of spirituality in the context of self and patient care. The reflection guide that schools are using is based on the verbatim used in CPE education (see Part II of this Chapter). Medical schools in the USA are currently implementing these rounds and looking at student outcomes, such as burn-out, depression, spiritual wellbeing, and being patient centred. By focusing on a student's inner life or spirituality it is anticipated that these outcomes will improve, with less student burnout and depression, and increased spiritual wellbeing and patient centredness.[15] GWish is also piloting a reflection mentor programme as a part of professionalism in which students will have a group reflection process, based on group spiritual direction led by a trained reflection mentor. The goal of these two programs is to focus on formation of students as future physicians integrating their inner life or spiritual development as part of their professional development.

Nursing

Most nursing theories are based on a dynamic and holistic view of the human individual as a biological, psychological, social, and spiritual being. Nursing theories include aspects of spirituality in patient care, directly or indirectly, including caring,[16] interpersonal relationship,[17] and spiritual variables.[18] In addition, one of six essential features of professional nursing practice is the establishment of a caring relationship to facilitate health and healing.[19] Spirituality has actually been described as the 'cornerstone of holistic nursing practice',[20] and as 'the integrating aspect of human wholeness . . .integral to quality care'.[21] In 1978, the

#	Competency	Observed Behaviors	Pedagogical Methods (see page 2)	Performance Assessments (see page 2)
HCS1	Health Care Systems	Describe the importance of incorporating spiritual care into a healthcare system	Health Care Systems: 8, 10, 15, 18, 19, 22, 24, 31, 32, 33, 34, 35, 36, 41, 44, 49	Health Care Systems: 1, 2, 3, 4, 8, 13, 14, 15, 16, 20
HCS2	Health Care Systems	Describe and evaluate spiritual resources in a healthcare system and a community		
HCS3	Health Care Systems	Compare and contrast spiritual resources in different healthcare systems		
HCS4	Health Care Systems	Discuss the ways in which healthcare systems may complicate spiritual care		
HCS5	Health Care Systems	Describe methods of reimbursement for spiritual care, including funding for other disciplines (e.g., nursing, chaplains, counseling)		
HCS6	Health Care Systems	Discuss how the legal, political and economic factors of healthcare influence spiritual care		
HCS7	Health Care Systems	Explain how effective spiritual care impacts the overall quality of and improvements to patient care		
HCS8	Health Care Systems	Describe how spiritual care is provided by interdisciplinary team members and community resources		
HCS9	Health Care Systems	Apply advocacy skills to spiritual care within healthcare systems (e.g., local, regional, national)		
K1	Knowledge	Compare and contrast spirituality (broadly defined) and religion	Knowledge: 8, 18, 20, 22, 24, 34, 36, 41, 43, 44, 46, 48, 49	Knowledge: 2, 4, 7, 8, 9,11,12, 13, 15, 20, 23
K2	Knowledge	Discuss the relationships between spirituality, religious beliefs, and cultural traditions		
K3	Knowledge	Describe how spirituality interrelates with complementary and alternative medicine		
K4	Knowledge	Discuss major religious traditions as they relate to patient care and patient decision making		
K5	Knowledge	Differentiate between a spiritual history, spiritual screening, and spiritual assessment		
K6	Knowledge	Describe common religious/spiritual problems that arise in clinical care		
K7	Knowledge	Compare and contrast sources of spiritual strength and spiritual distress		
K8	Knowledge	Differentiate between spirituality and psychological factors (e.g., grief, hope, meaning)		
K9	Knowledge	Describe boundary issues in providing spiritual care		
K10	Knowledge	Outline key findings of spirituality-health research		
K11	Knowledge	Locate and evaluate spiritual/religious information resources (online and hard copy)		
K12	Knowledge	Describe how a patient's spirituality may affect his/her context-specific clinical care		
CP1	Comp Presence	Discuss why it is a privilege to serve the patient	Compassionate Presence: 1, 5, 8, 8, 11, 12, 16, 18, 20, 21, 22, 26, 27, 31, 32, 34, 35, 36,38, 39, 40, 41, 42, 43, 44, 45, 46, 47	Compassionate Presence: 1, 2, 3, 4, 7, 13, 14, 16, 19, 20
CP2	Comp Presence	Describe personal and external factors that limit your ability to be fully "present" with a given patient		
CP3	Comp Presence	Discuss why the illness experience of the patient is an essential element of the physician-patient relationship		
CP4	Comp Presence	Discuss how you as a provider may be changed by your relationship with the patient		
CP5	Comp Presence	Demonstrate the ability to be engaged and fully "present" with a patient		
CP6	Comp Presence	Describe strategies to be more present with patients		
PC1	Patient Care	Appropriately utilize patients' spiritual network and supports	Patient Care: 1, 2,4, 5, 7, 8, 9, 11, 12, 13, 14, 15, 16, 17, 18, 20, 22, 23, 24,25, 26, 27, 2, 29, 32, 34, 45, 36, 40, 41, 42, 43, 44, 45, 46, 47, 48, 49	Patient Care: 2, 4, 5, 7, 8, 10, 12, 13, 18, 20, 23
PC2	Patient Care	Perform a detailed spiritual history at appropriate times (e.g., complete medical history, giving bad news)		
PC3	Patient Care	Perform spiritual screening at appropriate time		
PC4	Patient Care	Perform ongoing assessment of patient's spiritual distress		
PC5	Patient Care	Integrate patient's spiritual issues and resources into ongoing treatment and discharge plans		
PC6	Patient Care	Collaborate with staff, family, pastoral care and other members of healthcare team to address patient's spiritual care		
PC7	Patient Care	Invite patients to identify and explore their own spirituality or inner life		
PC8	Patient Care	Respond appropriately to verbal and nonverbal signs of spiritual distress		
PC9	Patient Care	Make timely referral to chaplain or spiritual counselor		

PC10	Patient Care	Respect patients' spiritual/religious belief systems		
#	**Competency**	**Observed Behaviors**	**Pedagogical Methods**	**Performance Assessments**
PPD1	Pers/Prof Develop	Explain the reasons and motives that drew you to the medical profession	Professional Development: 1, 2, 3, 4, 5, 6, 8, 13, 17, 18, 20, 21, 24, 30, 37, 38, 39, 40, 41, 43, 44, 36, 47	Professional Development: 2, 4,7, 8, 10, 14, 15, 20, 21
PPD2	Pers/Prof Develop	Explore the role that spirituality plays in your professional life		
PPD3	Pers/Prof Develop	Reflect on signs of personal spiritual crisis & methods of intervening		
PPD4	Pers/Prof Develop	Identify your sources of spiritual strengths		
PPD5	Pers/Prof Develop	Describe how spirituality functions as a way of connecting with healthcare team, family and patients		
PPD6	Pers/Prof Develop	Identify your personal and professional support communities		
C1	Communication	Practice deep listening—hearing what is being communicated through and between the words, the body language, and the emotions	Communication: 1, 4, 7, 8, 14, 15, 18, 20, 23, 25, 26, 27, 35, 36, 42, 43, 45, 47, 48, 49	Communication: 2, 3, 4, 5, 7, 8, 10, 12, 13, 14, 18, 20
C2	Communication	Practice curious inquiry—a sincere, attentive, non-directed, nonjudgmental exploration of the patient's perspective		
C3	Communication	Practice perceptive reflections—mirroring for the client what you hear or perceive, but always checking the "truth" of your reflection with the patient		
C4	Communication	Communicate professionally with spiritual care providers and other team members about the patient's spiritual distress or resources of strength		
C5	Communication	Use appropriate nonverbal behaviors to signal interest in the patient		
C6	Communication	Demonstrate the use of silence in patient communication		

Teaching Methods

1	Arts (music, visual/theatre)	26	Motivational interviewing
2	Bioethics course	27	Patient interviewing/practice
3	Careers in medicine (understanding yourself) program	28	Patient logbooks/student documentation
4	Case studies	29	Patient speakers/teachers
5	Case-based learning	30	Portfolio
6	Centering ritual	31	Student presentations
7	Communication Skills Course/Doctoring/Intro to Clinical Skills	32	Problem-based learning sessions/theme oriented (e.g., advance dirs)
8	Electives/selectives with spirituality curriculum/content	33	Quality improvement projects
9	Exercises in listening and being present	34	Reading/directed
10	Experiential/local politicians	35	Role modeling
11	Experiential/mentors & pastoral care	36	Role playing
12	Experiential (e.g.,practicing being in a wheelchair)	37	Personal well-being log
13	Feedback/patient	38	Self-awareness/self-care/spiritual experiences
14	Feedback/trained faculty observers giving feedback w SPs	39	Self-reflective writing
15	Feedback/trained faculty observers giving feedback w/o SPs	40	Narrative writing
16	Guided observation	41	Service learning
17	Interdisciplinary team training w chaplain participation	42	Shadow chaplain/other 'expert' at addressing spiritual needs
18	Lecture/interactive & didactic	43	Simulations
19	Living will/do your own	44	Small group discussion/debates
20	Mentoring w clinician &/or chaplain	45	Small groups/dyads with facilitators
21	Mindfulness training	46	Standardized patients
22	Observe preceptors/mentors	47	Video interviews w review
23	OSCEs/developmental/w checklists & guidelines	48	Videos/films
24	Panel discussions	49	Web searches/webcasts
25	Parallel charting/case studies with spiritual issues		

Performance Assessments

1	Assessment of narratives/journal entries
2	Assessment of student present/write ups
3	Assessment/pastoral care
4	Case-based learning/PBL
5	Chart review
6	Checklist evaluation live/recorded performance
7	Feedback or evaluation/faculty/mentor/precept/expert
8	Exam/MCQs/written
9	Exam/short answer
10	Feedback or evaluation/360-degree
11	Exam/essay
12	Feedback or evaluation/Mini-CEX
13	Feedback or evaluation/patients
14	Feedback or evaluation/peer
15	Feedback or evaluation/self
16	Feedback or evaluation/tutor
17	Global ratings of live/recorded performance
18	Objective structured clinical exams
19	Observation of performance/various settings
20	Portfolios
21	Pre/post testing (written/video)
22	Simulation/virtual patient
23	Standardized oral exams

Figure 56.1 The National Initiative to Develop Competencies in Spirituality for Medical Education.

first nursing diagnosis related to spirituality, spiritual distress, was established in the North American Nursing Diagnosis Association (NANDA) and remains today.[22] The Code of Ethics for professional nurses in the United States recognizes the importance of spirituality and health, illustrated by Provision 1 of the code, which states, 'the nurse in all professional relationships practices with compassion and respect for the inherent dignity, worth, and uniqueness of each individual unrestricted by considerations of social and economic status, personal attributes, or the nature of health problems.'[23] Interpretive statements for this provision of the code further asserts that 'the measures nurses take to care for the patients enable the patients to live with as much physical, psychological, social and spiritual wellbeing as possible.'[24] The International Council of Nurses also has a Code for Nurses which states, 'The nurse promotes an environment in which the human rights, values, customs and spiritual beliefs of the individual, family and community are respected.'[25]

Although nursing education teaches spirituality as a basic and essential element of the individual, there is too limited scholarly development of the nursing process in relation to this concept to make it a standard part of nursing education. In other words, there is not widespread acceptance of a standardized method to assess, plan, intervene and evaluate spiritual care in nursing. In 2004, a survey of 132 baccalaureate nursing programs in the US found that few defined spirituality or spiritual nursing care.[26] However, in the most recent iteration of the Essentials of Baccalaureate Education for Professional Nursing Practice, developed and published by American Association of Colleges of Nursing in 2008, spirituality was integrated throughout this document.[27] As a result, current nursing schools are integrating spirituality more fully in their curricula.

Social work

The US National Association of Social Workers' Code of Ethics declares that a social worker must include spirituality when completing an assessment.[28] Recognition of the relevance of spirituality to social work practice has led to recommendations that spirituality and religion be included in the Master of Social Work curriculum. Social work's earliest roots in the US were religious; religions sponsored the first social services programmes. The first Council on Social Work Education Curriculum Policy Statement (1953) used as its standard for accreditation that the 'physical, mental and emotional growth should be considered with due regard to social, cultural and spiritual influences upon the development of the individual.'[29] However, in the 1970 and 1984 Curriculum Policy Statements, references to spirituality and religion were not included. As with medical education, resurgence in the interest in spirituality, religion, and social work occurred in the 1990s and continues to the present day. The concepts of spirituality and religion have been reintroduced into the Council on Social Work Education's curriculum guidelines in 1995.[30] The guidelines state that programmes 'must provide curriculum about difference and similarities in experiences, needs and beliefs of people.' The standards also state that practice content include approaches and skills for practice with clients from different social religious spiritual backgrounds.[30]

Social work education is also focused on the relationship aspect of care. Social workers are trained to be a compassionate presence—to listen with empathy, assess a person's psychosocial network, and help draw in appropriate resources to help the patient do as well as possible. They are trained to be partners with the patient, open to the patient's agenda, and know how to listen to the patient's fears, hopes, and dreams.[31]

Physician assistants

Physician Assistants (PA) programmes, like medical schools in the US, have seen an increase in the number of spirituality and health courses. Paramount in the education of physician assistants is recognition, respect, and non-judgemental attitude for diversity which includes spiritual, cultural and ethnic diversity. Mandated content in curricula for accreditation listed in the Standards of the Accreditation Review Commission include respect for diversity of patients, including beliefs and values.[32]

Psychology

The American Psychological Association (APA) has funded post-doctoral fellowships for PhD psychologists in which they rotate with all members of an interdisciplinary team, including chaplains. Fellows learn to identify and address spiritual and religious concerns related to chronic illness and death and dying, and how to collaborate with other disciplines. Additionally, APA funded a programme for continuing education focused on end-of-life care, which includes the spiritual and religious issues facing dying patients, and how to conduct a spiritual screening.[33]

Physical therapy and occupational therapy

The physical therapy profession currently does not require the integration of spirituality in patient care in the physical therapy curriculum, and it is unclear how physical therapy faculty and practitioners view its inclusion. There is limited research on the integration of spirituality in the field of physical therapy or within its academic environment. A recent study investigated this further and found that more than half of the respondents indicated that they believed that spirituality concepts should be included in physical therapy education and that every physical therapy programme should include it in its curriculum. Response patterns indicated that respondents felt that spirituality concepts should be integrated into the physical therapy curriculum, rather than having specific courses focused on spirituality. In particular, effects on the older patient were cited as having potential benefit of inclusion of spirituality for the older patient.[34] There are programmes in physical therapy that include some material on spirituality, especially how to do a spiritual screening.

Occupation therapists also include spirituality as an important aspect of care. There has been a large body of research in this area in Canada. The Canadian Association of Occupational Therapists (CAOT) has recognized spirituality as an integral component of occupational performance in client-centred practice.[35] Despite acknowledging the influence of personal crisis, illness, and disability on a client's spirituality, occupational therapists have debated whether spirituality should be addressed within their scope of practice.[36] Utilizing a national sample of occupational therapists to investigate the current role of spirituality in practice, Engquist *et al.* found that the majority of therapists affirmed that spirituality was a critical dimension of the health and rehabilitation of their clients.[36] Nevertheless, many therapists neglected to address the spiritual dimension with their clients. Kirsh recommended a narrative approach to assessing a patient's spiritual needs in relation to his/her occupational therapy performance.[37]

Although spirituality is recognized as important, education in spirituality is minimal.[38] Methods of addressing spirituality varied and were limited to case studies, workshops, and guest speakers without any formal curriculum.

In other countries the situation is similar. Much is written of the importance of spirituality in occupational and physical therapy yet curricula do not exist or are limited to a lecture, case study or workshop.

Pharmacy

The American Association of Colleges of Pharmacy has recently held meetings to consider integrating spirituality into their curriculum. At their annual conference, in 2010 there were presentations on the importance of addressing spiritual issues with patients and clients and the need for this material to be covered in the curriculum. There are some courses in several of the Schools of Pharmacy in the United States which are beginning to teach this material. One such programme, in Western School of Osteopathy, developed a course on Spirituality and Health jointly between the Schools of Osteopathy and Pharmacy that was taught by faculty from both schools for students from both schools.

Chaplains, pastoral counsellors, and spiritual directors

Professional chaplains in the United States receive their clinical training in Clinical Pastoral Education (CPE) programmes, and generally have a master's level degree such as a Master of Divinity or clinical masters as indicated in Part II of this section. There are other training programmes that are not CPE, however, the standard in US hospitals and palliative care programmes is for Board Certification which requires a minimum of 1600 hours of CPE.

Pastoral counselling providing psychologically sound therapy that integrates the religious and spiritual dimension. Under the auspices of American Association of Pastoral Counseling, pastoral counselling adheres to rigorous standards of excellence, including education and clinical training, professional certification and licensure. Typical education for the AAPC-certified pastoral counsellor consists of study that leads to:

- a bachelor's degree from an accredited college or university
- a three-year professional degree from a seminary
- a specialized masters or doctoral degree in the mental health field.

A significant portion of this education is spent in clinical training. Post-graduate training involves completion of at least 1375 hours of supervised clinical experience (that is, the counsellor provides individual, group, marital, and family therapy) and 250 hours of direct approved supervision of the therapist's work in both crisis and long-term situations.

Spiritual direction is the process of accompanying people on a spiritual journey and inviting the directee into a deeper relationship with the spiritual aspect of being human. Spiritual direction offers a place to explore spiritual experiences, prayer practices, meditation, and the significant or sacred. Spiritual direction is not counselling or psychotherapy. Spiritual directors training includes one year of academic and practicum in study of theology, spirituality, and psychology. Practicums are supervised by peers and supervisors. At the end of the training the person receives a certificate of completion, but most training programmes do not 'certify' a person as a spiritual director.[39]

The ancient tradition of spiritual direction, as shown in the early practices of the Deserts Fathers of Egypt, indicated that spiritual directors were usually the wise men and women of the community.[40] The process of arriving at being a spiritual director is more of listening to a calling than practicing a profession. However, St Teresa of Avila stated that, based on her experiences, she would like a spiritual director that is more holy and learned, but if the two qualities are not present in the person she would rather have a learned director.[41] The learned director will be more able to direct people in any walk of life. Therefore, the programmes that presently train spiritual directors have this same focus in mind: that their studies and their learning will be great assets to any spiritual director the director may undertake. While in the past spiritual directors originated within Christianity, today spiritual directors may come from many of the religious and spiritual traditions of the contemporary world. Within the Christian tradition there are, of course, a spread of spiritualities including those from the Catholic, Orthodox, and Protestant traditions that all shape particular understandings and practices of spiritual direction—e.g. Ignatian, Franciscan, the Quaker practice of spiritual guidance, etc. Other religious traditions have different approaches to spiritual direction, such as in Buddhism where the relationship is more teacher/pupil. Increasingly there are also non-religious spiritual directors such as secular humanist directors. Organizations such as Spiritual Directors International network spiritual direction courses, centres, and directors.

UK perspectives

Training healthcare professionals

In the UK the NHS is devolved across the four countries of England, Scotland, Wales, and Northern Ireland and whilst there are country specific features and structures, the training of health professionals broadly follows a similar path of undergraduate training courses, graduate entry into a profession followed by postgraduate and specialist training programmes. Curricula and courses generally combine the interrelated demands of achieving competent clinical practice, academic standards, and the requirements of professional regulation. The content of training is therefore shaped by the workforce demands of the national health services; the knowledge, skills, and behaviours that professional bodies expect students to learn, and the academic criteria of higher education institutions.

The countries of the UK are also within the European Higher Education Area that provides a common frame of reference for higher education and comparable qualifications to support student mobility and employability. Member states of the European Union are also subject to antidiscrimination laws that include eliminating discrimination on the grounds of religion and belief (Article 19 of the Treaty of Lisbon). In the UK, the NHS is therefore required to respect the human rights of individuals, ensure it understands the particular needs of patient groups and achieve equal outcomes. This is an important basis for spirituality and spiritual care, but training about diversity in beliefs and religious practice is inadequate in itself. For example, the standards of proficiency required to register as an occupation therapist in the UK include the knowledge, understanding and skill to 'recognize the value of the diversity and complexity of human behaviour through the exploration of different physical, psychological, environmental, social, emotional and spiritual perspectives.'[42] No other competences are specified despite the relevance of religion and spirituality to the occupational behaviour of an individual and the holistic philosophy of occupational therapy.[43]

A common expectation of health professionals is that they will provide high quality person-centred care that is responsive to individual needs. This means that students should be capable of understanding and responding to the comprehensive needs of patients. For example, graduate medical doctors are required to, 'Interpret findings from the history, physical examination and mental-state examination, appreciating the importance of clinical, psychological, spiritual, religious, social and cultural factors.'[44] Similarly to meet the requirement for registration all nurses must acquire the competence 'to carry out comprehensive, systematic nursing assessments that take account of relevant physical, social, cultural, psychological, spiritual, genetic and environmental factors, in partnership with service users and others through interaction, observation and measurement.'[45] At the higher specialist level of training the content of the syllabus may be more specific, for example to be registered on the Specialist Register in Palliative Medicine a doctor must 'have the knowledge and skills to elicit spiritual concerns, recognize and respond to spiritual distress and demonstrate respect for differing religious beliefs and practice and accommodation of these in patient care.'[46]

Courses

The extent to which courses within the UK reflect the aspirations of curricula is variable and inconsistent. A survey of members of the Royal College of Nursing (UK) found that nearly four out of five of the nurses surveyed ($n = 4054$) agreed that they received insufficient training in this area and that it should be addressed within programmes of education.[47] In UK medical schools it has been estimated that between 31 and 59% are likely to provide teaching on the subject, which could be as little as a single tutorial, much of it optional, and with 'little uniformity between medical schools with regards to the content, form, amount or type of person delivering teaching on spirituality.'[48] In 2008, Neely and Minford investigated the current status of teaching on spirituality in medicine in United Kingdom medical schools.[48] They e-mailed contacts within the medical education unit (deans and associate deans of medical education and senior lecturers in medical education) of each medical school. As a result, 59% of respondents stated that there are at least some topics on spirituality in their curricula. A person trained in spirituality, or a medical practitioner with a special interest in spirituality, were the professionals most likely to teach this issue. Of the respondents that teach spirituality, 50% included compulsory teaching on spirituality in medicine, 80% included as optional components. Teaching about different faiths and cultures and about the link between spirituality and health is delivered in 70 and 80%, respectively, of the medical schools that deliver teaching on spirituality. However, only 40% of these schools include spiritual history taking and only 30% include spiritual counselling.

Variability arises from the discretion that training providers have in how they achieve learning outcomes, course designs and resources, and the personal and professional interests of faculty members. An evidence-based UK consensus statement on clinical communication illustrates some of the problem: it states that communication teaching should include issues related to spirituality, but purposively avoids describing competency levels because these are 'school-specific' and the approach allows the inclusion of areas that 'resist easy measurement, such as integrity and respect.'[49] Consequently, statements and curricula guidelines about spirituality and spiritual care remain recommendations that generally lack specificity, and add little to how teaching, learning, and assessment on this subject can be inter-related.

Learning opportunities

Spirituality and spiritual care provide subjects for a wide range of learning opportunities in the UK that include special study modules available as options within training programmes, inter-professional modules and short courses, conferences and knowledge sharing through specialist discussion and interest groups. A prominent example of the latter is the Spirituality and Psychiatry Special Interest Group (SPSIG), which is a forum for psychiatrists to discuss spirituality in relation to mental healthcare.[50]

Healthcare chaplains

Eligibility for a training post as a healthcare chaplain in the UK usually depends upon candidates demonstrating a level of prior pastoral formation, knowledge, and skills through a period of general training and supervised practice. For Christian candidates this is typically attained through a ministerial degree programme (ordination training) and completion of first training post with mentorship (post-ordination training phase). Candidates from other faith communities may have analogous learning and there are some opportunities provided by institutes of higher education for certificate-level and foundation degrees in chaplaincy subjects.

The UK Board of Healthcare Chaplaincy has set standards for training, education, and continuing professional development. In particular, it has published a framework of capabilities and competences that extend beyond knowledge and skills of professional practice to include core values and personal spiritual development.[51] Chaplains can access CPD programmes for healthcare professionals and there are a small number of chaplaincy-specific postgraduate programmes. A distinctive feature of training in the UK is that Clinical Pastoral Education (CPE) has not become an established model, instead academic and professional training combined with methods of reflective practice and pastoral supervision[52] have emerged that draw upon practices including theological reflection, clinical supervision and professional development.

Australian perspectives

Education of healthcare professionals in Australia is predominantly based in public universities. Some healthcare support disciplines are trained through the Technical and Further Education (TAFE) system at Certificate IV and Diploma level. TAFE qualifications have some limited articulation with the university system.[53] Professional awards are developed by the universities in consultation with professional peak bodies and are approved by those bodies, which in turn have direct accountability to the commonwealth (federal) government.

Religion is taught as an academic discipline in many of Australia's 39 public universities, but the secular charters of these universities mean that religious vocational training is provided through theological schools, many sponsored by a specific Christian denomination. Most of these schools now cooperate to provide degree programmes accredited by various state governments. These awards in theology articulate with university programmes, but are administered separately.

Curricula in spirituality and health

Unlike the UK and USA, there are no published studies of spiritual care content in the awards offered by Australian public universities. A survey of university websites undertaken for the purposes of this chapter found that a clear majority of universities offer spirituality subjects, and that these are taught in a range of faculties, mainly arts, education and health. Where spiritual care subjects are listed in health sciences courses they are usually part of a nursing programme and/or with a particular focus in ageing, indigenous health or palliative care. Of Australia's 19 medical schools which listed a full subject in spiritual care, only one has a full subject on Spirituality and Health. In 2007 at the medical school in Sydney, Spirituality and Health was accepted as one of the learning areas; 2008 a steering committee was formed for this subject, and in 2009 Spirituality was integrated into the curriculum. The process was based, in part, on the curriculum development in this subject in the USA. Mandatory sessions include an introduction to chaplaincy, meaning in medicine, definition of spirituality, and a review of the research. Methodologies include case discussion, didactics, use of film and literature, group discussion and individual projects (K. Curry, 2011, personal communication).

This does not mean that spiritual care is not taught as part of the healthcare qualifications in the universities that do not provide any spiritual care listing, but it does imply that such teaching is incidental—a lecture or a small module, embedded in general instruction about patient care. It also reflects that teaching spiritual care is not mandated by any profession's accrediting body. For example, although a number of subjects in spiritual care are offered in Schools of Nursing, there is no mention of spiritual care in the national framework for accreditation of nursing and midwifery courses,[54] while in the standards and criteria for accrediting courses leading to registration the only mention of spiritual care occurs in the context of cultural safety.[55] It is difficult to escape the conclusion that, where spiritual care is taught, this is more due to the initiative of particular university staff members, or perhaps departments, than to the professions themselves. However, spirituality interest groups are affiliated with many professional associations.

It is worth noting that competencies identified by a report of the Australia and New Zealand Deans of Medical Schools for the commonwealth government includes the need for spiritual and religious care of practitioners and patients.[56] How this might translate into curriculum is not as yet indicated. In the health sciences more broadly, La Trobe University currently is considering a proposal to establish a Grad Cert Spiritual Care that would be embedded in a spiritual care stream of the Master of Health Sciences degree.

Medical humanities

In the UK and USA, medical humanities programmes offer a learning environment open to considering spiritual need and spiritual care. The focus of such programmes is upon creating settings conducive to human development.[57,58] An Australian Association for Medical Humanities has been formed,[59] although the only specific awards to date are offered by the University of Sydney's Centre for Medical Humanities. This Centre, which has links with the Centre for Medical Humanities, University of Durham, UK, offers a Grad Cert Med Hum and Master of Medical Humanities, including this year a subject 'Spirituality, Consumerism and Healthcare'.[60] The University of Newcastle's Artshealth Centre for Research and Practice,[61] offers a medical humanities subject (albeit infrequently) in addition to developing interdisciplinary research in arts and medicine. The University of Melbourne Medical School, through the Medical Humanities Unit in conjunction with the Centre for Health and Society, offers an elective programme in medical humanities/ethics research.[62]

Healthcare chaplaincy training

Chaplaincy training is largely carried out in Clinical Pastoral Education (CPE) programmes based, for the most part, in acute care institutions. CPE is independent and self-accredited through the Association for Supervised Pastoral Education in Australia or cognate bodies.[63] Credit may be given into academic awards at the discretion of course coordinators at theological schools or university.

Some of those training as chaplains have prior theological qualifications, while others may commence theological studies during their CPE training. Chaplains also undertake studies at postgraduate level in various education and health sciences programmes. Spiritual Care Australia[64] is moving to position itself as a national accrediting body in conjunction with the recently-established Australian Health Practitioner Regulation Agency.[65]

Pastoral counsellors and spiritual directors

There is some limited intersection between healthcare practice at the community level and accredited pastoral counsellors or spiritual directors. These practitioners are trained through theological schools for the most part, and accredited by professional bodies such as Australian Association of Spiritual Care and Pastoral Counselling and Christian Counsellors Association are affiliated with the Psychotherapy and Counselling Federation of Australia,[66] while the Australian Ecumenical Council of Spiritual Directors[67] networks spiritual direction courses, centres and directors across the country.

Medical education in spirituality in other parts of the world

A literature review was undertaken to look at published articles in spirituality and health education globally.[68] The studies in this review indicate a predominance of studies related to health/medicine and spirituality in USA and Canadian medical schools. Few studies were found in Europe, Latin America, and Asia, and none in Africa and Australia. New studies and curriculum development in spirituality and health outside North America are needed to further investigate the role of spirituality and health globally, and how best to address this important issue in global medical education.[67]

In a number of countries 'spirituality' is incorporated through Traditional Complementary and Alternative Medicine (TCAM) that is taught in parallel with western medical programmes or in integrated form.[69] In analogous fashion, spirituality is an integral component of medical training developed for indigenous or First Nation practitioners. The International Council of Nurses called for spiritual assessment of patients to be seen as a professional standard for nurses.[25] To address this requirement in Korea, Yong develeoped a spiritual training programme for middle manager nurses to understand and develop their own spirituality in order to be able to care for their patients.[70] This programme had a significant influence in terms of their own spiritual and emotional wellbeing.

Continuing education for healthcare professionals in spirituality and health

There has been, in response to growing community interest in spirituality and health, a proliferation of workshops and training modules for in-service education of healthcare professionals, staff and volunteers. In some clinical setting, volunteers and staff are trained together, to essentially the same level, in screening skills. Often, although by no means always, these short courses are offered by educators who also teach spiritual care in the tertiary sector. There are numerous conferences, and presentations integrated into professional association annual conferences such as the American Psychiatric Association, the Association of American Medical Colleges, American Academy of Hospice and Palliative Medicine, the International Congress on Palliative Care, International Asian Conference of Palliative Care, the Asian Pacific Organization for Cancer Prevention's Middle East Cancer Consortium (MECC) Workshop on Cancer Pain, Suffering and Spirituality in Turkey, and the Australian Conference on Spirituality and Health to name a few.

Discussion

Clearly, there are differences in the level of teaching in spirituality and health in the different health professions, as well as different countries. Some of the barriers that have been cited in the literature include diverse definitions of spirituality, disparity of rigor of research used as an evidence base and lack of practical models and tools. As can been seen from other chapters in this book, these models and tools are now being developed and the body of research is more rigorous and continually expanding. However, most clinicians and healthcare providers note that spirituality is important in the lives of patients. Thus, we anticipate the area of curriculum development to grow over the next few years.

How spirituality is taught is another challenge for some programmes. More successful models include taking advantage of major trends in health education, for example, humanizing healthcare with the increase in humanities courses, and integrate spirituality into those subject areas. Courses that are vertically integrated and required have a greater likelihood of impact. Integrating board certified chaplains as faculty, as well as pastoral counsellors and spiritual directors is key to excellence in education in this topic area.

It is also critical to teach spirituality in the clinical years and to include a focus on the spirituality of the health profession students' lives. Formats that include personal reflection may be a powerful way to convene and experience the fuller dimension of spirituality as it pertains to the students' lives so that they in turn can have a greater appreciation for spirituality in their patients' lives. Translating theory into practice requires more than the assimilation of knowledge and skills and needs supporting with formation through reflective practice and learning from the wisdom and tacit knowledge of a community of practice.

References

1 Fortin, A., Barnett, K. (2004). Medical school curricula in spirituality and health. *J Am Med Ass* **29**(23): 2883.

2 Puchalski, C.M., Larson, D. (1998). Developing curricula in spirituality and medicine. *Acad Med* **73**(9): 970–4.

3 Puchalski, C.M. (2006). Spirituality and medicine: curricula in medical education. *J Cancer Educ* **21**(1): 14–18.

4 Association of American Medical Colleges (1999). Learning objectives for medical student education-guidelines for medical schools: report I of the Medical School Objectives Project. *Acad Med* **74**(1): 13–18.

5 Anandarajah, G., Mitchell, M. (2007). A spirituality and medicine elective for senior medical students: 4 years' experience, evaluation, and expansion to the family medicine residency. *Fam Med* **39**(5): 313–15.

6 Association of American Medical Colleges. (1999). *Contemporary Issues in Medicine: Communication in Medicine*, Report III. Washington, DC: Medical School Objectives Project (MSOP).

7 Puchalski, C.M., Larson, D.B., Lu, F.G. (2001). Spirituality in psychiatry residency training programs. *Int Rev Psychiat* **13**(2): 131–8.

8 Baetz, M., Griffin, R., Bowen, R., Marcoux, G. (2004). Spirituality and psychiatry in Canada: psychiatric practice compared with patient expectations. *Can J Psychiat* **49**(4): 265–71.

9 The George Washington Institute for Spirituality and Health (2005). Medical Education in Spirituality and Health in Canadian Medical Schools Needs Assessment. unpublished results.

10 Fortin, A.H., Barnett, K.G. (2004). Medical school curricula in spirituality and medicine. *JAMA* **291**(23): 2883.

11 Hebert, R.S., Levine, R.B., Smith, C.G., Wright, S.M. (2003). A systematic review of resident research curricula. *Acad Med* **78**, 61–8.

12 Green, M.L. (1999). Graduate medical education training in clinical epidemiology, critical appraisal and evidence-based health: a critical review of curricula. *Acad Med* **74**: 686–94.

13 Association of American Medical Colleges. (2006). *AAMC Statement on Physician Workforce*, p. 7. Washington, DC: AAMC.

14 The Accreditation Council for Graduate Medical Education (ACGME), (2011) Program Director Guide to the Common Program Requirements. Available at: http://www.acgme.org/acWebsite/navPages/commonpr_documents/CompleteGuide_v2%20.pdf (accessed 6 February 2012).

15 Puchalski, C., Blatt, B., Kogan, M., *et al.* (2012). *The National Initiative to Develop Competencies in Spirituality for Medical Education.* (In preparation).

16 Watson, J. (1999). Becoming aware: knowing yourself to care for others. *Home Healthcare Nurse* **17**: 317–22.

17 Travelbee, J. (1971). *Interpersonal Aspects of Nursing*, 2nd edn. Philadelphia: Davis.

18 Newman, B. (1995). *The Neuman Systems Model*, 3rd edn. Stamford: Appleton & Lange.

19 American Nurses Association (2003). *Nursing's Social Policy Statement*, 2nd edn. Silver Spring: ANA.

20 Nagai-Jacobson, M.G., Burkhardt, M.A. (1989). Spirituality: cornerstone of holistic nursing practice. *Holist Nurs Pract* **3**(3): 18–26.

21 Clark, C.C., Cross, J.R., Deane, D.M., Lowry, L.W. (1991). Spirituality: integral to quality care. *Holist Nurs Pract* **5**(3): 67–76.

22 North American Nursing Diagnosis Association. (2007). *NANDA-1-nursing Diagnosis: Definitions and Classification, 2007–2008.* Philadelphia: NANDA International.

23 American Nurses Association. (2003). *Nursing's Social Policy Statement*, 2nd edn. Silver Spring: ANA.

24 American Nurses Association. (2003). *Nursing's Social Policy Statement*, 2nd edn. Silver Spring: ANA.

25 International Council of Nurses. (2005). *Code of Ethics for Nurses.* Available at: http://www.icn.ch/images/stories/documents/about/icncode_english.pdf (accessed 6 February 2012).

26 Callister, L.C., Bond, A.E., Matsumura, G., Mangum, S. (2004). Threading spirituality throughout nursing education. *Holist Nurs Pract* **18**(3): 160–6.

27 American Association of Colleges of Nursing. (2008). *Essentials of Baccalaureate Education for Professional Nursing Practice*. Available at: http://www.aacn.nche.edu/Education/pdf/BaccEssentials08.pdf (accessed 8 August 2011).

28 National Association of Social Workers (1996). *Code of Ethics*. Available at: http://www.socialworkers.org/pubs/code/code.asp (accessed 8 August 2011).

29 Spencer, S. (1961). What place has religion in social work education? *Soc Serv Rev* **35**: 161–70.

30 Russel, R. (1998). Spirituality and Religion in Graduate Social Work Education. In: Canda E.R. (ed.) *Spirituality in Social Work: New Directions*, pp. 15–30. New York: Haworth Pastoral Press.

31 Puchalski, C.M., Lunsford, B., Harris, M.H., Miller, R.T. (2006). Interdisciplinary spiritual care for seriously ill and dying patients: a collaborative model. *Cancer J* **12**(5): 398–416.

32 Puchalski, C.M., Ferrell, B. (2010). *Making Healthcare Whole: Integrating Spirituality into Patient Care*, p.162. West Conshohocken: Templeton Press.

33 [32], pp.161–2.

34 Pitts, J. (2008). Spirituality in the physical therapy curriculum: effects on the older adult. *Top Geriat Rehab* **24**(4): 281–94.

35 Law, M., Polatajko, H., Baptiste, S., Townsend, E. (1997). Core concepts of occupational therapy, in Canadian Association of Occupational Therapists (eds) *Enabling Occupation: An Occupational Therapy Perspective*, pp. 29–56. Ottawa: CAOT Publications ACE.

36 Engquist, D.E., Short-DeGraff, M., Gliner, J., Oltjenbruns, K. (1997). Occupational therapists' beliefs and practices with regard to spirituality and therapy. *Am J Occup Ther* **51**: 173–80.

37 Kirsh, B. (1996). A narrative approach to addressing spirituality in occupational therapy: exploring personal meaning and purpose. *Canad J Occup Ther* **63**: 55–61.

38 Kirsh, Dawson, Antoliova, Reynolds. (2001). Developing awareness of spirituality in occupational therapy students: are our currila up to the task? *Occup Ther Int* **8**(2): 119–25.

39 Australian Ecumenical Council for Spiritual Direction (2011). Homepage. Available at: http://spiritualdirection.org.au/(accessed 8 August 2011).

40 Waddell, H. (1998). *The Desert Fathers*, Vintage Spiritual Classics. New York: Random House.

41 Kavanaugh, K., Rodriguez, O. (1976). *The Collected Works of St. Teresa of Avila*, Vol. 1. Washington, DC: ICS Publications.

42 Council, H.P. (2007). *Standards of Proficiency*. London: Occupational Therapists.

43 Belcham, C. (2004). Spirituality in occupational therapy: theory in practice? *Br J Occup Ther* **67**: 39–46.

44 Council, G.M. (2009). *Tomorrow's Doctors*. London: GMC.

45 Nursing & Midwifery Council (2010). *Standards for Pre-registration Nursing Education: Essential Skills Clusters*. London: NMC.

46 Joint Royal Colleges of Physicians Training Board. (2010). *Specialty Training Curriculum for Palliative Medicine*. London: RCPTB.

47 McSherry W (2011). *RCN Spirituality Survey 2010*. London: RCN.

48 Neely D, Minford EJ (2008). Current status of teaching on spirituality in UK medical schools. *Med Educ* **42**(2): 176–82.

49 von Fragstein, M., Silverman, J., Cushing, A., Quilligan, S., Salisbury, H., Wiskin, C. (2008). UK consensus statement on the content of communication curricula in undergraduate medical education. *Med Educ* **42**(11): 1100–7.

50 The Royal College of Psychiatrists: Spirituality and Psychiatry Special Interest Group. Available at: http://www.rcpsych.ac.uk/members/specialinterestgroups/spirituality.aspx (accessed 8 August 2011)

51 UK Board of Healthcare Chaplaincy. (2009). *Spiritual and Religious Care Capabilities and Competences for Healthcare Chaplains.* Cambridge.

52 Leach, J., Paterson, M. (2010). *Pastoral Supervision: a Handbook.* London: SCM.

53 Australian Qualifications Framework. (2011). *Australian Qualifications Framework*, Final 21 April, 2011. Available at: www.aqf.edu.au (accessed 8 August 2011).

54 Australian Nursing and Midwifery Council (ANMC). (2007). *The National Framework for the Accreditation of Nursing and Midwifery Courses Leading to Registration, Enrolment, Endorsement and Authorization in Australia.* Canberra: ANMC. Available at: http://www.anmc.org.au/userfiles/file/ANMC_Framework%20-%20Final.pdf (accessed 6 February 2012).

55 ANMC. (2009). *The Standards and Criteria for the Accreditation of Nursing and Midwifery Courses Leading to Registration, Enrolment, Endorsement and Authorization in Australia—With Evidence Guide, Registered Nurses.* Canberra: ANMC. Available at: http://www.anmc.org.au/userfiles/file/ANMC_Registered_Nurse%281%29.pdf (accessed 6 February 2012).

56 Australia and New Zealand Medical Deans (2011). *Developing a Framework of Competencies for Medical Graduate Outcomes: Final Report.* Sydney: Medical Deans Australia and New Zealand Inc. Available at: www.medicaldeans.org. au (accessed 23 November 2011).

57 Gordon, J. (2005). Medical humanities: to cure sometimes, to relieve often, to comfort always. *Med J Aust* **182**(1): 5–8.

58 Gordon, J.J. (2008a). Humanising doctors: what can the medical humanities offer? *Med J Aust* **189**(8): 420–1.

59 Gordon, J.J. (2008b). Medical humanities: state of the heart. *Med Educ* **42**: 333–7.

60 University of Sydney, Centre for Medical Humanities (2011). Medical Humanities Program. Available at: http://sydney.edu.au/medicine/humanities/ (accessed 23 November 2011).

61 University of Newcastle. (2011). The humanities/creative arts and medical sciences. Available at: http://www.newcastle.edu.au/research-centre/artshealth/ (accessed 23 November 2011).

62 University of Melbourne. (2011). Medical humanities unit, Centre for Health and Society. Available at: http://www.medicine.unimelb.edu.au/ams/ (accessed 6 Feb 2012).

63 Association for Supervised Pastoral Education in Australia. Available at: www.aspea.org.au (accessed 23 November 2011).

64 Spiritual Care Australia. Available at: http://www.spiritualcareaustralia.org.au/website/home.html(accessed 23 November 2011).

65 Australian Health Practitioner Regulation Agency. (2011). Available at: www.ahpra.gov.au (accessed 23 November 2011).

66 Psychotherapy and Counselling Federation of Australia. Available at: http://www.pacfa.org.au/ (accessed 8 August 2011).

67 Australian Ecumenical Council for Spiritual Direction. Available at: http://spiritualdirection.org.au/ (accessed 8 August 2011).

68 Lucchetti, G., Granero, A.L., Puchalski, C. (2011). *Spirituality in Medical Education. Global reality? J Relig Health.* 2011 Dec 1. [Epub ahead of print] Available at: http://www.springerlink.com/content/7r14821nt3471n64/fulltext.pdf (accessed 6 Feb 2012).

69 Bodeker, G., Burford, G. (2007) (Eds.), *Traditional, Complementary and Alternative Medicine: Policy and Public Health Perspectives.* London: Imperial College Press.

70 Yong, J., Kim, J., Park, J., Seo, I., Swinton, J. (2011). Effects of a spirituality training program on the spiritual and psychosocial wellbeing of hospital middle manager nurses in Korea. *J Contin Educ Nurs* **42**(6): 280–8.

CHAPTER 56B

Curriculum development

Part II: Clinical Pastoral Education

Angelika A. Zollfrank and Catherine F. Garlid

Introduction

The spiritual wellbeing of persons dealing with a healthcare crisis demands the attention of religious professionals and healthcare providers. There is growing consensus in the USA that professional board certified chaplains bring special expertise to spiritual care in the area of chronic illness, palliative care, and traumatic medical events. For optimal care the Palliative Care Consensus Report recommends interdisciplinary spiritual care models that enable health care professionals to identify spiritual issues and concerns. Multiple training modalities and programs offer education in compassionate spiritual care, particularly for healthcare providers. There is awareness that a Clinical Pastoral Education (CPE)-trained board-certified chaplain, as part of an inter-professional team is well-suited to provide expertise and guidance relative to the spiritual diagnosis and corresponding spiritual care.[1] In this chapter the focus will be on CPE as a distinct pathway to spiritual care competence.

CPE is closely supervised, experiential, clinical training for professional spiritual care givers of multiple religious and spiritual (R/S) backgrounds. Guided by patients' and families' needs, CPE trains spiritual care givers to provide respectful R/S care to patients, families, staff, and healthcare institutions. The CPE process deepens spiritual care givers' emotional and spiritual self-awareness and professional identity formation. CPE trains religious leaders, clergy, seminarians, lay persons and healthcare providers to translate effectively between[2] and become literate in the languages of modern Western medicine, multiple ancient belief and value systems, and the intersecting experiences of illness and faith.

Training healthcare chaplains in the USA

The training of healthcare chaplains in the USA includes 3–8 years of graduate education or an equivalent, specialized preparation for faith specific R/S leadership. Competencies acquired prior to or simultaneous with CPE include critical thinking skills, facility with metaphor and narrative, study, and interpretation of religious texts and their historical contexts, leadership development, and extensive understanding of human motivations and behaviours. Additionally, those engaged in clinical training towards healthcare chaplaincy have attained intimate knowledge of how humankind has responded throughout the ages to questions like 'Why is there suffering?' 'Where do we come from?' 'Where are we going?' 'What is the purpose of human existence?' 'Who and what is the Divine?' 'How is human life related to an ultimate reality?'

Reflecting the experiential and clinical nature of learning in CPE, the following case study illustrates the collaboration between a healthcare provider and a chaplain intern in providing spiritual care, informed by their concurrent participation in CPE.

Case Study

Diagnosed with sarcoma in 2005, Paul, a 61-year-old married man, was treated with chemotherapy and surgery. In 2008, Paul relapsed and received chemotherapy again. Two years later he was diagnosed with leukaemia caused by the sarcoma treatment. After induction therapy, complicated by several infections, Paul underwent a stem cell transplant. The treatment was successful. However, 4 months later Paul relapsed again. He and his wife Mildred were devastated. The years of caring for her husband had made Mildred fearful. She was at Paul's bedside as much as possible. Paul and Mildred had found each other later in life and their life together revolved around their relationship as a childless couple.

Leah, Paul's oncology nurse, had long observed that, for many of her patients, religion and spirituality offered a resource for coping. A person of mature Protestant faith, she decided to enroll in a Clinical Pastoral Education (CPE) programme for training in spiritual care-giving. In CPE, Leah learned to include spiritual assessment, listening and communication skills, and knowledge about different religious and spiritual belief systems in her practice. Leah found out that Paul and Mildred were originally Roman Catholic. After Paul's diagnosis with leukaemia in 2010 they had joined a conservative, evangelical Protestant Church. Leah learned that Paul believed that God gave him signs that indicated that God intended him to do well. Given that the chances for positive outcomes of his hospitalization in May 2011 were slim, Leah anticipated spiritual distress. If the leucocyte infusion did not work, would Paul feel let down not only by his healthcare providers, but also by God? Leah brought these concerns to her clinical supervisor in CPE. The CPE supervisor encouraged her to involve the unit chaplain, and to continue to monitor and listen closely to Paul's R/S coping with the goal of choosing an opportunity to explore how he imagined that people and God might be with him if the treatment were not successful. After a week, Leah reported in supervision that such an opportunity had not come up. However, Leah had communicated her concerns to Carol, the chaplain intern peer, who was assigned to her Oncology unit as part of completing an advanced unit of training in the same interdisciplinary CPE program.[3] Leah, who had excellent rapport with the couple, introduced Carol, a candidate for ordination in the Unitarian Universalist Church.

In a long conversation Carol listened to the couple, offered emotional support, completed a comprehensive spiritual assessment, and acknowledged Mildred's wish for a miracle. She also offered prayer sensitive to their R/S language asking God for strength in uncertainty. Carol confirmed Leah's sense that Paul and his wife struggled significantly with religious conflict about God's interventions in Paul's treatments. She concurred with the sense that such conflict would likely lead to greater spiritual struggle. She was also concerned about the lack of community support. The case discussion in the CPE group highlighted the importance of an interdisciplinary spiritual care plan: while Leah continued to listen to the couple's ongoing concerns, it was Carol's goal to help Paul develop a sense of God's presence independent of treatment outcomes; to address Mildred's anxiety through pastoral presence, scripture reading, and prayer; to explore and extend the couple's relationship to their church. In the last weeks of Carol's participation in CPE, her experiences of her own leave-taking of the training group and the hospital became instructive. In a role play on 'How to say good-bye' Carol rehearsed a conversation with Paul and Mildred, in which she began to transition their spiritual care to another chaplain. Subsequently, Carol explored with them their fears that Paul might not get better. Carol facilitated the couple in talking to each other about their distinctive perspectives. Paul was concerned about Mildred's life after his death, giving her permission to move on and to find a different partner. Mildred began to think about living life without Paul, even as he was still by her side. Eventually, Carol, Paul, and Mildred spoke openly about his death, subsequent arrangements, and his funeral. Upon discharge Paul and Mildred expressed gratitude for his successful medical care. They also stated that they were more intentional and hopeful about supporting each other whatever lay ahead. CPE helped Leah to feel comfortable in offering spiritual care appropriate to her role as a nurse. The cross-disciplinary learning improved Carol's effectiveness as part of the care team. Overall, the outcome of cross-disciplinary CPE learning was a higher quality of spiritual care.

In the above clinical case a healthcare provider offered initial screening and daily spiritual accompaniment. Due to her involvement in CPE the nurse not only did the screening that any healthcare provider should be equipped to do, she also assessed and anticipated potential spiritual concerns and made an informed referral to the chaplain intern. In concert with the overall medical care for Paul their collaboration made a significant difference in Paul and Mildred's lives. The nurse learned in CPE to use her own R/S understanding and practices to cope better with the accumulative grief related to her clinical practice. The chaplain intern utilized the CPE programme for professional identity formation and competency development towards board certification in healthcare chaplaincy. It is significant that her interventions were guided primarily by her understanding of clinical realities and R/S dynamics, aided by her knowledge of faith specific characteristics different from her own R/S identity.

Goals of clinical pastoral education

Religious and spiritual leaders have always reached out to suffering persons beyond their own communities. The disciplines of healthcare chaplaincy and CPE refrain from proselytizing or persuasion of patients in R/S matters.[4] This principle is reflected in the competencies and the professional code of ethics for healthcare chaplains and clinical pastoral education supervisors. The main goal of a chaplain is to support patients, families, and staff in *their* R/S practice, coping, and development. CPE prepares R/S leaders and future healthcare chaplains for this task.

In CPE, future R/S leaders and healthcare chaplains learn to:

- develop a R/S care plan that respects the patient's R/S background and journey
- support and intervene towards positive R/S coping through conversation, prayer, meditation, ritual, and worship
- collaborate with R/S communities and their leaders
- offer education regarding R/S principles and healthcare
- contribute expertise regarding the ways that religion and spirituality influence patient and family treatment decisions and support clinical ethics consultation processes.[5]

History

CPE has its roots in the early 1920s. The three persons credited as founders are Anton Boisen, a Protestant minister in the Christian tradition, and two physicians, Dr Richard Cabot of Massachusetts General Hospital (MGH) in Boston, and Dr William S. Keller of Cincinnati, Ohio. Dr Keller extended clinical training to seminarians in the context of mental hospitals and social service agencies. Anton Boisen, using William James's work in the psychology of religion, devoted himself to studying religious experience through his own mental illness, having suffered recurring psychotic episodes beginning in his twenties. Having studied the clinical case method with Dr Cabot at Harvard Medical School, a method developed for the close observation and reporting of patient behaviour and experience, Boisen was hired at Worcester State Hospital and began bridging the academic training of clergy and the world of Western medical practice.[6] At the centre of his educational focus was the thorough study of 'the living human document.'[7]

After having been hospitalized at MGH in 1933,[8] Russell Dicks, a Methodist minister, caught the attention of Dr Cabot and was hired as the first chaplain in a general hospital. Dicks pioneered the use of the verbatim as a tool for documenting a spiritual care visit for subsequent peer and supervisory critique.[9] As the discipline developed further, Dicks and his colleagues recognized the need for professional organizations to support and certify institutional chaplains and CPE supervisors.[10] Today, in the USA, the primary certifying organization for chaplains is the Association for Professional Chaplains (APC) and for supervisors, the Association for Clinical Pastoral Education (ACPE). Additional certifying bodies in North America are the National Association for Catholic Chaplains (NACC), the National Association for Jewish Chaplains (NAJC), the American Association of Pastoral Counselors (AAPC), and the Canadian Association for Spiritual Care (CASC). CPE is international in scope. Although begun in North America (in the United States and soon thereafter in Canada), CPE also took root during post-World War II years in Northern Europe, Southeast

Asia, New Zealand, Australia, Africa, and South America.[11] The CPE programmes offered in these international settings are accredited through organizations other than the ACPE, but their general structure is similar to that outlined below for ACPE programmes.

Theoretical foundations

The theoretical underpinnings of CPE and chaplaincy fall into four categories: theology, psychology, educational theory, and group dynamics. Given its roots in twentieth century Protestant Christianity, the influence of theologians such as Paul Tillich, Reinhold Niebuhr, and Karl Barth contributed heavily to the conceptual understandings of pastoral care and counseling, including CPE.[12] These theologians helped frame the existential suffering and spiritual longing of the persons chaplains encounter on a daily basis. In the 1970s and early 1980s the impact of civil rights, the women's movement, and an increasingly pluralistic society forced pastoral care organizations to confront the biases and blind spots of a Christocentric worldview. For example, the use of the word 'pastoral' carries meaning primarily for Christians. Work and debate over inclusive language will continue as healthcare and religious organizations engage with diverse theologies, religious expression, and spiritual practice. As Jews, Buddhists, Hindus, Muslims, and others are trained and certified, the programmes and contexts in which they learn and develop as professionals are required to examine the richness and impact of cultural and religious diversity, and make changes accordingly.[13] Among the organizational issues raised in training chaplains of diverse backgrounds is the need to accept legitimate equivalencies for the academic component required for certification.[14]

From the beginning, with its roots in psychiatric and medical settings, CPE has been informed by the work of Sigmund Freud and his followers, with a growing awareness that the personal history and social context of the chaplain, in addition to those of the patient, had an impact on his or her motivations and perceptions. Over the years CPE supervision has been influenced by many schools of thought including humanistic psychology, self-psychology, developmental and behavioural psychology, to name but a few.[15]

Educational theories underlying the training of chaplains in CPE are shared by medicine and social work. The term 'reflective practice' has roots in the pioneering work of John Dewey who provided a foundation for an experiential and practical approach to learning.[16] Adult learning theories,[17,18] an emphasis on self-directed learning,[19] and, more recently, models of transformative learning[20] have had a strong impact on the discipline of clinical pastoral supervision.

One of the unique aspects of CPE training and curriculum is the emphasis on learning in the context of a peer group reinforced by the intentional study of group dynamics. The focus on the group itself emerged through other pieces of the curriculum, such as the case study or verbatim seminar experienced by a small group of students over time. As group therapy emerged as a psychotherapeutic treatment modality, CPE supervisors, and religious leaders became interested in its application to work in religious communities, clinical training, and organizational development. Under the influence of the human potential movement there was a continuous shift from focus on the patient to focus on interpersonal relationships and group dynamics, with growing tensions among the differing goals of education for ministry, self-help groups and group therapy.[21] Theoretical foundations for group work in CPE were adopted from Wilfred Bion, A.K. Rice, Irvin Yalom, and Murray Bowen. While theoretical underpinnings for individual CPE programmes vary, the ACPE has developed rigorous standards for national certification of supervisors and CPE programme accreditation.

CPE programmes are open to religious leaders, seminarians, theological students, lay persons, and healthcare providers. Different CPE programmes are geared towards the different learning needs of their participants. CPE programmes consist of a total of 400 hours of clinical and educational work. Groups of up to ten students participate in didactic presentations, peer group consultation, individual clinical supervision, and supervised process groups. Didactic presentations span topics of:

- spiritual assessment tools
- reflective listening and communication skills
- initiating and ending meaningful spiritual care relationships and spiritual support in crisis
- issues related to health and spirituality in different religions
- theological reflection, loss and grief
- group dynamics
- specialized spiritual care related to clinical service lines.

Group consultations focus on case presentations, discussion of verbatims, role plays, and simulation lab practica.[22] Another programme element is the shared presentation of CPE participants' experiences of faith about core R/S themes. All CPE components and methods are designed to enable spiritual caregivers to engage and respond compassionately to emotional and life experiences that are expressed through the wide variety of belief systems and cultures.

CPE programmes are offered at three distinct levels. To meet the requirements of Level I CPE programmes one must be able to demonstrate the following:

- to articulate how R/S life experiences have shaped one's belief system
- to differentiate between one's own R/S experience and that of patients
- to offer entry level spiritual care, including spiritual assessment, basic spiritual care-giving skills and effective use of prayer, ritual and R/S resources
- a beginning awareness of transference and counter-transference issues in extensive and intensive spiritual care relationships
- to engage in constructive peer consultation; to reflect on one's functioning in professional teams
- intentionality in offering spiritual care to persons of a variety of religious, spiritual, ethnic, racial, and socioeconomic backgrounds, as well as persons of different gender, age, and sexual identity.[23]

For Level II CPE programmes one must be able to demonstrate the following:

- to provide effective spiritual care and to engage with humility across difference

- to engage in reflective practice leading to interventions within and across patient care units, services, departments, institutions without imposing one's own perspective
- to utilize several different assessment tools
- to operationalize realistic clinical judgment leading to effective use of a multitude of spiritual care skills, including confrontation, conflict resolution, management of crisis in context, anticipation of R/S needs
- to draw on an intellectual and emotional understanding of professional boundaries and a demonstrated ability to stay within the boundaries of the spiritual care giver's role as related to goal and context
- to integrate knowledge in the behavioral sciences
- to demonstrate competence in theory and research in spirituality and health
- to affect change and take leadership relative to R/S care.[24]

At least four units of CPE and demonstrated ability to work consistently on an advanced level are required for a certification review through one of six primary professional organizations in North America—the Association for Professional Chaplains (APC), the American Association of Pastoral Counselors (AAPC), the National Association of Catholic Chaplains (NACC), the Association for Clinical Pastoral Education (ACPE), the National Association of Jewish Chaplains (NAJC), and the Canadian Association for Spiritual Care (CASC).

The third level of CPE is designed to train religious leaders to become competent in clinical pastoral supervision, program development and evaluation. Within 3–5 years of additional training future supervisors undergo a rigorous national review of their clinical supervision practice and their theoretical expertise in the discipline. The certifying body is the ACPE.

Recent developments

In the late 1980s Larry VandeCreek and others challenged the fields of spiritual care and counseling to engage in research.[25] Initial empirical research focused on the positive impact or efficacy of spiritual care.[26] In the 1990s, the psychologist Ken Pargament began publishing his research on religious coping.[27] In the late 1990s chaplain George Fitchett and others began studying religious coping and R/S struggle.[28] This research has received the attention of physicians and other health care colleagues who may not have attended to questions such as, 'How does belief in a punishing diety affect the course of my patient's illness?'[29] Recently, George Fitchett and colleagues have challenged chaplains to develop a body of published case studies to strengthen the foundation of evidence based spiritual care.[30]

Conclusion

The discipline of CPE supervision must also demonstrate its efficacy. What are the particular contributions of CPE to spiritual care giving? Are CPE methods in fact improving the quality of spiritual care? Studies show that CPE aided participants' ability to use relational and counselling resources, as well as non-judgmental presence.[31] CPE also leads to increased emotional intelligence and improved spiritual care giving skills.[32] Many of the available studies are based on students' self-report. Additional data remains unpublished. For example, evaluation data from 12 alumni of two units of CPE implemented at Massachusetts General Hospital in 2009 indicate that 73% of participants felt that pastoral diagnostic skills learned in CPE continue to be very helpful. 73% of alumni in the same time period reported that CPE was very helpful in the development of basic learning and counselling skills related to spiritual care giving.[33] Additionally, data gathered in a pre and post CPE questionnaire from 45 healthcare providers, who participated in CPE, reported that CPE improved their ability to address existential and spiritual issues and increased their efficacy in providing spiritual care to a diverse population.[34] Furthermore, findings in an eleven week intensive CPE programme for chaplain interns suggest that CPE group learning was effective in helping students to empathize with others, rather than to act on the impulse 'to fix' things. The data also suggests that CPE helped these chaplain interns to assume their role as chaplains in their clinical areas.[35] Further research is needed to address how CPE contributes to improved spiritual care to patients, families, and staff, as well as which CPE methods are particularly useful in improving spiritual care giving in clinical care.[36,37]

References

1 Puchalski, C., Ferrell, B., Virani, R., Otis-Green, S., Baird, P., Bull, J., *et al.* (2009). Improving the quality of spiritual care as a dimension of palliative care: the report of the Consensus Conference. *J Palliat Med* **12**(10): 891–4.

2 DeVries, R., Berlinger, N., Cadge, W. (2008). Lost in translation: sociological observations and reflections on the practice of hospital chaplaincy. *Hastings Cent Rep* **38**(6): 9–13.

3 The Chaplaincy at Massachusetts General Hospital has offered CPE programs for healthcare providers since 1998. Since 2010 two units of CPE annually combine three to five advanced chaplain interns with three to four health care providers. This interdisciplinary approach to CPE offers a unique approach to training in spiritual care.

4 Association of Professional Chaplains. (2011). *Reading Room.* Available at: http://www.professionalchaplains.org/index.aspx?id=207#Common_Standards (accessed 5 August, 2011).

5 Fitchett, G., King, S.D.W., Vandenheck, A. (2010). Education of chaplains in psychooncology. In: J.C. Holland, W.S. Breitbart, P.B. Jacobsen, M.S. Lederberg (eds) *Psychooncology*, 2nd edn, pp. 605–9. New York: Oxford University Press.

6 Asquith, G.H. Jr (ed.) (1992). *Vision From a Little Known Country: A Boisen Reader*. Decatur: Journal of Pastoral Care Publications, Inc.

7 Hemenway, J.E. (1996). *Inside the Circle: A Historical and Practical inquiry Concerning Process Groups in Clinical Pastoral Education*, pp. 1–26. Decatur: Journal of Pastoral Care Publications, Inc.

8 Zollfrank, A.A. (2011). *CPE Handbook*. Boston: Massachusetts General Hospital, Partners Healthcare CPE Center.

9 Cabot, R.C., Dicks, R.L. (1936). *The Art of Ministering to the Sick*. New York: Macmillian Company.

10 Hall, C.E. (1992). *Head and Heart: The Story of the Clinical Pastoral Education Movement*. Decatur: Journal of Pastoral Care Publications, Inc.

11 International Association of Christian Chaplains (2011). *Clinical Pastoral Education*. Available at: http://www.christianchaplains.com/pages.php?pagina=pg_cpe.php (accessed 5 August, 2011).

12 Holifield, E.B. (1983). *A History of Pastoral Care in America: From Salvation to Self-realization*. Nashville: Abingdon Press.

13 Thiel, M.M. (2009). Contextualizing CPE: developing a Jewish Geriatric Program. In: C.F. Garlid, A.A. Zollfrank, G. Fitchett (eds) *Expanding the Circle*, pp. 137–60. Decatur: Journal of Pastoral Care Publications, Inc.

14 Board of Chaplaincy Certification (2011). *BCCI Certification*. Available at: http://www.professionalchaplains.org/bcci/index.aspx?id=1262 (accessed 8 August, 2011).

15 [14]

16 Schön, D.A. (1987). *Educating the Reflective Practitioner: Toward A New Design for Teaching and Learning in the Professions*, pp. 16–17. San Francisco: John Wiley & Sons.

17 Knowles, M.S. (1970). *The Modern Practice of Adult Education: Androgogy Versus Pedagogy*. New York: Association Press.

18 Kolb, D.A. (1984). *Experiential Learning: Experience as a Source of Learning and Development*. Englewood Cliffs: Prentice-Hall.

19 Rogers, C.R. (1961). *On Becoming a Person*. Boston: Houghton Mifflin.

20 Click, E. (2005). Transformative educational theory in relation to supervision and training in ministry. *J Supervis Train Minist* **25**: 8–25

21 [7], 145–66.

22 Tartaglia, A., Dodd-McCue, D. (2010). Enhancing objectivity in pastoral education: use of standardized patients in video simulation. *J Past Care Counsel* **64**(2): 1–10.

23 Since CPE is offered in multiple settings, the objectives and outcomes are deliberately vague in describing necessary competencies. Here, the authors' paraphrase the objective and outcomes of the ACPE Standards and Manuals, 2010 Standards, Association for Clinical Pastoral Education, Inc. 1549 Clairmont Road, Suite 103, Decatur GA 30033: (Outcomes of Level I/Level II CPE, 14). www.acpe.edu (accessed 1 August, 2011).

24 [23], p. 15.

25 VandeCreek, L. (1988). *A Research Primer for Pastoral Care and Counseling*. Decatur: Journal of Pastoral Care Publications, Inc.

26 VandeCreek, L. (ed.) (1995). *Spiritual Needs and Pastoral Resources: Readings in Research*. Decatur: Journal of Pastoral Care Publications, Inc.

27 Pargament, K.I. (1997). *The Psychology of Religion and Coping: Theory, Research, Practice*. New York: Guilford Press.

28 Fitchett, G., Rybarczyk, B.D., DeMarco, G.A., Nicholas, J.J. (1999). The role of religion in medical rehabilitation outcomes: a longitudinal study. *Rehab Psychol* **44**(4): 333–53

29 Fitchett, G., Risk, J. (2009). Screening for spiritual struggle. *J Past Care Counsel* [Online] **63**: 1–2.

30 Fitchett, G. (2011). Making our case(s). *J Hlth Care Chaplaincy* **17**(1–2): 1–18.

31 Fitchett, G., Gray, G.T. (1994). Evaluating the outcome of clinical pastoral education: a test of the Clinical Ministry Assessment Profile. *J Supervis Train Minist* **15**: 3–22.

32 O'Connor, T.S.J., Healey-Ogden, M., Meakes, E., Empey, G., Edey, L., Klimek, S., *et al.* (2001). The Hamilton SPE Evaluation Tool (HSET): is it any good? *J Past Care* **55**(1): 17–33.

33 Jankowski, K.R.B., Vanderwerker, L.C., Murphy, K.M., Montonye, M., Ross, A.M. (2008). Change in pastoral skills, emotional intelligence, self-reflection, and social desirability across a unit of CPE. *J Hlth Care Chaplaincy* **15**(2): 132–48.

34 Data from alumni questionnaires (unpublished).

35 Data from an 88-item pre- and post-questionnaire completed by participants in the CPE for healthcare providers program between 2003 and 2009 at Massachusetts General Hospital (unpublished).

36 Zollfrank, A.A. (2009). Functional subgrouping in CPE. In: C.F. Garlid, A.A. Zollfrank, G. Fitchett (eds) *Expanding the Circle*, pp. 137–60. Decatur: Journal of Pastoral Care Publications, Inc.

37 Derrickson, P.E. (1990). Instruments used to measure change in students preparing for ministry: a summary of research on clinical pastoral education students. *J Past Care* **44**(4): 343–56.

38 ACPE Research Network (2011). Available at: http://www.acperesearch.net/jul11.html (accessed 5 August, 2011).

CHAPTER 57

Competences in spiritual care education and training

Ewan Kelly

Introduction

This chapter will explore the significance of competences as one of several relevant aspects of education and training that are required to ensure spiritual care and practice is person-centred, timely, effective, and safe in the particular context that it is delivered, and whose overall aim is to enhance patient wellbeing. Utilising a competences-based learning methodology helps to provide healthcare professionals with the relevant knowledge, skills and attitudes necessary to practice with some degree of confidence.[1] However, an educational or training programme focused solely on this dimension of learning will not fully equip practitioners to meet the complex spiritual needs of patients, carers, colleagues, and themselves in the messy and paradoxical experience of dealing with suffering and loss, relief, and recovery that is working in healthcare; even if they possess the natural abilities conducive to the provision of meaningful relationship-based care. Other approaches are also required to ensure pre- and post-registration education and training facilitates informed and intuitive spiritual care practice by self-aware and motivated practitioners which improves patient experience and outcome as well as offering opportunities for personal fulfilment and vocational satisfaction. The example of competences being part of a wider educational framework to help shape the continuing professional development of healthcare staff, in particular chaplains in Scotland, is one which will be utilized to ground the discussion. Reference will also be made to the use of competences in the education and training of other healthcare disciplines.

Historical

The development of competences in education originated in the creation of technical and vocational training in different parts of the globe, including New Zealand, Australia, the USA, and the UK, motivated by seeking to make national workforces more competitive within a global economy. The predominant model utilized was to create separate competencies for each particular task undertaken by an employee, following detailed functional analysis. Each of these competences was then translated into a measurable outcome and the performance of the trainee monitored in relation to each specific task or role involved.[2, 3]

Within healthcare in the UK, a competency-based approach to the education of healthcare professionals came to the fore in the late 1990s as part of the government's drive to deliver quality assurance or clinical governance in response to the public demand for safe, competent, and accountable healthcare practice.[4] Competences were first used in the UK health service as part of the professional development and oversight of managers, but have subsequently become influential in shaping the education and training of clinical staff at all stages of their formation and ongoing development as practitioners.

Benefits of a competences-based approach

First, competences provide clarity regarding what a healthcare professional from a particular discipline needs to know to perform their role consistently and effectively. This enables educationalists and trainers to:

- construct curricula and programmes which are grounded in students' and practitioners' real needs
- create clear learning aims and outcomes for courses delivered
- assess what they deliver in terms of relevance, and impact on, practice.

An excellent example of such a competences-orientated methodology is found in undergraduate and postgraduate medical curricula across the globe—examination of the competency of trainees to perform certain tasks by clinical objective structured clinical examinations (OSCES). For the past 30 years, medical students and doctors have been assessed at different times in their training by OSCES; examination at a series of stations that they rotate around, being given an allotted time to carry out a particular task at each station. For example, at one station a student may have to demonstrate competency in the ability to listen to a patient's chest and at the next to examine a chest X-ray. What is being examined is the trainees' ability to carry out each task in a manner that complies with prescribed standards, as well as what the individual must know and understand to carry out that task, ensuring safe and competent practice.

For practitioners, a significant benefit of such clarity in terms of the knowledge and skills they need to acquire to perform their specific role, and being educated and trained to carry out required tasks competently is developing confidence in their ability to do so. Education and training that is focused and clearly relates to the real tasks practitioners have to perform on a regular basis within healthcare, not only equips them for the job they are paid to do, but enhances their motivation and job satisfaction in doing so.[6] In turn, experiencing a competent and consistent quality provision of care helps develop trust and instill confidence not only in patients, but in their families and friends who entrust their loved ones into a practitioner's care.

Secondly, competences provide a benchmark against which 'shared expectations around performance' may be measured.[7] They can helpfully be used in appraisal as part of continuing professional development to elicit learning needs an individual can work towards, within an agreed timescale. McManus, employed in public health in south east England, helpfully puts it this way:

> Many recent advances in training and development, especially professional training and development, identify that there is a need to ensure both a 'knows how' element of knowledge and range of 'shows how' domains of competency in real life practice to what health professionals do.[8]

Thirdly, competencies not only act as a tool to aid individual flexible work-based learning. They can also be linked to career progression and to remuneration frameworks where achievement of further knowledge and skills means movement up a nationally agreed pay scale.[9] In the UK, the Knowledge and Skills Framework (KSF) has been developed for this purpose.[10]

Limitations of a predominantly competency based approach

Whilst offering obvious benefits, an educational curriculum predominantly based on competency, is not a panacea in equipping practitioners for working in twenty-first century healthcare. The following are limitations of programmes where the emphasis on developing and maintaining competency predominates.

First, a competences-based approach tends to be rather atomistic in nature. Utilizing such a methodology means a particular vocational role is broken down into different domains of required knowledge and skills, and then into individual competences, which describe each discrete task considered relevant to that role. However, what is not highlighted by such a perspective is how such tasks are integrated. In practice, tasks in healthcare are seldom performed in discrete silos or vacuums, but are often intimately interwoven in a pressured environment. This includes the necessity for healthcare professionals to juggle and prioritize tasks and yet simultaneously keep an overarching perspective on their role and how it relates to the roles of others in the delivery of holistic healthcare. In addition, educational and training programmes dominated by competences do not adequately help healthcare practitioners to explore the meaning informing and underpinning each task they are asked to perform as well as the significance of the relationships between them.[11] Healthcare practitioners need to think about the overall process of what they and their multi-disciplinary colleagues are involved in, rather than just outcomes or the satisfactory performance of the tasks that make up their particular role in the system. A competences based approach does not encourage practitioners to ask such 'meta-questions'.[12] Other educational approaches require to be utilized alongside competences to ensure pre- and post-registration healthcare professionals are equipped to deal with the complexity of people, situations, and systems, while working in either community or institutional settings.

Secondly, a competency-based model for healthcare education and training is rather reductionist in approach and sits more comfortably with the view that healthcare provision is a technical science that applies acquired knowledge utilizing a relevant skill set to cure, alleviate, and care. As an educational methodology, it does not do justice to the art of healthcare where intuition, discernment, and creativity are significant to a practitioner's decision-making and performance in their role. A competency-based educational curriculum may produce safe clinical technicians, but does not encourage professional artistry in healthcare. The title of medical educationalist Martin Talbot's article critiquing competency-based methods encapsulates such shortcomings: 'Monkey see, monkey do; a critique of the competency model in graduate medical education.'[13] Moreover, such a reductionist method within education encourages students to learn what they need to learn to pass exams, rather than to engage critically with complex situations and to seek baseline competence rather than excellence in the service they will provide.[14]

Thirdly, within healthcare there has recently developed a deeper understanding of the importance of the impact of not just what is done to, or with, patients but the quality of the relationship between healthcare professionals and patients influencing outcome. It not just how skillfully a task is done or whether a relevant piece of knowledge is shared, but how the task is performed and the practitioner's way of relating to and being with patients which is significant for patient experience as well as vocational fulfillment. For example, patients with advanced cancer and non-malignant disease reported in one UK study that they were most able to utilize their inner resources to help deal with their situation when they felt affirmed and valued by the health professional involved in their care.[15] In addition, the acknowledgement in healthcare education and training of the significance of a doctor's ability to relate genuinely and empathetically for patient wellbeing can be seen in the development of tools to assess their level of empathy for patients in clinical encounters.[16,17]

Development of competences within spiritual care provision

The first competency frameworks informing the delivery of spiritual care were developed in 2003 by Marie Curie Cancer Care in the UK[18] and by nurse educators in the Netherlands in 2004.[19] The development of such frameworks to shape education and practice was an indication of the increasing interest in spiritual care as a core dimension of healthcare provision. By this time, the use of the term competences in healthcare education and training had begun to broaden and infer that ongoing reflection on practice is required, as well as acquiring the right knowledge and skill to enable best practice in the delivery of spiritual care.

Marie Curie Cancer Care's development of a competences model to aid spiritual needs assessment and provision of care was not only significant in raising the profile of spiritual care and helping its further integration into all holistic care within a palliative care context. Their competency framework also recognizes that different healthcare workers and volunteers operate at various levels of spiritual care competency. These levels range from one, which relates to all who have casual contact with patients and their carers, to level four, for those whose primary responsibility is spiritual and religious care for all in healthcare communities (Box 57.1).[20]

Box 57.1 The Marie Curie Cancer Care competency framework for spiritual and religious care

Level 1: All staff and volunteers who have casual contact with patients and their families

This level seeks to ensure that all staff and volunteers understand that all people have spiritual needs, and distinguishes spiritual and religious needs. It seeks to encourage basic skills of awareness, relationships and communication, and an ability to refer concerns to members of the multidisciplinary team

Level 2: Staff and volunteers whose duties require contact with patients and families/carers

This level seeks to enhance the competences developed at level 1 with an increased awareness of spiritual and religious needs and how they may be identified and responded to. In addition to increased communication skills, identification and referral of difficult needs should be achievable along with an ability to identify

Level 3: Staff and volunteers who are members of the multi-disciplinary team

This level seeks to further enhance the skills of levels 1 and 2. It moves into the area of assessment of spiritual and religious need, developing a plan for care and recognizing complex spiritual, religious, and ethical issues. This level also introduces confidentiality and the recording of sensitive and personal patient information.

Level 4: Staff or volunteers whose primary responsibility is for the spiritual and religious care of patients, visitors, and staff

Staff working at level 4 are expected to be able to manage and facilitate complex spiritual and religious needs in patients, families/carers, staff and volunteers, in particular the existential and practical needs arising from the impact on individuals from issues in illness, life, dying and death. In addition, they should have a clear understanding of their own personal beliefs and be able to journey with others focused on those persons' needs and agendas. They should liase with external resources as required. They should also act as a resource for support, training, and education of healthcare professionals and volunteers, and seek to be involved in professional and national initiatives.

Reproduced with permission of the author Rev. David Mitchell.

Gordon and Mitchell (the hospice chaplains involved in the creation of the Marie Curie Cancer Care spiritual care competences) recommend staff develop an awareness of their particular level of competence and the process by which they refer patients and carers, whose spiritual needs they cannot meet, to others better equipped to deal with complex issues. In addition, they importantly affirm that assessment and delivery of spiritual care is not only about applying learnt knowledge and skills, but also involves the consideration and development of practitioners' natural instincts and experience in discerning, identifying and responding to spiritual need.[21] Their work done on spiritual care competences in palliative care contexts laid the foundation for the formation of the *Spiritual and Religious Care Capabilities and Competences for Healthcare Chaplains* published by NHS Education for Scotland four years later.[22]

Following extensive literature review, Dutch educationalists van Leeuwen and Cusvellar formed a spiritual care competency profile for use in undergraduate nurse education which consisted of the following three core domains of spiritual care and six sub-domains of nursing competencies (Box 57.2).[23]

In order to perform competently, capably and sensitively the tasks outlined by both Dutch and British frameworks, nurses (or any other healthcare practitioner) would be not adequately equipped to provide relevant person-centred spiritual care by a narrowly defined competences-based educational approach (as described at the beginning of the chapter). These spiritual care frameworks reinforce the fact that healthcare staff require not only to assimilate the appropriate knowledge and skills to provide person centred spiritual care, but need regular reflection on their

Box 57.2 Van Leeuwen's and Cusveller's nursing competencies for spiritual care

Domain 1: Awareness and self-handling

Competency 1: Nurses handle their own values and convictions and feelings in their professional relationships and with patients of different beliefs and religions

Competency 2: The nurse addresses the subject of spirituality with patients from different cultures in a caring manner

Domain 2: Spiritual dimensions of nursing

Competency 3: The nurse collects information about patient spirituality and identifies patient needs

Competency 4: The nurse discusses with patients and team members how spiritual care is provided, planned and reported

Competency 5: The nurse provides spiritual care and evaluates it with the patient and team members

Domain 3: Assurance of quality and expertise

Competency 6: The nurse contributes to quality assurance and improving expertise in spiritual care within the organization

Journal of Advanced Nursing, Volume 48, Issue 3, René Van Leeuwen and Bart Cusveller, *Nursing competencies for spiritual care*, pp. 234–46, November 2004.

practice to explore their relational skills, their values and beliefs, and their ongoing level of self-awareness.

In 2006, within a Maltese context, using open-ended questionnaires and in-depth interviews, the competency of nurses in delivering spiritual care was investigated.[24] In this study, Baldacchino confirmed the first two domains of the Dutch competency project but not the third. In its place she offered two alternative domains:

- nurses' competency in communication with patients, the interdisciplinary team and educators
- safeguarding ethical issues in care.

More recently, utilizing their original work on nursing competences Van Leeuwen *et al.* developed and tested a spiritual care competency scale, as an instrument to assess student nurses' competency in spiritual care provision.[25] The tool not only may be used in this way but also to assess the areas in which nurses require further training to provide sensitive and competent spiritual care. However, education and training in spiritual care should not just be informed by the training needs of staff (as the work in Scotland, the Netherlands, and Malta proposes), but also by listening to the opinions of service users who cannot only help shape learning objectives, but also the means by which they may be achieved.[26] There are clear indications of the need for research to help identify the best educational and training methods to utilize in order to enhance competent, sensitive, and insightful spiritual care provision within healthcare for the future.[27]

Patient and carer involvement in such research or consultation would enhance the relevance of spiritual care education and training, grounding it in meeting the actual or real needs of service users. Such involvement could also inform the process of creating spiritual care competences themselves. This would follow the precedent set by general practitioners in the UK whose competences, which inform their continual professional development, are shaped through creative consultation utilizing a range of methodologies. In this particular healthcare role, competency development has involved the triangulation of results from focus groups with primary care physicians, behavioural coding of general practitioners' clinical encounters, and patient interviews.[28]

Competences, capabilities, and occupational standards

Increasingly in healthcare training and education, competences are utilized with other learning approaches and standards to help shape a more rounded and nuanced formation and ongoing continual professional development of practitioners. Staff require more than a set of defined competences to equip them to deal with complexity, and make meaningful connections between different aspects of their role and with others in a variety of healthcare settings. This necessitates training in developing capability, as well as competency through ongoing regular and effective reflective practice, prior to, and after registration. Capability is 'the extent to which individuals can adapt to change, generate new knowledge and continue to improve their performance.'[29] A capable practitioner has an ability to confidently:

- take effective and appropriate action
- explain what they are about
- work effectively with others
- continue to learn from their experiences and in association with others in a diverse and changing society.[30]

Capability is often equated with terms such as 'transferable skills', 'self-reliance skills' and 'enterprise skills'.[31] In order to perform capably and with competence, healthcare professionals require a framework of values, attitudes and knowledge to inform their practice along with an ability to discern how and when to utilize such resources in a manner that is applicable both to a particular patient and context.[32] Recognition of the limitations of a predominantly competences based approach to training and education is far from new and an interest in integrating 'reflection-on action' and 'reflection about-action' into continual professional development began in the 1980s.[33] Curricula developed to educate capable, as well as competent practitioners, which attended to the process of learning as well as the creation of defined educational and training outcomes.

> capability cannot be taught or passively assimilated; it is reached through a transformational process in which existing competences are adapted and tuned to new circumstances. Capability enables one to work effectively in unfamiliar contexts.[34]

Educational and training programmes for pre- and post-registration healthcare students, therefore, require a degree of flexibility ensuring a blended learning approach. For example, to equip trainees adequately for practice there needs to be room for students to be able to shape some of their own learning goals, receive regular feedback, and have time to reflect on and review what they have learnt, as well as aiming to help learners perform an identified range of tasks related to their vocational role at a required level.

Stephenson helpfully uses the example of a cartoon in which a group of sheep are at a cocktail party, depicted by the illustrator Gary Larson, to explore the relationship between competence and capability.[35] The sheep at the party are uncertain about where to stand and when to eat. 'Thank goodness,' one says, 'here comes a Border collie'. Sheep have all the skills and knowledge required for being sheep—they are competent at both eating and standing. In fact they do both at the same time, most of the day. However, put them in alien surroundings, like a cocktail party, and they are totally bewildered, absolutely dependent upon the arrival of a canine supervisor to guide them. They have the skills but not the discernment or insight to utilize appropriately when the context is alien. If these sheep were capable they would possess:

- the ability to be able to learn for themselves by reflection on previous experience and quickly review and get the measure of the different circumstances
- the confidence to adapt to perform in new situations having spotted the appetizing feed laid out for guests (and to respond appropriately by nibbling in a socially acceptable way)
- powers of judgement (they might even question whether it was appropriate for themselves as sheep to be at the party and simply leave).[36]

Healthcare professionals need to be equipped able to deal with situations and relationships which are not just socially awkward but which challenge them to utilize acquired knowledge and skills, innate abilities and make reference to previous experience which has been reflected on, and learnt from, to inform decision making and performance in the here and now. What healthcare educators are seeking to help form are professional artists (to use my colleague

Mark Stobert's term), as well as competent practitioners. The ancient Greek term *phronesis* sums up the optimum combination of these dimensions of healthcare practice which James Fowler, an American developmental psychologist, cited by British practical theologians Willows and Swinton, describes as:

> [A] knowing in which skill and understanding cooperate; a knowing in which experience and critical reflection work in concert; a knowing in which the disciplined improvisation, against the backdrop of reflective wisdom, marks the virtuosity of the competent practitioner.[37]

A healthcare practitioner who practices with *phronesis* is an expert in her field, working at the height of her powers, possessing the ability to work effectively, compassionately and competently in a range of different contexts with people from different backgrounds to deal with complex situations.

A variety of educational approaches, experiences and methods of assessing an individual's degree of learning and performance is, therefore, needed. This is especially true in the education and training of practitioners in spiritual care where the therapeutic use of self contributes significantly to the provision of compassionate and effective person-centred care. Spiritual care, significantly, being not so much about what tasks are done to, and with, a patient, but how they are performed and the quality of relationship established between carer and cared for.[38] Clearly, practitioners require to be knowledgeable of what spiritual, including religious, care may involve and its potential importance to those they work with. In addition, courses in communication skills can help individuals to utilize their natural abilities, such as empathy, warmth, and humour with greater insight and effectiveness. However, ongoing training methods which involve individuals and inter-disciplinary groups asking questions of themselves, and each other of their own and corporate practice are required. This necessitates effective pre- and post-registration programmes, which afford practitioners a varied range of opportunities to explore the beliefs, values and perceptions of experience that inform their practice. Such regular intentional occurrences enable reflection on how involvement in particular encounters, events, and processes, for example, decision-making, may potentially touch, indeed transform, these dimensions of personhood. Continual professional and personal development programmes, which involve combinations of supervision, mentorship, group reflective practice on case studies or verbatums, regular de-briefing, and critical event analysis facilitate such reflection on the complexity of clinical situations, teamwork and self. Journaling and maintaining a portfolio of learning experiences participated in are also tools that aid ongoing reflection on practice. In such activities the critical dialogue between learnt theory and technique, and the often harsh and complex nature of real experience in healthcare practice can be intentionally engaged with in an ongoing way.[39] Assessments for pre and post registration professionals can be performed by offering feedback on written reflections about specific topics or events or on portfolios or journals.[40] Oral feedback can be offered by mentors and line managers involved in annual appraisal and supporting colleagues with their personal development plans. Such blended learning activities and methods of feedback are not only significant for enhanced delivery of competent and person-centred patient care but for long term maintenance of a motivated and fulfilled workforce.

Utilizing capabilities and competencies together in one framework can help to inform work-based and life long learning programmes in particular areas of healthcare practice, for example, healthcare chaplaincy. Such frameworks enable 'practice learning outcomes to detail what practitioners should be able to achieve and to capture the notion of capability as current competence combined with the development of future potential competence.'[41]

A capability framework uses broad brushstrokes to outline different domains of activity involved in a particular vocational role. The development of particular competences for each domain and the creation of occupational standards describe the knowledge and skills specifically required to perform the different elements of the role and the level of service provision desired. Competences or practice learning outcomes describe the level of expertise expected within each domain of capability. Occupational standards, on the other hand, 'act as a performance measure of competence within the workplace environment'.[42] These are benchmark levels of service delivery to which patients, carers and colleagues can expect a particular healthcare profession to operate to.[43]

In order to help the reader envisage the relationship between capability domains and related competences in specialist spiritual care provision—those operating at level four of the Marie Curie Cancer Care competency framework[44]—the *Spiritual and Religious Care Capabilities and Competences for Healthcare Chaplains* recently developed in Scotland and now utilized throughout the UK will be summarized in Box 57.3 below.[45] Furthermore, one particular capability domain (2.1. Spiritual assessment and intervention) will be described in detail. By necessity and building on the work already done for nursing and other healthcare practitioners, this spiritual care framework is more nuanced and developed than those previously created. In this document, key contents are included to outline the knowledge base required to achieve the practice learning outcomes or competences in each capability domain.

Box 57. 3 The structure of NHS Education for Scotland's healthcare chaplaincy capabilities and competences framework. The framework is presented under four capability domains with a number of elements to each domain

1. *Knowledge and skills for professional practice*
   - Knowledge and skills for practice
   - Practicing ethically
   - Communication skills
   - Education and training
2. *Spiritual and religious assessment and intervention*
   - Spiritual assessment and intervention
   - Religious assessment and intervention
3. *Institutional practice*
   - Teamworking
   - Staff support
   - Chaplain to the hospital or unit
4. *Reflective practice*
   - Reflective practice
   - Personal spiritual development

Reproduced with permission from NHS Education for Scotland.

Capability Domain 2.1 of the framework outlines spiritual assessment and intervention: the chaplain, in partnership with the individual and the healthcare team, assesses the spiritual needs and resources of the individual and their family/carers, and responds with interventions, which can include referral to other internal and external care providers.

Key content

- Literature relating to needs, especially spiritual needs
- Knowledge of internal and external sources of spiritual support
- Local and national directory of sources of spiritual support.

The first three practice learning outcomes or competences (of seven) relating to this capability domain are:

The chaplain demonstrates an ability to:

1. *Assess the spiritual needs and resources of an individual*

   For example:

   - exploring the individual's sense of meaning and purpose in life
   - exploring attitudes, beliefs, ideas, values and concerns around ill-health, life, and death
   - affirming life and worth by encouraging reminiscing and narrative
   - exploring the individual's hopes and fears regarding the present and the future
   - exploring existential questions relating to life, death, illness, and suffering.
2. *Respond to assessed spiritual needs with spiritual care*
3. Assess *and* respect the experience and expression of an individual's spiritual wellbeing without necessarily endorsing the beliefs, religious or otherwise, and their observance, held by the individual.

Each capability domain is linked to a related aspect of the career progression and remuneration framework, the Knowledge and Skills Framework. Occupational standards to aid quality assurance activity have been developed by healthcare chaplains working in acute contexts in the USA, but not yet in the UK.[46]

Conclusion

Competences have a significant role in the development of educational and training programmes for healthcare staff in different dimensions of their practice, including the delivery of spiritual care. However, in order for practitioners to be able to aspire to practicing healthcare as an art, as well as a science other educational and training methods are required to be utilized alongside them. The development of competency (and capability) frameworks to inform the education and training of healthcare professionals in spiritual care has helped profile this aspect of healthcare practice as being core rather than peripheral or simply being the remit of religious functionaries. Further involvement of service users as well as a wider range of practitioners from different disciplines in the development of such frameworks is required. This would enable educational and training programmes become more focused on meeting the real learning needs of staff and, thus, in turn meeting the actual (and not the assumed) spiritual needs of patients and carers.

References

1 NHS Education for Scotland. (2008). *Spiritual and Religious Care Capabilities and Competences for Healthcare Chaplains*. Edinburgh: NHS Education for Scotland.

2 Macleod, C. (2005). Postgraduate medical education—competency or expertise. *J Roy Coll Physic Edin* **35**: 108–9.

3 Leung, W.C. (2002). *Competency Based Medical Training: Review*. Available at: http://www.bmj.com/content/325/7366/693 (accessed 30 September 2010).

4 Kerry, M. (2001). Towards competence: a narrative and framework for spiritual caregivers. In: H. Orchard (ed.) *Spirituality in Healthcare Contexts*, pp. 118–32. London: Jessica Kingsley Publishers.

5 Skills for Health. (2011). *Competences*. Available at: http://skillsforhealth.org.uk/competences.aspx (accessed 12 October 2011).

6 Skills for Health. (2011). *Competences*. Available at: http://skillsforhealth.org.uk/competences.aspx (accessed 12 October 2011).

7 Kerry, M. (2001). Towards competence: a narrative and framework for spiritual caregivers. In: H. Orchard (ed.) *Spirituality in Healthcare Contexts*, pp. 118–32. London: Jessica Kingsley Publishers.

8 McManus, J. (2006). What training should be required as an education standard for healthcare and hospital chaplains? *Sthn Med J* **99**(6): 665–70.

9 Department of Health (2004). *The Ten Essential Shared Capabilities: A Framework for the Whole of Mental Health Workforce*. London: Department of Health.

10 Department of Health (2004). *The NHS Knowledge and Skills Framework (NHS KSF) and the Development Review Process*. Leeds: Department of Health.

11 [3].

12 Shapiro, J., Coulehan, J., Wear, D., Montello, M. (2009). Medical humanities and their discontents: definitions, critiques, and implications. *Acad Med* **84**(2): 192–8.

13 Talbot, M. (2004). Monkey see, monkey do: a critique of the competency model in graduate education. *Med Educ* **38**(60): 580–1.

14 [3].

15 Grant, E., Murray, S., Kendall, M., Boyd, K., Tilley, S., Ryan, D. (2004). Spiritual issues and needs: perspectives from patients with advanced cancer and non-malignant disease. A qualitative study. *Palliat Support Care* **2**: 371–8.

16 Mercer, S., Murphy, D. (2008). Validity and reliability of the CARE measure in secondary care. *Clin Govern Int J* **13**(2): 261–83.

17 Mercer, S., Reynolds, W. (2002). Empathy and quality of care. *Br J GP* 52 (Supplement): S9–12.

18 Marie Curie Cancer Care. (2003*). Spiritual and Religious Care Competencies for Specialist Palliative Care*. London: Marie Curie Cancer Care.

19 van Leeuwen, R., Cusveller, B. (2004). Nursing competencies for spiritual care. *J Adv Nurs* **48**: 234–46.

20 Marie Curie Cancer Care. (2003) *Spiritual and Religious Care Competencies for Specialist Palliative Care*. London: Marie Curie Cancer Care.

21 Gordon, T., Mitchell, D. (2004). A competency model for the assessment and delivery of spiritual care. *Palliat Med* **18**: 646–51.

22 NHS Education for Scotland. (2008). *Spiritual and Religious Care Capabilities and Competences for Healthcare Chaplains*. Edinburgh: NHS Education for Scotland.

23 van Leeuwen, R., Cusveller, B. (2004). Nursing competencies for spiritual care. *J Adv Nurs* **48**: 234–46.

24 Baldacchino, D. (2006). Nursing competencies for spiritual care. *J Clin Nurs* **15**(7): 885–96.

25 van Leeuwen, R., Tiesings, L., Middel, B., Post, D., Jochemsen, H. (2009). The validity and reliability of an instrument to assess nursing competencies in spiritual care. *J Clin Nurs* **18**(20): 2857–69.

26 Yardley, S., Walshe, C., Parr, A. (2009). Improving training in spiritual care: a quality study exploring patient perceptions of professional educational requirements. *Palliat Med* **23**: 601–7.

27 Ross, L. (2006). Spiritual care in nursing: an overview of research to date. *J Clin Nurs* **15**(7): 852–62.

28 Patterson, F., Ferguson, E., Lane, P., Farrell, K., Martlew, J., Wells, A. (2000). A competency model for general practice: implications for selection, training, and development. *Br J Gen Practice* **50**, 188–93.

29 Fraser, S., Greenhalgh, T. (2001). Coping with complexity: educating for capability. *Br Med J* **323**: 799–803.

30 Stephenson, J. (1998). The concept of capability and its importance in higher education. In: J. Stephenson, M. Yorke (eds) *Capability and Quality in Higher Education*, pp. 1–13. London: Kogan Page.

31 Holmes, L. (1999). Competence and capability from 'confidence trick' to the construction of the graduate identity. In: D. O'Reilly, L. Cunningham, S. Lester (eds) *Developing the Capable Practitioner: Professional Ability Through Higher Education*, pp. 83–98. London: Kogan Page.

32 Sainsbury Centre for Mental Health. (2001). *The Capable Practitioner*. London: Sainsbury Centre.

33 Schoen, D. (1987). *Educating the Reflective Practitioner*. San Francisco: Jossey Bass.

34 Fraser, S., Greenhalgh, T. (2001). Coping with complexity: educating for capability. *Br Med J* **323**: 799–803.

35 Stephenson, J. (1998). The concept of capability and its importance in higher education. In: J. Stephenson and M. Yorke (eds) *Capability and Quality in Higher Education*, pp. 1–13. London: Kogan Page.

36 [35], pp. 1–13.

37 Willows, D., Swinton, J. (2000). Introduction. In: D. Willows, J. Swinton (eds) *Spiritual Dimensions of Pastoral Care*, pp. 11–16. London: Jessica Kingsley.

38 Kelly, E. (2007). *Marking Short Lives: Constructing and Sharing Rituals Following Pregnancy Loss*. Oxford: Peter Lang.

39 Cobb, M. (2005). *The Hospital Chaplain's Handbook*. Norwich: Canterbury Press.

40 Howe, A., Barrett, A., Leinster, S. (2009). How medical students demonstrate their professionalism when reflecting on experience. *Med Educ* **43**(10): 942–51.

41 NHS Education for Scotland. (2008). *Spiritual and Religious Care Capabilities and Competences for Healthcare Chaplains*, p. 8. Edinburgh: NHS Education for Scotland.

42 Sainsbury Centre for Mental Health. (2001). *The Capable Practitioner*, p. 6. London: Sainsbury Centre.

43 NHS Education for Scotland. (2007). *Standards for NHS Scotland Chaplaincy Services*. Edinburgh: NHS Education for Scotland.

44 Marie Curie Cancer Care. (2003). *Spiritual and Religious Care Competencies for Specialist Palliative Care*. London: Marie Curie Cancer Care.

45 NHS Education for Scotland. (2008). *Spiritual and Religious Care Capabilities and Competences for Healthcare Chaplains*. Edinburgh: NHS Education for Scotland.

46 Standards of Practice for Professional Chaplains in Acute Settings (2011). Available at: http://www.professionalchaplains.org (accessed 27 October 2010).

CHAPTER 58

Guidance from the humanities for professional formation

Nathan Carlin, Thomas Cole, and Henry Strobel

Introduction

The term 'professional formation' is being used increasingly in the context of medical education.[1] One reason for this seems to be that there is a growing dissatisfaction with the idea of professionalism in medical education, because professionalism is often reduced to mere compliance[2] and, perhaps as any 'ism' implies, to indoctrination. As Fred Hafferty, a prominent and passionate writer on the topic, has cautioned, 'The image of cohorts of medical students marching lock-step to the normative chant of their professors has a certain disquieting and Fascist ring to it.'[3] We support such concerns. Professional formation should be seen more as a process of development—a process of becoming a professional—and not equated with, as professionalism so often is, lists of 'do's' and 'don't's' or lists of behaviours that will lead to expulsion.

While we support the use of the term professional formation, we do not think that the term has been fully conceptualized.[4] There are two major reasons for this lack of conceptualization. First, there is little agreement on what the term 'professionalism' in medical education means, let alone the term 'professional formation,' despite the plethora of articles on professionalism[5,6] and the Physician Charter on Professionalism.[7] Indeed, to name only a few examples, professionalism has been conceptualized as a comprehensive entity; as a composite of separate elements, such as humanism, altruism, empathy, and more; and as one component of clinical competence.[8,9] Secondly, there has not been sufficient attention given to what *formation* means in professional formation. Who or what is being formed by whom and toward what ends?

The term professional formation, we suggest, needs further conceptual elaboration and clarification. We do not think that it is possible to do all of this intellectual work in a single article or chapter, and it seems likely that this work will be carried out step-by-step by various groups of scholars, precisely as literature on medical professionalism has grown over the past few decades.[5]

The purpose, argument, and organization of this chapter

The purpose of this chapter is to take steps to elaborate and to clarify, and to further justify, the term professional formation by focusing on the question of formation. We do so by locating the question of formation in the humanities and by focusing on what it might mean to take the soul seriously, though in a metaphorical and non-dogmatic way, when conceptualizing the work of professional formation. Another way of putting this—and this is our central argument—is to say that the humanities, and the recent field of spirituality and healthcare, ought to inform how we think about professional formation because these perspectives can help to overcome the pitfalls of professionalism, as these perspectives insist on a focus on meaning.

This chapter has several parts. We begin by introducing the concept of professional formation in medical education, a concept that we believe holds much promise. We then move to a discussion of various humanistic traditions to contextualize and to develop the idea of formation more fully. Here, we draw on the Renaissance notion of the personal self and its growth through humanistic study (*studia humanitatis*), and we briefly intimate its evolution in the thought of Matthew Arnold and Lionel Trilling. We next orient this chapter toward the subject matter of this volume—spirituality in healthcare—as we turn to a discussion of the soul in the social sciences. We draw on the experiences of medical students to demonstrate, concretely, what matters of the soul in medical education involve. Finally, we advocate the educational philosophy of Carl Rogers, a humanistic psychologist, as a way to safeguard against the dangers of professionalism and as a way to attend to the souls of medical students.

What is professional formation?

In the context of medical education, it seems that the term 'professional formation' was first used by Thomas Inui[10] in his report to the Association of American Medical Colleges, 'A Flag in the Wind: Educating for Professionalism in Medicine.' Inui noted that 'the most difficult challenge of all is for students and educators to understand that medical education is 'a special form of personal and professional *formation*.'[11] Recently, Inui, along with several others, further developed the concept of professional formation in an article titled: 'Professional Formation: Extending Medicine's Lineage of Service into the Next Century.'[1] These authors note that, while the Flexner Report, published by the Carnegie Foundation, is 'widely recognized' as having transformed medical education in terms of laboratory and clinical education, it is less widely known that the Flexner Report also advocated the teaching of the liberal arts in medical education. The authors write,

'On the 100th anniversary of the Flexner Report, we are challenged to reconsider Flexner's vision of an educational focus broader than the acquisition of cognitive and technical skills in order to ensure that physicians are prepared to lead lives of compassion and service.'[12] Advocating the notion of professional formation is their way of reclaiming a forgotten part of Flexner's vision. We, too, are also following in this vision by advocating the liberal arts in medical education.

What is professional formation? Rabow *et al.* define professional formation as 'the moral and professional development of students, the integration of their individual maturation with growth in clinical competency, and their ability to stay true to values which are both personal and core values of the profession.'[13] They note that, while professional formation goes by many names (such as professional development, professionalism education, identity formation, values education, and so forth), the basic rationale for such training is the same and is analogous to, they suggest, spiritual formation in clerical training. 'The goal of professional formation,' the authors write, 'is to tether or anchor students to their personal principles and the core values of the profession and help them navigate through the inevitable conflicts that arise in training and practice.'[13] Their article does not provide new models for professional formation, but rather reviews the status of professional formation in medical education and concludes by describing two commonly used educational programmes—namely, the Healer's Art and Appreciative Inquiry.

A shortcoming of Rabow *et al.*'s article is that it does not explain why the term professional formation is needed. It seems to us that simply re-labelling current practices in medical education with the term 'professional formation' is not enough to justify the use of the term in place of the more common term 'professionalism.' In other words, the authors do not provide a critique of 'professionalism,' as Coulehan[2] and Hafferty[3] do, to explain why they are advocating 'professional formation'. This critique is essential.

Other shortcomings of Rabow *et al.*'s article include that they could have articulated a broader context of professional formation as well as a deeper vision of what the humanities have to offer professional formation. The advantage of discussing two specific educational programmes, the Healer's Art and Appreciative Inquiry, is that Rabow *et al.* [1] were able to offer concrete examples of what they envision professional formation to be in practice, but the shortcoming is that these discussions do not convey the depth of what the humanities have to offer. We now turn to a brief discussion of this broader context and we attempt to convey the depth of the humanities.

Toward a broader context of and a deeper vision for professional formation

In the mid-1970s, medical humanities and bioethics emerged in academic medicine as a response to widely perceived dehumanization and to new ethical dilemmas inherent in high-tech medicine. Though there remains considerable debate about what the outcomes of medical humanities should be, the infusion of literature, history, philosophy, and the arts into medical education has been a slow but steady process.[14,15] In contrast to medical humanities, bioethics has become virtually ubiquitous in education, hospital practice, and public discourse. Knowledge in bioethics is most often concerned with identifying and resolving ethical conflicts that arise in clinical practice, traditionally in end-of-life care. Bioethics has evolved into standardized processes for making decisions, which are institutionalized in hospital ethics committees, institutional review boards, and various protocols. To oversimplify, bioethics is primarily concerned with 'doing,' while medical humanities is more concerned with 'being.'

Making morally sound decisions alone is an important but not a sufficient goal for the humanities in medicine.[16] Patients and students alike are confronted daily with questions of meaning, unexplained suffering, and the need for healing. Ethics and philosophy have been broadened by other humanities disciplines aimed at cultivating compassion and other dimensions of caring for patients. Medical humanists read literature, interpret films, view art, examine historical context, and study cultural differences in order to shape the moral imagination of students. More specifically, the humanities in medical education aim to strengthen the capacity to care, to enhance empathy, to help students attend to suffering, and to open them to the finitude and the mystery at the core of human experience. In other words, the humanities are taught *to* students in order to evoke the humanity *of* students. Evoking the humanity of students means feeding their hearts and their minds, helping them to develop a personal and professional identity.

The humanities, then, assist in the formation of the self—a goal that should be understood as part of an educational tradition which long pre-dates the birth of the university in late medieval Europe or of modern professional medical education in the early twentieth century. In ancient Greece and in ancient Rome, the original liberal arts or *artes liberales* were designed to give men (not, of course, women slaves, or those without property) the intellectual and practical tools to pursue life in the *polis*—a free, public, urban arena. The ancients understood that it is one thing to be a human being; it is another thing to be *human*. That is, one can be more or less human and the goal of a liberal arts curriculum is to help an individual know and aspire to the highest ideals of humanity, as well as to know and to experience its depth.

The word 'humanities' today refers to a range of disciplines and fields taught in colleges and universities by faculty who are credentialled in those disciplines or fields, such as history, philosophy, religious studies, literature, the human sciences, and so forth. Since the rise of the research university in the late nineteenth century, the primary focus of these disciplines and fields has been on research and the expansion of knowledge. However, the linguistic roots of 'humanities' reveal a much broader educational intent. The Latin word *humanitas* originally meant 'humane feeling' and gradually came to be understood as an educational ideal involving humane feeling, expert knowledge, and practical action in the world. The English word 'humanities' is also derived from the *studia humanitatis*, or the study of humanity. Put another way, the humanities are the study of ourselves and each other.

Why does it matter that we study ourselves, as well as the world of nature? It matters because self-knowledge and self-development are key components of living a good life. The self, however, is not a static and universal entity, but rather a historically-mediated concept and experience. When ancient authors referred to the self, they understood the self not as a separate entity but as part of the larger worlds of the polis and the cosmos. When Cicero, for example, was suffering from the death of his daughter Tullia, he removed himself from a highly public life in Rome and took to his little villa south of Rome to recover from intense grief. There, he struggled to recover by means of writing and reading, as well as by means of friendship. His restoration, he wrote in the *Tusculan Disputations*, depended on training and focusing his mind on its proper identity with the unchanging heavens.

During the Renaissance, which began in fourteenth century Italy, the modern concept of the inward-turning autonomous self emerged first in the writing of Petrarch, the founder of the *studia humanitatis*. Like Cicero, Petrarch suffered often from intense grief from the loss of friends and family in the Black Death and in the violent world of Italian city-state. Petrarch found no solace in the prevailing scholastic theology propounded by university faculties in Paris and Rome. Instead, he was inspired and comforted by returning to writings of ancient Greek and ancient Roman authors. Petrarch was a statesman and diplomat, not a professional classicist. He was no less a Christian than any university theologian. However, he could not find relief from grief and anxiety through faith or theological speculation alone. Instead, he turned inward and sought to cultivate a self strong enough to withstand the violent blows of Fortune. Reading Vergil, Horace, and Cicero was a deep inner experience for Petrarch. Their words provided a kind of healing and strengthening to a vulnerable self: 'These writings have entered into me so intimately ... and have become one with my mind, that even if I were never to read them again they would remain embedded in me, having set their roots in the deepest part of my soul.'[17]

Taking their cue from Petrarch, colleagues and successors developed a new version of the *studia humanitatis* that involved the study of grammar, rhetoric, history, poetry, and moral philosophy. These literary disciplines focused on ancient Greek and ancient Roman thought to contain the moral and spiritual wisdom required for the development of a unique, personally integrated self.

Although this original humanist impulse was often lost as these studies moved into the universities and evolved into a narrow philological focus, the goal of shaping an ideal self survived and reappeared in the vision of a liberal arts education in the nineteenth and twentieth centuries. In the English-speaking world, Matthew Arnold's (1869) *Culture and Anarchy*[18] was the prototypical expression of the ideal of humanistic education as a perfecting and shaping of one's self. A century later the Columbia English professor Lionel Trilling[19] commented on 'The Uncertain Future of the Humanistic Educational Ideal.' Under attack from a generation of students protesting the dominance of the traditional Western canon, Trilling defended the value of literary study for its ability to shape the moral imagination, to purge the mind from prejudice, and to contribute to the development of one's higher self.

However, while broadening the mind and deepening the inner life of students remained an ideal in undergraduate liberal arts education, humanistic education was deliberately separated from graduate and professional education. This meant that undergraduates had little exposure or connection to the world outside the academy and that professional students had little or no exposure to the liberal arts. Modern medical education, which took shape in the early twentieth century, followed this pattern and, hence, was ill-equipped to respond to the moral and spiritual crises which accompanied the high-tech biomedicine of the latter part of the twentieth century. Our technological capabilities outstripped our moral bearings as new questions began to be posed by life-sustaining treatment and complex market forces. The professionalism movement, Coulehan[2] notes, emerged in this context, as did bioethics and medical humanities.

Professional formation seems to be an attempt at recovering an older model of education, where technical skills are not the only goal, but rather the development of an inner life is a goal as well. What the humanities have to offer is not simply journaling or a discussion of this or that poem or short story. What the humanities offer is much deeper than this: They offer the only resources we have to inquire what it means to be human. Any serious vision of professional formation must draw on the full wealth of the humanities.

The language of the soul

We want to shift the focus of this essay, and now turn our attention to the soul as a way of orienting this discussion toward the field of spirituality and healthcare. We believe that introducing the language of the soul can enrich discussions of spirituality and healthcare in two primary ways: (1) soul-language brings to the fore the sufferings of health professionals—in terms of this essay, medical students; and (2) in terms of professional formation, soul-language, with its emphasis on local experience, provides a spiritual vocabulary for understanding the personal histories of medical students—a richer understanding, that is to say, of *who* is being formed in professional formation.

It is important to point out that, just as discussions of spirituality in healthcare are not intended to be some kind of evangelizing enterprise, our advocating of soul-language is not an attempt to privilege any particular faith commitment or dogmatic position. Soul-language here is, rather, an attempt to speak metaphorically about the human condition in ways that scientific discourse simply cannot. In *On Losing the Soul*, Richard Fenn and Donald Capps[20] offer an edited volume that attempts to recover soul language in social scientific discourse. In making the case for soul-language in the social sciences, Fenn quotes, with approval, Bernice Martin:

> The word 'soul' suggests to me the possibility of recognizing—hinting at—a level of discourse which accords some ultimate significance to the person beyond what can be said by the expert social scientific disciplines. The metaphysical and theological connotations of 'soul' suggest a dimension of the integrity of persons, which is not fully captured by the vocabulary of 'self' or 'selfhood.' The death of the soul is of greater moment than the death of the self. The poetic language of love and its corruption says more than, and different from, the scientific analysis of 'the self in relationship.'[21]

Fenn states that in this volume they are 'proposing to use the soul as an end-term: a word that comes at the end of a series of terms like the individual, individuality, the person, personality, self, selfhood, and even beyond the inner or essential self'. 'The soul,' he continues, 'represents a hypothetical point in the individual's subjectivity.'[21] It is in this sense that we advocate soul-language.

Distinguishing the spirit and the soul

Professionalism, at its best, focuses on forming the self and helping medical students forge a professional identity, what Rabow *et al.* [1] call professional formation. However, as this textbook in spirituality in healthcare is articulating, human beings also have spiritual dimensions. Human beings, we believe, have spirits and they have souls. Professional formation, we suggest, should not only focus on the self, but it should also focus on the spirit and the soul.

The model of the person that we are drawing on comes from the distinctions observed by Donald Capps, who writes:

> [T]he spirit is associated with the heart and one's aspirations toward the 'beyond and the above,' and the soul is linked to the liver and one's rootedness in the local, circumscribed realities in which we live our daily lives. … [T]he self is associated with the brain and specifically with its memory function that enables us to maintain a sense or awareness of ourselves as being the self-same person over a lifetime, despite changes in physical appearance due to aging.[22]

We realize that many in the medical context might view the idea of the soul being located in the liver with a great deal of scepticism, but it was actually a physician, Richard Selzer, that has informed Capps's thinking on this model of the person. In any case, the point here is that these vocabularies are metaphorical ways of talking about the complexity of personhood. Since this is a volume on spirituality, we focus here on the spirit and the soul in Capps's model of the person.

What is the difference between the spirit and the soul? In 'Enrapt Spirits and the Melancholy Soul,' Capps[23] discusses this distinction. He notes there have been two main enemies of the soul in the modern period: 'reductionists' and 'inflators.' Reductionists seek to take soul-language out of academic discussions, replacing, for example, the notion of the soul with terms like 'the self' or 'the psyche.' For example, following the work of Bruno Bettelheim, Capps notes that the word soul (*die Seele*) has been systematically removed from *The Standard Edition* of Freud's works, and that it was replaced with words such as 'mental apparatus.' This is an example of reducing the soul.

Drawing on the work of James Hillman, Capps also suggests that talk about spirituality often undermines our thinking about the soul, because all-too-often matters of the spirit become emphasized at the expense of the soul. As Capps puts it, 'the spiritual perspective inflates the spirit, and, in doing so, obscures the soul's depths of suffering.'[24] This is not, to be sure, the intent of those who write in the area or field of spirituality and healthcare. Indeed, as Christina Puchalski writes, 'Spirituality can be defined as that part of people that seeks ultimate meaning in life, especially in suffering.'[25] The spirit attempts to overcome suffering, to transcend it, to make meaning out of it, but in contrast, as Capps[22] writes, '[u]nlike spirit, which extracts meanings (insights) and puts them into action, soul sticks to the realm of experience and to reflections within experience.'[24] Following Hillman, Capps suggests that the spirit seeks peaks and meaning, while the soul, in contrast, remains in vales and in local experience.

Early Christian writers, Capps[23] notes, have contributed to soul-loss in contemporary discourse by confusing soul-talk with spirit-talk. Already by the organizing of the New Testament, Capps points out, the soul is rarely spoken of, as Paul, instead, writes about the spirit (*pneuma*) and things of the spirit, such as speaking in tongues and in prophecies. While the spirit looks upward, and is associated with sublimation and ecstasy, the soul looks downward, and is associated with the realm of the dead and the moon [23, p. 143]. The spirit is active and takes us places by means of visions and ecstasy and is associated with such words as fast, far, and high. The soul, however,

> moves indirectly in circular reasonings, where retreats are as important as advances, preferring labyrinths and corners, giving a metaphorical sense to life through such words as *close*, *near*, *slow*, and *deep*. … It is the 'patient' part of us. Soul is vulnerable and suffers; it is passive and remembers.[26]

However, in Christianity, the soul became usurped by the spirit at the Council of Constantinople in 869. Previously, human beings were conceived of as body, spirit, and soul, but at this council, the human being became defined as flesh and spirit.[26]

Capps points out that Hillman takes Abraham Maslow—and Maslow's notion of 'peak experiences'—to be representative of those who would inflate of the spirit. One problem with the inflating of the soul by means of peak experiences, Capps notes, is that:

> [b]y turning away from [the soul's] pathologizings they turn away from its full richness. By going upward towards spiritual betterment they leave its afflictions, giving them less validity and less reality than spiritual goals. In the name of the higher spirit, the soul is betrayed.[27]

While experiences of suffering may lead to spiritual experiences and moments of transcendence—such as a near-death experiences in the operating room or during car accidents—often times they do not. When such suffering does not lend itself to transcendence, such suffering is a matter of the soul and not a matter of the spirit—such experiences are not 'peak experiences' at all, but rather dark nights of the soul.

Why does the distinction between the soul and the spirit matter? This distinction gives us a richer vocabulary for thinking about the spiritual dimensions of personhood—human beings not only have goals, aspirations, and experiences of transcendence (spirit), but they also have histories, sufferings, and experiences of regeneration (soul). In terms of professional formation, students need to be able to connect where they have come from (soul) with where they are going (spirit). Professional formation also needs to focus not only on aspiration (spirit), but also on the frustrations of aspiration and how one recovers from such frustration (soul).

The souls of medical students

With regard to the distinction between the spirit and the soul that we outlined above, there are many common experiences in medical education that involve both the spirit and the soul. Matters of the spirit, for example, might involve the aspirations that led one to medical school in the first place, the experience of delivering a baby for the first time, and the 'high' one might experience on account of working for 30 straight hours during a clinical rotation. Matters of the soul, in contrast, might involve the uncanny emotions one feels when cutting into a cadaver for the first time, when holding an eyeball, or when witnessing a vast amount of suffering in the emergency room with no way of making meaning of senseless suffering. We contend that attending to the souls of medical students is just as important as attending to the spirits of medical students in writing and in teaching about spirituality in healthcare.

In *Surviving Medical School*, Robert Coombs[28] addresses common issues that medical students face, drawing on student interviews and student journal writing. He notes two such experiences that we believe are related to the souls of medical students: (1) the transition to a more difficult workload; and (2) the experience of the medical hierarchy.

One common issue that Coombs identified, as noted, is that students, when they arrive at medical school, have to adjust to new academic and social pressure to master difficult material. If a medical student measures how he or she is doing by looking at others around himself or herself, he or she is often left with a feeling of being 'average' or, sometimes, even 'below average.' When students arrive at medical school, Coombs points out, they are accustomed to being considered the best and the brightest, because, both in high school and in college, they distinguished themselves from their cohort. As one student described, 'I've never considered myself conceited, but it was a real ego buster to suddenly not be effortlessly at the top of the heap. I had to deal with some Bs instead of straight As. I learned to forgive myself.'[29] The fact that one has to 'forgive oneself' for receiving a 'B' intimates both the difficulty of the subject material for talented students and the difficulty of emotionally adjusting to a new environment. The fact that medical school is considerably harder than college leads some to be ultra-competitive, and this can sometimes create a hostile culture among medical students. One student described the destructive nature of such competition in medical school by relaying an incident where, to get an edge, some students would steal dissecting atlases and damage the cadavers of other students.

Some students react with mild bouts of disillusionment in response to these frustrations. 'This is not what I signed up for,' or 'This is not what I thought it was going to be like,' students tell us, with the underlying fear seeming to be, 'I'm not good enough to excel in medicine,' or, more deeply, 'I do not *want* a life in medicine if it is going to be like this, or if a life in medicine means being with people like this.' We take these anxieties and meanderings and questions and frustrations to be ruminations of the soul. They are matters of ordinary experience, having to do more with the vales of medicine rather than the peaks of medicine—but they are also ultimate in some way, as students struggle over the question, *What is becoming of me?* It seems as though the very souls of medical students are at stake in these meanderings.

Another issue that Coombs identified, as noted, is that students discover and experience the medical hierarchy very early. They notice the constant pecking order of the medical hierarchy: first year medical student, second year medical student, third year medical student, fourth year medical student, intern, resident, chief resident, fellow, residency director, attending—with each rank looking down on lower ranks. One medical student contrasted her experience with her husband's experience as a graduate student:

> His situation is more of a peer relationship between the professors and graduate students. Classes consist of meeting at each other's houses, having dinner, and sitting around and talking for a couple of hours. The faculty are his friends. It isn't a heavily structured situation like medical school. Here, we are not only treated like children, but also there is this rigid hierarchy and a somber authoritarian attitude that I just can't take seriously. Not only do they expect us to absorb all this technical information, but also they act like we don't know how to think, dress, or react in social situations. It's like we are coming in as blind slaves.[30, with permission Sage Publications]

The medical hierarchy reduces relationships to matters of rank, this student seems to be saying. Medical students, it seems, are not given permission to be human in the same way that graduate students are permitted.

Another medical student put it this way: 'Some residents, and even some nurses, expect medical students to do a substantial amount of scut work, much of it of the 3 a.m. variety.' Another medical student concurred: 'Residents take a bit of advantage, calling you late at night to start an IV. It might take you half an hour to get to the hospital and do it—something he or she could do in five or ten minutes—but for whatever reason, the call comes.'[31] The medical hierarchy constantly reinforces the fact that you have not quite made it yet, and even upon graduating from medical school with an MD, you then move on to residency to become what Coombs refers to as an 'R.D.'—that is, 'a real doctor.'[32]

Why are these matters of the soul? The soul is the part of us that, as Capps writes, involves 'the depressions and objections that come with spirit's rejections.'[33] While receiving the white coat was most likely an elevation of the spirit—perhaps even a moment of transcendence and an indication of how far one has come and how high one is going—the spirit is deflated when one experiences the fact that it is a *short* white coat that one is wearing. And when interns and residents remind medical students of this with their 3 a.m. calls for scut work, the spirit is deflated and the soul suffers.

There are other problems with the medical hierarchy that, we believe, affect the souls of medical students. In our conversations with medical students and in our reading, we know that medical students, from time to time, witness harsh and demeaning treatment of patients. The range of such episodes is wide. In its milder forms, such episodes may involve the unsympathetic announcement of impending death due to a cancer for which no treatment is offered, but in its more vicious forms such episodes may involve an announcement to a patient with AIDS that he deserves 'what he gets' because of his so-called 'lifestyle choice.' Other times comments from superiors are directed at students themselves. In this category fall comments with covert or explicit sexual overture or frank sexual harassment. Such pressures create a hostile environment and as such are illegal, but unfortunately are not always absent. Likewise, comments about race, sexual orientation, economic status, and the like can cause a troubling of the soul.

These points are made much more eloquently in works by authors such as Sam Shem,[34] Abraham Verghese,[35] and Richard Selzer,[36] and we can confirm such experiences in our own experience. In any case, we suggest that another way that the soul can be damaged is by witnessing various assaults on the humanity of patients or trainees repeatedly and without correction. It seems that this repetitive observation dulls the senses to outrage, perhaps reducing the ability even to recognize the offense at some point, let alone to respond to it appropriately. Interestingly and unfortunately, this could be a partial explanation of the conclusions of many studies that have indicated that empathy decreases in medical school.[37]

A pedagogy for the whole person

We noted above that the introduction of humanities teaching and research in the context of medical education during the last quarter of the twentieth century aimed at helping students to develop professional identities capable of grappling with moral and spiritual challenges. A major way that these initiatives made their way into medical schools was under the banner of professionalism, but in recent years, it has been felt, ironically, that these initiatives have engaged the mind but not the emotions—this has been a professionalism without substantial engagement with the humanities, a professionalism based, as it were, on rules, compliance, and assessment. As a corrective to what Coulehan[2] has called a 'rule-based professionalism,' we suggest turning to a modern day humanist psychologist who was interested in educating the whole person—including the spiritual dimension—and who was also deeply sceptical of any indoctrination: Carl Rogers.

Carl Rogers (1902–1987) was an American psychologist who helped to create humanistic psychology. He is most widely known for his person-centred approach to psychotherapy. While other dominant psychologies of the time, such as psychoanalysis and behaviourism, focused on 'fixing' individuals by means of offering expertise, Rogers believed that individuals themselves were the experts, that they themselves had the resources for growth in them—this was the guiding assumption of his person-centred approach. His views, while widely influential, were nevertheless quite controversial, because they challenged hierarchy and authority in virtually all of its forms. Rogers applied his views, as we will see, to fields outside of psychology as well, such as education.

Rogers's philosophy of interpersonal relationships

In 'My Philosophy of Interpersonal Relationships and How It Grew,' Rogers[38] writes about his time at Union Theological Seminary in New York City, and how they influenced his thought. He notes that he gradually became turned off by courses on religion. While he does not explain why he became turned off by such courses, a plausible explanation would be that the abstract and dogmatic nature of many religion courses turned him off, but if so this would be striking because Union Theological Seminary in New York City is often regarded as the most freethinking seminary in the United States. In any case, Rogers describes a very powerful experience that he had during his seminary training: 'a self-organized, self-directed seminar of students with no faculty leader.'[39] He notes that the students in the course took complete responsibility for how the course would run, and what the content would entail. They shared doubts and personal problems. His experience in this course—his experience of freedom—would come to influence his views on psychotherapy and education. Another course that Rogers took at Union Theological Seminary was titled 'Working with Young People.' This course prompted him to think about working with individuals (i.e., counseling) as opposed to ministry, and it actually led to him leaving seminary for graduate school.

In graduate school, he learned the standard methods of the day in clinical psychology—diagnostic testing and advice giving. He also learned about psychoanalysis. The therapeutic interview became the most interesting part of the whole process for Rogers, and he attributed this interest to the lack of close interpersonal relationships that had previously characterized his life. These interviews afforded him the opportunity to become close, intimately close, with persons in a very short period of time, something that he struggled with in his personal life.[40] A metaphor that was inculcated in him—a metaphor that he later came to reject—involved the notion that going to therapy was like going to the auto-mechanic shop: one goes there to be 'fixed' by an expert. The expert takes an elaborate history, evaluates what the problem is, and offers advice about how to fix the problem. To be an effective fixer, one needs, of course, to be warm so as to increase compliance, but these were merely matters of technique.

However, as noted, Rogers came to reject all of this. He eventually learned, almost by accident, that simply listening to clients—letting them take the lead, without judging them, without evaluating them, and even without offering advice—was really all that was needed. He found that trusting his clients enabled them to trust themselves. This approach, which took various names over the years, was called the non-directive technique, where he viewed his clients with 'unconditional positive regard.' Human beings, Rogers believed, have a self-actualizing tendency. Just as plants will grow if given sunlight, human beings will grow if they are given acceptance and validation. Just as plants do not need to be told how to grow, human beings do not need to be instructed either—these capacities are innate. Human beings, Rogers believed, can be trusted.

Rogers's philosophy of education

'If I [trust] my clients,' Rogers wonders, 'why [don't] I trust my students?'[41] He therefore continued to develop his ideas, as he gradually applied them to education.

In 'Can Learning Encompass Both Ideas and Feelings?' Rogers[42] argues that learning must include the *whole* person. He suggests that much of the excitement has fallen out of education, that professors have become anxious about whether they can keep going for a full 50 minutes, and that students have become bored. There is no energy in education—it is reduced to a requirement, something one has to do before one moves onto the real thing, a hoop to jump through—and Rogers dreams about closing all schools and creating a situation in which the only learning that takes place is out of freedom and curiosity.

Rogers describes four characteristics that enable learning. The first is a 'realness' in the facilitator of learning. Facilitators must be present, aware of their feelings, and able to communicate their feelings, if appropriate. Another characteristic is acceptance—a non-possessive caring for the learner and a basic trust of the learner. Such facilitators can accept the fear and uncertainty of students. A third characteristic is empathetic understanding—an understanding of learning experiences from the point of view of the students themselves, without judgment and evaluation. A fourth characteristic is that the students must believe that these attitudes genuinely exist in the teacher—that they are not being 'conned.'[43]

In 'Beyond the Watershed,' Rogers contrasts conventional education with his student-centred approach. In conventional education, Rogers points out, teachers are the possessors of knowledge, and students are the recipients. The lecture is the central means of conveying this knowledge, and exams assess whether the knowledge has been received. Teachers have the power, and they rule by authority and by means of fear. Students cannot be trusted to learn on their own—they need strict oversight. There is no democracy in learning, and learning is only for the intellect, not the emotions. Student-centred learning, in contrast, turns conventional education on its head. For effective student-centred learning, the facilitators must be self-aware and secure, and they must have a basic trust in the ability of others to learn for themselves. Facilitators share the responsibility for the learning process; they provide learning resources—books and illustrations from their own learning—but the students themselves develop the agenda and programme of learning. The primary goal of the facilitator is to cultivate an open environment, *not* to convey knowledge, and the only means of assessment is made by students themselves, based on whether students have found the learning *significant*. We do not have space here to spell out what student-centred learning in medical education might look like, but we can tell you what it is not: a crowded curriculum with virtually no space for electives and for inquiry for its own sake.

Permission to be human

The problem with professionalism is that it has no soul. It is not rooted in local experience; it is, rather, abstract and boring. As

Coulehan[2] puts it, the problem with professionalism is that it educates the mind, but fails to engage the heart. Rogers might put it this way: professionalism, as it is currently taught, does not engage the whole person, so it is unlikely that students would ever find themselves engaging in significant learning when reading about professionalism. It is hard to imagine, for example, students spending a Friday evening reading the ABIM charter on professionalism because they find it deeply meaningful.

If professional formation has a future, it must focus on educating whole persons—it must focus on the self, on the spirit, and on the soul. To do so effectively, professional formation, wherever possible, should employ strategies of student-centred learning for two reasons: (1) student-centred learning subverts the medical hierarchy, which contributes to the damaging of the souls of medical students; and (2) student-centred learning, by definition, cannot be reduced to compliance and to indoctrination—the central problems of professionalism—as such learning will provide a venue for medical students to explore what it is that they think they need, what it is that they feel is significant, what troubles their souls and raises their spirits.

What if professional formation could give medial students permission to be free, to be excited, to be average, to be great, to be interested, to be bored, to succeed, to fail, to be afraid, to be angry, to be confused, to be hungry, to be spiritual, to be tired, to be sorrowful, and to be soulful? It seems to us that if we could give medical students such freedom and such permission that they might become what the most reflective of us strive to become: human. This, in any case, is our lofty and local hope for professional formation.

References

1 Rabow, M., Remen, R., Parmelee, D., Inui, T. (2010). Professional formation: extending medicine's lineage of service into the next century. *Acad Med* **85**: 310–17.

2 Coulehan, J. (2005). Viewpoint: today's professionalism: engaging the mind, but not the heart. *Acad Med* **80**(10): 892–8.

3 Hafferty, F. (2006). Measuring professionalism: a commentary. In: D. Stern (ed.) *Measuring Medical Professionalism*, pp. 281–306. Oxford: Oxford University Press.

4 The authors are working on further developing the concept of professional formation.

5 Stern, D. (ed.) (2006). *Measuring Medical Professionalism.* Oxford: Oxford University Press.

6 Arnold, L., Stern, D. (2006). What is medical professionalism? In: D. Stern (ed.) *Measuring Medical Professionalism*. pp. 15–37. Oxford: Oxford University Press.

7 ABIM Foundation, ACP-ASIM Foundation, European Federation of Internal Medicine (2002). Medical professionalism in the new millennium: a physician charter. *Ann Intern Med* **136**: 243–6.

8 Arnold, L. (2002). Assessing professional behaviour: yesterday, today, and tomorrow. *Acad Med* **77**: 502–15.

9 Veloski, J., Fields, S., Boex, J., Blank, L. (2005). Measuring professionalism. *Acad Med* **80**: 366–70.

10 Inui, T. (2003). *A Flag in the Wind: Educating for Professionalism in Medicine.* Washington, DC: American Association of Medical Colleges.

11 [2].

12 [1].

13 [1].

14 Campo, R. (2005). The medical humanities, for lack of a better term. *J Am Med Ass* **294**: 1009–11.

15 Shapiro, J., Coulehan, J., Wear, D., Montello, M. (2009). Medical humanities and their discontents: definitions, critiques, and implications. *Acad Med* **84**: 192–8.

16 Belkin, G. (2004). Moving beyond bioethics: history and the search for medical humanism. *Perspect Biol Med* **47**: 372–85.

17 Proctor, R. (1988). *Education's Great Amnesia.* Bloomington: Indiana University Press.

18 Arnold, M. (1966). *Culture and Anarchy.* Cambridge: Cambridge University Press.

19 Trilling, L. (1982). The uncertain future of the humanistic educational ideal. In: D. Trilling (ed.) *The Last Decade: Essays and Reviews, 1965–75*, pp. 160–76. New York: Oxford University Press.

20 Fenn, R., Capps, D. (1995). *On Losing the Soul: Essays in the Social Psychology of Religion.* Albany: SUNY.

21 Fenn, R. (1995). Introduction: Why the soul? In: R. Fenn, D. Capps (eds) *On Losing the Soul: Essays in the Social Psychology of Religion*, pp. 1–20. Albany: SUNY.

22 Capps, D. (2005). *A Time to Laugh: The Religion of Humor*, p. 109. New York: Continuum.

23 Capps, D. (1995). Enrapt spirits and the melancholy soul: the locus of division in the Christian self and American society. In: R. Fenn, D. Capps (eds) *On Losing the Soul: Essays in the Social Psychology of Religion*, pp. 137–69. Albany: SUNY.

24 [23], pp. 137–69.

25 Puchalski, C. (2007). Foreword. In: E. Taylor (ed.) *What Do I Say? Talking with Patients about Spirituality*, p. ix. Philadelphia: Templeton Foundation Press.

26 [23], p. 143.

27 [23], p. 142.

28 Coombs, R. (1998). *Surviving Medical School.* Thousand Oaks: SAGE Publications.

29 [28], p. 14.

30 [28], p. 17.

31 [28], p. 104.

32 [28], p. 176.

33 [22], p. 106.

34 Shem, S. (1981). *The House of God.* New York: Dell.

35 Verghese, A. (1995). *My Own Country: a Doctor's Story.* New York: Vintage.

36 Selzer, R. (2001). *Confessions of a Knife.* East Lansing: Michigan State University.

37 Spiro, H. (1992). What is empathy and can it be taught? *Ann Intern Med* **116**(10): 843–6.

38 Rogers, C. (1980). My philosophy of interpersonal relationships and how it grew. In: C. Rogers (ed.) *A Way of Being*, pp. 27–45. Boston: Houghton Mifflin.

39 [38], p. 32.

40 [38], p. 34.

41 [38], p. 37.

42 Rogers, C. (1980). Can learning encompass both ideas and feelings? In: C. Rogers (ed.) *A Way of Being*, pp. 263–291. Boston: Houghton Mifflin.

43 [42], pp. 271–3.

CHAPTER 59

Training and formation: a case study

Fiona Gardner

Introduction

What's important in training and formation for those in health and human services wanting to engage in conversations about spirituality? While there is clearly an increasing interest in spirituality in the health and human service professions, there continues to be little training in how to work with spirituality in practice. This chapter focuses on the experience of a specific project to illustrate the centrality of a critically reflective approach to training and formation in spiritual practice for health and human service workers.

Background

The rapid increase in literature related to spirituality in health and related professions demonstrates the increasing interest in spirituality in the community and this has been well documented elsewhere in this book. Including the spiritual is often seen as particularly legitimate in times of loss and grief, trauma or death. Holloway's[1] studies, for example, with social workers in the US and the UK found that they saw spirituality as particularly relevant in three areas 'related to loss and death—terminal illness, bereavement and in the situation of natural disaster.' Abbas and Panjwani,[2] argue 'spirituality is a core human concern at the time of death,' and that it is important for healthcare workers to gain 'some understanding of patients' spirituality early on, as it would be difficult to accomplish this solely near the time of death.'

Others argue the need to include spirituality throughout life: Gale, Bohan and McRae-McMahon,[3] for example, identify people in the helping professions working with spiritual practices from Hinduism to Wicca and in fields of practice from domestic violence to mental health. Forman[4] and Kavanagh[5] identify the vast range of ways that people and communities experience and express spiritualty as an important part of their lives, both within religious traditions and outside them. Holloway and Moss[6] suggests increased migration means greater need to respond to different cultures with their own religious preferences. There is also the influence of demonstrated positive impacts of spirituality for health,[7] the search for meaning[8] and greater understanding of the spirituality of ageing.[9]

This, of course, raises the question of what is meant by spirituality. There is considerable variation in how spirituality is defined. Rumbold[10] points out the challenge of maintaining a holistic definition in systems that easily become overly focused on 'individualism and problem-oriented reductionism'. The terms spirituality and religion are often used interchangeably, but don't necessarily mean the same[11] as suggested in the following definition: 'Spirituality means something different for everybody and consequently there can be no single all-encompassing definition. It relates to how we find meaning and connection, and the resources we use to replenish ourselves and cope with adversity. Spirituality may be part of religious beliefs or another shared belief system or something entirely personal and self-developed.'[12]

Whatever definition is being used, much of the literature suggests that medical and health practitioners working in this field have 'little preparation or education for responding to patient's spiritual needs' such as finding meaning in life and death.[13] Puchalski and McSkimming's research[14] found that ' healthcare providers are ill equipped to care for the spiritual dimension in patients'. Similarly, other research in a hospital setting found staff recognized the value of spirituality and religion, but were able to 'acknowledge that they seldom ask patients about spirituality/religion, they lack confidence in responding to patients' comments on the subject and they do not currently have strategies for integrating spirituality/religion into their practice.'[15] D'Souza[16] comments that healthcare education in the Western world has revolved around the more easily measured physical aspects of patients and their care and 'learning how to deal with the spiritual aspects of medical care is not a typical part of medical school or college curricula.'[16]

Related to issues about training and strategies of definition are questions about who should be responsible for providing spiritual care: should all healthcare professionals be involved or is this a specialist role for chaplains or trained pastoral care workers or volunteers? Barletta and Witteveen[17] suggest three levels of care: the first level the pastoral care visitor with the ability to provide spiritual, pastoral and emotional support—a role that could be taken on by all professionals with some basic training. Their second level is a Pastoral Carer/Chaplain who is also able to provide worship experience and thirdly a Chaplaincy or Pastoral Care Coordinator who coordinates the service, providing support, supervision and ongoing training to those on the other levels. Kuin *et al.*[18] raise the issue of who on a team sees the spiritual as relevant; they found that 'Consultants who are nurses and nursing home physicians identified spiritual issues as relevant more often than medical specialists', but concluded that: 'consultants of all disciplines have specific expertise about spiritual issues and their influence on the wellbeing of patients'. Others ask how working with spiritual issues is to be assessed, measured and audited, and what types of knowledge and skills are needed.[19]

How to train practitioners to assess spiritual needs or issues is also contested in the literature with some concern about the tendency to see the development of assessment tools or scales of spiritual needs as 'the answer'. Chaplin and Mitchell[20] conclude that assessment tools and competency levels that are too specific are of limited value: 'spiritual care does not easily conform to recognized methods of assessment and care planning.' Cobb[21] reinforces this saying it is 'Important not to lose sight of dimensions that can't be measured: The enthusiastic and uncritical use of assessment tools and instruments to measure need must not make us indifferent to . . .the wider considerations of care which are recognized not so much by diligence or genius as by compassion and wisdom'. However, others have found that a broad assessment tool or set of questions can be helpful if used in as part of a continuing conversation to gain a holistic understanding of the person.[22,23] This means including the person's view of what is important to them, particularly in terms of how they express their spirituality, relationships with family, friends and community and then to varying degrees the environment, sense of transcendence and links to places and things.

There is, of course, substantial literature in the religious traditions that relates to spiritual formation and training and some writers in health and human services make connections to this.[24–26] Many writers address theological issues; others write about religious traditions and what is distinctive about each as well as what is shared. There is also much literature about stages of religious or spiritual development[27] and about varieties of religious experience.[28,29] Any training programme needs to make decisions about which of this knowledge to use and what to make explicit or implicit.

Why training and formation for healthcare professionals?

Overall, the literature supports both the value of encouraging professionals to explore spirituality with their clients and for themselves, but also the need for caution about how this happens. This implies the importance of professionals being adequately trained and supported. Clearly, there are dangers of unethical practice if healthcare professionals are not adequately trained such as the imposition of the professional's values and/or preferred religious practices on their clients. Winslow & Wehtje-Winslow,[30] remind healthcare workers to be mindful of patient vulnerability and 'ethical boundaries of spiritual care'. McCurdy[31] mentions how 'some caregivers, consciously or not, attempt to impose their beliefs on patients and families while they're most vulnerable, which is always inappropriate' and that caregivers must 'strive to allow patients to find and travel their own paths to meaning at the end of life'. There is also the concern that professionals assume that their own spiritual experience is sufficient for working with other people on theirs, without being sufficiently conscious of the assumptions they are making about what is 'normal.'[32]

Given that spirituality is part of life, it makes sense that all professionals have the capacity to explore spiritual issues with their clients at least at a beginning level when it is relevant to do so with the knowledge and skill to refer on as needed.[33] Currently, what training is included in professional courses varies significantly. While there is an increased recognition of the value of including spirituality in training,[34] some professions are more reluctant than others to actively include it.[35] As well as the debates about who should receive what kind of training, there is also debate about what to include. A Consensus Conference held in the United States involved a wide-ranging group of health professionals connected with palliative care in exploring how to improve the quality of spiritual care in palliative care.[36] The conference concluded that the first issue was convincing healthcare professionals that spiritual care was an integral part of healthcare. Secondly, they affirm that healthcare providers form deeper and more meaningful connections with the patients by developing an awareness of their own values, beliefs, and attitudes, particularly regarding their own mortality and that therefore spiritual development is part of professional development.[36]

This sense of awareness is one of the key common aspects of suggested training for spirituality in professional practice, primarily an awareness for professionals of their own 'spiritual formation'—the influence of their own spiritual history and current practices, their beliefs and values, their assumptions about what makes life meaningful and how this might impact on their interaction with others. Conscious use of their own spiritual practices can also enable health practitioners to manage more effectively the stresses of much work in organizations. Puchalski *et al.*[37] also suggest the need for continuing reflective work 'in order to gain insight into one's own sense of spirituality, meaning, and professional calling in order to have the capacity to provide compassionate and skillful care.'

Role of critical reflection in training and formation

This suggests the need for training in working with the spiritual from a critically reflective perspective which is increasingly seen as an integral part of health and social care generally [38, 39]. It is important to notice that terms such as critical reflection, reflective practice, and reflexivity are often used interchangeably, but can also have distinct meanings.[40] Given agreement about how it is defined, critical reflection can provide a common approach to practice across disciplines, providing a shared language for understanding practice issues and dilemmas and processes for working through these.

Some writers are also making the link between working with spirituality and the importance of a critically reflective approach.[41] Holloway and Moss,[6] for example, say that in the UK the focus has been on a cultural competence model, but needs to be more reflective concerned with 'with where the student starts from and how they, and their practice, develop'. Practitioners too affirm the need for a critically reflective approach: a nurse interviewed about working with spirituality says 'we have these, kind of a cultural awareness day ... I was sent on one recently and it's the same old stuff. This is a Sikh and this is a Jew! ... Surely we should be talking now actually about what is racism? And I think we should be getting underneath that and exploring our own ideas rather than sort of, you know, talking about differences that people have?'[42] White[43] says that reflective practice is an important way to explore spirituality and can offer a 'safe space,' which 'encourages the integration of theory with practice, while the opportunity to learn with others offers challenge and support.'

The definition of critical reflection as used in this chapter is that 'critical reflection involves the unsettling of fundamental and (socially dominant and often hidden) individually held assumptions about the social world, in order to enable a reworking of these, and associated actions, for changed professional practice.'[44] Essentially, critical reflection is about using specific experiences to articulate implicit assumptions and values combined with an understanding of how these are influenced by a person's own history and the broader social context, including their spiritual history and how it relates to the spiritualities expressed around them. The aim of critical reflection as a process is to be able to make conscious and active choices about whether these are the values that we want to operate from, those which have meaning and integrity for us.[45] The underlying theories in critical reflection encourage awareness of how the main ways of thinking in our culture influences the expression of spirituality and affirms the need to be inclusive: to allow difference and enable individuals to find their own meaning, while also promoting attitudes and actions that are socially just. Critical reflection then combines the expectation of self-awareness with the capacity to stand back from the immediate to see what is happening from a broader social perspective. The assumption is that increasing awareness of their own spirituality will enable professionals to recognize and respect the different spirituality of others. The use of a critically reflective approach clearly addresses some of the concerns raised about the dangers of working with spirituality.

A model of professional training and formation

To make explicit how critical reflection can be used in training and formation, I will explore here a training and formation process that was piloted with health professionals in a project funded by the Federal Government Department of Health and Ageing in Australia in February, 2006, as part of a broader programme of pilot projects exploring pastoral care in palliative care.[46] This particular project: the Pastoral Care Networks Project (PCNP) had a population health, community capacity building approach and aimed to develop, resource, strengthen, and evaluate pastoral care networks supporting palliative care services, and health and community providers in two Victorian health regions. Funding for chaplaincy or spiritual care services was minimal in both regions. Before the project began, health professionals, healthcare workers, and volunteers were attempting to fill the gaps in providing spiritual or pastoral care support with little or no training. Both regions had been exploring ways of improving pastoral and spiritual care, and had identified a need to develop community-based approaches to care, and willingness at the community level to be involved in pastoral/spiritual care. Two project workers were employed, who both had experience in providing education in spirituality in other contexts. Bruce Rumbold, a member of the coordinating group for the project, also contributed to the provision of the training. Altogether, 115 people completed training, from six rural areas in Victoria, Australia, including two provincial cities. Those involved included a wide range of palliative care and related professionals: primarily palliative care nurses, but also acute care nurses, social workers, bereavement counsellors, chaplains, psychologists, palliative care volunteer coordinators, and of course, the palliative care volunteers.

The project workers started by asking local service providers and volunteers in six local advisory groups whether they thought training was needed and if so: 'What's important in providing training for people wanting to engage in conversations about spirituality?' We were surprised how consistent their answers were—and how much they connected to what we had been thinking. All six groups suggested a combination of:

- Knowledge about spirituality and religion, particularly definitions of spirituality and religion
- Encouragement of self-awareness of own values in relation to spirituality/pastoral care and how they might be different from other people's
- Practice in listening
- Awareness of the roles of other team members
- Consciousness of when to refer on
- The ability to care for yourself.

The groups to varying degrees affirmed both their interest in spirituality/pastoral care and their concern about training being of good enough quality. Two of the advisory groups, which contained some people trained in pastoral care, were also concerned about the potential erosion of their specialized role and whether training would be adequate for those including spirituality in their general professional work.

How to manage these issues was discussed, as well as how to include the desired aspects of training, and the project workers compared this with their other experiences of spiritual formation and training, both personally and professionally. They also became clear that how the training was provided would be as important as the content. What potential participants felt they needed implied a mainly reflective and experiential approach. Given that the time available for training was limited to 3 days, it focused on providing an overview in terms of content about spirituality, with an emphasis on self-awareness and reflection, and also looked for ways to have each task or experience achieve more than one aspect of what was to be learnt or practiced. Many of the exercises were carried out in pairs or threes with time for individual reflection built in. Moving into smaller groups then back to the larger group for feedback and discussion helped build a sense of mutual understanding, but also generated affirming of difference as the range of views became clear.

Key elements of training and formation

These are divided into six main themes, with a common understanding of critically reflective theory and processes. The themes are: the centrality of experience, understanding the influence of history and social context, the use of language, valuing difference and working holistically, acknowledging values and assumptions and the capacity to reflect and act on reflections. Each of these will be explored below:

Theme one

The centrality of experience

Critical reflection emphasizes the importance of experience as a way of knowing and understanding, as well as the value of learning from experience. The training in the Project addressed this in two ways: first, emphasizing the use of participants' own experiences for learning, something that they had suggested themselves would be essential. This was reinforced by our own experience and that of related training,[47,48] which meant that learning needed to be conducted in an environment that felt safe and encouraged openness and sharing. Because of this it was decided to limit the size of groups to an absolute maximum of twenty, but with a preferred size of 12–15 participants. Early in the first day of training, the group was asked to explore what culture or expectations they needed in order to feel safely able to share with each other. It was made clear before the training that much of it would be experiential and that all participants would be expected to participate.

Secondly, the training demonstrated that how people experience spirituality varies enormously. A distinction often made in religious writing is between those who experience spirituality in a more mystical or 'transcendent' way—compared to those who experience the spiritual in the every day. Cronk[49] adds another way—'via moderna'—experiencing spirituality from 'service in the world ... involvement with others, and working to change the world so that it manifests more fully God's love and justice'. This may be particularly relevant to workers in health and human services. Heelas and Woodhead[50] found that people often express the spiritual in what they called the 'holistic milieu', practices like yoga or the use of complementary health therapies. The provision of spiritual care requires awareness that people are at 'different places in their spiritual development even though they might have comparable spiritual needs.'[51] These differences became clear to participants as they shared their very diverse experiences and perceptions of the spiritual and religious.

The training was also run in a way that offered the possibility of spiritual experience. We used some guided meditations as part of the process, including a Buddhist loving kindness mediation as preparation for deep listening. An exercise that asked people to sit with what it would feel like to have a life-threatening illness, encouraged them to sit with their perceptions of what made life meaningful for them.

Theme two: understanding the influence of history and social context

A critically reflective approach affirms the need for awareness of the social context: such as living in a culturally diverse community or a rural community isolated from spiritual support as well as awareness of changing social attitudes that might mean more or less acceptance of spiritual practices. Awareness of organizational policies would be part of this: recognizing how spirituality is viewed and how much it is, for example, seen as part of everyone's role or a more specialised role.

Understanding social context also includes awareness of the influence of history including current changes in understanding. In this project, an historical overview was presented which compared three phases in terms of spirituality, community, and attitudes to death: traditional society, modern society, and contemporary society. In a traditional society, at times of crisis the church and community would have had a shared religious understanding of the meaning of life and death that would have sustained them. In more modern times, as people moved away from a religious tradition to a greater belief in science, faith moved to professionals, the dying person might well move to a hospital or hospice, rather than being cared for as part of their community. Finally, in our current society we have the continuation for some of both of these, but also the development for others of a new desire to express spirituality differently and also to reconnect to ideas of community, exploring how we might create a new version of communities that care for those who are dying.

This exploration enabled participants to stand back from their immediate experience and to see how much we are influenced by both current and historical context. This can also raise issues about the limits of acceptable spiritual practices: the importance of people not limiting each other's expression unless it is harmful. Participants recognized that these contextual issues have implications for work with individuals and families, but also for access to support and supervision, ongoing training as well as knowledge and skill in using local networks for referral. The training ended with participants exploring implications for their particular communities.

Theme three: the use of language

The theory underlying critical reflection theory suggests the importance of language, particularly the need to understand how differently words may be understood. The question of how to talk about spirituality had been a significant issue in the development of the project. Initially, the project was identified as a 'pastoral care' project, but this language was alienating for many of the people involved. For some, there was a sense of unease until the facilitator explained the breadth of spirituality meant by pastoral care. It was impossible, however, to find a word or phrase that everyone felt comfortable with: there were strong positive and negative reactions to pastoral care, spirituality, and religion. In the end we agreed to talk about pastoral care/spirituality.

This issue was then explored further in the first day of training: what different ways of thinking are there about spirituality and religion and how language reflects that. Our starting point fitted with the view that 'no consensus has been reached on a formal definition of spirituality. However, the assumption common to (many writers) is that spirituality enables people to transcend their immediate circumstances and live constructively within them.'[52] We presented the use of the word 'spirituality' as a broad umbrella, which included religion, this provided a framework where participants could see how their own and others' spirituality fitted. For many it was liberating to have such a framework presented, it allowed for diversity in a constructive and accepting way. They described it as a 'relief' or 'a wonderful expansion' of their perceptions of spirituality with one saying: 'Better understanding of pastoral care today rather than when I was younger, helpful to understand how spiritual care crosses all areas and is part of all of us'. This connects to the next theme.

Theme four: valuing difference and working holistically

This is another key theme in a critically reflective approach: acknowledging and valuing difference. This was made explicit in using an inclusive definition of spirituality and acknowledging varieties of spiritual experience and change over time. One of the ways we did this was by asking people to select one or two 'Signpost' cards[53]—cards with images and a word relating to spirituality. After sharing why they had chosen these, participants did some journaling or drawing about their own experience of spirituality. This quickly and sometimes dramatically demonstrated difference.

Affirming such difference reinforced seeing the person as a whole, rather than as someone who is ill or, worse, as their illness. Critical reflection reinforces this, suggesting the need to understand the complexity of each person and their multiple roles. When asked what how they would want to be treated if they were dying, most participants said to be treated as a whole person, someone who still had the same interests and desires, the capacity to laugh as well as be sad. Seeing the differences in how people might want to be treated reinforced the need to see the person in their context: how their friends, family, and community might matter to them.

Theme five: acknowledging values and assumptions

The sharing of perspectives and experiences in exercises like these heightened awareness for participants of their own assumptions about spirituality, as well as expanding understanding of how different other people's assumptions might be. An exercise on awareness of values and value preferences helped with participants saying, for example: 'It is important to start with values—looking at our own 'stuff' and how that may influence others'. The Signposts exercise reinforced how different reactions could be and the need 'not to make assumptions'.

For an exercise about practicing listening, participants using examples from their own experience to explore either their own spirituality or something else that mattered to them. The feedback and discussion session reinforced how much people operated from their own assumptions and values and participants often mentioned their surprise at how different these were. An exercise using a number of scenarios relating to spirituality including a refugee from Sudan, an older man and a woman practicing Buddhism again provoked different reactions and consolidated understanding of the influence of social values and beliefs and the danger of making assumptions for others. One participant said: 'I have learnt about accepting people where they are at and I'm learning not to judge or become frustrated. I've noticed quite a profound change'.

Theme six: developing the capacity to reflect and act on reflections

Reflecting critically means seeking a deeper understanding and also an expectation of change. The sixth theme in training was becoming more able to reflect, but also to put the implications into practice.

Part of learning to reflect in this training involved listening in a particular way about spiritual matters. Lohring[54] calls this 'listening in the spirit' and suggests it is challenging to listen without specific goals or the desire to be helpful or wise or give advice, but simply to be open to hearing what it is that the other person wants to say. This capacity to listen deeply for the spiritual can then be thought of as an attitude of mind rather than a separate activity, something that permeates the working relationship what Johns[55] calls a 'way of being'; sitting with the person in the 'mystery of experience'.

The session on listening deeply began with a Buddhist loving kindness meditation, to encourage a sense of being present. Each pair of participants was asked then to listen to each other in turn, with the listener simply listening not responding in any way, but actively being present. Next each pair listened to each other with minimal responding. This experience generated a lot of discussion. Participants reported realizing how powerful it could be simply to listen and be listened to in this deeper, more present way, encouraging deeper reflection for both. As a nurse said: 'we're great if someone has a pain, but when people want to go on to more difficult places, we felt we should be saying something and didn't know what to say, the education gave permission just to sit and listen, which is what people want'.

We also assumed being more reflective implied the capacity to care more effectively for yourself: to see more readily how you might need to pay attention to your own sense of meaning and act on it. Those who work in a way that embraces spirituality often forget that in order to do this well, they need to care for themselves. The findings from the literature review confirm the value of recognizing workers' own spirituality. Puchalski and McSkimming,[56] for example, found that providing training in using a spiritualty assessment framework gave staff 'permission to be present to spiritual issues for ourselves and each other' and also led to better interdisciplinary relationships. Building spiritual experience into the workplace was also affirmed as sustaining staff in working in end of life care.[57] Wasner *et al.*[58] found that spiritual care education had a positive influence on the spiritual wellbeing and the attitudes of participating palliative care professionals.

What emerged from the project and implications for future training

A more detailed exploration of the impact of the project is available elsewhere.[59] Overall, there was a high degree of satisfaction expressed by participants in the training, with the pre and post evaluation questionnaire identifying a significant increase in knowledge related to spirituality in palliative care and in confidence in working with spirituality. In the thirty evaluation interviews, all of the participants indicated a change in awareness of spirituality, particularly of their own attitudes and values and, for some, of new ways of understanding. Over a third were more open to difference, and/or felt more able to have conversations about spirituality as part of their practice. Participants also affirmed their capacity to act differently as a result of the training: a typical comment was: 'Now I'll ask something like what's meaningful to you in your life? It's an easy question to ask now and document'. Others mentioned change in their awareness of their own spirituality, increased care for themselves and the development of more mutually supportive networks.

In terms of the training itself, the experiential and reflective nature of the training was particularly valued. Connected to this was the opportunity to share with others and the clear connections to practice. Increased understanding of the breadth of spirituality was also raised frequently. There were very few suggestions for change in relation to the training and many suggested providing more opportunities for others to have the same training. However, several participants raised the need to more formally engage their organization in the project, so that the new confidence and knowledge of staff could be recognized in their practice. One palliative care nurse commented: 'this isn't seen as part of the role—more what pastors do, might be included in music therapy, volunteer role doing massage, not part of everybody's role'. She, and others, considered that the project team needed to engage healthcare management in the project, so that they understood the greater capacity of their professionals and volunteers.

This attitude translated into action: a volunteer gave an example of now feeling comfortable with how differently her two clients wanted her to be: one wanted purely a 'listener', the other a more mutual conversation. One of the training groups continued to meet for mutual support and training.

Conclusions

The pressure is increasing for health professionals to be able to communicate effectively and appropriately about spirituality. Those they work with lead complex lives that include their own particular search for meaning expressed in many different ways. These may well have an impact on healthcare, and on how people want to be cared for. Professionals need training as well as ongoing support to be able to embark on holistic care that includes working with spirituality.

This chapter affirms the value of a critically reflective approach to training and formation. Six themes are identified that are integral to critically reflective training for those engaging with spirituality in their practice. The six themes overlap to some degree rather than being distinct categories, but do provide a way of ensuring that each aspect needed in training is included. The themes can be thought about to some extent as focusing on the inner or outer worlds: the centrality of experience and identification of core assumptions and values combined with an awareness of social context.

What is also identified is the value of the *process* of critically reflective learning, Implicit in critical reflection is the valuing of different perspectives including both specialist knowledge as well as experiential or practice knowledge. In this example, the input from a range of professional practitioners and volunteers was validated as offering useful insights. Healthcare practitioners heard other ways of seeing a situation from volunteers, how to recognize the need simply 'be with' someone. Volunteers understood more fully how the changing attitudes to spirituality might impact on their role and how to respond more flexibly to individual spiritual differences. The process also creates a space for learning within which participants can recognize the influence of their own past experience and knowledge, and can develop their own goals for learning within the one training process. This avoids separating what is essentially a team of people into separate strands of training to deliver 'right' training to the 'right' people. It means that team members have a greater clarity about each other and their different roles and gifts and so further strengthens the team's capacity to provide a community of care. Using a critically reflective approach to training and formation can affirm working with spirituality in appropriate ways that are life-enhancing for professionals and volunteers and those they work with.

Some resources for training

Fook, J., Gardner, F. (2007). *Practising Critical Reflection: A Handbook*. London: Open University Press. For more detail about critical reflection theory and processes.

The Janki Foundation for Global Healthcare (2004). *Resource Manual Values in Healthcare: A Spiritual Approach* This contains suggestions for workshops and includes a series of meditations on CD. Available at: www.jankifoundation.org/

Signposts Cards: Have an image and word or phrase such as an image of candles with the phrase: 'Honouring the sacred'; another has fireworks and says: 'Sparking with creativity'. These sets of cards and many others available through St Luke's Innovative Resources Available at: www.innovativeresources.org/

References

1 Holloway, M. (2006). Spiritual Need and the Core Business of Social Work. *Br J Soc Work* Advance Access [Online].

2 Abbas, S.Q., Panjwani, S. (2008). The necessity of spiritual care towards the end of life. *Eth Med* **24**(2): 113–18.

3 Gale, F., Bohan, N., McRae-McMahon, D. (eds) (2007). *Spirited Practices Spirituality and the Helping Professions*. Crows Nest: Allen & Unwin.

4 Forman, R. (2004). *Grassroots Spirituality*. Exeter: Imprint Academic.

5 Kavanagh, J. (2007). *The World is Our Cloister: A Guide to the Modern Religious Life*. Winchester: John Hunt Publishing.

6 Holloway, M., Moss, B. (2010). *Spirituality and Social Work*, p. 168. Houndmills: Palgrave MacMillan.

7 Lamberton, H. (2004). The resurgence of interest in spirituality and health. In: S.A. Sorajjakool, H.E. Lamberton (eds) *Spirituality, Health and Wholeness: An Introductory Guide for Healthcare Professionals*, pp. 1–14 New York: Haworth Press.

8 Tacey, D. (2003). *The Spirituality Revolution*. Sydney: HarperCollins.

9 MacKinlay, E. (2001). *The Spiritual Dimension of Ageing*. London: Jessica Kingsley Publishers.

10 Rumbold, B. (ed.) (2002). *Spirituality and Palliative Care*, p. 19. Melbourne: Oxford University Press.

11 Moss, E.L., Dobson, K.S. (2006). Psychology, Spirituality, and End-of-Life Care: An Ethical Integration? *Canad Psychol* **47**(4): 284–99.

12 Haynes,A., Hilbers, J., Kivikko, J., Ratnatvyuha, (2007). *Spirituality and Religion in Healthcare Practice: a person-centred resource for staff at the Prince of Wales Hospital*. Sydney: South Eastern Sydney Illawarra Area Health Service.

13 Wasner, M., Longaker, C., Fegg, M.J., Borasio, G.D. (2005). Effects of spiritual care education for palliative care professionals. *Palliat Med* **19**: 99–104.

14 Puchalski, C.M., McSkimming, S. (2006). Creating healing environments. *Hlth Progr* **87**(3): 30–3.

15 [12], 1.

16 D'Souza, R. (2007). The importance of spirituality in medicine and its application to clinical practice. *Med J Aust* **186**(10): S57-9.

17 Barletta, J., Witteveen. (2005). *The Development of Roles and Education for Pastoral Care Workers in Queensland Health: A Research Report*. Brisbane: Queensland Health.

18 Linden, B., van der Wal, G. (2006). Spiritual issues in palliative care consultations in the Netherlands. *Palliat Med* **20**(6): 585–92.

19 Gordon, T., Mitchell, D. (2004). A competency model for the assessment and delivery of spiritual care. *Palliat Med* **18**(7): 648–51.

20 Chaplin, J.A., Mitchell, D. (2002). *Spirituality in Palliative Care*. Edinburgh: Elsevier Churchill Livingstone, p. 190.

21 Cobb, M. (2001). *The Dying Soul: Spiritual Care at the End of Life*, p. 70. Buckingham: Open University.

22 Bryson, K.A. (2004). Spirituality, meaning and transcendence. *Palliat Support Care* **2**: 321–8.

23 Rumbold, B. (2007). A review of spiritual assessment in healthcare practice. *Med J Aust* **186**(10): S60–2.

24 Trelfa, J. (2005). Faith in reflective practice. *Reflect Pract* **6**(2): 205–12.

25 Canda E (2005). Transpersonal theory. In: S.P. Robbins, P. Chatterjee, E.R. Canda (eds) *Contemporary Human Behavior Theory: A Critical Perspective for Social Work,* 2nd edn. Boston: Pearson.

26 Cox, R.H., Ervin-Cox, B., Hoffman, L. (2005). *Spirituality and Psychological Health*. Colorado Springs: Colorado School of Professional Psychology Press.

27 Fowler, J.W. (1981). *Stages of Faith: the Psychology of Human Development and the Quest for Meaning.* San Francisco: Harper & Row.
28 Cronk, S. (1991). *Dark Night Journey.* Wallingford: Pendle Hill Publications.
29 Fox, M. (1983). *Original Blessing.* Santa Fe: Bear.
30 Winslow, G.R., Wehtje-Winslow, B. (2007). Ethical boundaries of spiritual care. *Med J Aust* **186**(10): S63-6.
31 McCurdy D (2008). Ethical spiritual care at the end of life. *Am J Nurs* **108**(5): 11–12.
32 Hoffman, L., Cox, R.H., Ervin-Cox, B., Mitchell, M. (2005). Training issues in spirituality and psychotherapy: a foundational approach. In: R.H. Cox, B. Ervin-Cox, L. Hoffman (eds) *Spirituality and Psychological Health.* Colorado Springs: Colorado School of Professional Psychology Press.
33 Gardner, F. (2011). *Critical Spirituality: a Holistic Approach to Contemporary Practice.* Farnham: Ashgate.
34 Puchalski, C.M., Ferrell, B., Virani, R., Otis-Green, S., Baird, P., Bull, J., *et al.* (2009). Improving the quality of spiritual care as a dimension of palliative care: the report of the Consensus Conference. *J Palliat Med* **12**(10): 885–904.
35 [3].
36 [34], 900.
37 [34], 900.
38 Fook, J., Gardner, F. (2007). *Practising Critical Reflection: A Resource Handbook.* Maidenhead: Open University Press.
39 Rolfe, G., Jasper, M., Freshwater, D. (2011). *Critical Reflection in Practice: Generating Knowledge for Care.* Houndmills: Palgrave Macmillan.
40 White, S., Fook, J., Gardner, F. (eds) (2006). *Critical Reflection in Health and Social Care.* London: Open University Press.
41 [33].
42 McSherry, W. (2007). *The Meaning of Spirituality and Spiritual Care within Nursing and Healthcare Practice*, p.198. London: Quay Books.
43 White, G. (2006). *Talking about Spirituality in Healthcare Practice*, p. 64. London: Jessica Kingsley.
44 [38], 21.
45 Gardner, F. (2009). Affirming values: using critical reflection to explore meaning and professional practice. *Reflect Pract* **10**(2): 179–90.
46 Rumbold, B., Gardner, F., Nolan, I. (2011). Spirituality and community practice. In: S. Conway (ed.) *Governing Death and Loss Empowerment, Involvement and Participation*, pp. 139–47. Oxford: Oxford University Press.
47 [26].
48 [12].
49 [28], p. 25.
50 Heelas, P.A., Woodhead, L. (2005). *The Spiritual Revolution: Why Religion is Giving Way to Spirituality.* Oxford: Blackwell Publishing.
51 Sorajjakool, S.A., Lamberton, H.E. (2004). *Spirituality, Health and Wholeness: An Introductory Guide for Healthcare Professionals*, p. 8. New York: Haworth Press.
52 Rumbold, B. (2003). Attending to Spiritual Care. *Hlth Iss* **77**(Summer): 14–17.
53 Signpost cards: see Resources.
54 Lohring, P. (1997). *Listening Spirituality Volume One: Personal Spiritual Practice.* Maryland: Openings Press.
55 Johns, C. (2005). Balancing the winds. *Reflect Pract* **6**(1): 67–84.
56 [14], 32.
57 Holland, J.M., Neimeyer, R.A. (2005). Reducing the risk of burnout in end-of-life care settings: the role of daily spiritual experiences and education. *Palliat Support Care* **3**: 173–81.
58 [13].
59 [46].

CHAPTER 60

Interdisciplinary teamwork

Peter Speck

Introduction

When a person becomes ill, whether physically or mentally, they begin a process of trying to discern both cause and remedy which will bring them into contact with a variety of people in both their social and healthcare setting. Having explored symptoms in their own mind, and consulted with family and friends, the person will then usually seek help from a family or primary care doctor or an advanced practice nurse in their community medical practice. The problems may be diagnosed and treated at that point or may lead to referral to a local hospital, specialist centre, or specialist in a different field. Here, the person may be seen at an out-patient clinic and then return home, or they may be admitted into the hospital for further investigation leading to medical, surgical or other forms of treatment and care. If the illness is the result of an accident or major collapse then the first contact with healthcare will be the Accident & Emergency department. The result of the various interventions may be complete cure and restoration to previous good health, or partial restoration with residual problems or disability, or death. Throughout this process the person will have met a variety of health professionals.

Most of these encounters will have focused on the physical and pathological aspects of disease, and the prescription of appropriate remedies to eradicate or minimize the disease process. However, the person who is on this illness journey is also experiencing an 'inner' journey in which they find themselves facing a variety of questions that are either familiar to them or they face for the first time. These questions are often associated with discerning the cause of their illness ('Why me? This is unfair'), the timing of this event ('Why now'?), the possible outcomes ('What if they can't sort it? What if I die') or 'If I'm going to die then what's my life been about?' Questions which may affect recovery and any sense of wellbeing.

This inner dialogue can raise issues of an existential and philosophical nature which many healthcare practitioners may not feel is their remit to address. However, in recent years the importance of addressing these issues has become more widely recognized in healthcare, especially in the fields of care of the elderly and palliative care, where there is a stronger emphasis on holistic approaches to care.[1,2] Addressing these issues, and the needs that can arise from them, requires a range of skills that any one individual may not possess and are usually best provided for by the development of a multi/inter-disciplinary team approach.

Teamwork

For many years it has been recognized that the changing needs of patients can best be met by a team approach in which a variety of health professionals, with different skills, can collaborate to meet the range of needs presented by people being treated in the community or the hospital.[2] A review of the literature, however, indicates that the form and success of that collaboration varies greatly and is reflected in the adjectives used to describe the team: multidisciplinary, multi-professional, interdisciplinary, trans-disciplinary, etc. So often, the nature and effectiveness of the team will be influenced by the relationships that exist, the leadership style, and the trust and respect engendered between those involved in providing consultation or hands-on care to the patient. It can also depend on the extent to which the patient is part of that team, especially in respect of decision-making.

A team is a group of people brought together, from within or outside of the organization, for a specific purpose or task. Whether the team's existence is long or short term, it is expected that they will work together interdependently and take some ownership for the outcome. Leadership and clarification of task are key and will affect the skill mix of the team, how well they work together and satisfactory outcomes for any interventions made by the team. In terms of a healthcare system the task may be variously defined by those in leadership positions. An orthopaedic surgeon may see the primary task of his team in terms of assessing the degree of damage to a patient's skeletal structure and the range of options open to him/her to reduce the damage or replace the damaged part. He may perceive this as primarily a task of reconstruction which would necessitate medical, nursing, and physiotherapy skills being properly deployed—in other words, a bio-mechanical model. The surgeon's intervention may also result in psychosocial-spiritual changes, such as altered body image, identity, and life style, which may, or may not, be seen as part of the remit of the surgeon.

An elderly care physician may define their primary task as enabling the elderly patient to retain as independent a life style as possible for as long as possible. To this end he/she may draw upon a range of medical, nursing, physiotherapy, occupational therapy, social work, and psycho-spiritual resources to achieve a positive outcome. In palliative care, like care of the elderly, a range of skilled resources may be drawn upon in order to enhance the quality of life for the patient with a life-threatening illness and ensure a more holistic approach.

The multi-disciplinary team

In a general acute hospital most teams are medically led and the various specialist skills are brought into play as required. Frequently, professionals will enter the 'team' make their contribution and then return to their own professional base. The association is often quite loose and under the direction of the medical leadership. Legally, the medical consultant has accountability for the care and management of patients admitted to hospital under his/her care. While such collaboration between professionals is often called teamwork, it is really better described as an example of multi-professional working and frequently operates in a hierarchical structure. The affiliation of members is primarily to their own profession and only secondarily to the team. In terms of the spiritual care provider, they would normally be asked to see a particular patient with a view to assessment and/or intervention. They would later report back to the multi-professional team meeting directly, or via the medical record, complete their intervention, and then return to their own professional base. This model of working means that some patients will only receive spiritual input if that need is discerned by the lead clinician and/or colleagues, whereas others who also have spiritual need may be missed. This irregular appearance of the spiritual care provider means that spiritual issues will not feature strongly on the team's radar unless an individual team member is alert to the importance and relevance of spirituality. Within community care access to, and knowledge of, spiritual care resources may also limit the degree of collaboration. Community staff may not know local faith leaders sufficiently well to confidently suggest referral to a patient. The training of faith leaders may also have not adequately prepared them for some of the pastoral challenges, which both religious and non-religious people may pose when experiencing serious illness.[3]

In those specialties that focus more clearly on an holistic approach to care, especially care of the elderly and palliative care, there is frequently a greater awareness of biopsychosocial-spiritual issues. This awareness does not necessarily translate into action to meet such needs as shown in the UK Liverpool Care Pathway (LCP) audits. Assessing and meeting spiritual and religious need is a key aspect of the pathway as a person moves towards the end of their life. However, the Round 2 audit of 2009[4] showed that only 30% (34% in 2007 audit) of patients had their *religious* needs assessed and results were not documented for 48% (40% in 2007 audit) of cases. Given that the LCP is widely disseminated across hospitals, hospices and nursing homes in the UK this is a worrying result, especially as the LCP highlights specific religious need as well as broader spiritual need. Other work by Ross,[5] McSherry,[6] and Baldacchino[7] indicate that one reason for poor rates of assessment may be the health professional's own belief system, and lack of adequate training, which may inhibit engaging in this aspect of care.

Where spiritual care needs are identified the usual default for staff is to refer to chaplaincy rather than explore or address issues themselves. Walter,[8] over 20 years ago, considered various approaches to the delivery of spiritual care within a hospice population. While he saw 'calling in the chaplain' as the norm, especially in hospitals, he also saw advantages in describing spirituality as a search for meaning in that it would allow doctors and nurses, and others to engage with spiritual care as part of holistic care, even in a secular setting. The absence of someone in the care team with a specific remit for spiritual care may also contribute to spiritual needs not being identified or met within a multi-disciplinary team.

Where professionals move to a more inter-disciplinary team structure some of these problems may be overcome, provided there is someone designated to attend to these concerns.

Inter-disciplinary teams

The hallmarks of an inter-disciplinary team are described by Cummings,[9] where 'the identity of the team supersedes individual personal identities. Members share information and work interdependently together to develop goals. Leadership is shared among team members depending on the task at hand. Because the team is the vehicle of action, the interaction process is vital to success.'[9, p. 19]

The interaction within the team is required to produce the final product, in this case high quality holistic care for patients and families, with the team achieving more than the sum total of the individuals involved. The interaction can have the effect of enabling individual practitioners to learn from each other, and so extend and enhance their own skills, while acknowledging the limits of their ability. For example, a doctor or nurse who has developed a wider understanding of spiritual care may feel more able to discuss existential and spiritual issues with patients who want to explore these areas. There may come a point where the doctor or nurse recognizes that the conversation is moving to the edges of their own personal experience, or their ability to assist the patient, and would then involve another team member more skilled or specialized in providing spiritual/existential support such as a healthcare chaplain or local community faith leader. The greater flexibility, and less hierarchical style of working, can allow team members to extend the range of support they can give personally to the patient and family and enhance choice for the patient as to who they share issues with. This also frees the chaplain/spiritual care provider to offer support to the staff member to continue the conversation with the patient/family, rather than replacing the staff member. If the need is more religious or liturgical then it may be possible to share the care role, rather than 'take over'.

There will be limits to the extent to which team members can 'cover' for each other, but there may also be greater scope for team members to offer general patient support with a range of needs until it is clear another resource person is required. That resource person (e.g. spiritual care provider/chaplain) may, as indicated, then work direct with the patient or may offer support to the team member who has the primary relationship with the patient and support them in continuing their exploration of issues with the patient. Within an inter-disciplinary team there is a high level of mutual accountability, which will require good documentation, effective communication skills and trust, and clarity and commitment to the primary task, in order to ensure continuity of care. Failure to achieve this can result in confused, delayed or clumsy referrals to team colleagues and reduced quality of care for the patient.

Inter-disciplinary working can be very creative for problem-solving and is especially relevant to specialist areas of care where ethical concerns abound. However, it is important that the contributions of individual members of the team are respected and valued. Studies of issues relating to team dynamics show that feeling respected and valued is a key component of effective teamworking.[10] In acute hospital medicine and primary healthcare, in contrast to many palliative care/hospice teams, inter-disciplinary teamwork is rare. Even within palliative care teams, which have evolved into inter-disciplinary working, changes of personnel within the team can move them back along the spectrum towards multi-disciplinary working for a while.

Irrespective of the style of team working a dynamic will develop and operate at an unconscious level within the team. This dynamic may enhance team effectiveness if the team leader can help members address issues of competitiveness or rivalry, etc., which have the potential to move individuals away from the primary task/focus of the team. Regular team meetings are essential to maintain a healthy team and develop an awareness of dynamic processes that develop within any team over time.[10]

Ethical and legal issues

Any healthcare team will be made up of people who will hold different personal, as well as professional values. Teamwork, whether multi-professional or inter-professional, will require the individual to balance their personal moral viewpoint with those required by their professional role and membership of the team. Health professionals, by virtue of their training and experience, value their autonomy, especially when it comes to making decisions. Patients also value autonomy and ethical debate often centres around balancing the autonomy held by different people in the healthcare setting. Working collaboratively requires consideration of this balance. Farsides argues that the autonomy of individuals working within palliative care teams (and I would suggest other healthcare teams also) is an issue we cannot ignore.[11] She states that the 'more sophisticated concepts of autonomy take realistic account of our associations with others. They also acknowledge that we construct our moral lives in such a way as to preclude that possibility of always acting independently.'[11, p. 169]

If a team is a group of people who have come together in order to fulfill a common task, in this case to provide for the health needs of patients in their care, then they will need to be bound together by this common purpose. At times, there may be tensions between personally held values and beliefs, the values held collectively by the team, and those held by the individual's primary professional group. Some members will be able to contain and manage these tensions better than others, but the team leader will need to be aware and able to deal with times when these tensions may become disruptive to the effective working of the team. In extreme cases, a member who holds views that are very opposed to those held by the team as a whole may need to forfeit their membership of the team if the tension cannot be resolved. This does not mean that individuals cannot express personally held views on the care and management of patients, but will need to be able to accept the final decision of the team leader following appropriate discussion and consultation. Once again, the issue of respect and value of each other's contribution to care is important, together with mutual accountability.

In addition to ethical concerns, teamwork can also raise legal concerns. The law may reserve some activities to certain team members (e.g. prescribing rights, ultimate responsibility for treatment decisions) and ecclesiastical law may restrict some religious rituals to only be performed by authorized members of particular religious groups (e.g. provision of holy communion or anointing with oil by Christian priests). For any team to function effectively there needs to be a sense of collective responsibility which is usually expressed as a 'duty of care,' but may lead to problems as to how one balances the priorities of duties. Thus, as Montgomery[12] indicates 'we may have a responsibility towards carers to help them deal with the death of someone they love, and this would point to sharing information about the patient's prognosis. However, that duty to the carers is outweighed by the patient's right to confidentiality unless they have waived it by giving consent to disclosure. Thus, there is not liability to relatives for distress caused by refusing to disclose information without the patient's agreement'[12, p. 185]

In terms of spiritual care, the spiritual care provider may not be at liberty to share the content of a pastoral encounter with other members of the care team, but could share themes (e.g. coping with uncertainty, fears of death, relationship with God). Where the content might affect clinical decision-making a spiritual care provider would usually explain the relevance to the patient and seek their permission to share relevant facts with the clinical team. In the UK, access to confidential information concerning a patient is strictly controlled and sharing is often dependant upon the extent to which a spiritual care provider is integrated into the work of the care team. It can be easier in an inter-disciplinary team where the spiritual care provider is perceived as a full member of the team. However, in multi-disciplinary teams the spiritual care provider may only enter the team following a specific request. Here, staff may feel unable to share information other than that the patient has requested to speak to a chaplain. If one adopts a 'need to know' basis then it should not be too difficult for the spiritual care provider to obtain the patient's permission for staff to share more openly. The success of this approach will depend on the degree of trust and respect which the chaplain/spiritual care provider has been able to build with the other health professionals on the team and the patient.

Accountability within teams is also important and relates very much to defining and understanding the roles and spheres of responsibility held by team members. Registered practitioners are subject to disciplinary action by their professional body if they fail to provide care in accordance with the law and the professional standards set down in their code of practice. Failure can lead to withdrawal of their license to practice. For medical, nursing, and other professions allied to medicine there are clear procedures to identify professional misconduct. However, it may be difficult to discipline lay members of a team unless they have some form of contract for the work they undertake (e.g. contract issued to lay volunteers within a spiritual care department). Clergy employed by a health Trust or contracted to provide a professional service to patients will be subject to discipline by the hospital Trust, and/or by the appropriate ecclesiastical authority, as well as any professional regulatory body to which they may belong.

Who should provide spiritual care?

In recent years there has been much discussion of who should be responsible for assessing and meeting the spiritual and religious needs of people entering a healthcare setting. To some extent it is acknowledged that if a holistic approach is adopted then spiritual care becomes the concern of everyone who comes into contact with patients. However, when something is the concern of everyone it can quickly become the concern of no-one. While healthcare chaplains have traditionally taken the lead their perceived religious identity has sometimes been seen as a barrier to providing spiritual care to non-religious people. Where chaplains are integrated into a healthcare team, and known and trusted, other team members are more able to introduce them to patients and families as people who are able to work with religious and non-religious need. For the chaplain this means that they must adopt an open and exploratory approach to spiritual care, as well as being able to provide for specific religious need, or be able to make an appropriate referral if the religious ritual is outside of their own tradition or faith. There is thus a clear training requirement to equip those entering healthcare chaplaincy to be able to work in this broader way and to develop teamwork skills appropriate to a multi or inter-professional setting.

Puchalski and colleagues assert that spiritual care is an example of the benefits of an interdisciplinary approach, with each member of the team having responsibility to provide spiritual care.[13] They see the chaplain as the trained spiritual care expert on the team holding key responsibility for ensuring team members interact with each other, to develop and implement a spiritual care plan for the patient, within a fully collaborative interdisciplinary model.[13, p. 414] Their model identifies four main components: compassionate presence, relationship-centred care, spirituality of the healthcare professional, extrinsic spiritual care which incorporates assessment and development of the spiritual care plan. The model has been developed against the background of chaplaincy training and accreditation in the USA and the greater integration of chaplains into the clinical hospital teams in that country. There is a danger with this model that spiritual care provision becomes another treatment model, whereby assessment tools are used to 'diagnose' problems, a 'treatment' plan is created, which can then lead to measurable outcomes and demonstrated effectiveness of the intervention. However, in 2009 a National Consensus Conference was held in Pasadena, California, which outlined two newer models of spiritual care: a biopsychosocial-spiritual model and an interprofessional spiritual care model.[14]

The biopsychosocial-spiritual model sees illness as disturbing the unity and integrity of what we know to be a human being. Thus, Sulmasy states that 'illness disturbs more than relationships inside the human organism; it disrupts families and workplaces, shatters pre-existing patterns of coping, and raises questions about one's relationship with the significant and the sacred.'[15] According to this model each person has a spiritual history that will unfold in various ways that are not necessarily explicitly religious. It is important that we discover this personal spiritual history for each person who enters a clinical setting. This leads into the second and interprofessional model. Here, it is the healthcare professional who is charged with taking the personal spiritual history and then identifying the presence of spiritual issues (whether distress or sources of spiritual strength). They should then make appropriate referral to spiritual care providers–usually board-certified chaplains within the US setting. The interdisciplinary team rounds are seen as including the chaplain as a spiritual care expert. In this report, however, the implementation model does refer to the chaplain establishing a 'treatment plan' (See Figure 1 of the *National Concensus Report*),[14] as distinct from what in the UK would be described as an 'intervention'. Whatever term is used, it is important that chaplains and spiritual care providers value the importance of a more exploratory, journeying-together, pastoral counselling approach where the outcomes may not be evident or measurable for many months or years. This aspect of spiritual care is highly valued by patients as shown in Hanson's study,[16] which is discussed below.

Within the UK chaplaincy formation and development has not always attained the same level of integration, especially within acute hospital clinical teams. Hospice and palliative care teams are more likely to have a closer working relationship with chaplaincy. In other specialties the degree of integration can depend on the relationship and skills of the individual chaplain, and the willingness of staff to recognize and value the contribution a chaplain can make to the patient's wellbeing. While there are several guidance documents in the NHS which emphasize the importance of spiritual care in various aspects of care they remain guidance and self-governing trusts are free to decide for themselves how they provide for spiritual care. This led initially to a period of expansion of chaplaincy in the UK and the development of a clearer UK evidence base to underpin the focus on spiritual care.[2,17] There is a professional code of conduct for healthcare chaplains[18] and a clearer training trajectory, some of which is at postgraduate level. Within the USA there is a common code of ethics for chaplains, pastoral counsellors, pastoral educators, and students, which has been affirmed by a Council for Collaboration in 2004 on behalf of six major chaplaincy bodies in the US and Canada.[19] The main professional training leading to certification is provided by Clinical Pastoral Education (CPE). Through a process of pastoral formation, reflection and acquired competence chaplains can obtain Board Certification as a professional chaplain.[20] They may then, as in the UK, continue to extend their knowledge and skills through a variety of academic and/or practical training opportunities. In spite of demonstrating the benefits of a viable chaplaincy, the changed economic climate and need to make funding cuts within the UK has led to several instances of chaplaincy reduction which has an effect on spiritual care provision. This change has the potential to reduce the opportunity, and the time available, for chaplains to attend multi- or inter-disciplinary team meetings and integrate more closely with the variety of teams existing in acute NHS hospitals.

Few studies have been undertaken to examine who actually provides spiritual care, and still less, the efficacy of the care offered.[21] Hanson *et al.*[16] examined the spiritual care experiences of 103 recipients of care, of whom 38 were seriously ill patients and 65 family caregivers. The 103 recipients received care from 237 spiritual care providers: 41% were family and friends, 17% were clergy, 29% were healthcare providers and two-thirds of the providers shared the same faith tradition as the recipients. The remainder of the sample cited God or a higher power as one of their sources of spiritual support. Of the various activities undertaken helping to cope with the illness was the most common (87%) together with helping to support positive relationships with significant people and with God (over 70%), and helping recognition of value and significance of life (73%). The least common activity was intercessory prayer (4%). This study shows that family, friends and healthcare workers were important in meeting spiritual need, but that outcome did not differ if the provider was family, healthcare worker, or clergy. Satisfaction level with spiritual care was around a modest 50%, but help with understanding and ability to cope with the illness led to greatest satisfaction. The benefits of this may not be seen for some time after the encounter.

Breitbart, in an editorial,[22] reflects on the findings of the 2009 National Consensus Conference on improving the quality of spiritual care within palliative care, and the National Consensus Project for Quality Palliative Care [23]. He suggests that two questions arise: Which of the many professional disciplines involved in palliative care are appropriate to be spiritual care professionals and what training and expertise is required for spiritual care as opposed to religious or existential care? The various domains of care identified in the NCP have the effect, according to Breitbart, of excluding many categories of staff from the spiritual domain, and raising questions about the role of nurses and physicians in dealing with spiritual and existential issues. The effect of this has been to create a tension between chaplains and other health professionals in the USA as to who is qualified and suitable to offer religious, spiritual and existential care. The National Consensus Conference report[14] addresses this issue when it recommends that all trained healthcare professionals should do spiritual screening and history-taking, and then plan appropriate care with a board-certified chaplain working with the interprofessional team as the spiritual care expert. The tension may continue, however, if the chaplain is not able to work effectively with non-religious people and this may represent a training issue for clergy. Certainly, the survey by Lloyd Williams *et al.* [3] indicates that while many of the Christian clergy interviewed felt adequately prepared to offer religious and liturgical care to dying people, 26% acknowledged the inadequacy of their pastoral skills in terms of supporting dying patients and bereaved families. This is seen as an issue to be addressed in pre- and post-ministerial training and, I believe, would benefit from opportunities for multi-professional training. Many of the problems that one encounters in teamwork arise from misunderstanding or mistrust of the stance taken by different professionals, and the theoretical basis of their approach to issues. Collaborating across the disciplines in research and training can aid team-building, and the development of greater respect and understanding of each other's discipline. In terms of providing for spiritual care it also allows individuals to explore their own understanding and that of colleagues, and so encourage a more collaborative, and less competitive, style of working. Payne sees team-building as an ongoing process which we should engage with every day. '... build your team however and wherever you can, in everything you do. Trying to enhance the quality of what we do means calling effectively on the whole range of services and care that might benefit our patients and service users, and coordinating it so that every element of works together well.' [24, p. 117] This is as important for the provision of spiritual care as it is for clinical need. Meader[25] asserts that 'the best spiritual care for the dying patient is most likely to be delivered in the same way other types of care are best provided, through partnerships with the team of persons caring for the patient'. This use of the term 'partnership' is interesting and important because it underlines the importance of seeing the patient as in partnership with the care team. Whereas some medical and surgical procedures may require the patient (after ethical consent has been obtained) to be a more passive recipient of care, spiritual care is intrinsically an interactive process.

User involvement is actively encouraged within research and in the development of services in the UK, but little research has been undertaken to discover what patients themselves wish for by way of spiritual care. In 2006, Holmes and colleagues[26] explored the spiritual concerns of 65 seriously ill outpatients and the spiritual care practices of 67 primary care physicians in the USA. Over 60% of both the patients and the physicians felt it important that physicians attend to patients' spiritual concerns. However, few patients actually received such care and few physicians practiced such care. The authors recognize the complexity of addressing spiritual concerns in the context of serious illness within an outpatient setting. They suggest their findings indicate the most appropriate role of the physician is to ask about and listen to spiritual concerns and leave the more active roles to others who have specific training in this area, such as chaplains or those with closer relationships such as family and friends. Yardley *et al.*[27] have conducted a qualitative study of patients in a UK hospice to discover their perspective on spiritual care and suggestions for the training of staff. Twenty patients were interviewed and the results showed that patients expected opportunities to arise for discussion of spiritual concerns. They felt staff needed to develop a non-judgemental attitude, show an interest in individuals and provide integrated care. 'Actions which patients felt would facilitate conversations are those used in communication skills training: considering atmosphere and environment, explaining motivation, asking questions naturally and giving permission to patients to share without risking judgement. Participants were also keen to learn from others' experiences and felt these could be a source of ideas which they could evaluate the usefulness of for themselves.' [27, p. 605] What patients were clear about was not wanting spiritual assessment to be a 'tick box' approach, but allowing them to set the pace and agenda. This study is an interesting example of the importance of seeing patients as 'partners', able to contribute to the life and work of the care team and not people to be 'processed' by the team. One way in which team members could explore spiritual needs with patients is through the use of some broad questions such as: 'what is really important to you at present?' 'When life has been difficult for you, what has helped you to cope?' and 'Do you have a way of making sense or understanding why things happen to us in life?'[28] These questions do not pre-suppose a religious or spiritual answer, but could also lead to an exploration of social or psychological needs. It is important in teamwork to avoid making decisions or assumptions without appropriate consultation with the patient and the adoption of a more exploratory approach, which invites the patient to be a more active participant in the identification of need. This is especially true for patients in Northern Europe, but can present a problem in Southern Europe where, culturally, the family claim the right to all information and consultation prior to their deciding what the patient shall be told.[29]

Walter[30] questions the belief that all patients have a spiritual dimension and that all staff can offer spiritual care. He suggests that there are different kinds of believing/belonging and that life-threatening events may lead people to use different types of discourse and we must beware the danger of imposing the language of spirituality onto people for whom it may have little meaning. It may, therefore, be important for carers to accompany the patient on their illness journey. This, in turn, raises the question of how far each carer can walk with each patient? Walter suggests that we drop the idea that any healthcare professional can offer spiritual care to any patient and, instead, focus more on the differences between and among patients and staff. He believes that this can relieve staff of what he perceives of as the burden of feeling obliged to accompany each and every patient. One implication of Walter's conclusion is to emphasize the importance of a team approach which allows for patients to be seen as individuals and for their perceived needs to be met by the most appropriate member of the team. This would be true within a hospice or a palliative care team and could be attainable within a hospital setting if the various specialties were able to evolve an effective approach to teamwork and adopt a holistic approach to care.

Conclusion

Spiritual care, wherever it is offered, requires the caregiver to focus on, and relate to, the whole person who is before them. The essence of the encounter is the ability to create a safe space within which the person can explore such issues as personal worth and value, the possible purpose of what is being experienced, the opportunity to access strength and support to transcend the here and now experience and sustain hope for a future. Whatever style of team the caregiver works within, whatever time pressures team members may experience, we shall fail in our attempts to offer holistic care if we do not give sufficient time and energy to this aspect of care which is clearly of importance to a large number of patients entering a healthcare setting. Spiritual care is integral to holistic care and all members of inter- or multi-disciplinary teams[2] should, therefore, address and respond to the spiritual needs of patients within their care.

References

1 Department of Health. (2000). *The NHS Plan. A Plan for Investment. A Plan for Reform*. London: HMSO.

2 National Institute for Clinical Excellence. (2004). *Improving Supportive and Palliative Care for Adults with Cancer*. London: NICE. www.nice.org.uk

3 Lloyd-Williams, M., Cobb, M., Taylor, F. (2006). How well trained are clergy in care of the dying patient and bereavement support? *J Pain Sympt Manage* **32**(1): 44–51.

4 MCPCIL. (2009). *National Care of the Dying Audit Hospitals Generic Report Round 2*. Available at: www.mcpcil.org.uk (accessed 24 November 2011).

5 Ross, L.A. (1996). Teaching spiritual care to nurses. *Nurse Educ Today* **16**: 38–43.

6 McSherry, W. (2006). The principal components model: a model for advancing spirituality and spiritual care within nursing and healthcare practice. *J Clin Nurs* **15**: 905–17.

7 Baldacchino, D.R. (2006). Nursing competencies for spiritual care. *J Clin Nurs* **15**(7): 885–96.

8 Walter, T. (1997). The ideology and organization of spiritual care: three approaches. *Palliat Med* **11**: 21–30.

9 Cummings, I. (1998). The interdisciplinary team. In: D. Doyle, G.W.C. Hanks, N. MacDonald (eds) *Oxford Textbook of Palliative Medicine*, 2nd edn. Oxford: Oxford University Press.

10 Speck, P. (2006). Maintaining a healthy team. In: P. Speck (ed.) *Teamwork in Palliative Care: Fulfilling or Frustrating?* Oxford: Oxford University Press.

11 Farsides, B. (2006). Ethical issues in multidisciplinary teamwork within palliative care. In: P. Speck (ed.) *Teamwork in Palliative Care: Fulfilling or Frustrating*. Oxford: Oxford University Press.

12 Montgomery, J. (2006). Legal issues of multiprofessional teamwork. In P. Speck (ed.) *Teamwork in Palliative Care: Fulfilling or Frustrating*. Oxford: Oxford University Press.

13 Puchalski, C.M., Lunsford, B., Harris, M.H., Miller, T. (2006). Interdisciplinary spiritual care for seriously ill and dying patients: a collaborative model. *Cancer J* **12**(5): 398–416.

14 Puchalski, C., Ferrell, B., Virani, R., Otis-Green, S., Baird, P. Bull J., *et al.* (2009). Improving the quality of spiritual care as a dimension of palliative care: the report of the consensus conference. *J Palliat Med* **12**(10): 885–904.

15 Sulasy, D.P. (2002). A biopsychosocial-spiritual model for the care of patients at the end of life. *Gerontologist* **42**(Spec no.3): 24–33.

16 Hanson, L.C., Dobbs, D., Usher, B.M., Williams, S., Rawlings, J., Daaleman, T.P. (2008). Providers and types of spiritual care during serious illness. *J Palliat Med* **11**(6): 907–14.

17 Speck, P. (2005). The evidence base for spiritual care. *Nurs Manage* **12**: 28–31.

18 UKBHC. (2010). *Code of Conduct for Healthcare Chaplains*. Available at: www.ukbhc.org.uk (accessed 24 November 2011).

19 US Chaplains. *Code of Ethics*. Available at: www.professionalchaplains.org (accessed 24 November 2011).

20 US Board. (2011). *Certification for Professional Chaplains*. Available at: www.acpe.edu (accessed 24 November 2011).

21 Mowat, H. (2008). *The Potential for Efficacy of Healthcare Chaplaincy and Spiritual Care Provision in the NHS (UK): a scoping review of recent research*. York: NHS Yorkshire & Humber.

22 Breitbart, W. (2009). Editorial: the spiritual domain of palliative care: who should be 'spiritual care professionals'? *Palliat Support Care* **7**: 139–41.

23 National Consensus Project for Quality Palliative Care (2009). *Clinical Practice Guidelines for Quality Palliative Care*, Second Edition. http://www.nationalconsensusproject.org

24 Payne, M. (2006). Team building: how, why and where? In: P. Speck (ed.) *Teamwork in Palliative Care: Fulfilling or Frustrating?* Oxford: Oxford University Press.

25 Meader, K.G. (2004). Spiritual care at the end of life: what is it and who does it? *NC Med J* **65**(4): 226–8.

26 Holmes, S.M., Rabow, M.W., Dibble, S.L. (2006) Screening the soul: communication regarding spiritual concerns among primary care physicians and seriously ill patients approaching the end of life. *Am J Hospice Palliat Med* **23**(1): 25–33.

27 Yardley, S.J., Walshe, C.E., Parr, A. (2009). Improving training in spiritual care: a qualitative study exploring patient perceptions of professional educational requirements. *Palliat Med* **23**: 601–7.

28 Speck, P. (2003). Spiritual/religious issues in care of the dying. In: J. Ellershaw, S. Wilkinson (eds) *Care of the Dying: a Pathway to Excellence*. Oxford: Oxford University Press.

29 Speck, P. (1998). Power and autonomy in palliative care: a matter of balance. Editorial. *Palliat Med* **12**(3): 145–6.

30 Walter, T. (2002). Spirituality in palliative care: opportunity or burden? *Palliat Med* **16**: 133–9.

CHAPTER 61

Ethical principles for spiritual care

Daniel P. Sulmasy

Introduction

Why should there be an ethics of spiritual care? Some readers will be so convinced of the generally beneficent nature of spiritual care that the idea that an ethic should be required might seem outlandish. Such enthusiasm notwithstanding, there is deep scepticism in many quarters about the moral justification for the spiritual care of the sick and injured, particularly the involvement of healthcare professionals in spiritual assessment and spiritual intervention. Even were there no such scepticism, however, wise chaplains and others involved in the spiritual care of the sick and injured must recognize that the deeply interpersonal nature of spiritual care and the predicament of the patient mark a moral terrain that requires ethical guidance if it is to be successfully navigated. This terrain is less well mapped than the domain of pastoral counselling or the domain of congregational pastoring: little has been written explicitly about the ethics of the spiritual care of the sick and injured. This chapter is an attempt to rectify that situation.

The ethical justification of spiritual care

The proper starting place for an ethics of spiritual care is the establishment of a moral warrant for spiritual intervention. Sceptics will need to be convinced of its necessity, but even those already convinced of the overall value of spiritual care need to reflect on its ethical justification. The establishment of such a justification will provide a foundation for the ethical practice of spiritual care for the sick and injured.

Some have tried to ground the moral warrant for spiritual care of patients on empirical data.[1,2] They cite studies demonstrating that many patients (a majority in most surveys) want their physicians and nurses to address spiritual issues with them. This might seem to provide a warrant for spiritual intervention, but these data do not constitute a sufficient moral grounding for spiritual care. One can readily grant that consent by the patient is a *necessary* moral condition for spiritual intervention, but a patient's preference for an intervention is not a *sufficient* moral warrant for any intervention in healthcare. For example, the bare fact that a patient desires to be treated with antibiotics for a viral upper respiratory infection or with hyperbaric oxygen for depression is not a sufficient moral justification for a physician to prescribe such treatment. Individual patient consent is necessary before embarking on any medical intervention, but that intervention only warrants being offered for the patient's consideration if it has been justified on other grounds. Consent alone is not enough.

Nor are data demonstrating an association between patient spiritual practices and salutary healthcare outcomes a moral warrant for spiritual intervention.[3] This is not because these data are invalid. Several well-done, long-term epidemiological studies, controlling carefully for many possible confounding factors have established that, independent of denomination, those who attend religious services on a regular basis live longer than those who do not. Religious practices and attitudes have also been associated with better mental health outcomes. However, one must be cautious regarding the scientific and ethical interpretation of these findings. These data do not establish that it is religious practice *per se* that brings these health benefits. It might be the case that these effects are mediated through a complex mixture of 'secular' explanations, such as social support, stress-reduction, etc. All that has been established by these retrospective studies is a statistical association, and association is not causation. The only real proof that attending religious services is, of itself, the cause of the observed lower mortality would require a controlled clinical trial assigning half the patients randomly to attend religious services and the other half to attend some sort of secular event as a 'control.' Such a trial, of course, would be immoral and absurd.

Furthermore, such data could not even in principle constitute a moral warrant to 'prescribe' religion the way a physician might 'prescribe' regular physical exercise. While these data associating good health outcomes with religious practice might be true:

- there is no definitive causal proof that religious practice per se improves health outcomes
- attending religious services for the 'extrinsic' reason of improving health might not confer the health benefits because they might only be associated with 'intrinsic' religiosity
- on purely religious grounds, no pastor would want a congregation filled with people who were there for the health benefits.

Authentic religious practice requires a commitment of one's whole person—heart, mind, body, and soul—in a manner more akin to marriage than to cardiovascular exercise. There is a profound moral difference between a physician recommending that a patient eat a low fat diet and recommending that a patient attend religious services.

While it is true that married people live longer, a physician is not justified urging a single patient to become married 'for the health benefits.' Likewise, there is no justification for a physician urging patients to attend religious services 'for the health benefits.'

The moral justification for attending to the spiritual needs of patients is not based upon healthcare outcomes. Such a view distorts the meaning of spirituality. Spirituality's role in human experience is more concerned with process than it is with outcomes. Religious belief can be bad for one's health, as is demonstrably evident in even a cursory view of the lives of figures such as Jesus of Nazareth, Mohandas Gandhi, or Martin Luther King, Jr From a spiritual point of view, better health is not the goal of spirituality. Spirituality concerns a person's relationship with questions of transcendence. The primary spiritual questions are truly universal, and comprise questions of meaning, value, and relationship. [4] Questions such as 'Why me?' or 'Do I still have value now that illness has rendered me unproductive?' or 'Can I bring myself to forgive those who have wronged me?' are the sorts of spiritual interrogatives that arise spontaneously and ubiquitously in the experiences of illness, injury, and death. Spirituality is concerned with how one lives one's life, and faces illness and death in light of whether one sees answers to these questions that transcend the finitude of human space and time.

The moral warrant for spiritual intervention lies not in patient preferences or in healthcare outcomes, but in the nature of healthcare and the nature of spirituality. Medicine and religion alike attend to some of the most central human experiences, such as birth, death, development, suffering, and sex. Physicians, nurses, and other healthcare professionals commit themselves, often by oaths that they have sworn, to care for patients as whole persons. Because illness and injury disrupt patients' lives in ways that extend beyond the body, encompassing families, communities, and religious experiences, a commitment to caring for whole persons must entail going beyond the care of the body. Human being is spiritual being. When injured or ill, human beings naturally ask transcendent questions about meaning, value, and relationship. If holistic care is a moral duty, then that duty extends to spiritual, as well as to physical care. Therefore, attending to the spiritual needs of patients is not just a moral option, but a moral imperative. Attending to the spiritual needs of patients is justified not because of patient preferences or healthcare outcomes, but because spirituality is intrinsic to nature of being sick and caring for the sick. It is this imperative that grounds the ethics of spiritual care.

The ethical principles of spiritual care

Despite the fact that clinical bioethics has been in existence for more than three decades, and despite the fact that pastoral care has been provided to the sick for millennia, no set of general, theoretically justified ethical principles has heretofore been proposed for the spiritual care of patients. As was the case for medicine until very recently,[5] codes of ethics have been promulgated for spiritual care,[6] but no critically evaluated and theoretically justified system of spiritual care ethics has been proposed. Since clinical care and spiritual care are inter-related but substantively different practices, the ethical principles that govern spiritual care will necessarily differ from the principles of clinical bioethics. This chapter proposes five ethical principles for spiritual care. These principles overlap in part with those of clinical bioethics, diverge in part from those of clinical bioethics, and also represent a set of aspirations by which clinical bioethics might incorporate a deeper concern for the spiritual aspects of patient care.

Patient-centredness

The first ethical principle of spiritual care is patient-centeredness. The point of all pastoral care is the person, and the point of clinical spiritual care is the patient, who is first and foremost a person. Spiritual care must focus on the spiritual needs of the sick person. Since persons are social, this focus on the person does not deny the familial, social, and ecclesiastical relationships of the patient, but places the individual patient at the centre of this nexus of relationships. The ethics of spiritual care must be focused on the service of the sick person, in his or her spiritual journey, in the face of illness, injury, and death. This means that spiritual care is directed by the patient's dignity, needs, and desires, the patient's perception of the highest good, and the patient's religious and spiritual relationships and commitments. Patients are whole persons: biologically, psychologically, socially, and spiritually constituted. As Pellegrino and Thomasma have pointed out, a duty of beneficence towards patients, considered as whole persons, requires a recognition that the patient's conception of the transcendent good is the overriding determinant of the patient's good.[7] This means that the biomedical good of the patient is at the service of the spiritual good of the patient and not vice-versa. Thus, for instance, there is a duty to respect a refusal of blood transfusion by committed Jehovah's Witness for whom the violation of divine law regarding blood would entail an overall harm for him or her as a whole person, despite the fact that it might entail even the loss of all biological value, i.e. death.

Patient-centeredness requires both competence and compassion. Those who would provide spiritual care to the sick require specific training that goes beyond what is ordinarily provided in general seminary education.

The commitment to patient-centeredness also concretely requires that anyone providing spiritual care must follow the patient's lead in bedside discourse. Patients are free to refuse spiritual intervention in general, as well as any and every aspect of spiritual care that might be offered. Patients should never be manipulated or cajoled into any spiritual conversation or practice. The first duty of those providing spiritual care is to listen—to hear the patient's story and how the patient's narrative history intersects, confronts, or is entwined with the patient's illness narrative.

Patient-centredness also requires confidentiality. Just as the Hippocratic Oath obliges physicians never to 'publish abroad' what patients have divulged to them,[8] so spiritual care professionals must respect patient confidentiality. Nonetheless, the ethical commitment to team care described below circumscribes this duty of confidentiality in ways that will be discussed in detail later in this chapter.

Holism

Spiritual care requires a respect for patients as persons integrally considered and this requires attention to the totality of their needs as whole persons. This sort of care is encompassed by a biopsycho-social-spiritual model of care, which recognizes the many distinct aspects of the needs that patients present as whole persons, but also attends to the interrelatedness of the biological, psychological, social, and spiritual aspects of the patient.[9] Those who provide spiritual care must commit themselves to a deeper understanding of medicine and psychology than the average pastor. Likewise, physicians and nurses ought to commit themselves to a greater knowledge of religion and spirituality than would be expected of a veterinarian. A major corollary of this principle of holism is a commitment to a team-approach to the care of patients. No one can be the master of the entire spectrum of the biopsychosocial-spiritual model of patient care. It takes a team of professionals, aware of the contributions that other distinct disciplines make to the care of the patient as a whole person, and a willingness to call upon the expertise of other members of the team to provide that care. This commitment requires communication skills, respect, and humility.

Discretion

Spiritual care is discrete in its interventions with patients. The aim is to provide no more spiritual care than is needed for a particular patient and a willingness to defer to the expertise of others when those others might be better suited to meeting the patient's needs. For example, some patients might require intensive pastoral counseling, but others will require just one visit for spiritual assessment and then limited visits or even, perhaps, no further visits. Some patients will present with denominationally specific needs, and while competent providers of spiritual care should be able to assess the spiritual needs of a patient regardless of the patient's religious background or lack thereof, that spiritual care provider must be ready to muster the denominationally specific resources necessary to meet the needs of patients, whether by deferring to chaplains, the patient's own clergy, or the provision of denominationally specific sacred texts or sacred objects. Discretion also implies respect for one's own limitations in expertise. This implies a moral requirement to refer patients when one lacks expertise. In the case of spiritual care, this implies a willingness on the part of clinicians to refer to chaplains or clergy in order best to meet the spiritual needs of patients. Discretion also implies that clergy should recognize when they need to refer to physicians, social workers, or psychiatrists when it appears that the patient's needs cannot be met through pastoral care or counselling. In turn, this mutual recognition of limits in expertise and a commitment to appropriate referral means that the principle of discretion also reinforces the need for a team approach to patient care.

Accompaniment

Non-abandonment is an important ethical principle in the provision of spiritual care. Those who are sick are already socially isolated. Among their greatest fears are of abandonment and alienation. As stated above, spiritual care begins with active listening. That listening constitutes the beginning of a relationship. Those providing spiritual care must continue that relationship for as long as it is desired and helpful to the patient. The journey of illness is not a path human beings were meant to walk alone.

Tolerance

The globalized world has produced a globalized need for tolerance and respect for a variety of religious commitments and communities. Western nations, particularly the United States, but to an increasing degree many other nations, are becoming highly religiously pluralistic. And even within the world's great religions, the specific inculturations of those religions and the particularities of the various sects within each religion result in differences that must be tolerated, especially as individuals and families migrate from their nations of origin.

If spirituality is correctly defined as the characteristics of a person's life in relationship with questions of transcendence, then spiritual needs will be universal—encompassing even those who profess no religious belief. Medicine cannot be hostile to spirituality if it is committed to care for patients as whole persons. Spiritual care providers cannot be hostile to patients who profess no religion. Spiritual care providers must be respectful and attentive to the spiritual needs of patients whose religious beliefs and practices differ from their own.

Note that this principle of tolerance does not imply that there is no truth. It would make little sense for anyone to profess religious beliefs that he or she did not think were true. Tolerance requires not agnosticism about religious truth, but a degree of epistemic humility—an acknowledgement that one's own beliefs require faith and that one might lack convincing evidence or arguments for persuading another person that one's own beliefs are true. This interfaith respect demands that healthcare never be made conditional upon the profession of any religious beliefs, and commands attention to the spiritual needs of patients of no beliefs and of all systems of belief.

Selected specific ethical issues

Against proselytizing

From these principles, one can derive further, more specific moral rules to govern the ethical practice of spiritual care. Chief among these is an absolute prohibition on proselytizing in the healthcare setting.[10] Certain clinicians and clergy, motivated to proselytize patients by virtue of zealous devotion to their own faith commitments, might ask, for example, 'If I have what I believe is the answer to all human concerns, how can I, morally, not share that with everyone I meet, including my patients?' I want to argue that this position is seriously misguided. Even those who have an intuitive sense that it is wrong for clinicians to proselytize their patients, however, might need assistance in understanding exactly why their intuitions are justified.

The first explanation for why such proselytizing is wrong is that it is not patient-centred. The power imbalance between clinician and patient, or chaplain and patient, coupled with the vulnerability of the patient, limit the power of the patient to assent freely to the invitation to convert. To the extent that any such wished-for 'conversion' were successful, one could not be sure that the patient would not be acceding to the proselytizer's demands out of fear, whether justifiable or not, of a diminution in level of clinical care, or even a loss of esteem in the eyes of the powerful clinician. Such a 'conversion' would not be free, but coerced and therefore false, and the clinician or chaplain would actually then have been frustrated in his or her aims. Secondly, proselytizing violates the principle of interfaith respect. Such tolerance need not diminish one's own convictions regarding the truth, but is necessary for peaceful and respectful pluralism. Thirdly, from the viewpoint of religious belief, the attempt to take advantage of the patient's predicament as an 'opportunity' for proselytizing is really an act of hubris, usurping a prerogative that belongs properly to God. God, the believer must suppose, freely gave human beings the gift of freedom and can only really be loved if a person comes to faith wholly and freely. If God risks rejection in order that human love of God be free, a believing clinician cannot justly claim the right to take advantage of a patient's weakness in order to manipulate an act of faith. Fourthly, the intimacy of religious belief and practice makes religion qualitatively different from other attitudes and behaviours a clinician might suggest to patients, such as exercising regularly and eating a low-fat diet. In this sense, religious conversion is more akin to sex. Even if it is true that sex might be good for a particular patient, a clinician is not justified in taking advantage of the clinical relationship as pretext for sexual relations, even if deemed 'therapeutic.' Similarly, a clinician is not justified advising patients to 'get religion,' even if his or her intent is beneficent.

Confidentiality

The principle of patient-centredness demands confidentiality. There are doubtless some things that patients want to tell clergy that they do not wish to disclose to their physicians and vice-versa. Yet, spiritual care providers such as chaplains are also committed, by the principle of holism, to a policy of teamwork. This apparent conflict of principles would seem to pose a dilemma.

The application of informed consent procedures provides a serviceable way to traverse this terrain. Chaplains and physicians should present themselves as members of a team that generally shares information unless the patient raises a particular objection. Clinical judgment, however, may dictate the need for more explicit consent conversations. Clinicians, for instance, may uncover serious patient spiritual issues, and, if so, should ask patients' permission to disclose sensitive information with the chaplain. For instance, the attending physician might say, 'Thanks for sharing all that with me. It sounds as if you are struggling with many serious spiritual issues in the midst of your illness. Would it help if I asked our chaplain, Rev. Jones, to see you, and would it be OK if I shared with her a little of what we've just been talking about?' Similarly, chaplains may uncover spiritual issues of significant clinical importance, and should ask patients' permission before sharing the content of these discussions with clinicians.

Exceptions to patient confidentiality arise for all members of the team when they uncover serious psychiatric problems such as suicidal or homicidal ideation. The moral duty then is to report these findings to nurses or physicians who can act upon these findings to prevent harm to the patients themselves or to others.

Clinical notes

Related to the issue of confidentiality is the question of whether chaplains should write notes in the chart. While the practice is currently uncommon, the principle of holism would suggest that team care is the optimal model, and that teams work best when lines of communication, such as the chart, are wide open and broadly utilized. The chart ideally functions in just this way for both clinicians and chaplains. Spiritual care notes should therefore be the morally preferable norm. The writing of notes, however, should be tempered by due regard for patient confidentiality across the various disciplines participating in the care team.

Spiritual assessment

The principle of holism suggests that all patients have potential spiritual needs. Treating patients as whole persons requires an assessment of the spiritual needs of patients, not merely as an option, but as a moral obligation. The team care approach that derives from the principles of holism and discretion does not require, however, that each and every member of the team assess the spiritual needs of all patients. Primary responsibility for this commitment can be delegated to individual members of the team. Nonetheless, to a certain extent, all members of the team play some role in the spiritual assessment of the patient. A patient who may have declined a visit from a chaplain early in a visit may be denying spiritual needs that only the physicians and nurses will be able to ascertain. New spiritual needs may also arise in the course of the patient's clinical condition and treatment. All must play a part even if formal assessment is delegated.

Some patients might initially resist or even refuse spiritual assessment or care in the face of a clinical-pastoral judgment that the patient would really benefit from a visit by a chaplain or clergy. Just as patients may be re-approached even if they initially refuse the offer of a clinical medical intervention, so it is ethically permissible to re-approach a patient to confirm that the refusal is truly informed and genuinely reflects the patient's considered judgment about spiritual care. This approach is perfectly consistent with the principle of patient-centredness. It would not be permissible, however, to force spiritual care on a patient, or to 'badger' patients who have consistently refused such care.

The ethics of team care

This chapter has emphasized a team approach to the care of all patients, often best exemplified by hospice care teams, in which physicians, nurses, chaplains, psychiatrists, social workers, and others work jointly to assure optimal patient care. Working in teams, however, raises its own set of ethical issues.[11]

First, how accountability is to be divided is itself an ethical issue. Certain responsibilities may be assigned to individual members relative to their function in the team, but there may be true collective responsibility in which each team member shares responsibility for the whole team's actions.

While the physician is ultimately responsible for the patient's care, nurses, chaplains, social workers, and psychiatrists are all professionals, and have codes of ethics that make them responsible for the care they provide. No member of the team can ask another member of the team to violate his or her professional ethics. Any member who cooperates in, or fails to object to, any harmful act is a moral accomplice. On occasion, if team members are unable to resolve serious moral disagreements within the team, they may need to resort to outside assistance such as an ethics consult. At the limit, in extraordinarily rare circumstances, each must be prepared to take on the role of 'whistle-blower.' Every team member shares collective moral responsibility for the care provided by the whole team.

Another complicating factor is the considerable overlap of roles and responsibilities. While each member has special professional expertise, it would be artificial to confine the physician to the technical, the nurse to the caring, the social worker to the social, the psychiatrist to the mental, and the chaplain to the spiritual. Each team member has a responsibility for patient care, which, unlike medical or other technical procedures, can never be discontinued or abandoned or neglected by any team member.

Another set of issues involves team dynamics. In the interest of team harmony, members can become overly eager to be seen as members of a team. They might lose the ability to see alternative ways of caring for patients or might never challenge the plan put forth by the majority of the team's members. Others might be lulled by group dynamics into paying more attention to their own 'moral distress' than to the anguish of the patient. Self-righteousness and self-pity are subtle tendencies in teams that care for the sick, and both should be eschewed.

Finally, the team leader bears particular moral responsibilities. This will generally be the physician, who should be careful to avoid acting autocratically, but more as a servant-leader. As always, the ethical imperative must be the impact of any team decision on the comprehensive care of the patient as a whole person.

Family and loved ones

Humans are social beings, and most patients experience illness in the context of their relationships with family, friends, congregations, workplaces, and other social networks. Holism requires attention to this nexus of relationships. Sometimes issues regarding these relationships are central themes in the spiritual struggles of patients. In most cases, with the patient's permission, spiritual care will also involve caring for those who care about the patient and whose reactions to the predicament of the patient may induce profound spiritual needs. When the patient lacks capacity, the focus of palliative care may shift more directly to family and other loved ones, but the principle of accompaniment requires that patients lacking decisional capacity never be thought to lack spiritual needs. They still have needs for prayer, presence, touch, and the rituals of their faith traditions.

Praying with patients

The spiritual care of patients will often involve praying with them. The principle of patient-centeredness, however, requires that anyone, whether chaplain or other team member, follow the patient's lead with respect to prayer. Prayer must never be forced on patients, but invited by the patient or offered in a non-coercive manner in response to appropriate clinical clues and consented to by the patient.

Although it may most commonly be done by chaplains, prayer with patients need not be a role limited to chaplains. Other members of the team may choose to be present while a chaplain and a patient pray, or to be present while a patient prays, or to pray with the patient as individual members of the patient care team. While there is an obligation on the part of all members of the team to assure proper spiritual assessment and spiritual care, however, there is no obligation that members of the team who are of a different faith from the patient or have no religious faith or are in any way uncomfortable praying with patients ever be forced to do so or be made to feel obligated to do so.

There would not seem to be any equivalent moral cautions for any member of the care team praying privately for the health and wellbeing of any patient or for that of all patients. Nor should there be any concerns with chaplains or clergy praying publically for the welfare of groups of patients or for all patients provided none are named specifically. By the principle of patient-centeredness, however, such public prayers should not be directed towards the conversion of patients. Pressing moral concerns would also arise with respect to any public prayers that would name patients without their permission or would impose prayers or rituals on patients in their presence and without their consent.

Miracles

An overwhelming number of Americans believe in miracles.[12] It is rare, however, that such beliefs develop into moral problems in the clinical arena.[13–15] An ethical problem arises only when such beliefs appear to conflict with the best-interests of the patient considered as a whole person. The most stressful cases for families and the healthcare team are those in which patients are unable to speak for themselves and families are demanding the continuation of life-sustaining treatments that the healthcare professionals have deemed biomedically futile. Such cases are extraordinarily complicated and delicate and a detailed approach to these cases has been described elsewhere. While there is no clear consensus on the proper clinical-pastoral approach to such cases, the following can be considered general guidelines.[16]

First, the expressed belief in miracles cannot be considered sacrosanct—not considered any more immune to challenge than any other deeply held beliefs of patients or families. Sometimes serious psychiatric illness can be expressed in religious language, and if all religious expression were considered immune to investigation, one would, in principle, have accepted the view that religious belief and mental illness cannot be distinguished. That view seems false. Secondly, spiritual care professionals have an obligation to probe carefully and gently into the reasons that lie behind the refusal to forgo treatment and the belief in miracles. Families may be expressing distrust of the medical system, harbouring false beliefs about the tenets of their own faith traditions, expressing anticipated grief, experiencing the psychological syndrome of denial, or expressing an authentic faith in miracles. Authentic faith in miracles lets God be God, and not the physician. As one Christian ethicist has put it, 'God is not ventilator-dependent.'[17] Spiritual care has an important role to play in sorting out the underlying issues through attentive listening and mustering the appropriate resources to help the patient and family. Thirdly, attempts by members of the team to 're-frame' the patient's or family's beliefs or interpret their religion for them when not members of the clergy of their religion are almost always bound to do more harm than good. Fourthly, a judgment will be necessary as to when such beliefs are helpful coping strategies and when such beliefs have actually become harmful to the patient as a whole person, such that some intervention might be necessary. Fifthly, the only defensible standard of futility that could be invoked in order to justify the unilateral withholding or withdrawing of life-sustaining treatments in such cases would be a standard of 'biomedical' futility, such that the treatment either will not work, or will be either repeatedly or continuously required even though the patient will die in a very short period of time regardless of any medical intervention. By contrast, the so-called 'subjective' standard of biomedical futility, according to which the biomedical effectiveness of the treatment cannot be appreciated by the patient as a benefit due to profound neurological impairment is overly broad, usurps judgments about quality of life that properly belong to patients and their families, and has not held up in the courts.[18]

Above all, such cases should be handled with patience, compassion, and respect. More can be accomplished by attentive listening than by rigidity.

Life-long learning

All members of the care team have a moral obligation to engage in continuing professional education. This is grounded in the principles of patient-centeredness and holism, since optimal care requires competence. Chaplains certainly need to keep abreast of developments in theology and pastoral care techniques, but they also have an obligation to keep up on basic developments in medicine. As medical technology advances, spiritual care inevitably changes. The questions patients ask, the ethical issues that emerge, the kinds of suffering patients encounter, and their options all depend importantly on what medicine has to offer. Likewise, physicians, nurses, and other members of the team need to keep abreast of the changing face of spiritual care and their own roles in the spiritual care of patients. Being grounded solidly in one's own discipline, but aware of developments in the care rendered by other members of the team is essential for well-ordered team care.

Personal spiritual development

Abraham Heschel once told the American Medical Association that 'to heal a person, you must first be a person.'[19] Heschel's insight seems to be that it is important for good spiritual care of patients that all members of the healthcare team be attentive to their own spiritual needs and spiritual development. This will obviously take unique forms for each member of the team, in his or her spiritual journey, but the principle of holism seems to apply to each member of the team as much as it does to patients. To render patient-centred and holistic care, those professionals who serve the sick will be better equipped if their own lives are centred and they pursue their own lives as whole persons.

Conclusions

This chapter has provided an ethical justification for spiritual care based on the nature of healing and the nature of spirituality rather than patient preferences or healthcare outcomes. Five ethical principles to guide spiritual care were set forth: patient-centredness, holism, discretion, accompaniment, and tolerance. A number of specific ethical issues were then addressed and approaches offered based upon these principles. Good spiritual care will always be ethical, and it is hoped that these considerations will help to shape such care.

References

1 Matthews, D.A., Clark, C. (1998). *The Faith Factor: Proof of the Healing Power of Prayer*, pp. 269–88. New York: Viking.

2 Koenig, H.G. (2007). Physician's role in addressing spiritual needs. *Sth Med J* **100**: 932–3.

3 Sulmasy, D.P. (2006). *The Rebirth of the Clinic: an Introduction to Spirituality and Healthcare*, pp. 161–85. Washington, DC: Georgetown University Press.

4 Sulmasy, D.P. (2006). Spiritual issues in the care of dying patients: it's ok between me and God. *J Am Med Ass* **296**: 1385–92.

5 Pellegrino, E.D. (1993). The metamorphosis of medical ethics. A 30-year retrospective. *J Am Med Ass* **269**: 1158–62.

6 ACPE Code (2011). *Common Code of Ethics for Chaplains, Pastoral Counselors, Pastoral Educators and Students*. Available at: http://www.acpe.edu/NewPDF/2010%20Manuals/2010%20Standards.pdf (accessed 16 January 2012).

7 Pellegrino, E.D., Thomasma, D. (1988). *For the Patient's Good: the Restoration of Beneficence in Healthcare*, pp. 73–91. New York: Oxford University Press.

8 Hippocrates. (1984). The oath. In: *Hippocrates*, pp. 298–301. W.H.S. Jones, transl. I.. Cambridge: Loeb Classical Library.

9 Sulmasy, D.P. (2002). A biopsychosocial-spiritual model for the care of patients at the end of life. *Gerontologist.* **42**(Suppl. 3): 24–33.

10 Puchalski, C.M., Ferrell, B. (2010). *Making Healthcare Whole: Integrating Spirituality into Patient Care*, pp. 44–5. West Conshohocken: Templeton Press.

11 Pellegrino, E.D. (1982). The ethics of collective judgments in medicine and healthcare. *J Med Philos* **7**: 3–10.

12 A Pew Forum On Religion & Public Life Report (2010). *Religion Among the Millennials: Less Religiously Active Than Older Americans, But Fairly Traditional In Other Ways*. Available from: http://pewforum.org/uploadedFiles/Topics/Demographics/Age/millennials-report.pdf. (accessed 16 January 2012).

13 La Puma, J., Stocking, C.B., Darling, C.M., Siegler, M. (1992). Community hospital ethics consultation: evaluation and comparison with a university hospital service. *Am J Med* **92**: 346–51.

14 DuVal, G., Sartorius, L., Clarridge, B., Gensler, G., Danis, M. (2001). What triggers requests for ethics consultations? *J Med Eth* **27**(Suppl 1): i24–9.

15 DuVal, G., Clarridge, B., Gensler, G., Danis, M. (2004). A national survey of US internists' experiences with ethical dilemmas and ethics consultation. *J Gen Intern Med*.**19**: 251–8.

16 Sulmasy, D.P. (2007). Distinguishing denial from authentic faith in miracles: a clinical-pastoral approach. *Sth Med J* **100**: 1268–72.

17 Orr, R.D. (2009). *Medical Ethics and the Faith Factor: a Handbook for Clergy and Healthcare Professionals*, p. 27. Grand Rapids: WB Eerdmans.

18 Sulmasy, D.P. (1997). Futility and the varieties of medical judgment. *Theor Med* **18**: 63–78.

19 Heschel, A.J. (1966). *The Insecurity of Freedom*, p. 24–38. New York: Noonday Press/Farrar, Strauss, Giroux.

SECTION VI

Challenges

CHAPTER 62

Contemporary spirituality

David Tacey

Will the world, perhaps, be able to discover an answer which, as yet, can only be guessed at? (Gadamer)[1]

Spirituality as a dynamic and contested field

The trends of contemporary spirituality are difficult to discern because what we find depends on what we are looking for. However, a definite trend in the English-speaking world and Western-style democracies is to see spirituality pulling further away from religion and becoming an autonomous field in its own right. This is reflected, at the popular level, in individuals claiming to be 'spiritual, but not religious,' and, at the academic level, in an increasing literature on spirituality which has no connection with religion as such.[2] Sandra Schneiders puts the situation well:

> Spirituality has rarely enjoyed such a high profile, positive evaluation, and even economic success as it does among Americans today. If religion is in serious trouble, spirituality is in the ascendancy and the irony of this situation evokes puzzlement and anxiety in the religious establishment, scrutiny among theologians, and justification among those who have traded the religion of their past for the spirituality of their present.[3]

In one sense this direction could be called 'progressive' and might be said to point to an imminent spiritual revival.[4] In another sense it might be said to point to a loss of historical sensibility, continuity, and cultural memory.[5] Spirituality could be said to be suffering from a kind of amnesia, insofar as many individuals think they are the first ones to have had spiritual feelings for nature, community, and soulful interiority. What we can say about the current epoch is that spirituality is coming back to public awareness, but because it is emerging in a primarily secular context it is often unaware of its religious background.

What this shows is that the break with the past represented by modernity and post-modernity is so profound that some think the history of religions has stopped, or is starting all over again as people grapple with the spiritual dimension of experience. Spirituality itself, as a term, has radically changed its meaning in the last few decades. It used to refer to those who were 'very' religious, namely, monastics, monks, and nuns, who were not content with the public demonstrations of faith, but wanted to appropriate faith at a personal and inward level. In the Catholic tradition, those who were rigorous in their lifestyle and disciplined in their prayers and rituals were referred to as 'spiritual'. Now it seems that those who are 'not very' religious are claiming the term and asking to be seen as spiritual. William Johnston writes:

> To the surprise of many, the term *spirituality* has become democratized since monastics first disseminated it. Ideals that for centuries an elite viewed as virtually unattainable now prompt spiritual growth in everyone. In a word, a 'spirituality revolution' during the past thirty years has democratized pursuit of holiness.[6]

Spirituality still exists as the inner life of religious tradition, but this use of the term is starting to seem marginal, as vast numbers of secular people are appropriating the term in a different way. Spirituality in religion refers to the capacity to enter into the core of a tradition and to weld it to experience. Spirituality outside religion refers to the capacity to intuit or bear witness to a depth dimension of experience, which has been lacking during the period of high secularism.

It has been argued that the emergence of spirituality indicates that our time is post-secular, insofar as spirituality is becoming mainstream.[7] Secular or non-religious spirituality is a force to be reckoned with, and one can see it arising in a range of social contexts. It is increasingly evident in the arts and music, in ecology and the appreciation of nature, in workplace cultures and industrial relations, in health and wellbeing, in psychiatry and medicine, in education theory and practice, in business and law, in urban design and architecture, in land-use and gardening, in discourses about community, world peace and the future.[8] It does seem, on the surface, to point to a spiritual revival, but secular spirituality may find it is not as resilient as it imagines once it recognizes it has no past, history, or memory. I often imagine it as a lovely flower in a vase on the table, but, lacking any roots, it will fade quickly and vanish from view. The flower of spirituality might wilt and die when its day passes, unless it can find its way back to the sources from which it arose. In my reckoning, those sources must include the religious and metaphysical traditions of the past. In denying its origins in religion, modern spirituality might be cutting itself off from its own continued survival.

However advocates of secular spirituality claim that the roots of spirituality are found in human experience, and not in religious traditions.[9] Spiritual experience, they claim, is 'prior' to religion, and need not go back to religion to find its deeper source.[10] As such, the cry that spirituality cannot exist without religion is seen by this school of thought as scare-mongering from a conservative religious lobby. However, the debate about whether or not religious traditions are dispensable represents one of the important tensions in the spirituality field at the present time. Those who argue that spirituality is indelibly tied to religion and cannot flourish without it include Schneiders,[3] Dreyer and Burrows,[11] Koenig,[12] Philip Sheldrake,[5] and David Ranson.[13] Those who argue the contrary case, that spirituality is able to exist without religious traditions and is perhaps even better off without it, include Daryl Paulson,[7] Robert Forman,[14] Heelas and Woodhead,[4] and Neville Drury.[15] There are others who argue that spirituality can exist independently, but religious tradition is an optional direction in which it can move, and in this category are David Hay,[16] David Tacey,[8] Bruce Rumbold,[17] and Diarmuid O'Murchu.[18]

Any survey of contemporary spirituality would have to include the conservative religious position, which holds that spirituality without religion is heresy or wrong-headed.[19–22] However, because the term 'spirituality' is being favoured above 'religion', this position is in the business of repackaging old-style religion as 'spirituality.' This position sponsors conferences on 'Spirituality and Health,' and 'Spirituality and Business,' which attract large numbers due to the fashionable terms, but what is offered may be unreconstructed religiosity. This discourse has a habit of referring to everything other than itself as 'New Age', with the implication of inauthenticity. Buddhism in the West, ecological, secular, feminist, and recovery programme spiritualities—all are dismissed as New Age and reprehensible. At the other end of the spectrum, but with strangely similar results, are the materialists, including Marxists and Freudians, who claim that spirituality in any context—religious or non-religious, old age or new—is a hoax perpetrated by businesses and institutions that seek to oppress and delude.[23,24] There may be a hoax element in some of the commercialized attempts to produce spirituality, but the signs of exploitation do not annul the integrity of the field. There are also revisionist Marxists who argue that spirituality can no longer be seen as negative by political and social progressives.[25] Some post-Freudians argue that Freud's negative view of spirituality[26] must be overcome as psychoanalysis moves into the post-modern era.[27,28]

It seems to me that contemporary spirituality is defined by the contrary voices and movements expressed within it. The fact that there are so many conflicting views, and a number of contested positions, is a sign that the field is dynamic and alive. There is every reason to believe that spirituality is destined to rise to the status of an academic discipline in its own right,[29] and there is some discussion about this at the moment.[11] The irony is that conferences are appearing in numerous cities and countries simultaneously, each claiming to be the first major interdisciplinary conference in the field. Until the field is ordered and regulated, we can expect this to continue for some time. The emerging discipline will have to be strongly interdisciplinary, and will need to be informed by medicine and psychiatry, psychology, psychotherapy, sociology, philosophy, literary and cultural studies, religious studies, and theology. It may look like a baggy monster, but I see no alternative other than to invite the concert of many voices. In future years, spirituality studies will rise like a new star on the horizon of academic life, representing the newest discipline to emerge since sociology.

Contemporary spirituality as an exploration of the heart

Spirituality is becoming more popular not because we want it, but because we need it. In the West the needs of the spirit have been relegated to the margins of society and the religions are felt to be increasingly out of touch with mainstream interests and desires. We live in a paradoxical time in many ways, because while many of us continue to discount religion and criticize its values and assumptions, we nevertheless complain of a spiritual emptiness and a God-shaped hole. The fact that an obsessive criticism of religion might have something to do with the modern sense of emptiness rarely seems to occur to people. Nevertheless, we face the conundrum that, although we need spiritual sustenance, many do not accept the traditional forms in which it is presented. There is a sense of revolution and ferment, and it is too early to tell where the unrest will lead. The statistics indicate that we are not heading toward a rebirth of the old religions, but that something new might be on the horizon, about which we can only guess at the present time.[4,14]

Although the term 'spirituality' has become fashionable and acquired a certain appeal, there is not a lot of glamour in what spirituality demands of us. In a secular world, with widespread repression of the spiritual life, when we go in search of this buried life it is rarely in a wonderful condition. After all, it has been neglected and hidden, and as Freud knew, any content of the psyche that has been badly treated is not going to express itself in an entirely positive way. The human spirit today is half-starved, under-nourished, desiccated, and full of anxiety, so when it finally appears it comes with considerable claims and a baggage of historical neglect. Signs of its poor condition are found in extremist positions, fundamentalism, and violence.[30] I think the New Age production of 'spirituality' as a consumer item is an attempt to defend against the reality of spirit, and pretend that it is about fun times and pleasures. The New Age shops are full of images of sunsets, peaceful oceans, dolphins, crystals, flowers, and North American Indians. However, the industries that manufacture these images are suffering from a loss of memory and moral proportion, since the Amerindian peoples carry a terrible history and great pain in their souls. It is the final insult to depict such peoples as the symbols of spirit when the colonizing cultures, which now idealize them have worked systematically to crush their spirit.

Spirituality is not merely a flight from the real or an escape from history, but a movement more deeply into history. In our personal lives, spirituality is an attempt to find something authentic and genuine in the human psyche. Thomas Merton speaks about spirituality as a quest for the true self,[31] and Jung sees it as a search for that which is beyond or outside the normal ego.[32] In either case, the search will involve us in turmoil, angst, and the recovery of a new equilibrium. If people realized how difficult spirituality is they would not idealize it or pretend it is some kind of fun park for the soul. To become spiritual is to encounter forces that are outside the control of the ego and beyond the pleasure principle. To encounter spirit is to discover an authentic self, which is likely to make real demands on us.

It is not for nothing that the search for spirituality in the monasteries and religious orders required a lifetime of patience, discipline, and regulated living. To adjust our lives, our egotistical existence, to something genuinely spiritual involves what used to be called 'metanoia,' a turning-around of the person. Today, we pursue spirituality for what benefits it might bestow or what we will get out of it, but we are reminded by the life within that it is *we* who have to make the adjustment. To accept spirit into our lives demands, as always, sacrifice and devotion. The problem with our age is that it has forgotten that the things of the spirit are beyond the ego and ask a great deal of us.

Spirituality involves us in a wrestling match with the heart and our inner demons. The poet W. B. Yeats wrote in his last poem:

> Now that my ladder's gone
> I must lie down where all the ladders start
> In the foul rag and bone shop of the heart.[33]

For Yeats the 'ladder' refers to cosmologies that once transported us from the mundane to the heavenly realm. The loss of this ladder, the vertical pathway to the transcendent, would not be replaced in the short-term by a new ladder, but by psychological experience in 'the foul rag and bone shop of the heart'. In other words, after the collapse of religious culture and the so-called 'death of God', we find ourselves having to deal with psychological experience.[34] As Yeats suggests, destiny has condemned us to this activity, since we have been thrown into the heart—or what psychology calls the unconscious—against our will and not from our own choosing. We need a way of connecting with the divine, which is not an upward pathway to moral perfection, but a deepening path toward the body, psyche, and the wholeness of personality.

Contemporary spirituality as soul-making

Contemporary spirituality is perhaps more about the exploration of 'soul' than of 'spirit', if by *soul* we mean the Greek *psyche*, or interiority. In the classical tradition, spirit is masculine (Latin: animus), ethereal, aspirational, and sublime. Soul is feminine (anima), embodied, a bridge between heaven and earth. Soul is the vessel that contains the universal spirit and makes it personal. Soul draws spirituality into a different key, making it earthly and holistic. A spirituality that is shaped by soul is akin to 'individuation', that is, the making of the personality. Some recent classics on the spiritual life do not refer to spirit as such, but to soul, and were written by secular psychologists.[35–37] Although secular in orientation, the psychotherapies find themselves, often in spite of their stated intentions, dealing with spiritual themes such as connecting to the heart, locating the inner self, relating to cosmic forces and attending to guiding dreams.

This may be one reason why religious traditionalists fail to understand what contemporary people mean by 'spirituality', and denounce it as fraudulent. In the past, the term referred to the activity by which the self was bypassed, transcended, or overcome in acts of humility, self-surrender, and compassion for others. Today, however, spirituality refers not to the overcoming of the self, but to the *fulfilment* of the self, and this gives contemporary spirituality its 'narcissistic' character, as claimed by traditionalists.[20,21] However, although some 'spirituality' is guilty as charged, and might be said to represent a form of navel-gazing, genuine spirituality is the discovery of an objective life within the self, which is akin to what the mystics and visionaries of various traditions call the God Within.[38,39]

To outsiders, this may look like narcissism in that it is inwardly focused, but the modern search is for the divine spark within the human personality. This places modern spirituality in the tradition of gnosticism, mysticism, and esotericism. In this case, 'self-transcendence' has effectively been redefined. It used to refer to the abnegation of self through surrender to God and good works, but today it has a psychological meaning. It refers to the art of transcending ego by exploring deeper regions of the personality. One 'overcomes' not self, but ego, and in so doing one liberates the spirit within. For those for whom spirituality must be extraverted, active, and socially committed, this introverted spirituality is frowned upon, as we see in the Vatican's denunciation of the post-modern spiritual quest.[40] The problem with the Vatican's attack is that it fails to appreciate that the self is not the same as the ego; the self is more complex and multi-layered. The self is a 'small infinity,' which has the capacity to reach the divine. This is old news in the East, where it has long been said that Atman (the divine within the human) and Brahman are one. However, it is a recent discovery in the West, where God has been kept well apart from human interiority by the major traditions.

Here, we can discern different theologies at work behind traditional and contemporary approaches to spirituality. The traditional approach seems firmly based on the doctrine of original sin, in which the human self is corrupt and unreliable. The self has to be overcome in order to reach the divine. Contemporary spirituality, however, has an Eastern-leaning emphasis. It adopts the view that man and woman are created in the image of God, even though this original likeness may have been radically altered by history. To seek God through the contemplation and deepening of the self is not considered delusional or wrong, but a logical consequence of the 'original blessing' bestowed upon humanity.[41] The self is not an obstacle to God, as it is in original sin doctrines, but a way toward God, albeit a way in which discernment and caution are required.[42] Contemporary spirituality is readily able to fashion itself as an 'ecological' or 'creation' spirituality, because the emphasis is not on the fallenness of creation, but on its potential to reveal and contain the sacred. Similarly, contemporary spirituality does not drive a wedge between spirit and body, nor does it represent sexuality as evil or degraded. For it, spirit and body co-exist and sexuality is claimed to be a part of one's spirituality.[43]

Post-Christianity and the hunger for experience

In these and other ways, contemporary spirituality in the West is appearing post-Christian, or at least, it is seeking to link with mystical and holistic sources that have not been mainstream. Western traditions are still unfamiliar with the unconscious and do not know how to guide us through it. This is not true for Eastern religions, which have long understood the interior domain and have developed sophisticated methods for exploring it through yoga, meditation, contemplation, and introspection. Western religions, if they want to survive, must befriend the soul and attempt to guide people into the human experience of God. God has been presented as so far away that the ordinary person can at most aspire to living a good moral life, after which God may be met in the next life. However, modern people are impatient with this theology, and want to have an experience of God in this life, and let the next look after itself. Consequently, there has been widespread defection in

Western societies to Eastern spiritual pathways, because the West has been perceived as incapable of leading people to life-changing experiences. Western religious leaders see this as an indulgent interest in self-absorption and personal development, while those who defect claim that Western religious traditions are not spiritual enough.

Church leaders say to such people: What is it that makes you so hungry and demanding? Why do you want what was once reserved for monastics and saints? Why are you so impatient with us and with God? Why not wait for the grace of God to come to you, rather than storm the transcendent with your spiritual desire? To us, your hunger for 'God' seems unholy. We are not even sure it is God you are seeking, because the God of our traditions asks us to wait and be contrite. In reply, post-modern people say: we don't want God talk or preaching, but an experience of transcendence. Christianity claims to be about Christ, but it is not of Christ. We want to experience what he experienced and not emulate him from afar. We don't want to obey an old moral code, but to live a fully embodied spirituality. This asks us to take risks, and, if necessary, to throw out the moralism of the past. If we have to go to the East, or back to nature, or to psychotherapy to find our transcendence, then so be it. The keynote of contemporary spirituality is experience, and traditions that fail to offer a pathway of experience can expect to decline or diminish.

My guess is that Western religions will eventually accept this passion for experience and be able to satisfy it with their traditional resources. However, the West will have to dust off the late medieval tomes on the interior life, dig up the lost and forgotten traditions of mysticism, and make these available to the starving masses. The way forward for Western religions is to bring the monastic traditions out of the cloisters and into the streets. Secularism has alienated us so fully from religious forms that when the spirit stirs again we will not be content with hearing stories about holy people, but we will want to taste holiness ourselves. Spirituality has acquired an urgent, personal, needy character that embarrasses the religions and seems to them to be the opposite of composure, patience and humility. However, when religions understand that people want experience and not preaching, transcendence and not God-talk, a bridge between contemporary spirituality and traditional religion will be found.

Spirituality redefined for our time

These reflections cause me to wonder if 'spirituality' is the right term for what contemporary people are seeking. The term is entrenched and widely used, but the holistic and experiential direction of contemporary aspiration is at odds with the term's historical background. The *Collins Dictionary* refers to the spiritual as 'not material; unworldly', and as 'the fact or state of being incorporeal.'[44] The *Macquarie Dictionary* defines the spiritual as 'pertaining to the spirit or soul as distinguished from the physical nature; standing in a relationship of the spirit; non-material.'[45] Dictionaries define the term in a dualistic manner, opposing spirit to the body, to matter and nature. However the momentum in contemporary spirituality is toward non-dualism and wholeness.

'Spirituality' carries a perfectionist legacy which is hard to shake off. Either the term has to be redefined and the dictionaries changed, or the contemporary project has to find another term to designate what it is looking for. There is something odd about the fact that the worldwide movement toward soul-making and individuation has chosen a term in which the integration of body and spirit is called into question. In seventeenth-century France, 'spiritualité' referred to ascetical and body-denying practices,[6] and yet what takes place under this term today bears little resemblance to these historical antecedents. In the past, the *other* to which spiritualité pointed was perfect, heavenly and sublime, but the *other* to which post-modern spirituality points is radically different.

In *Spirituality and the Secular Quest* Peter Van Ness defines spirituality as 'the desire to relate oneself as a personal whole to reality as a cosmic whole.'[46] He does not use religious language, but there is a religious dimension to this nevertheless. The 'cosmic whole' implies a new image of God. The image of God, the ultimate other, has changed from a figure of perfection to a symbol of wholeness. The new God-image no longer demands moral perfection, but invites us into an experience of embodied integration. Perhaps we are witnessing a theology that takes the incarnation of the holy into flesh and matter more seriously. Progressive religious thinkers are keen to redefine spirituality in light of this new direction. In both Protestant and Catholic traditions, the keynotes of contemporary spirituality are embodiment, earthly existence, and immanentalism. We see this in the Protestant 'ecological theology' of Sally McFague[47] and in the Catholic 'spirituality studies' of Sandra Schneiders:

> I define spirituality as the experience of conscious involvement in the project of life integration through self-transcendence toward the ultimate value one perceives. It is an effort to bring all of life together in an integrated synthesis of ongoing growth and development.[48]

Schneiders admits that spirituality means something different today to what it did in the past:

> The term 'spirituality' no longer refers exclusively or even primarily to prayer and spiritual exercises, much less to an elite state or superior practice of Christianity. Rather, from its original reference to the 'interior life' of the person, usually a cleric or religious, who was 'striving for perfection', for a life of prayer and virtue that exceeded in scope and intensity that of the 'ordinary' believer, the term has broadened to connote the whole of the life of faith and even the life of the person as a whole, including its bodily, psychological, social, and political dimensions.[49]

This is one of the best descriptions I have read of the 'sea change' that spirituality has undergone in recent decades. It no longer refers to the old world in which moral perfection and piety were of paramount importance. In advocating 'spirituality', contemporary people are not saying they wish to become angelic, devout or pure. They have wholeness on their minds, and this includes all aspects of our existence, including aspects previously shunned or moralized against. In using the word 'spirituality' today, we are apparently seeking to indicate that a power or force beyond ourselves is urging us to become more whole, and this power is supporting us as we attempt to bring together the incommensurable parts that were once divided. Philip Rieff calls this the 'triumph of the therapeutic,'[50] that is, the influence of the therapeutic goal of integration into all spheres of contemporary life, including the spiritual. The triumph of therapy is that it has made the old-fashioned quest for perfection seem abnormal, suspect or even pathological, and 'wholeness' is the new ideal of our moral existence.

The contemporary resurgence

Sociologists and cultural analysts are becoming more courageous in their recognition that 'spirit' is returning in the postmodern era. Historian William Johnston writes: 'Postmodernism and the study of spirituality go together. What modernism in homage to rationality discards, postmodernism in homage to spirituality revives.'[6] It is true that spirituality has prospered in the post-modern era, an unlikely prospect when one considers that post-modernism was at first greeted as an extreme form of modernism, promoting nihilism and the absence of meaning. However, the post-modern has an affirmative or positive side, in which meanings forgotten or rejected in the modern era have been revived.[51,52] This revival of spirit has seemingly been accompanied by the continuing secularization process. This appears contradictory, until we realize that although society continues on its secularizing course, individual consciousness has experienced a reverse process, in which re-enchantment and resacralization have played major roles.[53]

In *The Desecularization of the World* sociologist Peter Berger writes:

> Secularization on the societal level is not necessarily linked to secularization on the level of individual consciousness. Certain religious institutions have lost power and influence in many societies, but both old and new religious beliefs and practices have nevertheless continued in the lives of individuals.[54]

The earlier sociological view held out little hope for religion and adhered to the theory of secularization, which argued that as we became more educated, belief in God and the spiritual would disappear. However, the contemporary view has refuted this theory, in keeping with the fact that religion is not going away, but is changing its shape and reappearing as 'spirituality'. Contemporary philosophers are making similar kinds of comments. Gianni Vattimo writes:

> In spirit, something that we had thought irrevocably forgotten is made present again, a dormant trace is reawakened, a wound re-opened, the repressed returns and what we took to be an *Überwindung* (overcoming, realization and thus a setting aside) is no more than a *Verwindung*, a long convalescence that has once again to come to terms with the indelible trace of its sickness.[55]

Spirit for this philosopher is like an unhealed wound reopening at the centre of culture. Its long convalescence has not just been a sleep and a forgetting; it has been a sickness, a disease of the spirit, which we have to deal with today. We thought spirit would go away, but it did not. We can say that the repression of the sacred leads to its explosive return in degenerate and diseased forms.[56] It is for this reason that violence and religious fanaticism are found together in our time and to some extent they are indistinguishable from each other. We need to balance the modern idealization of spirit with the awareness that violence, fundamentalism, and social unrest are as much a part of 'the return of the repressed' as are the incense-smelling varieties of spirituality produced for the market economy.

Mircea Eliade put our situation well when he wrote:

> In a period of religious crisis one cannot anticipate the creative, and as such, probably unrecognisable, answers given to such a crisis. Moreover, one cannot predict the expressions of a potentially new experience of the sacred ... [which might] not be recognizable as such from a Judeo-Christian perspective.[57]

When the religious impulse is lost to culture and forced underground, it will resurface in unexpected and unpredictable ways. Eliade looked to fads and fashions, movies and popular novels, new social modes and lifestyles, to track the presence of the spirit in a godless time.[58] When the sacred returns, it does not come wearing the mask of the holiness of former times. To read the signs of the new sacred requires imagination and vision, and it is often artists, poets and writers who get there first.

There are many areas of scientific and artistic pursuit in which *spirit* is being included as a new and dynamic element in human experience, and these include the physical sciences of quantum mechanics, the new biology, medicine and neuroscience, transpersonal psychology, postmodern philosophy, political theory, education theory, the arts, music and ecology. These fields can hardly be dismissed as 'New Age', because they are serious pursuits within established fields of knowledge. Holmes Rolston put the situation memorably:

> So the secular, this present, empirical epoch, this phenomenal world, studied by science, does not eliminate the sacred after all; to the contrary, it urges us on a spiritual quest.[59]

Spirit is back, and, to the surprise of religious and secular commentators alike, it looks like being here to stay. However, spirit is in a free, unbounded and ill-defined condition. Historically, we have not seen it in this state for a long time. What we are seeing today are the primal stirrings of spirit, without the social institutions or forms into which spirit can be clearly recognized. The secular and religious are irritated by this inchoate condition of spirit, because it unsettles established orders. The times are ominous, pregnant with future possibilities, and there is a sense of anticipation, but also of dread in our present time. Matthew Arnold read the complexity of our age correctly when he said: 'We wander between two worlds, one dead, the other powerless to be born.'[60] It is as if a new continent of experience has emerged in the last couple of generations, ironically propelled into our awareness by the demise of the religions.

The phobic response that some religious people feel toward the newly arising spirituality is not just a matter of envy or resentment toward a new competitor in the spiritual landscape. There is something more basic: the appearance of spirit in the community, in the street, and outside traditional structures fills the conservative religious with a sense of panic. It makes them see that the old vessels have been shattered, and spirit or *pneuma* is let loose upon the world, suggesting the possibility of a return to chaos. This tone comes across in many of the pronouncements made by religious writers about the new spirituality.[19,22] In the new dispensation, everything is potentially filled with the sacred, whereas once it was safely contained and kept in order. The fact that the sacred is anarchic and abroad fills some of us with deep anxiety.

Primitive panic in the face of the uncontained numinous is expressed succinctly in John Updike's poem, 'Comp. Religion'.

In sixteen lines he offers a history of the West in its relations with the sacred. First there is the primal spirit, mysterious and uncanny, which Updike calls 'fear of mana.' Such fear drives us to invent various kinds of propitiatory rites and devices, to appease spirit and protect ourselves from contamination. From the humble forms of propitiation we developed fear and love for the holy, and these grew into systems of totemism, ancestor worship, and animism. The West graduated to polytheism and then to monotheism, but in post-modern times our monotheistic conception has collapsed and 'God is dead'.

Forces once contained in symbols are showered upon us in a storm of cosmic energies. There are few safe places, and we have brought this upon ourselves by neglecting to update and change our religion with as much energy as we have updated our science and technology. We are sophisticated in some respects, but in our spiritual lives we have been returned to the past, and as fearful of spirit as early humanity. We need to move closer to the spirit, so that our fear is able to be transformed into respect. We cannot make this change until we surrender some of our rationality and learn to submit to a mystery over which we have no control. Our consciousness has to become more receptive to spirit, but how can this be achieved if our age remains secular and resistant? Perhaps we need to take a cue from Derrida, who dismissed the notion that the modern mind is secular, and said 'secularization is only a manner of speaking.'[61]

References

1 Gadamer, H.G. (1998). Dialogues in Capri. In: J. Derrida, G. Vattimo (eds) *Religion*. Stanford: Stanford University Press.
2 Van Ness, P. (ed) (1996). *Spirituality and the Secular Quest*. New York: Crossroad.
3 Schneiders, S. (2000). Religion and Spirituality: Strangers, Rivals, or Partners? *The Santa Clara Lectures* **6**(2): 1.
4 Heelas, P., Woodhead, L. (2005). *The Spiritual Revolution: Why Religion is Giving Way to Spirituality*. Oxford: Blackwell.
5 Sheldrake, P. (1992). *Spirituality and History*. New York: Crossroad.
6 Johnston, W.M. (1996). *Recent Reference Books in Religion*, p.131. Illinois: InterVarsity Press Downers Grove.
7 Caputo, J. (2001). *On Religion*. London: Routledge.
8 Tacey, D. (2004). *The Spirituality Revolution: the Emergence of Contemporary Spirituality*. London, New York: Brunner-Routledge.
9 Huxley, A. (1946). *The Perennial Philosophy*. London: Chatto & Windus.
10 Paulson, D.S. (2005). Existential and transpersonal spirituality. In: R. Cox, L. Hoffman (eds) *Spirituality and Psychological Health*, pp. 151–66. Colorado Springs: Professional Psychology Press.
11 Dreyer, E.A., Burrows, M.S. (eds) (2005). *Minding the Spirit: the Study of Christian Spirituality*. Baltimore: Johns Hopkins University Press.
12 Koenig, H. (2002). *Spirituality in Patient Care*. Philadelphia: Templeton Foundation Press.
13 Ranson, D. (2002). *Across the Great Divide: Bridging Spirituality and Religion Today*. Sydney: St Pauls Publications.
14 Forman, R. (2004). *Grassroots Spirituality*. Boston: Academic Imprint.
15 Drury, N. (1999). *Exploring the Labyrinth: Making Sense of the New Spirituality*. Sydney: Allen & Unwin.
16 Hay, D. (2006). *Something There: The Biology of the Human Spirit*. London: Darton, Longman & Todd.
17 Rumbold, B. (ed) (2002). *Spirituality and Palliative Care: Social and Pastoral Perspectives*. Melbourne: Oxford University Press.
18 O'Murchu, D. (1997). *Reclaiming Spirituality*. Dublin: Gill and Macmillan.
19 Spink, P. (1991). *A Christian in the New Age*. London: Darton, Longman & Todd.
20 Pacwa, M. (1992). *Catholics and the New Age*. Ann Arbor MI: Servant Press.
21 Hanegraaff, W.J. (1996). *New Age Religion and Western Culture*. Esotericism in the Mirror of Secular Thought. Leiden: Brill.
22 Rhodes, R. (1990). *The Counterfeit Christ of the New Age Movement*. Michigan: Baker.
23 Carrette, J., King, R. (2005). *Selling Spirituality: the Silent Takeover of Religion*. London, New York: Routledge.
24 Faber, M.D. (1996). *New Age Thinking: a Psychoanalytic Critique*. Ottawa: University of Ottawa Press.
25 Kovel, J. (1991). *History and Spirit: an Inquiry into the Philosophy of Liberation*. Boston: Beacon Press.
26 Freud, S. (1927). The future of an illusion. In: J. Strachey (ed.) *The Standard Edition of the Complete Psychological Works of Sigmund Freud*, Vol. **21**, 2001. London: Vintage.
27 Symington, N. (1998). *Emotion and Spirit: Questioning the Claims of Psychoanalysis and Religion*. London: Karnac.
28 Eigen, M. (1998). *The Psychoanalytic Mystic*. New York: Free Association Books.
29 Schneiders, S. (1989). Spirituality in the academy. *Theolog Stud* **50**(2): 682–96.
30 Almond, G., Appleby, R., Sivan, E. (2003). *Strong Religion: the Rise of Fundamentalisms Around the World*. Chicago: University of Chicago Press.
31 Merton, T. (1961/1972). *New Seeds of Contemplation*. New York: New Directions.
32 Jung, C.G. (1928/1931). The spiritual problem of modern man. In: H. Read, M. Fordham, G. Adler, W. McGuire (eds) *The Collected Works of C. G. Jung*, Vol. **10**, 1964/1970. London: Routledge & Kegan Paul.
33 Yeats, W.B. (1939). The circus animals' desertion. In: T. Webb (ed.) *W. B. Yeats: Selected Poetry*, p. 224. Harmondsworth: Penguin.
34 Griffin, D.R. (ed.) (1988). *Spirituality and Society: Postmodern Visions*. Albany: State University of New York Press.
35 Moore, T. (1991). *Care of the Soul: A Guide for Cultivating Depth and Sacredness in Everyday Life*. New York: Harper Collins.
36 Moore, T. (1996). *Educating the Heart*. New York: Harper Collins.
37 Hillman, J. (1996). *The Soul's Code: In Search of Character and Calling*. New York: Warner Books.
38 Johnston, W. (1981). *The Mirror Mind: Spirituality and Transformation*. London: Collins.
39 Fox, M. (1981). *Western Spirituality: Historical Roots, Ecumenical Routes*. Sante Fe, New Mexico: Bear.
40 Pontifical Council for Culture and Pontifical Council for Interreligious Dialogue (2003) *Jesus Christ: The Bearer of the Water of Life: A Christian Reflection on the 'New Age'*. Rome: Vatican. Available at: http://www.vatican.va/roman_curia/pontifical_councils/interelg/documents/rc_pc_interelg_doc_20030203_new-age_en.html (accessed 24 November 2011).
41 Fox, M. (1983). *Original Blessing: A Primer in Creation Spirituality*. Santa Fe: Bear,
42 O'Donohue, J. (1997). *Anam Cara*. London: Bantam.
43 Ulanov, B., Ulanov, A. (1994). *Transforming Sexuality*. Boston: Shambhala.
44 Collins National Dictionary (1966). London, Sydney: Collins.
45 The Macquarie Dictionary (1983). Sydney: Doubleday.
46 Van Ness, P. (ed.) (1996). *Spirituality and the Secular Quest*, p. 5. New York: Crossroad.
47 McFague, S. (1993). *The Body of God: An Ecological Theology*. Minneapolis: Fortress Press.
48 Schneiders, S. (2000). Religion and spirituality: strangers, rivals, or partners? *The Santa Clara Lectures* **6**(2): 4–5.
49 Schneiders, S. (1989). Spirituality in the Academy. *Theolog Stud* **50**(2): 683.
50 Rieff, P. (1966). *The Triumph of the Therapeutic: Uses of Faith After Freud*. New York: Harper & Row.
51 Spretnak, C. (1991). *States of Grace: The Recovery of Meaning in the Postmodern World*. San Francisco: Harper.
52 Griffin, D.R. (ed.) (1989). *God and Religion in the Postmodern World*. Albany: State University of New York Press.
53 Tacey, D. (2000). *Re-enchantment: the New Australian Spirituality*. Sydney: HarperCollins.
54 Berger, P. (1999). *The Desecularization of the World*, p. 3. Grand Rapids: Eerdmans Publishing.
55 Vattimo, G. (1998). The trace of the trace. In: J. Derrida, G. Vattimo (eds) *Religion*, p. 79. Stanford: Stanford University Press.

56 Tacey, D. (2011). *Gods and Diseases*. Sydney: HarperCollins.
57 Eliade, M. (1969). *The Quest: History and Meaning in Religion*, pp. iii–iv. Chicago: University of Chicago Press.
58 Eliade, M. (1976). *Occultism, Witchcraft, and Cultural Fashions*. Chicago: University of Chicago Press.
59 Rolston, H. (1996). Scientific inquiry. In: P. Van Ness (ed.) *Spirituality and the Secular Quest*, p.411. New York: Crossroad.
60 Arnold, M. (1855/1945). Stanzas from the Grande Chartreuse. In: H. Milford (ed.) *The Poetical Works of Matthew Arnold*, pp. 1185–6. London: Oxford University Press.
61 Derrida, J. (2005). Epoché and faith: an interview with Jacques Derrida. In: Y. Sherwood, K. Hart (eds) *Derrida and Religion: Other Testaments*, p. 32. New York: Routledge.

CHAPTER 63

The future of religion

Grace Davie and Martyn Percy

Introduction

One point must be made clear at the outset: there is not one future for religion in relation to healthcare, but several. The European scenario is very different from the United States, and the developing world is different again. Each of these (and their internal variations) will be developed in the pages that follow. A second point follows from this. In all of these cases, the futures of religion are related to the futures of healthcare, remembering that the relationship takes different forms in different places: in some cases, healthcare 'replaces' religion; in others religion substitutes for healthcare. Contacts, moreover, can be formal or informal, mutually supportive or mutually suspicious, collaborative, or conflictual.

With this in mind this chapter will be structured as follows. The first section will outline the futures of religion in Europe, the United States, and (skeletally) the developing world. For practical reasons, the discussion will be limited to Christianity. This is not to imply that other faith communities are not important in this context—they most certainly are. They present, however, a very different set of examples, which cannot all be discussed in a relatively short chapter. The second section considers these various futures in relation to healthcare concentrating on the subtle and continuing connections between the two spheres. Crucial to this discussion is the role of the state and the manner in which this entity is conceptualized. Both state churches and welfare states depend on how the state itself is understood. The third section is a little different in both content and tone. It looks at the significance of religion in relation to healthcare in terms of two concepts, which are central to both spheres: values and vocation, recognizing the changing role of religion in late modern societies that, at one and the same time, are both increasingly secular and religiously plural. The discourse in this section is philosophical (theological even), rather than sociological.

Throughout, the authors of this chapter start from the position that in modern Western democracies religion should neither dominate nor disappear. How, though, should religious people and religious agencies play their part in debates that relate to healthcare in its broadest sense? And what happens if religious voices do not concur with the voices of other people, be they religious or secular?

The future of religion: some possible scenarios

It is a common place to contrast the continuing religiousness of the United States with the relative secularity of Europe.[1] The difference between the two remains however a crucial point in the understanding of religion in the modern world, in that it raises a deeper question: what is the relationship between religion and modernity? Is it the case that modern societies are necessarily secular societies? Or is this relationship contingent—in the sense that it pertains in some part of the world and not in others? The following paragraphs will set out the barebones of the European and the American cases, arguing that the former, the more, rather than less secular example, should be considered distinctive; it is not a global prototype.

Religion in Europe is complex; it is best understood by taking into account a variety of factors that are currently shaping the religious life of this part of the world.[2,3] The crucial point to grasp is that these factors not only change and adapt over time, but push and pull in different directions. The six factors are:

1. The role of the historic churches in forming European culture. This is easily illustrated in the sense that the Christian tradition has had an irreversible effect on time (calendars, seasons, festivals, holidays, weeks, and weekends) and space (the parish system and the dominance of Christian buildings) in this part of the world. The notion of a state church is part of this legacy.

2. An awareness that the historic churches still have a place at particular moments in the lives of modern Europeans, although they are no longer able to discipline the beliefs and behaviour of the great majority of the population. Despite their relatively secularity, Europeans are likely to return to their churches at moments of celebration or grief (whether individual or collective).

3. An observable change in the churchgoing constituencies of the continent, which operate increasingly on a model of choice, rather than a model of obligation or duty. As a result, membership of the historic churches is changing in nature; increasingly, it is chosen rather than inherited, although more so in some places than in others.

4. The arrival into Europe of groups of people from many different parts of the world. This is primarily an economic movement,

but the implications for the religious life of the continent are immense. The growing presence of Christians from the global South alongside significant other faith communities has altered the religious profile of Europe. Quite apart from this, some of these communities are—simply by their presence—challenging some deeply held European assumptions, notably the notion that religion should be considered a private matter.

5. Rather different are the sometimes vehement reactions of Europe's secular elites to this shift, i.e. to the increasing significance of religion in public, as well as private life. Such elites did not anticipate a change of this nature, but see it as their duty to question what is happening, sometimes aggressively, sometimes less so.
6. A gradual, but growing realization that the patterns of religious life in modern Europe should be considered an 'exceptional case'—they are not a global prototype. In short, Europeans are beginning to realize that Europe is secular not because it is modern, but because it is European. It is equally true that some Europeans welcome this insight; others are disconcerted by it.

It is important to consider these factors alongside one another in order to assess the current situation. Two rather different things are happening at once. On the one hand, religion has re-entered the public square and demands a response. Barely a day passes without a religious issue finding its way into the news (see points 4 and 5 above). On the other, a largely unchurched population has difficulty dealing with these questions in the sense that Europeans are rapidly losing the concepts, knowledge, and vocabulary that are necessary to talk about religion. The two tendencies are unrelated to each other; the fact that they have occurred at the same time is a paradox. For this reason alone, the future of religion in this part of the world is very hard to predict.

In many respects the American case is more straightforward. Here, a vibrant religious market established itself at the moment when the nation became a federal state and continues to exist. American denominations thrived, rather than contracted, as the nation industrialized and urbanized: wave after wave of immigrants arrived in America's nascent cities bringing with them their own forms of (mostly) Christianity. The situation was entirely different from that in Europe where a territorially-based state church was unable to respond to the needs of a rapidly changing society. Its parishes (both plant and personnel) were locked into pre-modern and primarily rural ways of living and were unable to follow the population to the cities where increasingly they now lived.

In the United States, the free-standing congregation, rather than the parish, is the core unit of religious life. Congregations, moreover, are far more flexible than parishes—not only do they have the capacity to migrate geographically, they can also mutate socially, meaning that they are much more able than parishes to respond to changing needs. Congregations, moreover, belong to denominations (rather than state churches), all of which have equal status in the United States—a situation enshrined in the First Amendment to the American Constitution. The First Amendment has two clauses, known as the establishment clause and the freedom clause, which read as follows: 'Congress shall make no law respecting an establishment of religion or prohibiting the free exercise thereof'. Both are fundamental to American self-understanding.

The 'establishment' clause proscribes a dominant or state church, of whatever nature. The notion of 'free exercise' captures a second crucial contrast between Europe and the United States. In the former, the Enlightenment (especially in its French forms) was largely conceived as a 'freedom from belief,' notably from the hegemonic grip of the Catholic Church. Such thinking was markedly less clear-cut (i.e. less anti-religious) in the Protestant countries of Europe, and by the time that Enlightenment ideas crossed the Atlantic they had acquired a rather different connotation: not so much a 'freedom from belief' as a 'freedom to believe.' In America, moreover, these innovative proposals were carried by, not against, the growing numbers of Protestant churches.

There is nothing particularly new in this analysis. Indeed, it was precisely these features of American life—the vitality of religious life and the commitment to voluntary associations (both religious and secular)—that formed the core of De Tocqueville's observations about American democracy in the mid-nineteenth century.[4] The implications, however, go very deep. They reveal an entirely different trajectory from that found in Europe. It is an upward, rather than downward spiral—nation building, economic expansion, rapid urbanization, and an influx of new people interacted positively to promote growth rather than decline in the religious sector. Each of these factors supported the others—a far cry from the vicissitudes of Europe's state churches in the same historical period.

Which of these models is likely to dominate in the twenty-first century? In his recent writing on Pentecostalism in the global South, David Martin draws a contrast between what he calls transnational voluntarism, on the one hand, and forms of religion that are based not on the idea of free competition, but on the notion of territory.[5] The former are market-based; the latter regard particular parts of the world as their exclusive domain—an attitude that affects a whole range of factors (among them, land, kin, ethnicity, and faith). In such a situation, joining or leaving the religion in question is to embrace or to break with rather more than a particular system of belief. Religious choice, in other words, means different things in different places. Martin puts this as follows: '[T]he global variations run along a scale from North America, where it is normal, to Western European and Australasia where it is accepted, but not all that frequent, to the Arabian Peninsula, which is by definition Islamic territory where even foreigners cannot establish their own sacred buildings.'[6]

The contrast between Europe and the United States is clear. Martin, however, develops the argument further in his analyses of Pentecostalism (the quintessential form of transnational voluntarism) in the current period. Specifically, he seeks to explain why Pentecostalism grows exponentially in the global South, but less so elsewhere. In Europe, the Westphalian (territorial) model, although changing, continues to sustain a diffuse form of religiousness, which is there at the point of need for all citizens; in the United States, the voluntary sector is already fully developed. Pentecostalism is present in both cases, but modestly so. In the global South, in contrast, the spaces for new forms of religiousness are larger, permitting Pentecostalism to become the fastest-growing form of Christianity in the modern world (notably in Latin America, sub-Saharan Africa and the Pacific Rim). Conservative estimates suggest circa 250 million adherents.

How then should we envisage the future of religion? Even a modest survey, limited to various forms of Western Christianity, indicates that the relatively secularity of Europe is unlikely to become the global norm, a conclusion that is amply reinforced if the net is cast more widely. Both quantitative and qualitative data from the Middle East, from the Muslim world more generally, from the Indian sub-continent, and most interestingly of all, from twenty-first century China all point to the wisdom of taking religion seriously as a significant factor in both human and global affairs.

Relating the futures of religion to the futures of healthcare

Recent, empirically-based work on religion and welfare in Europe reveals that the great majority of Europeans have well-established views not only about welfare as such, but about the responsibilities of the state for this.[8,9] Using—almost certainly unconsciously—a religious metaphor, they consider the state responsible for the care of its citizens 'from the cradle to the grave.' A full account of the development of the welfare state, and within this some form of publically-funded healthcare, goes well beyond the limits of this chapter. A more limited, but nonetheless crucial point for the argument presented here, however, is that the welfare states of Europe very largely mirror the state churches that, on some readings of the data, they have come to replace.

The essential point can be made by taking Gøsta Esping-Andersen's analyses of welfare-regimes of Western Europe in one hand and David Martin's work on secularization in the other, noting especially Martin's magisterial *A General Theory of Secularization*.[9,10] Social policy experts are very familiar with the former; scholars of religion continue to engage with the latter. Very seldom, however, are the two bodies of material brought together.

Martin's central thesis is easily summarized. The process of secularization—strongly associated in the European case with the onset of industrialization and urbanization—is common to the continent as a whole, but unfolds differently within particular economic, social, and cultural contexts.[11] These contexts are determined by identifiable factors, for example the precise timing and the nature of what Martin terms 'crucial events,' namely the English Civil War, the American, French, and Russian Revolutions, and the place of religion in these. Did these cataclysmic struggles occur over religion, against religion, or through religion? The absence of such an event in the Lutheran countries of Northern Europe is just as significant. The details are complex, but the underlying idea is simple enough. Emerging, in the fullness of time, from these various upheavals, are specific—and up to a point predictable—variations in the secularization process.

The connection with welfare lies in the following. These variations mirror very closely the regime-types initially identified by Esping-Andersen. The pathways of secularization on the one hand 'match' the distinctive patterns of welfare that emerge on the other, namely the liberal model of the Anglo-Saxon countries, the conservative model of continental Europe, and the social democratic model of the Nordic countries. It is simply that the story is told from different points of view. One scholar documents the influence and the adjustments of a territorially-based church to the upheavals and dislocations of the industrialization process; another observes the emergence of the secular institutions required by a modern industrial society. The reasons for this parallel thinking are clear enough—they lie in the fact that both 'theories' (the contrasting processes of secularization and the very different welfare regimes that have emerged in different parts of Europe) draw on the same underlying alignments and cleavages in European society, initially identified by political sociologists in their work on the nineteenth century. Especially significant in this respect is the pioneering research of Lipset and Rokkan.[12] Such cleavages are, in turn, determined by the 'crucial events' already outlined.

One element in this transformation is the process of institutional separation or differentiation, in which tasks or areas of activity traditionally undertaken by the churches move bit by bit into the secular sphere.[10,13] Such areas of activity include education, welfare, and of course, healthcare. In each situation, a particular variant of the welfare state emerges, as a similar goal (the separating out of welfare from the influence of the churches and the creation of an autonomous sphere with its own institutional norms) is achieved, or semi-achieved, in somewhat different ways. Interestingly, the role of both theology and ecclesiology in determining these pathways, albeit as one factor among many, is increasingly recognized in the literature.[14]

In short European *state* churches find parallels in European welfare *states*, remembering that both effectively are public utilities. What, however, of the American case where there is no state church and where state-funded welfare (including healthcare) is highly contentious? The first observation concerns the state itself. This is understood differently in Europe and in the United States, bearing in mind that the British case is something of hybrid. Americans perceive the state primarily as a regulator, not a provider. For this reason, they resist what they call 'big government.' Indeed, there is a profound mistrust of such a thing—a view that sees the welfare state as the source of Europe's economic ills, rather than the basis of mutual solidarity. It is something to be avoided at all costs. The majority of Europeans have a different view (as, it should be said, do many Americans); they are not only supportive, but proud of their welfare states, as they are of the political values that these represent.

It is not true, however, that there is no public welfare in America; it is simply that it is organized differently. Once again, a full account of such provision, including the details of American healthcare is not possible in this chapter. It is, however, important to recognize the role of faith-based organizations in such provision. George W. Bush introduced the notion of 'faith-based initiatives' in his first term (in 2001); this included a programme of government funding for churches and other houses of worship, by means of which social services would be offered to Americans in need. With certain modifications it has been continued by Barack Obama.[15] From the outset, the programme has been controversial—markedly so. For a start, it constitutes a bold challenge to the principle of church–state separation, in the sense that it removes the restrictions that normally apply to funding attached to any religious institution (i.e. that an individual should attend a worship service in order to receive aid from a particular organization). But, quite apart from questions of constitutionality, the notion of faith-based initiatives has provoked a wide-ranging debate about welfare provision in American society and the place of the churches in this.

On the one hand, it is possible to see such programmes as a natural extension of what the hundreds and thousands of American congregations do every day. Much of what is normally considered welfare is already taking place amongst groups of people who come together for primarily religious reasons, so why not encourage this? Others, however, are more wary, recognizing that faith-based initiatives raise difficult moral as well as constitutional questions–among them the links between government policies and religious values. To what extent should one be allowed to influence the other? Always assuming that the moral issues can be satisfactorily resolved, how should faith-based initiatives be put into practice? Should government-funded faith-based organizations employ only individuals who share their religious beliefs? More importantly, would such a policy endorse a notion of funding that, consciously or not, discriminates on religious grounds?

In terms of healthcare *per se*, two points are particularly important. The first concerns the substantial proportion of religious hospitals in the not-for-profit sector in the United States and the implications of this situation for certain types of medical care.[16] On what grounds, for instance, are difficult decisions regarding policy and treatment taken? Are these medical or religious? The second is to appreciate the intensity of the debates surrounding Barack Obama's 2010 healthcare reforms and the reasons for resistance in this area. It is all too easy for Europeans to cast the United States in a negative light for their opposition to reform. It is more sensible to recognize the genuine antipathy of American people to a solution that extends the power of the state. Once again, the parallels with religion are clear. Religion is not the only thing in American life that should be free from state interference.

That said, both the European and the American situations are changing. In Europe, the market is beginning bit-by-bit to encroach on both religion and healthcare (see below); and in the United States, the state is gradually–if controversially–extending its reach. So far, however, both clauses of the First Amendment remain sacrosanct. An effective and highly competitive market in religion continues to flourish in almost every part of the United States.

Historically, Latin America is an extension of Latin Europe in religious terms. The majority of Latin Americans are and remain Catholic, noting the wide variety of native religions and spirit cults that intermingle with more popular forms of Catholicism. The spread of Pentecostalism in the 1960s challenged this hegemony.[17] This is a fascinating and still unfinished story which has attracted considerable attention. For the purposes of this chapter, two very different elements of Pentecostalism are worth noting, both of which relate to healthcare. The first is to appreciate the very practical aspects of this form of Christianity: it grows fastest among groups of people who find in Pentecostalism, both a vision for themselves and an effective means of support for their families. In the fragile economies of the developing world, where alternative sources of care are conspicuous by their absence, this has proved a winning combination. At the same time, the immediate presence of the spirit and the possibility of miraculous healing complement the deficiencies of conventional healthcare in a very different way.

Articulating religion in a secular society: values and vocation in healthcare

The previous sections have demonstrated the uneven persistence of religion in different parts of the modern world and its continuing relationship to systems of healthcare. Here, a different point requires attention: it is memorably articulated by Charles Taylor in what has become an iconic text.[18] In modern Western societies, we take for granted—more in some places than in others—the right to believe and to practice religious alterity. Nothing can be imposed anymore; religion, along with other creeds and ideologies, has become a matter of individual choice. As part and parcel of this process, agnosticism or atheism has become enshrined, such that it is an endemic dimension of our freedom. The frames of reference and ideological paradigms that individuals and groups choose to live by are, therefore, a matter of selection, rather than non-negotiable imposition. Faith is not enforceable.

The seeds of initial disenchantment and subsequent disengagement from religion were carried in the (if you will) DNA of the Reformation. And in the fullness of time this would lead, as Charles Taylor puts it, to a seismic shift in the capacity of religion to form sociality:

> Once disenchantment has befallen the world, the sense that God is an indispensable source for our spiritual and moral life migrates. From being the guarantor that good will triumph, or at least hold its own, in a world of spirits and meaningful forces, he becomes (1) the essential energizer of that ordering power through which we disenchant the world, and turn it to our purposes. As the very origin of our being, spiritual and material, he (2) commands our allegiance and worship, a worship which is now purer through being disintricated from the enchanted world.[19]

Of course, the Reformation could not possibly have brought about such a change by itself, and so quickly. Bit by bit, however, religion receded into the realm of the private and the sentiments; public space, conversely, became something in which religion could participate, but which God no longer ordered. Modern societies were no longer polities that could not have conceived of their origins and ethos without God as the fundamental point of reference; they had become instead states and nations that were their own guarantors of social flourishing and human freedom.

Granted, this is not the only way of looking back over several centuries of Christianity: there are more positive alternatives to this kind of 'history of subtraction', as Taylor calls it. Indeed it is worth noting that Taylor himself, in narrating this history of the secular age, does not capitulate to the kind of reactionary nostalgia that some scholars might be tempted to indulge in. Nor does he look back to an (imagined) age of Christendom and call for its immediate restoration. Rather, he suggests that faith will have to find its way in modernity through a subtle mixture of challenge and reformation; picking its way through pluralism, as it were, but with renewed hope and confidence. Specifically, and alongside many others, it must find new ways to contribute to the complex and difficult issues that are part and parcel of modern healthcare. In short, it must engage the question of values.

The early work of Philip Selznick, notably his contrast between organizations and institutions, offers a second approach to this question.[20] Selznick argues that organizations primarily exist for utilitarian purposes, and when they are fulfilled, the organization may become expendable. Institutions, in contrast, are 'natural communities' with roots that are embedded in the very fabric of society. They incorporate various groups that may contest with each other over the very nature of the institution and its values. Following Selznick, a hospital is much more like an institution, thereby requiring a particular kind of skills, values, and practices from its staff (doctors, nurses, carers, etc.) rather than (mere) management. For Selznick, the very term 'organization' suggests a certain rudimentary bareness; a kind of lean, no-nonsense system of consciously co-ordinated activities. It refers to an expendable and rational instrument engineered to do a job. An institution, on the other hand, is more of a natural product of the prevailing social needs and pressures. In effect, it is a responsive, adaptive organism that serves a wider body.

Of course, Selznick's characterization of difference is a matter of analysis, rather than of direct description. No single body or given enterprise need be wholly one or the other. While extreme cases may closely approximate to either an 'ideal' organization or an 'ideal' institution, most living associations resist such easy classifications. They are complex mixtures of both designed and responsive behaviours. There are, however, tensions between the identity and behaviour of institutions and organizations. Both models of association carry hidden assumptions and values, which can at times rise to the surface, either through competition or through synergy. The distinction, moreover, allows us to reflect on what might be lost and gained in the competition and synergy between organizational and institutional identity. What happens, for example, to the concept of vocation in an organization as against an institution? Is the language and practice of vocation better-suited to one type of environment than the other, and if so, what impact does this have on the offering of services such as care-taking, nursing, healthcare, and education?

In terms of healthcare, a parallel dialectic emerges between spirituality and religion. In recent years, two predominant approaches to spiritual care have taken root within the medical profession. One has been to associate it closely with religion, and to assume that anyone articulating an explicit spirituality requires a religious resource. The other has been to detach 'spirituality' from religion, and re-describe many forms of care-delivery, education, and healthcare as having a 'spiritual dimension'. Both approaches have their problems, perhaps best generalized as being 'too narrow' and 'too broad'. Yet this chasm of definition and delivery has opened up precisely because of the small revolutions that that have taken place in healthcare in the post-war era. The following examples are taken from the British case.

The Hospice Movement, particularly through Dame Cicely Saunders, borrowed its initial concept of spirituality from Victor Frankl. It was Frankl who had sought 'meaning-centred' contexts for care: patients would address life as it slowly turned to death, not simply stave it off with whatever medicine was to hand. Similarly, a number within the nursing profession have also come to adopt echoes of Frankl's ideology, developing a more holistic approach to care alongside prevention and cure. It follows that the demand for 'spiritual' needs in *The Patient's Charter* can no longer be read as simply belonging to the portfolio of the Chaplain.[21] Increasingly, National Health Service Trusts claim their own distinctive definitions of what it means to offer 'spiritual services' to its client community. Beyond meeting 'traditional' religious needs and those that are best described as 'implicit' or 'folk', healthcare deliverers are beginning to recognize a deeper spiritual pulse that may permeate many areas of practice that have no obvious religious connection.

Yet this shift risks losing sight of the collective and the common good. In *Saving Lives: Our Healthier Nation*[22] the Labour government in Britain (1997–2010), amongst many others, recognized that there was a persistent relationship between longevity, where individuals live, and their employment or position in life. The root causes of ill health often remain stubbornly 'social'. Following this line of thought, spirituality is not simply an individual's collection of feelings, sentiments, aspirations, and religious desires. Spirituality needs to be treated as something that flows from the individual to be sure, but as something that has implications for the wider body politic.

For example, an older person in a nursing or residential home who complains of loneliness at meal times is probably asking for that home to re-evaluate what a meal is: namely, turning it from a nutritional exercise into some kind of social event. This is much more demanding than it first appears, for it requires the re-ordering of space, time, priorities and resources and to take seriously the spiritual meaning of a word like 'home.' Attention to the elderly can sharply focus the proper and full relationship between healing and spirituality. Clearly, those who are advanced of years, and are losing their faculties and independence, are not going to be healed, as such. Physically, they are becoming frail. However, what of their spiritual needs? How best can they be expressed in practice? It is questions such as these that throw into relief, not only the fundamental values of care, but the setting in which they are expressed. Is a care home, in Selznick's terms, an institution or an organization?

If they are to restore the balance between an individual with needs and the wider society, healthcare systems may need to recover a sense of vocation. However, before one can do this, it is important to acknowledge that the sense of vocation has indeed been mislaid: that the ontological has given way to the functional, that a sense of 'calling' has been subjugated, or lost to forces of bureaucracy, capitalism, and professionalization. The point is nicely illustrated by a rather different example. The case, moreover, reflects the contradictory tendencies that co-exist in modern healthcare. On the one hand, is the growing recourse to spirituality as person-centred medicine gains in favour over the bio-medical model (see above). On the other is an increased awareness that religion can divide as well as unite and must therefore be kept from public view. In the spring of 2010, an English nurse of long-standing was asked either to remove or to hide a cross while working with patients. Tellingly, the argument for removal was couched in terms of health and safety, rather than religion. The nurse refused to comply arguing that she had worked in the NHS for 30 years and on no occasion had her cross caused herself or anyone else any injury. She was nonetheless moved to a desk job. Unhappy with this decision, she took her case to an industrial tribunal, which found against her.[23] Rightly or wrongly comparisons were made with Muslims who are allowed to wear the hijab when working for the NHS.

Motivations in this case were openly Christian, but fell foul of the law. What then does this tell us about vocation? On the one hand, the idea is still valued and even cherished, but on the other the content of that ideal has become hopelessly fragmented and attenuated. As MacIntyre noted in *After Virtue*,[24] when it comes to morality and spirituality, we may be handling the fragments of a broken pot that society cannot re-make. Whilst the echo of vocation is still strong enough to evoke all kinds of wistful memories, it appears to be too weak and diffuse to suggest any clear way forward. In a situation marked primarily by ambiguity, an explicit expression of Christian vocation is considered controversial.

Underpinning the same ambiguity is confusion about the sources of values, and their authorities (both secular and religious). Are values given or chosen and by whom? Are they fixed or changing, public or private? Do definitions of vocation mutate differently in particular contexts? How exactly is vocation valued? Interestingly, one of the most telling comments on the current situation comes not from a theologian, but a sociologist—Zygmunt Bauman. The welfare state, he claims, institutionalizes the principle of universally shared responsibility for individual weal and woe, whereas private provision institutionalizes diversity of fate. In buying out of collective provision, we buy out of collective responsibility.

Conclusion

The above discussion clearly reflects the continuing connections between religion, spirituality and healthcare in the British case, bearing in mind that the latter hovers—at times uneasily—between the European and the American models. Britain has advanced further towards the market than most of continental Europe—a fact applauded by some and resisted by others. The crucial point, however, is the following: the need to consider carefully the issues outlined above and the values that lie behind them in whatever context they present: the primarily public provision of Europe's historic churches and the welfare state, the religious, and healthcare markets of the United States, or the burgeoning religiousness, but relative precariousness of the developing world. In each case, the role of religion remains significant and at every 'level' of the system—structures, institutions, organizations, communities, cultures, and individuals (be they providers or patients). But, as Charles Taylor reminds us, we do this in societies that are profoundly altered. Specifically, we have moved from a context 'in which it was virtually impossible not to believe in God, to one in which faith, even for the staunchest believer, is one human possibility among others.'[25] The future of religion and its contribution to healthcare must adapt accordingly.

References

1 Berger, P., Davie, G. and Fokas, F. (eds) (2008). *Religious America, Secular Europe: A Theme and Variations.* Farnham: Ashgate.
2 Davie, G. (2006). Is Europe an exceptional case? *Hedgehog Rev* **8** (1–2), 23–34.
3 Davie, G. (2006) Religion in Europe in the 21st century: the factors to take into account. *Eur J Sociol* **XLVII**(2): 271–96.
4 See Pierson, G.W. (1938). *Tocqueville and Beaumont in America.* New York: Oxford University Press.
5 Martin, D. (2011). *Pentecostalism: a dramatic expression of the transnational voluntary principle.* Unpublished paper Religion and Globalization Conference. Antwerp: St. Ignatius University.
6 [5].
7 Bäckström, A., Davie, G., with Edgardh, N., Pettersson, P. (eds) (2010). *Welfare and Religion in 21st Century Europe: Volume 1.* Configuring the connections. Farnham: Ashgate.
8 Bäckström, A., Davie, G., Edgardh, N., Pettersson, P. (eds) (2011). *Welfare and Religion in 21st Century Europe: Volume 2. Gendered, Religious and Social Change.* Farnham: Ashgate.
9 Esping-Andersen, G. (1990). *The Three Worlds of Welfare Capitalism.* Polity Press, Cambridge.
10 Martin, D. (1978). *A General Theory of Secularization.* Oxford: Blackwell.
11 [10], pp. 4–5.
12 Lipset, S.M., Rokkan, S. (eds) (1964). *Party Systems and Voter Alignments.* New York: Free Press.
13 Casanova, J. (1994). *Public Religions in the Modern World.* Chicago: University of Chicago Press.
14 Van Kersbergen, K., Manow, P. (eds) (2009). *Religion, Class Coalitions and Welfare State Regimes.* Cambridge: Cambridge University Press.
15 Further details are available at: http://www.whitehouse.gov/the_press_office/ObamaAnnouncesWhiteHouseOfficeofFaith-basedandNeighborhoodPartnerships/(accessed 22 March 2011).
16 Uttley, L., Pawelko, R. (2002). *No Strings Attached: Public Funding of Religiously-Sponsored Hospitals in the United States.* New York: MergerWatch. Available at http://www.mergerwatch.org/storage/pdf-files/bp_no_strings.pdf (accessed 23 August 2011).
17 Martin, D. (1990). *Tongues of Fire: The Explosion of Protestantism in Latin America.* Oxford: Blackwell.
18 Taylor, C. (2007). *A Secular Age.* Cambridge: Harvard University Press.
19 [18], p. 233.
20 Selznick, P. (1957). *Leadership in Administration: A Sociological Interpretation.* New York: Harper.
21 The Patient's Charter for England: Putting the Citizen's Charter into practice in the National Health Service. Initially published 1991.
22 Secretary of State for Health (1999). *Saving Lives: Our Healthier Nation.* Available at: http://www.archive.official-documents.co.uk/document/cm43/4386/4386.htm (accessed 23 March 2011).
23 This case was widely reported in the press. See, for example: http://www.independent.co.uk/opinion/faith/nurse-to-go-to-tribunal-in-row-over-cross-1929691.html (accessed 25 November 2011).
24 MacIntyre, A. (1984). *After Virtue: A Study in Moral Theory.* Notre Dame: University of Notre Dame Press.
25 [18], p. 3.

CHAPTER 64

The future of spirituality and healthcare

Mark Cobb, Bruce Rumbold, and Christina M. Puchalski

Introduction

A chapter that comes at the end of an extensive collection of work on spirituality and healthcare might be expected to be conclusive, gathering the many colourful threads running through the book, and weaving them into a coherent whole. However, as many of the contributors to the book have mentioned, spirituality and healthcare is a dynamic field where the attainment of perfect control and order is a misleading goal regardless of tempting it appears. The discourse of spirituality and healthcare is open at the edges, orientated around core organizing principles, but containing levels of disorder, indeterminacy and tension that provide meaningful interactions and suggest creative opportunities. This chapter therefore looks forward and suggests points for future development, rather than issues brought to closure; questions rather than conclusions.

Spirituality and healthcare share, in their most humane forms and practices, attributes of insightfulness, imagination, discipline, skill, and enrichment; in other words, each is an art. Healthcare professions have to some extent made claims about what constitutes the art of their practice and how this can be learnt and fostered. However, there is some controversy as to the exact role of spirituality in the practice of healthcare. Spirituality sits on the margins of institutional recognition, conventional discourse and the health agenda: a position some might argue is not a weakness, but strength. Others firmly believe it is an ethical mandate to include spirituality as foundational in healthcare. One reason for this apparent polarization could be that spirituality presents with something of a Mona Lisa smile: it rejoices in ambiguity and by avoiding simple resolutions maintains the elusive qualities of the human condition. This leaves spirituality open to the charge that almost anything can be considered as spiritual, in a similar way that anything can be considered a work of art.

Spirituality in the context of healthcare is highly mutable and transgressive. It shows every sign of wanting to move beyond classical forms of religion and medicine, and hence has trouble clarifying its relationship with either. This re-positioning circumvents boundary limitations and opens the possibility of ubiquity: it is now almost axiomatic in healthcare circles that 'all people are spiritual, but only some are religious.' Despite a largely unexamined anthropology being assumed here spirituality is being used as a vehicle for introducing issues such as identity, community, meaning, and purpose into the clinical encounter; in other words, all those things that we carefully extract in order to produce high-order evidence, then try to return in selective ways through the remedial strategy of translational research.

One of the broad movements that have assisted the emergence of spiritual interest is a shift in western culture from orthodoxy toward orthopraxis, represented in medicine by the rise of evidence-based medicine. This is the idea that interventions should be judged on their effectiveness, not primarily by their theoretical underpinnings or lack thereof. If spirituality has the potential to 'work,' then, of course, it has relevance to the care of patients, and some patients expect and permit clinicians to include spirituality. Similarly, if spirituality has a role in the health of communities then it has relevance to the social and political determinants of health. The constraint here is that evidence is created through funding, and here the playing field tilts sharply toward orthodoxy once again.

Asking how spirituality relates to heath and healthcare is a radical enquiry. It means exploring what may have been marginalized or excluded when, in the early nineteenth century, medicine, responding to the advances in science, reframed medicine as a scientific field. Through a new capacity to diagnose and prognosticate medicine gained a status that initially was out of all proportion to its capacity to effect anything by way of cure. When performance began to match knowledge the partnership between medicine and biology appeared complete. For much of the twentieth century, medicine's comprehensive and welcome expertise in illness seems to have intimidated and quenched attempts to talk about health as something other than the absence of disease. Theology retreated to inner and other-worldly rhetoric about wholeness that carefully avoided the idea of incarnation (even the Pentecostal groups that did go for alternative healing strategies were actually, like medicine, really only interested in cure). Philosophy fell silent, only now beginning to talk in some places about human flourishing. Sociology has sniped around the edges of the medical enterprise and psychology began to focus on the biology of mental functions.

In the present context, spirituality functions as a Trojan horse. The beauty of the *S* word is that it cannot readily be claimed by any single discipline. That is what gives it its contemporary power: no-one can dictate its use or exercise the power to define and control it. We can either ignore it, or we can negotiate around it. It is like 'health,' which has a certain wildcard status even though medicine continues to have proprietary rights over illness. There are also similarities with 'education' in an age where teaching and learning have been rendered as information and techniques, losing sight of the essential formative character of the enterprise. Consequently, because spirituality is untamed there are many attempts to capture and control it, but as yet spirituality continues to be a countervailing discourse.

Spirituality in the context of healthcare therefore looks for a broadening of the conversation, as we hope this book has demonstrated. This means more specifically a re-engagement of the humanities (or the 'spiritual disciplines' as Husserl called them) around questions of health in particular and the good life in general; and a creative and critical dialogue with the natural sciences, some of whom have entered the field to discover and explain. From where we stand it therefore seems that the time is passing when spirituality could be ignored or dismissed. This is a good thing for both those who embrace spirituality and those who would prefer to ignore it. The pro-spirituality lobby needs the reasoned critique of sceptics, for there is a romantic, idealistic, individualistic, uncritical utopian edge to some of the literature. And those who would rather ignore spirituality need the destabilizing perspective of the spirituality 'movement' to remind them that their disciplines too are human constructions, needing to remain open to possibility, and not just on their own terms. Science is also a relatively new field open to huge possibilities with emerging questions that will need innovative methods beyond what we have seen to date.

Understanding spirituality

We therefore come to our points for development in this expanding conversation, and our first one concerns a philosophical question: how should we understand spirituality in healthcare? In attempting to answer the question we would do well to learn from philosophy itself and consider what is central to its enterprise and enquiry, philosophy after all is a sibling of theology and a parent of science. Philosophy tries to make sense of human thought and experience, including attempts to answer the enduring moral question about how we should live our lives. As a discipline, philosophy is guided by the coordinates of clarity and sound argument and whilst it can become obsessed by analysis, at its best it can help formulate critical questions, expose our claims to the truth, uncover what underpins our arguments, and make us think more rigorously about our assumptions and normative positions.

Philosophy can help us consider the intelligibility of what we describe as spirituality: it can help us examine claims to our knowledge of this subject, and it can prompt us to formulate questions that help sustain dialogue and the exploration of answers. In this way we may be able to make progress beyond persuasion and influence by learning how to discuss spirituality in ways that are adequately informed and described so that a conversation can be shared and an agenda fashioned that shapes future debates and lines of enquiry. Williams provides us with a helpful reminder that, '... although philosophy is worse than natural science at some things, such as discovering the nature of the galaxies ... it is better than natural science at other things, for instance making sense of what we are trying to do in our intellectual activities.'[1]

The sometimes-fractious debates between the humanities (religion specifically) and the natural sciences are another area where philosophy has been reluctant to tread. Spirituality too has been caught in this fray as it has attempted to engage with healthcare. Healthcare has made dramatic advances through the discoveries of the natural sciences to the extent that healthcare practice seems in thrall to the labs. However, the apparent primacy of the bio-medical sciences is not a complete answer to the questions of healthcare and to the challenges of how we should respond to people who are ill and suffering. The abstract knowledge of science is helpful in understanding diabetes (why it occurs, what its consequences are for the body and how these might be controlled), but the humanistic disciplines are needed to make sense of what diabetes means to someone living with the condition. The former is responding to a different question from the latter, their answers therefore differ, and one is not inferior to the other. Some philosophical commentaries and enquiries could prove informative guides and critical companions in developing this enquiry.

Spirituality in healthcare may be a way of acknowledging and providing space for human expressions and experience that are no longer registered on bio-medical scales or measured by healthcare systems as deliverables. Even apparent exceptions to this can be misleading; for example, studies into the neural correlates of spirituality are generally attempts to provide materialist explanations of spiritual experiences. The philosopher Nagel offers the following insightful commentary:

> The concepts of physical science provide a very special, and partial, description of the world that experience reveals to us. It is the work with all subjective consciousness, sensory appearances, thoughts, value, and purpose and will left out; what remains is the mathematically describable order of things and events in space and time ... The reductionist project usually tries to reclaim some of the originally excluded aspects of the world, by analysing them in physical (e.g. behavioural or neurophysiological) terms, but it denies reality to what cannot be so reduced.[2]

Arguments concerning the role of spirituality in healthcare need philosophical clarity. This is a long-term project, but it will assist proponents of spirituality in developing a self-critical stance and conducting their critical dialogues with the other disciplines contributing to healthcare. It is not, however, a *de novo* task because the historical spiritual traditions and communities of practice have well-developed philosophical commitments and positions that have perhaps been left on the shelf for too long. These traditions are a reminder that in order to make sense of ourselves we need, in addition to whatever abstract or propositional knowledge offers, perspectives of location, culture, history, and understandings of the particular ways people have come to apprehend the world and their place in it, and what they name as sacred and holy.

Ways of knowing, evidence and research

Healthcare's apologists would have it that healthcare is at the apogee of a scientifically driven evidence-based process diligently applying research findings without fear or prejudice to the benefit of the ill and injured. However, the practice of healthcare cannot be limited to an intellectual problem, and practitioners cannot be isolated from all the social entanglements, personal commitments, beliefs, and influences that make them human:

> Evidence-based decision models may be very powerful, but are like computer-generated symphonies in the style of Mozart—correct, but lifeless. The art of caring for patients, then, should flourish not merely in the theoretical or abstract grey zones where scientific evidence is incomplete or conflicting, but also in the recognition that what is black and white in the abstract often becomes grey in practice,

> as clinicians seek to meet their patients' needs. In the practice of clinical medicine, the art is not merely part of the 'medical humanities,' but is integral to medicine as an applied science.[3]

Studies into spirituality in the context of healthcare frequently attempt to follow the evidence-based approaches of the natural sciences and consequently produce results that are correct according to the methodologies used, but have little life and few applications. If these types of studies serve any purpose it is a political one of putting a marker down for spirituality in the forums that decide what counts as clinical reality and is therefore worthy of attention. This leads us to another point for development, in this case an epistemological issue concerning the ways we know about spirituality, what should be considered as evidence and which research designs and methods can contribute to our understanding.

The spirituality encountered in people with health needs, like spirituality in general, is a lived dimension of the person expressed in beliefs, values, actions, and commitments and experienced through our engagement with the world and those around us. The way we know about spirituality is therefore not like knowing an object of cognition, it is more like a form of practical knowing, learnt from participating in the world as both embodied individuals and persons entangled in a web of social and cultural meaning. Importantly, this participation is not at random nor is it directionless, but orientated by a particular inclination or view of the world that is often referred to as faith, meaning, or inner life. This presents challenges to the way a third-party may acquire knowledge of the spirituality of a particular person, for spirituality is clearly more than a simple attribute or characteristic.

There are measurable quantities that relate to spirituality that we may consider to be matters of fact (examples include spiritual practices and observances), but there are also beliefs, meanings, expectations, and lived experiences of a transcendent reality that may be less susceptible to conventional empirical measurement. In this case we may be dealing with highly humanized symbols and metaphors that are likely to be marginalized or excluded by many health research methods. We need therefore research methods and paradigms that are congruent with the spiritual realities being investigated. Modes of research that take narrative seriously may provide a way forward and counterbalance the limitations of empiricism. Personal, social, and cultural narratives of spirituality in relation to illness, health, and healing are sources of human understanding and meaning that require hermeneutic ways of knowing and comprehending, rather than abstraction and deduction. And narrative representations can be understood as including a wide range of forms—music, painting, drawing, film, dance—as well as story. However, we must also look to the neurosciences, to physics, to anthropology and other growing areas of biomedical research as possible partners in developing approaches to understanding spirituality particularly in relation to health. Trans-disciplinary approaches may likely provide the paths to greater understanding particularly in that part of spiritual experiences and understandings that impact health. Spirituality, by the questions it raises, may provide a useful critical perspective on the social discourses and practices tacit in many accepted research methods.

While medicine and healthcare are therefore challenged to be less biomedical and reductionist, and integrate humanism, spirituality, and the narrative of human beings into their care, religious organizations and philosophical communities are challenged to integrate the findings and capacities of the sciences into their research and discourse. The ultimate question is about mystery that encompasses the spirit, the sacred and the soul. Many would say that the spiritual part of the person is hidden, private, and inaccessible, and certainly not to be studied or researched. This limited stance maybe based on fear, but what would happen if theoretically, innovative research methodology did uncover the mysteries of the spirit? Would that make us less sacred? Perhaps the answer lies in the biomedical community being more open to the story and being creative in how they approach spiritual studies and questions. However, it also lies in the philosophical and religious communities being more open to scientific progress in their fields. Thus chaplains should come to the biomedical table, so to speak, to provide direction for research, and models of care.

Practice and practitioners

Many clinicians today would agree that spirituality should be an essential part of caring for the patient and families. However, a point of contention and an enduring question for healthcare spirituality relates to who should be involved in the delivery of spirituality within the healthcare system. Too often chaplains are not an integral part of healthcare teams. Patients would like their clinicians to address spiritual issues with them, but continue to respond in surveys that this does not occur. It is incumbent upon all healthcare professionals to work together and learn from each other so that the best models of interprofessional care can be developed. This requires chaplains, clergy and other spiritual professionals to explain in clear ways what they do and how they are trained and certified. And it requires the other healthcare professionals to broaden their thinking beyond the science of healthcare to the art of healthcare, and in so doing being more comfortable with narrative approaches. It also requires the development of outcome measures as well as measures by which all members of the healthcare team, including spiritual care professionals, can be held accountable for discipline appropriate spiritual care. Finally, it requires all healthcare professionals to integrate personal and professional formation as part of their professional development.

The unquestioned axiom that 'all are spiritual' could imply that all healthcare practitioners have some access to this human dimension and therefore some capacity for responding to it. Not everyone does consider him- or herself spiritual, some are indifferent and some directly oppose the notion. Even for those who profess a spiritual dimension to their lives a further set of questions follow such as what form does this take, how developed is it, is it a positive contribution to their lives, how does it frame their experience of the world, and how do they view other people's spirituality? Spirituality in healthcare is, too often, an uncritical reference to a simple benign concept, but in reality it is polysemant and refers to diverse beliefs, experiences and practices not all of which have health benefits or promote the wellbeing of individuals or communities. This provides spirituality with a conundrum that researchers or practitioners frequently solve by appealing to our 'common humanity'. Whilst there is much to be said for this as an ethical stance in relation to healthcare and the equality of persons, it does not allow for genuine differences, problematic disagreements, and the enrichment that can come from diversity. This point for development is therefore about the profession and practice of spirituality in healthcare.

It may be instructive to consider briefly how healthcare professions in general attain their privileged positions as accredited practitioners. In a similar fashion to other professions, healthcare students are selected for courses on their potential to learn a discrete body of knowledge and to develop the cognitive and technical skills to perform their professional duties. Professional courses for physicians, nurses, physiotherapists, and the like also aim to develop the person in terms of their capacity to relate to patients, to understand their particular circumstances and to act with humanity and compassion. This aspect of professional education is often referred to as formation (a term found in seminaries) and relates to the development of a person's professional identity and '... the maturation of moral sensibility and the integration of personal values with professional expertise.'[4] Typically, professional formation is supported by the development of reflective practices and experiential learning that draws upon the humanities and liberal arts. Ongoing assessment of knowledge, practice, and behaviours culminate in a qualification and licensure in the chosen profession followed by a form of apprenticeship that furthers the development of identity and advanced practice through shared learning among peers and coaching by experts.

Professional schools for healthcare professions have historical roots in the professional schools for clergy (seminaries) that also seek to develop the knowledge, skill and vocation of their students that results in an authorized public function and identity. Like other professional schools, seminaries and their equivalents teach a discrete body of knowledge related to their faith tradition, and 'Seminary educators seek to form dispositions and the intuitive knowledge, or *habitus*, of a given religious or intellectual tradition in students.'[5] Seminaries not only cultivate learning and practice to prepare people for their professional role, but they also foster the pastoral imagination that equips trainees to engage with the sacred and holy and be attuned to its significance and meaning in individuals and communities.

Where then does this leave healthcare spirituality and those we expect to be its agents? It seems reasonable to require all healthcare professionals to have a basic understanding of how spirituality operates in people's lives so that they avoid offence, show respect, and can facilitate relevant resources. There is evidence that some educators are providing learning opportunities to enable healthcare professionals to acquire this level of understanding. However, we should not expect our podiatrist, nurse, social worker, or psychiatrist to have attained levels of spiritual practice and wisdom that we would expect of say a rabbi, priest or minister (unless our healthcare practitioner is dual qualified). More significantly, traditional forms of spirituality are deeply contextualized within their respective religious traditions and their communities of practice. Paradoxically, it is when someone is deeply rooted in a tradition and *habitus* that they have the freedom to relate to those outside of the tradition without imposing beliefs or feeling threatened by the other.

We can locate religious professionals on our social maps as easily as we can locate healthcare professionals by the knowledge they bear, their accountability to the public, their professed ethic to act on behalf of others, and the uncertainties and limitations they deal with. However, what of those who are not anchored in a spiritual tradition, whose learning bears no accreditation and whose practices are largely unaccountable? Spirituality, unlike many other aspects of healthcare, requires little technical competence, but its practices can be harmful and limiting, it can undermine hope and destabilize established meanings and beliefs. There are, therefore, ethical limitations to what is acceptable on the one hand, and the limited number of specialist spiritual care professionals we know as healthcare chaplains on the other. Much that lies in between these two remains largely uncharted, which is why there are beginning to be consensus-driven attempts at recommendations and guidelines in some healthcare systems. We need to develop generosity in our multidisciplinary practices, to learn from each other and grow, to stretch beyond our own expertise, to accept the mentoring and coaching of others with greater experience and skills than our own, and to become in due course mentors and coaches ourselves. Healthcare systems and practitioners also have much to learn from disciplines and communities outside of the traditional domain who also address matters of spiritual health and wellbeing. Only when all disciplines come together can spirituality be fully integrated into care systems and not be on the fringes. The research and the resulting clinical guidelines should be rigorous and thorough, but should always honor the mystery and sacredness of people.

Beyond the clinic

It has long been recognized that the determinants of health extend beyond the individual body to the wider social and contextual circumstances in which the person lives. However, the way spirituality has been applied in healthcare contexts has been criticized for attending to the individual to such an extent that the bigger social and cultural picture is disregarded and spiritual care becomes a form of detached personal therapy. An over-reliance on psychology and counselling may be a cause of this individualist bias, which has gone uncorrected despite a flourishing of approaches in pastoral and practical theology informed and influenced by the challenges and practices of liberation and contextual theology. These seek to understand and address wider and more systemic determinants of personhood. Graham is representative of this outward move whose basic thesis is:

> ... to care for persons is to create new worlds; to care for the world is to build a new personhood. The destiny of persons and the character of the world are intertwined. Each is made poorer or richer by the quality of the other and of the forces uniting or dividing them. Thus, the call to care for persons is simultaneously a call to care for the world.[6]

The discourses and practices of healthcare spirituality are typically concentrated within clinical institutions and the practitioners organized to function within them. There is a fringe of alternative and informal practice outside of the official healthcare system, such as that offered within communities or by complementary and alternative health practitioners, but these are not afforded the approval and authority of clinical institutions. This raises interesting questions about the role, status and location of faith communities in terms of their pastoral functions and in relation to clinical institutions. It also suggests another point for development that we describe as spirituality and healthcare beyond the clinic. The clinical model has obvious benefits within the biomedical paradigm of disease and healing, but there is much human wisdom and practice about health and wholeness that operates beyond institutional walls. Perhaps a wider dialogue that includes social and cultural voices can help develop more holistic systems of care.

Health is found beyond the health system in the ways we live our lives together, and spirituality is one discourse that can make the links between health and illness. Wilson's observation is pertinent that, 'There is no way to health through the cure of illness ... Rather than trying to reach health by understanding illness, we must first try to understand health, in the light of which we may be able to say something about being well or ill.'[7] Health, as the World Health Organization reminds us, is not merely the absence of disease or infirmity, but a state of complete wellbeing.[8] The project to attain wellbeing in this case is not an idealistic vision of holism, but the development of capacities and capabilities that nurture purpose, meaning, value, identity and connectedness. This approach also provides a critique of those things that diminish or actively harm the wellbeing of people.

The convergence of spirituality and health sets an ethical, political, and theological agenda that presents some real challenges to both spirituality and healthcare in the ways they understand persons, the interplay between the individual and the community, and the ways they can contribute to creating a healthy world.

One location in which this agenda can be addressed is in faith communities and their role in the spiritual formation and development of communities that promote wellbeing. It is possible that spirituality can provide a bridge between the patient in the clinic and the person in the community. This presents the opportunity for dialogue about how what is learnt through spiritual care in the clinic can inform health promoting spiritual practices in the community, and how what is learnt and known in communities can inform clinical practices so that they are less myopic and more holistic. However, this is not without difficulties given the differences that exist in many health systems between the clinic and the community in terms of resources, value and authority. What may shift this position are two drivers that question the current dominance of clinical institutions.

The first driver results from recognition in developed countries that current models and systems of healthcare are unsustainable. The many factors contributing to this realization include fiscal constraints, increasing lifespans, lower fertility rates and therefore a reduced workforce, the impact of chronic and degenerative diseases, ageing populations, urbanization and globalization, and citizens who expect choice and prefer home care to institutional care. Health inflation appears difficult to limit, as innovation fuels expectation and patients demand individualized care of the highest quality. Rationing is a crude and ultimately inadequate response and new approaches are emerging that focus on deinstitutionalized care and health systems dispersed across resourced communities. Traditional models still dominate the picture, but there is evidence of movement at the level of health policy where it is observed that there is a:

> ... a shifting of emphasis: from sickness to prevention, from epidemic disease to chronic illness, from prescriptive healthcare systems to systems that encourage more independence and choice. It's possible to see how those changes of focus could permanently alter the ways in which healthcare will work in the future, leading it away from a paternalistic approach to one in which citizens take more responsibility for their own health. Institutional care will give way to community-based care, and, in turn, healthcare professionals will become less independent, and work within collaborative teams.[9]

Discussions of spirituality in healthcare lack a coherent community health strand, with the likely exceptions of mental health, primary care, and palliative care. A concern for human flourishing and spiritual development that fosters resilience and wellbeing requires community-based initiatives and partnerships with community organizations. Faith groups need to recognize that pastoral and spiritual skills developed in clinical settings could complement theirs and they could be partners in developing networks of community-based schemes that build pastoral capacity and capabilities to promote community wellbeing, enable healthy lifestyles and empower citizens to participate actively in the health agenda.

The second driver comes from a global recognition that health is a public good, and health systems can contribute to social justice through promoting health for all and ensuring equity of access. The reforms promoted by the primary health care movement describe the realignment of healthcare systems needed in response to population challenges. These include the reorganization of services to make them more socially relevant, able to secure healthier communities and operate with more inclusive and participatory models of leadership. This signals a shift identified by the World Health Organization in the very premise of healthcare and highlights differences between conventional clinical models and the primary health model (Table 64.1) [10]. The primary care model demonstrates that addressing health problems requires understanding the whole person which itself requires more participatory models of healthcare that can respond to the many dimensions of personhood. Person-centred care (or people-centred care in recent WHO developments) is a core value and principle of healthcare spirituality. Those involved in advocating for and practicing spiritual care are likely to be natural allies in

Table 64.1 Features of different healthcare models

Conventional ambulatory medical care in clinics or outpatient departments	Disease control programmes	People-centred primary care
Focus on illness and cure	Focus on priority diseases	Focus on health needs
Relationship limited to the moment of consultation	Relationship limited to programme implementation	Enduring personal relationship
Episodic curative care	Proramme-defined disease control interventions	Comprehensive, continuous and person-centred care
Responsibility limited to effective and safe advice to the patient at the moment of consultation	Responsibility for disease-control targets among the target population	Responsibility for the health of all in the community along the life cycle; responsibility for tacking determinants of ill-health
Users are consumers of the care they purchase	Population groups are target of disease-control interventions	People are partners in managing their own health and that of their community

World Health Organization (2008). *Primary Health Care: Now More than Ever*, p. 43 Geneva © World Health Organization.

promoting people-centred care, and in developing the practice skills needed to implement it. Spirituality will be an important framework through which to understand how people experience and respond to their health problems. Insights gained through spiritual care within the healthcare system can also be linked with diverse spiritual resources and services in the community. Primary care teams should be expected to recognize spiritual health needs and resources, and attend respectfully to the suffering of their patients. Where these are beyond their level of competence they should be able to mobilize resources external to the team or direct people to other resources.

Conclusion

This book could not have been envisaged 25 years ago. While many of the principal issues faced by healthcare systems today were already being discussed in the 1980s, spiritual care as an integral aspect of healthcare was not among them. That a conversation between spirituality and healthcare has emerged is not due to concerted advocacy from lobby groups, but rather is a consequence of changed consciousness in society at large. Western culture is in transition, and one of the many signs is the emergence of a spiritual discourse that challenges both religious and medical authority. This discourse has engaged not only healthcare, but also other social institutions, particularly education. One of the challenges ahead of spiritual care practitioners in healthcare is to develop conversations with practitioners in these other fields. Interdisciplinary solidarity will be important both in resisting some of the unjust and dehumanizing policies that issue from political and economic self-interest and in developing a more coherent public conversation about spirituality and eventually a healthcare system that recognizes and treats all aspects of the patient and not just the disease.

It seems clear that health has been a catalyst for a significant part of the public discussion of spirituality. Cancer survivors attribute their remission and recovery to finding their spirituality, while people living with chronic illness name as a major coping resource their spiritual beliefs and practices. It may be that health crises are the most common biographical disruptions experienced by comparatively-privileged citizens of the west. However, other crises loom that will require a spiritual response, not least the massive social changes precipitated by demographic shift, economic instability, food insecurity, and of course climate change. Developing just social action to enable appropriate sharing of global resources will bring to the fore questions of responsibility, generosity and compassion. The spiritual care experienced by many in their encounters with the health system could be one plank for building just and compassionate public and health policy in the decades that lie ahead.

References

1 Williams, B.A.O., Moore, A.W. (2006). *Philosophy as a Humanistic Discipline*, p. 186. Princeton: Princeton University Press.

2 Nagel, T. (2010). *Secular Philosophy and the Religious Temperament: Essays 2002–2008*, p. 25. New York: Oxford University Press.

3 Saunders, J. (2000). The practice of clinical medicine as an art and as a science. *Med Human* **26**(1): 18–22.

4 Rabow, M.W., Remen, R.N., Parmelee, D.X., Inui, T.S. (2010). Professional formation: extending medicine's lineage of service into the next century. *Acad Med* **85**(2): 310–17.

5 Foster, C.R. (2006). *Educating Clergy: Teaching Practices and the Pastoral Imagination*, 1st edn, p. 23. San Francisco: John Wiley/ Chichester: Jossey-Bass.

6 Graham, L.K. (1992). *Care of Persons, Care of Worlds: a Psychosystems Approach to Pastoral Care and Counseling*, pp. 13–14. Nashville: Abingdon Press.

7 Wilson, M. (1975). *Health is for People*, p. 55. Longman & Todd, London: Darton.

8 World Health Organization. (1946). Preamble to the Constitution of the World Health Organization as adopted by the International Health Conference, New York, 19–22 July 1946. Zürich: World Health Organization.

9 Economist Intelligence Unit. (2009). Fixing Healthcare: The professionals' perspective. *Economist*, London, p. 24.

10 World Health Organization. (2008). *Primary Health Care: Now More than Ever*, p. 43. Geneva: World Health Organization.

Index

Page numbers in *italics* denote figures or tables.